Infectious Disease

Vassil St. Georgiev
Series Editor

For other titles published in this series, go to
www.springer.com/series/7646

Antimicrobial Drug Resistance

Volume 2

Clinical and Epidemiological Aspects

Edited by
Douglas L. Mayers

Section Editors
Stephen A. Lerner, Marc Ouellette, Jack D. Sobel

Humana Press

Editors

Douglas L. Mayers, MD
Executive Vice President
    and Chief Medical Officer
Idenix Pharmaceuticals
Cambridge
Massachusetts

Marc Ouellette, Ph.D
Professor
Canada Research Chair
in Antimicrobial Resistance
Centre de recherche en Infectiologie
Université Laval
Quebec City, Canada

Stephen A. Lerner, MD
Professor of Medicine
Wayne State University School
    of Medicine
Detroit Medical Center
Detroit, Michigan

Jack D. Sobel, MD
Professor of Medicine
Chief Division of Infectious Diseases
Wayne State University School of Medicine
Detroit Medical Center
Detroit, Michigan

ISBN: 978-1-60327-594-1   e-ISBN: 978-1-60327-595-8
DOI: 10.1007/978-1-60327-595-8
Springer Dordrecht Heidelberg London New York

Library of Congress Control Number: 2008944287

Springer is part of Springer Science+Business Media (www.springer.com)

Preface

This first edition of *Antimicrobial Drug Resistance* grew out of a desire by the editors and authors to have a comprehensive resource of information on antimicrobial drug resistance that encompassed the current information available for bacteria, fungi, protozoa and viruses. We believe that this information will be of value to clinicians, epidemiologists, microbiologists, virologists, parasitologists, public health authorities, medical students and fellows in training. We have endeavored to provide this information in a style which would be accessible to the broad community of persons who are concerned with the impact of drug resistance in our clinics and across the broader global communities.

Antimicrobial Drug Resistance is divided into Volume 1 which has sections covering a general overview of drug resistance and mechanisms of drug resistance first for classes of drugs and then by individual microbial agents including bacteria, fungi, protozoa and viruses. Volume 2 addresses clinical, epidemiologic and public health aspects of drug resistance along with an overview of the conduct and interpretation of specific drug resistance assays. Together, these two volumes offer a comprehensive source of information on drug resistance issues by the experts in each topic.

We are very grateful to the 175 international experts who have contributed to this textbook for their patience and support as the work came together. The editors would like to especially thank Shelley Crim for her administrative assistance in pulling the book together. The staff at Humana and Springer including Renata Hutter, Kathleen Lyons, Jenny Wolkowicki, and Harvey Kane have provided exceptional support and encouragement to the editors over several years required to develop this textbook. Finally, the book would never have been completed without the patience and support of our wives and families.

Douglas L. Mayers, MD
Jack D. Sobel, MD
Marc Ouellette, PhD
Stephen A. Lerner, MD

Table of Contents
Antimicrobial Drug Resistance
Volume 2

Table of Contents
Antimicrobial Drug Resistance
Volume 1

Section A   General Overview
Douglas L. Mayers

Section B   General Mechanisms of Drug Resistance
Stephen A. Lerner

Contributors

Robert A. Akins, Ph.D.
Biochemistry & Molecular Biology, Wayne State University,
School of Medicine, Detroit, MI, USA

Barbara D. Alexander, M.D.
Associate Professor of Medicine, Duke University Medical Center, Durham, NC, USA

Samir Ali, Ph.D.
Research Scientist, Viral Diseases Biology Area, Roche Palo Alto, LLC, Palo Alto, CA, USA

Sevtap Arikan, M.D.
Department of Microbiology and Clinical Microbiology,
Hacettepe University Medical School, Ankara, Turkey

Maja Babic, M.D.
Fellow, Division of Infectious Diseases and HIV Medicine,
University Hospitals Case Medical Center, Cleveland, OH, USA

Yanina Balabanova, M.D., Ph.D.
Research Associate, Institute of Cell and Molecular Sciences,
Barts and the London School of Medicine, Queen Mary College, London, UK

Fernando Baquero, Ph.D.
Ramón y Cajal Research Professor, FiBio-RYC, Department of Microbiology,
Ramón y Cajal University Hospital, Madrid, Spain
Laboratory for Microbial Evolution, Center for Astrobiology (CAB CSIC-NTA-NASA),
Madrid, Spain

Margaret C. Bash, M.D., M.P.H.
Center for Biologics Evaluation and Research,
U.S. Food and Drug Administration, Silver Spring, MD, USA

Gonzalo Bearman, M.D., M.P.H.
Virginia Commonwealth University Medical Center, Richmond, VA, USA

Thomas Benfield, M.D., D.M.Sci.
Department of Infectious Disease, Hvidovre University Hospital, Copenhagen, Denmark

Michael L. Bennish, M.D.
Department of Population, Family and Reproductive Health,
Bloomberg School of Public Health, Johns Hopkins University, Baltimore, MD,
Mpilonhle, Mtubatuba, South Africa

Michel G. Bergeron, O.Q., M.D., F.R.C.P.C.
Centre de Recherche en Infectiologie of Université Laval, Québec City, QC, Canada

Hiranmoy Bhattacharjee, Ph.D.
Associate Professor, Department of Cellular Biology and Pharmacology,
Florida International University College of Medicine, Miami, FL, USA

Giancarlo A. Biagini
Research Fellow, Liverpool School of Tropical Medicine, Liverpool, UK

John S. Blanchard, Ph.D.
Department of Biochemistry, Albert Einstein College of Medicine, Bronx, NY, USA

Guy Boivin, M.D.
Centre de Recherche en Infectiologie of Université Laval, Québec City, QC, Canada

Pierre R. Bonneau, Ph.D.
Boehringer Ingelheim (Canada) Ltd., Research and Development, Laval, QC, Canada

Robert A. Bonomo, M.D.
Research Service, Louis Stokes Cleveland Veterans Affairs Medical Center,
Case Western Reserve University, Cleveland, OH, USA

Charles A.B. Boucher, M.D., Ph.D.
Department of Virology, Eijkman-Winkler Center for Microbiology, Infectious Diseases
and Inflammation, University Medical Center, Utrecht, The Netherlands

Patrick G. Bray, Ph.D.
Reader, Liverpool School of Tropical Medicine, Liverpool, UK

Michelle D. Brazas, Ph.D.
Manager, Bioinformatics Education, Research Associate, Ontario Institute for Cancer
Research, Toronto, ON, Canada

Itzhak Brook, M.D., M.Sc.
Department of Pediatrics, Georgetown University School of Medicine, Washington, DC, USA

Nathaniel A. Brown, M.D.
Antiviral Development Consultants LLC, Weston, MA, USA

Robert W. Buckheit, Jr., Ph.D.
ImQuest BioSciences, Inc., Frederick, MD, USA

Karen Bush, Ph.D.
Johnson & Johnson Pharmaceutical Research & Development, Raritan, NJ, USA

Nick Cammack, Ph.D.
Vice President, Viral Diseases, Roche Pharmaceuticals, Palo Alto, CA, USA

Gerard A. Cangelosi, Ph.D.
Department of Global Health, Seattle Biomedical Research Institute, University
of Washington, Seattle, WA, USA

Rafael Canton, Ph.D.
Department of Microbiology, Ramón y Cajal University Hospital, Madrid, Spain
Department of Microbiology, Faculty of Pharmacy, Complutensis University,
Madrid, Spain

Annie Canu, Ph.D.
Professor of Microbiology, UFR Sciences Pharmaceutiques, University of Caen
Basse-Normandie, Caen, France

Henry F. Chambers, III, M.D.
Professor, Department of Medicine, Division of Infectious Diseases,
University of California, San Francisco, CA, USA
Chief, Infectious Diseases, San Francisco General Hospital, San Francisco, CA, USA

Jyotsna Chandra, Ph.D.
Research Associate, Center for Medical Mycology and Mycology Reference Laboratory,
Department of Dermatology, University Hospitals of Cleveland and Case Western Reserve
University, Cleveland, OH, USA

P.H. Chandrasekar, M.D.
Division of Infectious Diseases, Department of Internal Medicine, Wayne State University
School of Medicine, Harper University Hospital, Detroit, MI, USA

Anne Chen, M.D.
Clinical Assistant Professor of Medicine, Wayne State University School of Medicine,
Henry Ford Health System, Detroit, MI, USA

Gerald C. Coles, M.A., Ph.D.
Department of Clinical Veterinary Science, University of Bristol, Bristol, UK

Patricia Connolly, M.Sc.
Director of Research & Development, MiraVista Diagnostics/MiraBella Technologies,
Indianapolis, IN, USA

J. William Costerton, Ph.D., F.R.C.S.
Director, Center for Biofilms, School of Dentistry, University of Southern California,
Los Angeles, CA, USA

Patrice M. Courvalin, M.D.
Institut Pasteur, Unité des Agents Antibactériens, Paris, France

Clyde S. Crumpacker, II, M.D.
Professor of Medicine, Harvard Medical School, Division of Infectious Diseases,
Beth Israel Deaconess Medical Center, Boston, MA, USA

Sarah L. Cudmore, B.Sc.
Ph.D. Candidate, Department of Biochemistry, Microbiology and Immunology,
Faculty of Medicine, University of Ottawa, Ottawa, ON, Canada

Vanessa D'Costa, Ph.D.
Department of Biochemistry & Biomedical Sciences, M.G. DeGroote Institute for Infectious
Disease Research, McMaster University, Hamilton, ON, Canada

Saskia Decuypere, L.Sc.
Postdoctoral Researcher, Institute of Tropical Medicine, Antwerpen, Belgium

Abhay Dhand, M.D.
Assistant Professor of Medicine, New York Medical College, Valhalla, NY, USA

Carlos A. DiazGranados, M.D., M.S.C.R.
Assistant Professor of Medicine and Infectious Diseases, Emory University School
of Medicine, Atlanta, GA, USA

Michael J. Doenhoff, B.Sc., Ph.D.
School of Biology, University of Nottingham, University Park, Nottingham, UK

Cameron M. Douglas, Ph.D.
Merck Research Laboratories, Rahway, NJ, USA

Louise Doyon, Ph.D.
Senior Scientist (previous affiliation), Boehringer Ingelheim (Canada), Ltd.,
Research & Development, Laval, QC, Canada

W. Lawrence Drew, M.D., Ph.D.
Professor, Laboratory Medicine and Medicine, Director, Clinical Virology Laboratory,
University of California – San Francisco, San Francisco, CA, USA

Francis A. Drobniewski, M.D., Ph.D.
Professor, Institute of Cell and Molecular Sciences, Barts and the London School of Medicine,
Queen Mary College, London, UK

George L. Drusano, M.D.
Ordway Research Institute, Albany, NY, USA

Jean-Claude Dujardin, D.Sc.
Professor, Vrije Universiteit Brussell, Prince Leopold Institute of Tropical Medicine,
Molecular Parasitology, Antwerpen, Belgium

Herbert L. DuPont, M.D.
University of Texas – Houston School of Public Health, St. Luke's Episcopal Hospital and
Baylor College of Medicine, Houston, TX, USA

Manoj T. Durasingh, Ph.D.
Department of Immunology & Infectious Diseases, Harvard School of Public Health,
Boston, MA, USA

George M. Eliopoulos, M.D.
Professor of Medicine, Harvard Medical School, Division of Infectious Diseases,
Beth Israel Deaconess Medical Center, Boston, MA, USA

Robert Elston, Ph.D.
Roche Products Ltd., Hexagon Place, Welwyn Garden City, UK

Matthew E. Falagas, M.D., M.Sc., D.Sc.
Alfa Institute of Biomedical Sciences (AIBS), Marousi, Greece

Christoph A. Fux, M.D.
Division of Infectious Disease, University Hospital of Bern, Bern, Switzerland

Gary E. Garber, M.D., F.R.C.P.C., F.A.C.P.
Division of Infectious Diseases, Ottawa Hospital, General Campus, Ottawa, ON, Canada

Stanny Geerts, D.V.M., Ph.D.
Professor, Prince Leopold Institute of Tropical Medicine, Department of Animal Health,
Antwerpen, Belgium

Mahmoud A. Ghannoum, Ph.D.
Center for Medical Mycology, Department of Dermatology, University Hospitals
of Cleveland, Case Western Reserve University, Cleveland, OH, USA

Consuelo Gomez, Ph.D.
Professor, Programa Institucional de Biomedicina Molecular, Escuela Nacional
de Medicina y Homeopatia, Instituto Politecnico Nacional, Mexico, D.F., Mexico

Michael L. Greenberg, Ph.D.
b3bio, Research Triangle Park, NC, USA

Robert E.W. Hancock, Ph.D.
Centre for Microbial Diseases and Immunity Research, University of British Columbia,
Vancouver, BC, Canada

Kimberly E. Hanson, M.D., M.H.S.
Associate in Medicine and Pathology, Associate Director, Molecular Microbiology,
Duke University Medical Center, Durham, NC, USA

Frederick G. Hayden, M.D.
Department of Medicine, University of Virginia School of Medicine, Charlottesville, VA, USA

Daria J. Hazuda, Ph.D.
Merck Research Labs, West Point, PA, USA

Leonid Heifets, M.D.
Mycobacterial Reference Laboratory, National Jewish Medical and Research Center,
Denver, CO, USA

Gabrielle M. Heilek, Ph.D.
Principal Research Scientist, Roche Pharmaceuticals, Palo Alto, CA, USA

Jannik Helweg-Larsen, M.D., D.M.Sci.
Department of Infectious Diseases, Rigshospitalet, Copenhagen University Hospital,
Copenhagen, Denmark

David K. Henderson, M.D.
Clinical Center, National Institutes of Health, Bethesda, MD, USA

Kathleen Horan, M.D.
Attending Physician, Pulmonary and Critical Care Medicine, Virginia Mason Medical
Center, Seattle, WA, USA

Marleen C.D.G. Huigen, Ph.D.
Department of Medical Microbiology, University Medical Center, Utrecht, Utrecht,
The Netherlands

Ann Huletsky, Ph.D.
Centre de Recherche en Infectiologie of Université Laval, Québec City, QC, Canada

Michael R. Jacobs, M.D., Ph.D.
Case Western Reserve University School of Medicine, University Hospitals Case Medical
Center, Cleveland, OH, USA

George A. Jacoby, M.D.
Lahey Clinic, Burlington, MA, USA

Jari Jalava, Ph.D.
Department of Bacterial and Infectious Diseases, National Public Health Institute,
Turku, Finland

Glenn W. Kaatz, M.D.
Division of Infectious Diseases, Wayne State University School of Medicine,
Detroit, MI, USA

Petros C. Karakousis, M.D.
Assistant Professor of Medicine and International Health,
Johns Hopkins University Center for Tuberculosis Research, Baltimore, MD, USA

Efthymia A. Karveli, M.D.
Research Fellow, Alfa Institute of Biomedical Sciences (AIBS), Athens, Greece

Wasif A. Khan, M.B.B.S., M.H.S.
Associate Scientist, International Centre for Diarrhoeal Disease Research,
Bangladesh (ICDDR, B), Dhaka, Bangladesh

Keith P. Klugman, M.D., Ph.D.
William H. Foege Professor of Global Health, Hubert Department of Global Health, Rollins
School of Public Health, Professor, Division of Infectious Diseases, School of Medicine,
Emory University, Atlanta, GA, USA

Joseph Kovacs, M.D.
Senior Investigator, CCMD, National Institutes of Health, Bethesda, MD, USA

George Kukolj, Ph.D.
Boehringer Ingelheim (Canada) Ltd., Research and Development, Laval, QC, Canada

Roland Leclercq, M.D., Ph.D.
CHU de Caen, Service de Microbiologie, Caen, France

Kimberly D. Leuthner, Pharm.D.
Infectious Diseases Clinical Specialist, University Medical Center of Southern Nevada,
Las Vegas, NY, USA

Shawn Lewenza, Ph.D.
Assistant Professor, Department of Microbiology and Infectious Diseases,
University of Calgary, Calgary, AB, Canada

Stephen Locarnini, M.B.B.S., B.Sc.(Hon.), Ph.D., F.R.C.(Path.)
Victorian Infectious Diseases Reference Laboratory, North Melbourne, VIC, Australia

Cesar Lopez-Camarillo, Ph.D.
Professor, Programa de Ciencias Genomicas, Universidad Autonoma de la Ciudad de Mexico,
Mexico, D.F., Mexico

Jose L. Lopez-Ribot, Pharm. D., Ph.D.
Professor, Department of Biology and South Texas Center for Emerging Infectious Diseases,
The University of Texas at San Antonio, San Antonio, TX, USA

R. Dwayne Lunsford, Ph.D.
Director, Antimicrobial Services, ImQuest BioSciences, Inc., Frederick, MD, USA

Caron A. Lyman, Ph.D.
Research Scientist, Immunocompromised Host Section, Pediatric Oncology Branch,
National Cancer Institute, Bethesda, MD, USA

Pauline Macheboeuf, Ph.D.
Postdoctoral Scholar, Department of Chemistry & Biochemistry, University of California,
San Diego, La Jolla, CA, USA

Maria L. Magalhaes
Graduate Student, Department of Biochemistry, Albert Einstein College of Medicine,
Bronx, NY, USA

Gabrielle Maitland, B.V.Sc.
Ph.D. Research Student, Parasitology Department, Faculty of Veterinary Science,
University of Sydney, Sydney, NSW, Australia

Elias Manavathu, Ph.D.
Division of Infectious Diseases, Department of Internal Medicine, Wayne State University
School of Medicine, Detroit, MI, USA

Laurence A. Marchat, Ph.D.
Professor, Programa Institucional de Biomedicina Molecular, Escuela Nacional de Medicina
y Homepatia, Instituto Politecnico Nacional, Mexico, D.F., Mexico

Jorge L. Martinez-Cajas, M.D.
Postdoctoral Fellow, McGill University AIDS Centre, Jewish General Hospital,
Montreal, QC, Canada

Pascal Mäser, Ph.D.
Professor of Molecular Biology, Institute of Cell Biology, University of Bern,
Bern, Switzerland

Henry Masur, M.D.
Chief, Critical Care Medicine Department, National Institutes of Health,
Bethesda, MD, USA

Douglas L. Mayers, M.D.
Executive Vice President & Chief Medical Officer, Idenix Pharmaceuticals,
Cambridge, MA, USA

Patrick F. McDermott, M.S., Ph.D.
Director, Division of Animal and Food Microbiology, Office of Research, Center
for Veterinary Medicine, U.S. Food and Drug Administration, Laurel, MD, USA

Lesley McGee, Ph.D.
Hubert Department of Global Health, Rollins School of Public Health,
Emory University, Atlanta, GA, USA

John E. McGowan, Jr., M.D.
Department of Epidemiology, Rollins School of Public Health, Atlanta, GA, USA

Durrie L. McKnew, M.D.
Pediatrician, Pasadena, MD, USA

Joseph B. McPhee, Ph.D.
Postdoctoral Fellow, Center for Infectious Disease, State University of New York – Stony Brook,
Stony Brook, NY, USA

Honorè Méda, M.D., Ph.D.
Catholic Relief Services, Kigali, Rwanda

Thomas Melby, M.S.
Senior Medical Writer, i3 statprobe, Ann Arbor, MI

Sotohy Mohammad, Ph.D.
Postdoctoral Fellow, Center for Medical Mycology and Mycology Reference Laboratory,
Department of Dermatology, University Hospitals of Cleveland and Case Western Reserve
University, Cleveland, OH, USA

Stephen A. Morse, M.S.P.H., Ph.D.
Associate Director for Environmental Microbiology,
National Center for Preparedness, Detection, and Control of Infectious Diseases,
Centers for Disease Control and Prevention, Atlanta, GA, USA

Varsha V. Moudgal, M.D.
Assistant Professor of Medicine, Wayne State University School of Medicine,
St. Joseph Mercy Hospital, Ypsilanti, MI, USA

Rita Mukhopadhyay, Ph.D.
Department of Molecular Microbiology and Infectious Diseases,
Florida International University College of Medicine, Miami, FL, USA

Esther Orozco, Ph.D.
Departamento de Infectomica y Patogenesis Molecular, CINVESTAV IPN,
México, D.F., Mexico

Elizabeth M. O'Shaughnessy, M.D.
Research Fellow, Immunocompromised Host Section, Pediatric Oncology Branch,
National Cancer Institute, Bethesda, MD, USA

Neil Parkin, Ph.D.
Monogram Biosciences, South San Francisco, CA, USA

David L. Paterson M.D., Ph.D.
Professor of Medicine, University of Queensland, Centre for Clinical Research,
Royal Brisbane and Women's Hospital, Brisbane, QLD, Australia

Thomas F. Patterson, M.D., F.A.C.P., F.I.D.S.A.
Professor of Medicine and Chief, Division of Infectious Diseases,
The University of Texas Health Science Center and the South Texas Veterans Healthcare
System, San Antonio, TX, USA

Anton Y. Peleg, M.B., B.S.
Research Fellow, Beth Israel Deaconess Medical Center, Boston, MA, USA

Jacque Pepin, M.D., F.R.C.P.C., M.Sc.
Center for International Health, University of Sherbrooke, Sherbrooke, QC, Canada

D. Guillermo Perez, Ph.D.
Professor, Programa Institucional de Biomedicina Molecular, Escuela Nacional de Medicina
y Homeopatia, Instituto Politecnico Nacional, Mexico, D.F., Mexico

John Perfect, M.D.
Acting Chief, Division Infections Diseases, Duke University Medical Center,
Durham, NC, USA

Bruno Périchon, Ph.D.
Institut Pasteur, Unité des Agents Antibactériens, Paris, France

Marco Petrella, Ph.D.
Postdoctoral Fellow, McGill University AIDS Centre, Jewish General Hospital,
Montreal, QC, Canada

Livia Pica-Mattoccia, Ph.D.
Institute of Cell Biology, Monterotondo, Rome, Italy

Roger K. Prichard, Ph.D.
Institute of Parasitology, Macdonald Campus, McGill University, Ste. Anne de Bellevue,
QC, Canada

Steven J. Projan, Ph.D.
Vice President; Global Head, Infectious Diseases, Novartis Institutes for BioMedical Research,
Cambridge, MA, USA

Madhukar Rai, M.D., D.M.
Professor, Department of Medicine, Institute of Medical Sciences, Banaras Hindu University,
Varanasi, India

John H. Rex, M.D.
Infection Clinical Vice President, Oncology & Infection Therapy Area,
AstraZeneca Pharmaceuticals, Macclesfield, UK
Adjunct Professor of Medicine, University of Texas Medical School – Houston,
Houston, TX, USA

Louis B. Rice, M.D.
Louis Stokes Cleveland Department of Veterans Affairs Medical Center and Case Western
Reserve University, Cleveland, OH, USA

Marilyn C. Roberts, Ph.D.
Department of Environmental & Occupational Health Sciences,
School of Public Health and Community Medicine, University of Washington,
Seattle, WA, USA

P. David Rogers, Pharm.D., Ph.D.
Assistant Professor of Pharmacy, Pharmaceutical Sciences and Pediatrics,
Colleges of Pharmacy and Medicine, University of Tennessee, Children's Foundation
Research Center of Memphis, Le Bonheur Children's Medical Center,
Memphis, TN, USA

Marleen H. Roos, Ph.D.
Director, RoosProjectConsult, Hulshorst, The Netherlands

Barry P. Rosen, Ph.D.
Associate Dean for Basic Research and Graduate Studies, Florida International University,
College of Medicine, Miami, FL, USA

Philip J. Rosenthal, M.D.
Department of Medicine, San Francisco General Hospital, University of California,
San Francisco, CA, USA

Paul H. Roy, Ph.D.
Département de Biochimie et de Microbiologie, Centre de Recherche en Infectiologie,
Université Laval, Québec, QC, Canada

William A. Rutala, Ph.D., M.P.H.
Director, Hospital Epidemiology, Occupational Health and Safety Program,
UNC Health Care System, Chapel Hill, NC, USA
Professor of Medicine, UNC School of Medicine, Chapel Hill, NC, USA
Director, Statewide Program in Infection Control and Epidemiology,
UNC School of Medicine, Chapel Hill, NC, USA

Michael J. Rybak, Pharm.D., M.P.H.
Associate Dean for Research, Professor of Pharmacy & Adjunct, Professor of Medicine,
Director, Anti-Infective Research Laboratory, Eugene Applebaum College of Pharmacy &
Health Sciences, Wayne State University, Detroit, MI, USA

Debasish Saha, M.B.B.S., M.S.
Clinical Epidemiologist, Bacterial Diseases Programme,
Medical Research Council Laboratories, The Gambia, West Africa

Nicholas C. Sangster, B.Sc.(Vet.), B.F.Sc., Ph.D.
School of Animal and Veterinary Sciences, Charles Sturt University, Wagga Wagga,
NSW, Australia

Michael A. Saubolle, Ph.D.
Department of Clinical Pathology, Banner Good Samaritan Medical Center,
Phoenix, AZ, USA

Stefan Schwarz, D.V.M.
Institut für Nutztiergenetik, Friedrich-Loeffler-Institut (FLI), Neustadt-Mariensee, Germany

Thomas Seebeck, Ph.D.
Institute of Cell Biology, University of Bern, Bern, Switzerland

Helena Seppala, M.D., Ph.D.
Ophthalmologist, Docent in Medical Bacteriology, Department of Ophthalmology,
Turku City Hospital, Turku, Finland

Dean Shinabarger, Ph.D.
Micromyx, LLC, Kalamazoo, MI, USA

Mark E. Shirtliff, Ph.D.
Assistant Professor, Department of Biomedical Sciences, Dental School,
University of Maryland – Baltimore, Baltimore, MD, USA
Adjunct Professor, Department of Microbiology and Immunology, School of Medicine,
University of Maryland – Baltimore, Baltimore, MD, USA

David M. Shlaes, M.D., Ph.D.
Anti-infectives Consulting, LLC, Stonington, CT, USA

Joanne L. Simala-Grant, B.Sc., Ph.D.
Research Facilitator, Faculty of Medicine and Dentistry,
University of Alberta, Edmonton, AB, Canada

Paul F.G. Sims, Ph.D.
Manchester Interdisciplinary Biocentre, University of Manchester, Manchester, UK

Ola E. Skold, M.D., Ph.D.
Department of Medical Biochemistry and Microbiology, Biomedical Center,
Uppsala University, Uppsala, Sweden, Uppsala, Sweden

Melinda Smedema, B.Sc.
Research Associate, Mira Vista Diagnostics/MiraBella Technologies, Indianapolis, IN, USA

David R. Snydman, M.D., F.A.C.P.
Chief, Division of Geographic Medicine and Infectious Diseases, Tufts Medical Center,
Boston, MA, USA
Professor of Medicine, Tufts University School of Medicine, Boston, MA, USA

Jack D. Sobel, M.D.
Division of Infectious Diseases, Harper University Hospital, Detroit, MI, USA

Kathryn A. Stafford
Research Assistant, Department of Clinical Veterinary Science, University of Bristol,
Langford, Bristol, UK

Paul Stoodley, Ph.D.
Associate Professor, Immunology & Microbiology, Singer Research Institute,
Drexel University College of Medicine – Pittsburgh Campus, Allegheny General
Hospital, Pittsburgh, PA

Boris Striepen, Ph.D.
Center for Tropical and Emerging Global Diseases & Department of Cellular Biology,
University of Georgia, Paul Coverdell Center, Athens, GA, USA

Shyam Sundar, M.D., F.R.C.P., F.N.A.
Professor, Department of Medicine, Institute of Medical Sciences, Banaras Hindu University,
Varanasi, India

Sandeep Tamber, Ph.D.
Postdoctoral Fellow, Dartmouth College Medical School, Dartmouth College,
Hanover, NH, USA

John W. Tapsall, M.B., B.S., F.R.C.P.A., M.D.
Director, WHO Collaborating Centre for STD and HIV, The Prince of Wales Hospitals,
Sydney, NSW, Australia

Diane E. Taylor, B.Sc., Ph.D.
Professor Emeritus, Department of Medical Microbiology and Immunology,
University of Alberta, Edmonton, AB, Canada

Fred C. Tenover, Ph.D., D(ABMM)
Senior Director, Scientific Affairs, Cepheid, Sunnyvale, CA, USA

Margaret Tisdale, Ph.D.
GlaxoSmithKline Medicines Research Centre, Stevenage, Hertfordshire, UK

Jacqueline Anne Upcroft, B.Sc. Hons., Ph.D.
The Queensland Institute of Medical Research, Brisbane, QLD, Australia

Peter Upcroft, B.Sc. Hons., Ph.D.
Associate Professor, The Queensland Institute of Medical Research,
Brisbane, QLD, Australia

Thierry Vernet, Ph.D.
Laboratoire d'Ingénierie des Macromolécules, Institut de Biologie, Structurale,
Grenoble, France

Mark A. Wainberg, Ph.D.
McGill University AIDS Centre, Jewish General Hospital, Montréal, QC, Canada

Adrian R. Walmsley, Ph.D.
School of Biological and Biomedical Sciences, Durham University, Durham, UK

Thomas J. Walsh, M.D.
Pediatric Oncology Branch, National Cancer Institute, Bethesda, MD, USA

Stephen A. Ward, Ph.D.
Liverpool School of Tropical Medicine, Liverpool, UK

David J. Weber, M.D., M.P.H.
Professor of Medicine, Pediatrics, and Epidemiology, Associate Chief of Staff,
UNC Health Care, Chapel Hill, NC, USA
Medical Director, Hospital Epidemiology and Occupational Health,
UNC Hospitals, Chapel Hill, NC, USA

Linda M. Weigel, Ph.D.
Antimicrobial Resistance Laboratory, Division of Healthcare Quality Promotion,
Centers for Disease Control and Prevention, Atlanta, GA, USA

Richard P. Wenzel, M.D., M.Sc.
William Branch Porter Professor and Chair, Department of Medicine,
Virginia Commonwealth University Medical Center, Richmond, VA, USA

L. Joseph Wheat, M.D.
MiraVista Diagnostics/MiraBella Technologies, Indianapolis, IN, USA

Katherine Wheatcroft-Francklow, Ph.D.
School of Biological Sciences, University of Wales Bangor, Bangor, Gwynedd, UK

Lisa G. Winston, M.D.
Department of Medicine, Division of Infectious Diseases, University of California,
San Francisco, Hospital Epidemiologist, San Francisco General Hospital,
San Francisco, CA, USA

Gerard D. Wright, Ph.D.
M.G. DeGroote Institute for Infectious Disease Research, Antimicrobial Research Centre,
Department of Biochemistry and Biomedical Sciences, McMaster University,
Hamilton, ON, Canada

Andre Zapun, Ph.D.
Research Scientist, CNRS, Laboratory for Macromolecular Engineering,
Institut de Biologie Structurale (CEA, CNRS, UJF), Grenoble, France

Marcus J. Zervos, M.D.
Wayne State University School of Medicine, Division Head, Infectious Diseases,
Henry Ford Health System, Detroit, MI, USA

Chapter 47
Resistance in *Streptococcus pneumoniae*

Lesley McGee and Keith P. Klugman

1 Introduction

Streptococcus pneumoniae (the pneumococcus) has been an important human pathogen for over 100 years and continues to cause a wide variety of infections, ranging from mild infections to serious lower respiratory infections, as well as life-threatening invasive infections such as meningitis. It is the most common bacterial cause of acute otitis media and pneumonia and an important cause of childhood mortality. The World Health Organization estimates that more than 1.6 million people die every year from pneumococcal infections – primarily pneumonia and meningitis – including more that 800,000 children under 5 years of age (1). As well as affecting the young, *S. pneumoniae* is an important cause of morbidity and mortality in the elderly; it is the most common etiological agent of community-acquired pneumonia, often resulting in hospitalization of previously healthy individuals.

Infections caused by *S. pneumoniae* were for many years traditionally treated with penicillin or ampicillin, to which this species was exquisitely sensitive when penicillin was first introduced in the 1940s. However, resistance which was first seen in the 1960s has continued to increase throughout the world in more recent decades. The emergence of resistance to penicillin and other beta-lactam antibiotics in pneumococci in the 1980s and 1990s led to increased use of macrolides, fluoroquinolones, and other non-beta-lactam antibiotics for pneumococcal infections. Efforts to treat pneumococcal disease in both adults and children have been complicated by this increasing resistance to antimicrobials. The increase in antimicrobial resistance rates is in part due to the selective pressures associated with the widespread use of antibiotics (2, 3) and the clonal expansion and spread of multiresistant *S. pneumoniae*.

L. McGee (✉)
Hubert Department of Global Health, Rollins School of Public Health, Emory University, Atlanta, GA, USA
lmcgee@sph.emory.edu

The total population of antibiotic-resistant pneumococci increasingly is dominated by a small number of highly successful clones (4) and understanding the genetic basis of resistance in these clones may provide insights that lead to effective strategies to reduce transmission of multiple resistant pneumococci.

This chapter focuses on the emergence and incidence of antibiotic resistance in pneumococci, mechanisms and the clinical implications of this resistance.

2 Epidemiology of the Pneumococcus and Risk Factors for Resistance

The incidence of pneumococcal disease is the highest in children <2 years of age and in adults >65 years of age. Other important risk factors include underlying medical conditions such as chronic heart and lung disease, cigarette smoking, and immunodeficiency states such as asplenia, HIV, and sickle cell disease.

S. pneumoniae colonizes the upper respiratory tract and is part of the normal flora of healthy individuals. A particular serotype can be carried for many months before being eradicated or replaced by a different serotype. Carriage increases in the first few months of life and the highest asymptomatic colonization rates (exceeding 40%) are observed in young children. Factors associated with increased carriage include winter season, day care attendance, and living in crowded conditions (5). Carriage in adults is approximately 10–20% and the duration of carriage is generally shorter. Investigations of serotype prevalence from various parts of the world have shown that serotype distribution varies with geographical location and age (6). The distribution of serotypes also varies between carriage isolates and invasive disease and antibiotic resistance is most frequent in pneumococcal serotypes that are carried by children (types/groups 6, 9, 14, 19, and 23) (6). The probable reason is the frequent use of antibiotic therapy in small children and hence exposure of strains of these serotypes to antimicrobial drugs, providing a selective advantage to resistant mutants (7).

There are multiple risk factors for acquisition of infection with antibiotic-resistant pneumococci. Most of these factors have a commonality in exposure to the drugs that select the resistance. This exposure to β-lactams can be at the level of a country (8); province (9); day care (10); family (11); or individual (12). Macrolide resistance is also a function of exposure, particularly of long-acting drugs such as azithromycin (13). The selection of resistant strains is complicated by multiple resistance where macrolides appear to be better selectors of multiresistant strains than do β-lactam drugs (12). The issue of cross-resistance extends to treatment of such diverse organisms as the malaria parasite, where treatment with fansidar selects trimethoprim–sulfamethoxazole resistance in pneumococci (14).

Most resistance is selected as mentioned above in children, but the exception is fluoroquinolone resistance which is selected in adults (15–17) as these agents are not usually given to children.

Little is known about the impact of drug dose on the selection of resistant strains, but there is a prospective study that suggests that high dose and short duration of amoxicillin therapy may select less resistance than the same total dose given over a longer period of time (18).

Nosocomial acquisition is a major risk for resistant pneumococci (19) and the first multiple resistant strains were selected in hospitals (20).

HIV infection is a risk for increased resistance in pneumococcal infections due to the frequent exposure of these patients to antibiotic prophylaxis and the hospital environment (21–23) as well as the fact that these patients, especially HIV-infected women are at risk due to the antibiotic-resistant serotypes carried by children (24).

3 The Role of Clones in Resistance

The spread of antibiotic resistance and the development of new vaccines have focused attention on the epidemiology of *S. pneumoniae* over recent years. While antimicrobial susceptibility patterns and serotyping remain important methods for characterizing pneumococci, molecular typing techniques add greater discrimination and complementary information. A major challenge to delineating the epidemiology of pneumococcal isolates is the determination of clonality. To this end, the Pneumococcal Molecular Epidemiology Network (PMEN) was established in 1997 with the aim of standardizing laboratory methods and epidemiological definitions to identify clones of antimicrobial-resistant *S. pneumoniae*. The use of typing methods like PFGE, BOX-PCR, and MLST and

fingerprinting of penicillin-binding protein (*pbp*) genes, combined with serotyping and antimicrobial resistance patterns have allowed isolates from different epidemiological regions to be examined for potential relationships and the identification of persistent local and global clones ((4), www.sph.emory.edu/PMEN).

Molecular typing of data from numerous studies over the past few decades has added to our knowledge by showing, that although there is considerable diversity among resistant strains within most serotypes, a small number of highly successful clones have emerged within countries and in some cases have achieved massive geographical spread (4, 25). Isolates belonging to some of these clones also represent a very large proportion of resistant strains in a given epidemiological setting. These clones have been isolated from pediatric as well as from adult disease and also as pneumococci colonizing the nasopharyngeal flora of healthy children.

The best characterized, and most widely spread of these international clones is the Spain[23F]-1 originally described in Spain during the 1980s. Intercontinental spread of this clone to the United States was described in 1991 (25) and strains belonging to this genotype continue to be isolated in many countries all over the world. As these global clones have spread, they have been exposed to new selective pressures applied by regional variations in the use of different antibiotics. This has led to the further selection of strains belonging to these clones with varying antimicrobial resistance patterns. Studies have shown that recombinational exchanges at the capsular biosynthetic locus are responsible for the emergence of serotype variants of these clones (26). A penicillin-resistant serotype 9V clone (Spain[9V]-3) detected in Spain and France has become widely disseminated and the variants in its serotype 14 appear to have a marked predilection to cause invasive disease (27). This clone has emerged as one of the dominant serotype 14 clones particularly common in parts of South America (28). Erythromycin-resistant serotype 14 pneumococci in the United Kingdom are primarily associated with a single clone, which has remained the dominant cause of the serotype 14 disease for the past two decades (29). This England[14]-9 clone has spread intercontinentally and is one of the major serotype 14 clones associated with penicillin and erythromycin-resistant invasive strains in the United States (30) and elsewhere. Molecular epidemiology studies have also shown that some resistant clones recovered in different countries are completely distinct and have almost certainly emerged separately in each of these countries (4).

There is extensive documentation of the importance of clonal spread as a mechanism for the dissemination of penicillin-resistant and macrolide-resistant pneumococci. The rapid emergence and spread of macrolide resistance associated with strains carrying both the *erm*(B) and *mef*(A) genes over the past decade, is primarily associated with the clonal expansion of the Taiwan[19F]-14 genotype. Pneumococcal isolates containing both these genes are thought to have evolved from early isolates of this clone which contained only the *mef*(A) (4, 31). Of 366 *erm(B)* + *mef(A)* isolates from the PROTEKT global study (1999–2003), 83.3% were the Taiwan[19F]-14 clonal complex, with the highest prevalence seen in South Africa, South Korea, and the United States (32). This and other studies (31, 33) confirm the increasing global emergence and rapidly increasing prevalence of this multidrug-resistant pneumococcal clone in many regions of the world. There have also been reports of the emergence of resistance to newer drug classes such as the fluoroquinolones (34, 35) and the evolution of strains with resistance to higher concentrations of antimicrobial agents already in use (36). Globally most of the FQ-resistant strains of *S. pneumoniae* arise form heterogeneous mutations and are not clonal. However clonal spread of FQ resistance has been documented and resistance to FQs has been reported in several international clones including Spain[23F]-1, Spain[9V]-23, England[14]-9, - Taiwan[19F]-14, and others (37). The emergence and dissemination of resistance to new antimicrobials via international clones is plausible and is likely to accelerate the spread of resistance in countries characterized by high use of these antibiotics.

4 Laboratory Detection of Resistance

Bacterial culture and phenotypic susceptibility tests remain the gold-standard approaches for the detection of antibacterial resistance in pneumococci in clinical laboratories. Because it is a fastidious organism, however, specific methods and interpretative criteria developed by a variety of professional bodies such as the Clinical and Laboratory Standards Institute (CLSI, formerly the National Committee for Clinical Laboratory Standards, NCCLS), the British Society for Antimicrobial Chemotherapy (BSAC), and the European Committee on Antimicrobial Susceptibility testing (EUCAST) must be used to ensure accurate and consistent results (38). Because the breakpoints are determined on the basis of the outcome of microbiological, pharmacological and clinical data, and since patterns of resistance to antimicrobial drugs continue to evolve, changes to breakpoints can occur during the lifetime of an antibiotic.

Rapid tests based mainly on immunological or molecular techniques have gained importance for the detection of antibacterial resistance over the last two decades. Molecular assays for several resistance markers are reliable, such as *mec*A in staphylococci and *van*A in enterococci (39). For other resistance markers, there is currently a lack of field testing. Du Plessis et al. developed a semi-nested PCR assay for the detection of penicillin-resistant and -susceptible pneumococci in cerebrospinal fluid and their PCR results were 100% concordant with MIC data (40). Another study by the same investigators differentiated intermediate- and high-level penicillin resistance and PCR results were in agreement with MIC data for 98.3% (180 of 183) of these isolates (41). Additional assays using conventional PCR (42) and real-time PCR (43) have been developed for the detection of penicillin resistance in clinical isolates of *S. pneumoniae*.

Although genotypic-based methods hold promise for the rapid and accurate detection or confirmation of antimicrobial resistance, phenotypic methods will continue to have an advantage when resistance to the same antimicrobial agent may be caused by several different mechanisms. Genotypic assays have the ability to detect resistance genes, but not necessarily their level of transcription and translation; so susceptibility and clinical studies will be required to validate the genotypic approach to detection of antimicrobial resistance. In addition, direct detection of pneumococcal genetic resistance loci from clinical specimens must be interpreted with caution since streptococci in the normal flora may also harbor the same loci.

5 Resistance to β-Lactams

With the advent of penicillin G therapy in the 1940s, the case fatality rate for pneumonia fell dramatically (44). Pneumococcal isolates were initially extremely sensitive to the drug with MICs of ≤0.01 mg/L. Penicillin resistance was demonstrated in laboratory mutants soon after the introduction of penicillin G into clinical use but was not reported in clinical strains until 20 years later when investigators in Boston reported penicillin resistance in 2 of 200 strains (45). Initially, the observation was not considered relevant, until Hansman and Bullen (46) gave a report describing a penicillin-resistant strain (MIC 0.6 mg/L) isolated in Australia from the sputum of a patient with hypogammaglobulinemia. Subsequently, resistant strains were identified in New Guinea and Australia and in 1974 the first clinical infection due to a penicillin non-susceptible strain was reported in the Unites States (47, 48). In 1977 pneumococci resistant to penicillin began to appear in South Africa and in 1978, the first multidrug-resistant pneumococci were documented in Johannesburg, South Africa (20, 49). In between and after these initial reports, detection of penicillin-resistant pneumococci among clinical isolates began to be reported with increasing frequency in the clinical and microbiological setting. Today, penicillin-resistant strains are encountered in all countries in which adequate surveys are conducted and an increasing number of countries are reporting a high prevalence of penicillin-resistant pneumococci.

In two recent multinational studies, the prevalence of penicillin resistance among *S. pneumoniae* isolates ranged from 18.2 to 22.1% (50, 51).

β-lactam antibiotics inhibit the growth of pneumococci by inactivation of cell-wall synthesizing penicillin-binding proteins (PBPs). β-lactam resistance in pneumococci occurs by alterations in the key cell wall of PBPs and the creation of *pbp* genes with decreased affinities for these antimicrobials. Six PBPs have been identified in *S. pneumoniae* (PBPs 1a, 1b, 2a, 2b, 2x, 3), of which PBP2X and PBP2B have been confirmed to be essential for cell growth (52, 53). Little data exist for the role of PBPs 1b, 2a and 3 (54, 55) as resistance determinants and altered PBPs 2x, 2b, and 1a are the major players in the development of β-lactam resistance in most clinical isolates. The altered PBPs are encoded by genes with a mosaic structure and can undergo inter- and intraspecies recombination so that parts of the genes are replaced by allelic variants that differ by up to 25% in DNA sequence. In general, the resistance profile of particular isolates results from interactions between various combinations of altered PBPs, in conjunction with a functional *murMN* operon which encodes enzymes involved in the synthesis of branched structured muropeptides.

Resistance to penicillin is associated with some degree of non-susceptibility to all β-lactam antibiotics. Mutations in PBP2x confer low-grade penicillin resistance and may be sufficient for the cell to become nonsusceptible to oral cephalosporins. Alterations in PBP2b result in even higher MICs to penicillin (56) while changes in PBP1a are required for high-level penicillin resistance (55, 57) and extended-spectrum cephalosporin resistance (58, 59). Isolates with very high levels of penicillin resistance (MICs ≥ 8 mg/L) require changes in all three PBPs (i.e. 1a, 2b, and 2x) and sometimes also in additional non-PBP resistance determinants such as MurM (60).

Resistance rates reported for amoxicillin are relatively low (<5%) as a result of the favorable pharmacodynamic properties of this agent (61, 62). Generally, MICs to amoxicillin are equal to, or two to four times less than the MIC of penicillin (63). In the past few years there have been numerous reports of strains with amoxicillin MICs (4–16 mg/L) higher than penicillin MICs (2–8 mg/L) (36, 62, 64, 65). In particular, PBP2b appears to play a significant role in mediating the expression of this resistance phenotype (66). In addition to typical changes in PBP1a and PBP2x, these strains have unique mutations in the 590–641 region of the PBP2b gene in close proximity to the active binding site (62, 65, 66).

Resistance to cephalosporins may develop with mutations in the pbp1a and pbp2x genes and the close linkage of these two genes on the chromosome is conducive to the transfer of both genes in a single transformation step (58, 67). PBP2b is not a target for cephalosporins; so would remain unaltered in isolates expressing cephalosporin resistance and susceptibility to penicillin (68). Most, but not all, extended-spectrum cephalosporin-resistant strains are also penicillin-resistant and as with amoxicillin, the MICs of cefotaxime and ceftriaxone are usually lower than the MICs of penicillin. In the early 1990s in the United States, pneumococci with high-level cefotaxime and ceftriaxone (2–32 mg/L) resistance were detected (69) and this high-level resistance was due to alterations in PBPs 1A and 2X (59). The cephalosporin MICs were in excess of the MICs of penicillin for these isolates and specific point mutations (Thr$_{550}$Ala) in the *pbp2x* gene were associated with this phenotype (59). These cephalosporin-resistant strains emerged within a few preexisting clones and demonstrate that point mutations as well as recombinational events are important in the development of resistance to β-lactam antibiotics in pneumococci.

6   Resistance to Macrolides

The macrolides have been used extensively to treat community-acquired respiratory tract infections worldwide and in recent years resistance to macrolide antibiotics (e.g. erythromycin, clarithromycin, and azithromycin) in *S. pneumoniae* has escalated dramatically. Macrolide-resistant *S. pneumoniae* are now more common than penicillin-resistant *S. pneumoniae* in many parts of the world (70). However, both macrolide resistance rates and resistance mechanisms may vary considerably depending on location (71). Erythromycin resistance rates range from <4 to >70% in worldwide surveillance studies (51, 72) and these differences probably reflect, in part, the variation in antibiotic-prescribing behavior between different countries.

Macrolide resistance in *S. pneumoniae* is mediated primarily by two mechanisms: target modification and active efflux. The most common form of target modification is usually the result of dimethylation of the adenine residue at position 2058 on the 23S rRNA by a methylase enzyme (73). This mechanism confers constitutive high-level resistance (MIC, >256 mg/L) to 14-, 15-, and 16-member macrolides, lincosamides, and streptogramins B, the so called MLS$_B$ phenotype. In *S. pneumoniae*, methylation is *erm*(B) mediated in almost all cases, although, more rarely, a methylase encoded by *erm*(A) subclass *erm*(TR) has been implicated (74). Target modification by point mutations in domain II and V of 23S rRNA and in the genes encoding riboproteins L4 and L22 can also confer macrolide resistance and have been documented in clinical isolates from widely distributed global sites (75–77).

In certain countries, such as the United States (78), active efflux is the major mechanism for macrolide resistance. It confers low-level resistance (MIC, 1–16 mg/L) to 14- and 15-member macrolides but not to 16-member macrolides, lincosamides, and streptogramin B and is phenotypically referred to as the M phenotype. This efflux in *S. pneumoniae* is due to acquisition of the *mef* gene, originally described in *Streptococcus pyogenes* as *mef*(A) and then identified as the *mef*(E) gene in *S. pneumoniae* (79, 80). As homology between these two genes is >80%, the two genes were originally grouped as a single class, *mef*(A) (81). Important differences however exist between these two variants and recent data shows that the two genes have disseminated differently and are being recognized in an ever-growing number of microbial species (82, 83). In addition, the two *mef* variants exist on different genetic elements – *mef*(A) on Tn1207.1 and *mef*(E) on mega (84, 85). An additional efflux mechanism, mediated by the *msr*(D) or the *mel* gene, has been found on Tn1207.1 and the mega element, respectively (84, 86). *msr*(D) and *mel* are homologues of the ATP-binding cassette gene *msr*(A), found in staphylococci and known to be responsible for efflux of macrolides and streptogramins (87).

Worldwide *erm*(B) and *mef* (A or E) mechanisms account for the majority of macrolide resistance among pneumococci and the prevalence of these genes varies considerably among countries. Some macrolide-resistant *S. pneumoniae* contain both *erm*(B) and *mef* genes. Corso et al. in a 1996–1997 US study, found a prevalence of 7% (88). McGee et al. (31) identified 30.5% of erythromycin-resistant pneumococci with dual mutations and showed that the majority (83%) of these isolates were clonally related to a serotype 19F strain originating in Taiwan (31). Data from the PROTEKT US surveillance study (32) show an increase in the prevalence of resistant isolates containing both *erm*(B) and *mef*(A) from 9.7% in 2000–2001 to 16.4% in 2002–2003, with substantial regional variability. The majority of these isolates exhibited multidrug resistance and >90% were clonally related to the multidrug-resistant international Taiwan[19F]-14 clonal complex. It appears that the global increase in macrolide resistant strains carrying both the *erm*(B) and *mef* genes is being driven in part by the expansion of this Taiwan[19F]-14 clone.

7 Resistance to Fluoroquinolones

Due to the increased rates of resistance to β-lactam and macrolide antibiotics among pneumococcal strains, fluoroquinolones (FQs) are now included among the choices for first-line therapy in clinical guidelines for the treatment of pneumonia. However, there has been growing concern about the emergence of FQ-resistant strains and there have been numerous reports of treatment failures due to infection with FQ-resistant pneumococci (89).

Fluoroquinolone resistance in *S. pneumoniae* remains relatively low worldwide (<1%), but it is nonetheless increasing, particularly in some countries. Large surveillance studies conducted over the past decade suggest that the prevalence of levofloxacin-resistant strains in North America remains <2% (34, 35, 90). Higher rates have been reported in Spain (7%), Sri Lanka (9.5%), the Philippines (9.1%) and Korea (6.5%) (91–93). The highest prevalence of levofloxacin resistance has been reported from Hong Kong (15.2%) and this rapid increase in resistance has been associated with the dissemination of strains related to the Spain[23F]-1 clone (94).

Two mechanisms that decrease susceptibility to FQs in pneumococci have been identified: target alteration and reduced accumulation due to efflux. Resistance associated with target modification requires a combination of mutations in the quinolone resistance-determining region (QRDR) of the genes encoding the DNA gyrase and DNA topoisomerase IV subunits. First-step mutants generally result from spontaneous mutations in the preferential target for a given FQ, ParC for ciprofloxacin and levofloxacin or GyrA for moxifloxacin, gatifloxacin, and gemifloxacin (95, 96). Some isolates with a first-step mutation in *parC* gene have ciprofloxacin MICs that would indicate that they are clinically susceptible (MIC, <4 mg/L) and these strains would not be identified using routine antibiotic susceptibility testing (97). The population of isolates with first-step mutations is important because, compared with strains without these first-step mutations, they are more likely to develop high-level resistance during therapy with the acquisition of a second-step mutation (98, 99). In the second-step mutants, amino acid substitutions are present in both topoisomerase IV and gyrase, most frequently affecting ParC and GyrA, and less so ParE and GyrB (100). Using a PCR-RFLP method to determine mutations known to confer resistance, Pletz et al. (101) screened 286 clinically susceptible isolates with levofloxacin MICs of 1 mg/L and 142 isolates with MICs of 2 mg/L. The prevalence of first step mutants among those strains with MICs of 1 mg/L was very low at 0.35%. Among those with a levofloxacin MIC of 2 mg/L, 16.2% of isolates recovered from nursing home residents and 6.4% from non-nursing home residents had first-step mutations. This data supports previous studies from large surveillance sites in Canada (102) and the US (103, 104) that report low prevalence of first-step mutants, ranging from 0.8 to 1.4% among strains with levofloxacin MICs of 1 mg/L. Although the actual numbers of isolates is smaller, there is however a higher prevalence of QRDR mutations among isolates with MICs of 2 mg/L, ~50–70% reported from the TRUST surveillance study (105).

Another mechanism underlying non-susceptibility to FQs in some pneumococcal isolates, is an increase in active efflux which affects quinolones such as ciprofloxacin (106). This efflux mechanism has primarily been demonstrated in isolates with low-level quinolone resistance (96). The role of interspecies recombination in FQ resistance among pneumococci has been described but appears to be minor (107–109).

Five of 46 (11%) ciprofloxacin-resistant strains from Spain showed evidence of the transfer of resistance genes from viridans streptococci to *S. pneumoniae* (107). But in a study from Canada (108) only 1 of 71 resistant isolates showed interspecies recombination and a recent study of 49 isolates from the USA (109) found no role played by recombination.

8 Resistance to New Classes of Antibiotics

Telithromycin, the first available ketolide drug, was developed to overcome macrolide resistance and was introduced into clinical practice in Germany in 2001, followed shortly by Italy, Spain, Mexico, Brazil, and France. The global surveillance project PROTEKT (Prospective Resistant Organism Tracking and Epidemiology for the Ketolide Telithromycin) reported that over 4 years, 21 out of 20 750 (0.1%) of *S. pneumoniae* isolates demonstrated low-level resistance (MICs 4–8 mg/L) to telithromycin (110). A low occurrence of telithromycin-nonsusceptible pneumococci has also been reported in other studies (111, 112). Thus, although ketolide resistance is rare, resistant isolates have nonetheless been documented. Mutations in the resistance determinant *erm*(B) have been suggested to confer telithromycin resistance (112, 113). In addition, mutations at macrolide and ketolide binding sites, such as domains II and V of 23S rRNA and ribosomal proteins L4 and L22, have been reported to be associated with an elevated telithromycin MIC (113).

Linezolid is the first in the class oxazolidinone that was approved for clinical use in 2000 for the treatment of nosocomial and community-acquired pneumonia. Reports of nonsusceptibility to linezolid have been sporadic among clinical isolates of staphylococci and enterococci and resistance has been found to be conferred by mutations in domain V of 23S rRNA (114). To date, linezolid nonsusceptible pneumococcal strains are extremely rare (115, 116). Wolter et al. (117) recently described two clinical isolates with decreased susceptibility to linezolid (MICs 4 mg/L) which were found to contain 6-bp deletions in the gene encoding the riboprotein L4. The L4 deletions were also found to confer a novel mechanism of simultaneous resistance to macrolides, oxazolidinones, and chloramphenicol.

Resistance to quinupristin–dalfopristin among Grampositive cocci has been very uncommon. Two clinical isolates among 8,837 (0.02%) *Streptococcus pneumoniae* isolates were discovered in 2001–2002 with MICs of 4 µg/mL. Each had a 5-amino-acid tandem duplication (RTAHI) in the L22 ribosomal protein gene (rplV) preventing synergistic ribosomal binding of the streptogramin combination (118).

9 Resistance to Other Agents

One class of antimicrobial agents previously used often in clinical practice is the tetracyclines, which are broad-spectrum bacteriostatic drugs shown to be active against pneumococci. Reflecting patterns of past usage, in some countries, reported rates of non-susceptibility to tetracyclines remain the most frequently observed resistance phenotype (119, 120). In *S. pneumoniae* tetracycline resistance is due to the protection of the bacterial 30S ribosome subunit against antibiotic binding by the TetM or TetO (121, 122) proteins, with the *tet*(M) gene being far more common than the *tet*(O)gene in pneumococci (123). In streptococci, *tet*(M) is usually associated with highly mobile conjugative transposons of the Tn*916*–Tn*1545* type and large composite structures like Tn*5253* and Tn*3872*. These transposons often carry other resistance genes, such as *erm*(B) coding for resistance to macrolides, lincosamides, and streptogramins B (124) which explains the persistence of tetracycline resistance (these transposons continue to be selected by macrolides). Comparison of *tet*(M) sequences in isolates of multidrug-resistant isolates, reveal a high degree of allelic variation (125). There is evidence of clonal distribution of selected alleles as well as horizontal movement of the mobile elements carrying *tet*(M) (126, 127).

The use of rifampin combined with either β-lactam antibiotics or vancomycin has been recommended for the treatment of meningitis caused by multiresistant pneumococci (128). Rifampin has been used in combined therapy to treat tuberculosis and resistant staphylococci (129), and it is extensively used in the prophylaxis of *Neisseria menigitidis* and *Haemophilus influenzae* type b exposure (130, 131). The prevalence of rifampin resistance among pneumococcal isolates is low at present and reported rates vary between 0.1 and 1.5% (132, 133). Rifampin resistance has been described in several bacterial species and is caused by an alteration of the β subunit of RNA polymerase, the target for the antibiotic. Resistance to rifampin in pneumococci has been linked to mutations in clusters N, I, II, and III of the *rpo*B gene, which encodes the β subunit (134, 135).

Resistance to chloramphenicol in *S. pneumoniae* is due to the acetylation of the antibiotic by the production of a chloramphenicol acetyltransferase (CAT) (136). The cat gene in pneumococcal isolates is carried on the conjugative transposon Tn*5253*, a composite transposon consisting of the tetracycline resistance transposon, Tn*5251*, and Tn*5252* which carries the chloramphenicol resistance determinant (137). Chloramphenicol-resistant strains have been shown to contain sequences homologous to cat$_{pC194}$ and other flanking sequences from *S. aureus* plasmid pC194 (138, 139).

Trimethoprim and sulfamethoxazole are used extensively in combination as the drug 'co-trimoxazole'. Cotrimoxazole has been used in the treatment of a range of *S. pneumoniae* diseases, especially in children, because it is inexpensive and generally effective. Resistance to cotrimoxazole has increased dramatically in many regions of the world and recent surveillance studies show rates ranging from 19% in Europe to around 50% associated with HIV infection in Africa and >60% in Asia (22, 140, 141). Resistance to cotrimoxazole is often associated with resistance to other antibiotics, especially to penicillin. Trimethoprim resistance in pneumococci has been reported to result from a single amino acid substitution (Ile-100→Leu) in the dihydrofolate reductase (DHFR) protein (142). Additional mutations have also been reported which seem to enhance resistance and modulate the effects of existing alterations on the affinity of DHFR for its natural substrates (143). In many cases, resistance to sulfonamides is associated with chromosomal mutations within the gene encoding dihydropteroate synthase (DHPS). Different studies have reported the occurrence of single and/or multiple amino acid mutations in the DHPS of sulfonamide-resistant clinical isolates of *S. pneumoniae* (144–146). The use of fansidar therapy for malaria in Africa has been shown to increase cotrimoxazole resistance in pneumococci (14).

Optochin, a quinine analogue, was introduced early in the twentieth century as a chemotherapeutic agent for the treatment of lobar pneumonia. However, serious side effects coupled with treatment failures quickly terminated the therapeutic use of this agent (147). During the first 30 years of its use for differentiating pneumococci from other α -hemolytic streptococci, there were no reports of optochin-resistant pneumococci. Since then, there have been sporadic reports of optochin-resistant pneumococci (148, 149). Investigators from Spain identified a gene responsible for the optochin susceptibility/resistance phenotype (150). They found that point mutations in amino acid residues 48, 49, or 50 of the H^+-ATPase c-subunit confer optochin resistance.

10 Clinical Relevance of Antibiotic Resistance

When penicillin-resistant pneumococci were first isolated from adults, there was an implicit assumption that such strains would fail intravenous penicillin therapy (151, 152). As our appreciation of pharmacodynamics has allowed the understanding of the time-based mode of action of β-lactams it is clear that the very high levels of penicillin achieved by intravenous therapy exceed the MICs of strains up to 8 μg/mL for most of the short 4–6 h dosing interval for high-dose intravenous penicillin (153). Such highly penicillin-resistant strains remain rare and there is little evidence for the failure of intravenous penicillin, amoxicillin, cefotaxime, or ceftriaxone (154, 155) due to penicillin resistance. It is possible that less active intravenous agents such as cefuroxime (156) may fail to treat penicillin-resistant infections and β-lactams with a more Gram-negative spectrum such as ticarcillin (151) and ceftazidime (157) should not be used to treat penicillin-resistant pneumococcal infections. It is likely that oral β-lactam therapy may fail in the management of pneumococcal infections such as otitis media when the strains become intermediately (MIC ≥ 0.1 μg/mL) resistant to penicillin. Poorly active cephalosporins such as cefaclor fail more often than cefuroxime (158, 159) and high-dose amoxicillin is the most active oral agent available against penicillin- resistant pneumococcal otitis media (160). It is likely that the inferences made for otitis will be similar for sinusitis (161). β-lactam resistance is clinically important for meningitis treatment where penicillin has been shown to fail (162) even for intermediately resistant strains because of the poor penetration of penicillin through the blood–brain barrier. Extended-spectrum cephalosporins fail too when there is full penicillin resistance in meningitis (MIC ≥ 2 μg/mL; associated with cefotaxime or ceftriaxone MIC's ≥ 1 μg/mL) (163, 164). The empiric therapy therefore of penicillin-resistant pneumococcal meningitis is cefotaxime plus vancomycin or ceftriaxone plus vancomycin, based on the observation that these drugs in combination are able to eradicate cephalosporin-resistant pneumococci from the CSF better (165) than either drug alone (165, 166).

Macrolide resistance is associated in most instances with MICs >2 μg/mL regardless of the mechanism of macrolide resistance, and treatment of these strains with macrolides has been shown to fail (71, 167), both in the management of otitis media (158, 159) and of pneumonia (168). These failures are in keeping with our knowledge of the pharmacodynamics of these agents (169).

Trimethoprim–sulfmethoxazole has been shown to not be able to eradicate from the middle ear, strains resistant to that agent (170).

Fluoroquinolones fail to successfully treat pneumococcal infections when pre-existing resistant strains are present, or even when first-step mutations in the *parC* gene are present (171). Immunocompromised patients may be most at risk for repeated infections due to fluoroquinolone-resistant strains (172).

11 Impact of Conjugate Vaccine

The introduction of conjugate pneumococcal vaccine has not only reduced the burden of invasive disease in children (173), but has impacted on carriage and thus on the burden of disease in adults (174) by preventing the spread of vaccine-type resistant strains to adults (175). Direct demonstration of the impact of conjugate vaccine on antibiotic-resistant invasive disease was demonstrated in the 9-valent conjugate vaccine trial in South Africa (176) while effectiveness studies both in individual states (177–179) and in multi-state studies (180) have demonstrated a significant reduction in the proportion and absolute incidence of antibiotic-resistant pneumococci isolated from blood. There is however less impact of the vaccine on isolates from the otitis media, as serotype replacement is far more common in the respiratory tract than in blood isolates. Antibiotic resistance is emerging in non-vaccine-type pneumococci causing ear infections (181) and a number of studies in the US post licensure of the conjugate vaccine, have failed to demonstrate an impact of the vaccine on nasopharyngeal or otitis isolates (182–184). Introduction of conjugate vaccine into a day care center in Portugal showed that antibiotic-resistant non-vaccine types emerged in that day-care center compared to a control day-care where children did not receive the vaccine (185).

12 Concluding Remarks

The multiple resistant pneumococcus now has a global distribution. Attempts to reduce the burden of resistance in this pathogen are frustrated by widespread empiric therapy for respiratory infections. Both appropriate and inappropriate antibiotic use continue to select resistance in this pathogen. Although the conjugate vaccine has reduced the burden of resistance in invasive isolates, continued antibiotic exposure is leading to the emergence of resistance in non-vaccine types.

References

1. WHO. Pneumococcal vaccines. Wkly Epidemiol Record 2003; 14:110–119
2. Castanheira M, Gales AC, Mendes RE, Jones RN, Sader HS. Antimicrobial susceptibility of *Streptococcus pneumoniae* in Latin America: results from five years of the SENTRY Antimicrobial Surveillance Program. Clin Microbiol Infect 2004; 10:645–651
3. Reinert RR, Reinert S, van der Linden M, Cil MY, Al-Lahham A, Appelbaum P. Antimicrobial susceptibility of *Streptococcus pneumoniae* in eight European countries from 2001 to 2003. Antimicrob Agents Chemother 2005;49:2903–2913
4. McGee L, McDougal L, Zhou J, et al. Nomenclature of major antimicrobial-resistant clones of *Streptococcus pneumoniae* defined by the pneumococcal molecular epidemiology network. J Clin Microbiol 2001;39:2565–2571
5. Zenni MK, Cheatham SH, Thompson JM, et al. *Streptococcus pneumoniae* colonization in the young child: association with otitis media and resistance to penicillin. J Pediatr 1995;127:533–537
6. Hausdorff WP, Feikin DR, Klugman KP. Epidemiological differences among pneumococcal serotypes. Lancet Infect Dis 2005;5:83–93
7. Klugman KP, Friedland IR. Antibiotic-resistant pneumococci in pediatric disease. Microb Drug Resist 1995;1:5–8
8. Bronzwaer S, Cars O, Buchholz U, et al. A European Study on the relationship between antimicrobial use and antimicrobial resistance. Emerg Infect Dis 2002;8:278–282
9. Arason VA, Kristinsson KG, Sigurdsson JA, Stefansdottir G, Molstad S, Gudmundsson S. Do antimicrobials increase the carriage rate of penicillin resistant pneumococci in children? Cross sectional prevalence study. Br Med J 1996;313:387–391
10. Levine OS, Farley M, Harrison LH, Lefkowitz L, McGeer A, Schwartz B. Risk factors for invasive pneumococcal disease in children: a population-based case-control study in North America. Pediatrics 199;103:E28
11. Samore MH, Magill MK, Alder SC, et al. High rates of multiple antibiotic resistance in *Streptococcus pneumoniae* from healthy children living in isolated rural communities: association with cephalosporin use and intrafamilial transmission. Pediatrics 2001;108:856–865
12. Vanderkooi OG, Low DE, Green K, Powis JE, McGeer A, Toronto Invasive Bacterial Disease Network. Predicting antimicrobial resistance in invasive pneumococcal infections. Clin Infect Dis 2005;40:1288–1297
13. Dias R. Emergence of invasive erythromycin-resistant *Streptococcus pneumoniae* strains in Portugal: contribution and phylogenetic relatedness of serotype 14. J Antimicrob Chemother 2004;54: 1035–1039
14. Feikin DR, Dowell SF, Nwanyanwu OC, et al. Increased carriage of trimethoprim/sulfamethoxazole-resistant *Streptococcus pneumoniae* in Malawian children after treatment for malaria with sulfadoxine/pyrimethamine. J Infect Dis 2000;181:1501–1505
15. Chen DK, McGeer A, de Azavedo JC, Low DE. Decreased susceptibility of *Streptococcus pneumoniae* to fluoroquinolones in Canada. Canadian Bacterial Surveillance Network. N Engl J Med 1999;341:233–239
16. Ho PL, Tse WS, Tsang KW, et al. Risk factors for acquisition of levofloxacin-resistant *Streptococcus pneumoniae*: a case-control study. Clinical Infect Dis 2001;32:701–707
17. Kupronis BA, Richards CL, Whitney CG, Active Bacterial Core Surveillance Team. Invasive pneumococcal disease in older adults residing in long-term care facilities and in the community. J Am Geriatr Soc 2003;51:1520–1525
18. Schrag SJ, Pena C, Fernandez J, et al. Effect of short-course, high-dose amoxicillin therapy on resistant pneumococcal carriage: a randomized trial. JAMA 2001;286:49–56
19. Bedos JP, Chevret S, Chastang C, Geslin P, Regnier B. Epidemiological features of and risk factors for infection by *Streptococcus pneumoniae* strains with diminished susceptibility to penicillin: findings of a French survey. Clin Infect Dis 1996;22:63–72
20. Jacobs MR, Koornhof HJ, Robins-Browne RM, et al. Emergence of multiply resistant pneumococci. N Engl J Med 1978;299: 735–740
21. Crewe-Brown HH, Karstaedt AS, Saunders GL, et al. *Streptococcus pneumoniae* blood culture isolates from patients with and without human immunodeficiency virus infection: alterations in penicillin susceptibilities and in serogroups or serotypes. Clin Infect Dis 1997;25:1165–1172
22. Madhi SA, Petersen K, Madhi A, Wasas A, Klugman KP. Impact of human immunodeficiency virus type 1 on the disease spectrum of *Streptococcus pneumoniae* in South African children. Pediatr Infect Dis J 2000;19:1141–1147
23. Jordano Q, Falco V, Almirante B, et al. Invasive pneumococcal disease in patients infected with HIV: still a threat in the era of highly active antiretroviral therapy. Clin Infect Dis 2004;38:1623–1628
24. Buie KA, Klugman KP, von Gottberg A, et al. Gender as a risk factor for both antibiotic resistance and infection with pediatric

serogroups/serotypes, in HIV-infected and –uninfected adults with pneumococcal bacteremia. J Infect Dis 2004;189:1996–2000

25. Munoz R, Coffey TJ, Daniels M, et al. Intercontinental spread of a multiresistant clone of serotype 23F *Streptococcus pneumoniae*. J Infect Dis 1991;164:302–306

26. Coffey TJ, Dowson CG, Daniels M, et al. Horizontal transfer of multiple penicillin-binding protein genes, and capsular biosynthetic genes, in natural populations of *Streptococcus pneumoniae*. Mol Microbiol 1991;5:2255–2260

27. Hanage WP, Kaijalainen TH, Syrjänen RK, et al. Invasiveness of serotypes and clones of *Streptococcus pneumoniae* among children in Finland. Infect Immun 2005;73:431–435

28. Vela MC, Fonseca N, Di Fabio JL, Castaneda E. Presence of international multiresistant clones of *Streptococcus pneumoniae* in Colombia. Microb Drug Resist 2001;7:153–164

29. Brueggemann AB, Griffiths DT, Meats E, Peto T, Crook DW, Spratt BG. Clonal relationships between invasive and carriage *Streptococcus pneumoniae* and serotype- and clone-specific differences in invasive disease potential. J Infect Dis 2003;187:1424–1432

30. Gertz Jr RE, McEllistrem MC, Boxrud DJ, et al. Clonal distribution of invasive pneumococcal isolates from children and selected adults in the United States prior to 7-valent conjugate vaccine introduction. J Clin Microbiol 2003;41:4194–4216

31. McGee L, Klugman KP, Wasas A, Capper T, Brink A. Serotype 19F multiresistant pneumococcal clone harboring two erythromycin resistance determinants (*erm*(B) and *mef*(A)) in South Africa. Antimicrob Agents Chemother 2001;45:1595–1598

32. Farrell DJ, Jenkins SG, Brown SD, Patel M, Lavin BS, Klugman KP. Emergence and spread of *Streptococcus pneumoniae* with *erm*(B) and *mef*(A) resistance. Emerg Infect Dis 2005;11: 851–858

33. Ko KS, Song JH. Evolution of erythromycin-resistant *Streptococcus pneumoniae* from Asian countries that contains *erm*(B) and *mef*(A) genes. J Infect Dis 2004;190:739–747

34. Pletz MWR, McGee L, Jorgensen JH, et al. Levofloxacin-resistant invasive *Streptococcus pneumoniae* in the United States: evidence for clonal spread and impact of the pneumococcal conjugate vaccine. Antimicrob Agents Chemother 2004;48:3491–3497

35. Richter SS, Heilmann KP, Beekmann SE, Miller NJ, Rice CL, Doern GV. The molecular epidemiology of *Streptococcus pneumoniae* with quinolone resistance mutations. Clin Infect Dis 2005;40:225–235

36. Schrag SJ, McGee L, Whitney CG, et al. Emergence of *Streptococcus pneumoniae* with very-high-level resistance to penicillin. Antimicrob Agents Chemother 2004;48:3016–3023

37. McGee L, Goldsmith CE, Klugman KP. Fluoroquinolone resistance among clinical isolates of *Streptococcus pneumoniae* belonging to international multiresistant clones. J Antimicrob Chemother 2002;49:173–176

38. Edson DC, Glick T, Massey LD. Susceptibility testing practices for *Streptococcus pneumoniae*: results of a proficiency testing survey of clinical laboratories. Diagn Microbiol Infect Dis 2006;55:225–230

39. Metan G, Zarakolu P, Unal S. Rapid detection of antibacterial resistance in emerging Gram-positive cocci. J Hosp Infect 2005;61:93–99

40. du Plessis M, Smith AM, Klugman KP. Rapid detection of penicillin-resistant *Streptococcus pneumoniae* in cerebrospinal fluid by a seminested-PCR strategy. J Clin Microbiol 1998;36:453–457

41. du Plessis M, Smith AM, Klugman KP. Application of pbp1A PCR in identification of penicillin-resistant *Streptococcus pneumoniae*. J Clin Microbiol 1999;37:628–632

42. Zettler EW, Scheibe RM, Dias CA, et al. Determination of penicillin resistance in *Streptococcus pneumoniae* isolates from southern Brazil by PCR. Int J Infect Dis 2006;10:110–115

43. Kearns AM, Graham C, Burdess D, Heatherington J, Freeman R. Rapid real-time PCR for determination of penicillin susceptibility in pneumococcal meningitis, including culture-negative cases. J Clin Microbiol 2002;40:682–684

44. Austrian R, Gold J. Pneumococcal bacteremia with special reference to bacteremic pneumococcal pneumonia. Ann Intern Med 1964;60:759–776

45. Kislak JW, Razavi LM, Daly AK, Finland M. Susceptibility of pneumococci to nine antibiotics. Am J Med Sci 1965;250:261–268

46. Hansman D, Bullen MM. A resistant pneumococcus. Lancet 1967;1:264–265

47. Hansman D, Glasgow H, Sturt J, Devitt HL, Douglas R. Increased resistance to penicillin of pneumococci isolated from man. N Engl J Med 1971;284:175–177

48. Naraqi S, Kirkpatrick GP, Kabins S. Relapsing pneumococcal meningitis: isolation of an organism with decreased susceptibility to penicillin G. J Pediatr 1974;85:671–673

49. Appelbaum PC, Bhamjee A, Scragg JN, Hallett AF, Bowen AJ, Cooper RC. *Streptococcus pneumoniae* resistant to penicillin and chloramphenicol. Lancet 1977;2:995–997

50. Felmingham D. Evolving resistance patterns in community-acquired respiratory tract pathogens: first results from the PROTEKT global surveillance study. Prospective Resistant Organism Tracking and Epidemiology for the Ketolide Telithromycin. J Infect Dis 2002;44:3–10

51. Jacobs MR, Felmingham D, Appelbaum PC, Grüneberg RN, the Alexander Project Group. The Alexander Project 1998–2000: susceptibility of pathogens isolated from community-acquired respiratory tract infection to commonly used antimicrobial agents. J Antimicrob Chemother 2003;52:229–246

52. Hakenbeck R, Ellerbrok H, Briese T, Handwerger S, Tomasz A. Penicillin-binding proteins of penicillin-susceptible and -resistant pneumococci: immunological relatedness of altered proteins and changes in peptides carrying the β-lactam binding site. Antimicrob Agents Chemother 1986;30:553–558

53. Kell CM, Sharma UK, Dowson CG, Town C, Balganesh TS, Spratt BG. Deletion analysis of the essentiality of penicillin binding proteins 1A, 2B and 2X of *Streptococcus pneumoniae*. FEMS Microbiol Lett 1993;106:171–175

54. Smith AM, Feldman C, Massidda O, McCarthy K, Ndiweni D, Klugman KP. Altered PBP2A and its role in the development of penicillin, cefotaxime and ceftriaxone resistance in a clinical isolate of *Streptococcus pneumoniae*. Antimicrob Agents Chemother 2005;49:2002–2007

55. Reichmann P, Koning A, Marton A, Hakenbeck R. Penicillin-binding proteins as resistance determinants in clinical isolates of *Streptococcus pneumoniae*. Microb Drug Resist 1996;2:177–181

56. Grebe T, Hakenbeck R. Penicillin-binding proteins 2b and 2x of *Streptococcus pneumoniae* are primary resistance determinants for different classes of β-lactam antibiotics. Antimicrob Agents Chemother 1996;40:829–834

57. Dowson CG, Johnson AP, Cercenado E, George RC. Genetics of oxacillin resistance in clinical isolates of *Streptococcus pneumoniae* that are oxacillin resistant and penicillin susceptible. Antimicrob Agents Chemother 1994;38:49–53

58. Munoz R, Dowson CG, Daniels M, et al. Genetics of resistance to third-generation cephalosporins in clinical isolates of *Streptococcus pneumoniae*. Mol Microbiol 1992;6:2461–2465

59. Coffey TJ, Daniels M, McDougal LK, Dowson CG, Tenover FC, Spratt BG. Genetic analysis of clinical isolates of *Streptococcus pneumoniae* with high-level resistance to expanded-spectrum cephalosporins. Antimicrob Agents Chemother 1995;39:1306–1313

60. Smith AM, Klugman KP. Alterations in MurM, a cell wall muropeptide branching enzyme, increase high-level penicillin and cephalosporin resistance in *Streptococcus pneumoniae*. Antimicrob Agents Chemother 2001;45:2393–2396

61. Vanhoof R, Brouillard J, Damee S, et al. High prevalence of penicillin resistance and comparative in vitro activity of various antibiotics in clinical isolates of *Streptococcus pneumoniae* isolated in the Province of Hainaut during winter 2004. Acta Clin Belg 2005;60:345–349

62. Cafini F, del Campo R, Alou L, et al. Alterations of the penicillin-binding proteins and *mur*M alleles of clinical *Streptococcus pneumoniae* isolates with high-level resistance to amoxicillin in Spain. J Antimicrob Chemother 2006;57:224–229

63. Butler DL, Gagnon RC, Miller LA, Poupard JA, Felmingham D, Gruneberg RN. Differences between the activity of penicillin, amoxycillin, and co-amoxyclav against 5,252 *Streptococcus pneumoniae* isolates tested in the Alexander Project 1992–1996. J Antimicrob Chemother 1999;43:777–782

64. Doit C, Loukil C, Fitoussi F, Geslin P, Bingen E. Emergence in France of multiple clones of clinical *Streptococcus pneumoniae* isolates with high-level resistance to amoxicillin. Antimicrob Agents Chemother 1999;43:1480–1483

65. Kosowska K, Jacobs MR, Bajaksouzian S, Koeth L, Appelbaum PC. Alterations of penicillin-binding proteins 1A, 2X and 2B in *Streptococcus pneumoniae* isolates with amoxicillin MICs are higher than penicillin MICs. Antimicrob Agents Chemother 2004;48:4020–4022

66. Du Plessis M, Bingen E, Klugman KP. Analysis of penicillin-binding protein genes of clinical isolates of *Streptococcus pneumoniae* with reduced susceptibility to amoxicillin. Antimicrob Agents Chemother 2002;46:2349–2357

67. Gasc AM, Kauc L, Barraillé P, Sicard M, Goodgal S. Gene localization, size, and physical map of the chromosome of *Streptococcus pneumoniae*. J Bacteriol 1991;173:7361–7367

68. Smith AM, Botha RF, Koornhof HJ, Klugman KP. Emergence of a pneumococcal clone with cephalosporin resistance and penicillin susceptiblity. Antimicrob Agents Chemother 2001;45:2648–2650

69. McDougal LK, Rasheed JK, Biddle JW, Tenover FC. Identification of multiple clones of extended-spectrum cephalosporin-resistant *Streptococcus pneumoniae* isolates in the United States. Antimicrob Agents Chemother 1995;39:2282–2288

70. Felmingham D, Reinert RR, Hirakata Y, Rodloff A. Increasing prevalence of antimicrobial resistance among isolates of *Streptococcus pneumoniae* from the PROTEKT surveillance study, and comparative in vitro activity of the ketolide telithromycin. J Antimicrob Chemother 2002;50(Suppl Sl):25–37

71. Klugman KP, Lonks JR. Hidden epidemic of macrolide-resistant pneumococci. Emerg Infect Dis 2005;11:802–807

72. File Jr TM, Tan JS. International guidelines for the treatment of community-acquired pneumonia in adults: the role of macrolides. Drugs 2003;63:181–205

73. Weisblum B. Erythromycin resistance by ribosome modification. Antimicrob Agents Chemother 1995;39:577–585

74. Syrogiannopoulos GA, Grivea IN, Tait-Kamradt A, et al. Identification of an *erm*(A) erythromycin resistance methylase gene in *Streptococcus pneumoniae* isolated in Greece. Antimicrob Agents Chemother 2001;45:342–344

75. Farrell DJ, Douthwaite S, Morrissey I, et al. Macrolide resistance by ribosomal mutation in clinical isolates of *Streptococcus pneumoniae* from the PROTEKT 1999–2000 study. Antimicrob Agents Chemother 2003;47:1777–1783

76. Doktor SZ, Shortridge VD, Beyer JM, Flamm RK. Epidemiology of macrolide and/or lincosamide resistant *Streptococcus pneumoniae* clinical isolates with ribosomal mutations. Diagn Microbiol Infect Dis 2004;49:47–52

77. Davies TA, Bush K, Sahm D, Evangelista A. Predominance of 23S rRNA mutants among non-erm, non-mef macrolide-resistant clinical isolates of *Streptococcus pneumoniae* collected in the United States in 1999–2000. Antimicrob Agents Chemother 2005;49:3031–3033

78. Farrell DJ, Jenkins SG. Distribution across the USA of macrolide resistance and macrolide resistance mechanisms among *Streptococcus pneumoniae* isolates collected from patients with respiratory tract infections: PROTEKT US 2001–2002. J Antimicrob Chemother 2004;54(Suppl S1):17–22

79. Clancy J, Petitpas J, Dib Hajj F, et al. Molecular cloning and functional analysis of a novel macrolide-resistance determinant, *mef*A, from *Streptococcus pyogenes*. Mol Microbiol 1996;22: 867–879

80. Tait-Kamradt A, Clancy J, Cronan M, et al. *mef*E is necessary for the erythromycin-resistant M phenotype in *Streptococcus pneumoniae*. Antimicrob Agents Chemother 1997;41:2251–2255

81. Roberts MC, Sutcliffe P, Courvalin P, Bogo Jensen L, Rood J, Seppala H. Nomenclature for macrolide and macrolide-lincosamide-streptogramin V resistance determinants. Antimicrob Agents Chemother 1999;43:2823–2830

82. Klaassen CHW, Mouton JW. Molecular detection of the macrolide efflux gene: to discriminate or not to discriminate between *mef*(A) and *mef*(E). Antimicrob Agents Chemother 2005;9:1271–1278

83. Klomberg DM, de Valk HA, Mouton JW, Klaassen CH. Rapid and reliable real-time PCR assay for detection of the macrolide efflux gene and subsequent discrimination between its distinct subclasses *mef*(A) and *mef*(E). J Microbiol Methods 2005;60:269–273

84. Gay K, Stephens DS. Structure and dissemination of a chromosomal insertion element encoding macrolide efflux in *Streptococcus pneumoniae*. J Infect Dis 2001;184:56–65

85. Del Grosso M, Iannelli F, Messina C, et al. Macrolide efflux genes *mef*(A) and *mef*(E) are carried by different genetic elements in *Streptococcus pneumoniae*. J Clin Microbiol 2002;40:774–778

86. Santagati M, Iannelli F, Oggioni MR, Stefani S, Pozzi G. Characterization of a genetic element carrying the macrolide efflux gene *mef*(A) in *Streptococcus pneumoniae*. Antimicrob Agents Chemother 2000;44:2585–2587

87. Ross JI, Eady EA, Cove JH, Cunliffe WJ, Baumberg S, Wooton JC. Inducible erythromycin resistance in staphylococci is encoded by a member of the ATP-binding transport super-gene family. Mol Microbiol 1990;4:1207–1214

88. Corso A, Severina EP, Petruk VF Mauriz YR, Tomasz A. Molecular characterization of penicillin-resistant *Streptococcus pneumoniae* isolates causing respiratory disease in the United States. Microb Drug Resist 1998;4:325–337

89. Fuller JD, Low DE. A review of *Streptococcus pneumoniae* infection treatment failures associated with fluoroquinolones resistance. Clin Infect Dis 2005;41:1181–21

90. Powis J, McGeer A, Green K, et al. In vitro antimicrobial susceptibilities of *Streptococcus pneumoniae* clinical isolates obtained in Canada in 2002. Antimicrob Agents Chemother 2004;48:3305–3311

91. Song JH, Jung SI, Ko KS, et al. High prevalence of antimicrobial resistance among clinical *Streptococcus pneumoniae* isolates in Asia (an ANSORP study). Antimicrob Agents Chemother 2004;48:2101–2107

92. Perez-Trallero E, Fernandez-Mazarrasa C, Garcia-Rey C, et al. Antimicrobial susceptibilities of 1,684 *Streptococcus pneumoniae* and 2,039 *Streptococcus pyogenes* isolates and their ecological relationships: results of a 1-year (1998–1999) multicenter surveillance study in Spain. Antimicrob Agents Chemother 2001;45:3334–3340

93. Canton R, Morosini M, Enright MC, Morrissey I. Worldwide incidence, molecular epidemiology and mutations implicated in fluoroquinolone-resistant *Streptococcus pneumoniae*: data from the global PROTEKT surveillance programme. J Antimicrob Chemother 2003;52:944–952

94. Ho PL, Que TL, Chiu SS, et al. Fluoroquinolone and other antimicrobial resistance in invasive pneumococci, Hong Kong, 1995–2001. Emerg Infect Dis 2004;10:1250–1257

95. Pan XS, Ambler J, Mehtar S, Fisher LM. Involvement of topoisomerase IV and DNA gyrase as ciprofloxacin targets in *Streptococcus pneumoniae*. Antimicrob Agents Chemother 1996;40:2321–2326

96. Bast DJ, Low DE, Duncan CL, et al. Fluoroquinolone resistance in clinical isolates of *Streptococcus pneumoniae*: contributions of type II topoisomerase mutations and efflux to levels of resistance. Antimicrob Agents Chemother 2000;44:3049–3054

97. Lim S, Bast D, McGeer A, de Azavedo J, Low DE. Antimicrobial susceptibility breakpoints and first-step *parC* mutations in *Streptococcus pneumoniae*: redefining fluoroquinolones resistance. Emerg Infect Dis 2003;9:833–837

98. Li X, Zhao X, Drlica K. Selection of *Streptococcus pneumoniae* mutants having reduced susceptibility to moxifloxacin and levofloxacin. Antimicrob Agents Chemother 2002;46:522–524

99. Gillespie SH, Voelker LL, Ambler JE, Traini C, Dickens A. Fluoroquinolone resistance in *Streptococcus pneumoniae*: evidence that *gyrA* mutations arise at a lower rate and that mutation in *gyrA* or *parC* predisposes to further mutation. Microb Drug Resist 2003;9:17–24

100. Perichon B, Tankovic J, Courvalin P. Characterization of a mutation in the *pare* gene that confers fluoroquinolone resistance in *Streptococcus pneumoniae*. Antimicrob Agents Chemother 1997;41:1166–1167

101. Pletz MW, Shergill AP, McGee L, et al. Prevalence of first-step mutants among levofloxacin-susceptible invasive isolates of *Streptococcus pneumoniae* in the United States. Antimicrob Agents Chemother 2006;50:1561–1563

102. Schurek KN, Adam HJ, Siemens CG, Hoban CJ, Hoban DJ, Zhanel GG. Are fluoroquinolone-susceptible isolates of *Streptococcus pneumoniae* really susceptible? A comparison of resistance mechanisms in Canadian isolates from 1997 and 2003. J Antimicrob Chemother 2005;56:769–772

103. Doern GV, Richter SS, Miller A, et al. Antimicrobial resistance among *Streptococcus pneumoniae* in the United States: have we begun to turn the corner on resistance to certain antimicrobial classes? Clin Infect Dis 2005;41:139–148

104. Davies TA, Yee YC, Goldschmidt R, Bush K, Sahm DF, Evangelista A. Infrequent occurrence of single mutations in topoisomerase IV and DNA gyrase genes among US levofloxacin-susceptible clinical isolates of *Streptococcus pneumoniae* from nine institutions (1999–2003). J Antimicrob Chemother 2006;57:437–442

105. Davies TA, Evangelista A, Pfleger S, Bush K, Sahm DF, Goldschmidt R. Prevalence of single mutations in topoisomerase type II genes among levofloxacin-susceptible clinical strains of *Streptococcus pneumoniae* isolated in the United States in 1992 to 1996 and 1999 to 2000. Antimicrob Agents Chemother 2002;46:119–124

106. Zeller V, Janoir C, Kitzis MD, Gutmann L, Moreau NJ. Active efflux as a mechanism of resistance to ciprofloxacin in *Streptococcus pneumoniae*. Antimicrob Agents Chemother 1997;41:1973–1978

107. Balsalobre L, Ferrandiz MJ, Linares J, Tubau F, de la Campa AG. Viridans group streptococci are donors in horizontal transfer of toposiomerase IV genes to *Streptococcus pneumoniae*. Antimicrob Agents Chemother 2003;47:2072–2081

108. Bast DJ, de Azavedo JC, Tam TY, et al. Interspecies recombination contributes minimally to fluoroquinolone resistance in *Streptococcus pneumoniae*. Antimicrob Agents Chemother 2001;45:2631–2634

109. Pletz MWR, McGee L, Beall B, Whitney CG, Klugman KP. Interspecies recombination in type II topoisomerase genes is not a major cause of fluoroquinolones resistance in invasive *Streptococcus pneumoniae* isolates in the United States. Antimicrob Agents Chemother 2005;49:779–780

110. Farrell DJ, Felmingham D. The PROTEKT global study (year 4) demonstrates a continued lack of resistance development to telithromycin in *Streptococcus pneumoniae*. J Antimicrob Chemother 2005;56:795–797

111. Bingen E, Doit C, Loukil C, et al. Activity of telithromycin against penicillin-resistant *Streptococcus pneumoniae* isolates recovered from French children with invasive and noninvasive infections. Antimicrob Agents Chemother 2003;47:2345–2347

112. Rantala M, Huikko S, Huovinen P, Jalava J. Prevalence and molecular genetics of macrolide resistance among *Streptococcus pneumoniae* isolates collected in Finland in 2002. Antimicrob Agents Chemother 2005;49:4180–4184

113. Hisanaga T, Hoban DG, Zhanel GG. Mechanisms of resistance to telithromycin in *Streptococcus pneumoniae*. J Antimicrob Chemother 2005;56:447–450

114. Meka VG, Gold HS. Antimicrobial resistance to linezolid. Clin Infect Dis 2004;39:1010–1015

115. Farrell DJ, Morrissey I, Bakker S, Buckridge S, Felmingham D. In vitro activities of telithromycin, linezolid, and quinupristin–dalfopristin against *Streptococcus pneumoniae* with macrolide resistance due to ribosomal mutations. Antimicrob Agents Chemother 2004;48:3169–3171

116. Draghi DC, Sheehan DJ, Hogan P, Sahm DF. In vitro activity of linezolid against key Gram-positive organisms isolated in the United States: Results of the LEADER 2004 surveillance program. Antimicrob Agents Chemother 2005;49:5024–5032

117. Wolter N, Smith AM, Farrell DJ, et al. Novel mechanism of resistance to oxazolidinones, macrolides, and chloramphenicol in ribosomal protein L4 of the pneumococcus. Antimicrob Agents Chemother 2005;49:3554–3557

118. Jones RN, Farrell DJ, Morrissey I. Quinupristin–dalfopristin resistance in *Streptococcus pneumoniae*: novel L22 ribosomal protein mutation in two clinical isolates from the SENTRY antimicrobial surveillance program. Antimicrob Agents Chemother 2003;47:2696–2698

119. Schmitz FJ, Perdikouli M, Beeck A, Verhoef J, Fluit AC. Molecular surveillance of macrolide, tetracycline and quinolone resistance mechanisms in 1191 clinical European *Streptococcus pneumoniae* isolates. Int J Antimicrob Agents 2001;18:433–436

120. Jones ME, Blosser-Middleton RS, Thornsberry C, Karlowsky JA, Sahm DF. The activity of levofloxacin and other antimicrobials against clinical isolates of *Streptococcus pneumoniae* collected worldwide during 1999–2002. Diagn Microbiol Infect Dis 2003;47:579–586

121. Burdett V, Inamine J, Rajagopalan S. Heterogeneity of tetracycline resistance determinants in *Streptococcus*. J. Bacteriol 1982;149:995–1004

122. Widdowson CA, Klugman KP, Hanslo D. Identification of the tetracycline resistance gene, *tet*(O), in *Streptococcus pneumoniae*. Antimicrob Agents Chemother 1996;40:2891–2893

123. Luna VA, Roberts MC. The presence of the tetO gene in a variety of tetracycline-resistant *Streptococcus pneumoniae* serotypes from Washington State. J Antimicrob Chemother 1998;42:613–619

124. McDougal LK, Tenover FC, Lee LN, et al. Detection of *Tn*917-like sequences within a *Tn*916-like conjugative transposon (*Tn*3782) in erythromycin-resistant isolates of *Streptococcus pneumoniae*. Antimicrob Agents Chemother 1998;42:2312–2318

125. Oggioni MR, Dowson CG, Smith JM, Provvedi R, Pozzi G. The tetracycline resistance gene *tet*(M) exhibits mosaic structure. Plasmid 1996;35:156–163

126. Doherty N, Trzcinski K, Pickerill P, Zawadzki P, Dowson CG. Genetic diversity of the *tet*(M) gene in tetracycline-resistant

clonal lineages of *Streptococcus pneumoniae*. Antimicrob Agents Chemother 2000;44:2979–2984

127. Dzierzanowska-Fangrat K, Semczuk K, Gorska P, et al. Evidence for tetracycline resistance determinant *tet*(M) allele replacement in a *Streptococcus pneumoniae* population of limited geographical origin. Int J Antimicrob Agents 2006;27:159–164

128. Bradley JS, Scheld WM. The challenge of penicillin-resistant *Streptococcus pneumoniae* meningitis: current antibiotic therapy in the 1990s. Clin Infect Dis 1997;24(Suppl 2):S213–S221

129. Chambers H. Methicillin-resistant staphylococci. Clin Microbiol Rev 1988;1:173–186

130. Deal W, Sanders E. Efficacy of rifampicin in treatment of meningococcal carriers. N Engl J Med 1969;281:641–645

131. Band J, Fraser D, Ajello G. Prevention of *Haemophilus influenzae* type b disease. JAMA 1984;251:2381–2386

132. Doern GV, Brueggemann A, Holley HP Jr, Rauch AM. Antimicrobial resistance of *Streptococcus pneumoniae* recovered from outpatients in the United States during the winter months of 1994 to 1995: results of a 30-center national surveillance study. Antimicrob Agents Chemother 1996;40:1208–1213

133. Marchese A, Mannelli S, Tonoli E, Gorlero F, Toni M, Schito GC. Prevalence of antimicrobial resistance in *Streptococcus pneumoniae* circulating in Italy: results of the Italian Epidemiological Observatory Survey (1997–1999). Microb Drug Resist 2001;7:277–287

134. Padayachee T, Klugman KP. Molecular basis of rifampin resistance in *Streptococcus pneumoniae*. Antimicrob Agents Chemother 1999;43:2361–2365

135. Ferrandiz MJ, Ardanuy C, Linares J, et al. New mutations and horizontal transfer of *rpo*B among rifampin-resistant *Streptococcus pneumoniae* from four Spanish hospitals. Antimicrob Agents Chemother 2005;49:2237–2245

136. Dang-Van A, Tiraby G, Acar JF, Shaw WV, Bonanchaud DH. Chloramphenicol resistance in *Streptococcus pneumoniae*: enzymatic acetylation and possible plasmid linkage. Antimicrob Agents Chemother 1978;13:557–583

137. Ayoubi P, Kilic AO, Vijayakumar MN. *Tn*5253, the pneumococcal omega (*cat tet*) BM6001 element, is a composite structure of two conjugative transposons, *Tn*5251 and *Tn*5252. J Bacteriol 1991;173:1617–1622

138. Pepper K, de Cespedes G, Horaud T. Heterogeneity of chromosomal genes encoding chloramphenicol resistance in streptococci. Plasmid 1988;19:71–74

139. Widdowson CA, Adrian PV, Klugman KP. Acquisition of chloramphenicol resistance by the linearization and integration of the entire staphylococcal plasmid pC194 into the chromosome of *Streptococcus pneumoniae*. Antimicrob Agents Chemother 2000;44:393–395

140. Jones ME, Blosser-Middleton RS, Critchley IA, Karlowsky JA, Thornsberry C, Sahm DF. In vitro susceptibility of *Streptococcus pneumoniae*, *Haemophilus influenzae* and *Moraxella catarrhalis*: a European multicenter study during 2000–2001. Clin Microbiol Infect 2003;9:590–599

141. Johnson DM, Stilwell MG, Fritsche TR, Jones RN. Emergence of multidrug-resistant *Streptococcus pneumoniae*: report from the SENTRY Antimicrobial Surveillance Program (1999–2003). Diagn Microbiol Infect Dis 2006;56:69–74

142. Adrian PV, Klugman KP. Mutations in the dihydrofolate reductase gene of trimethoprim-resistant isolates of *Streptococcus pneumoniae*. Antimicrob Agents Chemother 1997;41:2406–2413

143. Maskell JP, Sefton AM, Hall LM. Multiple mutations modulate the function of dihydrofolate reductase in trimethoprim-resistant *Streptococcus pneumoniae*. Antimicrob Agents Chemother 2001;45:1104–1108

144. Lopez P, Espinosa M, Greenberg B, Lacks S. Sulfonamide resistance in *Streptococcus pneumoniae*: DNA sequence of the gene encoding dihydropteroate synthase and characterization of the enzyme. J Bacteriol 1987;169:4320–4326

145. Maskell JP, Sefton AM, Hall LM. Mechanism of sulfonamide resistance in clinical isolates of *Streptococcus pneumoniae*. Antimicrob Agents Chemother 1997;41:2121–2126

146. Padayachee T, Klugman KP. Novel expansions of the gene encoding dihydropteroate synthase in trimethoprim–sulfamethoxazole-resistant *Streptococcus pneumoniae*. Antimicrob Agents Chemother 1999;43:2225–2230

147. Moore HF, Chesney AM. A study of ethylhydrocuprein (optochin) in the treatment of acute lobar pneumonia. Arch Intern Med 1917;19:611–82

148. Borek AP, Dressel DC, Hussong J, Peterson LR. Evolving clinical problems with *Streptococcus pneumoniae*: increasing resistance to antimicrobial agents, and failure of traditional optochin identification in Chicago, Illinois, between 1993 and 1996. Diagn Microbiol Infect Dis 1997;29:209–214

149. Pikis A, Campos JM, Rodriguez WJ, Keith JM. Optochin resistance in *Streptococcus pneumoniae*: mechanism, significance, and clinical implications. J Infect Dis 2001;184:582–590

150. Fenoll A, Muñoz R, García E, de la Campa AG. Molecular basis of the optochin-sensitive phenotype of pneumococcus: characterization of the genes encoding the F_0 complex of the *Streptococcus pneumoniae* and *Streptococcus oralis* H$^+$-ATPases. Mol Microbiol 1994;12:587–98

151. Feldman C, Kallenbach JM, Miller SD, Thorburn JR, Koornhof HJ. Community-acquired pneumonia due to penicillin-resistant pneumococci. N Engl J Med 1985;313:615–617

152. Pallares R, Gudiol F, Linares J, et al. Risk factors and response to antibiotic therapy in adults with bacteremic pneumonia caused by penicillin-resistant pneumococci. N Engl J Med 1987;317:18–22

153. Bryan CS, Talwani R, Stinson MS. Penicillin dosing for pneumococcal pneumonia. Chest 1997;112:1657–1664

154. Kaplan SL, Mason Jr EO, Barson WJ, et al. Outcome of invasive infections outside the central nervous system caused by *Streptococcus pneumoniae* isolates nonsusceptible to ceftriazone in children treated with beta-lactam antibiotics. Pediatr Infect Dis J 2001;20:392–396

155. Pallares R, Capdevila O, Linares J, et al. The effect of cephalosporin resistance on mortality in adult patients with nonmeningeal systemic pneumococcal infections. Am J Med 2002;113:120–126

156. Yu VL, Chiou CC, Feldman C, et al. An international prospective study of pneumococcal bacteremia: correlation with in vitro resistance, antibiotics administered, and clinical outcome. Clin Infect Dis 2003;37:230–237

157. Daum RS, Nachman JP, Leitch CD, Tenover FC. Nosocomial epiglottitis associated with penicillin- and cephalosporin-resistant *Streptococcus pneumoniae* bacteremia. J Clin Microbiol 1994;32:246–248

158. Dagan R, Leibovitz E, Fliss DM, et al. Bacteriologic efficacies of oral azithromycin and oral cefaclor in treatment of acute otitis media in infants and young children. Antimicrob Agents Chemother 2000;44:43–50

159. Dagan R, Leibovitz E. Bacterial eradication in the treatment of otitis media. Lancet Infect Dis 2002;2:593–604

160. Dagan R, Hoberman A, Johnson C, et al. Bacteriologic and clinical efficacy of high dose amoxicillin/clavulanate in children with acute otitis media. Pediatr Infect Dis J 2001;20:829–837

161. Brook I, Gooch WMI et al. Medical management of acute bacterial sinusitis. Recommendations of a clinical advisory committee on pediatric and adult sinusitis. Ann Otol Rhinol Laryngol 2000;109:2–20

162. Friedland IR, Klugman KP. Failure of chloramphenicol therapy in penicillin-resistant pneumococcal meningitis. Lancet 1992;339:405–408

163. Bradley JS, Connor JD. Ceftriaxone failure in meningitis caused by *Streptococcus pneumoniae* with reduced susceptibility to beta-lactam antibiotics. Pediatr Infect Dis J 1991;10:871–873

164. Klugman KP. Pneumococcal resistance to the third-generation cephalosporins: clinical, laboratory and molecular aspects. Int J Antimicrob Agents 1994;4:63–67

165. Klugman KP, Friedland IR, Bradley JS. Bactericidal activity against cephalosporin-resistant *Streptococcus pneumoniae* in cerebrospinal fluid of children with acute bacterial meningitis. Antimicrob Agents Chemother 1995;39:1988–1992

166. Friedland IR, Klugman KP. Cerebrospinal fluid bactericidal activity against cephalosporin-resistant *Streptococcus pneumoniae* in children with meningitis treated with high-dosage cefotaxime. Antimicrob Agents Chemother 1997;41:1888–1891

167. Musher DM, Dowell ME, Shortridge VD, et al. Emergence of macrolide resistance during treatment of pneumococcal pneumonia. N Engl J Med 2002;346:630–631

168. Lonks JR, Garau J, Gomez L, et al. Failure of macrolide antibiotic treatment in patients with bacteremia due to erythromycin-resistant *Streptococcus pneumoniae*. Clin Infect Dis 2002;35:556–564

169. Jacobs MR, Bajaksouzian S, Windau A, et al. Susceptibility of *Streptococcus pneumoniae*, *Haemophilus influenzae*, and *Moraxella catarrhalis* to 17 oral antimicrobial agents based on pharmacodynamic parameters: 1998–2001 U S Surveillance Study. Clin Lab Med 2004;24:503–530

170. Leiberman A, Leibovitz E, Piglansky L, et al. Bacteriologic and clinical efficacy of trimethoprim–sulfamethoxazole for treatment of acute otitis media. Pediatr Infect Dis J 2001;20:260–264

171. Davidson R, Cavalcanti R, Brunton JL, et al. Resistance to levofloxacin and failure of treatment of pneumococcal pneumonia. N Engl J Med 2002;346:747–750

172. Anderson KB, Tan JS, File TM Jr, DiPersio JR, Willey BM, Low DE. Emergence of levofloxacin-resistant pneumococci in immunocompromised adults after therapy for community-acquired pneumonia. Clin Infect Dis 2003;37:376–381

173. Whitney CG, Farley MM, Hadler J, et al. Decline in invasive pneumococcal disease after the introduction of protein-polysaccharide conjugate vaccine. N Engl J Med 2003;348:1737–1746

174. CDC. Direct and indirect effects of routine vaccination of children with 7-valent pneumococcal conjugate vaccine on incidence of invasive pneumococcal disease – United States, 1998–2003. MMWR Mortal Wkly Rep 2005;54:893–897

175. Whitney CG, Klugman KP. Vaccines as tools against resistance: the example of pneumococcal conjugate vaccine. Semin Pediatr Infect Dis 2004;15:86–93

176. Klugman KP, Madhi SA, Huebner RE, et al. A trial of a 9-valent pneumococcal conjugate vaccine in children with and those without HIV infection. N Engl J Med 2003;349:1341–1348

177. Black S, Shinefield H, Baxter R, et al. Postlicensure surveillance for pneumococcal invasive disease after use of heptavalent pneumococcal conjugate vaccine in Northern California Kaiser Permanente. Pediatr Infect Dis J 2004;23:48548–9

178. Talbot TR, Poehling KA, Hartert TV, et al. Reduction in high rates of antiobiotic-nonsusceptible invasive pneumococcal disease in Tennessee following introduction of the pneumococcal conjugate vaccine. Clin Infect Dis 2004;39:641–648

179. Stephens DS. Incidence of macrolide resistance in *Streptococcus pneumoniae* after introduction of the pneumococcal conjugate vaccine: population-based assessment. Lancet 2005;365:855–863

180. Kyaw MH, Lynfield R, Schaffner W, et al. Effect of introduction of the pneumococcal conjugate vaccine on drug-resistant *Streptococcus pneumoniae*. N Engl J Med 2006;354:1455–1463

181. Porat N, Arguedas A, Spratt BG, et al. Emergence of penicillin-nonsusceptible *Streptococcus pneumoniae* clones expressing serotypes not present in the antipneumococcal conjugate vaccine. J Infect Dis 2004;190:2154–2161

182. Block SL, Hedrick J, Harrison CJ, Tyler R, Smith A, Findlay R, Keegan E. Community-wide vaccination with the heptavalent pneumococcal conjugate significantly alters the microbiology of acute otitis media. Pediatr Infect Dis J 2004;23:829–833

183. Moore MR, Hyde TB, Hennessy TW, et al. Impact of a conjugate vaccine on community-wide carriage of nonsusceptible *Streptococcus pneumoniae* in Alaska. J Infect Dis 2004;190:2031–2038

184. Pelton SI, Loughlin AM, Marchant CD. Seven valent pneumococcal conjugate vaccine immunization in two Boston communities: changes in serotypes and antimicrobial susceptibility among Streptococcus pneumoniae isolates. Pediatr Infect Dis J 2004;23:1015–1022

185. Frazao N, Brito-Avo A, Simas C, et al. Effect of the seven-valent conjugate pneumococcal vaccine on carriage and drug resistance of *Streptococcus pneumoniae* in healthy children attending day-care centers in Lisbon. Pediatr Infect Dis J 2005;24:243–252

Chapter 48
Antibiotic Resistance of Non-Pneumococcal Streptococci and Its Clinical Impact

Jari Jalava and Helena Seppälä

1 Characteristics of Non-pneumococcal Streptococci

1.1 Viridans Streptococci

Viridans streptococci (VGS) form a phylogenetically heterogeneous group of species belonging to the genus *Streptococcus* (1). However, they have some common phenotypic properties. They are alfa- or non-haemolytic. They can be differentiated from *S. pneumoniae* by resistance to optochin and the lack of bile solubility (2). They can be differentiated from the *Enterococcus* species by their inability to grow in a medium containing 6.5% sodium chloride (2). Earlier, so-called nutritionally variant streptococci were included in the VGS but based on the molecular data they have now been removed to a new genus *Abiotrophia* (3) and are not included in the discussion below. VGS belong to the normal microbiota of the oral cavities and upper respiratory tracts of humans and animals. They can also be isolated from the female genital tract and all regions of the gastrointestinal tract (2, 3). Several species are included in VGS and are listed elsewhere (2, 3). Clinically the most important species belonging to the VGS are *S. mitis*, *S. sanguis* and *S. oralis*.

1.2 Beta-Hemolytic Streptococci

Beta-hemolytic streptococci can be differentiated from the heterogeneous group of streptococci by the pattern of hemolysis on blood agar plates, antigenic composition, growth characteristics, biochemical reactions and genetic analyses. Beta-hemolytic streptococci commonly produce hemolysins, which cause complete lysis (beta-hemolysis) of red blood cells when cultivated on blood agar plates. Non-hemolytic strains can also be pathogenic. Traditional subdividing into serological groups is based on the detection of group-specific antigenic differences in cell wall carbohydrates using the serologic scheme of classification by Lancefield (4). Serogroups A, B, C, D, F and G are those most commonly found in humans (5).

1.3 Group A Streptococcus (Streptococcus pyogenes)

Group A streptococcus (GAS, *Streptococcus pyogenes*) is an important pathogen confined almost exclusively to human hosts. Transmission occurs from persons with acute infections or from asymptomatic carriers usually through hand contact and respiratory droplets, but food- and waterborne outbreaks have also been documented (6).

GAS is a common cause of bacterial infections especially in children of more than 3 years of age, and also in other age groups. Most commonly the diseases are self-limiting, localized infections of the pharynx and skin (e.g. pharyngitis and impetigo). However, invasion especially from the skin can lead to septicaemia or severe deep-seated tissue infections, such as necrotizing fasciitis and myositis. Other clinical manifestations of GAS include scarlet fever, peritonsillar and retropharyngeal abscesses, otitis media, sinusitis, myositis, lymphangitis, meningitis, suppurative arthritis, endocarditis, osteomyelitis, pneumonia, erysipelas, cellulites, streptococcal toxic shock syndrome, vaginitis, and balanitis (7–10). Primary suppurative infections may also lead to serious nonsuppurative sequelae, acute rheumatic fever and acute glomerulonephritis (11, 12).

Serologic typing of the M (13) and T proteins (14) has traditionally been used in epidemiologic typing of GAS (15). Nowadays, molecular typing methods such as *emm* sequence

J. Jalava (✉)
Department of Bacterial and Infectious Diseases,
National Public Health Institute, Turku, Finland
jari.jalava@ktl.fi

D.L. Mayers (ed.), *Antimicrobial Drug Resistance*,
DOI 10.1007/978-1-60327-595-8_48, © Humana Press, a part of Springer Science+Business Media, LLC 2009

typing, multilocus sequence typing, pulse field gel electro-phoresis, inversion gel electrophoresis, restriction length polymorphism analysis of the *mga*-regulon (vir-typing) and random amplified polymorphic DNA analysis, have provided more discriminatory power for studying the clonal relation-ships between GAS strains.

1.4 Group B Streptococcus (Streptococcus agalactiae)

Group B streptococci (GBS, *Streptococcus agalactiae*) is one of the primary causes of bacteremia and meningitis in neonates and infections in pregnant women (16, 17). It is also an important cause of invasive infections in the elderly and in non-pregnant adults with underlying or chronic dis-eases. The clinical spectrum of invasive GBS disease in adults includes skin and soft tissue infections, primary bacte-remia, urosepsis, pneumonia, osteomyelitis, peritonitis, sep-tic arthritis, meningitis, endocarditis, and intravenous catheter infection. Vaginal colonization of non-pregnant and pregnant women is the principal source of GBS. GBS has been classi-fied into different serotypes on the basis of different chain structures of its capsular polysaccharide.

1.5 Groups C and G Beta-Hemolytic Streptococci

Most of the Lancefield group C streptococci (GCS) produce beta-haemolysis on blood agar although non-hemolytic strains also exist. GCS are mainly animal pathogens. Group C beta-hemolytic streptococci have been isolated from human normal microbiota of nasopharynx, skin and genital tract. Of the four group C streptococci species *S. equisimilis* is the most common human isolate (2). Most of the group G streptococci (GGS) are beta-haemolytic. As GCS, they are also found in human normal microbiota of nasopharynx, skin and genital tract. Both GCS and GGS cause pharyngitis and a variety of severe infections in humans (2).

2 Antimicrobial Resistance in VGS

2.1 Beta-Lactam Resistance

Penicillin and beta-lactam resistance in general, among streptococci is mediated by point mutations in the penicillin-binding proteins (PBPs). PBPs are membrane-bound trans-peptidases, active-site serine hydrolases, which catalyse cross-linking of the peptidoglycan subunits during the bacte-rial cell wall synthesis (18, 19). Beta-lactam antibiotics serve as substrates for PBPs. The active-site serine reacts with the beta-lactam ring and generates a covalently linked enzyme-beta-lactame intermediate. This acyl enzyme intermediate is not able to catalyse cross-linking of the peptidoglycan sub-units (18). In streptococci there are low- and high-molecular-weight PBPs (20, 21). Both of these enzymes are important for cell wall synthesis, but only the high-molecular-weight PBPs are important for the bacterial killing activity of the beta-lactam antibiotics (19). In VGS there are two kind of high-molecular-weight PBPs: PBP1 (PBP1a and PBP1b) and PBP2 (PBP2a, PBP2b, PBP2x) (20). Homologous molecules can be found from *S. pneumoniae* and naming conventions for PBPs of the VGS are adapted from *S. pneumoniae* (19–21).

VGS with wild-type PBSs are susceptible to beta-lactam antibiotics (22). In order to become resistant, they have to decrease the affinity of beta-lactams to the high-molecular-weight PBPs. This can be achieved by amino acid substitu-tions in the transpeptidase domain of the PBPs (19, 22). One point mutation can result in slight increase in the penicillin MIC. Normally more than one mutation is needed for inter-mediate-level beta-lactam resistance. Highly resistant strains have accumulated several mutations in the PBPs. Based on the data obtained from *S. pneumoniae*; these highly resistant strains may also need mutations other than PBP (19). Accumulation of several mutations in the PBPs may also lead to lethal mutations. Streptococci have overcome this problem by horizontal transfer of functional mutated PBP-coding genes or gene fragments. Transformation and subse-quent homologous recombination has produced beta-lactam-resistant VGS with mosaic PBP genes. In these mosaics of PBP genes there are gene regions obtained from resistant strains dispersed through the wild-type PBP genes (23).

Penicillin resistance among VGS isolated from blood has been extensively studied (Table 1). These results indicate that low-level penicillin resistance is quite a common charac-ter in blood isolates (up to 56%). However, highly resistant VGS strains can also be found, and the resistance rates vary between 2 and 24%. There are small differences in the resis-tance levels in different countries (Table 1). Only few reports are available of the resistance among VGS isolated from human normal microbiota (33, 35). Penicillin resistance of these VGS strains is at the same level as among the strains isolated from blood samples (Table 1).

VGS strains, that have increased MICs for penicillin, have typically decreased susceptibility to all beta-lactams includ-ing piperzillin, cephalosporins and carbapenems (24). Of the third-generation cephalosporins, ceftriaxone is the most active against VGS in vitro (24). The NCCLS resistance

Table 1 Beta-lactam resistance of viridans group streptococci

Number of strains	Isolation site	Antibiotic resistance %[a]							Year	Country[d]	References
		Penicillin R	Penicillin I + R	Ceftriaxone R[c]	Ceftriaxone I + R[c]	Cefepime I+R[c]	Cefepime R[c]				
410	Blood	9	33.6						1988–1993	Spain	(24)
65	Blood	3.1	38.5						1989–1993	Denmark	(25)
352	Blood	13.4	56.3	17(R ≥ 2)	18(S ≤ 0.5)				1993–1994	USA	(26)
98	Blood	9.2	39		23(S ≤ 0.5)				1994–1996	USA	(27)
235	Blood		32.3			12.3(≤0.5)			1997–1999	USA	(28)
438	Blood	5.9	33.8			13.9(≤ 0.5)			1997–1999	America	(28)
62	Cancer patients	11.3	33.9	11.3(R ≥ 2)	16.1(S ≤ 0.5)	24.2(≤0.5)	11.3 (≥2)		1998	USA	(29)
68	Blood	7.4	48.5						1997	USA	(219)
89	Blood	22	39	12.7	26.6	41.9	19.4		1986–1996	Spain	(30, 31)
162	Invasive[b]	10							1995–1997	Taiwan	(32)
45	Non-invasive[b]	16							1995–1997	Taiwan	(32)
161	Normal flora	0	16.8						1999–2001	Finland	(33)
108	Blood	5	29						1998–2001	Finland	(34)
200	Pharyngeal	14.5	44							Greece	(35)
77	Blood	23.4	40.3						1986–1996	Spain	(36)
66	Blood	24.3	36.4						1988–1994	Spain	(37)
191	Blood	7	37	4	8				2000	Canada	(38)
211	Blood	9	38	0(R ≥ 2)	0(S ≤ 0.5)				1988–1991	South Africa	(39)
451	Endocarditis	1.3	13						1996–2000	UK	(40)
418	Blood	6	28	6.5(R ≥ 2)	12.4(S ≤ 0.5)				1995–1997	Canada	(41)
57	Blood	2	21						1995–1998	Germany	(42)

[a] Breakpoints (mg/L) used for calculating the percentage of R (resistant), intermediately resistant (I) and susceptible (S) strains: cefepime S ≤ 1 R ≥ 4; ceftriaxone S ≤ 1 R ≥ 4; penicillin S ≤ 0,_25 R ≥ 4

[b] *Invasive* = blood, pleural infusion, ascites, abscess aspirate; non-invasive = pus, urine, and in cancer patients = blood or sterile-site

[c] Old breakpoints that were used in studies, are in parenthesis (mg/L).

[d] America = USA, Canada, Latin America

breakpoint for ceftriaxone was 2 mg/L until 2002 when it changed to 4 mg/L (43, 44). Using the old breakpoint for ceftriaxone, penicillin and ceftriaxone resistance levels are similar (Table 1). In different studies, resistance percentages of VGS for ceftriaxone vary between 0 and 27% (Table 1). As expected, cefotaxime is almost as active as ceftriaxone against VGS although there is not as much resistance data available (24, 34). It is of worth to note that a third-generation cephalosporin, ceftazidime, although very active against various Gram-negative bacteria, is not as active as penicillin, cefotaxime or ceftriaxone against VGS (8, 12). As presented in Table 1, most of the blood isolates have a reduced susceptibility to ceftazidime with up to 70% resistance. Resistance levels of the fourth-generation cephalosporin, cefepime, vary between 11 and 42% (Table 1). However, the new NCCLS breakpoint for cefepime is 4 mg/L and if that is used the highest level of resistance is 19% (30). Whatsoever, all this data indicate that penicillin is in vitro as effective as cephalosporins against VGS although ceftriaxone has, in vitro, lower resistance figures than penicillin if the new NCCLS breakpoints are used (43, 44).

Imipemen, a carbapenem antibiotic, is in vitro active against VGS (45). Most of the VGS strains have low imipenem MIC values, i.e. less than 0.5 mg/L (24, 31). However, strains, highly penicillin resistant, can have elevated MICs (1–2 mg/L) (24). Marron et al., have found that 20% of the VGS blood isolates of neutropenic cancer patients can have imipenem MIC of 1 mg/L or more (31). Similarly, Diekema et al. reported that 11% of VGS strains had imipenem MICs equal to or higher than 0.5 mg/L (29). The problem with imipenem is that there are no NCCLS breakpoints for non-pneumococcal streptococci (44). Streptococci are in vitro highly susceptible to another carbapenem compound, meropenem. Only few resistant strains with MICs as high as 2 mg/L have been found (46).

2.2 Resistance to Macrolides, Lincosamides and Ketolides

Macrolides, ketolides, lincosamides and streptogramin B antibiotics, although having different kind of chemical structure, all have similar although not identical antimicrobial activity against VGS. The resistance mechanisms developed by bacteria against these antimicrobials are also similar. All these antibiotics inhibit protein synthesis by binding to bacterial ribosomes. Macrolides can be divided into different groups according to the number of carbon atoms in their lactone ring. 14- and 15-membered ring macrolides, like erythromycin and azithromycin, have similar antibacterial properties. Sixteen-membered ring macrolides, like spiramycin, differ from 14- and 15-membered ring macrolides in

their antimicrobial activity against VGS. Also lincosamides (clindamycin) and streptogramins have some differences in their activity against bacteria, when compared to macrolides.

In streptococci, there are two well-characterised macrolide resistance mechanisms: target site modification and active drug efflux. Target site modification is mediated by methylases encoded by the *erm* (erythromycin ribosome methylation) genes or by mutations at the 23S ribosomal RNA or ribosomal proteins L4 and L22. Methylation of adenine 2058 of the peptidyl transferase loop of 23S rRNA causes resistance to macrolides as well as to lincosamides and streptogramin B antibiotics (47). The active efflux mechanism, encoded by the *mef* (macrolide efflux) genes, is more specific and causes resistance only to 14- and 15-membered-ring macrolides (48). Mutations at the macrolide-binding domains of the 23S ribosomal RNA and at the ribosomal proteins L4 and L22 lower the affinity of macrolides to ribosomes (39). Mutations can cause several different kinds of resistance phenotypes. Both *erm* and *mef* genes can be horizontally transferred between different streptococci (49).

2.3 Erythromycin Resistance

Erythromycin A has similar *in vitro* activity against VGS strains as other 14- and 15-membered ring macrolides including azithromycin (33). The resistance against erythromycin is quite common among clinical VGS isolates. In the blood isolates, the resistance level is between 27 and 40% (Table 2). The VGS strains isolated from normal microbiota (Table 2) are also often resistant to erythromycin, the resistance levels being at the same level as among the blood isolates (33, 50, 53). The most common erythromycin resistance mechanism is mediated by *mef*(A) genes (33, 53). Roughly 70–80% of the erythromycin resistant VGS strains carry *mef*(A) gene and about 16–20% carry *erm*(B) gene (33, 38, 53). However, the situation may vary. There is one report from France, where *erm*(B) gene was reported to be much more common than *mef*(A) gene among blood isolates of VGS (49).

2.4 Clindamycin Resistance

Resistance against clindamycin is much less frequent among blood and normal microbiota VGS than resistance to erythromycin. Resistance figures vary between 2 and 10%. Resistance levels are similar among both blood and the normal microbiota isolates (Table 2). The reason for lower resistance levels

Table 2 Erythromycin, clindamycin, ketolide and tetracycline resistance of viridans group streptococci

Number of strains	Isolation site	Antibiotic resistance %[a]							Year	Country	References
		Erythromycin R	Erythromycin I+R	Clindamycin R	Clindamycin I+R	Telithromycin R	Tetracycline R	Tetracycline I+R			
200	Oropharynx	38.5	43.5	7.5	8		23	25.5		Greece	(35)
84	Oral and nasal	17								Japan	(50)
161	Normal flora	22.4	27	3.7			27.3		1999–2001	Finland	(33)
108	Blood	27		2		0			1998–2001	Finland	(34)
77	Blood	35.1	39.4			0			1986–1996	Spain	(36)
66	Blood	34.8				0			1988–1994	Spain	(37)
191	Blood	40	42.4	9.9	9.9	0			2000	Canada	(38)
211	Blood							41	1988–1991	South Africa	(45)
90	Blood		30						1988–1995	France	(49)
77	Blood	27	31	6.8					1996–1999	Germany	(51)
418	Blood	28	29.2		4		23.4	26.6	1995–1997	Canada	(41)
57	Blood	32					39		1995–1998	Germany	(42)
107	Blood			9					1999–2000	Europe	(52)
352	Blood	38.0	40.9				26.4	34.1	1993–1994	USA	(26)
68	Blood		39.7						1997	USA	(27)
438	Blood		39.7		8.4				1997–1999	America	(28)

[a]Breakpoints (mg/L) used for calculating the percentage of R (resistant), intermediately resistant (I) and susceptible (S) strains: erythromycin $S \leq 0.25$, $R \geq 1$; clindamycin $S \leq 0.25$, $R \geq 1$; telithromycin $S \leq 1$, $R \geq 4$; tetra $S \leq 2$, $R \geq 8$

is that the efflux mechanism mediated by *mef*(A) resistance gene, does not confer resistance to clindamycin(54).

2.5 Ketolide Resistance

Ketolides, represented here by telithromycin – the first ketolide on the market, are new-generation macrolides, in which a 3-keto group replaces L-cladinose in the lactone ring. Ketolides have shown to be in vitro more active than macrolides against the erythromycin-resistant *S. pneumoniae* and *S. pyogenes* strains (55). NCCLS does not yet offer telithromycin breakpoint values for other streptococci than *S. pneumoniae* (44). If the estimation of telithromycin resistance is done based on the breakpoint values of *S. pneumoniae*, telithromycin-resistant clinical VGS strains do not exist (Table 2). The binding of telithromycin to the bacterial ribosomes is much stronger than the binding of the erythromycin. This is the reason why methylation of the ribosomal RNA does not increase the MIC values as much as it does for erythromycin (56). Neither do the Mef(A) efflux pumps transport telithromycin out of the bacterial cell as well as they pump erythromycin. However, in streptococci, Mef(A) efflux does elevate telithromycin MIC when compared to the strains without *mef*(A) gene (55). In every case, telithromycin seems to be the most active macrolide group antimicrobial on the market at the moment.

2.6 Streptogramin Resistance

Quinupristin–dalfopristin (Synercid^R), a combination of streptogramin B and streptogramin A antibiotics, is available for intravenous use. It has rather good in vitro activity against VGS. However, resistance rates between different studies vary a lot (Table 3). In some studies, resistant strains have not been found at all, but in other studies 70% of the strains have showed reduced susceptibility and 28% have been resistant (26, 52). Also VGS strains, which have quinupristin–dalfopristin MIC of 16 mg/L have been described (26). Resistance against quinupristin–dalfopristin combination is linked to the streptogramin A (dalfopristin) resistance, so that in order to be resistant against the antibiotic combination, a strain must be resistant to streptogramin A. Streptogramin B resistance is not necessary. Streptogramin A resistance is mediated by *vga*(A), *vga*(B), *lsa* and various *vat* genes. Thus far, these genes have been found in clinical *Staphylococcus* and *Enterococcus* strains, but the presence of the genes in VGS has not been reported (57). Although not studied in detail (26, 37), it is possible that the resistance is mediated by ribosomal mutation like in *S. aureus* (58).

2.7 Tetracycline and Trimethoprim– Sulfamethoxazole Resistance

Tetracycline resistance among VGS is quite common. 23–39% of the strains are tetracycline resistant (33, 41, 45, 53, 59). Tetracycline resistance rates are similar as are the erythromycin resistance rates. Trimethoprim–sulfamethoxazole is not used for treatment of VGS infections but is commonly used for prophylaxis of neutropenic patients (60). Reduced susceptibility against it is quite common among VGS strains (Table 2).

2.8 Fluoroquinolone Resistance

In streptococci, there are two fluoroquinolone resistance mechanisms: mutations at the quinolone resistance-determining regions (QRDRs) of the topoisomerase IV and DNA gyrase molecules, and an efflux mechanism (61–63). In streptococci, toposisomerase IV molecule has two subunits coded by *par*C and *par*E genes. The DNA gyrase has also two subunits GyrA and GyrB coded by corresponding genes. Topoisomerase IV is the primary target for fluoroquinolones in VGS (61). Mutations at the topoisomerase IV genes confer low-level resistance (MIC 4 mg/L). A combination of topoisomerase IV mutations and fluoroquinolone efflux mechanism is needed for high-level fluoroquinolone resistance (MIC of 16 mg/L or more). Fluoroquinolone resistance determinants can be horizontally transferred between VGS and *S. pneumoniae* strains (61, 64–66).

New fluoroquinolones levofloxacin and moxifloxacin are active against Gram-positive bacteria. Levofloxacin is active against both VGS strains of normal microbiota (33) and blood isolates (38, 41). Only few levofloxacin resistant strains have been found thus far (33, 38, 41). NCCLS does not have interpretive standards for moxifloxacin yet, and therefore resistance rates cannot be determined. However, the activity of the moxifloxacin is somewhat better than that of levofloxacin. MIC$_{90}$ values for moxifloxacin and levofloxacin are 0.25 mg/L and 0.5 mg/L, respectively (38). In addition, all VGS strains studied for their in vitro susceptibility for moxifloxacin so far have had MIC of equal or less than 2 mg/L (33, 38) (Table 3). Ciprofloxacin is less active than levofloxacin or moxifloxacin. About 8% of the VGS blood isolates are resistant to ciprofloxacin (38).

2.9 Activity of Glycopeptides and Aminoglycosides

Vancomycin, a glycopeptide antibiotic, has retained its activity against VGS. Not a single vancomycin-resistant VGS has been reported thus far (25, 27, 31–33, 40, 51, 59). MICs

Table 3 Fluoroquinolone, quinupristin–dalfopristin and trimethoprim–sulfamethoxazole resistance of viridans group streptococci

Number of strains	Isolation site	Antibiotic resistance %[a]								Year	Country	References
		Levofloxacin R	Levofloxacin I + R	Moxifloxacin R	Moxifloxacin I + R	QD R	QD (I + R)	Trim/sulfa (R)	Trim/sulfa (I + R)			
200	Oropharynx					0	33.8				Greece	(35)
84	Oral and nasal										Japan	(50)
161	Normal flora	1.9	3.1	1.9		13	38.5			1999–2001	Finland	(33)
108	Blood	0	16							1998–2001	Finland	(34)
77	Blood									1986–1996	Spain	(36)
66	Blood					12				1988–1994	Spain	(37)
191	Blood	4.2	2.1	0	2.1			11.0	45.0	2000	Canada	(38)
211	Blood									1988–1991	South Africa	(45)
90	Blood									1988–1995	France	(49)
77	Blood						4.1			1996–1999	Germany	(51)
418	Blood	1.3	5.1					13.9	33.7	1995–1997	Canada	(41)
57	Blood					0				1995–1998	Germany	(42)
107	Blood					0	5.7			1999–2000	Europe	(52)
352	Blood					27.6	70.1	16.5	33.2	1993–1994	USA	(26)
68	Blood		2.9				14.7			1997	USA	(27)
438	Blood						2.7		20.1	1997–1999	America	(28)

[a]Breakpoints (mg/L) used for calculating the percentage of R (resistant), intermediately resistant (I) and susceptible (S) strains: levofloxacin S ≤ 2, R ≥8; linezolid S ≤ 2; moxifloxacin S ≤ 1, R ≥ 4; quinupristin–dalfopristin (QD) S ≤ 1, R ≥ 4; trimethoprim–sulfamethoxazole (trim/sulfa) S ≤ 0.5/9.5, R ≥ 4/76

for vancomycin are typically between 0.125 and 1 mg/L (27, 30–32, 51) and MIC_{90} values between 0.5 and 1 mg/L (27, 51). Teicoplanin, another glycopeptide antibiotic, is also active against VGS, although there are no NCCLS breakpoints available for this antibiotic (44). MIC_{90} values for teicoplanin are 0.25 mg/L or less (25, 32, 40, 51).

In general, the activity of the aminoglycosides against VGS is limited (67). Aminoglycosides like gentamycin, amikacin, streptogramin and netilmicin, are used in combination with penicillin or a cephalosporin for the treatment infective endocarditis (68) and sepsis in neutropenic patients (69). High-level gentamicin resistance (MIC of 500 mg/L or more) to VGS is very rare. This is true with VGS isolates of blood origin (25, 32, 40) as well as with VGS strains from the normal microbiota (35). MIC values are typically between 0.25 and 96 mg/L (25, 32, 45) and the MIC_{90} values between 0.5 and 32 mg/L (32, 35). However, few high-level aminoglycosides-resistant *S. mitis* strains have been detected. In these strains gentamicin MICs have been as high as 1,000 mg/L (45).

2.10 Activity of Linezolid

Linezolid is an antibacterial agent belonging to the new oxazolidinone group of antibacterials. Oxazolidinones are not related to any other antibacterials in use (70). Linezolid has been used in the treatment of vancomycin-resistant *Enterococcus faecium* infections, hospital-acquired pneumonia and complicated skin infections (71). The activity of linezolid against VGS strains has not been studied well. However, in those few studies the in vitro activity of linezolid has been good. Only one VGS strain of the 298 strains studied have had linezolid MIC of 4 mg/L (38, 52).

3 Antimicrobial Resistance in Beta-Hemolytic Streptococci

3.1 Resistance to Macrolides

3.1.1 Incidence of Macrolide Resistance in GAS

In 1959 Lowburry and Hurst (72) reported the first isolate of erythromycin-resistant GAS from burns of four patients in the United Kingdom. During the following years in Europe, mainly sporadic cases and small epidemics of erythromycin-resistant GAS were reported from the United Kingdom, Sweden, Italy and Spain (72–77). Also in the United States and Canada low proportions, 5% or less, were reported (78–80) except in a study with 22% of erythromycin-resistant GAS in Florida in 1980

(81). In the 1970s the largest outbreak of erythromycin-resistant GAS occurred in Japan, where the proportion of resistant strains increased from 12% in 1971 to 82% in 1977 (82). These strains were characterized as highly resistant (MICs > 100 mg/L) to macrolides and lincomycin and they were often resistant also to tetracycline and chloramphenicol and were exclusively of T12 serotype. In 1985–1987, an increase from 1 to 17.6% in the frequency of erythromycin-resistant GAS was seen in Australia Fremantle area (83). These strains represented different serotypes and exhibited low-level resistance to erythromycin (MICs (2–8 mg/L) and resistance to clindamycin and tetracycline was rare. In 1988–1989 sporadic isolates and family outbreaks with 22% of erythromycin-resistant GAS was reported from the Dundee area in the United Kingdom with predominance of T4M4 serotype (84). Thereafter, in 1990 a nationwide increase of erythromycin-resistant GAS of multiclonal origin was reported from Finland, where the frequencies reached 24%, 20% and 31% among blood culture, pharyngeal and pus isolates, respectively (75). Since the beginning of 1990s increased frequencies has been reported from several countries. Today macrolide resistance in GAS is a worldwide problem. Increased figures include the following frequencies of macrolide-resistant GAS: In Europe, frequencies of 20–29% in 1996–2001 have been reported from Spain (85–87), 15–42% in 1996–2001 in Greece (88–93), 8–14% in Germany in 1996–2001 (94–97), 43–51% in 1997 in Italy (98, 99), 6–10% in 1996–1999 in France (100, 101) and 16–25% in Croatia, Czech Republic and Slovakia (102). An average frequency of 11% of macrolide-resistant GAS in 2000–2001 was recorded in isolates from different parts of Russia; the frequency (25%) was highest among Siberian isolates (103). In Asian countries the frequency of erythromycin-resistant GAS was 53–71% between 1985 and 1998 in Taiwan (104, 105), 41% in 1998 in Korea (106) and 31% in 1998–2000 in Hong Kong (107). In North America, an increase of erythromycin-resistant GAS occurred from 2.1% in 1997 to 14% in 2001 in Toronto, Canada, with a predominace of a M4 serotype clone (108), and from 0% in 1998 to 38–48% in 2000–2001 among school children in Pittsburgh, PA, the United States, where the increase was caused by one single clone of emm6 (M6 serotype) (109). In South America, frequencies of 7% of erythromycin-resistant GAS have been reported from Chile in 1994–1998 (110) and 8% in Argentina (111).

3.1.2 Incidence of Macrolide Resistance in GBS

Resistance to erythromycin has been reported in GBS since 1962. The first description was from the United States (112) and in the same country an increase in the rate of macrolide resistance in GBS from 1.2% among isolates collected in 1980–1993 to 18% in 1997–1998 was reported (113). Increasing frequencies have been reported also from other countries. In Spain, the frequency of macrolide resistance in GBS increased from 2.5 to 5.6% in 1993–1996 to 14.5–18% in 1998–2001 (114) and in Taiwan from 19% in 1994 to 46% in 1997 (115). Since the end of the 1990s frequencies of 15–21% have been reported in France (116–118), 13–18% in Canada (119, 120), 40% in Korea (121) and 22% in Turkey (122).

3.1.3 Incidence of Macrolide Resistance in GCG and GGS

Macrolide resistance among group C and G streptococci varies a lot among different countries. In Finland resistance has not been very common. 3.6% and 1.0% of the GCS have been resistant to erythromycin and clindamycin, respectively. The most common macrolide resistance mechanism has been *mef*(A) (123). Similarly 3.5% and 0.3% of the GGS have been resistant to erythromycin and clindamycin, respectively. Most of these strains have had *erm*(TR) resistance gene and only one have had *erm*(B) (123). A bit higher numbers of erythromycin resistance among GCS and GGS have been reported from Turkey. Ergen et al. (23) reported that 1.4% and 16.2% of GCS and GGS were resistant to erytromycin respectively. In Taiwan, erythromycin resistance among GCS and GGS has been more common, 41.7% and 53.3% of the GCS and GGS isolates being erythromycin resistant (124).

3.1.4 Mechanisms of Macrolide Resistance in Beta-Hemolytic Streptococci

The macrolide resistance mechanism by ribosomal methylation encoded my *erm* genes, which was first identified in 1956 in *Staphylococcus aureus* (125), affects macrolides, linconamides and streptogramin B (MLSb) antibiotics. The inducible and constitutive forms of MLSb resistance has been found in beta-hemolytic streptococci since the early 1970s (126–128). The *erm*(B) methylase gene was the only *erm* gene class found in streptococci (129–131) until 1998, when the sequence of *erm*(TR) in *S. pyogenes* was published (132). Its nucleotide sequence is 82.5% identical to staphylococcal *erm*(A) and 58% identical to *erm*(B) and therefore *erm*(TR) belongs to *erm*(A) methylase gene class (133). The inducible or constitutive production of the methylase is dependent on the sequence of the regulatory region situated upstream from the structural methylase gene. It has been shown that in clindamycin, highly resistant mutants of *S. pyogenes* harbouring inducible *erm*(TR) and originally susceptible to clindamycin could be selected by 0.12–1 mg/L concentrations of clindamycin. Resistance was associated to structural changes in the regulatory sequence (134). The phenotypic expression of macrolide resistance in strepto-

cocci has been commonly studied by MIC determinations and induction tests including the double-disk test (erythromycin and clindamycin disks placed in vicinity on inoculated agar). Analysis of the Finnish GAS strains isolated in 1990 indicated a new erythromycin resistance phenotype with low- or moderate-level resistance (MICs 1–32 mg/L) to 14- and 15-membered macrolides only (M-phenotype). Thirty-four percent of the studied isolates represented the new phenotype (76). Subsequently, the active efflux mechanism causing this phenotype and the encoding *mef*(A) and *mef*(E) (macrolide efflux) genes were characterized in *S. pyogenes* and *S. pneumoniae* (48, 135, 136) and isolates with this mechanism have been found among beta-haemolytic streptococci in different parts of the world. Countries, where strains of GAS carrying *mef*(A) have been observed to account nowadays for the majority of macrolide-resistant isolates, include Spain (86, 137), Germany (97) and Greece (93), Finland (138), Taiwan (105), the United States (139), Chile (110) and Argentina (111). Predomination of GAS strains carrying *erm*(A) have been reported from Russia, Slovakia, Czech Republic and Croatia (103, 140). In GBS isolates with MLS resistance caused by *erm*(B) and *erm*A predominate in most reports in Canada and other parts of the Western Hemisphere (120, 141), France (116, 117, 142), Spain (114, 143, 144) and Taiwan (115). So far, GBS and GCS with the highest proportion of isolates carrying *mef*(A), 37% and 95%, have been reported from Taiwan and Finland, respectively (145, 146).

In addition to macrolide resistance determinants of *erm*(B), *erm*(A) and *mef*(A), all of which have been found from beta-haemolytic streptococci all over the world, a more rare mechanism, i.e. mutations in the *S. pyogenes* ribosomal protein L4 and in positions 2611 and 2058 of 23S rRNA encoding genes have been recently shown to cause resistance to macrolides. Mutations in positions 2611 and 2058 of the 23S rRNA gene cause resistance to clindamycin and streptogramin B (quinupristin), and also mutation at 2058 to telithromycin (147–149). The presence of a putative novel efflux system associated with *erm*(TR) in *S. pyogenes* has also recently been found (150). Another gene, *mre*A, which was originally described as a macrolide efflux gene in *S. agalactiae* (151), is encoding riboflavin kinase and is found also in erythromycin-susceptible GBS strains (152). Strains with two different macrolide resistance mechanisms (*mef* and *erm*) within a single bacterial cell also exist among GAS and more commonly among GBS (86, 100, 116, 122, 143, 152, 153). The phenotype of these strains is usually that determined by the *erm* gene.

While *mef*(A) and constitutively expressed *erm*(B) and *erm*(A) determinants provide constant and predictable phenotypes in beta-haemolytic streptococci, the phenotypes of inducible expressed *erm*(B) and especially *erm*(A) may vary. Isolates with *mef*(A) have low- or moderate-level resistance to 14- and 15-membered macrolides and isolates with either of the *erm* genes with constitutive expression have commonly high-level resistance to 14-, 15- and 16-membered macrolides, lincosamides and streptogramin B antibiotics. Inducible strains, especially those with *erm*(A) are often susceptible to 16-membered macrolides and clindamycin, but become highly resistant (MICs > 128 mg/L) to clindamycin and moderately or highly resistant to 16-membered macrolides after induction with subinhibitory concentrations of erythromycin. Also low-level resistance to ketolides can be induced (76, 153). Beta-haemolytic streptococci with inducible *erm*(B) are more commonly associated to high-level resistance to MLSb-antibiotics than isolates with inducible *erm*(A) gene(122, 153). In epidemiological studies the distribution of the resistance mechanisms, the expression of *erm*(A) has more often been inducible and that of *erm*(B) has more often been constitutive in GAS, but among GBS constitutive *erm*(A) and inducible *erm*(B) are also rather common (122, 144), e.g. in Turkey, isolates with inducible *erm*(B) accounted for majority of macrolide resistance in GBS (122).

erm(B) has been shown to be either plasmid or chromosome borne in streptococci (133). In earlier studies conjugative plasmids with the erythromycin resistance determinants were found from group A, B, C and G streptococci and they were shown to transfer by conjugation between streptococcal species (154) and among GAS also by transduction (155, 156). However, most antibiotic resistance genes are nowadays thought to be chromosomal in streptococci, and beta-haemolytic streptococci belonging to groups A, B, C and G have been shown to transfer their chromosomal macrolide resistance determinants by conjugation (152, 157–159). A composite chromosomal conjugative element Tn3701, encoding resistance to erythromycin and tetracycline has been described in GAS (160). Within this element the resistance genes are carried by a Tn*916*-like transposon. The presence of Tn916-Tn1545-like conjugative transposons carrying *erm*(B) and *tet*(M) has been verified later in GAS in other studies (161, 162) and an association of chromosomal *erm*(A) with *tet*(O) has been noted in some strains of GAS (161). An unusual chimeric genetic element containing DNA identical to *Tn*1207.1, a transposable element carrying *mef*(A) in macrolide-resistant *S. pneumoniae*, has also been found in different GAS strains. The mechanism of horizontal transfer in these strains was suggested to be transduction (163). Furthermore, analysis of the genetic environments of the *mef*(A) and *erm*(B) genes by Southern blot experiments have indicated a remarkable heterogeneity of genetic elements carrying these genes, especially *erm*(B), suggesting that different mobile elements can be recruited into the chromosomes of the circulating GAS population and that genetic rearrangement may also occur after a strain has acquired the resistance determinant (162).

3.1.5 Epidemiology of Macrolide-Resistant Beta-Haemolytic Streptococci

A large variety of clones of GAS are mediating macrolide resistance (105, 162, 164, 165). Increased resistance rates may be caused by clonal spread of resistant strains and by horizontal transfer of resistance determinants among the circulating microbial population. Macrolide-resistant GAS of the same clone have been found from different countries and even different continents (164) and the same clones have been found among susceptible isolates, but in general the heterogeneity of GAS clones seems to be lower among resistant than susceptible isolates (162, 164, 165). Single clones of GAS with a macrolide-resistant determinant may become regionally or nationally widely predominant or cause outbreaks (100, 108, 109, 166). For example, in Finland, 82% of isolates of erythromycin-resistant GAS collected all over the country in 1994 expressed the M-phenotype; although multiple clones were found among these isolates, increased regional resistance rates were clearly associated to a clone of T4M4 serotype with *mef*(A) (138, 158). In Taiwan, 33% of the erythromycin-resistant GAS collected in 1992–1995 and 1997–1998 carried constitutive *erm*(B) and were of one clonal origin. Sixty-four percent carried *mef*(A) of which only 23% were of one clonal origin and 16 other clones were found among the rest of these isolates (105). In Russia, 87% of erythromycin-resistant GAS collected in 2000–2001 carried inducible *erm*(TR) and 86% of these were of one clonal origin (103). In the United States, Pittsburgh, isolates carrying *mef*(A) of an emm6 (M6 serotype) clone that caused an epidemic among school children in 2001 were not at all found in the region within a two-month period in April–May in 2002, when the resistance rate was again at a high level (35% of isolates were resistant to erythromycin); this time an emm75 (M75 serotype) clone predominated (109, 139). In Italy, Cresti et al. found that a steady increase of erythromycin-resistant GAS from 9% in 1992 to 53% in 1997 in an area in central Italy was caused by an increase of the proportion of strains carrying inducible and constitutive *erm*(B) and *erm*(TR) determinants. These strains were of multiclonal origin. Correlation of the erythromycin-resistant GAS clones to the heterogeneity of genetic elements carrying the *erm*(B) indicated identical genetic environments of *erm*(B) in clonally unrelated strains, but on the other hand also indicated considerable diversity of these genetic elements both among clonally unrelated and within clonally identical strains (162). The increase of resistance, therefore, includes a complex genetic interaction within circulating streptococcal population and maybe between streptococci and other species (167). Macrolide consumption and different immunity status and other host factors of populations are also possible factors that contribute to this interplay and spread of resistance determinants and resistant clones (168–170).

3.2 Resistance to Clindamycin

Clindamycin resistance is almost exquisitely related to MLS resistance in beta-haemolytic streptococci and is thus mediated by *erm* genes. However, in some studies among GBS the frequency of clindamycin resistance exceeds that of macrolide resistance suggesting another mechanism of clindamycin resistance (114, 121, 171). In one isolate of GBS from Canada, the *linB* gene encoding a lincosamide-inactivating nucleotidyltransferase, was found (120). This gene has previously been identified in *Enterococcus faecium*.

3.3 Resistance to Telithromycin

Resistance to telitromycin is so far rare. Only a few strains, with such high MIC values for telithromycin that they can be considered as resistant, have been isolated. These isolates have constitutively expressed *erm*(B) gene or they have adenine-to-guanine mutation at the position 2058 (55, 149).

3.4 Resistance to Tetracycline

Resistance to tetracycline is common among beta-haemolytic streptococci, especially among macrolide resistant strains. As much as 80% of the beta-haemolytic streptococci in Korea, have been reported to be resistant to tetracycline (121). However, only 16.1% and 0.5% of GAS isolated in Germany and Canada respectively, are shown to be resistant to tetracycline (97, 172). Resistance is caused by tetracycline resistance to ribosomal protection proteins encoded by *tet*(M) or *tet*(O). The *tet*(M) gene is the most widely distributed and is found in GAS often in linkage with *erm*(B) on mobile elements (161), but in GBS it is found both among macrolide-susceptible and macrolide-resistant organisms with all different macrolide resistance determinants (143). *Tet*(O) has been found in GAS carrying chromosomal *erm*(A) or *mef*(A) and it can transfer with or without *erm*(A) and with *mef*(A) (161).

4 Clinical Significance of Resistance

4.1 Infections Caused by VGS

4.1.1 Infective Endocarditis

Infective endocarditis, despite proper treatment, is a life-threatening condition (173). The etiology of infective endocarditis varies according to the age of patients and the clinical nature of the disease (173–176). VGS cause about 28% of all cases (173, 176). The proportion of VGS among native valve endocarditis varies between 11 and 43% (174, 177), and VGS are the most common cause of late prosthetic-valve endocarditis (174, 175, 177). Several different VGS species have been reported to cause endocarditis, *S. sanguis* (68, 174), *S. mitis*, *S. oralis* and *S. gordonii* (177) being the most common species isolated from blood or infected valves. Among intravenous drug abusers, the VGS do not have as important a role as they have in general (174). In the point of view of the treatment and prophylaxis, penicillin resistance is a cause of concern.

The treatment recommendation for infective endocarditis caused by penicillin-susceptible (MIC ≤0.1 mg/L) streptococci is intravenous penicillin G for 4 weeks combined with intravenous gentamicin for 2 weeks (68, 178, 179). Instead of penicillin, ceftriaxone also can be used in combination with gentamicin (68, 178). Streptococcal strains with reduced susceptibility to penicillin (MIC > 0.1 mg/L) can be treated with penicillin G in combination with gentamicin. However, higher dose of penicillin and longer treatment times (4–6 weeks) are recommended (68, 178, 179). Low-level penicillin resistance among VGS isolated either from blood samples or normal microbiota is quite common. From 17 up to 56% show penicillin MIC of 0.125 mg/L or higher (Table 1). Although, there is not much data available in the literature, this low-level penicillin resistance seem not to be a significant clinical problem. Penicillin and aminoglycoside, most often penicillin and gentamicin, combination has synergistic activity against VGS (178). In the literature there are a few documented cases where patients with endocarditis caused by intermediately penicillin-resistant streptococcus were treated successfully with penicillin-gentamicin or in one case a penicillin-streptomycin combination (180). Also penicillin therapy alone followed by cephalotin and vancomycin therapies has been successfully used for treatment of endocarditis caused by low-level penicillin resistant streptococci (180).

High-level penicillin resistance (MIC of 4 mg/L of more) rates among VGS vary between 2 and 24% (Table 1). Among VGS from endocarditis patients, high-level penicillin resistance is rare. Only a few strains with MICs higher than or equal to 4 mg/L, have been reported (40, 179–183). Decreased susceptibility among VGS strains from normal microbiota is common. In the future, penicillin non-susceptible streptococci will more often cause endocarditis infections, and it is also likely that high-level penicillin resistance will increase. This is a challenge because optimal treatment regimens have not yet been determined in endocarditis caused by highly penicillin-resistant VGS. Thus far, all VGS strains tested have been susceptible to vancomycin (68, 178). There are reports where vancomycin alone (182) and vancomycin, ceftriaxone and gentamicin in combination (183) has been successfully used for treatment of endocarditis caused by highly resistant streptococci. However, some reports show that treatment of endocarditis caused by highly penicillin-resistant streptococci can be difficult. In one study, neither vancomycin treatment alone, nor a cefotaxime-gentamicin combination, was enough to completely cure endocarditis caused by a highly penicillin-resistant *S. mitis* strain in a human immunodeficiency virus positive individual (181). Also the vancomycin-gentamicin combination failed to cure endocarditis caused by highly penicillin-resistant *S. sanguis* in a 65-year-old woman with multiple medical problems (180). This indicates that other antibiotic regimens may be needed. Possible new candidates are levofloxacin, moxifloxacin, quinupristin/dalfopristin and linezolid. Resistance against these antibiotics is rare. However, the usage of these agents may select resistant strains especially among streptococci in the normal microbiota. For example, point mutations causing resistance to quinupristin/dalfopristin combination have already been described in other bacterial species (58). The same is true with fluoroquinolones, where point mutations are able to cause low-level resistance among streptococci (38, 61, 64). Linezolid-resistant strains are very rare, although one strain with linezolid resistance (MIC 4 mg/L) has been reported (38). Oxazolinones are bacteriostatic antibiotics and in that sense their usage for treatment of infective endocarditis may be compromised (70). However, linezolid has been successfully used for treatments of endocarditis caused by vancomycin-resistant enterococci and methicillin-resistant staphylococci (71, 184). At the moment there is no information of the efficacy of linezolid in the treatment of endocarditis caused by VGS.

Increasing numbers of penicillin-resistant VGS strains among normal microbiota may also challenge the prevention therapies of infective endocarditis. Amoxicillin or ampicillin is recommended for endocarditis prophylaxis (68). The prophylactic use of these antibiotics may select penicillin-resistant VGS strains among normal microbiota and these strains may be able to cause infective endocarditis (181). Clindamycin, which is recommended for prophylaxis for patients allergic to penicillin (68), might be, from the point of view of resistance, a better choice at the moment (Table 2). However, use of macrolides can also select clindamycin-resistant strains among normal microbiota streptococci, because Erm(B) methylase is able to cause both macrolide and clindamycin resistance. So, it is possible that in the future the clindamycin resistance rates are also higher than now. Telithromycin is very active against VGS strains of normal microbiota. *erm*(B) and *mef*(A) resistance genes do not mediate telithromycin resistance among VGS (33), although the presence of *mef*(A) gene in streptococci is increasing the MIC values (55). So, just from the resistance point of view, prophylactic use of telithromycin might be a better choice than the use of clindamycin.

4.1.2 Septic Infections Due to VGS in Neutropenic Patients

Infections are an important cause of morbidity and mortality among neutropenic patients, although the mortality caused by infections has significantly decreased during recent years (185, 186). There have been changes in the aetiology of bacteremia in febrile neutropenic patients. Earlier, Gram-negative bacteria were the most common cause. Nowadays, up to 70% of the bacteremia in neutropenic patients is caused by Gram-positive bacteria (185–188). Possible reasons for this shift in the aetiology are the use of antibiotic prophylaxis, increased use of intravenous catheters and aggressive chemotherapies with prolonged neutropenia and mucositis (186, 187, 189, 190). VGS are an important cause of bacteremia among neutropenic patients. Depending on the study the proportion of VGS as a cause of bacteremia ranges between 3 and 30% (31, 187, 188, 191–193). *S. mitis* followed by *S. oralis* or *S. sanguis* are the most commonly isolated species (24, 188, 193–195). Bacteremias caused by VGS strains originate from the oral mucosa (42, 196). Predisposing factors for VGS infections are severe and prolonged neutropenia, prophylactic antibiotic treatments with quinolones or trimethoprim–sulfamethoxazole, mucositis and treatment of chemotherapy-induced gastritis with antacids or histamine type 2 antagonists (189, 195). VGS infections can be associated with a high morbidity and mortality. Range of overall mortality of VGS bacteremia is between 6 and 18%, but this does not differ from the mortality rate of bacteremia caused by other bacteria (185, 194, 197). VGS infections can be rather asymptomatic, fever being the most common symptom (189, 194, 197–199). 4 to 26% of the patients with VGS infections develop serious complications, like septic shock, acute respiratory distress syndrome (ARDS) or both (31, 189, 194, 197, 198). Mortality among patients that develop ARDS is high, up to 60–100% (31, 189, 194).

Adequate empirical antimicrobial therapy of neutropenic patients with fever is essential, because infection may progress rapidly. The empirical therapy should cover both Gram-positive and Gram-negative bacteria (200–202). Especially important is that empirical treatment cover VGS and *Pseudomonas aeruginosa* strains (201). Recommendation for empirical therapy depend on the risk of the of neutropenic patients to develop serious complication during the febrile episode (200). Empiric antibacterial treatment for low-risk neutropenic patients relies on ciprofloxacin or levofloxacin with or without amoxicillin-clavulanate (200–202). In addition, fluoroquinolones with clindamycin has been suggested (200). Monotherapy with new fluoroquinolones, which show better activity against Gram-positive bacteria is not yet suggested for empirical treatment of low-risk neutropenic patients (200). Empirical antibacterial treatment of high-risk neutropenic patient relies on broad-spectrum parenteral antibiotics. Third- (ceftazidime) or fourth- (cefepime) generation cephalosporin alone or together with an aminoglycoside, or carbapenem either alone or in combination with aminoglycoside are the first choice of drugs (201, 202). Also, piperacillin-tazobactam either alone or in combination with aminoglycoside is recommended (185). Glycopeptides should be avoided in order to reduce the development of glycopeptide-resistant bacterial strains (185). It has also shown that empirical addition of vancomycin to the therapy would not give any benefit, when compared to piperacillin-tazobactam therapy (203).

Antimicrobial resistance of streptococci isolated from neutropenic patients have been widely studied. These studies indicate that low-level penicillin resistance is common. 21 to 39% of the VGS strains isolated from neutropenic patients present reduced susceptibility against penicillin (28, 30, 36, 42, 51). However, as much as 57% of the VGS strains have been reported to be non-susceptible to penicillin (204). Highly resistant VGS strains (MIC≥4 mg/L) can also be found, the resistance rates varying typically between 2 and 24% (30, 36, 42, 51). Penicillin and especially highly penicillin resistant VGS strains are often resistant to cephalosporins and also express reduced susceptibility to imipenem (30). In these cases ceftazidime is not active (29, 30). Despite the high rates of penicillin resistance among VGS strains, penicillin resistance has not been associated with the development of severe complications, like ARDS (30, 31, 189) or the overall mortality (30). However, there are few reports, which indicate that increasing rates of penicillin resistance might cause problems in the empirical treatment of neutropenic patients with VGS bacteremia. For example, Marron et al. (30) reported a breakthrough bacteraemia of ceftazidime-resistant VGS strains among patients receiving ceftazidime treatment. Similarly, Elting et al. (188) reported that neutropenic patients with VGS infections who did not receive vancomycin in the initial empiric therapy, died more often than-patients who received initial vancomycin therapy. Also in the same study it was shown that patients with penicillin-susceptible VGS infections responded to the initial therapy better than patients with penicillin-resistant VGS, although the final outcome was not affected by penicillin resistance (188).

Carbapenems are active against VGS in vitro (46) and are recommended for empirical treatment of neutropenic patients (200–202). However, VGS strains with elevated (1–2 mg/L) MICs for carbapenems have been isolated from neutropenic patients (24, 29, 30). Whether resistance among VGS strains will in the future compromise the use of carbapenems for monotherapy of neutropenic patients will be seen.

Glycopeptides, linezolid and quinupristin/dalfopristin are not used alone for empirical treatment of febrile neutropenic patients because of their low activity against Gram-negative bacteria. However, glycopeptides are in vitro very effective against VGS and are widely used as a combination with other antibacterials (203). Linezolid has been shown to be as effective as teicoplanin for treatment of Gram-positive infections (205, 206). The same is true with quinupristin/dalfopristin (207). However, there is lack of data as to how well these new drugs are suited for treatment of streptococcal infections. At the moment they are not recommended for empirical therapy of febrile neutropenic patients (200).

The combined use of both fluoroquinolones and penicillin as prophylaxis for bacterial infections in neutropenic patients has reduced bacteremic, especially streptococcal, episodes (199, 208, 209). However, this kind of prophylaxis does not reduce the overall morbidity or mortality. Penicillin resistance among VGS strains may affect the efficiency of penicillin prophylaxis. Whether this will affect the morbidity or mortality of neutropenic patients will be seen.

4.2 Beta-Hemolytic Streptococci

The importance of identifying antimicrobial resistance in beta-hemolytic streptococci is dependent upon whether these antimicrobials are used for treatment and whether the in vitro resistance leads to clinical treatment failure. Penicillin is the drug of choice for treatment of streptococcal infections and macrolides are considered as an alternative treatment for penicillin-allergic patients. In the treatment of pharyngitis caused by GAS, it has been shown that the eradication rate is lower (38–60%) when 14- and 15-membered macrolides are used against macrolide-resistant strains in comparison to the eradication rate (80–92%) when these agents are used against macrolide-susceptible organisms (99, 210, 211). The use of a macrolides for the treatment of macrolide-resistant GAS pharyngitis is also associated with a significantly lower clinical cure rate compared to that achieved with amoxicillin, amoxicillin-clavulanate or cefaclor (211). In addition, it has been shown that regardless of the macrolide resistance mechanism and of epidemiological origin, the erythromycin-resistant isolates harbour the prtF1 gene, more often, encoding a protein that enhances the ability to enter respiratory cells, than erythromycin-susceptible organisms (212). Macrolide-resistant GAS strains are so far mostly susceptible to telithromycin, which is a better choice than macrolides. However, few resistant strains exist and the knowledge of resistance and resistance mechanisms is important. The same is true with clindamycin. Use of clindamycin against an erythromycin-resistant isolate requires knowledge of the result of both the susceptibity testing and the determination of the macrolide resistance phenotype for a given isolate, because clindamycin should not be used against isolates with the MLSb-phenotype (134). Since we lack many alternatives for macrolides, and beta-hemolytic streptococci, especially GAS and GBS, may cause serious infections and non-suppurative sequelae, limiting the use of macrolides should be encouraged (213, 214). The selective pressure caused by the amount of macrolides used in the community has been shown to correlate to the level of macrolide resistance in GAS in the community (168–170, 215) and reduction of use of these agents has been shown to lead to reduction of macrolide resistance (213, 214).

Because GBS is the leading cause of neonatal infections, intrapartum antibiotic prophylaxis is recommended for colonized women with increased risk factors, such as low gestational age. For those at risk, intrapartum penicillin therapy is recommended, with ampicilin, clindamycin, erythromycin and vancomycin as acceptable alternative treatments (CDC), with penicillin G being the drug of choice (216).

There has been debate of the remarkable state of susceptibility to penicillin in GAS and other beta-hemolytic streptococci and of the probability of this state to continue. Resistance to penicillin occurs in related species, such as *S. pneumoniae*, VGS and enterococci. Among the reasons for the continuing susceptibility to penicillin in GAS, the following have been suggested: the pathogens inefficient mechanisms for genetic transfer or barriers to DNA uptake and replication and the findings that low-affinity PBPs expressed by penicillin-resistant laboratory mutants of GAS have a potentially defective performance in the cell-wall biosynthesis, thus decreasing the viability of the penicillin-resistant organism (28, 217).

References

1. Kawamura, Y., Hou, X. G., Sultana, F., Miura, H. & Ezaki, T. (1995) Determination of 16S rRNA sequences of *Streptococcus mitis* and *Streptococcus gordonii* and phylogenetic relationships among members of the genus *Streptococcus*. *Int. J. Syst. Bacteriol.* 45, 406–408

2. Johnson, C. C. & Tunkel, A. R. (2000) Viridans streptococci and groups C and G streptococci. In: *Mandell, Douglas, and Bennett's Principles and Practice of Infectious Diseases* (Mandell, G. L., Bennett, J. E. & Dolin, R., eds.), Chapter 191, pp. 2167–2173, 2 vols. Churchill Livingstone, Philadelphia

3. Whiley, R. A. & Beighton, D. (1998) Current classification of the oral streptococci. *Oral Microbiol. Immunol.* 13, 195–216

4. Lancefield, R. C. (1933) A serological differentiation of human and other groups of hemolytic streptococci. *J. Exp. Med.* 57, 571–595

5. Bisno, A. L. & van de Rijn, I. (1995) Classification of streptococci. In: *Principles and Practice of Infectious Diseases* Fourth edition (Mandell, G. L., Bennett, J. E. & Dolin, R., eds.), pp. 1784–1785. Churchill Livingstone Inc., New York

6. Farley, T. A., Wilson, S. A., Mahoney, F., Kelso, K. Y., Johnson, D. R. & Kaplan, E. L. (1993) Direct inoculation of food as the cause of an outbreak of group A streptococcal pharyngitis. *J. Infect. Dis.* 167, 1232–1235

7. Donald, F. E., Slack, R. C. B. & Colman, G. (1991) *Streptococcus pyogenes* vulvovaginitis in children in Nottingham. *Epidemiol. Infect.* 106, 459–465

8. Bisno, A. L. & Stevens, D. L. (1996) Streptococcal infections of skin and soft tissues. *N. Engl. J. Med.* 334, 240–245

9. Orden, B., Martin, R., Franco, A., Ibañez, G. & Mendez, E. (1996) Balanitis caused by group A beta-hemolytic streptococci. *Pediatr. Infect. Dis. J.* 15, 920–921

10. Bisno, A. L. (1995) *Streptococcus pyogenes*. In: *Principles and Practice of Infectious Diseases*, Fourth edition (Mandell, G. L., Bennett, J. E. & Dolin, R., eds.), pp. 1786–1799. Churchill Livingstone Inc., New York

11. Stollerman, G. H. (1993) Variation in group A streptococci and the prevalence of rheumatic fever: a half-century vigil. *Ann. Intern. Med.* 118, 467–469

12. Weinstein, L. & Le Frock, J. (1971) Does antimicrobial therapy of streptococcal pharyngitis or pyoderma alter the risk of glomerulonephritis? *J. Infect. Dis.* 124, 229–231

13. Lancefield, R. C. (1962) Current knowledge of type-specific M antigens of group A streptococci. *J. Immunol.* 89, 307–313

14. Griffith, M. B. (1934) The serological classification of *Streptococcus pyogenes*. *J. Hyg.* 34, 542–584

15. Maxted, W. R., Widdowson, J. P., Fraser, C. A. M., Ball, L. C. & Bassett, D. C. J. (1973) The use of the serum opacity reaction in the typing of group-A streptococci. *J. Med. Microbiol.* 6, 83–90

16. Poyart, C., Quesne, G., Couloun, S., Berche, P. & Trieu-Cuot, P. (1998) Identification of streptococci to species level by sequencing the gene encoding the manganese-dependent superoxide dismutate. *J. Clin. Microbiol.* 36, 41–47

17. Edwards, M. S. & Baker, C. J. (1995) *Streptococcus agalactiae* (group B streptococcus). In: *Principles and Practice of Infectious Diseases*, Fourth edition (Mandell, G. L., Bennett, J. E. & Dolin, R., eds.), pp. 1835–1845. Churchill Livingstone, New York

18. Walsh, C. (2003) *Antibiotics: Actions, Origins, Resistance*. ASM Press, Washington, DC

19. Chambers, H. F. (1999) Penicillin-binding protein-mediated resistance in pneumococci and staphylococci. *J. Infect. Dis.* 179, S353–S359

20. Ajdic, D., McShan, W. M., McLaughlin, R. E., Saviæ, G., Chang, J., Carson, M. B., Primeaux, C., Tian, R., Kenton, S., Jia, H., Lin, S., Qian, Y., Li, S., Zhu, H., Najar, F., Lai, H., White, J., Roe, B. A. & Ferretti, J. J. (2002) Genome sequence of *Streptococcus mutans* UA159, a cariogenic dental pathogen. *Proc. Natl. Acad. Sci. U.S.A.* 99, 14434–14439

21. Hoskins, J., Alborn, W. E. J., Arnold, J., Blaszczak, L. B., Burgett, S., DeHoff, B. S., Estrem, S. T., Fritz, L., Fu, D. J., Fuller, W., Geringer, C., Gilmour, R., Glass, J. S., Khoja, H., Kraft, A. R., Lagace, R. E., LeBlanc, D. J., Lee, L. N., Lefkowitz, E. J., Lu, J., Matsushima, P., McAhren, S. M., McHenney, M., McLeaster, K., Mundy, C. W., Nicas, T. I., Norris, F. H., O'Gara, M., Peery, R. B., Robertson, G. T., Rockey, P., Sun, P. M., Winkler, M. E., Yang, Y., Young-Bellido, M., Zhao, G., Zook, C. A., Baltz, R. H., Jaskunas, S. R. & Rosteck, P. R., Jr. (2001) Genome of the bacterium *Streptococcus pneumoniae* Strain R6. *J. Bacteriol* 183, 5709–5717

22. Dowson, C. G., Hutchison, A., Woodford, N., Johnson, A. P., George, R. C. & Spratt, B. G. (1990) Penicillin-resistant viridans streptococci have obtained altered penicillin-binding protein genes from penicillin-resistant strains of *Streptococcus pneumoniae*. *Proc. Natl. Acad. Sci. U.S.A.* 87, 5858–5862

23. Ergin, A., Ercis, S. & Hascelik, G. (2003) In vitro susceptibility, tolerance and MLS resistance phenotypes of Group C and Group G streptococci isolated in Turkey between 1995 and 2002. *Int. J. Antimicrob. Agents* 22, 160–163

24. Alcaide, F., Liñares, J., Pallares, R., Carratalà, J., Benitez, M. A., Gudiol, F. & Martin, R. (1995) In vitro activities of 22 β–lactam antibiotics against penicillin-resistant and penicillin-susceptible viridans group streptococci isolated from blood. *Antimicrob. Agents Chemother*. 39, 2243–2247

25. Renneberg, J., Niemann, L. L. & Gutschik, E. (1997) Antimicrobial susceptibility of 278 streptococcal blood isolates to seven antimicrobial agents. *J. Antimicrob. Chemother*. 39, 135–140

26. Doern, G. V., Ferraro, M. J., Brueggemann, A. B. & Ruoff, K. L. (1996) Emergence of high rates of antimicrobial resistance among viridans group streptococci in the United States. *Antimicrob. Agents Chemother*. 40, 891–894

27. Pfaller, M. A., Jones, R. N., Marshall, S. A., Edmond, M. B., Wenzel, R. P. & SCOPE Hospital Study Group (1997) Nosocomial streptococcal blood stream infections in the SCOPE program: species occurrence and antimicrobial resistance. *Diagn. Microbiol. Infect. Dis*. 29, 259–263

28. Diekema,D.J.,Beach,M.L.,Pfaller,M.A.,Jones,R.N.&Group,T.S.P. (2001) Antimicrobial resistance in viridans group streptococci among patients with and without the diagnosis of cancer in the USA, Canada and Latin America. *Clin. Microbiol. Infect*. 7, 152–157

29. Diekema, D. J., Coffman, S. L., Marshall, S. A., Beach, M. L., Rolston, K. V. & Jones, R. N. (1999) Comparison of activities of broad-spectrum beta-lactam compounds against 1,128 gram-positive cocci recently isolated in cancer treatment centers. *Antimicrob. Agents Chemother*. 43, 940–943

30. Marron, A., Carratalà, J., Alcaide, F., Fernández-Sevilla, A. & Gudiol, F. (2001) High rates of resistance to cephalosporins among viridans-group streptococci causing bacteraemia in neutropenic cancer patients. *J. Antimicrob. Chemother*. 47, 87–91

31. Marron, A., Carratalà, J., González-Barca, E., Fernández-Sevilla, A., Alcaide, F. & Gudiol, F. (2000) Serious complications of bacteremia caused by viridans streptococci in neutropenic patients with cancer. *Clin. Infect. Dis*. 31, 1126–1130

32. Teng, L. J., Hsueh, P. R., Chen, Y. C., Ho, S. W. & Luh, K. T. (1998) Antimicrobial susceptibility of viridans group streptococci in Taiwan with an emphasis on the high rates of resistance to penicillin and macrolides in *Streptococcus oralis*. *J. Antimicrob. Chemother*. 41, 621–627

33. Seppälä, H., Haanperä, M., Al-Juhaish, M., Järvinen, H., Jalava, J. & Huovinen, P. (2003) Antimicrobial susceptibility patterns and macrolide resistance genes of viridans group streptococci from normal flora. *J. Antimicrob. Chemother*. 52, 636–644

34. Lyytikainen, O., Rautio, M., Carlson, P., Anttila, V. J., Vuento, R., Sarkkinen, H., Kostiala, A., Vaisanen, M. L., Kanervo, A. & Ruutu, P. (2004) Nosocomial bloodstream infections due to viridans streptococci in haematological and non-haematological patients: species distribution and antimicrobial resistance. *J. Antimicrob. Chemother*. 53, 631–634

35. Ioannidou, S., Tassios, P. T., Kotsovili-Tseleni, A., Foustoukou, M., Legakis, N. J. & Vatopoulos, A. (2001) Antibiotic resistance rates and macrolide resistance phenotypes of viridans group streptococci from the oropharynx of healthy Greek children. *Int. J. Antimicrob. Agents* 17, 195–201

36. Alcaide, F., Benítez, M. A., Carratalà, J., Gudiol, F., Liñares, J. & Martín, R. (2001) In vitro activities of the New Ketolide HMR 3647 (Telithromycin) in comparison with those of eight other antibiotics against viridans group streptococci isolated from blood of neutropenic patients with cancer. *Antimicrob. Agents Chemother*. 45, 624–626

37. Alcaide, F., Carratala, J., Linares, J., Gudiol, F. & Martin, R. (1996) In vitro activities of eight macrolide antibiotics and RP-59500 (quinupristin–dalfopristin) against viridans group streptococci isolated from blood of neutropenic cancer patients. *Antimicrob. Agents Chemother*. 40, 2117–2120

38. Gershon, A. S., de Azavedo, J. C., McGeer, A., Ostrowska, K. I., Church, D., Hoban, D. J., Harding, G. K., Weiss, K., Abbott, L., Smaill, F., Gourdeau, M., Murray, G. & Low, D. E. (2002) Activities of new fluoroquinolones, ketolides, and other antimicrobials against blood culture isolates of viridans group streptococci from across Canada, 2000. *Antimicrob. Agents Chemother*. 46, 1553–1556

39. Pihlajamaki, M., Kataja, J., Seppälä, H., Elliot, J., Leinonen, M., Huovinen, P. & Jalava, J. (2002) Ribosomal mutations in *Streptococcus pneumoniae* clinical isolates. *Antimicrob Agents Chemother* 46, 654–658

40. Johnson, A. P., Warner, M., Broughton, K., James, D., Efsratiou, A., George, R. C. & Livermore, D. M. (2001) Antibiotic susceptibility of streptococci and related genera causing endocarditis: analysis of UK reference laboratory referrals, January 1996 to March 2000. *Br. Med. J*. 322, 395–396

41. de Azavedo, J. C., Trpeski, L., Pong-Porter, S., Matsumura, S. & Low, D. E. (1999) In vitro activities of fluoroquinolones against antibiotic-resistant blood culture isolates of viridans group streptococci from across Canada. *Antimicrob. Agents Chemother*. 43, 2299–2301

42. Wisplinghoff, H., Reinert, R. R., Cornely, O. & Seifert, H. (1999) Molecular relationships and antimicrobial susceptibilities of viridans group streptococci isolated from blood of neutropenic cancer patients. *J. Clin. Microbiol*. 37, 1876–1880

43. NCCLS. (1999) *Performance Standards for Antimicrobial Susceptibility Testing; Ninth Informational Supplement, M100-S9, 19*

44. NCCLS. (2004) *Performance Standards for Antimicrobial Susceptibility Testing; Fourteenth Informational Supplement, M100-S14*

45. Potgieter, E., Carmichael, M., Koornhof, H. J. & Chalkey, L. J. (1992) In vitro antimicrobial susceptibility of viridans streptococci isolated from blood cultures. *Eur. J. Clin. Microbiol. Infect. Dis* 11, 543–546

46. Pfaller, M. A. & Jones, R. N. (2000) MYSTIC (meropenem yearly susceptibility test information collection) results from the Americas: resistance implications in the treatment of serious infections. *J. Antimicrob. Chemother*. 46(Suppl B), 25–37

47. Weisblum, B. (1995) Erythromycin resistance by ribosome modification. *Antimicrob. Agents Chemother*. 39, 577–585

48. Sutcliffe, J., Tait-Kamradt, A. & Wondrack, L. (1996) *Streptococcus pneumoniae* and *Streptococcus pyogenes* resistant to macrolides but sensitive to clindamycin: a common resistance pattern mediated by an efflux system. *Antimicrob. Agents Chemother*. 40, 1817–1824

49. Arpin, C., Canron, M. H., Maugein, J. & Quentin, C. (1999) Incidence of *mefA* and *mefE* genes in viridans group streptococci. *Antimicrob. Agents Chemother*. 43, 2335–2336

50. Ono, T., Shiota, S., Hirota, K., Nemoto, K., Tsuchiya, T. & Miyake, Y. (2000) Susceptibilities of oral and nasal isolates of *Streptococcus mitis* and *Streptococcus oralis* to macrolides and PCR detection of resistance genes. *Antimicrob. Agents Chemother*. 44, 1078–1080

51. Reinert, R. R., von Eiff, C., Kresken, M., Brauers, J., Hafner, D., Al-Lahham, A., Schorn, H., Lutticken, R., Peters, G. & The Multicenter Study on Antibiotic Resistance in Staphylococci and Other Gram-Positive Cocci (Mars) Study Group (2001) Nationwide German multicenter study on the prevalence of antibiotic resistance in streptococcal blood isolates from neutropenic patients and comparative in vitro activities of quinupristin–dalfopristin and eight other antibiotics. *J. Clin. Microbiol*. 39, 1928–1931

52. Fluit, A. C., Schmitz, F. J., Verhoef, J. & Milatovic, D. (2004) Daptomycin in vitro susceptibility in European Gram-positive clinical isolates. *Int. J. Antimicrob. Agents* 24, 59–66

53. Ioannidou, S., Papaparaskevas, J., Tassios, P. T., Foustoukou, M., Legakis, N. J. & Vatopoulos, A. C. (2003) Prevalence and

characterization of the mechanisms of macrolide, lincosamide and streptogramin resistance in viridans group streptococci. *Int. J. Antimicrob. Agents* 22, 626–629

54. Leclercq, R. (2002) Mechanisms of resistance to macrolides and lincosamides: nature of the resistance elements and their clinical implications. *Clin. Infect. Dis.* 34, 482–492

55. Jalava, J., Kataja, J., Seppälä, H. & Huovinen, P. (2001) In vitro activities of the novel ketolide telithromycin (HMR 3647) against erythromycin-resistant Streptococcus species. *Antimicrob. Agents Chemother.* 45, 789–793

56. Liu, M. & Douthwaite, S. (2002) Activity of the ketolide telithromycin is refractory to Erm monomethylation of bacterial rRNA. *Antimicrob. Agents Chemother.* 46, 1629–1633

57. Thal, L. A. & Zervos, M. J. (1999) Occurrence and epidemiology of resistance to virginiamycin and streptogramins. *J. Antimicrob. Chemother.* 43, 171–176

58. Malbruny, B., Canu, A., Bozdogan, B., Fantin, B., Zarrouk, V., Dutka-Malen, S., Feger, C. & Leclercq, R. (2002) Resistance to quinupristin–dalfopristin due to mutation of L22 ribosomal protein in *Staphylococcus aureus. Antimicrob. Agents Chemother.* 46, 2200–2207

59. Aracil, B., Minambres, M., Oteo, J., Torresb, C., Gómez-Garcésa, J. L. & Alósa, J. I. (2001) High prevalence of erythromycin-resistant and clindamycin-susceptible (M phenotype) viridans group streptococci from pharyngeal samples: a reservoir of *mef* genes in commensal bacteria. *J. Antimicrob. Chemother.* 48, 592–594

60. Kern, W. & Kurrle, E. (1991) Ofloxacin versus trimethoprim–sulfamethoxazole for prevention of infection in patients with acute leukemia and granulocytopenia. *Infection* 19, 73–80

61. Ferrándiz, M. J., Oteo, J., Aracil, B., Gómez-Garcés, J. L. & De La Campa, A. G. (1999) Drug efflux and *parC* mutations are involved in fuoroquinolone resistance in viridans group streptococci. *Antimicrob. Agents Chemother.* 43, 2520–2523

62. González, I., Georgiou, M., Alcaide, F., Balas, D., Liñares, J. & de la Campa, A. G. (1998) Fluoroquinolone resistance mutations in the *parC, parE*, and *gyrA* genes of clinical isolates of viridans group streptococci. *Antimicrob. Agents Chemother.* 42, 2792–2798

63. Guerin, F., Varon, E., Hoï, A. B., Gutmann, L. & Podglajen, I. (2000) Fluoroquinolone resistance associated with target mutations and active efflux in oropharyngeal colonizing isolates of viridans group streptococci. *Antimicrob. Agents Chemother.* 44, 2197–2200

64. Ferrándiz, M. J., Fenoll, A., Liñares, J. & De La Campa, A. G. (2000) Horizontal transfer of *parC* and *gyrA* in fluoroquinolone-resistant clinical isolates of *Streptococcus pneumoniae. Antimicrob. Agents Chemother.* 44, 840–847

65. Balsalobre, L., Ferrándiz, M. J., Liñares, J., Tubau, F. & de la Campa, A. G. (2003) Viridans group streptococci are donors in horizontal transfer of topoisomerase IV genes to *Streptococcus pneumoniae. Antimicrob. Agents Chemother.* 47, 2072–2081

66. Janoir, C., Podglajen, I., Kitzis, M. D., Poyart, C. & Gutmann, L. (1999) In vitro exchange of fluoroquinolone resistance determinants between *Streptococcus pneumoniae* and viridans streptococci and genomic organization of the *parE-parC* region in *S. mitis. J. Infect. Dis.* 180, 555–558

67. Phillips, I. & Shannon, K. P. (1997) Aminoglycosides and aminocyclitols. In: *Antibiotic and Chemotherapy: Anti-infective Agents and Their Use in Therapy*, Seventh edition. (O'Grady, F., Lambert, H. P., Finch, R. G. & Greenwood, D., eds.), pp. 164–201. Churchill Livingstone Inc., New York

68. Horstkotte, D., Follath, F., Gutschik, E., Lengyel, M., Oto, A., Pavie, A., Soler-Soler, J., Thiene, G., von Graevenitz, A., Priori, S. G., Garcia, M. A., Blanc, J. J., Budaj, A., Cowie, M., Dean, V., Deckers, J., Fernandez Burgos, E., Lekakis, J., Lindahl, B., Mazzotta, G., Morais, J., Smiseth, O. A., Vahanian, A., Delahaye, F., Parkhomenko, A.,

Filipatos, G., Aldershvile, J. & Vardas, P. (2004) Guidelines on prevention, diagnosis and treatment of infective endocarditis executive summary; The task force on infective endocarditis of the European society of cardiology. *Eur. Heart J.* 25, 267–276

69. Cometta, A., Zinner, S., de Bock, R., Calandra, T., Gaya, H., Klastersky, J., Langenaeken, J., Paesmans, M., Viscoli, C. & Glauser, M. P. (1995) Piperacillin–tazobactam plus amikacin versus ceftazidime plus amikacin as empiric therapy for fever in granulocytopenic patients with cancer. *Antimicrob. Agents Chemother.* 39, 445–452

70. Eliopoulos, G. M. (2003) Quinupristin–dalfopristin and linezolid: evidence and opinion. *Clin. Infect. Dis.* 36, 473–481

71. Birmingham, M. C., Rayner, C. R., Meagher, A. K., Flavin, S. M., Batts, D. H. & Schentag, J. J. (2003) Linezolid for the treatment of multidrug-resistant, gram-positive infections: experience from a compassionate-use program. *Clin. Infect. Dis.* 36, 159–168

72. Lowbury, E. J. & Hurst, L. (1959) The sensitivity of staphylococci and other wound bacteria to erythromycin, oleandomycin, and spiramycin. *J. Clin. Pathol.* 12, 163–169

73. Kohn, J. & Evans, A. J. (1970) Group A streptococci resistant to clindamycin. *Br. Med. J.* 2, 423

74. Betriu, C., Sanchez, A., Gomez, M., Cruceyra, A. & Picazo, J. J. (1993) Antibiotic susceptibility of group A streptococci: a 6-year follow-up study. *Antimicrob. Agents Chemother.* 37, 1717–1719

75. Seppälä, H., Nissinen, A., Järvinen, H., Huovinen, S., Henriksson, T., Herva, E., Holm, S. E., Jahkola, M., Katila, M. L., Klaukka, T. & et al. (1992) Resistance to erythromycin in group A streptococci. *N. Engl. J. Med.* 326, 292–297

76. Seppälä, H., Nissinen, A., Yu, Q. & Huovinen, P. (1993) Three different phenotypes of erythromycin-resistant *Streptococcus pyogenes* in Finland. *J. Antimicrob. Chemother.* 32, 885–891

77. Seppälä, H. (1994) *Streptococcus pyogenes*; erythromycin resistance and molecular typing, Turku University

78. Dixon, J. M. & Lipinski, A. E. (1972) Resistance of group A beta-hemolytic streptococci to lincomycin and erythromycin. *Antimicrob. Agents Chemother.* 1, 333–339

79. Istre, G. R., Welch, D. F., Marks, M. I. & Moyer, N. (1981) Susceptibility of group A beta-hemolytic *Streptococcus* isolates to penicillin and erythromycin. *Antimicrob. Agents Chemother.* 20, 244–246

80. Arthur, J. D., Keiser, J. F., Brown, S. L., Higbee, J. & Butler, C. E. (1984) Erythromycin-resistant group A beta-hemolytic streptococci: prevalence at four medical centers. *Pediatr. Infect. Dis.* 3, 489

81. Gentry, J. L. & Burns, W. W. (1980) Antibiotic-resistant streptococci. *Am. J. Dis. Child.* 134, 801

82. Mitsuhashi, S., Inoue, M., Saito, K. & Nakae, M. (1982) Drug resistance in *Streptococcus pyogenes* strains isolated in Japan. In: *Microbiology* (Schlessinger, D., ed.), pp. 151–154. American Society of Microbiolgy, Washington DC

83. Stingemore, N., Francis, G. R. J., Toohey, M. & McGechie, D. B. (1989) The emergence of erythromycin resistance in *Streptococcus pyogenes* in Fremantle, Western Australia. *Med. J. Aust.* 150, 626–627, 630–621

84. Phillips, G., Parratt, D., Orange, G. V., Harper, I., McEwan, H. & Young, N. (1990) Erythromycin-resistant *Streptococcus pyogenes. J. Antimicrob. Chemother.* 25, 723–724

85. Perez-Trallero, E., Fernandez-Mazarrasa, C., Garcia-Rey, C., Bouza, E., Aguilar, L., Garcia-de-Lomas, J. & Baquero, F. (2001) Antimicrobial susceptibilities of 1,684 *Streptococcus pneumoniae* and 2,039 *Streptococcus pyogenes* isolates and their ecological relationships: results of a 1-year (1998–1999) multicenter surveillance study in Spain. *Antimicrob. Agents Chemother.* 45, 3334–3340

86. Portillo, A., Lantero, M., Gastanares, M. J., Ruiz-Larrea, F. & Torres, C. (1999) Macrolide resistance phenotypes and mechanisms of resistance in *Streptococcus pyogenes* in La Rioja, Spain. *Int. J. Antimicrob. Agents* 13, 137–140

87. Alos, J. I., Aracil, B., Oteo, J. & Gomez-Garces, J. L. (2003) Significant increase in the prevalence of erythromycin-resistant, clindamycin- and miocamycin-susceptible (M phenotype) *Streptococcus pyogenes* in Spain. *J. Antimicrob. Chemother.* 51, 333 337

88. Ioannidou, S., Tassios, P. T., Kotsovili-Tseleni, A., Foustoukou, M., Legakis, N. J. & Vatopoulos, A. (2001) Antibiotic resistance rates and macrolide resistance phenotypes of viridans group streptococci from the oropharynx of healthy Greek children. *Int. J. Antimicrob. Agents* 17, 195–201

89. Stamos, G., Bedevis, K., Paraskaki, I., Chronopoulou, A., Tsirepa, M. & Foustoukou, M. (2001) Emergence of group A beta-hemolytic streptococci resistant to erythromycin in Athens, Greece. *Eur. J. Clin. Microbiol. Infect. Dis.* 20, 70–71

90. Tzelepi, E., Kouppari, G., Mavroidi, A., Zaphiropoulou, A. & Tzouvelekis, L. S. (1999) Erythromycin resistance amongst group A beta-haemolytic streptococci isolated in a paediatric hospital in Athens, Greece. *J. Antimicrob. Chemother.* 43, 745–746

91. Syrogiannopoulos, G. A., Grivea, I. N., Fitoussi, F., Doit, C., Katopodis, G. D., Bingen, E. & Beratis, N. G. (2001) High prevalence of erythromycin resistance of *Streptococcus pyogenes* in Greek children. *Pediatr. Infect. Dis. J.* 20, 863–868

92. Ioannidou, S., Tassios, P. T., Zachariadou, L., Salem, Z., Kanelopoulou, M., Kanavaki, S., Chronopoulou, G., Petropoulou, N., Foustoukou, M., Pangalis, A., Trikka-Graphakos, E., Papafraggas, E. & Vatopoulos, A. C. (2003) In vitro activity of telithromycin (HMR 3647) against Greek *Streptococcus pyogenes* and *Streptococcus pneumoniae* clinical isolates with different macrolide susceptibilities. *Clin. Microbiol. Infect.* 9, 704–707

93. Petinaki, E., Kontos, F., Pratti, A., Skulakis, C. & Maniatis, A. N. (2003) Clinical isolates of macrolide-resistant *Streptococcus pyogenes* in Central Greece. *Int. J. Antimicrob. Agents* 21, 67–70

94. Arvand, M., Hoeck, M., Hahn, H. & Wagner, J. (2000) Antimicrobial resistance in *Streptococcus pyogenes* isolates in Berlin. *J. Antimicrob. Chemother.* 46, 621–624

95. Brandt, C. M., Honscha, M., Truong, N. D., Holland, R., Hovener, B., Bryskier, A., Lutticken, R. & Reinert, R. R. (2001) Macrolide resistance in *Streptococcus pyogenes* isolates from throat infections in the region of Aachen, Germany. *Microb. Drug Resist.* 7, 165–170

96. Reinert, R. R., Lutticken, R., Bryskier, A. & Al-Lahham, A. (2003) Macrolide-resistant *Streptococcus pneumoniae* and *Streptococcus pyogenes* in the pediatric population in Germany during 2000–2001. *Antimicrob. Agents Chemother.* 47, 489–493

97. Sauermann, R., Gattringer, R., Graninger, W., Buxbaum, A. & Georgopoulos, A. (2003) Phenotypes of macrolide resistance of group A streptococci isolated from outpatients in Bavaria and susceptibility to 16 antibiotics. *J. Antimicrob. Chemother.* 51, 53–57

98. Savoia, D., Avanzini, C., Bosio, K., Volpe, G., Carpi, D., Dotti, G. & Zucca, M. (2000) Macrolide resistance in group A streptococci. *J. Antimicrob. Chemother.* 45, 41–47

99. Varaldo, P. E., Debbia, E. A., Nicoletti, G., Pavesio, D., Ripa, S., Schito, G. C. & Tempera, G. (1999) Nationwide survey in Italy of treatment of *Streptococcus pyogenes* pharyngitis in children: influence of macrolide resistance on clinical and microbiological outcomes. Artemis-Italy Study Group. *Clin. Infect. Dis.* 29, 869–873

100. Bingen, E., Fitoussi, F., Doit, C., Cohen, R., Tanna, A., George, R., Loukil, C., Brahimi, N., Le Thomas, I. & Deforche, D. (2000) Resistance to macrolides in *Streptococcus pyogenes* in France in pediatric patients. *Antimicrob. Agents Chemother.* 44, 1453–1457

101. Weber, P., Filipecki, J., Bingen, E., Fitoussi, F., Goldfarb, G., Chauvin, J. P., Reitz, C. & Portier, H. (2001) Genetic and phenotypic characterization of macrolide resistance in group A strep-

tococci isolated from adults with pharyngo-tonsillitis in France. *J. Antimicrob. Chemother.* 48, 291–294

102. Bozdogan, B., Appelbaum, P. C., Ednie, L., Grivea, I. N. & Syrogiannopoulos, G. A. (2003) Development of macrolide resistance by ribosomal protein L4 mutation in *Streptococcus pyogenes* during miocamycin treatment of an eight-year-old Greek child with tonsillopharyngitis. *Clin. Microbiol. Infect.* 9, 966–969

103. Kozlov, R. S., Bogdanovitch, T. M., Appelbaum, P. C., Ednie, L., Stratchounski, L. S., Jacobs, M. R. & Bozdogan, B. (2002) Antistreptococcal activity of telithromycin compared with seven other drugs in relation to macrolide resistance mechanisms in Russia. *Antimicrob. Agents Chemother.* 46, 2963–2968

104. Hsueh, P. R., Teng, L. J., Lee, L. N., Yang, P. C., Ho, S. W., Lue, H. C. & Luh, K. T. (2002) Increased prevalence of erythromycin resistance in streptococci: substantial upsurge in erythromycin-resistant M phenotype in *Streptococcus pyogenes* (1979–1998) but not in *Streptococcus pneumoniae* (1985–1999) in Taiwan. *Microb. Drug Resist.* 8, 27–33

105. Yan, J. J., Wu, H. M., Huang, A. H., Fu, H. M., Lee, C. T. & Wu, J. J. (2000) Prevalence of polyclonal mefA-containing isolates among erythromycin-resistant group A streptococci in Southern Taiwan. *J. Clin. Microbiol.* 38, 2475–2479

106. Cha, S., Lee, H., Lee, K., Hwang, K., Bae, S. & Lee, Y. (2001) The emergence of erythromycin-resistant *Streptococcus pyogenes* in Seoul, Korea. *J Infect Chemother* 7, 81–86

107. Ip, M., Lyon, D. J., Leung, T. & Cheng, A. F. (2002) Macrolide resistance and distribution of erm and mef genes among beta-haemolytic streptococci in Hong Kong. *Eur. J. Clin. Microbiol. Infect. Dis.* 21, 238–240

108. Katz, K. C., McGeer, A. J., Duncan, C. L., Ashi-Sulaiman, A., Willey, B. M., Sarabia, A., McCann, J., Pong-Porter, S., Rzayev, Y., de Azavedo, J. S. & Low, D. E. (2003) Emergence of macrolide resistance in throat culture isolates of group a streptococci in Ontario, Canada, in 2001. *Antimicrob. Agents Chemother.* 47, 2370–2372

109. Martin, J. M., Green, M., Barbadora, K. A. & Wald, E. R. (2002) Erythromycin-resistant group S streptococci in schoolchildren in Pittsburgh. *N. Engl. J. Med.* 346, 1200–1206

110. Palavecino, E. L., Riedel, I., Berrios, X., Bajaksouzian, S., Johnson, D., Kaplan, E. & Jacobs, M. R. (2001) Prevalence and mechanisms of macrolide resistance in *Streptococcus pyogenes* in Santiago, Chile. *Antimicrob. Agents Chemother.* 45, 339–341

111. Martinez, S., Amoroso, A. M., Famiglietti, A., de Mier, C., Vay, C. & Gutkind, G. O. (2004) Genetic and phenotypic characterization of resistance to macrolides in Streptococcus pyogenes from Argentina. *Int J. Antimicrob. Agents* 23, 95–98

112. Eickhoff, T. C., Klein, J. O., Daly, A. K., Ingall, D. & Finland, M. (1964) Neonatal sepsis and other infections due to group B beta-hemolytic streptococci. *N. Engl. J. Med.* 271, 1221–1228

113. Morales, W. J., Dickey, S. S., Bornick, P. & Lim, D. V. (1999) Change in antibiotic resistance of group B streptococcus: impact on intrapartum management. *Am. J. Obstet. Gynecol.* 181, 310–314

114. Betriu, C., Culebras, E., Gomez, M., Rodriguez-Avial, I., Sanchez, B. A., Agreda, M. C. & Picazo, J. J. (2003) Erythromycin and clindamycin resistance and telithromycin susceptibility in *Streptococcus agalactiae*. *Antimicrob. Agents Chemother.* 47, 1112–1114

115. Hsueh, P. R., Teng, L. J., Lee, L. N., Ho, S. W., Yang, P. C. & Luh, K. T. (2001) High incidence of erythromycin resistance among clinical isolates of *Streptococcus agalactiae* in Taiwan. *Antimicrob. Agents Chemother.* 45, 3205–3208

116. De Mouy, D., Cavallo, J. D., Leclercq, R. & Fabre, R. (2001) Antibiotic susceptibility and mechanisms of erythromycin resistance in clinical isolates of *Streptococcus agalactiae*: French multicenter study. *Antimicrob. Agents Chemother.* 45, 2400–2402

117. Fitoussi, F., Loukil, C., Gros, I., Clermont, O., Mariani, P., Bonacorsi, S., Le Thomas, I., Deforche, D. & Bingen, E. (2001) Mechanisms of macrolide resistance in clinical group B streptococci isolated in France. *Antimicrob. Agents Chemother.* 45, 1889–1891

118. Poyart, C., Jardy, L., Quesne, G., Berche, P. & Trieu-Cuot, P. (2003) Genetic basis of antibiotic resistance in *Streptococcus agalactiae* strains isolated in a French hospital. *Antimicrob. Agents Chemother.* 47, 794–797

119. Andrews, J. I., Diekema, D. J., Hunter, S. K., Rhomberg, P. R., Pfaller, M. A., Jones, R. N. & Doern, G. V. (2000) Group B streptococci causing neonatal bloodstream infection: antimicrobial susceptibility and serotyping results from SENTRY centers in the Western Hemisphere. *Am. J. Obstet. Gynecol.* 183, 859–862

120. de Azavedo, J. C., McGavin, M., Duncan, C., Low, D. E. & McGeer, A. (2001) Prevalence and mechanisms of macrolide resistance in invasive and noninvasive group B streptococcus isolates from Ontario, Canada. *Antimicrob. Agents Chemother.* 45, 3504–3508

121. Uh, Y., Jang, I. H., Hwang, G. Y., Yoon, K. J. & Song, W. (2001) Emerging erythromycin resistance among group B streptococci in Korea. *Eur. J. Clin. Microbiol. Infect. Dis.* 20, 52–54

122. Acikgoz, Z. C., Almayanlar, E., Gamberzade, S. & Gocer, S. (2004) Macrolide resistance determinants of invasive and non-invasive group B streptococci in a Turkish hospital. *Antimicrob. Agents Chemother.* 48, 1410–1412

123. Kataja, J., Seppälä, H., Skurnik, M., Sarkkinen, H. & Huovinen, P. (1998) Different erythromycin resistance mechanisms in group C and group G streptococci. *Antimicrob. Agents Chemother* 42, 1493–1494

124. Wu, J. J., Lin, K. Y., Hsueh, P. R., Liu, J. W., Pan, H. I. & Sheu, S. M. (1997) High incidence of erythromycin-resistant streptococci in Taiwan. *Antimicrob. Agents Chemother.* 41, 844–846

125. Chabbert, Y. A. (1956) Antagonisme in vitro entre l'erythromycine et la spiramycine. *Ann. Inst. Pasteur* 90, 787–790

126. Hyder, S. L. & Streitfeld, M. M. (1973) Inducible and constitutive resistance to macrolide antibiotics and lincomycin in clinically isolated strains of *Streptococcus pyogenes*. *Antimicrob. Agents Chemother.* 4, 327–331

127. Dixon, J. M. & Lipinski, A. E. (1974) Infections with beta-hemolytic *Streptococcus* resistant to lincomycin and erythromycin and observations on zonal-pattern resistance to lincomycin. *J. Infect. Dis.* 130, 351–356

128. Horodniceanu, T., Bougueleret, L., El-Solh, N., Bouanchaud, D. H. & Chabbert, Y. A. (1979) Conjugative R plasmids in *Streptococcus agalactiae* (group B). *Plasmid* 2, 197–206

129. Weisblum, B., Holder, S. B. & Halling, S. M. (1979) Deoxyribonucleic acid sequence common to staphylococcal and streptococcal plasmids which specify erythromycin resistance. *J. Bacteriol.* 138, 990–998

130. Horinouchi, S., Byeon, W. H. & Weisblum, B. (1983) A complex attenuator regulates inducible resistance to macrolides, lincosamides, and streptogramin type B antibiotics in *Streptococcus sanguis*. *J. Bacteriol.* 154, 1252–1262

131. Shaw, J. H. & Clewell, D. B. (1985) Complete nucleotide sequence of macrolide-lincosamide-streptogramin B- resistance transposon Tn*917* in *Streptococcus faecalis*. *J. Bacteriol.* 164, 782–796

132. Seppälä, H., Skurnik, M., Soini, H., Roberts, M. C. & Huovinen, P. (1998) A novel erythromycin resistance methylase gene (*ermTR*) in *Streptococcus pyogenes*. *Antimicrob. Agents Chemother.* 42, 257–262

133. Roberts, M. C., Sutcliffe, J., Courvalin, P., Jensen, L. B., Rood, J. & Seppala, H. (1999) Nomenclature for macrolide and macrolide-lincosamide-streptogramin B resistance determinants. *Antimicrob. Agents Chemother.* 43, 2823–2830

134. Fines, M., Gueudin, M., Ramon, A. & Leclercq, R. (2001) In vitro selection of resistance to clindamycin related to alterations in the attenuator of the erm(TR) gene of *Streptococcus pyogenes* UCN1 inducibly resistant to erythromycin. *J. Antimicrob. Chemother.* 48, 411–416

135. Clancy, J., Petitpas, J., Dib-Hajj, F., Yuan, W., Cronan, M., Kamath, A. V., Bergeron, J. & Retsema, J. A. (1996) Molecular cloning and functional analysis of a novel macrolide-resistance determinant, *mefA*, from *Streptococcus pyogenes*. *Mol. Microbiol.* 22, 867–879

136. Clancy, J., Petitpas, J., Dib-Hajj, F., Yuan, W., Cronan, M., Kamath, A. V., Bergeron, J. & Retsema, J. A. (1996) Molecular cloning and functional analysis of a novel macrolide-resistant determinant, mefA, from *Streptococcus pyogenes*. *Mol. Microbiol.* 22, 867–879

137. Betriu, C., Redondo, M., Palau, M. L., Sanchez, A., Gomez, M., Culebras, E., Boloix, A. & Picazo, J. J. (2000) Comparative in vitro activities of linezolid, quinupristin-dalfopristin, moxifloxacin, and trovafloxacin against erythromycin-susceptible and -resistant streptococci. *Antimicrob. Agents Chemother.* 44, 1838–1841

138. Kataja, J., Huovinen, P., Muotiala, A., Vuopio-Varkila, J., Efstratiou, A., Hallas, G. & Seppälä, H. (1998) Clonal spread of group A streptococcus with the new type of erythromycin resistance. Finnish Study Group for Antimicrobial Resistance. *J. Infect. Dis.* 177, 786–789

139. Green, M., Martin, J. M., Barbadora, K. A., Beall, B. & Wald, E. R. (2004) Reemergence of macrolide resistance in pharyngeal isolates of group a streptococci in southwestern Pennsylvania. *Antimicrob. Agents Chemother.* 48, 473–476

140. Bozdogan, B. & Appelbaum, P. C. (2004) Macrolide resistance in streptococci and *Haemophilus influenzae*. *Clin. Lab. Med.* 24, 455–475

141. Diekema, D. J., Andrews, J. I., Huynh, H., Rhomberg, P. R., Doktor, S. R., Beyer, J., Shortridge, V. D., Flamm, R. K., Jones, R. N. & Pfaller, M. A. (2003) Molecular epidemiology of macrolide resistance in neonatal bloodstream isolates of group B streptococci. *J. Clin. Microbiol.* 41, 2659–2661

142. Poyart, C., Quesne, G., Acar, P., Berche, P. & Trieu-Cuot, P. (2000) Characterization of the Tn916-like transposon Tn3872 in a strain of abiotrophia defectiva (*Streptococcus defectivus*) causing sequential episodes of endocarditis in a child. *Antimicrob. Agents Chemother.* 44, 790–793

143. Culebras, E., Rodriguez-Avial, I., Betriu, C., Redondo, M. & Picazo, J. J. (2002) Macrolide and tetracycline resistance and molecular relationships of clinical strains of *Streptococcus agalactiae*. *Antimicrob. Agents Chemother.* 46, 1574–1576

144. Betriu, C., Culebras, E., Rodriguez-Avial, I., Gomez, M., Sanchez, B. A. & Picazo, J. J. (2004) In vitro activities of tigecycline against erythromycin-resistant *Streptococcus pyogenes* and *Streptococcus agalactiae*: mechanisms of macrolide and tetracycline resistance. *Antimicrob. Agents Chemother.* 48, 323–325

145. Wu, J. J., Lin, K. Y., Hsueh, P. R., Liu, J. W., Pan, H. I. & Sheu, S. M. (1997) High incidence of erythromycin-resistant streptococci in Taiwan. *Antimicrob. Agents Chemother.* 41, 844–846

146. Kataja, J., Seppälä, H., Skurnik, M., Sarkkinen, H. & Huovinen, P. (1998) Different erythromycin resistance mechanisms in group C and group G streptococci. *Antimicrob. Agents Chemother.* 42, 1493–1494

147. Bingen, E., Leclercq, R., Fitoussi, F., Brahimi, N., Malbruny, B., Deforche, D. & Cohen, R. (2002) Emergence of group A streptococcus strains with different mechanisms of macrolide resistance. *Antimicrob. Agents Chemother.* 46, 1199–1203

148. Malbruny, B., Nagai, K., Coquemont, M., Bozdogan, B., Andrasevic, A. T., Hupkova, H., Leclercq, R. & Appelbaum, P. C. (2002) Resistance to macrolides in clinical isolates of *Streptococcus pyogenes* due to ribosomal mutations. *J. Antimicrob. Chemother.* 49, 935–939

149. Jalava, J., Vaara, M. & Huovinen, P. (2004) Mutation at the position 2058 of the 23S rRNA as a cause of macrolide resistance in *Streptococcus pyogenes*. *Ann. Clin. Microbiol. Antimicrob.* 3, 5

150. Giovanetti, E., Brenciani, A., Burioni, R. & Varaldo, P. E. (2002) A novel efflux system in inducibly erythromycin-resistant strains of *Streptococcus pyogenes*. *Antimicrob. Agents Chemother*. 46, 3750–3755

151. Clancy, J., Petitpas, J., Dib-Hajj, F., Yuan, W., Cronan, M., Kamath, A. V., Bergeron, J. & Retsema, J. A. (1996) Molecular cloning and functional analysis of a novel macrolide-resistance determinant, mefA, from *Streptococcus pyogenes*. *Mol. Microbiol*. 22, 867–879

152. Portillo, A., Lantero, M., Olarte, I., Ruiz-Larrea, F. & Torres, C. (2001) MLS resistance phenotypes and mechanisms in beta-haemolytic group B, C and G streptococcus isolates in La Rioja, Spain. *J. Antimicrob. Chemother*. 47, 115–116

153. Giovanetti, E., Montanari, M. P., Mingoia, M. & Varaldo, P. E. (1999) Phenotypes and genotypes of erythromycin-resistant *Streptococcus pyogenes* strains in Italy and heterogeneity of inducibly resistant strains. *Antimicrob. Agents Chemother*. 43, 1935–1940

154. Buu-Hoi, A., Bieth, G. & Horaud, T. (1984) Broad host range of streptococcal macrolide resistance plasmids. *Antimicrob. Agents Chemother*. 25, 289–291

155. Malke, H. (1975) Transfer of a plasmid mediating antibiotic resistance between strains of *Streptococcus pyogenes* in mixed cultures. *Z. Allg. Mikrobiol*. 15, 645–649

156. Malke, H., Starke, R., Köhler, W., Kolesnichenko, G. & Totolian, A. A. (1975) Bacteriophage P13234 mo-mediated intra- and inter-group transduction of antibiotic resistance among streptococci. *Zentralbl. Bakteriol. [Orig A]* 233, 24–34

157. Horaud, T., De Cespedes, G., Clermont, D., David, F. & Delbos, F. (1991) Variability of chromosomal genetic elements in strep-tococci. In: *Genetics and Molecular Biology of Streptococci, Lactococci, and Enterococci* (Dunny, G. M., Cleary, P. P. & McKay, L. L., eds.), pp. 16–20. American Society for Microbiology, Washington, DC

158. Kataja, J., Huovinen, P., Skurnik, M. & Seppälä, H. (1999) Erythromycin resistance genes in group A streptococci in Finland. The Finnish Study Group for antimicrobial resistance. *Antimicrob. Agents Chemother*. 43, 48–52

159. Giovanetti, E., Magi, G., Brenciani, A., Spinaci, C., Lupidi, R., Facinelli, B. & Varaldo, P. E. (2002) Conjugative transfer of the erm(A) gene from erythromycin-resistant *Streptococcus pyogenes* to macrolide-susceptible *S. pyogenes*, *Enterococcus faecalis* and *Listeria innocua*. *J. Antimicrob. Chemother*. 50, 249–252

160. Le Bouguenec, C., de Cespedes, G. & Horaud, T. (1988) Molecular analysis of a composite chromosomal conjugative element (Tn*3701*) of *Streptococcus pyogenes*. *J. Bacteriol*. 170, 3930–3936

161. Giovanetti, E., Brenciani, A., Lupidi, R., Roberts, M. C. & Varaldo, P. E. (2003) Presence of the tet(O) gene in erythromycin- and tetracycline-resistant strains of *Streptococcus pyogenes* and linkage with either the mef(A) or the erm(A) gene. *Antimicrob. Agents Chemother*. 47, 2844–2849

162. Cresti, S., Lattanzi, M., Zanchi, A., Montagnani, F., Pollini, S., Cellesi, C. & Rossolini, G. M. (2002) Resistance determinants and clonal diversity in group A streptococci collected during a period of increasing macrolide resistance. *Antimicrob. Agents Chemother*. 46, 1816–1822

163. Banks, D. J., Porcella, S. F., Barbian, K. D., Martin, J. M. & Musser, J. M. (2003) Structure and distribution of an unusual chimeric genetic element encoding macrolide resistance in phy-logenetically diverse clones of group A streptococcus. *J. Infect. Dis*. 188, 1898–1908

164. Kataja, J., Huovinen, P., Efstratiou, A., Perez-Trallero, E. & Seppälä, H. (2002) Clonal relationships among isolates of erythromycin-resistant *Streptococcus pyogenes* of different geographical origin. *Eur. J. Clin. Microbiol. Infect. Dis*. 21, 589–595

165. Reinert, R. R., Lütticken, R., Sutcliffe, J. A., Tait-Kamradt, A., Cil, M. Y., Schorn, H. M., Bryskier, A. & Al-Lahham, A. (2004) Clonal relatedness of erythromycin-resistant *Streptococcus pyogenes* isolates in Germany. *Antimicrob. Agents Chemother*. 48, 1369–1373

166. Perez-Trallero, E., Marimon, J. M., Montes, M., Orden, B. & de Pablos, M. (1999) Clonal differences among erythromycin-resistant *Streptococcus pyogenes* in Spain. *Emerg. Infect. Dis*. 5, 235–240

167. Reig, M., Galan, J., Baquero, F. & Perez-Diaz, J. C. (2001) Macrolide resistance in *Peptostreptococcus* spp. mediated by ermTR: possible source of macrolide-lincosamide-streptogramin B resistance in *Streptococcus pyogenes*. *Antimicrob. Agents Chemother*. 45, 630–632

168. Granizo, J. J., Aguilar, L., Casal, J., Dal-Re, R. & Baquero, F. (2000) *Streptococcus pyogenes* resistance to erythromycin in relation to macrolide consumption in Spain (1986–1997). *J. Antimicrob. Chemother*. 46, 959–964

169. Seppälä, H., Klaukka, T., Lehtonen, R., Nenonen, E. & Huovinen, P. (1995) Outpatient use of erythromycin: link to increased erythromycin resistance in group A streptococci. *Clin. Infect. Dis*. 21, 1378–1385

170. Bergman, M., Huikko, S., Pihlajamaki, M., Laippala, P., Palva, E., Huovinen, P. & Seppälä, H. (2004) Effect of macrolide consumption on erythromycin resistance in *Streptococcus pyogenes* in Finland in 1997–2001. *Clin. Infect. Dis*. 38, 1251–1256

171. Ko, W. C., Lee, H. C., Wang, L. R., Lee, C. T., Liu, A. J. & Wu, J. J. (2001) Serotyping and antimicrobial susceptibility of group B streptococcus over an eight-year period in southern Taiwan. *Eur. J. Clin. Microbiol. Infect. Dis*. 20, 334–339

172. De Azavedo, J. C., Yeung, R. H., Bast, D. J., Duncan, C. L., Borgia, S. B. & Low, D. E. (1999) Prevalence and mechanisms of macrolide resistance in clinical isolates of group A streptococci from Ontario, Canada. *Antimicrob. Agents Chemother*. 43, 2144–2147

173. Hogevik, H., Olaison, L., Andersson, R., Lindberg, J. & Alestig, K. (1995) Epidemiologic aspects of infective endocarditis in an urban population. A 5-year prospective study. *Medicine (Baltimore)* 74, 324–339

174. Watanakunakorn, C. & Burkert, T. (1993) Infective endocarditis at a large community teaching hospital, 1980–1990. A review of 210 episodes. *Medicine (Baltimore)* 72, 90–102

175. Mylonakis, E. & Calderwood, S. B. (2001) Infective endocarditis in adults. *N. Engl. J. Med*. 345, 1318–1330

176. Alestig, K., Hogevik, H. & Olaison, L. (2000) Infective endocarditis: a diagnostic and therapeutic challenge for the new millennium. *Scand. J. Infect. Dis*. 32, 343–356

177. Eykyn, S. J. Bacteraemia, septicaemia and endocarditis, Vol. Chapter 16, pp. 277–298

178. Gutschik, E. (1999) New developments in the treatment of infective endocarditis infective cardiovasculitis. *Int. J. Antimicrob. Agents* 13, 79–92

179. Shanson, D. C. (1998) New guidelines for the antibiotic treatment of streptococcal, enterococcal and staphylococcal endocarditis. *J. Antimicrob. Chemother*. 42, 292–296

180. Levy, C. S., Kogulan, P., Gill, V. J., Croxton, M. B., Kane, J. G. & Lucey, D. R. (2001) Endocarditis caused by penicillin-resistant viridans streptococci: 2 cases and controversies in therapy. *Clin. Infect. Dis*. 33, 577–579

181. Lonks, J. R., Dickinson, B. P. & Runarsdottir, V. (1999) Endocarditis due to Streptococcus mitis with high-level resistance to penicillin and cefotaxime. *N. Engl. J. Med*. 341, 1239

182. Levitz, R. E. (1999) Prosthetic-valve endocarditis caused by penicillin-resistant *Streptococcus mitis*. *N. Engl. J. Med*. 340, 1843–1844

183. Sabella, C., Murphy, D. & Drummond-Webb, J. (2001) Endocarditis due to Streptococcus mitis with high-level resistance to penicillin and ceftriaxone. *JAMA* 285, 2195

184. Hamza, N., Ortiz, J. & Bonomo, R. A. (2004) Isolated pulmonic valve infective endocarditis: a persistent challenge. *Infection* 32, 170–175

185. Klastersky, J. (1998) Science and pragmatism in the treatment and prevention of neutropenic infection. *J. Antimicrob. Chemother.* 41(Suppl D), 13–24

186. Collin, B. A., Leather, H. L., Wingard, J. R. & Ramphal, R. (2001) Evolution, incidence, and susceptibility of bacterial bloodstream isolates from 519 bone marrow transplant patients. *Clin. Infect. Dis.* 33, 947–953

187. Ramphal, R. (2004) Changes in the etiology of bacteremia in febrile neutropenic patients and the susceptibilities of the currently isolated pathogens. *Clin. Infect. Dis.* 39, S25–S31

188. Elting, L. S., Rubenstein, E. B., Rolston, K. V. & Bodey, G. P. (1997) Outcomes of bacteremia in patients with cancer and neutropenia: observations from two decades of epidemiological and clinical trials. *Clin. Infect. Dis.* 25, 247–259

189. Elting, L. S., Bodey, G. P. & Keefe, B. H. (1992) Septicemia and shock syndrome due to viridans streptococci: a case-control study of predisposing factors. *Clin. Infect. Dis.* 14, 1201–1207

190. Picazo, J. (2004) Management of the febrile neutropenic patient: a consensus conference. *Clin. Infect. Dis.* 39, S1–S6

191. Kanamaru, A. & Tatsumi, Y. (2004) Microbiological data for patients with febrile neutropenia. *Clin. Infect. Dis.* 39, S7–S10

192. Gonzalez-Barca, E., Fernández-Sevilla, A., Carratalà, J., Grañena, A. & Gudiol, F. (1996) Prospective study of 288 episodes of bacteremia in neutropenic cancer patients in a single institution. *Eur. J. Clin. Microbiol. Infect. Dis* 15, 291–296

193. Bochud, P. Y., Calandra, T. & Francioli, P. (1994) Bacteremia due to viridans streptococci in neutropenic patients: a review. *Am. J. Med.* 97, 256–264

194. Villablanca, J., Steiner, M., Kersey, J., Ramsay, N. K. C., Ferrieri, P., Haake, R. & Weisdorf, D. (1990) The clinical spectrum of infections with viridans streptococci in bone marrow transplant patients. *Bone Marrow Transplant.* 6, 387–393

195. Bochud, P. Y., Eggiman, P., Calandra, T., Van Melle, G., Saghafi, L. & Francioli, P. (1994) Bacteremia due to viridans streptococcus in neutropenic patients with cancer: clinical spectrum and risk factors. *Clin. Infect. Dis.* 18, 25–31

196. Richard, P., Amador Del Valle, G., Moreau, P., Milpied, N., Felice, M. P., Daeschler, T., Harousseau, J. L. & Richet, H. (1995) Viridans streptococcal bacteraemia in patients with neutropenia. *Lancet* 345, 1607–1609

197. Kern, W., Kurrle, E. & Schmeiser, T. (1990) Streptococcal bacteremia in adult patients with leukemia undergoing aggressive chemotherapy. A review of 55 Cases. *Infection* 18, 138–145

198. Steiner, M., Villablanca, J., Kersey, J., Ramsay, N., Haake, R., Ferrieri, P. & Weisdorf, D. (1993) Viridans streptococcal shock in bone marrow transplantation patients. *Am. J Hematol.* 42, 354–358

199. Zinner, S., Calandra, T., Meunier, F., Gaya, H., Viscoli, C., Klastersky, J., Glauser, M. P., Langenaeken, J. & Paesmans, M. (1994) Reduction of fever and streptococcal bacteremia in granulocytopenic patients with cancer. *JAMA* 272, 1183–1189

200. Rolston, K. V. (2004) The infectious diseases society of America 2002 guidelines for the use of antimicrobial agents in patients with cancer and neutropenia: salient features and comments. *Clin. Infect. Dis.* 39, S44–S48

201. Masaoka, T. (2004) Evidence-based recommendations for antimicrobial use in febrile neutropenia in Japan: executive summary. *Clin. Infect. Dis.* 39, S49–S52

202. Tamura, K. (2004) Initial empirical antimicrobial therapy: duration and subsequent modifications. *Clin. Infect. Dis.* 39, S59–S64

203. Cometta, A., Kern, W. V., De Bock, R., Paesmans, M., Vandenbergh, M., Crokaert, F., Engelhard, D., Marchetti, O., Akan, H., Skoutelis, A., Korten, V., Vandercam, M., Gaya, H., Padmos, A., Klastersky, J., Zinner, S., Glauser, M. P., Calandra, T. & Viscoli, C. (2003) Vancomycin versus placebo for treating persistent fever in patients with neutropenic cancer receiving piperacillin-tazobactam monotherapy. *Clin. Infect. Dis.* 37, 382–389

204. Carratalà, J., Alcaide, F., Fernández-Sevilla, A., Corbella, X., Liñares, J. & Gudiol, F. (1995) Bacteremia due to viridans streptococci that are highly resistant to penicillin: increase among neutropenic patients with cancer. *Clin. Infect. Dis.* 20, 1169–1173

205. Cepeda, J. A., Whitehouse, T., Cooper, B., Hails, J., Jones, K., Kwaku, F., Taylor, L., Hayman, S., Shaw, S., Kibbler, C., Shulman, R., Singer, M. & Wilson, A. P. (2004) Linezolid versus teicoplanin in the treatment of Gram-positive infections in the critically ill: a randomized, double-blind, multicentre study. *J. Antimicrob. Chemother.* 53, 345–355

206. Wilcox, M., Nathwani, D. & Dryden, M. (2004) Linezolid compared with teicoplanin for the treatment of suspected or proven Gram-positive infections. *J. Antimicrob. Chemother.* 53, 335–344

207. Klastersky, J. (2003) Role of quinupristin/dalfopristin in the treatment of Gram-positive nosocomial infections in haematological or oncological patients. *Cancer Treat. Rev.* 29, 431–440

208. Cruciani, M., Rampazzo, R., Malena, M., Lazzarini, L., Todeschini, G., Messori, A. & Concia, E. (1996) Prophylaxis with fluoroquinolones for bacterial infections in neutropenic patients: a meta-analysis. *Clin. Infect. Dis.* 23, 795–805

209. Guiot, H. F., Peters, W. G., van den Broek, P. J., van der Meer, J. W., Kramps, J. A., Willemze, R. & van Furth, R. (1990) Respiratory failure elicited by streptococcal septicaemia in patients treated with cytosine arabinoside, and its prevention by penicillin. *Infection* 18, 131–137

210. Rondini, G., Cocuzza, C. E., Cianflone, M., Lanzafame, A., Santini, L. & Mattina, R. (2001) Bacteriological and clinical efficacy of various antibiotics used in the treatment of streptococcal pharyngitis in Italy. An epidemiological study. *Int. J. Antimicrob. Agents* 18, 9–17

211. Bassetti, M., Manno, G., Collida, A., Ferrando, A., Gatti, G., Ugolotti, E., Cruciani, M. & Bassetti, D. (2000) Erythromycin resistance in *Streptococcus pyogenes* in Italy. *Emerg. Infect. Dis.* 6, 180–183

212. Facinelli, B., Spinaci, C., Magi, G., Giovanetti, E. & Varaldo, E. P. (2001) Association between erythromycin resistance and ability to enter human respiratory cells in group A streptococci. *Lancet* 358, 30–33

213. Seppälä, H., Klaukka, T., Vuopio-Varkila, J., Muotiala, A., Helenius, H., Lager, K., Huovinen, P. & Finnish Study Group for Antimicrobial Resistance (1997) The effect of changes in the consumption of macrolide antibiotics on erythromycin resistance in group A streptococci in Finland. *N. Engl. J. Med.* 337, 441–446

214. Fujita, K., Murono, K., Yoshikawa, M. & Murai, T. (1994) Decline of erythromycin resistance of group A streptococci in Japan. *Pediatr. Infect. Dis. J.* 13, 1075–1078

215. Cizman, M., Pokorn, M., Seme, K., Orazem, A. & Paragi, M. (2001) The relationship between trends in macrolide use and resistance to macrolides of common respiratory pathogens. *J. Antimicrob. Chemother.* 47, 475–477

216. Commitee. (1997) Revised guidelines for prevention of early-onset group B streptococcal (GBS) infection. American Academy of Pediatrics Committee on Infectious Diseases and Committee on Fetus and Newborn. *Pediatrics* 99, 489–496

217. Horn, D. L., Zabriskie, J. B., Austrian, R., Cleary, P. P., Ferretti, J. J., Fischetti, V. A., Gotschlich, E., Kaplan, E. L., McCarty, M., Opal, S. M., Roberts, R. B., Tomasz, A. & Wachtfogel, Y. (1998) Why have group A streptococci remained susceptible to penicillin? Report on a symposium. *Clin. Infect. Dis.* 26, 1341–1345

218. Bryskier, A. (2000) Ketolides-telithromycin, an example of a new class of antibacterial agents. *Clin. Microbiol. Infect.* 6, 661–669

Chapter 49

Enterococcus: Antimicrobial Resistance in Enterococci Epidemiology, Treatment, and Control

Anne Y. Chen and Marcus J. Zervos

1 General Description

1.1 Microbiology

Enterococci are Gram-positive, facultative anaerobic cocci that are morphologically similar to streptococci on gram strain (1, 2). The normal habitat of these microorganisms is the gastrointestinal tract of human and other mammals, although they can be isolated from the oropharynx, female genital tract, and skin. Most recently, 36 species of enterococci have been described; however, 26 have been associated with human infection (2–4). *Enterococcus faecalis* is the most common human pathogen, but *Enterococcus faecium* has become increasingly prevalent in hospital-acquired infections. All the other enterococcal species together constitute less than 5% of enterococcal infections (2–4). These other species associated with human infections include *Enterococcus gallinarum*, *Enterococcus casseliflavus*, *Enterococcus avium*, *Enterococcus cecorum*, *Enterococcus durans*, *Enterococcus hirae*, *Enterococcus malodoratus*, *Enterococcus mundtii*, *Enterococcus pseudoavium*, and *Enterococcus raffinosus* (2–11).

1.2 Epidemiology

Enterococci are generally not as virulent as other Gram-positive cocci, and often occur as a component of a polymicrobial infection in debilitated hosts. Since the first description of person-to-person transmission of enterococci (12), their increasing resistance to antimicrobial agents has led to their emergence as superinfecting nosocomial pathogens in immune-compromised patients in the hospital setting (12–16). Resistance of enterococci to multiple antimicrobial agents, including vancomycin (VRE), occurs in both acute and long-term care settings. When first introduced into a facility, an outbreak of VRE infection may occur. In acute outbreaks, the VRE isolates typically represent a single clone or a limited number of clones, as identified by pulsed field gel electrophoretic analysis of bacterial DNA (14–16). The organisms are generally transmitted between patients by indirect contact on the hands of healthcare workers. After endemicity has become established, multiple clones of VRE are usually present (17–20). Patients with asymptomatic colonization of the gastrointestinal tract by VRE exceed those with clinically recognized infection by a ratio of 10:1 or greater (15). Thus, there is a potentially large reservoir of patients harboring VRE who may be a source of transmission to other patients. Unless these colonized patients are identified by appropriate surveillance procedures, they can continue to serve as reservoirs of VRE.

Risk factors for acquisition of or infection with VRE include admission to a critical care unit, severity of illness, exposure to other patients with VRE, duration of hospitalization, and exposure to antimicrobials (13–21). Vancomycin resistance is an independent risk factor for mortality in patients with enterococcal bacteremia (13, 21). Antimicrobials exposures epidemiologically linked to VRE acquisition include vancomycin, cephalosporins, quinolones, and agents with anti-anaerobic activity (12–30). Receipt of the latter group of agents leads to a marked increase in stool density of VRE, as well as persistence of VRE (30–33). It should be noted that a meta-analysis concluded that many prior studies finding an association between receipt of vancomycin and VRE suffered from a number of flaws, including selection of an inappropriate control group and failure to control for duration of hospitalization (27, 34). When these factors were taken into account, the association between VRE acquisition and antecedent vancomycin exposure was not statistically significant in some analyses.

Evidence is clear that with the consumption of antimicrobial agents that lack activity *in vitro* to enterococci administered to humans and food animals, there is an association with an increase in antimicrobial resistance. Evidence

M.J. Zervos (✉)
Wayne State University School of Medicine, Division Head,
Infectious Diseases, Henry Ford Health System, Detroit, MI, USA,
mzervos1@hfhs.org

D.L. Mayers (ed.), *Antimicrobial Drug Resistance*,
DOI 10.1007/978-1-60327-595-8_49, © Humana Press, a part of Springer Science+Business Media, LLC 2009

suggests a relationship between streptogramin, aminoglycoside, and glycopeptide resistance genes between humans and animals (35–38). Recent studies have also shown evidence for not only transmission of strains of resistant bacteria from animals to humans, but also transfer of genetic elements. The degree of risk to humans related to the administration of antimicrobial agents to animals remains very controversial (38).

1.3 Clinical Manifestations

Urinary tract infections and bacteremia are among the most common manifestations of enterococcal infection. Endocarditis is the most serious infection caused by enterococci, although it consists of only about 3% of enterococcal bacteremias (1). Enterococci are also commonly found in intraabdominal, pelvic, wound, and soft tissue infections, but in these cases they are often part of a mixed infection due to aerobic and anaerobic bacteria. Much less common are enterococcal meningitis, osteomyelitis, and septic arthritis.

1.4 Laboratory Diagnosis

Enterococci are Gram-positive cocci in pairs and short chains. On blood agar plates, they appear as grey colonies and are usually alpha-hemolytic. A quick biochemical test can rapidly identify colonies of enterococci within minutes, based on the ability of almost all enterococcal species to hydrolyze pyrrolidonyl-beta-naphthylamide (PYR). As all enterococci produce leucine aminopeptidase, this test is used on some rapid streptococcal identification panels. Other older tests that are used less frequently include the bile-esculin test, growth on broth containing 6.5% NaCl, and ability to grow at both 10°C and 45°C. For identification of newer species of enterococci, a combination of conventional biochemical tests and evaluation of DNA content is needed.

1.5 Pathogenesis

Enterococci are less virulent than many other bacteria that cause infections in humans. Some E. faecalis factors – such as cytolysin ("hemolysin"), aggregation substance, gelatinase, serine protease, enterococcal surface protein, Ace protein, and enterococcal polysaccharide antigen – have been associated with virulence in vitro and in animal models (39, 40). The pathogenic role of these factors in human infections has not been established.

2 Susceptibility In Vitro and In Vivo

Enterococci are resistant to many antibimicrobial agents that are active against Gram-positive cocci, including cephalosporins, macrolides, and clindamycin. Agents with varying degrees of in vitro activity against enterococci include the penicillins (especially penicillin, ampicillin, and piperacillin), glycopeptides (vancomycin and teicoplanin), carbapenems (imipenem and meropenem), aminoglycosides, tetracyclines (tetracycline and doxycycline), quinolones (including ciprofloxacin, moxifloxacin, and gatifloxacin), chloramphenicol, and rifampin. The streptogramin combination quinupristin/dalfopristin, glycolipopeptides (daptomycin), glycylcycline, tigecycline, and oxazolidinone (linezolid) are active in vitro versus most strains. The penicillins and the glycopeptides have the best activity, and ampicillin typically has greater in vitro killing ability than vancomycin (41, 42). Enterococci have intrinsic low-level resistance to the aminoglycosides due to the decreased ability of these agents to penetrate the cell wall, but this can be overcome by the addition of cell wall-active agents (such as the penicillins and glycopeptides) that result in synergistic killing of the organisms (42).

2.1 Aminoglycoside Resistance in Enterococci

High-level gentamicin resistance (MICs >500–2,000 mg/mL) in enterococci is usually due to the presence of the "bifunctional" aminoglycoside-modifying enzyme encoded by the aac(6′)-Ie-aph(2″)-Ia gene (43–45). This enzyme modifies the aminoglycoside and eliminates synergism between a cell wall-active agent (such as ampicillin or vancomycin) and gentamicin, plus essentially all clinically available aminoglycosides except streptomycin. High-level streptomycin resistance can be caused by a gene that encodes the streptomycin-modifying enzyme ANT(6′)-Ia or by a change in the ribosome binding site, and also eliminates synergism with the cell wall-active agents (46–48). Nosocomial isolates that possess genes for high-level resistance to both gentamicin and streptomycin are not uncommon (3, 49–51). Although high-level aminoglycoside resistance is synonymous with resistance to synergism, there are rare enterococci with gentamicin MICs <500 μg/mL that are also resistant to the synergistic effect of a cell wall-active agent plus gentamicin. Moellering and colleagues have detected several E. faecalis with gentamicin MICs of only 8 μg/mL that are resistant to ampicillin–gentamicin synergism, but susceptible to ampicillin–tobramycin synergism (52). Hayden and colleagues have reported five E. faecium with gentamicin MICs between 4 and 32 μg/mL that are resistant to ampicillin–gentamicin synergism (53). The mechanisms of these resistance phenotypes have not yet been determined. A new gentamicin resistance gene, aph(2″)-Ic, has been found in *E. faecalis*, *E. faecium*, and *E. gallinarum* isolates (54, 55). This gene compromises ampicillin–gentamicin synergism but typically confers a gentamicin MIC of only 256 μg/mL. If these three enterococcal phenotypes become more prevalent, synergy testing of a cell wall-active agent combined with gentamicin may be indicated in selected clinical situations, such as enterococcal endocarditis or meningitis, to confirm the efficacy of the antimicrobial combination utilized for therapy.

Until now, only gentamicin and streptomycin have been used for high-level aminoglycoside testing in enterococci, as the aac(6′)-Ie-aph(2″)-Ia gene confers high-level resistance to essentially all the clinically available aminoglycosides (including gentamicin, amikacin, tobramycin, netilmicin, and kanamycin) except streptomycin. A second gene, aph(2″)-Id, that confers high-level gentamicin resistance has been detected (56). This gene also confers resistance to tobramycin, netilmicin, and kanamycin, but not to amikacin. Studies performed on the *E. casseliflavus* from which the gene was isolated showed synergistic killing with the combination of ampicillin and amikacin (56). However, ampicillin plus amikacin did not achieve as much killing against several *E. faecium* isolates that possess the aph(2″)-Id gene (56). Therefore, only a small percentage of enterococcal isolates with high-level gentamicin resistance might be susceptible to the combination of a cell wall-active agent plus amikacin.

2.2 Penicillin Resistance

High-level penicillin resistance in enterococci is due predominantly to overexpression of penicillin-binding protein 5 (PBP 5), which has low affinity for the penicillins, but is able to substitute for the functions of the susceptible penicillin-binding proteins when they are inhibited by the beta-lactam agents (57–63). For an *E. faecium* strain resistant to penicillin (MIC = 200 μg/mL) but susceptible to gentamicin, no *in vitro* synergistic bactericidal activity was observed when penicillin was combined with gentamicin, and the combination did not significantly lower bacterial counts in vegetations in a rat endocarditis model when compared with no therapy (63). However, Torres and colleagues have found *in vitro* synergism when high levels of penicillin are combined with gentamicin against some *E. faecium* isolates with high-level penicillin resistance (MIC > 128 μg/mL), but low-level gentamicin resistance. Synergism was exhibited in nine of twelve strains (penicillin MIC = 200 μg/mL) when penicillin at 100 μg/mL was combined with gentamicin (5 μg/mL) (64). In addition, synergism was seen in all three strains for

which the penicillin MIC was 400 μg/mL when penicillin at 200 μg/mL was combined with gentamicin at 5 μg/mL (64).

2.3 Glycopeptide Resistance

Glycopeptide resistance in enterococci is due to the synthesis of modified peptidoglycan precursors that have decreased affinity for vancomycin and teicoplanin (65, 66). Most glycopeptide-resistant clinical isolates are of the VanA or VanB phenotype, although VanA to VanG phenotypes have been described. Strains with the VanA phenotype have high level resistance to both vancomycin (MICs = 64 to >1,024 μg/mL) and teicoplanin (MICs = 16–512 μg/mL), while strains with the VanB phenotype have varying levels of resistance to vancomycin (MICs = 4–1,024 μg/mL), but are susceptible to teicoplanin (65, 66). Heteroresistance to vancomycin has also been identified (67). *E. gallinarum*, *E. casseliflavus*, and *E. flavescens* strains are intrinsically resistant to vancomycin (MICs = 4–32 μg/mL), but remain susceptible to teicoplanin, and are of the VanC phenotype (66, 68, 69). Teicoplanin appears to be effective therapy against some enterococcal strains lacking glycopeptide resistance determinants. In a rat endocarditis model, teicoplanin was actually more efficacious than vancomycin against a beta-lactamase-producing strain with high-level gentamicin resistance (70). Teicoplanin's efficacy for the treatment of VanB-type VRE is not as promising. Teicoplanin plus gentamicin produced *in vitro* bactericidal synergism against an *E. faecalis* resistant to vancomycin, but susceptible to teicoplanin and gentamicin (71). However, teicoplanin resistance can be selected for *in vitro* with both *E. faecalis* and *E. faecium* strains (72), and teicoplanin-resistant *E. faecalis* mutants have arisen during teicoplanin therapy in a rabbit endocarditis model (72). The *in vivo* emergence of resistance to teicoplanin during vancomycin therapy for *E. faecium* (VanB phenotype) bacteremia has also been observed (72).

3 Antimicrobial Therapy

As the human reservoir is the gastrointestinal tract, polymicrobial infections involving the gastrointestinal tract, urinary tract, and female genital tract are the primary infections. Infections of the urinary tract, soft tissue, and intraabdominal infections, and perhaps some cases of septic arthritis, can be treated with a single antimicrobial agent, especially in patients with normal host defenses (1, 73, 74). For bacteremia (without endocarditis), combination antibiotic therapy is often used, but studies are not definitive. Some studies suggest that enterococcal bacteremia without endocarditis can be treated with a single agent (6, 75, 76), although the sources of bacteremia were not considered, which may be an important factor in determining outcome (77). Other studies suggest that for serious infections such as bacteremia, combination therapy may be more effective than monotherapy therapy (1, 73, 78). In one prospective, observational study of 110 serious enterococcal infections, 71% of patients who received appropriate combination therapy (cell wall-active agent + aminoglycoside) achieved clinical cure, compared to 53% of patients who received an active single agent only ($p = 0.08$) (79).

For monotherapy in patients without penicillin allergy, the drug of choice is ampicillin (MIC usually two- to fourfold lower than penicillin). Beta-lactamase-producing enterococci were a concern, as they are resistant to ampicillin but are not detected by routine ampicillin susceptibility testing (80–83). However, it appears now that they are rare, and many hospitals that have screened for beta-lactamase production in enterococci for several years have not found any (3). If isolated, they can be treated with ampicillin/sulbactam. If the organism is resistant to ampicillin, a glycopeptide such as vancomycin may be used for monotherapy. Imipenem offers no advantage over ampicillin against (beta-lactamase negative) enterococci *in vitro*, nor in animal endocarditis models (84–86). *E. faecalis* isolates that are susceptible to ampicillin (MIC = 0.5–1.0 μg/mL) but relatively resistant to imipenem (MIC > 8.0 μg/mL) have been identified, but are rare. However, in situations such as empiric therapy for complex intraabdominal infections, where coverage that includes enterococci may be prudent, imipenem (or piperacillin/tazobactam or ampicillin/sulbactam) might be substituted for regimens that contain ampicillin. A summary of treatment recommendations for enterococcal infection due to strains susceptible *in vitro* to glycopeptides is shown in Table 1.

3.1 Urinary Tract Infections

Urinary tract infections are the most common infection caused by enterococci, and are often associated with urinary catheters. Enterococcal urinary tract infections that are not accompanied by bacteremia generally require only single-drug therapy. If the organism is susceptible, ampicillin is the drug of choice. Vancomycin can be used if the organism is ampicillin-resistant. Linezolid or quinupristin/dalfopristin are reasonable alternatives if the enterococcus is resistant to both ampicillin and vancomycin.

For simple urinary tract infections, a quinolone with a low MIC for a particular isolate might be considered as an alternative, but caution must be exerted, as enterococcal superinfections have occurred in patients treated with ciprofloxacin for infections caused by other bacteria (87, 88). Complicated urinary tract infections such as prostatitis and pyelonephritis are less common. They can be treated with the same agents used for simple urinary tract infections, but the duration of therapy would be longer. A seriously ill patient with pyelonephritis or perinephric abscess may benefit from combination therapy with a beta-lactam agent plus an aminoglycoside. Nitrofurantoin and fosfomycin exhibit excellent activity *in vitro* versus urinary enterococcal isolates, including VRE strains (89, 90). Oral rifampin plus nitrofurantoin has cured a case of chronic prostatitis due to vancomycin-resistant *E. faecium* (90).

3.2 Intraabdominal Infections

The therapeutic recommendations outlined in this chapter are predominantly based on studies of *E. faecium* and *E. faecalis*. Optimal antimicrobial therapy for *E. gallinarum*, *E. casseliflavus*, *E. avium*, *E. cecorum*, *E. durans*, *E. hirae*, *E. malodoratus*, *E. mundtii*, *E. pseudoavium*, and *E. raffinosus* is not known. However, based on *in vitro* data and anecdotal reports, it would seem reasonable to suggest that therapy for these enterococcal species is the same as that for *E. faecium* and *E. faecalis*.

Intraabdominal infections are polymicrobial in origin, in which coverage for enteric bacteria (*E. coli*, *Klebsiella pneumonia*, etc.) and anaerobes (*Bacteroides fragilis*), including Enterococcus species, must be covered. Broad-spectrum

Table 1 Antimicrobial therapy for *Enterococcus faecalis* susceptible to glycopeptides

Infection	Antibiotic(s) primary:alternative	Comments
Urinary tract infection	Ampicillin: Vancomycin, Nitrofurantoin, Fosfomycin	Nitrofurantoin only for (cystitis) with isolates susceptible, not in sepsis or renal failure; usual duration 7–10 d
Intraabdominal infection	Ampicillin: Beta-lactamase inhibitors, Vancomycin	Not essential to treat for Enterococcus in all intraabdominal infection, unless organisms cultured, patient severely ill; duration 10–14 d
Endocarditis	Ampicillin or Penicillin plus Gentamicin: Streptomycin, Vancomycin (Penicillin allergy)	To be used in combination for the treatment of enterococcal endocarditis caused by organisms susceptible *in vitro* to either agent; streptomycin is used when gentamicin cannot be used because of high-level resistance. Ampicillin plus gentamicin for 4–6 weeks is treatment of choice for endocarditis
Intravenous catheter bacteremia	Ampicillin: Vancomycin	Duration 10–14 d, some patients (single positive blood culture) will respond to removal of the line alone

See Table 2 for drug dosages

therapy for the gastrointestinal flora mentioned above include ampicillin/sulbactam, piperacillin/tazobactam, and imipenem. A case-control study has suggested that empiric therapy for enterococci should be especially considered for hepatobiliary or pancreatic infection, where both the prevalence of entero-cocci and the rate of enterococcal bacteremia are high (91).

3.3 Endocarditis

The necessity for combination antibiotic therapy is well established for enterococcal endocarditis. Improved outcome has been demonstrated in patients who received a synergistic combination of a cell wall-active agent plus an aminoglyco-side, compared to patients who received monotherapy (1, 73, 92–97). Cell wall-active antimicrobial agents such as the penicillins and glycopeptides, when combined with amino-glycosides, produce a synergistic bactericidal effect against susceptible strains of enterococci due to the enhanced intra-cellular penetration and the use of the aminoglycoside in the presence of the cell wall-active agent (98). Penicillin (or ampicillin) plus gentamicin is the most commonly used com-bination for enterococcal endocarditis, although penicillin plus streptomycin has been the most studied combination regimen for enterococcal endocarditis. No direct compara-tive studies of efficacy between penicillin (or ampicillin) plus streptomycin versus penicillin plus gentamicin have been done, although streptomycin may be more effective than gentamicin in treatment of enterococcal endocarditis (99). In a study of streptomycin-resistant enterococcal endo-carditis, 16 of 20 (80%) patients treated with penicillin plus gentamicin were cured, compared with a cure in 33 of 36 (92%) patients treated with penicillin plus streptomycin for streptomycin-susceptible enterococci in the same study (99). This higher relapse rate in patients treated with penicillin plus gentamicin was also higher than the relapse rate among patients treated with penicillin plus streptomycin in previous studies (95, 96, 100). Streptomycin has traditionally been given intramuscularly, which involves greater pain for the patient, although intravenous streptomycin has been given to a few patients and seemed to be well-tolerated (101). Streptomycin is predominantly ototoxic, and gentamicin is primarily nephrotoxic; while nephrotoxicity is often revers-ible, ototoxicity is often not (97). Moreover, gentamicin serum levels are more readily available to aid in monitoring for potential toxicity, and gentamicin is less expensive than streptomycin. A sufficient number of patients have been treated successfully with penicillin (or ampicillin) plus gen-tamicin for this to be a well-accepted regimen (73, 96, 97, 102). For these reasons, gentamicin has replaced streptomy-cin as the more commonly used aminoglycoside in combina-tion regimens for enterococcal endocarditis.

The recommended streptomycin dosage in enterococcal endocarditis is 7.5 µg/kg IM every 12 h, with target peak serum levels of 15–30 µg/mL (96, 97). Gentamicin is usually given at 1 µg/kg IV every 8 h, with target peak serum levels of >3 µg/mL (96, 97). Treatment should continue for at least 4 weeks. Patients with symptoms for longer than 3 months duration before initiation of appropriate therapy and patients with prosthetic valve endocarditis should receive antimicro-bial therapy for at least 6 weeks (99, 102). Animal data do not support the use of once-daily dosing of aminoglycosides in enterococcal endocarditis (103, 104). However, one patient with E. faecalis pulmonic and tricuspid endocarditis was treated successfully with ampicillin and once-daily gentami-cin (105). The combination of vancomycin plus an amino glycoside has not been as extensively studied, so vancomycin should be used only when the patient has a significant history of allergy to the penicillins (97). The addition of ciprofloxa-cin to a regimen of ampicillin plus gentamicin was associ-ated with cure in a case of relapsing E. faecalis endocarditis (106, 107). In selected patients, a shortened course of amino-glycosides may be considered. A 5-year nationwide prospec-tive study in Sweden during 1995–1999 identified 881 definite episodes of infective endocarditis (108). Definite enterococcal endocarditis was diagnosed in 93 episodes (11%), the largest series of enterococcal endocarditis so far presented. Mortality during treatment was 16%, the relapse rate was 3%, and clinical cure was achieved in the remaining 81% of the episodes. Clinical cure was achieved with a median duration of cell wall-active antimicrobial therapy of 42 days combined with an aminoglycoside (median treat-ment time, 15 days). International guidelines generally rec-ommend a 4–6-week combined synergistic treatment course with a cell wall-active antibiotic and an aminoglycoside. Treatment regimens in Sweden often include a shortened aminoglycoside treatment course, to minimize adverse effects in older patients. In this study, fatal outcome seemed not to be due to the shortened aminoglycoside therapy course. In some enterococcal endocarditis episodes, shortening the duration of aminoglycoside therapy to 2–3 weeks requires further study.

Endocarditis due to vancomycin-resistant enterococcus is rare. The literature consists of limited experimental endocarditis data or single case reports, with most patients having serious underlying disease, including transplanta-tion, dialysis, and healthcare-associated infection (94, 97, 109–127). Most patients survived despite the lack of bacte-ricidal therapy and valve replacement. The optimal therapy for this infection remains undefined, as comparative data are not available; patients were treated with various and multiple agents, in combination and sequentially, over vary-ing periods of time. Bacteremia in the absence of endo-carditis without an identifiable focus is generally related to an indwelling venous catheter when it occurs in the hospital setting (128). Usually, removal of the line is sufficient for resolution.

3.4 Meningitis

Enterococcal meningitis is rare (129–136). Most experts would concur that treatment of enterococcal meningitis requires combination therapy, so that maximal bactericidal activity may be achieved (1, 73, 129). However, in contrast to endocarditis, there are scant clinical data available to state unequivocally that combination therapy is superior to monotherapy in meningitis. In a review of enterococcal meningitis, 30 of 32 cases had data on antibiotic therapy (130). The majority of patients (20 of 30) received penicillin or ampicillin plus an aminoglycoside (three patients also received intrathecal gentamicin); there was only one death in this group, compared with one death in the group of four patients who received penicillin or ampicillin alone. One patient failed his initial regimen of ampicillin plus chloramphenicol, but recovered when the chloramphenicol was replaced by gentamicin. One severely ill patient received chloramphenicol plus gentamicin, and subsequently died (130). Ciprofloxacin has been reported to cure one case of E. faecalis meningitis in an infant (131). The combination of quinupristin/dalfopristin plus chloramphenicol cured a case of neonatal E. faecium meningitis that had failed therapy with teicoplanin plus chloramphenicol (132). A child with E. faecium meningitis was treated successfully with chloramphenicol (10). Intrathecal teicoplanin has been used successfully to treat a case of E faecium meningitis (133). Intraventricular plus intravenous quinipristin/dalfopristin plus intravenous chloramphenicol sterilized the CSF of a patient with vancomycin-resistant E. faecium shunt infection, who had failed therapy with chloramphenicol alone (134). Linezolid used alone for 28 days cured vancomycin-resistant E. faecium meningitis in a patient who had failed therapy with chloramphenicol (135). Linezolid used for 3 weeks plus gentamicin for 5 days sterilized the CSF of a second patient with vancomycin-resistant enterococcal meningitis (136).

3.5 Therapy for Strains Resistant to Aminoglycosides

Treatment of patients with endocarditis caused by enterococci with high-level resistance to aminoglycosides is associated with a high incidence of failure or relapse (137). Therapy for strains resistant to all aminoglycosides is usually limited to the use of ampicillin alone. Vancomycin alone is potentially less efficacious. The optimal duration of therapy with ampicillin alone is not known, but the observation that valve cultures at surgery are positive after as much as 1 month of ampicillin therapy suggests that longer courses than the traditional 4–6 weeks, such as 8–12 weeks, should be strongly considered (92, 97, 138). Continuous, rather than intermittent, infusion of ampicillin may prove beneficial, as there are data showing its greater efficacy in sterilizing cardiac vegetations and improving survival in a rat endocarditis model (139). Cardiac valve replacement may well be required for a cure in many of these patients (92, 97, 102, 137). A patient with ampicillin- and vancomycin-susceptible but gentamicin- and streptomycin-resistant E. faecalis endocarditis was initially treated with ampicillin (4 g IV q6h) plus vancomycin. Both peak and trough serum bactericidal titers were 1:2. After imipenem was added (500 mg IV q6h), the peak and trough serum bactericidal titers increased to 1:128 and 1:64, respectively. A total of 6 weeks of antibiotics was given and the patient was cured (140). The authors suggest that the increased serum bactericidal activity seen after the addition of imipenem may be due to the saturation of different penicillin-binding proteins (140). The same regimen of ampicillin plus vancomycin plus imipenem was used successfully in treating a case of gentamicin-resistant enterococcal bacteremia without endocarditis (141).

3.6 Therapy for Strains Resistant to Penicillins and Glycopeptides, but Susceptible to Aminoglycosides

If the cell wall-active agents (penicillins and glycopeptides) are inactive against some enterococci, the antibiotic combinations of cell wall-active agents plus aminoglycosides will no longer be synergistic. Given the in vitro resistance for certain enterococcal strains discussed previously, synergism may be limited chiefly by the achievable penicillin serum concentration. As 5 million units of penicillin G infused intravenously can achieve a peak serum concentration of $135 \mu g/mL$, the authors conclude that some gentamicin-susceptible E. faecium strains with penicillin MICs between 50 and $200 \mu g/mL$ may be treated with high-dose penicillin plus gentamicin (64).

These findings for penicillin have been assumed to be true for ampicillin as well, because the two agents' mechanism of action is the same. As peak ampicillin serum levels from 109 to $150 \mu g/mL$ can be attained after a 2-g intravenous dose (142, 143), some enterococci with an ampicillin MIC up to 64 or even $128 \mu g/mL$ may prove to be susceptible to ampicillin–gentamicin synergism if high-dose ampicillin is used. A hemodialysis patient with ampicillin-resistant (MIC = $32 \mu g/mL$) and gentamicin-resistant (MIC = $1,000 \mu g/mL$) E. faecium bacteremia was treated successfully with ampicillin 2 g IV q6h and streptomycin (MIC = 32 µg/mL) 500 mg twice weekly, after failing therapy with doxycycline plus chloramphenicol (144). A patient with vancomycin-resistant *E. faecium* endocarditis had persistent bacteremia during therapy with 12 g of ampicillin (MIC = 64 µg/mL) per day plus gentamicin, and subsequently with quinupristin/dalfopristin. Blood cultures finally became sterile when therapy was changed to ampicillin 20 g per day plus gentamicin (144).

A patient with ampicillin-resistant (MIC = 64 µg/mL) *E. faecium* bacteremia failed therapy with continuous infusion ampicillin (20 g/day) plus gentamicin (MIC < 500 µg/mL) q12h, but was cured with continuous infusion ampicillin/sulbactam (20 g ampicillin/10 g sulbactam) plus gentamicin q12h (145). No bactericidal effect was seen when the patient was on ampicillin plus gentamicin (serum ampicillin concentration of 103 mg/mL), but a serum bactericidal titer of 1:2 was detected when the patient was on ampicillin/sulbactam plus gentamicin (serum ampicillin concentration of 130 mg/mL). It is possible that sulbactam may slightly enhance the activity of ampicillin against certain strains of enterococci via an unknown mechanism (145). In an open trial of teicoplanin therapy for enterococcal endocarditis, 5 of 7 patients treated with teicoplanin alone and 6 of 7 patients treated with teicoplanin plus an aminoglycoside were cured (146). In a study of teicoplanin therapy for endocarditis caused by Gram-positive bacteria, five patients with *E. faecalis* endocarditis were treated with teicoplanin alone, and all five were cured (147).

3.7 Therapy for Strains Resistant to Penicillins, Glycopeptides, and Aminoglycosides

The terms "VRE" and "VREF" are commonly used to describe these multiply resistant strains, which, to date, have been predominantly *E. faecium* (148). The optimal therapy for these infections is unsettled, and antibiotic selection is most problematic for these strains (Table 2). Currently, linezolid is approved for the treatment of VRE and is the drug of choice. Based on *in vitro* susceptibility results and anecdotal reports, daptomycin and quinupristin–dalfopristin also warrant consideration.

Various other bacteriostatic antimicrobials with less *in vitro* activity than the penicillins, glycopeptides, and aminoglycosides have been tried, either alone or in combination, against multiresistant enterococci. Oral rifampin plus nitrofurantoin has cured a case of chronic prostatitis due to vancomycin-resistant *E. faecium* (90). In one study, chloramphenicol therapy for multiresistant enterococci in 16 severely ill patients showed somewhat encouraging results (149). Of the 14 patients in whom a clinical response could be determined, 8 showed improvement; 4 patients were treated with rifampin in addition to chloramphenicol; most patients received other antibiotics that alone do not have activity against enterococci. Of the 16 patients, 11 had a drainage procedure or debridement performed. In a study of *E. faecium* infections in liver transplant recipients, chloramphenicol was

Table 2 Antimicrobial therapy for vancomycin-resistant enterococci (VRE)

Antibiotic(s)	Dose, duration	Comments
Primary		
Ampicillin	12 g/d IV	For rare ampicillin-susceptible isolates of *Enterococcus faecium*; vancomycin-resistant *E. faecalis* are usually susceptible
Gentamicin or Streptomycin	1 g/kg 8 h to achieve serum peaks of 3–4 µg/mL and trough <1 µg/mL for endocarditis, treat for at least 4–6 weeks	To be used in combination with ampicillin for the treatment of enterococcal endocarditis caused by organisms susceptible *in vitro* to either agent; streptomycin is used when gentamicin cannot be used because of resistance
Linezolid	600 mg PO or IV q 12 h	For linezolid-susceptible isolates of *E faecium* and *E faecalis*. An agent of choice for serious enterococcal VREF infections
Daptomycin	Use dose of 6 mg/kg/24 h for serious enterococcal infection; 6–8 weeks for endocarditis	Not approved for treatment of VRE infection. Not approved for treatment of endocarditis. Limited clinical information for VREF, but bactericidal activity makes therapy with this is agent a consideration for serious infections
Alternative		
Doxycycline	100 mg PO or IV q 12 h	Not a first-line therapy. For susceptible isolates, not bacteremia or endocarditis
Nitrofurantoin	100 mg PO Q 6 h	For urinary tract infections (cystitis) with isolates susceptible to nitrofurantoin; not indicated in renal failure
Fosfomycin	3 g X1	For urinary tract infections (cystitis) with isolates susceptible to fosfomycin
Chloramphenicol	50 mg/kg/d IV (in q 6 h divided doses)	For chloramphenicol-susceptible isolates of *E. faecium* and *E. faecalis*. Not a first-line therapy
Tigecycline	100 mg IV then 50 mg IV q 12 h	Not indicated for VRE, approved in US for skin soft tissue infection, excellent *in vitro* activity vs. VRE
Quinupristin/ dalfopristin	7.5 mg/kg Q8 h IV	For susceptible isolates of *E. faecium* only

used as monotherapy in 16 cases, and 6 patients died (150). Single cases of successful therapy using chloramphenicol alone or in combination with vancomycin or rifampin have also been reported (10, 79, 151). In another study of vancomycin-resistant Enterococcus bacteremia treated with chloramphenicol, 22 of 36 patients demonstrated a clinical response, and 34 of 43 patients showed a microbiological response (152). However, no significant effect on mortality by chloramphenicol usage could be demonstrated (152). Lynch and colleagues studied four strains of E. faecalis and one strain of E. faecium and demonstrated efflux of chloramphenicol in all the strains (153). Their results suggest that many wild-type strains of E. faecalis, and presumably also of E. faecium, possess endogenous efflux pumps that excrete chloramphenicol (153). Therefore, chloramphenicol use probably should be limited to those cases where no other agents are likely to be effective.

Intravenous doxycycline used alone for 2 weeks in a patient with catheter-related sepsis and probable endocarditis resulted in clearing of the bacteremia, but the patient subsequently died of congestive heart failure (151). Oral doxycycline for 2 weeks, plus removal of the Hickman catheter presumed to be the source of the bacteremia, was successful in treating a case of E. faecium bacteremia (154). An immunocompromised patient with vancomycin- and ampicillin-resistant E. faecium bacteremia who appeared to fail therapy with quinupristin/dalfopristin plus gentamicin was cured with five days of intravenous tetracycline, followed by 2 months of oral doxycycline, with occasional periods of intravenous tetracycline when he could not tolerate oral therapy (155).

The streptogramin combination quinupristin/dalfopristin has been used for treatment of E. faecium, but not E. faecalis, which are intrinsically resistant to the combination. Among 15 cases of multiresistant E. faecium infection treated with quinupristin/dalfopristin, 3 patients were cured of their infection, 5 had recurrence of the infection, and the outcome was indeterminate in 7 cases (156). Blood cultures became negative for enterococcus during treatment in all patients with bacteremia. However, catheters were removed in the patients with catheter-related bacteremia prior to therapy, so it is not known whether removal of catheters alone would have been curative (156). Vancomycin-resistant E. faecium-associated mortality was significantly lower in a group of 20 patients with vancomycin-resistant E. faecium bacteremia treated with quinupristin/dalfopristin, compared with an historical cohort of 42 patients with vancomycin-resistant E. faecium bacteremia treated with other agents (157). In another study, bacteriologic eradication occurred in 17 of 23 evaluable patients with serious E. faecium infections treated with quinupristin/dalfopristin (158). In a multicenter study of quinupristin/dalfopristin for vancomycin-resistant E. faecium infections, clinical success was achieved in 73.6% (142 of 193) of evaluable patients, and the bacteriological success rate was 70.5% (110 of 156),

resulting in an overall success rate of 65.4% (102 of 156) (159). Successful treatment with quinupristin/dalfopristin for E. faecium vertebral osteomyelitis, peritonitis, ventriculitis, aortic graft infection, and endocarditis has also been reported (127, 132, 156–164). Quinupristin/dalfopristin has also been used successfully in treating pediatric patients (160). As quinupristin/dalfopristin is not bactericidal against E. faecium, combining other agents with quinupristin/dalfopristin may be a reasonable approach in selected cases. A case of vancomycin-resistant E. faecium endocarditis, with persistently positive blood cultures after 2 weeks of therapy with quinupristin/dalfopristin, was cured after intravenous doxycycline and oral rifampin were added to the quinupristin/dalfopristin and therapy continued for 8 more weeks (165). As E. faecium strains resistant to quinupristin/dalfopristin can be selected in vitro without difficulty (166, 167), it is not surprising that emergence of increased resistance to quinupristin/dalfopristin has appeared during therapy for E. faecium infections (158, 159, 167–169). Resistance development to quinupristin/dalfopristin in vitro can be diminished with the addition of doxycycline (167). Superinfection with E. faecalis has occurred during quinupristin/dalfopristin therapy for E. faecium infections (158, 159, 170). The agent is only available by intravenous infusion. Myalgias in 6.6% of patients, arthralgias in 9.1%, and reports of antimicrobial resistance have been limiting features (160).

The oxazolidinones are a new class of antimicrobials that inhibit bacterial protein synthesis (171–173). Linezolid is a semisynthetic oxazolidinone agent that exhibits bacteriostatic in vitro and in vivo activity against enterococci (174–180). Although linezolid has in vitro activity against vancomycin-resistant E. faecalis, it has only received approval for vancomycin-resistant E. faecium infections because of the lack of patients with E. faecalis isolates in the phase III trials. In one case report, a neutropenic patient with ampicillin- and vancomycin-resistant E. faecium bacteremia was treated successfully with 14 days of linezolid (600 mg IV q12h) plus gentamicin. Time-kill studies with linezolid plus gentamicin did not show in vitro synergism (181). In another case report, a patient with acute myelogenous leukemia developed vancomycin-resistant E. faecium bacteremia after bone marrow transplantation. Blood cultures were persistently positive during 10 weeks of therapy with quinupristin/dalfopristin, despite the addition of chloramphenicol and doxycycline at various times (182). The source of the E. faecium bacteremia was deemed to be an extensive central venous thrombus. The E. faecium remained susceptible in vitro to quinupristin/dalfopristin during therapy. Antimicrobial therapy was changed to intravenous linezolid alone, and blood cultures became negative 8 days later, and all subsequent blood cultures were negative. The patient received 6 weeks of intravenous linezolid, followed by 6 weeks of oral linezolid, and had no further complications (182). In an open-label, non-comparative, non-randomized compassionate-use program for linezolid, in which 66% of 826 treatment courses were prescribed for the treatment of VRE, the clinical and microbiological cure rates were 81% and 86%, respectively (183). Sites of infection included the bloodstream, the intraabdominal region, complicated skin and soft tissue, the urinary tract, and bone.

In the largest case series published to date, 15 patients infected with vancomycin-resistant *E. faecium* were treated with linezolid after all other available therapeutic options had been tried (126). The median duration of therapy was 20.5 (+ 3.5) days. Microbiologic cure was achieved in all ten patients who survived and completed therapy, including a patient with infective endocarditis, who was treated for 42 days. All seven patients alive at long-term follow-up were free of infection. No deaths were attributable to the index infection (126). Linezolid use has been reported in immunosuppressed patients. In a prospective randomized study comparing quinupristin–dalfopristin with linezolid in 40 cancer patients infected with VREF, comparable clinical efficacy was seen (184). Clinical response was seen in 58% of patients treated with linezolid versus 43% treated with quinupristin–dalfopristin (184). Out of six liver recipients with sepsis secondary to intraabdominal VRE infection, five were cured at end of treatment, although a sixth patient relapsed with a linezolid-resistant *E. faecium* strain (185). Although no comparative trials of linezolid have been carried out in patients with endocarditis, osteomyelitis, or meningitis, multiple case reports have been described. Oral linezolid was successful in treating a case of vancomycin-resistant *E. faecium* endocarditis that failed sequential monotherapy with chloramphenicol and quinupristin/dalfopristin (110). Oral linezolid was successful in treating a case of vancomycin-resistant *E. faecium* endocarditis in a renal transplant recipient with HIV infection (111). Linezolid was also reported to be successful in treating cases of *E. faecalis* prosthetic valve endocarditis, with (186) and without (126) high-level gentamicin-resistance. Failure of therapy for endocarditis with linezolid was noted in another report (187). Intravenous linezolid was successful in treating a patient with MRSA and VRE bacteremias secondary to vertebral osteomyelitis, who failed therapy with intravenous vancomycin and oral amoxicillin and fusidic acid (188). Oral linezolid was reported to be successful in treating cases of *E. faecalis* (189) and *E. faecium* osteomyelitis (190). Although only bacteriostatic, there have been several case reports of successful treatment with linezolid in patients with VREF meningitis, including patients in the postoperative period, persons with infections associated with a device, and patients with infections in the setting of hyperinfection with *Strongyloides stercoralis* (135, 136, 191). The emergence of linezolid resistance during therapy is uncommon (192–196). Resistant mutants can be generated at a low frequency, having mutations involving the domain V peptidyltransferase center of 23S rRNA, which is the same

mutation as in linezolid-resistant MRSA. How stable the resistance is in these isolates is uncertain. Other centers have isolated increased numbers of linezolid-resistant VRE and have noted a higher incidence of linezolid resistance (1 of 45) emerging during therapy (193). However, prior use with linezolid is not necessary before the development of resistance (194). A case of linezolid-resistant *E. faecalis* was isolated in a cord blood stem cell recipient following treatment with linezolid for VRE bacteremia (195). Three cases of linezolid-resistant *E. faecalis* were reported after prolonged treatment with linezolid for VRE. One of these patients had been diagnosed with VRE aortic and mitral valve endocarditis that was sensitive to ampicillin. The patient was treated for 6 weeks with linezolid. Two weeks following treatment, the patient was readmitted with third-degree heart block and VRE bacteremia. The patient was desensitized to penicillin and treated successfully with ampicillin (196). Given the complexity in determining optimal antimicrobial therapy for multiply resistant enterococci (VRE/VREF), consultation with an infectious diseases specialist may be prudent in these cases.

Daptomycin is a novel cyclic lipopeptide that is a fermentation product of *Streptomyces roseosporus*, with a unique mechanism of action (197–204). It acts specifically at the bacterial cytoplasmic membrane, with multiple effects on cellular function, including inhibition of lipoteichoic acid synthesis, disruption of membrane potential, and inhibition of peptidoglycan synthesis. It displays rapid concentration-dependent killing, and is bactericidal even in the stationary phase of growth. The agent is currently FDA approved in the United States for management of complicated skin and soft tissue infection bacteremia and right-sided endocarditis due to *Staphylococcus aureus*. The current recommended dosage is 4 mg/kg once daily; however, in clinical trials of serious staphylococcal and enterococcal infection, doses of 6 mg/kg/24 h were used (197, 198). *In vitro* studies of 289 isolates of *E. faecalis* demonstrated MICs < = 2 μg/mL in all isolates to daptomycin (199). A large multicenter European study with *in vitro* studies of 40 isolates of vancomycin-resistant *E. faecalis* and 114 isolates of vancomycin-resistant *E. faecium* demonstrated MICs <2 in all isolates (200). *In vitro* activity of daptomycin against enterococci from the nosocomial and community environments in Portugal were studied. Of the 1,151 isolates that were obtained, all demonstrated MICs ≤4 μg/mL (201). Similarly, 89 strains of VRE were tested *in vitro*. Daptomycin MICs were ≤2 and ≤4 mg/L for *E. faecalis* and *E. faecium*, respectively (202). *In vitro* studies have demonstrated additive or indifferent interactions with other antibiotics. Antagonism, as determined by kill-curve studies, has not been observed. Daptomycin has been reported to show synergism *in vitro* with aminoglycosides, rifampin, and beta-lactams against some VRE (203, 204). In an *in vitro* study using 20 isolates of vancomycin-susceptible *E. faecalis*, daptomycin showed synergistic activity with ceftrioxone, cefepime, and imipenem against 65%, 35%, and 35% of the isolates, respectively (204). Unfortunately, very limited clinical data exists. A phase III trial comparing linezolid to daptomycin for the treatment of VRE was terminated early due to difficulty in enrolling patients (197, 198). Daptomycin-resistant strains are very difficult to generate *in vitro* (203, 205–207). Resistance to daptomycin during therapy with the agent is rare, having been reported in three patients with enterococcal infection. The emergence of resistance to daptomycin occurred in two of more than 1,000 (<0.2%) infected subjects across the entire set of Phase 2 and 3 clinical trials (one *S. aureus* and one *E. faecalis*). A case was reported where there was emergence of daptomycin resistance (MICs > 32) in *E. faecium* during daptomycin therapy (206). Furthermore, a case of daptomycin resistance that developed during daptomycin therapy for *E. faecalis* has also been reported (207). At this time, no mechanism of resistance to daptomycin has been identified, there are no known transferable elements, and cross-resistance has not been observed with any other class of antibiotic. Daptomycin appears to be a promising drug, with good *in vitro* bactericidal activity against enterococci, regardless of vancomycin susceptibility; however, data regarding clinical outcomes is lacking.

Tigecycline is a semisynthetic glycylcycline antimicrobial agent that is similar in structure to minocycline, but with excellent *in vitro* activity versus Gram-positive bacteria, including VRE (208–210). It is a bacteriostatic agent *in vitro* versus enterococci. The agent has been recently approved in the United States for therapy of complicated skin soft tissue and intraabdominal infection. It has linear pharmacokinetics, has a C_{max} of 0.87 μg/mL, a C_{min} of 0.13 μg/mL, and AUC0–24h of 4.7 μg/h/mL, a $t_{1/2}$ of 42 h, and significant tissue uptake (211). The drug is administered by intravenous infusion only and, in initial clinical trials, had nausea that was more common than comparators (212, 213). Antimicrobial agents undergoing development include dalbavancin and oritavancin, which are both new glycopeptides, the lipoglycopeptide telavancin, and iclaprim, which is a diaminopyrimidine inhibitor of microbial dihydrofolate reductase (211–221). Dalbavancin is an investigational semisynthetic, glycopeptide antibiotic with excellent *in vitro* activity against Gram-positive bacteria. It is active *in vitro* against vancomycin-susceptible enterococci and vancomycin-resistant enterococci containing the vanB phenotype (214–217). It is structurally related to teicoplanin, and therefore will likely be of limited utility for therapy of vancomycin-resistant enterococci (214, 215). Dalbavancin has a long half-life (9–12 days); a single infusion of 1,000 mg results in mean plasma concentrations of >35 mg/L for a 7-day period (215). It is being studied in skin soft tissue and catheter bloodstream infection, with preliminary results showing clinical and bacteriologic success rates similar to comparators (215–217). The oligosac-

charide, evernimicin, and fluoroquinolone clinafloxacin exhibited good *in vitro* enterococcal activity, but did not complete clinical trials (53, 211–213). The new aminoglycoside, arbekacin, shows preliminary promise in treating some high-level gentamicin-resistant enterococci (218–220). Arbekacin is currently available only in Japan, where it is used to treat gentamicin- and methicillin-resistant *Staphylococcus aureus* infections (221).

4 Adjunctive Therapy

Although infections by VRE and VREF appear to be increasing, such organisms are not necessarily highly virulent. There may be clinical settings where the patient will recover even when no appropriate antimicrobial therapy is available. For example, catheter-related bacteremias might sometimes be treatable with catheter removal alone (75, 161). Surgical site infections, skin and soft tissue infections, and intraabdominal abscesses may be manageable by surgical debridement and drainage, and treated with antibiotics active against other gastrointestinal flora (77, 91, 161).

5 Endpoints for Monitoring Therapy

Duration of antimicrobial therapy for enterococcal infections depends predominantly on the site of infection and the patient's clinical response to therapy. Treatment for simple urinary tract infections may require only a few days of oral or intravenous antibiotics. Bacteremia without endocarditis may require 10–14 days of antibiotics, and typically depends on how quickly the patient responds to therapy. If the source of infection cannot be removed, such as central venous catheters that must remain or abscesses that cannot be drained, the duration of antimicrobial therapy may naturally be longer. As mentioned previously, endocarditis in certain clinical situations can require a minimum of 6 weeks of antibiotics.

6 Vaccines

There are no vaccines for this bacterium.

7 Infection Control

Colonized patients are the primary reservoir of VRE. Patient-to-patient transmission occurs primarily via indirect transmission by healthcare workers (222). Although colonized patients are a major reservoir for infection, decolonization of patients is not recommended, as is likely to fail (222, 223).

Medical devices, such as electronic rectal thermometers, have also been implicated (224). VRE are relatively hardy, and can persist for prolonged periods in the environment, and the immediate surroundings of a colonized patient may be heavily contaminated (225). The role of environmental contamination in transmission remains to be precisely defined. The epidemiology of vancomycin-resistant *E. faecalis* is similar to that of vancomycin-resistant *E. faecium* (226).

The Hospital Infection Control Practices Advisory Committee (HICPAC) has published "Recommendations for Preventing the Spread of Vancomycin Resistance (222)." They are summarized in Tables 3 and 4.

Key principals underlying an effective control strategy include:

1. The hospital laboratory must be able to accurately identify VRE. Automated microtitre systems may be unreliable.
2. The number of asymptomatically colonized patients exceeds the number of clinically infected patients many-fold. The former group of patients is a reservoir for spread of VRE; surveillance via stool or rectal swab cultures of patients at risk is needed to detect VRE carriage.

3. VRE infected or colonized patients must be identified and placed into appropriate isolation as rapidly as possible.
4. As most transmission occurs via healthcare workers, hospital staff must be familiar with and must follow isolation and control procedures (Table 4).
5. Contamination of the environment and of medical equipment may play a role in transmission; effective disinfection procedures are necessary.
6. VRE carriers who are re-admitted or transferred to other facilities must be quickly identified and placed into isolation.
7. Antibiotic usage should be controlled. Although current CDC recommendations stress control of vancomycin usage, the strength of the association between VRE and vancomycin is controversial (see Sect. 2.3). Reduction in the use of cephalosporins and agents with potent anaerobic activity may be beneficial.

Implementation of a multi-faceted control strategy, such as that outlined in the HICPAC recommendations, has reportedly led to a reduction in the rate of VRE transmission in several acute care facilities. In the setting of an acute out-

Table 3 Summary of recommendations for preventing the spread of vancomycin resistance (adapted from CDC-HICPAC (222))

Appropriate use of vancomycin

Treatment of infection due to B-lactam-resistant Gram-positive organisms

Treatment of infection due to Gram-positive organisms in patients with serious beta-lactam allergy

Treatment of antibiotic-associated colitis in cases of metronidazole failure or potentially life-threatening illness

Endocarditis prophylaxis, as recommended by the American Heart Association (Dajani)

Prophylaxis for surgical procedures involving implantation of a prosthesis in institutions with a high rate of infection due to MRSA or methicillin-resistant *S. epidermidis*

Education program

Include physicians, nurses, pharmacy and laboratory personnel, students, and all other direct patient care providers

Program should include information on epidemiology of VRE, and impact of VRE on cost and outcome of patient care

Role of the microbiology laboratory

Laboratory should be able to identify and speciate enterococci

Fully automated methods of testing enterococci for susceptibility testing are unreliable; disk diffusion, gradient disk diffusion, agar dilation, or manual broth dilution are acceptable

Vancomycin resistance should be confirmed by repeating one of the above tests, or by streaking onto brain heart infusion containing 6 μg/mL of vancomycin. Preliminary and confirmatory identification of VRE should be immediately reported to patient care personnel and infection control

Screening for VRE should be conducted periodically in hospitals where VRE has not been previously detected

Prevention and control of nosocomial transmission of VRE

For all hospitals, including those with infrequent or no isolation of VRE

   Notify appropriate staff immediately when VRE is detected

   Educate clinical staff about hospital policies regarding VRE colonized or infected patients so that appropriate procedures can be implemented immediately

   Establish systems for monitoring process and outcome measures

   Isolation precautions to prevent patient-to-patient transmission of VRE: refer to Table 2

In hospitals with endemic VRE or continued VRE transmission despite implementation of above measures:

   Focus initial control efforts on critical care units and other areas where VRE transmission rates are highest

   Where feasible, cohort staff caring for VRE-positive and VRE-negative patients

   Carriage of enterococci by hospital staff is rarely implicated in transmission. Investigation and culturing of hospital staff should be at the direction of infection control staff

   Verify that environmental disinfection procedures are adequate and that procedures are correctly performed

   Consider sending representative VRE isolates to reference laboratories for strain typing as an aid in identifying reservoirs and patterns of transmission

Table 4 Isolation precautions to prevent patient-to-patient transmission of VRE (adapted from CDC-HICPAC (222))

Place VRE colonized or infected patients in single rooms, or cohort with other patients with VRE

Wear gloves when entering the room of a VRE-infected or colonized patient

Wear a gown when entering the room of a VRE-infected or colonized patient if

    Substantial contact with the patient or environmental surfaces in the room is anticipated

    The patient is incontinent

    The patient has an ileostomy, colostomy, or wound drainage not contained by dressing

Remove gloves and gown before leaving the patient's room, and wash hands immediately with an antiseptic soap or waterless antiseptic agent

Dedicate the use of non-critical items such as stethoscope, sphygmomanometer, or rectal thermometer to a single patient or cohort of isolated patients. Devices must be disinfected before use on other patients

Obtain stool or rectal swab cultures of roommates of patients newly found to be infected or colonized with VRE. Perform additional patient screening at the discretion of the infection control staff

Adopt a policy for determining when patients infected or colonized with VRE can be removed from isolation precautions. As VRE colonization may be prolonged, negative cultures from multiple sites on three separate occasions at least 1 week apart is recommended

The hospital should adopt a system by which infected and colonized patients can be recognized and placed into isolation promptly on transfer or re-admission

Develop a plan, in consultation with public health authorities, for discharge or transfer of colonized or infected patients to other health facilities, including nursing homes and home healthcare

---

break in a facility or unit in which VRE was previously present at low levels, vigorous implementation of such a strategy may lead to the elimination of VRE (16) or return it to baseline levels (15). Even after establishment of endemic VRE in a facility, transmission can be significantly reduced by a sustained and vigorous intervention that addresses key control issues (17). A coordinated, multi-institutional control strategy has resulted in a sustained reduction in the prevalence of VRE among hospitals and long-term care facilities in a large geographic region (222, 227). The majority of patients colonized with VRE in long-term care facilities appear to have acquired the organism during acute care hospitalization (94). Patient-to-patient transmission appears to occur at a much lower rate than in acute care facilities. This may be due to the lower level of medical care and infrequency of invasive procedures in long-term care. Thus, there is little justification for denying a patient colonized with VRE to a long-term care facility. Administration of antibiotics prolongs the duration of VRE carriage in long-term care patients; thus antibiotics should be administered only when clearly indicated. Recommendations for control of VRE in a long-term care facility have been published (Table 5).

Testing of the molecular relatedness of isolates is a well-established method for investigation of epidemics of hospital-acquired infection (228–234). Pulse field gel electrophoresis is the method of choice for delineation of the relatedness of strains; however, for evaluation of the possibility of gene dissemination, PCR methods are needed (228, 231, 232). These methods were essential in showing that various enterococcal resistance genes are capable of spread by clonal, transposon, and plasmid dissemination. Resistance can spread not only among enterococci, but also between different genera of bacteria, including staphylococci. This was an important mechanism for the recent description of vancomycin resistance in *Staphylococcus aureus* due to the acquisition of vanA

from enterococcus (232). The best use of molecular tests for endemic infection control requires further investigation (229–232). In one Chicago hospital system (229, 230), data on nosocomial infection was collected during a 24-month period before and a 60-month period after implementing a new program that included routine molecular testing of VRE, drug-resistant Gram-negative bacteria, and methicillin-resistant *Staphylococcus aureus*. During the intervention period, infections per 1,000 patient days fell 13%, and the percentage of hospitalized patients with nosocomial infections decreased 23%. The rate of infection fell to 43% below the US rate. Approximately 50 deaths were avoided in a 5-year period. The typing laboratory costs for the program were $400,000 per year, with a savings of $5.00 for each dollar spent in relation to nosocomial infection reduction. In this study, cost savings by use of molecular tests for endemic nosocomial infection were accomplished by a combination of establishment of clonality of isolates so that early intervention could be accomplished, and by determination of the unrelatedness of isolates, thereby avoiding unneeded and costly epidemic investigation. Cost reduction was also accomplished by earlier recognition of person-to-person spread of isolates as compared to traditional surveillance, and molecular testing was used to establish the presence of pseudoepidemics, also avoiding further epidemic investigation.

8 Summary and Conclusions

Although part of the normal intestinal flora and once felt to be innocuous endogenous pathogens, enterococci have proven to have much more complex interactions with the human host, having emerged in recent years as important nosocomial pathogens. Strains with resistance to multiple antimicrobials

Table 5 Recommendations for control of VRE in long-term care facilities

Patients colonized with VRE should not be denied admission to long-term care
Patients colonized with VRE should be placed in private rooms or cohorted with other colonized patients
Staff should wear gowns and gloves during patient activities likely to result in VRE transmission. This includes dressing changes, bathing, changing bed linen, toileting, and care of indwelling catheters
Hands must be washed after patient contact
Patients who are colonized with VRE who are continent of stool and who do not have wounds that cannot be contained by dressings may attend activities such as physical therapy and recreation
Antibiotic therapy should be given only when clearly indicated
If a patient colonized with VRE is transferred to another healthcare facility, the receiving institution should be notified of the patient's status

are on the rise, posing significant therapeutic and epidemiological challenges. In order to achieve the goal of minimizing the impact of resistance, a more comprehensive, multidisciplinary effort is needed, including a better understanding of the epidemiology and pathogenicity of these microorganisms, judicious use of antimicrobials, effective infection control measures in hospitals, and reduction of resistance in reservoirs, including the environment and animal husbandry.

References

1. Murray BE. The life and times of the *Enterococcus*. Clin Microbiol Rev 1990;3:46–65
2. Facklam RR, Collins MD. Identification of *Enterococcus* species isolated from human infections by a conventional test scheme. J Clin Microbiol 1989;27:731–734
3. Gordon S, Swenson JM, Hill BC, et al. Antimicrobial susceptibility patterns of common and unusual species of enterococci causing infections in the United States. J Clin Microbiol 1992;30:2373–2378
4. Ruoff KL, de la Maza L, Murtagh MJ, Spargo JD, Ferraro MJ. Species identities of enterococci isolated from clinical specimens. J Clin Microbiol 1990;28:435–437
5. De Baere T, Claeys G, Verschraegen G, et al. Continuous ambulatory peritoneal dialysis peritonitis due to *Enterococcus cecorum*. J Clin Microbiol 2000;38:3511–3512
6. Gullberg RM, Homann SR, Phair JP. Enterococcal bacteremia: analysis of 75 episodes. Rev Infect Dis 1989;11:74–85
7. Hsueh PR, Teng LJ, Chen YC, Yang PC, Ho SW, Luh KT. Recurrent bacteremic peritonitis caused by *Enterococcus cecorum* in a patient with liver cirrhosis. J Clin Microbiol 2000;38:2450–2452
8. Mellman RL, Spisak GM, Burakoff R. *Enterococcus avium* bacteremia in association with ulcerative colitis. Am J Gast 1992;87:337–338
9. Patel R, Keating MR, Cockerill FR III, Steckelberg JM. Bacteremia due to *Enterococcus avium*. Clin Infect Dis 1993;17:1006–1011
10. Pérez Mato S, Robinson S, Bégué RE. Vancomycin-resistant *Enterococcus faecium* meningitis successfully treated with chloramphenicol. Pediatr Infect Dis J 1999;18:483–484
11. Van Goethem GF, Louwagie BM, Simoens MJ, Vandeven JM, Verhaegen JL, Boogaerts MA. *Enterococcus casseliflavus* septicaemia in a patient with acute myeloid leukaemia. Eur J Clin Microbiol Infect Dis 1994;13:519–520
12. Zervos MJ, Kauffman CA, Therasse P, Bergman A, Mikesell TS, Schaberg DR. Nosocomial infection caused by gentamicin resistant *Streptococcus faecalis*: an epidemiologic study. Ann Intern Med 1987;106:687–691
13. Fridkin SK, Edwards JR, Courval JM, et al. The effect of vancomycin and third-generation cephalosporins on prevalence of vancomycin-resistant enterococci in 126 U.S. adult intensive care units. Ann Int Med 2001;135:175–183
14. Vergis EN, Hayden MK, Chow JW, et al. Determinants of vancomycin resistance and mortality rates in enterococcal bacteremia: a prospective multicenter study. Ann Intern Med 2001;135:484–492
15. Byers KE, Anglim AM, Anneski CJ, et al. A hospital epidemic of vancomycin-resistant *Enterococcus*: risk factors and control. Infect Control Hosp Epidemiol 2001;22:140–147
16. Falk PS, Winnike J, Woodmansee C, Desai M, Mayhall CG. Outbreak of vancomycin-resistant enterococci in a burn unit. Infect Control Hosp Epidemiol 2000;21:575–582
17. Montecalvo MA, Jarvis WR, Uman J, et al. Infection-control measures reduce transmission of vancomycin-resistant enterococci in an endemic setting. Ann Intern Med 1999;131:269–272
18. Morris JG Jr, Shay DK, Hebden JN, et al. Enterococci resistant to multiple antimicrobial agents, including vancomycin. Ann Intern Med 1995; 123:250–259
19. Malani PN, Thal L, Donabedian SM, et al. Molecular analysis of vancomycin-resistant *Enterococcus faecalis* from Michigan hospitals during a 10 year period. J Antimicrob Chemother 2002;49(5):841–843
20. Thal L, Donabedian S, Robinson-Dunn B, et al. Molecular analysis of glycopeptide-resistant *Enterococcus faecium* isolates collected from Michigan hospitals over a 6-year period. J Clin Microbiol 1998;36(11):3303–3308
21. Diaz Granados CA, Zimmer SM, Klein M, Jernigan JA. Comparison of mortality associated with vancomycin-resistant and vancomycin-susceptible enterococcal bloodstream infections: a meta-analysis. Clin Infect Dis 2005;41:327–333
22. Cetinkaya Y, Falk P, Mayhall CG. Vancomycin-resistant enterococci. Clin Microbiol Rev 2000;13:686–707
23. Edmond MB, Ober JF, Weinbaum DL, et al. Vancomycin-resistant *Enterococcus faecium* bacteremia: risk factors for infection. Clin Infect Dis 1995; 20:1126–1133
24. Hayden MK. Insights into the epidemiology and control of infection with vancomycin-resistant enterococci. Clin Infect Dis 2000;31:1058–1065
25. Tornieporth NG, Roberts RB, John J, Hafner A, Riley LW. Risk factors associated with vancomycin-resistant *Enterococcus faecium* infection or colonization in 145 matched case patients and control patients. Clin Infect Dis 1996;23:767–772
26. Zaas AK, Song X, Tucker P, Perl TM. Risk factors for development of vancomycin-resistant enterococcal bloodstream infection in patients with cancer who are colonized with vancomycin-resistant enterococci. Clin Infect Dis 2002;35:1139–1146
27. Carmeli Y, Eliopoulos GM, Samore MH. Antecedent treatment with different antibiotic agents as a risk factor for vancomycin-resistant *Enterococcus*. Emerg Infect Dis 2002;8:802–807
28. Harbarth S, Cosgrove S, Carmeli Y. Effects of antibiotics on nosocomial epidemiology of vancomycin-resistant enterococci. Antimicrob Agents Chemother 2002;46:1619–1628
29. Padiglione AA, Wolfe R, Grabsch EA, et al. Risk factors for new detection of vancomycin-resistant enterococci in acute-care hospitals that employ strict infection control procedures. Antimicrob Agents Chemother 2003;47:2492–2498
30. Stiefel U, Paterson DL, Pultz NJ, Gordon SM, Aron DC, Donskey CJ. Effect of the increasing use of piperacillin/tazobactam on the

incidence of vancomycin-resistant enterococci in four academic medical centers. Infect Control Hosp Epidemiol 2004;25:380–383

31. DiNubile MJ, Chow JW, Satishchandran V, et al. Acquisition of resistant bowel flora during a double-blind randomized clinical trial of ertapenem versus piperacillin–tazobactam therapy for intraabdominal infections. Antimicrob Agents Chemother 2005;49:3217–3221

32. Donskey CJ, Chowdhry TK, Hecker MT, et al. Effect of antibiotic therapy on the density of vancomycin-resistant enterococci in the stool of colonized patients. N Engl J Med 2000;343:1925–1932

33. Stiefel U, Pultz NJ, Helfand MS, Donskey CJ. Increased susceptibility to vancomycin-resistant *Enterococcus* intestinal colonization persists after completion of anti-anaerobic antibiotic treatment in mice. Infect Control Hosp Epidemiol 2004;25:373–379

34. Carmeli Y, Samore MH, Huskins WC. The association between antecedent vancomycin treatment and hospital-acquired vancomycin-resistant enterococci: a meta-analysis. Arch Intern Med 1999;159:2461–2468

35. Donabedian SM, Thal LA, Hershberger E, et al. Molecular characterization of gentamicin-resistant *Enterococci* in the United States: evidence of spread from animals to humans through food. J Clin Microbiol 2003;41:1109–1113

36. Hershberger E, Donabedian S, Konstantinou K, Zervos MJ. Quinupristin–dalfopristin resistance in gram-positive bacteria: mechanism of resistance and epidemiology. Clin Infect Dis 2004;38:92–98

37. Hershberger E, Oprea SF, Donabedian SM, et al. Epidemiology of antimicrobial resistance in enterococci of animal origin. J Antimicrob Chemother 2005;55:127–130

38. Jensen VF, Neimann J, Hammerum AM, Molbak K, Wegener HC. Does the use of antibiotics in food animals pose a risk to human health? An unbiased review? J Antimicrob Chemother 2004;54:274–275

39. Vergis EN, Shankar N, Chow JW, et al. Association between the presence of enterococcal virulence factors gelatinase, hemolysin, and enterococcal surface protein and mortality among patients with bacteremia due to *Enterococcus faecalis*. Clin Infect Dis 2002;35:570–575

40. Gilmore MS, Coburn PS, Nallapareddy SR, Murray BE. Enterococcal virulence. In: Gilmore MS, ed. The Enterococci. Pathogenesis, Molecular Biology, and Antibiotic Resistance. Washington, DC: ASM Press, 2002:301–354

41. Cercenado E, Eliopoulos GM, Wennersten CB, Moellering RC Jr. Influence of high-level gentamicin resistance and beta-hemolysis on susceptibility of enterococci to the bactericidal activities of ampicillin and vancomycin. Antimicrob Agents Chemother 1992;36:2526–2528

42. Moellering RC Jr, Weinberg AN. Studies on antibiotic synergism against enterococci. II. Effect of various antibiotics on the uptake of 14C-labelled streptomycin by enterococci. J Clin Invest 1971;50:2580–2584

43. Patterson JE, Zervos MJ. High-level gentamicin resistance in enterococci: epidemiology, microbiology and genetic basis. Rev Infect Dis 1990;12:644–652

44. Arduino RC, Murray BE. Enterococci: antimicrobial resistance. In: Mandell GL, Douglas RG, Bennett JE, eds. Update to Principles and Practice of Infectious Diseases. New York: Churchill Livingstone Inc, 1993:3–15

45. Ferretti JJ, Gilmore KS, Courvalin P. Nucleotide sequence analysis of the gene specifying the bifunctional 6′-aminoglycoside acetyltransferase 2′-aminoglycoside phosphotransferase enzyme in *Streptococcus faecalis* and identification and cloning of gene regions specifying the two activities. J Bacteriol 1986;167:631–638

46. Eliopoulos GM, Farber BF, Murray BE, Wennersten C, Moellering RC Jr. Ribosomal resistance of clinical enterococcal isolates to streptomycin. Antimicrob Agents Chemother 1984;25:398–399

47. Krogstad DJ, Korfhagen TR, Moellering RC Jr, et al. Aminoglycoside-inactivating enzymes in clinical isolates of *Streptococcus faecalis*: an explanation for antibiotic synergism. J Clin Invest 1978;62:480–486

48. Ounissi H, Courvalin P. Appendix B. Nucleotide sequences of streptococcal genes. In: Ferretti JJ, Curtis R III, eds. Streptococcal Genetics. Washington, DC. American Society for Microbiology, 1987:275

49. Coque TM, Arduino RC, Murray BE. High-level resistance to aminoglycosides: comparison of community and nosocomial fecal isolates of enterococci. Clin Infect Dis 1995;20:1048–1051

50. Silverman J, Thal LA, Perri MB, Bostic G, Zervos MJ. Epidemiologic evaluation of antimicrobial resistance in community acquired enterococci. J Clin Microbiol 1998;36:830–832

51. Watanakunakorn C. Rapid increase in the prevalence of high-level aminoglycoside resistance among enterococci isolated from blood cultures during 1989–1991. J Antimicrob Chemother 1992;30:289–293

52. Moellering RC Jr, Murray BE, Schoenbaum SC, Adler J, Wennersten CB. A novel mechanism of resistance to penicillin–gentamicin synergism in *Streptococcus faecalis*. J Infect Dis 1980;141:81–86

53. Hayden M, Koenig GI, Trenholme GM. Bactericidal activities of antibiotics against vancomycin-resistant *Enterococcus faecium* blood isolates and synergistic activities of combinations. Antimicrob Agents Chemother 1994;38:1225–1229

54. Chow JW, Zervos MJ, Lerner SA, et al. A novel gentamicin resistance gene in *Enterococcus*. Antimicrob Agents Chemother 1997;41:511–514

55. Chow JW, Donabedian SM, Clewell DB, Sahm DF, Zervos MJ. In vitro susceptibility and molecular analysis of gentamicin-resistant enterococci. Diagn Microbiol Infect Dis 1998;32:141–146

56. Tsai SF, Zervos MJ, Clewell DB, Donabedian SM, Sahm DF, Chow JW. A new high-level gentamicin resistance gene, aph(2′)-Id, in *Enterococcus* spp. Antimicrob Agents Chemother 1998;42:1229–1232

57. Al-Obeid S, Gutmann L, Williamson R. Modification of penicillin-binding proteins of penicillin-resistant mutants of different species of enterococci. J Antimicrob Chemother 1990;26:613–618

58. Fontana R, Aldegheri M, Ligozzi M, Lopez H, Sucari A, Satta G. Overproduction of a low-affinity penicillin-binding protein and high-level ampicillin resistance in *Enterococcus faecium*. Antimicrob Agents Chemother 1994;38:1980–1983

59. Grayson ML, Eliopoulos GM, Wennersten CB, et al. Increasing resistance to beta-lactam antibiotics among clinical isolates of *Enterococcus faecium*: a 22-year review at one institution. Antimicrob Agents Chemother 1991;35:2180–2184

60. Ligozzi M, Pittaluga F, Fontana R. Identification of a genetic element (psr) which negatively controls expression of *Enterococcus hirae* penicillin-binding protein 5. J Bacteriol 1993;175:2046–2051

61. Ligozzi M, Pittaluga F, Fontana R. Modification of penicillin-binding protein 5 associated with high-level ampicillin resistance in *Enterococcus fae*cium. Antimicrob Agents Chemother 1996;40:354–357

62. Signoretto C, Boaretti M, Canepari P. Cloning, sequencing and expression in *Escherichia coli* of the low-affinity penicillin-binding protein of *Enterococcus faecalis*. FEMS Microbiol Lett 1994;123:99–106

63. Bush LM, Calmon J, Cherney CL, et al. High-level penicillin resistance among isolates of enterococci. Ann Intern Med 1989;110:515–520

64. Torres C, Tenorio C, Lantero M, Gastañares MJ, Baquero F. High-level penicillin resistance and penicillin–gentamicin synergy in *Enterococcus faecium*. Antimicrob Agents Chemother 1993;37:2427–2431

65. Arthur M, Courvalin P. Genetics and mechanisms of glycopeptide resistance in enterococci. Antimicrob Agents Chemother 1993;37:1563–1571

66. Leclercq R, Courvalin P. Resistance to glycopeptides in enterococci. Clin Infect Dis 1997;24:545–556

67. Alam MR, Donabedian S, Brown W, et al. Heteroresistance to vancomycin in *Enterococcus faecium*. J Clin Microbiol 2001;39:3379–3381

68. Navarro F, Courvalin P. Analysis of genes encoding D-alanine-D-alanine ligase-related enzymes in *Enterococcus casseliflavus* and *Enterococcus flavescens*. Antimicrob Agents Chemother 1994;38:1788–1793

69. Reynolds PE, Snaith HA, Maguire AJ, Dutka-Malen S, Courvalin P. Analysis of peptidoglycan precursors in vancomycin-resistant *Enterococcus gallinarum* BM4174. Biochem J 1994;301:5–8

70. Yao JDC, Thauvin-Eliopoulos C, Eliopoulos GM, Moellering RC Jr. Efficacy of teicoplanin in two dosage regimens for experimental endocarditis caused by a beta-lactamase-producing strain of *Enterococcus faecalis* with high-level resistance to gentamicin. Antimicrob Agents Chemother 1990;34:827–830

71. Aslangul E, Baptista M, Fantin B, et al. Selection of glycopeptide-resistant mutants of VanB-type *Enterococcus faecalis* BM4281 in vitro and in experimental endocarditis. J Infect Dis 1997;175:598–605

72. Hayden MK, Trenholme GM, Schultz JE, Sahm DF. In vivo development of teicoplanin resistance in a VanB *Enterococcus faecium* isolate. J Infect Dis 1993;167:1224–1227

73. Moellering RC Jr. Emergence of *Enterococcus* as a significant pathogen. Clin Infect Dis 1992;14:1173–1178

74. Raymond NJ, Henry J, Workowski KA. Enterococcal arthritis: case report and review. Clin Infect Dis 1995;21:516–522

75. Graninger W, Ragette R. Nosocomial bacteremia due to *Enterococcus faecalis* without endocarditis. Clin Infect Dis 1992;15:49–57

76. Maki DG, Agger WA. Enterococcal bacteremia: clinical features, the risk of endocarditis, and management. Medicine (Baltimore) 1988;67:248–269

77. Hoge CW, Adams J, Buchanan B, Sears SD. Enterococcal bacteremia: to treat or not to treat, a reappraisal. Rev Infect Dis 1991;13:600–605

78. Noskin GA, Peterson LR, Warren JR. *Enterococcus faecium* and *Enterococcus faecalis* bacteremia: acquisition and outcome. Clin Infect Dis 1995;20:296–301

79. Patterson JE, Sweeney AH, Simms M, et al. An analysis of 110 serious enterococcal infections: epidemiology, antibiotic susceptibility, and outcome. Medicine (Baltimore) 1995;74:191–200

80. Murray BE. Beta-lactamase-producing enterococci. Antimicrob Agents Chemother 1992;36:2355–2359

81. Murray BE, Singh KV, Markowitz SM, et al. Evidence for clonal spread of a single strain of beta-lactamase-producing *Enterococcus (Streptococcus) faecalis* to six hospitals in five states. J Infect Dis 1991;163:780–785

82. Patterson JE, Masecar B, Zervos MJ. Characterization and comparison of two penicillinase-producing strains of *Streptococcus faecalis*. Antimicrob Agents Chemother 1988;32:122–123

83. Murray BE, Singh KV, Markowitz SM, Lopardo HA, Patterson JE, Zervos MJ, Rubeglio E, Eliopoulos G, Rice LB, Goldstein FW, Caputo G, Nasnas R, Moore LS, Wong ES, Weinstock G. Evidence for clonal spread of a single strain of beta-lactamase producing *Enterococcus faecalis* to five hospitals in four states. J Infect Dis 1991;163:780–785

84. Auckenthaler R, Wilson WR, Wright AJ, Washington JA II, Durack DT, Geraci JE. Lack of an in vivo and in vitro bactericidal activity of *N*-formimidoyl thienamycin against enterococci. Antimicrob Agents Chemother 1982;22:448–452

85. Eliopoulos GM, Eliopoulos CT. Therapy of enterococcal infections. Eur J Clin Microbiol Infect Dis 1990;9:118–126

86. Scheld WE, Keeley JM. Imipenem therapy of experimental *Staphylococcus aureus* and *Streptococcus faecalis* endocarditis. J Antimicrob Chemother 1983;12(Suppl D):65–78

87. Fang G, Brennen C, Wagener M, et al. Use of ciprofloxacin versus use of aminoglycoside for therapy of complicated urinary tract infection: prospective, randomized clinical and pharmacokinetic study. Antimicrob Agents Chemother 1991;35:1849–1855

88. Zervos MJ, Bacon AE III, Patterson JE, Schaberg DR, Kauffman CA. Enterococcal superinfection in patients treated with ciprofloxacin. J Antimicrob Chemother 1988;21:113–115

89. Perri MB, Hershberger E, Ionescu M, Lauter C, Zervos MJ. In vitro susceptibility of vancomycin-resistant enterococci (VRE) to fosfomycin. Diagn Microbiol Infect Dis 2002;42(4):269–271

90. Taylor SE, Paterson DL, Yu VL. Treatment options for chronic prostatitis due to vancomycin-resistant *Enterococcus faecium*. Eur J clin Microbiol Infect Dis 1998;17:798–800

91. Cooper GS, Shlaes DM, Jacobs MR, Salata RA. The role of *Enterococcus* in intraabdominal infections: case control analysis. Infect Dis Clin Pract 1993;2:332–339

92. Eliopoulos GM. Aminoglycoside resistant enterococcal endocarditis. Infect Dis Clin N Am 1993;7:117–133

93. Francioli P. Antibiotic treatment of streptococcal and enterococcal endocarditis: an overview. Eur Heart J 1995;16 (Suppl B):75–79

94. Konstantinov IE, Zehr KJ. Aortic root replacement in a patient with vancomycin-resistant *Enterococcus faecium* endocarditis and leukemia. Chest 2001;120:1744–1746

95. Mandell GL, Kaye D, Levison ME, Hook EW. Enterococcal endocarditis: an analysis of 38 patients observed at the New York Hospital-Cornell Medical Center. Arch Intern Med 1970;125.258–264

96. Megran DW. Enterococcal endocarditis. Clin Infect Dis 1992;15:63–71

97. Wilson WR, Karchmer AW, Dajani AS, et al. Antibiotic treatment of adults with infective endocarditis due to streptococci, enterococci staphylococci, and HACEK microorganisms. JAMA 1995;274:1706–1713

98. Moellering RC Jr, Wennersten C, Weinberg AN. Studies on antibiotic synergism against enterococci 1. Bacteriologic studies. J Lab Clin Med 1971;77:821–828

99. Wilson WR, Wilkowske CJ, Wright AJ, Sande MA, Geraci JE. Treatment of streptomycin-susceptible and streptomycin-resistant enterococcal endocarditis. Ann Intern Med 1984;100:816–823

100. Koenig MG, Kaye D. Enterococcal endocarditis: report of nineteen cases with long term follow up data. N Engl J Med 1961;264:257–264

101. Morris JT, Cooper RH. Intravenous streptomycin: a useful route of administration. Clin Infect Dis 1994;19:1150–1151

102. Rice LB, Calderwood SB, Eliopoulos GM, Farber BF, Karchmer AW. Enterococcal endocarditis: a comparison of prosthetic and native valve disease. Rev Infect Dis 1991;13:1–7

103. Fantin B, Carbon C. Importance of the aminoglycoside dosing regimen in the penicillin-netilmicin combination for treatment of *Enterococcus faecalis*-induced experimental endocarditis. Antimicrob Agents Chemother 1990;34:2387–2391

104. Marangos MN, Nicolau DP, Quintiliani R, Nightingale CH. Influence of gentamicin dosing interval on the efficacy of penicillin-containing regimens in experimental *Enterococcus faecalis* endocarditis. J Antimicrob Chemother 1997;39:519–522

105. Tam VH, Mckinnon PS, Levine DP, Brandel SM, Rybak MJ. Once-daily aminoglycoside in the treatment of *Enterococcus faecalis* endocarditis: case report and review. Pharmacotherapy 2000;20(9):1116–1119

106. Lee PYC, Das SS, Stevens PJ. Achieving bactericidal therapy and high-level aminoglycoside resistance. J Antimicrob Chemother 1993;31.608–609

107. Sacher HL, Miller WC, Landau SW, Sacher ML, Dixon WA, Dietrich KA. Relapsing native-valve enterococcal endocarditis:

a unique cure with oral ciprofloxacin combination drug therapy. J Clin Pharmacol 1991;31:719–721

108. Olaison L, Schadewitz K; Swedish Society of Infectious Diseases Quality Assurance Study Group for Endocarditis. Enterococcal endocarditis in Sweden, 1995–1999: can shorter therapy with aminoglycosides be used? Clin Infect Dis 2002;34:159–166

109. Ang JY, Lua JL, Turner DR, Asmar BI. Vancomycin-resistant *Enterococcus faecium* in a premature infant successfully treated with linezolid. Pediatr Infect Dis J 2003;22:1101–1103

110. Archuleta S, Murphy B, Keller MJ. Successful treatment of vancomycin-resistant *Enterococcus faecium* endocarditis with linezolid in a renal transplant recipient with human immunodeficiency virus infection. Transpl Infect Dis 2004;6:117–119

111. Babcock HM, Ritchie DJ, Christiansen E, Starlin R, Little R, Stanley S. Successful treatment of vancomycin-resistant *Enterococcus* endocarditis with oral linezolid. Clin Infect Dis 2001;32:1373–1375

112. Bishara J, Sagie A, Samra Z, Pitlik S. Polymicrobial endocarditis caused by methicillin resistant-*Staphylococcus aureus* and glycopeptide-resistant enterococci. Eur J Clin Microbiol Infect Dis 1999;18:674–675

113. Bohta PL, Struwig MC, de Vreis W, Hough J, Chalkey LJ. Enterococcal endocarditis – a case treated with teicoplanin and amoxycillin. S Afr Med J 1998;88:564–565

114. Brink AJ, van den Ende J, Routier RJ, Devenish L. A case of vancomycin-resistant enterococcal endocarditis. S Afr Med J 2000;90:1113–1115

115. Carfanga P, Tarasi A, Cassne M, Del Grosso MF, Bianco G, Venditti M. Prosthetic biologic valve endocarditis caused by a vancomycin-resistant (vanA) *Enterococcus faecalis*: case report. J Chemother 2000;12:416–420

116. Chien JW, Kucia ML, Salata RA. Use of linezolid, an oxazolidinone, in the treatment of multidrug-resistant gram-positive bacterial infections. Clin Infect Dis 2000;30:146–151

117. Furlong WB, Rakowski TA. Therapy with RP 59500 (quinupristin/dalfopristin) for prosthetic valve endocarditis due to enterococci with vanA/vanB resistance patterns. Clin Infect Dis 1997;25:163–164

118. Kapur D, Dorsky D, Feingold JM, et al. Incidence and outcome of vancomycin-resistant Enterococcal bacteremia following autologous peripheral blood stem cell transplantation. Bone Marrow Transplant 2000;25:147–152

119. Matsumura S, Simor AE. Treatment of endocarditis due of vancomycin-resistant *Enterococcus faecium* with quinupristin/dalfopristin, doxycycline, and rifampin: a synergistic drug combination. Clin Infect Dis 1998;27:1554–1556

120. Paterson DL, Dominguez EA, Chang F-Y, Snydman DR, Singh N. Infective endocarditis in solid organ transplant patients. Clin Infect Dis 1998;26:689–694

121. Thompson RL, Lavin B, Talbot GH. Endocarditis due to vancomycin-resistant *Enterococcus faecium* in an immunocompromised patient: cure by administering combination therapy with quinupristin–dalfopristin and high-dose ampicillin. South Med J 2003;96:818–820

122. Tiong IY, Novaro GM, Jefferson B, Monson M, Smedira N, Penn MS. Bacterial endocarditis and functional mitral stenosis: a report of two cases and literature review. Chest 2002;122:2259–2262

123. Tripodi MF, Locatelli A, Adinolfi LE, Andreana A, Utili R. Successful treatment with ampicillin and fluoroquinolones of human endocarditis due to high-level gentamicin-resistant enterococci. Eur J Clin Microbiol Infect Dis 1998;17:734–736

124. Venditti M, Biavasco F, Varaldo PE, et al. Catheter related endocarditis due to glycopeptide-resistant *Enterococcus faecalis* in a transplanted heart. Clin Infect Dis 1993;17:524–5164a

125. Vijayvargiya R, Veis JH. Antibiotic-resistant endocarditis in a hemodialysis patient. J Am Soc Nephrol 1996;7:536–542

126. Wareham DW, Abbas H, Karcher AM, Das SS. Treatment of prosthetic valve infective endocarditis due to multi-resistant Gram-positive bacteria with linezolid. J Infect 2006;52:300–304

127. Yelamanchili S, Cunliffe NA, Miles RS. Prosthetic valve endocarditis caused by a vancomycin-resistant *Enterococcus faecalis*. J Infect Dis 1998;36:348–349

128. Sandoe JA, Witherden IR, Au-Yeung HK, Kite P, Kerr KG, Wilcox MH. Enterococcal intravascular catheter-related bloodstream infection: management and outcome of 61 consecutive cases. J Antimicrob Chemother 2002;50(4):577–582

129. Bayer AS, Seidel JS, Yoshikawa TT, Anthony BF, Guze LB. Group D enterococcal meningitis: clinical and therapeutic considerations with report of three cases and review of the literature. Arch Intern Med 1976;136:883–886

130. Stevenson KB, Murray EW, Sarubbi FA. Enterococcal meningitis: report of four cases and review. Clin Infect Dis 1994;18:233–239

131. Krcméry V Jr, Filka J, Uher J, et al. Ciprofloxacin in treatment of nosocomial meningitis in neonates and in infants: report of 12 cases and review. Diagn Microb Infect Dis 1999;35:75–80

132. Gransden WR, King A, Marossy D, Rosenthal E. Quinupristin/dalfopristin in neonatal *Enterococcus faecium* meningitis. Arch Dis Child Fetal Neonatal Ed 1998;78:F235–F236

133. Losonsky GA, Wolf A, Schwalbe RS, Nataro J, Gibson CB, Lewis EW. Successful treatment of meningitis due to multiple resistant *Enterococcus faecium* with a combination of intrathecal teicoplanin and intravenous antimicrobial agents. Clin Infect Dis 1994;19:163–165

134. Tush GM, Huneycutt S, Phillips A, Ward JD. Intraventricular quinupristin/dalfopristin for the treatment of vancomycin-resistant *Enterococcus faecium* shunt infection. Clin Infect Dis 1998;26:1460–1461

135. Zeana C, Kubin CJ, Della-Latta P, Hammer SM. Vancomycin-resistant *Enterococcus faecium* meningitis successfully managed with linezolid: case report and review of the literature. Clin Infect Dis 2001;33:477–482

136. Hachem R, Afif C, Gokasian Z, Raad I. Successful treatment of vancomycin-resistant *Enterococcus meningitis* with linezolid. Eur J Clin Microbiol Infect Dis 2001;20:432–434

137. Moellering RC Jr. The enterococcus: a classic example of the impact of antimicrobial resistance on therapeutic options. J Antimicrob Chemother 1991;28:1–12

138. Kaye D. Treatment of infective endocarditis. Ann Intern Med 1996;124:606–608

139. Thauvin C, Eliopoulos GM, Willey S, Wennersten C, Moellering RC Jr. Continuous-infusion ampicillin therapy of enterococcal endocarditis in rats. Antimicrob Agents Chemother 1989;31:139–143

140. Antony SJ, Ladner J, Stratton CW, Raudales F, Drummer SJ. High-level aminoglycoside-resistant enterococcus causing endocarditis successfully treated with a combination of ampicillin, imipenem and vancomycin. Scand J Infect Dis 1997;29:628–630

141. Antony SJ, Matheren P, Stratton CW. Increased bactericidal activity as documented by serum bactericidal titers for a triple combination of cell wall active agents against gentamicin-resistant enterococci. Scand J Infect Dis 1995;27:401–403

142. Foulds G. Pharmacokinetics of sulbactam/ampicillin in humans: a review. Rev Infect Dis 1986;8(Suppl 5):S503–S511

143. Physicians' Desk Reference. 51st ed. Montvale, NJ: Medical Economics Company, Inc., 1997:2035

144. Dodge RA, Daly JS, Davaro R, Glew RH. High-dose ampicillin plus streptomycin for treatment of a patient with severe infection due to multiresistant enterococci. Clin Infect Dis 1997;25:1269–1270

145. Mekonen ET, Noskin GA, Hacek DM, Peterson LR. Successful treatment of persistent bacteremia due to vancomycin-resistant, ampicillin-resistant *Enterococcus faecium*. Microb Drug Resist 1995;1:249–253

146. Schmit JL. Efficacy of teicoplanin for enterococcal infections: 63 cases and review. Clin Infect Dis 1992;15:302–306

147. Presterl E, Graninger W, Georgopoulos A. The efficacy of teicoplanin in the treatment of endocarditis caused by Gram-positive bacteria. J Antimicrob Chemother 1993;31:755–766

148. Murray BE. Vancomycin-resistant enterococcal infections. N Engl J Med 2000;342:710–721

149. Norris AH, Reilly JP, Edelstein PH, Brennan PJ, Schuster MG. Chloramphenicol for the treatment of vancomycin-resistant enterococcal infections. Clin Infect Dis 1995;20:1137–1144

150. Papanicolaou GA, Meyers RR, Meyers J, et al. Nosocomial infections with vancomycin-resistant *Enterococcus faecium* in liver transplant recipients: risk factors for acquisition and mortality. Clin Infect Dis 1996;23:760–766

151. Lam S, Singer C, Tucci V, Morthland VH, Pfaller MA, Isenberg HD. The challenge of vancomycin-resistant enterococci: a clinical and epidemiologic study. Am J Infect Control 1995;23:170–180

152. Lautenbach E, Schuster MG, Bilker WB, Brennan PJ. The role of chloramphenicol in the treatment of bloodstream infection due to vancomycin-resistant *Enterococcus*. Clin Infect Dis 1998;27:1259–1265

153. Lynch C, Courvalin P, Nikaido H. Active efflux of antimicrobial agents in wild-type strains of enterococci. Antimicrob Agents Chemother 1997;41:869–871

154. Moreno F, Jorgensen JH, Weiner MH. An old antibiotic for a new multiple resistant *Enterococcus faecium*? Diagn Microbiol Infect Dis 1994;20:41–43

155. Howe RA, Robson M, Oakhill A, Cornish JM, Millar MR. Successful use of tetracycline as therapy of an immunocompromised patient with septicaemia caused by a vancomycin-resistant enterococcus. J Antimicrob Chemother 1997;40:144–145

156. Dever LL, Smith SM, DeJesus D, et al. Treatment of vancomycin-resistant *Enterococcus faecium* infections with an investigational streptogramin antibiotic (quinupristin/dalfopristin): a report of fifteen cases. Microbial Drug Resist 1996;2:407–413

157. Linden PK, Pasculle AW, McDevitt D, Kramer DJ. Effect of quinupristin/dalfopristin on the outcome of vancomycin-resistant *Enterococcus faecium* bacteraemia: comparison with a control cohort. J Antimicrob Chemother 1997;39(Suppl A):145–151

158. Winston DJ, Emmanouilides C, Kroeber A, et al. Quinupristin/dalfopristin therapy for infections due to vancomycin-resistant *Enterococcus faecium*. Clin Infect Dis 2000;30:790–797

159. Moellering RC, Linden PK, Reinhardt J, Blumberg EA, Bompart F, Talbot GH. The efficacy and safety of quinupristin/dalfopristin for the treatment of infections caused by vancomycin-resistant *Enterococcus faecium*. J Antimicrob Chemother 1999;44:251–261

160. Eliopoulos GM. Quinupristin–Dalfopristin and linezolid: evidence and opinion. Clin Infect Dis 2003;36:473–481

161. Lai KK. Treatment of vancomycin-resistant *Enterococcus faecium* infections. Arch Intern Med 1996;156:2579–2584

162. Nachtman A, Verma R, Egnor M. Vancomycin-resistant *Enterococcus faecium* shunt infection in an infant: an antibiotic cure. Microbial Drug Resist 1995;1:95–96

163. Sahgal VS, Urban C, Mariano N, Weinbaum F, Turner J, Rahal JJ. Quinupristin/dalfopristin (RP 59500) therapy for vancomycin-resistant *Enterococcus faecium* aortic graft infection: case report. Microbial Drug Resist 1995;1:245–247

164. Tan TY, Pitman I, Penrose-Stevens A, Simpson BA, Flanagan PG. Treatment of a vancomycin-resistant *Enterococcus faecium* ventricular drain infection with quinupristin/dalfopristin and review of the literature. J Infect 2000;41:85–97

165. Patel RM, Rouse S, Piper KE, Steckelberg JM. Linezolid therapy of vancomycin-resistant *Enterococcus faecium* experimental endocarditis. Antimicrob Agents Chemother 2001;45:621–623

166. Millichap J, Ristow RA, Noskin GA, Peterson LR. Selection of *Enterococcus faecium* strains with stable and unstable resistance to the streptogramin RP 59500 using stepwise in vitro exposure. Diagn Microbiol Infect Dis 1996;25:15–20

167. Aeschlimann JR, Zervos MJ, Rybak MJ. Treatment of vancomycin-resistant *Enterococcus faecium* with RP 59500 (quinupristin–dalfopristin) administered by intermittent or continuous infusion, alone or in combination with doxycycline, in an in vitro pharmacodynamic infection model with simulated endocardial vegetations. Antimicrob Agents Chemother 1998;42(10):2710–2717

168. Chow JW, Donabedian SM, Zervos MJ. Emergence of increased resistance to quinupristin/dalfopristin during therapy for *Enterococcus faecium* bacteremia. Clin Infect Dis 1997;24:90–91

169. Linden PK, Pasculle AW, Manez R, et al. Differences in outcomes for patients with bacteremia due to vancomycin-resistant *Enterococcus faecium* or vancomycin-susceptible E. faecium. Clin Infect Dis 1996;22:663–670

170. Chow JW, Davidson A, Sanford E III, Zervos MJ. Superinfection with *Enterococcus faecalis* during quinupristin/dalfopristin therapy. Clin Infect Dis 1997;24:91–92

171. Shinabarger DL, Marotti KR, Murray RW, et al. Mechanism of action of oxazolidinones: effects of linezolid and eperezolid on translation reactions. Antimicrob Agents Chemother 1997;41:2132–2136

172. Swaney SM, Aoki H, Ganoza MC, Shinabarger DL. The oxazolidinone linezolid inhibits initiation of protein synthesis in bacteria. Antimicrob Agents Chemother 1998;42:3251–3255

173. Moellering RC. Linezolid: the first oxazolidinone antimicrobial. Ann Intern Med 2003;138:135–142

174. Bostic GD, Perri MB, Thal LA, Zervos MJ. Comparative in vitro and bactericidal activity of oxazolidinone antibiotics against multidrug-resistant enterococci. Diagn Microbiol Infect dis 1996;173:909–913

175. Eliopoulos GM, Wennersten CB, Gold HS, Moellering RC Jr. In vitro activities of new oxazolidinone antimicrobial agents against enterococci. Antimicrob Agents Chemother 1996;40:1745–1747

176. Ford CW, Hamel JC, Wilson DM, et al. invivo activities of U-100592 and U-100766, novel oxazolidinone antimicrobial agents against experimental bacterial infections. Antimicrob Agents Chemother 1996;40:1508–1513

177. Noskin GA, Siddiqui F, Stosor V, Hacek D, Peterson LR. In vitro activities of linezolid against important Gram-positive bacterial pathogens including vancomycin-resistant enterococci. Antimicrob Agents Chemother 1999;43:2059–2062

178. Patel R, Rouse MS, Piper KE, et al. In vitro activity of linezolid against vancomycin-resistant enterococci, methicillin-resistant *Staphylococcus aureus* and penicillin-resistant *Streptococcus pneumoniae*. Diagn Microbiol Infect Dis 1999;34:119–122

179. Rybak MJ, Cappelletty DM, Moldovan T, Aeschlimann JR, Kaatz GW. Comparative in vitro activities and postantibiotic effects of the oxazolidinone compounds eperezolid (PNU-100592) and linezolid (PNU-100766) versus vancomycin against *Staphylococcus aureus*, coagulase-negative staphylococci, *Enterococcus faecalis*, and *Enterococcus faecium*. Antimicrob Agents Chemother 1998;42:721–724

180. Schülin T, Thauvin-Eliopoulos C, Moellering RC Jr, Elipopulos GM. Activities of the oxazolidinones linezolid and eperezolid in experimental intraabdominal abscess due to *Enterococcus faecalis* or vancomycin-resistant *Enterococcus faecium*. Antimicrob Agents Chemother 1999;43:2873–2876

181. Noskin GA, Siddiqui F, Stosor V, Kruzynski J, Peterson LR. Successful treatment of persistent vancomycin-resistant *Enterococcus faecium* bacteremia with linezolid and gentamicin. Clin Infect Dis 1999;28:689–690

182. McNeil SA, Clark NM, Chandrasekar PH, Kauffman CA. Successful treatment of vancomycin-resistant *Enterococcus faecium* bacteremia with linezolid after failure of treatment with Synercid (quinupristin/dalfopristin). Clin Infect Dis 2000;30:403–404

183. Birmingham MC, Rayner CR, Meagher AK, Flavin SM, Batts DH, Schentag JJ. Linezolid for the treatment of multidrug-resistant, gram-positive infections: experience from a compassionate-use program. Clin Infect Dis 2003;36(2):159–168

184. Raad I, Hachem R, Hanna H, et al. Prospective, randomized study comparing quinupristin–dalfopristin with linezolid in the treatment of vancomycin-resistant *Enterococcus faecium* infections. J Antimicrob Chemother 2004;53(4):646–649

185. Linden PK. Treatment options for vancomycin-resistant enterococcal infections. Drugs 2002;62(3):425–441

186. Rao N, White GJ. Successful treatment of *Enterococcus faecalis* prosthetic valve endocarditis with linezolid. Clin Infect Dis 2002;35(7):902–904

187. Zimmer SM, Caliendo AM, Thigpen MC, Somani J. Failure of linezolid treatment for enterococcal endocarditis. Clin Infect Dis 2003;37:e29–e30

188. Melzer M, Goldsmith D, Gransden W. Successful treatment of vertebral osteomyelitis with linezolid in a patient receiving hemodialysis and with persistent methicillin-resistant *Staphylococcus aureus* and vancomycin-resistant *Enterococcus* bacteremias. Clin Infect Dis 2000;31:208–209

189. Rao N, Ziran BH, Hall RA, Santa ER. Successful treatment of chronic bone and joint infections with oral linezolid. Clin Orthop Relat Res 2004;427:67–71

190. Till M, Wixson RL, Pertel PE. Linezolid treatment for osteomyelitis due to vancomycin-resistant *Enterococcus faecium*. Clin Infect Dis 2002;34(10):1412–1414

191. Steinmetz MP, Vogelbaum MA, De Georgia MA, Andrefsky JC, Isada C. Successful treatment of vancomycin-resistant *Enterococcus* meningitis with linezolid: case report and review of the literature. Crit Care Med 2001;29(12):2383–2385

192. Zurenko GE, Todd WM, Hafkin B, et al. Development of linezolid-resistant *Enterococcus faecium* in two compassionate use program patients treated with linezolid [abstract]. Abstracts of the 39th Interscience Conference on Antimicrobial Agents and Chemotherapy, San Francisco, CA, Sept 24–27, 1999. Washington, DC. American Society for Microbiology, 1999:118

193. Gonzales RD, Schreckenberger PC, Graham MB, Kelkar S, DenBesten K, Quinn JP. Infections due to vancomycin-resistant *Enterococcus faecium* resistant to linezolid. Lancet 2001;357:1179

194. Mutnick AH, Enne V, Jones RN. Linezolid resistance since 2001: SENTRY Antimicrobial Surveillance Program. Ann Pharmacother 2003;37:769–774

195. Dibo I, Pillai SK, Gold HS, et al. Linezolid-resistant *Enterococcus faecalis* isolated from a cord blood transplant recipient. J Clin Microbiol 2004;42(4):1843–1845

196. Burleson BS, Ritchie DJ, Micek ST, Dunne WM. *Enterococcus faecalis* resistant to linezolid: case series and review of the literature. Pharmacotherapy 2004;24(9):1225–1231

197. Carpenter CF, Chambers HF. Daptomycin: another novel agent for treating infections due to drug-resistant gram-positive pathogens. Clin Infect Dis 2004;38(7):994–1000

198. Shah PM. The need for new therapeutic agents: what is the pipeline? Clin Microbiol Infect 2005;11(Suppl 3):36–42

199. Hsueh PR, Chen WH, Teng LJ, Luh KT. Nosocomial infections due to methicillin-resistant *Staphylococcus aureus* and vancomycin-resistant enterococci at a university hospital in Taiwan from 1991 to 2003: resistance trends, antibiotic usage and in vitro activities of newer antimicrobial agents. Int J Antimicrob Agents 2005;26(1):43–49

200. Critchley IA, Draghi DC, Sahm DF, Thornsberry C, Jones Me, Karlowsky JA. Activity of daptomycin against susceptible and multidrug-resistant Gram-positive pathogens collected in the SECURE study (Europe) during 2000–2001. J Antimicrob Chemother 2003;51(3):639–649

201. Novais C, Sousa JC, Coque TM, Peixe LV. Portuguese Resistance Study Group. In vitro activity of daptomycin against enterococci from nosocomial and community environments in Portugal. J Antimicrob Chemother 2004;54(5):964–966

202. Johnson AP, Mushtaq S, Warner M, Livermore DM. Activity of daptomycin against multi-resistant Gram-positive bacteria including enterococci and *Staphylococcus aureus* resistant to linezolid. Int J Antimicrob Agents 2004;24(4):315–319

203. Cha R, Rybak MJ. Daptomycin against multiple drug-resistant staphylococcus and enterococcus isolates in an in vitro pharmacodynamic model with simulated endocardial vegetations. Diagn Microbiol Infect Dis 2003;47:539–546

204. Snydman DR, McDermott LA, Jacobus NV. Determination of synergistic effects of daptomycin with gentamicin or in vitro effect of beta-lactam antibiotics against *Staphylococcus aureus* and enterococci by FIC index and time kill kinetics. 41st Interscience Conference on Antimicrobial Agents and Chemotherapy 2001; Dec 16–19; Chicago, IL, Abstract no. E-533

205. Silverman JA, Oliver N, Andrew T, Li T. Resistance studies with daptomycin. Antimicrob Agents Chemother 2001;45(6):1799–1802

206. Lewis JS II, Owens A, Cadena J, Sabol K, Patterson JE, Jorgensen JH. Emergence of daptomycin resistance in *Enterococcus faecium* during daptomycin therapy. Antimicrob Agents Chemother 2005;49(4):1664–1665

207. Munoz-Price LS, Lolans K, Quinn JP. Emergence of resistance to daptomycin during treatment of vancomycin-resistant *Enterococcus faecalis* infection. Clin Infect Dis 2005;41(4):565–566

208. Muralidharan G, Micalizzi M, Speth J, Raible D, Troy S. Pharmacokinetics of tigecycline after a single and multiple doses in healthy subjects. Antimicrob Agents Chemother 2005;49:220–229

209. Noskin GA. Tigecycline: a new glycylcycline for treatment of serious infection. Clin Infect Dis 2005;41:S303–S314

210. Stein GE. Safety of the newer parenteral antibiotics. Clin Infect Dis 2005;41:S293–S302

211. Levine DP, Holley HP, Eiseman I, Willcox P, Tack K. Clinafloxacin for the treatment of bacterial endocarditis. Clin Infect Dis 2004;38:620–631

212. Shah P, Trostmann U, Tack K. Open-label, multicentre, emergency-use study of clinafloxacin (CI-960) in the treatment of patients with serious life-threatening infections. Int J Antimicrob Agents 2002;19:245–248

213. Tack KJ, Eiseman I, Zervos MJ. Clinafloxacin in serious infections caused by multiply resistant pathogens. Drugs 1999;58:260–262

214. Streit JM, Fritsche TR, Sader HS, Jones RN. Worldwide assessment of dalbavancin activity and spectrum against over 6,000 clinical isolates. Diagn Microbiol Infect Dis 2004;48:137–143

215. Malabarba A, Goldstein BP. Origin, structure, and activity in vitro and in vivo of dalbavancin. J Antimicrob Chemo 2005;55:ii15–ii20

216. Guay DRP. Dalbavancin: an investigational glycopeptide. Expert Rev Anti Infect Ther 2004;2:845–852

217. Raad I, Darouiche R, Vazquez J, et al. Efficacy and safety of weekly dalbavancin therapy for catheter-related bloodstream infection caused by gram-positive pathogens. Clin Infect Dis 2005;40:374–380

218. Inoue M, Nonoyama M, Okamoto R, Ida T. Antimicrobial activity of arbekacin, a new aminoglycoside antibiotic, against methicillin-resistant *Staphylococcus aureus*. Drugs Exp Clin Res 1994;22:233–240

219. Kak V, Donabedian SM, Zervos MJ, Kariyama R, Kumon H, Chow JW. Efficacy of ampicillin plus arbekacin in experimental rabbit endocarditis caused by an *Enterococcus faecalis* strain with high-level gentamicin resistance. Antimicrob Agents Chemother 2000; 44:2545–2546

220. Kak V, You I, Zervos MJ, Kariyama R, Kumon H, Chow JW. In-vitro synergistic activity of the combination of ampicillin and arbekacin against vancomycin- and high-level gentamicin-resistant *Enterococcus faecium* with the aph(2′)-Id gene. Diagn Microbiol Infect Dis 2000;37:297–299

221. Osakabe Y, Takahashi Y, Narihara K. The utility and dosage and administration of arbekacin in patients with MRSA infection. Antibiot Chemother 1996;12:120–127

222. Centers for Disease Control and Prevention. Recommendations for preventing the spread of vancomycin resistance. Recommendations of the Hospital Infection Control Practices Advisory Committee (HICPAC). MMWR Recomm Rep 1995;44(RR-12):1–13

223. Hachem R, Raad I. Failure of oral antimicrobial agents in eradicating gastrointestinal colonization with vancomycin-resistant enterococci. Infect Control Hosp Epidemiol 2002; 23:43–44

224. Livornese LL Jr, Dias S, Samel C, et al. Hospital-acquired infection with vancomycin-resistant *Enterococcus faecium* transmitted by electronic thermometers. Ann Intern Med 1992;117:112–116

225. Bonilla HF, Zervos MJ, Kauffman CA. Long term survival of vancomycin-resistant *Enterococcus faecium* on a contaminated surface. Infect Control Hosp Epidemiol 1996;17(12):770–772

226. Oprea SF, Zaidi N, Donabedian SM, Balasubramaniam M, Hershberger E, Zervos MJ. Molecular and clinical epidemiology of vancomycin-resistant *Enterococcus faecalis*. J Antimicrob Chemother 2004;53:626–630

227. Ostrowsky BE, Trick WE, Sohn AH, et al. Control of vancomycin-resistant enterococcus in health care facilities in a region. N Engl J Med 2001; 344:1427–1433

228. Donabedian S, Hershberger E, Thal LA, et al. PCR fragment length polymorphism analysis of vancomycin-resistant *Enterococcus faecium*. J Clin Microbiol 2000;38:2885–2888

229. Peterson LR, Noskin GA. New technology for detecting multi-drug-resistant pathogens in the clinical microbiology laboratory. Emerg Infect Dis 2001;7:1–12

230. Peterson LR, Petzel RA, Clabots CR, Fasching CE, Gerding DN. Medical technologists using molecular epidemiology as part of the infection control team. Diagn Microbiol Infect Dis 1993;16:303–311

231. Singh P, Goering RV, Simjee S, Foley SL, and Zervos MJ. Application of molecular techniques to the study of hospital infection. Clin Microbiol Rev 2006;19:512–530

232. Flannagan SE, Chow JW, Donabedian SM, et al. Plasmid content of a vancomycin-resistant *Enterococcus faecalis* isolate from a patient also colonized by *Staphylococcus aureus* with a VanA phenotype. Antimicrob Agents Chemother 2003;47:3954–3959

233. Sadfar AJ, Bryan CS, Stinson S, Saunders DE. Prosthetic valve endocarditis due to vancomycin resistant *Enterococcus faecium*: treatment with chloramphenicol and minocycline. Clin Infect Dis 2002;34:61–63

234. Fowler VG Jr, Boucher HW, Corey GR, Abrutyn E, Karchmer AW, Rupp ME, Levine DP, Chambers HF, Tally FP, Vigliani GA, Cabell CH, Link AS, DeMeyer I, Filler SG, Zervos M, et al., Daptomycin versus standard therapy for bacteremia and endocarditis caused by *Staphylococcus aureus*. N Engl J Med 2006;335:653–665

Chapter 50
Antimicrobial Resistance in Staphylococci: Mechanisms of Resistance and Clinical Implications

Lisa G. Winston and Henry F. Chambers

1 Introduction

Staphylococci are among the most important bacterial pathogens in humans. *Staphylococcus aureus* is the most common organism isolated from patients with clinically significant bacteremia (1). It produces a number of virulence factors that mediate its ability to adhere to host tissues. Thus, in the setting of bloodstream infections, metastatic complications such as arthritis, endocarditis, and osteomyelitis frequently ensue (2). *S. aureus* is also the leading cause of skin and soft tissue infections such as folliculitis and furunculosis, and it is the pathogen most often implicated in wound infections resulting from surgery or trauma. Thus, *S. aureus* is of major significance in both community-onset and healthcare-associated infections.

Coagulase-negative staphylococci less commonly cause invasive infections in healthy persons. However, these organisms are particularly associated with infections related to foreign material, such as venous catheters and prosthetic heart valves. Their role as pathogens has been increasingly appreciated in hospitalized patients (3). *S. epidermidis* is the species most frequently isolated and the best characterized of the coagulase-negative staphylococci, but other species – including *S. saprophyticus*, *S. lugdunensis*, and *S. schleiferi* – also play a role in human disease (4).

The length of time for antibiotic resistance to develop and then to become clinically significant is highly variable, and depends upon patterns of antimicrobial usage and the specific characteristics of the organism and antimicrobial in question. The development of resistance has had a dramatic impact on the antimicrobial agents used for both initial and definitive therapy of staphylococcal infections. Much of the work to elucidate mechanisms of resistance has been carried out using *S. aureus*, given the importance of this organism in human disease. Therefore, the resistance mechanisms discussed below largely reflect data obtained from *S. aureus*, but generally apply to coagulase-negative staphylococci.

2 Resistance to Specific Antimicrobial Agents

2.1 Natural Penicillins

Penicillin G resistance in staphylococci was reported in 1944, very early in clinical use (5). As was later seen with methicillin resistance, hospital strains were the first to develop penicillin resistance, and penicillin was used to treat community strains through the 1960s (6).

Penicillin exerts its effect by forming a covalent bond with penicillin-binding proteins (PBPs), which are critical for assembly of the cell wall. PBPs are involved in the final stages of peptidoglycan synthesis, and penicillin inhibits crosslinking of peptidoglycan chains. *S. aureus* usually has four PBPs, three of high molecular weight and one (PBP4) which is smaller. Penicillin resistance in staphylocci is mediated by the production of beta-lactamase, a type of PBP, which hydrolyzes the penicillin beta-lactam ring. The beta-lactamase produced by staphylococci is relatively narrow spectrum and acts primarily as a pencillinase. It is plasmid-encoded and generally inducible by beta-lactam antibiotics (7). Staphylococcal beta-lactamase is extracellular, and located at the cell membrane or released into the surroundings. It is encoded by the gene *blaZ* and regulated by two genes *blaR1-blaI* (8). BlaR1 is thought to act as a sensor-transducer protein, while BlaI acts as a repressor of *blaZ*.

Currently, more than 90% of unselected *S. aureus* and coagulase-negative staphylococci produce beta-lactamases. However, in one survey, approximately 15% of methicillin-susceptible staphylococci remained sensitive to penicillin (9),

L.G. Winston (✉)
Department of Medicine, Division of Infectious Diseases, University of California, San Francisco, Hospital Epidemiologist, San Francisco General Hospital, San Francisco, CA, USA
lisa.winston@ucsf.edu

D.L. Mayers (ed.), *Antimicrobial Drug Resistance*,
DOI 10.1007/978-1-60327-595-8_50, © Humana Press, a part of Springer Science+Business Media, LLC 2009

and penicillin may still be used in staphylococcal infections when susceptibility has been documented.

2.2 Methicillin and Other Beta-Lactams

Methicillin, the prototype penicillinase-resistant penicillin, became available in 1959 to treat staphylococci resistant to penicillin. Methicillin is one of several semisynthetic penicillins with bulky side chains, such that the antibiotic undergoes very slow hydrolysis by the staphylococcal beta-lactamase. However, in 1961, a few methicillin-resistant *S. aureus* (MRSA) isolates had already been reported in Britain (10). By the late 1960s, MRSA isolates were found in countries around the world. Methicillin is no longer in use clinically, having been replaced with nafcillin and oxacillin in the United States. However, the term MRSA persists to describe *S. aureus* isolates resistant to all currently available beta-lactam antibiotics, including cephalosporins and carbapenems.

Resistance to methicillin in staphylococci is mediated by the gene *mecA*. The *mecA* gene encodes a penicillin-binding protein, PBP2a (also known as PBP2′), which has low affinity for beta-lactam antibiotics (11). When beta-lactam antibiotics are present and bound to normal staphylococcal PBPs, PBP2a can substitute as a transpeptidase, even at high beta-

lactam concentrations. The *mecA* gene is regulated by two genes, *mecR1* and *mecI*. The *mecA* regulatory genes are highly related to the regulatory genes of *blaZ*, and BlaR1 and BlaI can also regulate *mecA* transcription (12, 13). The origin of *mecA* is not clear, but it remains highly conserved among human staphylococcal species (14–16), suggesting relatively recent acquisition of the gene. A gene similar to *mecA* has been found in methicillin-susceptible *S. sciuri*, a rodent staphylococcal species, and appears to be part of the normal chromosome (17, 18).

The *mecA* gene is carried on an element termed staphylococcal cassette chromosome *mec* (SCC*mec*). SCC elements without a *mec* determinant have been found in coagulase negative staphylococci (19, 20). In addition to *mecA*, SCC*mec* contains two site-specific recombinase genes: cassette chromosome recombinases A and B (called *ccrA* and *ccrB*) (21). The recombinase genes encode enzymes that mediate precise excision and site and orientation-specific insertion of SCC*mec* in the *S. aureus* chromosome. This is postulated to play a role in the horizontal transmission of *mecA* within and among staphylococcal species (21, 22).

Four types of SCC*mec* have been identified in *S. aureus*. Types I–III were identified in a worldwide collection of hospital strains, and range from approximately 34 to 67 kb in size (23). Types II and III may also carry genes encoding resistance to other antibiotics. Type IV SCC*mec*, the most recently described, is a smaller element (approximately

Table 1 Antimicrobial resistance genes and mechanisms in Staphylococci

Antimicrobial	Gene	Mechanism
Beta-lactams	*blaZ*	Hydrolysis of beta-lactam ring
	mecA	Low affinity PBP
Vancomycin	Several chromosomal mutations (?)	VISA: thickened cell wall (?)
	vanA	VRSA: alternate ligase produces altered peptidoglycan target
Macrolides	*msrA*	Efflux
	erm genes (inducible, constitutive)	Altered ribosomal target site
Clindamycin	*erm* genes (constitutive)	Altered ribosomal target site
	linA	Nucleotidyltransferase inactivates drug
Streptogramins A	*vgaA*, *vgaB*	Efflux
	vat genes	Acetylation of drug
Streptogramins B	*erm* genes (constitutive)	Altered ribosomal target site
	vgb	Lyase inactivates drug
Aminoglycosides	Multiple	Primarily drug inactivation
Sulfonamides	Chromosomal mutation DHPS	Altered DHPS target
Trimethoprim	*dfrA*, chromosomal mutation DHFR	Altered DHFR target
Tetracyclines	*tetK* (not minocycline)	Efflux
	tetL	Protection of ribosomal target
Fluoroquinolones	Point mutation *grlA* and/or *gyrA*	Altered topoisomerase IV target and/or altered DNA gyrase target
	norA (norfloxacin, ciprofloxacin)	Efflux
Rifampin	Point mutation *rpoB*	Altered target RNA polymerase
Linezolid	Point mutation 23S rRNA	Altered ribosomal target
Daptomycin	Unknown	Unknown

20–25 kb) initially found in strains associated with community-onset MRSA (24, 25). These community strains tend to be more susceptible to non-beta-lactam antibiotics than are healthcare-associated MRSA.

MRSA worldwide appear to be descended from a limited number of ancestral genotypes (26, 27). From studies using multilocus sequence typing, it is presumed that only a small number of genetic backgrounds are hospitable for *mecA* and can continue to disseminate widely after acquisition of the resistance gene (28).

2.3 Vancomycin

Vancomycin, a glycopeptide antibiotic, became available in the mid-1950s. Vancomycin inhibits synthesis of cell wall peptidoglycan by binding to the C-terminal of the cell wall precursor pentapeptide. After 40 years of use, the first isolate of *S. aureus* with reduced susceptibility to vancomycin was isolated from a child in Japan (29). The organism demonstrated a vancomycin minimum inhibitory concentration (MIC) of 8 μg/mL, placing it in the category of intermediate vancomycin resistance (VISA). By the guidelines of the National Committee for Clinical Laboratory Standards, intermediate resistance to vancomycin is defined as an MIC 8–16 μg/mL, and resistance is defined as an MIC ≥ 32 μg/mL. VISA isolates continue to be reported sporadically (30–33), but remain relatively uncommon.

The mechanism of resistance in VISA relates to changes in the cell wall. Electron microscopy has shown a thicker layer of extracellular material in VISA isolates, compared with MRSA controls (34). The cell wall components are less tightly cross-linked, and isolates have increased rates of autolysis (35, 36). Several loss-of-function mutations may explain the changes in peptidoglycan synthesis (37). The thickened cell wall may act to sequester vancomycin in its outer layers, away from the cytoplasmic membrane.

Coincident with the isolation of VISA, heterogeneous vancomycin-resistant *S. aureus* (hVISA) strains were described in Japan (38). The hVISA strains appear susceptible to vancomycin with conventional testing, but contain subpopulations with vancomycin MICs in the intermediately resistant range. VISA strains may arise from hVISA, usually in the presence of selective antibiotic pressure. Labor-intensive population analysis techniques are used to identify hVISA, but these tests have not been standardized and are not routinely performed (39). Most hVISA strains are methicillin-resistant, but the hVISA phenotype has also been described in methicillin-susceptible *S. aureus* (MSSA) (40). Challenges in detection of hVISA make precise estimates of prevalence difficult, but these strains are uncommon in most settings and currently account for a minority of clinical fail-

ures associated with vancomycin therapy for *S. aureus* (39, 41). Clinical vancomycin failure may be associated with the group II polymorphism at the accessory gene regulator (*agr*) locus in strains that appear vancomycin-susceptible, as well as in VISA and hVISA strains (42).

Although it was known that vancomycin resistance genes could be transferred in the laboratory from *Enterococcus faecalis* to *S. aureus* (43), high-level vancomycin-resistance in *S. aureus* (VRSA) was not reported until 2002 (44). Since the initial report, several other VRSA strains have been isolated (45, 46). The *vanA* gene complex, which mediates high-level glycopeptide resistance in enterococci, was detected in the VRSA isolates confirmed to date. VanA is a ligase that, in enterococci, allows the formation of a terminal D-alanyl-D-lactate in peptidoglycan, in place of the native D-ala-D-ala to which vancomycin binds. At least two of the patients from whom VRSA were isolated also harbored vancomycin-resistant enterococci (44, 46). The VRSA isolates detected to date in the United States are methicillin-resistant and contain the *mecA* gene. In *S. aureus*, the *vanA* gene complex appears to confer changes in the cell wall similar to those seen in vancomycin-resistant enterococci, and *mecA* and *vanA* seem to function independently (47).

To date, VRSA strains have been susceptible to other antibiotics, including linezolid, minocycline, quinupristin–dalfopristin, and trimethoprim/sulfamethoxazole. Person-to-person transmission of VRSA has not been identified, and the isolates do not appear to be epidemiologically linked. In at least one patient, VRSA arose in the absence of vancomycin selective pressure (48).

2.4 Macrolides, Lincosamides, and Streptogramins

Macrolides, lincosamides, and streptogramin B (MLS$_B$) antibiotics are structurally dissimilar, but are grouped together due to a common mechanism of action. Macrolides include the drugs erythromycin, clarithromycin, and azithromycin. Clindamycin is the only lincosamide used clinically at this time. Quinupristin, combined with streptogramin A dalfopristin, is the only streptogramin B antibiotic used in the United States. These drugs bind to the 50S ribosomal subunit in susceptible bacteria and inhibit protein synthesis by blocking transpeptidation or translocation. Three related erythromycin ribosomal methylase genes, *ermA*, *ermB*, and *ermC*, alter the ribosomal target site and confer MLS$_B$ resistance (49, 50).

The *erm* genes are carried on plasmids and transposable elements, and may be produced in an inducible or constitutive manner (51–53). When the methylase is constitutively produced, strains will demonstrate in vitro resistance to macrolides, clindamycin, and streptogramin B antibiotics. *S. aureus* strains with the inducible MLS$_B$ phenotype have traditionally been considered resistant to macrolides that induce *erm* expression, and susceptible to clindamycin and streptogramins B (54). However, strains with inducible *erm* production may also develop resistance to clindamycin and streptogramins B, and clindamycin failures have been reported (55, 56). The double-disk diffusion test (D test) can be used to distinguish MLS resistance from efflux mechanisms (55, 56) that do not confer resistance to clindamycin.

The *msrA* gene confers inducible resistance to macrolides and to streptogramins B via an efflux mechanism (57). This type of resistance appears to be more common in coagulase-negative staphylococci than in *S. aureus* (58). Specific resistance to clindamycin is conferred by the *linA* gene, the product of which acts as an *o*-nucleotidyltransferase, which inactivates lincosamides (59).

Resistance to streptogramin A antibiotics can be mediated by the *vgaA* and *vgaB* genes, which encode ATP-binding proteins that likely promote drug efflux (60,61). Streptogramin A resistance can also be due to genes *vatA*, *vatB*, and *vatC*, which encode drug-inactivating acetyltransferases (62–64). Streptogramin B antibiotics can be inactivated by a lyase produced by the *vgb* gene (65). At least one gene mediating streptogramin A resistance is required before in vitro resistance to the combination antibiotic quinupristin–dalfopristin develops (66). However, quinpristin–dalfopristin may be less efficacious when streptogramin B resistance is present (67).

2.5 Aminoglycosides

Aminoglycosides such as gentamicin are often used to treat serious staphylococcal infections in conjunction with other antimicrobial agents, particularly those active against the bacterial cell wall. These antibiotics bind to the bacterial 30S ribosomal subunit. Binding interrupts protein synthesis and may also cause aberrant protein sythesis (68).

Resistance to aminoglycosides is primarily mediated by drug modification and inactivation. Enzymes encoded by resistance genes include phosphotransferases, acetyltransferases, and adenyltransferases (69, 70). One protein with both acetyltransferase and phosphotransferase activities has been well characterized, and confers high-level resistance to all aminoglycosides (71). Aminoglycoside resistance genes are carried on plasmids and transposons, and may be integrated into the bacterial chromosome.

2.6 Trimethoprim–Sulfamethoxazole

Trimethoprim and sulfamethoxazole are most commonly used in combination, as they act synergistically to inhibit sequential steps in bacterial folic acid synthesis. Sulfamethoxazole, an analog of para-amino-benzoic acid, competitively inhibits the enzyme dihydropteroate synthase (DHPS), while trimethoprim competitively inhibits dihydrofolate reductase (DHFR).

Early in the use of these drugs, resistance to sulfonamides was described as resulting from an overproduction of para-amino-benzoic acid (72). More recently, chromosomal mutations resulting in altered DHPS have been reported (73, 74). High-level trimethoprim resistance is mediated by a single amino acid substitution in a DHFR gene, which is typically plasmid encoded. The trimethoprim-resistant DHFR seen in *S. aureus* and several species of coagulase-negative staphylococci, termed *dfrA*, probably evolved from *S. epidermidis* (75). Lower-level trimethoprim resistance may be mediated by a similar mutation in the *S. aureus* chromosomal DHFR gene (76).

2.7 Tetracyclines

Tetracyclines inhibit bacterial protein synthesis by binding to the 30S ribosomal subunit and blocking the association with aminoacyl-tRNA. Two general mechanisms of resistance to this class of drugs have been described, and may be present in the same isolate. Active efflux is mediated by the inducible genes *tetK* and *tetL*, which are typically located on plasmids. The *tetK* resistance gene may be found without other tetracycline resistance determinants, and these isolates are resistant to tetracycline but remain susceptible to minocycline (77). The chromosomally encoded *tetM* gene is also inducible (78), and confers resistance to all currently available tetracyclines by a proposed mechanism of ribosomal protection (79, 80). When resistance to tetracycline is demonstrated in vitro, resistance to doxycycline should also be assumed (77).

2.8 Fluoroquinolones

Systemically active fluoroquinolones became widely available in the mid-1980s, and staphylococcal resistance to this class is increasingly common. Fluoroquinolones inhibit two enzymes, DNA gyrase and topoisomerase IV, both of which are critical for DNA replication. In *S. aureus*, older fluoroquinolones primarily target topoisomerase IV, while some newer drugs, such as gatifloxacin and moxifloxacin, appear to target DNA gyrase and topoisomerase IV equally (81). DNA gyrase is composed of two subunits GyrA and GyrB, and topoisomerase IV is composed of homologous subunits ParC and ParE (also known as GrlA and GrlB in *S. aureus*) (82, 83). Most resistance mutations occur within the quinolone resistance-determining regions of the genes *gyrA* and *grlA*, and reduce drug binding to the target (84, 85). Single mutations in *grlA* confer detectable resistance to older fluoroquinolones such as ciprofloxacin, while more potent fluoroquinolones may appear susceptible, at least by laboratory criteria (83, 86). When mutations are present in both DNA gyrase and topoisomerase IV, resistance to all fluoroquinolones is likely (87). In *S. aureus*, moderate decreases in susceptibility to some fluoroquinolones, especially norfloxacin and ciprofloxacin, may be mediated by the gene product of *norA*, a multidrug efflux pump (88, 89).

2.9 Rifampin

Rifampin is a member of the rifamycin family of antimicrobials that inhibit the beta subunit of bacterial RNA polymerase, preventing chain initiation (90). The beta subunit is encoded by the *rpoB* gene, and point mutations in this gene occur at several sites after exposure to rifampin (91). Mutations develop rapidly when rifampin is used as a single agent, but can also develop when rifampin is used in combination therapy.

2.10 Linezolid

Linezolid is the first member of the oxazolidinone class of antibiotics to become available. Cross-resistance with other antibiotic classes has not been described. Linezolid binds to the bacterial 23S rRNA of the 50S ribosomal subunit and inhibits formation of the initiation complex, thereby blocking protein synthesis (92). At present, almost all *S. aureus* remain susceptible to linezolid. However, clinical resistance has developed after exposure to the drug, and is associated with point mutations in the domain V region of the 23S rRNA gene (93, 94). Bacteria contain multiple copies of the 23S rRNA gene, and loss of wild-type copies may also contribute to resistance (93).

2.11 Daptomycin

Daptomycin represents a new class of antibiotic agents with a unique mechanism of action. It is a cyclic lipopeptide, active against Gram-positive bacteria. Daptomycin binds to the cytoplasmic membrane and disrupts the membrane potential, probably via ion conduction (95). Most *S. aureus* are susceptible to daptomycin, and specific resistance mechanisms have not yet been described. Daptomycin may be more active against vancomycin-sensitive staphylococci than against strains with reduced vancomycin susceptibility. Results of in vitro susceptibility testing may vary, depending upon the calcium concentration in the media used (96, 97).

2.12 Small Colony Variants

Small colony variants (SCVs) have long been recognized in *S. aureus*, and may lead to organism persistence and relapse of infection, particularly in patients with osteomyelitis and cystic fibrosis (98). SCVs grow slowly in the laboratory as pinpoint colonies and can be difficult to isolate, especially when mixed with a normally growing *S. aureus* population (99). SCVs are defective in electron transport, and are selected in the presence of certain antibiotics, such as aminoglycosides, whose import into the organism is impaired (100). SCVs may be resistant to a number of antibiotic classes when adherent to a biopolymer surface or when organisms are intracellular (99).

3 Epidemiology of Antimicrobial Resistance

Estimates of the prevalence of staphylococcal resistance to selected antibiotics in the United States are shown in Table 2. It should be noted that resistance to any given antibiotic is not independent, and MRSA are much more likely than MSSA to be resistant to non-beta-lactam antibiotics. For example, in one large hospital-based survey, more than 95% of MSSA were susceptible to ciprofloxacin, while less than 10% of MRSA were susceptible (1). However, these trends are somewhat different in healthcare-associated versus community-associated MRSA isolates.

Until recently, MRSA was largely confined to the healthcare setting. Although community outbreaks were noted in the 1980s, they were typically associated with defined risk factors such as intravenous drug use, recent hospital admission, or recent use of antibiotics (101–104). Risk factors for isolation of MRSA in hospitalized patients were also well defined and

Table 2 Estimated prevalence of Staphylococcal resistance to selected antibiotics

	Staphylococcus aureus resistant (%)	Coagulase-negative staphylococci resistant (%)
Nafcillin	40–45	75–80
Erythromycin	50–55	60–70
Clindamycin	30–35	35–40
Trimethoprim–sulfamethoxazole	5–10	30–40
Ciprofloxacin	40–45	50–55
Later-generation fluoroquinolones	30–35	20–40
Gentamicin	10	20–25
Vancomycin	~0	~0
Quinupristin/dalfopristin	~0	~0
Linezolid	~0	~0

Estimates based on laboratory data from North American hospitals 2001–2002 (184, 185)

included prior exposure to antibiotics, recent surgery, and admission to an intensive care unit (105). Based on National Nosocomial Infections Surveillance (NNIS) data, average rates of MRSA in intensive care units continue to rise at a rapid pace, reaching nearly 60% in 2003 (106). Parallel to this rise in the healthcare arena, an increase in the prevalence of community MRSA has been appreciated.

In the 1990s, it became apparent that MRSA could be a true community pathogen. Attention was focused on this issue by a report of the deaths of four children without traditional risk for MRSA (107). In addition, these MRSA strains were noted to be susceptible to all antibiotics except beta-lactams. Other reports have confirmed that community strains of MRSA are more susceptible to non-beta-lactam antibiotics, compared with usually multidrug-resistant hospital strains (108, 109). Community MRSA have now been reported in a number of studies in adults and children without known risk factors for MRSA (110–112). Daycare center attendance and household spread are more recently implicated risk factors (113, 114). Although many studies suggest that MRSA is increasing in the community, the exact prevalence is unknown and may remain low among persons who have had no contact with the healthcare system (115).

Community MRSA strains have other biologic differences from healthcare-associated strains. As discussed above, community strains tend to carry SCC*mec* type IV, which is smaller than the other cassette types and does not carry with it other drug resistance determinants (24, 116). Community MRSA strains typically carry the locus for producing Panton-Valentine leukocidin (PVL) (117). PVL is associated with skin and soft tissue infections and necrotizing pneumonia, and is likely one of the virulence factors allowing community MRSA strains to affect otherwise healthy persons (118, 119).

4 Clinical Implications of Antimicrobial Resistance

The increasing frequency of antimicrobial resistance in staphylococci has had substantial effects on treatment of these common infections. Resistance to beta-lactams, in particular, has changed both the initial selection of antibiotics and definitive therapy. Beta-lactam agents are more effective than vancomycin in serious *S. aureus* infections in animals (120, 121), and the clinical response to vancomycin therapy in humans may be delayed and complicated by frequent relapses (122–124). Observational data have clearly demonstrated that nafcillin is more efficacious than vancomycin for therapy of MSSA bacteremia (125). However, at present, vancomycin is the drug of choice for treating most serious infections with methicillin-resistant staphylococci. Although not all studies are in agreement, outcomes in MRSA bacter-

emia are probably worse than those in MSSA bacteremia (126–129), and the inability to use beta-lactam drugs likely contributes to these observations.

4.1 Initial Therapy: S. aureus

Rates of methicillin resistance amongst staphylococci are high enough in most settings that non-beta-lactam antibiotics, such as vancomycin, are appropriate initial therapy when serious staphylococcal infections are suspected. A switch to a beta-lactam should be made if methicillin susceptibility is established. When oral therapy is desirable, usually for less serious conditions such as skin and soft tissue infections, multiple factors may be considered in the initial selection of therapy. In patients with few risk factors for MRSA, beta-lactam agents such as first-generation cephalosporins and dicloxacillin are preferred, as they are potent, well tolerated, and have excellent activity against beta-hemolytic streptococci, which also cause skin and soft tissue infections, especially cellulitis. The threshold to culture infected sites to obtain organism susceptibilities should be low, especially if patients are not responding to initial antimicrobial therapy.

In patients with risk factors for MRSA (e.g. previous hospitalization, receipt of antibiotics, known high-prevalence population) with infections amenable to oral antibiotics, initial non-beta-lactam agents can be considered. Most *S. aureus*, including MRSA, are susceptible to trimethoprim–sulfamethoxazole. Doxycycline and minocycline are alternatives. Fluroquinolones, erythromycin, and clinidamycin are less reliable in the absence of susceptibility data, especially against MRSA. At this time, essentially all *S. aureus* are susceptible to linezolid, but this drug is expensive and may be associated with thrombocytopenia, especially when used for an extended period.

4.2 Definitive Therapy: MSSA

For some serious staphylococcal infections, a penicillinase-resistant penicillin, e.g. nafcillin, appears to have the greatest efficacy. In animal models of endocarditis with *S. aureus*, penicillinase-resistant penicillins may reduce bacterial titers in vegetations more rapidly than first-generation cephalosporins (130, 131). Case series have reported failures of cephalosporin treatment in *S. aureus* endocarditis, often with later response to a penicillinase-resistant penicillin (132 134). However, outcomes with *S. aureus* osteomyelitis are similar when cefazolin or ceftriaxone is used, compared with a penicillinase-resistant pencillin, while vancomycin is not as effective (135). In general, a pencillinase-resistant

Table 3 Regimens for the treatment of serious *S. aureus* infections

Methicillin-sensitive

Uncomplicated bacteremia with removable focus of infection
Nafcillin 1.5–2 g IV every 4 h for 2 weeks
Cefazolin 1 g IV every 8 h for 2 weeks
(Shorter course may be considered with negative transesophageal echocardiogram)

Tricuspid valve endocarditis in an injection drug user
Nafcillin 2 g IV every 4 h + gentamicin 1 mg/kg IV every 8 h for 2 weeks
Nafcillin 2 g IV every 4 h for 4 weeks

Aortic or mitral native valve endocarditis
Nafcillin 2 g IV every 4 h for 4–6 weeks +/− gentamicin 1 mg/kg IV every 8 h for the first 5 days

Prosthetic valve endocarditis
Nafcillin 2 g IV every 4 h for 6 weeks + gentamicin 1 mg/kg IV every 8 h for 2 weeks + rifampin 300 mg orally every 8 h for 6 weeks

Osteomyelitis
Nafcillin 2 g IV every 4 h for 6 weeks +/− rifampin 600 mg orally every day for 6 weeks
Cefazolin 1–2 g IV every 8 h for 6 weeks +/− rifampin 600 mg orally every day for 6 weeks
Ceftriaxone 2 g IV every day for 6 weeks +/− rifampin 600 mg orally every day for 6 weeks
(Oral agents including fluoroquinolones, beta-lactams, and clindamycin are acceptable in many cases, particularly when the origin is not hematogenous spread. Longer therapy may be needed, especially in chronic osteomyelitis or if orthopedic hardware is present. Consider addition of rifampin, especially when foreign material is present and cannot be removed. Rifampin may help prevent the emergence of drug resistance during therapy, e.g. with fluoroquinolones.)

Methicillin-resistant

Uncomplicated bacteremia with removeable focus of infection
Vancomycin 15 mg/kg IV every 12 h for 2 weeks
(Shorter course may be considered with negative transesophageal echocardiogram)

Tricuspid valve endocarditis in an injection drug user
Vancomycin 15 mg/kg IV every 12 h for 4 weeks

Aortic or mitral valve native endocarditis
Vancomycin 15 mg/kg every 12 h for 4–6 weeks

Prosthetic valve endocarditis
Vancomycin 15 mg/kg IV every 12 h for 6 weeks + gentamicin 1 mg/kg IV every 8 h for 2 weeks + rifampin 300 mg orally every 8 h for 6 weeks

Osteomyelitis
Vancomycin 15 mg/kg IV every 12 h for 6 weeks +/− rifampin 600 mg orally every day for 6 weeks
(Please see comments regarding therapy for MSSA osteomyelitis. With oral therapy, careful attention should be paid to the drug susceptibility of the isolate, as many MRSA are also resistant to non-beta-lactam antibiotics. Clindamycin should be avoided when erythromycin resistance is present. Experience with linezolid is limited.)

penicillin is preferred when meningitis or endocarditis is confirmed or suspected. In other cases, cephalosporins with potent anti-staphylococcal activity, such as cefazolin, are also effective and may have superior tolerability and convenience. Appropriate oral regimens for less serious MSSA infections include first-generation cephalosporins (e.g. cephalexin) and penicillinase-resistant penicillins such as dicloxacillin.

4.3 Definitive Therapy: MRSA

Though vancomycin became available in the 1950s, it was little used for twenty years because it offered no advantage over other antimicrobials (136). In the late 1970s, its use was reevaluated as resistant Gram-positive infections emerged in hospital settings (137, 138). Today, vancomycin remains the standard of care for treating serious MRSA infections,

despite concerns regarding slow response and the potential for clinical failures (124, 125). Although most *S. aureus*, including MRSA, are susceptible to trimethoprim–sulfamethoxazole, limited data suggest that treatment with vancomycin leads to superior outcomes in hospitalized patients (139). Quinupristin–dalfopristin appears similar to vancomycin in treating Gram-positive nosocomial pneumonia and complicated skin and soft tissue infections (140, 141). Results in treating catheter-related staphylococcal bacteremia are also comparable, although few patients have been studied (142). However, use of quinupristin–dalfopristin is limited due to its high cost and side effects, including phlebitis and myalgias. Daptomycin is an effective agent in skin and soft tissue infections, but is not indicated for the treatment of pneumonia (143). Studies are ongoing to assess its efficacy in *S. aureus* bacteremia and endocarditis. For oral therapy in less serious infections, choices include trimthoprim–sulfamethoxazole, minocycline or doxycycline, and fluoroquinolones when susceptibility is confirmed.

Linezolid is the only one of the new anti-staphylococcal drugs that is available in an oral formulation, in addition to a parenteral formulation. It is nearly 100% bioavailable, and has the potential to allow for oral therapy for serious and/or resistant staphylococcal infections. Linezolid has similar efficacy to vancomycin in treating various MRSA infections in both adults and children (144, 145). It may be superior to vancomycin in treating hospital-acquired MRSA pneumonia (146, 147), but additional studies are needed for confirmation. Traditional teaching holds that only bactericidal agents should be used for certain infections such as meningitis and endocarditis, and linezolid is bacteriostatic. Linezolid has been successfully used in some cases of *S. aureus* endocarditis and central nervous system infections (148–150), but failures have also been reported (151). The disadvantages of linezolid include its cost and the potential development of resistance, especially if it is used inappropriately. Reversible myelosuppression, especially thrombocytopenia, is a known adverse effect (152), but the risk with vancomycin therapy may be comparable (153, 154).

4.4 Combination Therapy

Combination therapy is theoretically beneficial if it is more efficacious than single-drug therapy and/or it can prevent the development of resistance during therapy. For staphylococcal infections, combination therapy has relatively few confirmed indications. The addition of gentamicin to nafcillin in the treatment of *S. aureus* endocarditis has been shown to modestly decrease the duration of bacteremia, but did not otherwise improve morbidity or mortality (155). In patients with staphylococcal endocarditis who will be treated with an antistaphylococcal penicillin for 4–6 weeks (156), gentamicin may be added for the first three to five days. The combination of a penicillinase-resistant penicillin plus an aminoglycoside for 2 weeks has been shown to be effective therapy in *S. aureus* tricuspid valve endocarditis in injection drug users (122, 157, 158). However, one study suggested that most patients with tricuspid valve endocarditis will be cured after 2 weeks of therapy with an antistaphylococcal penicillin alone (159). Prosthetic valve endocarditis is a disease with high morbidity and mortality, and is difficult to cure with antibiotics alone. Triple-drug therapy with vancomycin, gentamicin, and rifampin is recommended for the treatment of methcillin-resistant coagulase-negative staphylococci causing prosthetic valve endocarditis (160, 161), and these data have been extrapolated to *S. aureus*. Rifampin is thought to penetrate infected foreign material and valve microabscesses, but must be used in combination to prevent the emergence of resistance.

The combination of a fluoroquinolone plus rifampin has been studied in several types of staphylococcal infections. In selected cases, infections of stable orthopedic implants may be cured without removing the hardware, by prolonged therapy with ciprofloxacin and rifampin (162, 163). Ciprofloxacin monotherapy has been less successful, and is associated with the development of fluoroquinolone resistance (163). This approach is indicated only in early infections managed with initial debridement, and data regarding MRSA are lacking. Ciprofloxacin plus rifampin may be an alternative for treating right-sided *S. aureus* endocarditis in injection drug users when patients can be closely monitored (164, 165). However, animal data have shown some potential for antagonism between ciprofloxacin and rifampin (166).

A variety of case reports document clearance of staphylococcal bacteremia and clinical response with the addition of rifampin or gentamicin in patients receiving monotherapy (156, 167–172). However, switches to alternative monotherapy may also be effective, and there are no compelling comparative data on which to base recommendations for specific regimens in the event of clinical failure.

4.5 Use of Fluoroquinolones

Fluoroquinolones are an option in several serious infections due to *S. aureus*, but their extensive usage for many indications may be one factor contributing to the increasing prevalence of MRSA. Although not every study has uncovered an association (173), evidence is accumulating that exposure to both ciprofloxacin and levofloxacin is a risk factor for isolation of MRSA (174–178). Part of the explanation may be that MRSA are much more likely to be fluoroquinolone-resistant than MSSA, so the drugs exert a selective pressure. *S. aureus* strains with heterogeneous resistance to oxacillin grown in the presence of a fluoroquinolone develop full oxacillin resistance, in addition to a modest increase in fluoroquinolone minimum inhibitory concentration. It is postulated that fluoroquinolones inhibit or kill oxacillin-susceptible subpopulations, leaving surviving populations that are more resistant to oxacillin and fluoroquinolones (179). Exposure to subinhibitory levels of ciprofloxacin also appears to induce expression of fibronectin-binding proteins in *S. aureus*, which may promote host colonization (180, 181). Thus, exposure to fluoroquinolones may lead to host colonization *S. aureus*, but fluroquinolone susceptible strains are selectively eliminated (174). Whether newer fluoroquinolones, such as moxifloxacin and gatifloxacin, will have the same effect is less clear.

4.6 Vancomycin Resistance

As described above, intermediate and full resistance to vancomycin is uncommon at present, and future prevalence is difficult to predict. Patients infected with *S. aureus* with reduced susceptibility to vancomycin may have worse outcomes than those infected with MRSA susceptible to vancomycin, but data are necessarily sparse, given the number of infections reported to date (30). Fortunately, *S. aureus* with reduced susceptibility to vancomycin are generally sensitive to several other antibiotics, including trimethoprim–sulfamethoxazole, quinupristin–dalfopristin, linezolid, tetracyclines, and probably daptomycin. Detection of VISA strains requires specific laboratory procedures (182), and clinicians must maintain a level of suspicion for *S. aureus* with reduced vancomycin susceptibility, so that patients receive appropriate therapy as quickly as possible.

4.7 Coagulase-Negative Staphylococci

Although coagulase-negative staphylococci are normal skin flora and frequent culture contaminants, they are also common causes of infections related to indwelling devices. *S. epidermidis* is the species most commonly identified in healthcare-associated infections. One of the key factors in *S. epidermidis* colonization of foreign bodies is the ability to attach to polymer surfaces and then to form a multilayered biofilm (4). Antimicrobial resistance has traditionally been more prevalent in coagulase-negative staphylococci than in *S. aureus*, perhaps because these organisms are usually isolated in the healthcare setting where antibiotic use is frequent. Indeed, coagulase-negative staphylococci were the first organisms in which acquired resistance to glycopeptide antibiotics was reported (136), but vancomycin resistance in coagulase-negative staphylococci is still uncommon. Susceptible coagulase-negative staphylococci can be treated with beta-lactam antibiotics, but vancomycin is commonly used due to widespread methicillin resistance. In most cases, an important feature of successfully treating infections associated with indwelling devices and implants is complete removal of the foreign material.

5 Conclusions

The increasing prevalence of resistance in staphylococci has changed the approach to the treatment of these organisms, and has raised questions about the adequacy of future therapy. Of particular concern is the recent dramatic rise of methicillin-resistance in community-associated *S. aureus*, and the emergence of *S. aureus* with reduced susceptibility and frank resistance to vancomycin. The durability of newly approved drugs is not yet clear, and the availability of new agents may not keep pace with the loss of traditional antimicrobials due to emerging resistance (183). Ideal new antibiotics would (1) have a high intrinsic barrier to resistance;

(2) would be effective in diseases such as endocarditis and meningitis where "bactericidal" activity is presumed to be required; (3) would not be prohibitively costly; (4) would be convenient to administer; and (5) would have few serious side effects. Unfortunately, it is unlikely that any new agent will fit all these criteria. At this time, methicillin resistance is common enough in most settings for it to be presumed in any patient with a reasonable potential for serious staphylococcal disease. The clinical implications of vancomycin resistance in *S. aureus* remain to be determined.

References

1. Diekema DJ, Pfaller MA, Jones RN, et al. Trends in antimicrobial susceptibility of bacterial pathogens isolated from patients with bloodstream infections in the USA, Canada and Latin America. SENTRY Participants Group. Int J Antimicrob Agents 2000;13:257–271
2. Fowler VG, Jr, Olsen MK, Corey GR, et al. Clinical identifiers of complicated *Staphylococcus aureus* bacteremia. Arch Intern Med 2003;163:2066–2072
3. Huebner J, Goldmann DA. Coagulase-negative staphylococci: role as pathogens. Annu Rev Med 1999;50:223–236
4. von Eiff C, Peters G, Heilmann C. Pathogenesis of infections due to coagulase-negative staphylococci. Lancet Infect Dis 2002;2:677–685
5. Kirby WMM. Extraction of a highly potent penicillin inactivator from penicillin resistant staphylococci. Science 1944;99:452–453
6. Chambers HF. The changing epidemiology of *Staphylococcus aureus*? Emerg Infect Dis 2001;7:178–182
7. Chambers HF. Penicillins. In: Mandell GL, Bennett JE, Dolin R, eds. *Mandell, Douglas, and Bennett's Principles and Practice of Infectious Diseases*. Philadelphia, PA: Churchill Livingstone, 2000:261–274
8. Asheshov EH, Dyke KG. Regulation of the synthesis of penicillinase in diploids of *Staphylococcus aureus*. Biochem Biophys Res Commun 1968;30:213–218
9. Marshall SA, Wilke WW, Pfaller MA, Jones RN. *Staphylococcus aureus* and coagulase-negative staphylococci from blood stream infections: frequency of occurrence, antimicrobial susceptibility, and molecular (mecA) characterization of oxacillin resistance in the SCOPE program. Diagn Microbiol Infect Dis 1998;30:205–214
10. Jevons MP. Celbenin-resistant staphylococci. Br Med J 1961;1:124–125
11. Reynolds PE, Brown DF. Penicillin-binding proteins of beta-lactam-resistant strains of *Staphylococcus aureus*. Effect of growth conditions. FEBS Lett 1985;192:28–32
12. Ryffel C, Kayser FH, Berger-Bachi B. Correlation between regulation of mecA transcription and expression of methicillin resistance in staphylococci. Antimicrob Agents Chemother 1992;36:25–31
13. Hackbarth CJ, Chambers HF. blaI and blaR1 regulate beta-lactamase and PBP 2a production in methicillin-resistant *Staphylococcus aureus*. Antimicrob Agents Chemother 1993;37:1144–1149
14. Ryffel C, Tesch W, Birch-Machin I, et al. Sequence comparison of mecA genes isolated from methicillin-resistant *Staphylococcus aureus* and *Staphylococcus epidermidis*. Gene 1990;94:137–138
15. Archer GL, Niemeyer DM, Thanassi JA, Pucci MJ. Dissemination among staphylococci of DNA sequences associated with methicillin resistance. Antimicrob Agents Chemother 1994;38:447–454
16. Ubukata K, Nonoguchi R, Song MD, Matsuhashi M, Konno M. Homology of mecA gene in methicillin-resistant *Staphylococcus*

haemolyticus and *Staphylococcus simulans* to that of *Staphylococcus aureus*. Antimicrob Agents Chemother 1990;34:170–172

17. Wu S, Piscitelli C, de Lencastre H, Tomasz A. Tracking the evolutionary origin of the methicillin resistance gene: cloning and sequencing of a homologue of *mecA* from a methicillin susceptible strain of *Staphylococcus sciuri*. Microb Drug Resist 1996;2:435–441

18. Couto I, de Lencastre H, Severina E, et al. Ubiquitous presence of a *mecA* homologue in natural isolates of *Staphylococcus sciuri*. Microb Drug Resist 1996;2:377–391

19. Katayama Y, Takeuchi F, Ito T, et al. Identification in methicillin-susceptible *Staphylococcus hominis* of an active primordial mobile genetic element for the staphylococcal cassette chromosome *mec* of methicillin-resistant *Staphylococcus aureus*. J Bacteriol 2003;185:2711–2722

20. Mongkolrattanothai K, Boyle S, Murphy TV, Daum RS. Novel non-*mecA*-containing staphylococcal chromosomal cassette composite island containing pbp4 and tagF genes in a commensal staphylococcal species: a possible reservoir for antibiotic resistance islands in *Staphylococcus aureus*. Antimicrob Agents Chemother 2004;48:1823–1836

21. Katayama Y, Ito T, Hiramatsu K. A new class of genetic element, staphylococcus cassette chromosome *mec*, encodes methicillin resistance in *Staphylococcus aureus*. Antimicrob Agents Chemother 2000;44:1549–1555

22. Hanssen AM, Kjeldsen G, Sollid JU. Local variants of staphylococcal cassette chromosome *mec* in sporadic methicillin-resistant *Staphylococcus aureus* and methicillin-resistant coagulase-negative staphylococci: evidence of horizontal gene transfer? Antimicrob Agents Chemother 2004;48:285–296

23. Ito T, Katayama Y, Asada K, et al. Structural comparison of three types of staphylococcal cassette chromosome *mec* integrated in the chromosome in methicillin-resistant *Staphylococcus aureus*. Antimicrob Agents Chemother 2001;45:1323–1336

24. Daum RS, Ito T, Hiramatsu K, et al. A novel methicillin-resistance cassette in community-acquired methicillin-resistant *Staphylococcus aureus* isolates of diverse genetic backgrounds. J Infect Dis 2002;186:1344–1347

25. Ma XX, Ito T, Tiensasitorn C, et al. Novel type of staphylococcal cassette chromosome *mec* identified in community-acquired methicillin-resistant *Staphylococcus aureus* strains. Antimicrob Agents Chemother 2002;46:1147–1152

26. Enright MC, Day NP, Davies CE, Peacock SJ, Spratt BG. Multilocus sequence typing for characterization of methicillin-resistant and methicillin-susceptible clones of *Staphylococcus aureus*. J Clin Microbiol 2000;38:1008–1015

27. Enright MC, Robinson DA, Randle G, Feil EJ, Grundmann H, Spratt BG. The evolutionary history of methicillin-resistant *Staphylococcus aureus* (MRSA). Proc Natl Acad Sci U S A 2002;99: 7687–7692

28. Robinson DA, Enright MC. Multilocus sequence typing and the evolution of methicillin-resistant *Staphylococcus aureus*. Clin Microbiol Infect 2004;10:92–97

29. Centers for Disease Control and Prevention. Reduced susceptibility of *Staphylococcus aureus* to vancomycin – Japan, 1996. MMWR Morb Mortal Wkly Rep 1997;46:624–626

30. Fridkin SK, Hageman J, McDougal LK, et al. Epidemiological and microbiological characterization of infections caused by *Staphylococcus aureus* with reduced susceptibility to vancomycin, United States, 1997–2001. Clin Infect Dis 2003;36:429–439

31. Centers for Disease Control and Prevention. *Staphylococcus aureus* with reduced susceptibility to vancomycin – United States, 1997. MMWR Morb Mortal Wkly Rep 1997;46:765–766

32. Centers for Disease Control and Prevention. *Staphylococcus aureus* with reduced susceptibility to vancomycin – Illinois, 1999. MMWR Morb Mortal Wkly Rep 2000;48:1165–1167

33. Ploy MC, Grelaud C, Martin C, de Lumley L, Denis F. First clinical isolate of vancomycin-intermediate *Staphylococcus aureus* in a French hospital. Lancet 1998;351:1212

34. Smith TL, Pearson ML, Wilcox KR, et al. Emergence of vancomycin resistance in *Staphylococcus aureus*. Glycopeptide-intermediate *Staphylococcus aureus* working group. N Engl J Med 1999;340:493–501

35. Hanaki H, Labischinski H, Inaba Y, Kondo N, Murakami H, Hiramatsu K. Increase in glutamine-non-amidated muropeptides in the peptidoglycan of vancomycin-resistant *Staphylococcus aureus* strain Mu50. J Antimicrob Chemother 1998;42:315–320

36. Cui L, Murakami H, Kuwahara-Arai K, Hanaki H, Hiramatsu K. Contribution of a thickened cell wall and its glutamine non-amidated component to the vancomycin resistance expressed by *Staphylococcus aureus* Mu50. Antimicrob Agents Chemother 2000;44:2276–2285

37. Avison MB, Bennett PM, Howe RA, Walsh TR. Preliminary analysis of the genetic basis for vancomycin resistance in *Staphylococcus aureus* strain Mu50. J Antimicrob Chemother 2002;49:255–260

38. Hiramatsu K, Aritaka N, Hanaki H, et al. Dissemination in Japanese hospitals of strains of *Staphylococcus aureus* heterogeneously resistant to vancomycin. Lancet 1997;350:1670–1673

39. Liu C, Chambers HF. *Staphylococcus aureus* with heterogeneous resistance to vancomycin: epidemiology, clinical significance, and critical assessment of diagnostic methods. Antimicrob Agents Chemother 2003;47:3040–3045

40. Bobin-Dubreux S, Reverdy ME, Nervi C, et al. Clinical isolate of vancomycin-heterointermediate *Staphylococcus aureus* susceptible to methicillin and in vitro selection of a vancomycin-resistant derivative. Antimicrob Agents Chemother 2001;45:349–352

41. Walsh TR, Howe RA. The prevalence and mechanisms of vancomycin resistance in *Staphylococcus aureus*. Annu Rev Microbiol 2002;56:657–675

42. Moise-Broder PA, Sakoulas G, Eliopoulos GM, Schentag JJ, Forrest A, Moellering RC, Jr. Accessory gene regulator group II polymorphism in methicillin-resistant *Staphylococcus aureus* is predictive of failure of vancomycin therapy. Clin Infect Dis 2004;38:1700–1705

43. Noble WC, Virani Z, Cree RG. Co-transfer of vancomycin and other resistance genes from *Enterococcus faecalis* NCTC 12201 to *Staphylococcus aureus*. FEMS Microbiol Lett 1992;72:195–198

44. Centers for Disease Control and Prevention. *Staphylococcus aureus* resistant to vancomycin – United States, 2002. MMWR Morb Mortal Wkly Rep 2002;51:565–567

45. Centers for Disease Control and Prevention. Vancomycin-resistant *Staphylococcus aureus* – New York, 2004. MMWR Morb Mortal Wkly Rep 2004;53:322–323

46. Centers for Disease Control and Prevention. Vancomycin-resistant *Staphylococcus aureus* – Pennsylvania, 2002. MMWR Morb Mortal Wkly Rep 2002;51:902

47. Severin A, Tabei K, Tenover F, Chung M, Clarke N, Tomasz A. High level oxacillin and vancomycin resistance and altered cell wall composition in *Staphylococcus aureus* carrying the staphylococcal *mecA* and the enterococcal *vanA* gene complex. J Biol Chem 2004;279:3398–3407

48. Whitener CJ, Park SY, Browne FA, et al. Vancomycin-resistant *Staphylococcus aureus* in the absence of vancomycin exposure. Clin Infect Dis 2004;38:1049–1055

49. Courvalin P, Ounissi H, Arthur M. Multiplicity of macrolide-lincosamide–streptogramin antibiotic resistance determinants. J Antimicrob Chemother 1985;16(Suppl A):91–100

50. Leclercq R, Courvalin P. Bacterial resistance to macrolide, lincosamide, and streptogramin antibiotics by target modification. Antimicrob Agents Chemother 1991;35:1267–1272

51. Oliveira SS, Murphy E, Gamon MR, Bastos MC. pRJ5: a naturally occurring *Staphylococcus aureus* plasmid expressing constitu-

tive macrolide-lincosamide–streptogramin B resistance contains a tandem duplication in the leader region of the *ermC* gene. J Gen Microbiol 1993;139(Pt 7):1461–1467

52. Catchpole I, Dyke KG. A *Staphylococcus aureus* plasmid that specifies constitutive macrolide-lincosamide–streptogramin B resistance contains a novel deletion in the *ermC* attenuator. FEMS Microbiol Lett 1990;57:43–47

53. Weisblum B. Inducible resistance to macrolides, lincosamides and streptogramin type B antibiotics: the resistance phenotype, its biological diversity, and structural elements that regulate expression – a review. J Antimicrob Chemother 1985;16(Suppl A): 63–90

54. Weisblum B. Insights into erythromycin action from studies of its activity as inducer of resistance. Antimicrob Agents Chemother 1995;39:797–805

55. Clarebout G, Nativelle E, Leclercq R. Unusual inducible cross resistance to macrolides, lincosamides, and streptogramins B by methylase production in clinical isolates of *Staphylococcus aureus*. Microb Drug Resist 2001;7:317–322

56. Siberry GK, Tekle T, Carroll K, Dick J. Failure of clindamycin treatment of methicillin-resistant *Staphylococcus aureus* expressing inducible clindamycin resistance in vitro. Clin Infect Dis 2003;37:1257–1260

57. Ross JI, Eady EA, Cove JH, Cunliffe WJ, Baumberg S, Wootton JC. Inducible erythromycin resistance in staphylococci is encoded by a member of the ATP-binding transport super-gene family. Mol Microbiol 1990;4:1207–1214

58. Lina G, Quaglia A, Reverdy ME, Leclercq R, Vandenesch F, Etienne J. Distribution of genes encoding resistance to macrolides, lincosamides, and streptogramins among staphylococci. Antimicrob Agents Chemother 1999;43:1062–1066

59. Brisson-Noel A, Delrieu P, Samain D, Courvalin P. Inactivation of lincosaminide antibiotics in *Staphylococcus*. Identification of lincosaminide *O* nucleotidyltransferases and comparison of the corresponding resistance genes. J Biol Chem 1988;263:15880–15887

60. Allignet J, Loncle V, el Sohl N. Sequence of a staphylococcal plasmid gene, *vga*, encoding a putative ATP-binding protein involved in resistance to virginiamycin A-like antibiotics. Gene 1992;117:45–51

61. Allignet J, El Solh N. Characterization of a new staphylococcal gene, *vgaB*, encoding a putative ABC transporter conferring resistance to streptogramin A and related compounds. Gene 1997;202:133–138

62. Allignet J, Liassine N, el Solh N. Characterization of a staphylococcal plasmid related to pUB110 and carrying two novel genes, *vatC* and *vgbB*, encoding resistance to streptogramins A and B and similar antibiotics. Antimicrob Agents Chemother 1998;42:1794–1798

63. Allignet J, Loncle V, Simenel C, Delepierre M, el Solh N. Sequence of a staphylococcal gene, *vat*, encoding an acetyltransferase inactivating the A-type compounds of virginiamycin-like antibiotics. Gene 1993;130:91–98

64. Allignet J, el Solh N. Diversity among the gram-positive acetyltransferases inactivating streptogramin A and structurally related compounds and characterization of a new staphylococcal determinant, *vatB*. Antimicrob Agents Chemother 1995;39:2027–2036

65. Mukhtar TA, Koteva KP, Hughes DW, Wright GD. Vgb from *Staphylococcus aureus* inactivates streptogramin B antibiotics by an elimination mechanism not hydrolysis. Biochemistry 2001;40:8877–8886

66. Hershberger E, Donabedian S, Konstantinou K, Zervos MJ. Quinupristin–dalfopristin resistance in gram-positive bacteria: mechanism of resistance and epidemiology. Clin Infect Dis 2004;38:92–98

67. Fantin B, Leclercq R, Merle Y, et al. Critical influence of resistance to streptogramin B-type antibiotics on activity of RP 59500 (quinupristin–dalfopristin) in experimental endocarditis due to *Staphylococcus aureus*. Antimicrob Agents Chemother 1995;39:400–405

68. Davies J, Gorini L, Davis BD. Misreading of RNA codewords induced by aminoglycoside antibiotics. Mol Pharmacol 1965;1:93–106

69. Shaw KJ, Rather PN, Hare RS, Miller GH. Molecular genetics of aminoglycoside resistance genes and familial relationships of the aminoglycoside-modifying enzymes. Microbiol Rev 1993;57:138–163

70. Lyon BR, Skurray R. Antimicrobial resistance of *Staphylococcus aureus*: genetic basis. Microbiol Rev 1987;51:88–134

71. Daigle DM, Hughes DW, Wright GD. Prodigious substrate specificity of AAC(6′)-APH(2″), an aminoglycoside antibiotic resistance determinant in enterococci and staphylococci. Chem Biol 1999;6:99–110

72. Landy M, Larkum NW, Oswald EJ, Streighoff P. Increased synthesis of *p*-amino-benzoic acid associated with the development of sulfonamide resistance in *Staphylococcus aureus*. Science 1943;97:265–267

73. Then RL, Kohl I, Burdeska A. Frequency and transferability of trimethoprim and sulfonamide resistance in methicillin-resistant *Staphylococcus aureus* and *Staphylococcus epidermidis*. J Chemother 1992;4:67–71

74. Hampele IC, D'Arcy A, Dale GE, et al. Structure and function of the dihydropteroate synthase from *Staphylococcus aureus*. J Mol Biol 1997;268:21–30

75. Dale GE, Broger C, Hartman PG, et al. Characterization of the gene for the chromosomal dihydrofolate reductase (DHFR) of *Staphylococcus epidermidis* ATCC 14990: the origin of the trimethoprim-resistant S1 DHFR from *Staphylococcus aureus*? J Bacteriol 1995;177:2965–2970

76. Dale GE, Broger C, D'Arcy A, et al. A single amino acid substitution in *Staphylococcus aureus* dihydrofolate reductase determines trimethoprim resistance. J Mol Biol 1997;266:23–30

77. Trzcinski K, Cooper BS, Hryniewicz W, Dowson CG. Expression of resistance to tetracyclines in strains of methicillin-resistant *Staphylococcus aureus*. J Antimicrob Chemother 2000;45:763–770

78. Nesin M, Svec P, Lupski JR, et al. Cloning and nucleotide sequence of a chromosomally encoded tetracycline resistance determinant, tetA(M), from a pathogenic, methicillin-resistant strain of *Staphylococcus aureus*. Antimicrob Agents Chemother 1990;34:2273–2276

79. Bismuth R, Zilhao R, Sakamoto H, Guesdon JL, Courvalin P. Gene heterogeneity for tetracycline resistance in *Staphylococcus* spp. Antimicrob Agents Chemother 1990;34:1611–1614

80. Burdett V. tRNA modification activity is necessary for Tet(M)-mediated tetracycline resistance. J Bacteriol 1993;175:7209–7215

81. Takei M, Fukuda H, Kishii R, Hosaka M. Target preference of 15 quinolones against *Staphylococcus aureus*, based on antibacterial activities and target inhibition. Antimicrob Agents Chemother 2001;45:3544–3547

82. Drlica K, Zhao X. DNA gyrase, topoisomerase IV, and the 4-quinolones. Microbiol Mol Biol Rev 1997;61:377–392

83. Hooper DC. Fluoroquinolone resistance among Gram-positive cocci. Lancet Infect Dis 2002;2:530–538

84. Tanaka M, Wang T, Onodera Y, Uchida Y, Sato K. Mechanism of quinolone resistance in *Staphylococcus aureus*. J Infect Chemother 2000;6:131–139

85. Sreedharan S, Oram M, Jensen B, Peterson LR, Fisher LM. DNA gyrase *gyrA* mutations in ciprofloxacin-resistant strains of *Staphylococcus aureus*: close similarity with quinolone resistance mutations in *Escherichia coli*. J Bacteriol 1990;172: 7260–7262

86. Schmitz FJ, Hofmann B, Hansen B, et al. Relationship between ciprofloxacin, ofloxacin, levofloxacin, sparfloxacin and moxifloxacin (BAY 12–8039) MICs and mutations in *grlA*, *grlB*, *gyrA* and *gyrB* in 116 unrelated clinical isolates of *Staphylococcus aureus*. J Antimicrob Chemother 1998;41:481–484

87. Ince D, Hooper DC. Mechanisms and frequency of resistance to gatifloxacin in comparison to AM-1121 and ciprofloxacin in *Staphylococcus aureus*. Antimicrob Agents Chemother 2001;45:2755–2764

88. Yu JL, Grinius L, Hooper DC. NorA functions as a multidrug efflux protein in both cytoplasmic membrane vesicles and reconstituted proteoliposomes. J Bacteriol 2002;184:1370–1377

89. Yoshida H, Bogaki M, Nakamura S, Ubukata K, Konno M. Nucleotide sequence and characterization of the *Staphylococcus aureus norA* gene, which confers resistance to quinolones. J Bacteriol 1990;172:6942–6949

90. Wehrli W, Knusel F, Schmid K, Staehelin M. Interaction of rifamycin with bacterial RNA polymerase. Proc Natl Acad Sci U S A 1968;61:667–673

91. Aubry-Damon H, Soussy CJ, Courvalin P. Characterization of mutations in the rpoB gene that confer rifampin resistance in *Staphylococcus aureus*. Antimicrob Agents Chemother 1998;42:2590–2594

92. Swaney SM, Aoki H, Ganoza MC, Shinabarger DL. The oxazolidinone linezolid inhibits initiation of protein synthesis in bacteria. Antimicrob Agents Chemother 1998;42:3251–3255

93. Meka VG, Pillai SK, Sakoulas G, et al. Linezolid resistance in sequential *Staphylococcus aureus* isolates associated with a T2500A mutation in the 23S rRNA gene and loss of a single copy of rRNA. J Infect Dis 2004;190:311–317

94. Tsiodras S, Gold HS, Sakoulas G, et al. Linezolid resistance in a clinical isolate of *Staphylococcus aureus*. Lancet 2001;358:207–208

95. Carpenter CF, Chambers HF. Daptomycin: another novel agent for treating infections due to drug-resistant gram-positive pathogens. Clin Infect Dis 2004;38:994–1000

96. Jevitt LA, Smith AJ, Williams PP, Raney PM, McGowan JE, Jr, Tenover FC. In vitro activities of daptomycin, linezolid, and quinupristin–dalfopristin against a challenge panel of staphylococci and enterococci, including vancomycin-intermediate *Staphylococcus aureus* and vancomycin-resistant *Enterococcus faecium*. Microb Drug Resist 2003;9:389–393

97. Silverman JA, Oliver N, Andrew T, Li T. Resistance studies with daptomycin. Antimicrob Agents Chemother 2001;45:1799–1802

98. von Eiff C, Proctor RA, Peters G. *Staphylococcus aureus* small colony variants: formation and clinical impact. Int J Clin Pract Suppl 2000;115:44–49

99. Proctor RA, Kahl B, von Eiff C, Vaudaux PE, Lew DP, Peters G. Staphylococcal small colony variants have novel mechanisms for antibiotic resistance. Clin Infect Dis 1998;27(Suppl 1):S68–S74

100. Balwit JM, van Langevelde P, Vann JM, Proctor RA. Gentamicin-resistant menadione and hemin auxotrophic *Staphylococcus aureus* persist within cultured endothelial cells. J Infect Dis 1994;170:1033–1037

101. Craven DE, Rixinger AI, Goularte TA, McCabe WR. Methicillin-resistant *Staphylococcus aureus* bacteremia linked to intravenous drug abusers using a "shooting gallery". Am J Med 1986;80:770–776

102. Levine DP, Cushing RD, Jui J, Brown WJ. Community-acquired methicillin-resistant *Staphylococcus aureus* endocarditis in the Detroit Medical Center. Ann Intern Med 1982;97:330–338

103. Saravolatz LD, Markowitz N, Arking L, Pohlod D, Fisher E. Methicillin-resistant *Staphylococcus aureus*. Epidemiologic observations during a community-acquired outbreak. Ann Intern Med 1982;96:11–16

104. Saravolatz LD, Pohlod DJ, Arking LM. Community-acquired methicillin-resistant *Staphylococcus aureus* infections: a new source for nosocomial outbreaks. Ann Intern Med 1982;97:325–329

105. Thompson RL, Cabezudo I, Wenzel RP. Epidemiology of nosocomial infections caused by methicillin-resistant *Staphylococcus aureus*. Ann Intern Med 1982;97:309–317

106. National Nosocomial Infections Surveillance (NNIS) System Report, data summary from January 1992 through June 2003, issued August 2003. Am J Infect Control 2003;31:481–498

107. From the Centers for Disease Control and Prevention. Four pediatric deaths from community-acquired methicillin-resistant *Staphylococcus aureus* – Minnesota and North Dakota, 1997–1999. JAMA 1999;282:1123–1125

108. Frank AL, Marcinak JF, Mangat PD, Schreckenberger PC. Community-acquired and clindamycin-susceptible methicillin-resistant *Staphylococcus aureus* in children. Pediatr Infect Dis J 1999;18:993–1000

109. Naimi TS, LeDell KH, Como-Sabetti K, et al. Comparison of community- and health care-associated methicillin-resistant *Staphylococcus aureus* infection. JAMA 2003;290:2976–2984

110. Groom AV, Wolsey DH, Naimi TS, et al. Community-acquired methicillin-resistant *Staphylococcus aureus* in a rural American Indian community. JAMA 2001;286:1201–1205

111. Herold BC, Immergluck LC, Maranan MC, et al. Community-acquired methicillin-resistant *Staphylococcus aureus* in children with no identified predisposing risk. JAMA 1998;279:593–598

112. Gorak EJ, Yamada SM, Brown JD. Community-acquired methicillin-resistant *Staphylococcus aureus* in hospitalized adults and children without known risk factors. Clin Infect Dis 1999;29:797–800

113. Dietrich DW, Auld DB, Mermel LA. Community-acquired methicillin-resistant *Staphylococcus aureus* in southern New England children. Pediatrics 2004;113:e347–e352

114. Adcock PM, Pastor P, Medley F, Patterson JE, Murphy TV. Methicillin-resistant *Staphylococcus aureus* in two child care centers. J Infect Dis 1998;178:577–580

115. Salgado CD, Farr BM, Calfee DP. Community-acquired methicillin-resistant *Staphylococcus aureus*: a meta-analysis of prevalence and risk factors. Clin Infect Dis 2003;36:131–139

116. Baba T, Takeuchi F, Kuroda M, et al. Genome and virulence determinants of high virulence community-acquired MRSA. Lancet 2002;359:1819–1827

117. Vandenesch F, Naimi T, Enright MC, et al. Community-acquired methicillin-resistant *Staphylococcus aureus* carrying Panton-Valentine leukocidin genes: worldwide emergence. Emerg Infect Dis 2003;9:978–984

118. Gillet Y, Issartel B, Vanhems P, et al. Association between *Staphylococcus aureus* strains carrying gene for Panton-Valentine leukocidin and highly lethal necrotising pneumonia in young immunocompetent patients. Lancet 2002;359:753–759

119. Lina G, Piemont Y, Godail-Gamot F, et al. Involvement of Panton-Valentine leukocidin-producing *Staphylococcus aureus* in primary skin infections and pneumonia. Clin Infect Dis 1999;29:1128–1132

120. Cantoni L, Wenger A, Glauser MP, Bille J. Comparative efficacy of amoxicillin–clavulanate, cloxacillin, and vancomycin against methicillin-sensitive and methicillin-resistant *Staphylococcus aureus* endocarditis in rats. J Infect Dis 1989;159:989–993

121. Wood CA, Wisniewski RM. Beta-lactams versus glycopeptides in treatment of subcutaneous abscesses infected with *Staphylococcus aureus*. Antimicrob Agents Chemother 1994;38:1023–1026

122. Chambers HF, Miller RT, Newman MD. Right-sided *Staphylococcus aureus* endocarditis in intravenous drug abusers: two-week combination therapy. Ann Intern Med 1988;109:619–624

123. Small PM, Chambers HF. Vancomycin for *Staphylococcus aureus* endocarditis in intravenous drug users. Antimicrob Agents Chemother 1990;34:1227–1231

124. Levine DP, Fromm BS, Reddy BR. Slow response to vancomycin or vancomycin plus rifampin in methicillin-resistant *Staphylococcus aureus* endocarditis. Ann Intern Med 1991;115:674–680

125. Chang FY, Peacock JE, Jr, Musher DM, et al. *Staphylococcus aureus* bacteremia: recurrence and the impact of antibiotic

treatment in a prospective multicenter study. Medicine (Baltimore) 2003;82:333–339

126. Selvey LA, Whitby M, Johnson B. Nosocomial methicillin-resistant *Staphylococcus aureus* bacteremia: is it any worse than nosocomial methicillin-sensitive *Staphylococcus aureus* bacteremia?. Infect Control Hosp Epidemiol 2000;21:645–648

127. Harbarth S, Rutschmann O, Sudre P, Pittet D. Impact of methicillin resistance on the outcome of patients with bacteremia caused by *Staphylococcus aureus*. Arch Intern Med 1998;158:182–189

128. Hershow RC, Khayr WF, Smith NL. A comparison of clinical virulence of nosocomially acquired methicillin-resistant and methicillin-sensitive *Staphylococcus aureus* infections in a university hospital. Infect Control Hosp Epidemiol 1992;13:587–593

129. Blot SI, Vandewoude KH, Hoste EA, Colardyn FA. Outcome and attributable mortality in critically Ill patients with bacteremia involving methicillin-susceptible and methicillin-resistant *Staphylococcus aureus*. Arch Intern Med 2002;162:2229–2235

130. Carrizosa J, Santoro J, Kaye D. Treatment of experimental *Staphylococcus aureus* endocarditis: comparison of cephalothin, cefazolin, and methicillin. Antimicrob Agents Chemother 1978;13:74–77

131. Carrizosa J, Kobasa WD, Kaye D. Effectiveness of nafcillin, methicillin, and cephalothin in experimental *Staphylococcus aureus* endocarditis. Antimicrob Agents Chemother 1979;15:735–737

132. Reymann MT, Holley HP, Jr, Cobbs CG. Persistent bacteremia in staphylococcal endocarditis. Am J Med 1978;65:729–737

133. Chambers HF, Mills J, Drake TA, Sande MA. Failure of a once-daily regimen of cefonicid for treatment of endocarditis due to *Staphylococcus aureus*. Rev Infect Dis 1984;6(Suppl 4):S870–S874

134. Bryant RE, Alford RH. Unsuccessful treatment of staphylococcal endocarditis with cefazolin. JAMA 1977;237:569–570

135. Tice AD, Hoaglund PA, Shoultz DA. Outcomes of osteomyelitis among patients treated with outpatient parenteral antimicrobial therapy. Am J Med 2003;114:723–728

136. Biavasco F, Vignaroli C, Varaldo PE. Glycopeptide resistance in coagulase-negative staphylococci. Eur J Clin Microbiol Infect Dis 2000;19:403–417

137. Cook FV, Farrar WE, Jr Vancomycin revisited. Ann Intern Med 1978;88:813–818

138. Esposito AL, Gleckman RA. Vancomycin. A second look. JAMA 1977;238:1756–1757

139. Markowitz N, Quinn EL, Saravolatz LD. Trimethoprim–sulfamethoxazole compared with vancomycin for the treatment of *Staphylococcus aureus* infection. Ann Intern Med 1992;117:390–398

140. Fagon J, Patrick H, Haas DW, et al. Treatment of gram-positive nosocomial pneumonia. Prospective randomized comparison of quinupristin/dalfopristin versus vancomycin. Nosocomial Pneumonia Group. Am J Respir Crit Care Med 2000;161:753–762

141. Nichols RL, Graham DR, Barriere SL, et al. Treatment of hospitalized patients with complicated gram-positive skin and skin structure infections: two randomized, multicentre studies of quinupristin/dalfopristin versus cefazolin, oxacillin or vancomycin. Synercid Skin and Skin Structure Infection Group. J Antimicrob Chemother 1999;44:263–273

142. Raad I, Bompart F, Hachem R. Prospective, randomized dose-ranging open phase II pilot study of quinupristin/dalfopristin versus vancomycin in the treatment of catheter-related staphylococcal bacteremia. Eur J Clin Microbiol Infect Dis 1999;18:199–202

143. Cubicin (daptomycin for injection) [package insert]. Lexington, MA: Cubist Pharmaceuticals, 2003

144. Stevens DL, Herr D, Lampiris H, Hunt JL, Batts DH, Hafkin B. Linezolid versus vancomycin for the treatment of methicillin-resistant *Staphylococcus aureus* infections. Clin Infect Dis 2002;34:1481–1490

145. Kaplan SL, Afghani B, Lopez P, et al. Linezolid for the treatment of methicillin-resistant *Staphylococcus aureus* infections in children. Pediatr Infect Dis J 2003;22:S178–S185

146. Kollef MH, Rello J, Cammarata SK, Croos-Dabrera RV, Wunderink RG. Clinical cure and survival in Gram-positive ventilator-associated pneumonia: retrospective analysis of two double-blind studies comparing linezolid with vancomycin. Intensive Care Med 2004;30:388–394

147. Wunderink RG, Rello J, Cammarata SK, Croos-Dabrera RV, Kollef MH. Linezolid vs vancomycin: analysis of two double-blind studies of patients with methicillin-resistant *Staphylococcus aureus* nosocomial pneumonia. Chest 2003;124:1789–1797

148. Bassetti M, Di Biagio A, Del Bono V, Cenderello G, Bassetti D. Successful treatment of methicillin-resistant *Staphylococcus aureus* endocarditis with linezolid. Int J Antimicrob Agents 2004;24:83–84

149. Pistella E, Campanile F, Bongiorno D, et al. Successful treatment of disseminated cerebritis complicating methicillin-resistant *Staphylococcus aureus* endocarditis unresponsive to vancomycin therapy with linezolid. Scand J Infect Dis 2004;36:222–225

150. Ravindran V, John J, Kaye GC, Meigh RE. Successful use of oral linezolid as a single active agent in endocarditis unresponsive to conventional antibiotic therapy. J Infect 2003;47:164–166

151. Ruiz ME, Guerrero IC, Tuazon CU. Endocarditis caused by methicillin-resistant *Staphylococcus aureus*: treatment failure with linezolid. Clin Infect Dis 2002;35:1018–1020

152. Gerson SL, Kaplan SL, Bruss JB, et al. Hematologic effects of linezolid: summary of clinical experience. Antimicrob Agents Chemother 2002;46:2723–2726

153. Rao N, Ziran BH, Wagener MM, Santa ER, Yu VL. Similar hematologic effects of long-term linezolid and vancomycin therapy in a prospective observational study of patients with orthopedic infections. Clin Infect Dis 2004;38:1058–1064

154. Nasraway SA, Shorr AF, Kuter DJ, O'Grady N, Le VH, Cammarata SK. Linezolid does not increase the risk of thrombocytopenia in patients with nosocomial pneumonia: comparative analysis of linezolid and vancomycin use. Clin Infect Dis 2003;37:1609–1616

155. Korzeniowski O, Sande MA. Combination antimicrobial therapy for *Staphylococcus aureus* endocarditis in patients addicted to parenteral drugs and in nonaddicts: A prospective study. Ann Intern Med 1982;97:496–503

156. Wilson WR, Karchmer AW, Dajani AS, et al. Antibiotic treatment of adults with infective endocarditis due to streptococci, enterococci, staphylococci, and HACEK microorganisms. American Heart Association. JAMA 1995;274:1706–1713

157. Fortun J, Perez-Molina JA, Anon MT, Martinez-Beltran J, Loza E, Guerrero A. Right-sided endocarditis caused by *Staphylococcus aureus* in drug abusers. Antimicrob Agents Chemother 1995;39:525–528

158. Torres-Tortosa M, de Cueto M, Vergara A, et al. Prospective evaluation of a two-week course of intravenous antibiotics in intravenous drug addicts with infective endocarditis. Grupo de Estudio de Enfermedades Infecciosas de la Provincia de Cadiz. Eur J Clin Microbiol Infect Dis 1994;13:559–564

159. Ribera E, Gomez-Jimenez J, Cortes E, et al. Effectiveness of cloxacillin with and without gentamicin in short-term therapy for right-sided *Staphylococcus aureus* endocarditis. A randomized, controlled trial. Ann Intern Med 1996;125:969–974

160. Karchmer AW, Archer GL, Dismukes WE. *Staphylococcus epidermidis* causing prosthetic valve endocarditis: microbiologic and clinical observations as guides to therapy. Ann Intern Med 1983;98:447–455

161. Whitener C, Caputo GM, Weitekamp MR, Karchmer AW. Endocarditis due to coagulase-negative staphylococci. Microbiologic, epidemiologic, and clinical considerations. Infect Dis Clin North Am 1993;7:81–96

162. Widmer AF, Gaechter A, Ochsner PE, Zimmerli W. Antimicrobial treatment of orthopedic implant-related infections with rifampin combinations. Clin Infect Dis 1992;14:1251–1253

163. Zimmerli W, Widmer AF, Blatter M, Frei R, Ochsner PE. Role of rifampin for treatment of orthopedic implant-related staphylococcal infections: a randomized controlled trial. Foreign-Body Infection (FBI) Study Group. JAMA 1998;279: 1537–1541

164. Dworkin RJ, Lee BL, Sande MA, Chambers HF. Treatment of right-sided *Staphylococcus aureus* endocarditis in intravenous drug users with ciprofloxacin and rifampicin. Lancet 1989;2:1071–1073

165. Heldman AW, Hartert TV, Ray SC, et al. Oral antibiotic treatment of right-sided staphylococcal endocarditis in injection drug users: prospective randomized comparison with parenteral therapy. Am J Med 1996;101:68–76

166. Kaatz GW, Seo SM, Barriere SL, Albrecht LM, Rybak MJ. Ciprofloxacin and rifampin, alone and in combination, for therapy of experimental *Staphylococcus aureus* endocarditis. Antimicrob Agents Chemother 1989;33:1184–1187

167. Aspinall SL, Friedland DM, Yu VL, Rihs JD, Muder RR. Recurrent methicillin-resistant *Staphylococcus aureus* osteomyelitis: combination antibiotic therapy with evaluation by serum bactericidal titers. Ann Pharmacother 1995;29:694–697

168. Tan TQ, Mason EO, Jr, Ou CN, Kaplan SL. Use of intravenous rifampin in neonates with persistent staphylococcal bacteremia. Antimicrob Agents Chemother 1993;37:2401–2406

169. Shama A, Patole SK, Whitehall JS. Intravenous rifampicin in neonates with persistent staphylococcal bacteraemia. Acta Paediatr 2002;91:670–673

170. Massanari RM, Donta ST. The efficacy of rifampin as adjunctive therapy in selected cases of staphylococcal endocarditis. Chest 1978;73:371–375

171. Faville RJ, Jr, Zaske DE, Kaplan EL, Crossley K, Sabath LD, Quie PG. *Staphylococcus aureus* endocarditis. Combined therapy with vancomycin and rifampin. JAMA 1978;240:1963–1965

172. Khatib R, Riederer KM, Held M, Aljundi H. Protracted and recurrent methicillin-resistant *Staphylococcus aureus* bacteremia despite defervescence with vancomycin therapy. Scand J Infect Dis 1995;27:529–532

173. Young LS, Perdreau-Remington F, Winston LG. Clinical, epidemiologic, and molecular evaluation of a clonal outbreak of methicillin-resistant *Staphylococcus aureus* infection. Clin Infect Dis 2004;38:1075–1083

174. Weber SG, Gold HS, Hooper DC, Karchmer AW, Carmeli Y. Fluoroquinolones and the risk for methicillin-resistant *Staphylococcus aureus* in hospitalized patients. Emerg Infect Dis 2003;9:1415–1422

175. Crowcroft NS, Ronveaux O, Monnet DL, Mertens R. Methicillin-resistant *Staphylococcus aureus* and antimicrobial use in Belgian hospitals. Infect Control Hosp Epidemiol 1999;20:31–36

176. Dziekan G, Hahn A, Thune K, et al. Methicillin-resistant *Staphylococcus aureus* in a teaching hospital: investigation of nosocomial transmission using a matched case-control study. J Hosp Infect 2000;46:263–270

177. Graffunder EM, Venezia RA. Risk factors associated with nosocomial methicillin-resistant *Staphylococcus aureus* (MRSA) infection including previous use of antimicrobials. J Antimicrob Chemother 2002;49:999–1005

178. Harbarth S, Liassine N, Dharan S, Herrault P, Auckenthaler R, Pittet D. Risk factors for persistent carriage of methicillin-resistant *Staphylococcus aureus*. Clin Infect Dis 2000;31:1380–1385

179. Venezia RA, Domaracki BE, Evans AM, Preston KE, Graffunder EM. Selection of high-level oxacillin resistance in heteroresistant *Staphylococcus aureus* by fluoroquinolone exposure. J Antimicrob Chemother 2001;48:375–381

180. Bisognano C, Vaudaux PE, Lew DP, Ng EY, Hooper DC. Increased expression of fibronectin-binding proteins by fluoroquinolone-resistant *Staphylococcus aureus* exposed to subinhibitory levels of ciprofloxacin. Antimicrob Agents Chemother 1997;41:906–913

181. Bisognano C, Vaudaux P, Rohner P, Lew DP, Hooper DC. Induction of fibronectin-binding proteins and increased adhesion of quinolone-resistant *Staphylococcus aureus* by subinhibitory levels of ciprofloxacin. Antimicrob Agents Chemother 2000;44:1428–1437

182. Centers for Disease Control and Prevention. Laboratory capacity to detect antimicrobial resistance, 1998. MMWR Morb Mortal Wkly Rep 2000;48:1167–1171

183. Wenzel RP. The antibiotic pipeline – challenges, costs, and values. N Engl J Med 2004;351:523–526

184. Jones ME, Karlowsky JA, Draghi DC, Thornsberry C, Sahm DF, Nathwani D. Epidemiology and antibiotic susceptibility of bacteria causing skin and soft tissue infections in the USA and Europe: a guide to appropriate antimicrobial therapy. Int J Antimicrob Agents 2003;22:406–419

185. Fritsche TR, Sader HS, Jones RN. Comparative activity and spectrum of broad-spectrum beta-lactams (cefepime, ceftazidime, ceftriaxone, piperacillin/tazobactam) tested against 12,295 staphylococci and streptococci: report from the SENTRY antimicrobial surveillance program (North America: 2001–2002). Diagn Microbiol Infect Dis 2003;47:435–440

Chapter 51
Resistance in Aerobic Gram-Positive Bacilli

David J. Weber and William A. Rutala

1 Overview

Aerobic Gram-positive bacilli comprise a variety of organisms, including *Bacillus, Listeria, Erysipelothrix, Lactobacillus, Corynebacterium, Gardnerella, Actinomyces, Nocardia*, and *Mycobacterium*. This chapter will focus on infections due to *Bacillus* spp. because of the threat of anthrax as a bioterrorist weapon, the significance of *Bacillus cereus* as an agent of foodborne illness, and *Bacillus* spp. as occasional but important pathogens. This genus is a diverse group of Gram-positive, spore-forming organisms (1, 2).

1.1 Microbiology

Members of the genus *Bacillus* are characterized as endospore-forming, aerobic, or facultatively anaerobic organisms. They are generally catalase positive, and may be motile by means of peritrichous flagella. Although usually Gram-positive, some species show a variable reaction, especially when the stain is prepared from samples taken from the later stages of growth. When viewed under the microscope, *Bacillus* may appear as single organisms or in chains of considerable length. The size of individual rods may range from small (0.5 × 1.2 mm) to large (2.5 × 10 mm), and rod ends may appear as rounded or square. Formation of a single endospore in the vegetative bacterium is a dominant feature of *Bacillus*. The spore may be oval or cylindrical, and may be located centrally, subterminally, or terminally. *Bacillus* is a large genus with approximately 70 species (2).

D.J. Weber (✉)
Professor of Medicine, Pediatrics, and Epidemiology,
Associate Chief of Staff, UNC Health Care, Chapel Hill, NC, USA
Medical Director, Hospital Epidemiology and Occupational Health,
UNC Hospitals, Chapel Hill, NC, USA
dweber@unch.unc.edu

1.2 Clinical Syndromes

Bacillus spp. are capable of causing a variety of clinical infections (Table 1). Clinical infections due to *Bacillus* spp. can be categorized into three groups: infections caused by *Bacillus anthracis*, including cutaneous infections, pneumonia, and disseminated infections such as meningitis; food poisoning due to *Bacillus cereus*; and invasive infections due to non-*B. anthracis* spp.

1.2.1 *Bacillus anthracis* Infection

B. anthracis is the causative agent of anthrax, which is primarily a worldwide epizootic or enzootic disease of herbivores (e.g., cattle, goats, and sheep) that acquire the disease from direct contact with contaminated soil (3–5). However, all mammals, including humans, are susceptible. In the United States, endemic anthrax is a rare disease, with only 29 cases reported between 1970 and 2000 (6). Anthrax is now recognized as a potential bioterrorist agent (7–9). It is classified as a Category A agent by the Centers for Disease Control and Prevention (CDC): easily disseminated or transmitted person-to-person; causes high mortality, with potential for major public health impact; might cause public panic and social disruption; and requires special action for public health preparedness (10). In 2003, the United States had 22 cases of anthrax as a result of an intentional release of *B. anthracis* (11, 12).

The ultimate reservoir of *B. anthracis* is the soil, where, under proper conditions, spores may persist for decades (13). Dormant spores are highly resistant to adverse environmental conditions, including heat, ultraviolet and ionizing radiation, pressure, and chemical agents (3, 14). Following the intentional release of *B. anthracis* on Gruinard Island, spores persisted for more than four decades (15, 16). In a suitable environment, spores reestablish vegetative growth. Vegetative bacteria have poor survival outside an animal or human host; colony counts decline to an undetectable level within 24 h after inoculation into water.

D.L. Mayers (ed.), *Antimicrobial Drug Resistance*,
DOI 10.1007/978-1-60327-595-8_51, © Humana Press, a part of Springer Science+Business Media, LLC 2009

Table 1 Classification of *Bacillus* infections

	Blood cultures	Prognosis
Infections due to *B. anthracis*		
Cutaneous (contact)	Rarely positive	Excellent with therapy
Pneumonia (inhalation)	Often positive	Frequently fatal
Gastrointestinal (ingestion)	Sometimes positive	
Metastatic (bacteremic)	Always positive	Frequently fatal
B. cereus food poisoning		
Short incubation	Always negative	Generally mild and self-limiting
Long incubation		
Infections due to "opportunistic" *Bacillus* spp.	Rarely positive	
Superficial		Good, occasional fasciitis or myositis
Wound (surgical, burn, traumatic)		
Skin (impetigo-like lesions)		
Closed space Panophthalmitis	Sometimes positive	Infection occasionally fatal, affected organ may be permanently damaged
Cholecystitis		
Soft tissue abscess		
Urogenital infection		
Osteomyelitis		
Septic arthritis		
Fasciitis		
Myositis		
Severe systemic infection	Frequently positive	Frequently fatal
Pneumonia		
Empyeme		
Meningitis		
Endocarditis		

Human anthrax is often a fatal bacterial infection that occurs when *Bacillus anthracis* endospores enter the body through abrasions in the skin, or by inhalation or ingestion (17, 18). The source of human anthrax is direct contact with infected animal products (e.g., wool, hides, bone) or soil, ingestion of contaminated meat, or inhalation of aerosolized endospores. Rarely, direct human-to-human spread may occur (19). The clinical manifestations of anthrax depend on the mode of acquisition being primarily cutaneous (20–23), respiratory (24–26), and gastrointestinal (27). Following initial infection, *B. anthracis* may spread via the bloodstream, resulting most commonly in sepsis and/or meningitis (28, 29). The virulence of the organism is variable, determined by at least two factors: the polysaccharide capsule that prevents

phagocytosis and an extracellular toxin. The anthrax toxin is comprised of three polypeptides: protective antigen (PA) binds to cellular receptors where it is cleaved by cellular furin, oligomerizes, and transports lethal factor (LF, a protease) and edema factor (EF, an adenyl cyclase) into cells (30–32). These toxins are sufficient to produce many of the symptoms of anthrax.

Cutaneous anthrax is the most common naturally occurring form, with an estimated 2,000 cases reported worldwide annually (8). Cutaneous anthrax follows deposition of the organisms into the skin via contamination of previous cuts or abrasions. An initial pruritic macule or papule enlarges into a round ulcer by the second day. This develops into a painless, black eschar, often with extensive local edema. In most cases, the eschar begins to resolve in about 10 days, with complete resolution by 6 weeks. However, lymphangitis and painful lymphadenopathy may occur with associated systemic symptoms. Without antibiotic therapy, the mortality rate has been reported to be as high as 20% (8). With appropriate therapy, the mortality rate is under 1%.

Although gastrointestinal anthrax is uncommon, outbreaks continue to be reported from Africa and Asia following ingestion of insufficiently cooked meat (33–35). The incubation period is 2–5 days. Two clinical forms of disease have been described: oral-pharyngeal and abdominal. The oral pharyngeal form of anthrax is characterized by an oral or esophageal ulcer and development of regional lymphadenopathy, edema, and sepsis. Disease in the lower gastrointestinal tract manifests as primary intestinal lesions, most commonly in the terminal ileum or cecum. Patients present with nausea, vomiting, and malaise, which rapidly progress to bloody diarrhea, development of an acute abdomen, or sepsis.

Inhalation anthrax causes deposition of spore-bearing particles into alveolar spaces. Spores are ingested by macrophages that are transported via the lymphatic vessels to mediastinal lymph nodes, where germination occurs after a period of spore dormancy of variable, and possibly extended, duration (8). Once germination occurs, clinical symptoms follow rapidly. Replicating *B. anthracis* bacilli release toxins that lead to hemorrhage, edema, and necrosis. The mortality of inhalation anthrax, even with antibiotic therapy, remains greater than 50%. Symptoms associated with inhalation anthrax commonly include fever and chills, sweats, fatigue, nonproductive cough, dyspnea, chest pain or pleuritic pain, and myalgias. Most patients demonstrate fever and tachycardia. Laboratory findings most commonly include a normal or slightly high white blood cell count, often with a left shift, elevated liver transaminases, and hypoxia. The classic radiographic finding of a widened mediastinum is found in approximately 70% of patients.

Chest radiographs often demonstrate a pleural effusion and infiltrates or consolidation. The finding of mediastinal widening or pleural effusion on chest radiography is 100% sensitive for inhalation anthrax, 71.8% specific compared with community-acquired pneumonia, and 95.6% specific compared with influenza-like illness (36). A chest computed tomography (CT) scan is more sensitive for detection of anthrax-associated pulmonary disease than a standard chest radiograph.

1.2.2 *Bacillus cereus* Food Poisoning

B. cereus is a well-described but uncommon cause of foodborne disease accounting for 0.5% of reported outbreaks (0.8% of reported cases) in the United States from 1993 to 1997 (37) and 0.6% of outbreaks (0.4% of cases) from 1998 to 2002 (38). Although the CDC reported no deaths in these cases, death from *B. cereus*-associated food poisoning has been reported (39). *B. cereus* strains can cause two types of food poisoning syndromes (1, 40–44). Type 1, "short incubation" or "emetic" syndrome, has an incubation period of 0.5–6 h; the predominant symptoms are vomiting, cramps and, less frequently, diarrhea. The duration of illness is usually 8–10 h (range, 6–24 h). "Short incubation" strains elaborate a heat-stable toxin, cereulide, that is capable of causing vomiting when fed to monkeys. Type 2, "long incubation" or "diarrhea" syndrome, has an incubation period of 6–24 h; the predominant symptoms are diarrhea, abdominal cramps and, less frequently, vomiting. The duration of illness is usually 20–36 h (occasionally, several days). "Long incubation" strains elaborate a heat-labile enterotoxin, tripartite hemolysin BL, which activates intestinal adenylate cyclase and results in intestinal fluid secretion. Clinical manifestations of both syndromes are usually mild and self-limited, and fever is uncommon. There is no seasonality to *B. cereus* food poisoning, and secondary cases do not occur. "Short incubation" disease has most commonly been associated with contaminated fried rice or pasta, and "long incubation" disease has most commonly been associated with contaminated meats or vegetables. The usual source of contamination is raw food, rather than food-handlers or the food preparation environment. Inadequate cooking is the most important factor leading to disease outbreak.

1.2.3 Opportunistic *Bacillus* Species Infections

Bacillus spp. have often been dismissed as contaminants in clinical specimens. However, it is now well recognized that non-*B. anthracis Bacillus* spp. are capable of causing serious human infections (1, 40, 45). Local and systemic infections are most commonly caused by *B. cereus* and *B. subtilis*.

Bacillus spp. have been isolated from surgical and traumatic wounds, often as part of mixed infections (46, 47). The clinical significance of *Bacillus* in such cases is often unclear. However, *Bacillus* spp. may cause severe fasciitis and myositis resembling gas gangrene. In addition, *Bacillus* spp. may colonize or infect burn wounds. Rarely, bacteremia may accompany cutaneous or burn infection. Nosocomial wound infections have resulted from the use of contaminated plaster (48) used for preparing casts or from contaminated incontinence pads (49).

Bacillus spp. may cause a variety of closed-space infections, especially ocular infections, including conjunctivitis, iridocyclitis, dacrocystitis, keratitis, and panophthalmitis (40, 50 55). *B. cereus* is a well-recognized cause of panophthalmitis following penetrating ocular trauma and in intravenous drug users. Exogenous *B. cereus* panophthalmitis is characterized by rapid onset (18–24 h after injury), severe pain, chemosis, proptosis, periorbital swelling, and fever. Infection often results in evisceration and blindness. Other closed-space infections include cholecystitis, septic arthritis, osteomyelitis, intra-abdominal infection, soft tissue abscesses, and urinary tract infections.

Serious systemic infections include central nervous system infection (56 58), lower respiratory tract infections (59), endocarditis (60) including prosthetic valve endocarditis (61), and primary bacteremia with clinical sepsis (62, 63). Most patients with meningitis have predisposing factors, including remote site infections, recent neurosurgery (often with use of a ventriculostomy), cancer, endocarditis, or intravenous drug use (56). The mortality with central nervous system infection is high, approximately 50%.

The prevalence of positive blood cultures for *Bacillus* spp. has ranged from 0.1 to 0.9%. *Bacillus* organisms are common laboratory contaminants due to their hardy growth characteristics. Sources of *Bacillus* pseudoinfections have included contaminated broth culture, syringes, alcohol swabs used to disinfect the tops of blood culture bottles, and gloves. Approximately, 10% of patients who have *Bacillus* isolated from a blood culture will have either recurrent *Bacillus* bacteremia or evidence of significant *Bacillus* infection. Most bacteremic patients will have underlying predisposing medical conditions, such as prematurity, intravenous drug use, indwelling central venous catheters, immunosuppressive medication, or neutropenia (64, 65). Bacteremia has been commonly associated with clinically significant foci of infection, such as meningitis and pneumonia. Endocarditis may accompany bacteremia, especially in intravenous drug users.

2 Therapy of *Bacillus* Infections

2.1 Infections due to Bacillus anthracis

2.1.1 In Vitro Antibiotic Susceptibility

Three caveats should be mentioned in evaluating the reports of the in vitro susceptibility of *B. anthracis* to antibiotics. First, multiple methods for determining in vitro susceptibility have been used. The Clinical and Laboratory Standards Institute (CLSI) currently recommends susceptibility testing be performed using cation-adjusted Mueller-Hinton broth (CAMHB) with incubation at 35 ± 2°C ambient air for 16–20 h (66). Second, CLIS provides an interpretative standard (i.e., break points) only for penicillin, tetracycline, and ciprofloxacin (66). Third, β-lactamase testing of clinical isolates of *B. anthracis* is unreliable, and should not be performed (66). Mohammed and colleagues compared the CLIS broth microdilution method to the Etest agar gradient diffusion method and reported no statistically significant differences between the results of these two methods for any of the tested antibiotics; however, results for penicillin obtained by the Etest method were 1–9 dilutions lower than those obtained by the broth microdilution method (67). In addition, they noted that reading the Etest results through the glass of a biologic safety cabinet was difficult.

Testing of clinical isolates of *B. anthracis* has revealed that strains are generally susceptible to first-generation cephalosporins, tetracyclines, quinolones, carbapenems, clindamycin, chloramphenicol, and vancomycin (Table 2) (68–78). Most strains are susceptible to penicillin, but clinical strains may produce a β-lactamase (see below). Most strains are resistant to second- and third-generation cephalosporins, aztreonam, and trimethoprim–sulfamethoxazole.

The rapidity of killing of antibacterials against selected strains of *B. anthracis* has been determined using the time-kill method (79). The most rapid bacterial killing was achieved by quinupristin–dalfopristin, rifampin, and moxifloxacin, with a 4-$\log_{10}$ reduction in 0.5–4 h. The β-lactams and vancomycin demonstrated a 2–4 $\log_{10}$ reduction within 5–15 h. The macrolides, tetracyclines, and linezolid demonstrated a lower kill rate, while chloramphenicol did not kill at all. In vitro synergy of antibiotics against *B. anthracis* has also been evaluated (80). Against two strains of *B. anthracis*, only the combination of rifampin and clindamycin were synergistic. All other combinations were either indifferent or antagonistic.

The post-antibiotic effects of a variety of antibiotics have been determined against two strains of *B. anthracis* (81). The post-antibiotic effects observed were as follows: fluoroquinolones 2–5 h; macrolides 1–4 h; clindamycin 2 h; tetracyclines 1–3 h; β-lactams (penicillin G, amoxicillin, ceftriaxone) and vancomycin, linezolid and chloramphenicol 1–2 h; and quinupristin–dalfopristin 7–8 h.

Table 2 In vitro susceptibility of *B. anthracis* to antimicrobials

Highly active	Variable activity	Often resistant
First-generation cephalosporins	Penicillins	Second-generation cephalosporins
Cefazolin	Macrolides	Cefuroxime
Cephalothin	Erythromycin	Cefamandole
Carbapenems	Azithromycin	Third-generation cephalosporins
Imipenem	Clindamycin	Cefotaxime
Meropenem	Aminoglycosides	Ceftazidime
Tetracyclines	Gentamicin	Ceftriaxone
Tetracycline	Netilmicin	Fourth-generation cephalosporins
Doxycycline	Amikacin	Cefepime
Ketolides		Aztreonam
Telithromycin		Trimethoprim–sulfamethoxazole
Quinolones		
Ciprofloxacin		
Levofloxacin		
Moxifloxacin		
Ofloxacin		
Macrolides		
Clarithromycin		
Chloramphenicol		
Vancomycin		

2.1.2 Antimicrobial Resistance in *Bacillus anthracis*

Surveys of clinical and soil-derived strains have revealed resistance to penicillin G in up to 16% of isolates tested (67–70, 74, 75). Human infection due to naturally occurring penicillin-resistant strains has been reported (82–84). Exposure to β-lactams has been reported to induce penicillin resistance in *B. anthracis* (67, 69, 71). The mechanism underlying β-lactam resistance in *B. anthracis* is due to the presence of two β-lactamases, bla1 and bla2 (85). These two β-lactamase genes were found in the Sterne strain of *B. anthracis*, and were evaluated by cloning into *E. coli* (86). Bla1 is a penicillinase that confers high-level resistance to ampicillin, amoxicillin, and penicillin G, while bla2 is a cephalosporinase that confers low-level resistance to ceftriaxone, cefazolin, cefoxitin, and cefotetan (86). More recent work has further characterized the β-lactamases of *B. anthracis* (87, 88). Bla1 was found to preferentially hydrolyze penicillins and to be inhibited by tazobactam and clavulanic acid. Bla2 exhibited carbapenem-, penicillin-, and cephalosporin-hydrolyzing activities as were inhibited by EDTA.

B. anthracis has variable in vitro susceptibility to macrolides. The inducible macrolide-lincoasmide–streptogramin B resistance determinant from *B. anthracis*, ermJ, has been cloned in *E. coli* (89).

Sequential subcultures in sub-inhibitory concentrations of antibiotics led to the development of resistance to quinolones and macrolides (90, 91). Although the MIC of tetracycline increased, it did not reach a level that yielded clinical resistance (91). A more recent study demonstrated that serial passages on brain-heart infusion agar led to the development of resistance to quinolones, macrolides, tetracyclines, clindamycin, vancomycin, linezolid, and a ketolide (92). Strains resistant to a quinolone exhibited cross-resistance to other quinolones, but not to doxycycline.

2.1.3 Recommended Therapy

Penicillin G has long been the standard therapy for anthrax, despite the fact that penicillin resistance has been well described (9, 18). Prior to the intentional anthrax release in the United States in 2003, the recommended therapy for anthrax included penicillin (provided the strain was penicillin-susceptible), tetracycline, doxycycline, erythromycin, and other macrolides, chloramphenicol, ciprofloxacin, streptomycin, first-generation cephalosporins, gentamicin, and vancomycin (7, 17, 93). The exact drugs, dose, and route depended on the clinical syndrome being treated (i.e., inhalation, cutaneous, or gastrointestinal).

Bacillus anthracis infections should be immediately reported to the local health department. The current therapy recommended for anthrax depends on the clinical syndrome being treated. It is important to note that there are no controlled studies for the treatment of inhalation anthrax in humans. Further, there are only limited animal data using primate models of inhalation anthrax to guide therapy decisions. Penicillin, doxycycline, and ciprofloxacin are approved by the FDA for the treatment of inhalation anthrax. Monkeys were shown to be protected from exposure to a lethal aerosol challenge (i.e., $8 LD_{50}$) of *B. anthracis* by penicillin, ciprofloxacin, and doxycycline (94).

Following the 2001 intentional release of anthrax, the CDC recommended that adult patients with inhalation anthrax initially should receive intravenous therapy with ciprofloxacin (400 mg IV every 12 h) or doxycycline (100 mg IV every 12 h) plus 1 or 2 additional antimicrobials (vancomycin, chloramphenicol, imipenem, clindamycin, or clarithromycin) (95). Because an inducible β-lactamase was present, treatment with penicillin was not advised. Similar drugs were advised for children (with appropriate dose adjustment), pregnant women, and immunocompromised persons (95–97). The total duration of recommended therapy was 60 days (IV and oral combined). The prolonged duration is based on evidence (such as the Sverdlovsk outbreak) that following point exposure to aerosolized anthrax, patients may not develop inhalation anthrax for up to 6 weeks postexposure (98). This is thought to be due to late germination of *B. anthracis* spores colonizing the upper respiratory tract. Management algorithms for the clinical assessment of patients with suspected inhalation or cutaneous anthrax have been published (99).

Several issues regarding therapy of inhalation anthrax bear further comments. First, essential elements of care include rapid institution of antibiotic therapy; supportive care (i.e., intravascular volume repletion, with vasopressor and ventilatory support as necessary); and drainage of large pleural effusions, usually with chest tubes (100). Second, therapy with corticosteroids should be considered for patients with inhalation anthrax associated with meningitis or for patients who have severe mediastinal edema (100). Third, currently the CDC recommends ciprofloxacin or doxycycline plus one or two additional antimicrobials, despite the fact that in vitro synergy has not been demonstrated (80). In fact, a recent animal experiment suggested that the combination of ciprofloxacin plus clindamycin increased mortality associated with *B. anthracis* infections, compared with ciprofloxacin therapy alone (101). Cephalosporins and trimethoprim–sulfamethoxazole should be avoided. Although clarithromycin has activity, erythromycin and azithromycin have borderline activity and should be avoided. Fourth, the recommended duration of therapy is at least 60 days. Prolonged therapy is supported by the observation that 5 of 29 monkeys treated for 30 days after inhalation challenge relapsed after antimicrobial therapy was discontinued (93). Further, after aerosol challenge, spores persisted in trace amounts in lung homogenates of monkeys for up to 100 days (102). For this reason, some treatment algorithms include recommendations for therapy for up to 100 days (100). Finally, animal challenge studies suggest that antibiotic therapy when combined with vaccine results in a higher success rate (93). A more recent inhalation challenge study using rhesus macaques demonstrated that only four of nine monkeys (44%) survived the challenge when provided 14 days of postexposure therapy with ciprofloxacin alone, while all ten monkeys (100%) treated with ciprofloxacin for 14 days plus vaccination survived (103). Similar data has been reported using an intranasally infected guinea pig model (104). A cost-effectiveness evaluation reported that post-attack prophylactic vaccination and antibiotic therapy is the most effective and least expensive method of protecting the public (105). Assessment of the safety of the anthrax vaccine in US military personnel has not revealed an unusual rate of serious adverse events (106–108).

The CDC has recommended that cutaneous anthrax in adults should be treated with ciprofloxacin 500 mg twice daily or doxycycline 100 mg twice daily, for 7–10 days. The duration of therapy should be extended to 60 days in the setting of bioterrorism with presumed aerosol exposure (95). If the strain is penicillin-susceptible, then amoxicillin may be used for therapy.

For anthrax meningitis, the recommendation is for the use of a fluoroquinolone (ciprofloxacin or levofloxacin) plus one or two agents with good penetration of the central nervous system, such as penicillin or ampicillin (provided the strain is susceptible), meropenem, rifampin, or vancomycin (106). The use of corticosteroids should be considered, if needed, for the management of cerebral edema (106).

2.1.4 Recommended Prophylaxis Following Inhalation Exposure

In 1999, the CDC recommended that postexposure prophylaxis should consist of chemoprophylaxis with ciprofloxacin (500 mg twice daily) and vaccination as soon as possible after exposure and at 2 and 4 weeks after exposure (109). If fluoroquinolones were not available or contraindicated, then doxycycline was acceptable. Following the 2001 anthrax release in the United States, the CDC amended its adult guidelines to recommend ciprofloxacin (500 mg twice daily) or doxycycline (100 mg twice daily) for 60 days (110). Other fluoroquinolones (i.e., moxifloxacin and gatifloxacin) likely would also be effective, but there is no clinical experience with these agents. Neither cephalosporins nor trimethoprim–sulfamethoxazole should be used. Vaccination was not included in the most current recommendations. Similar therapy was recommended for pregnant women (111) and children (96).

2.1.5 Adverse Events Following Anthrax Postexposure Prophylaxis and Therapy

Several articles have been published detailing the adverse events associated with postexposure prophylaxis and therapy following the intentional release of *B. anthracis* in the United States in 2001 (112–117). The frequency of at least one adverse event following 10 days of therapy with ciprofloxacin was 45%, and for doxycycline was 49%; after 30 days of therapy the frequency of at least one adverse event with ciprofloxacin was 77%, and with doxycycline it was 71% (115). Ciprofloxacin prophylaxis compared with doxycycline prophylaxis resulted in more neurologic toxicity (e.g., fainting, dizziness) but less gastrointestinal symptoms (e.g., nausea, vomiting, diarrhea). Serious side effects were rare (116).

2.2 Infections due to Bacillus Species Other than B. anthracis

2.2.1 In Vitro Antibiotic Susceptibility

Only recently has the Clinical and Laboratory Standards Institute (CLSI) issued guidelines for performing susceptibility testing of *Bacillus* spp. (other than *B. anthracis*) (118, 119). Susceptibility testing should be performed using broth microdilution using cation-adjusted Mueller-Hinton broth; disc diffusion testing is not recommended (118, 119). Break points have been provided by CLSI for selected penicillins (penicillin, ampicillin), cephalosporins (cefazolin, cefotaxime, ceftazidime, ceftriaxone), carbapenems (imipenem), glycopeptides (vancomycin), aminoglycosides (gentamicin, amikacin), macrolides (erythromycin), tetracyclines (tetracycline), quinolones (ciprofloxacin, levofloxacin), lincosamides (clindamycin), folate antagonists (trimethoprim–sulfamethoxazole), and miscellaneous agents (chloramphenicol, rifampin). Andrews and Wise reported that gradient tests for *Bacillus* spp. have been found to be unreliable (120). They also demonstrated a poor correlation between penicillin resistance and detection of β-lactamase. Detection of β-lactamase production by a double disc method was more reliable than nitrocefin or intralactam.

The in vitro antimicrobial susceptibility *of Bacillus* spp. has been evaluated in human isolate studies, as part of a comprehensive study of *Bacillus* spp. (121, 122), evaluation of specific clinical infections (45, 46, 123–128), and assessments of new antimicrobials (129, 130). *Bacillus* spp. are generally susceptible to vancomycin, imipenem, ciprofloxacin, and aminoglycosides (Table 3). They are generally resistant to β-lactams, including third-generation cephalosporins. Preliminary studies suggest that they are susceptible to daptomycin and linezolid (129). In vitro susceptibility testing of ten ocular isolates of *Bacillus cereus* demonstrated that vancomycin, clindamycin, and gentamicin were all active (131).

Table 3 Susceptibility of *Bacillus* to selected antibiotics

Bacillus spp.	Highly susceptible	Moderately susceptible	Rarely susceptible
B. cereus	Imipenem	Clindamycin	Penicillin
	Vancomycin	Erythromycin	Oxacillin
	Chloramphenicol	Azithromycin	Cefazolin
	Ciprofloxacin		Cefoxitin
	Gentamicin		Cefuroxime
			Cefotaxime
			Tetracycline
			Trimethoprim–sulfamethoxazole
			Amoxicillin–clavulanate
Other *Bacillus* spp.	Imipenem	Cefazolin	Penicillin
	Vancomycin	Cefoxitin	Oxacillin
	Erythromycin	Cefuroxime	Clindamycin
	Trimethoprim–sulfamethoxazole	Cefotaxime	
	Gentamicin	Chloramphenicol	
	Ciprofloxacin	Tetracycline	
		Piperacillin–tazobactam	

Highly susceptible, >95% strains susceptible; moderately susceptible, 70–95% strains susceptible; rarely susceptible, <70% strains susceptible

A clindamycin–gentamicin combination demonstrated a higher rate of bactericidal synergy than a vancomycin–gentamicin combination.

2.2.2 Antimicrobial Resistance

B. cereus typically produces β-lactamases and so is resistant to β-lactam antibiotics, including the third-generation cephalosporins (40, 132). Other *Bacillus* spp. also often produce β-lactamase (128). For example, Uraz and colleagues isolated 19 *Bacillus* strains from milk, of which five demonstrated β-lactamase activity (133). Little attention has been devoted to evaluating the β-lactamases of *Bacillus* spp., and little is known except that most strains are broadly resistant to penicillins and cephalosporins, including third-generation cephalosporins. Many strains are also resistant to antibiotics containing β-lactamase inhibitors (e.g., clavulanic acid) (78, 129, 130). However, most strains are susceptible to carbapenems.

2.2.3 Recommended Therapy

Vancomycin is generally considered the drug of choice for serious *Bacillus* infections. Alternatives include clindamycin, imipenem, or a fluoroquinolone. Endophthalmitis due to *Bacillus* usually requires both intravenous and intravitreal therapy. For patients with meningitis or endocarditis, a combination of vancomycin plus gentamicin has often been used in the past. A carbapenem would be a reasonable alternative, but there is only limited clinical experience. Whether monotherapy is adequate for serious *Bacillus* infections or combination therapy is superior has not been assessed in animal models or clinical trials.

The duration of therapy for most *Bacillus* infections ranges from 7 to 14 days, depending on the site of infection, severity of illness, and underlying host defense abnormalities. Catheter removal is often required for patients with catheter-related bloodstream infections. Patients with endocarditis and osteomyelitis require prolonged therapy. For bone and soft tissue infections, oral clindamycin or ciprofloxacin may be an appropriate choice for prolonged therapy.

3 Germicide Susceptibility of *Bacillus* spp.

The CDC has estimated that healthcare-associated infections (HAIs) account for an estimated 2 million infections, 90,000 deaths, and $4.5 billion in excess healthcare costs annually (134). Key interventions to control healthcare-associated infections include surveillance, isolation of patients with communicable diseases or multidrug-resistant pathogens, proper skin antisepsis and hand hygiene, and appropriate disinfection and sterilization of medical devices and environmental surfaces.

Multiple nosocomial outbreaks have resulted from inadequate antisepsis or disinfection. Inadequate skin antisepsis may result from lack of intrinsic antimicrobial activity of the antiseptic, a resistant pathogen, over-dilution of the antiseptic, or use of a contaminated antiseptic. Inadequate disinfection of medical devices or environmental surfaces may result from lack of intrinsic antimicrobial activity of the disinfectant, a resistant pathogen, over-dilution of the disinfectant, inadequate duration of disinfection, lack of contact between the disinfectant and the microbes, or use of a contaminated disinfectant.

Spore-forming bacilli such as *Bacillus* spp. are intrinsically resistant to alcohols (135). In a human challenge model, an alcohol-based hand hygiene agent did not have activity against *Bacillus atropheus* (a surrogate of *B. anthracis*) (136). Despite the attempted decontamination with alcohol of the outside of vials containing *B. anthracis*, in one instance these surfaces remained contaminated, resulting in cutaneous infection in a laboratory worker (137). The use of a 70% ethanol solution for skin disinfection led to a pseudo-outbreak of *Bacillus cereus* (138).

However, *Bacillus anthracis* has been demonstrated to be inactivated by chlorine (139–142), 4% formaldehyde (141), 2% glutaraldehyde (140, 142), ethylene oxide (142), and 0.025% peracetic acid (140, 142).

4 Infection Control

The CDC recommends that all patients, including those infected with *B. anthracis*, should be treated with standard precautions. However, because of rare person-to-person transmission (19), the University of North Carolina places patients with cutaneous lesions on contact precautions (4).

Patients infected with *Bacillus* strains other than *B. anthracis* do not require isolation. Clinicians should be aware that outbreaks and pseudo-outbreaks of *Bacillus* spp. infections have occurred, and should investigate clusters of such infections.

5 Conclusions

Several genera of Gram-positive bacilli, including *Bacillus*, *Listeria*, *Erysipelothrix*, *Lactobacillus*, *Corynebacterium*, *Gardnerella*, *Actinomyces*, and *Nocardia* are capable of causing human infection. This chapter focuses on *Bacillus* spp., because *B. anthracis* is considered one of the most important potential bioterrorist agents, *B. cereus* is an important cause of foodborne infections, and non-*B. anthracis* species are an unusual though important source of human infection, especially in immunocompromised patients.

Understanding the antibiotic spectrum of *Bacillus* spp. and their common mechanisms of antibiotic resistance is crucial to proper therapy for these pathogens.

References

1. Weber DJ, Rutala WA. *Bacillus* species. Infect Control Hosp Epidemiol 1988;9:368–373
2. Logan NG, Turnball PC. *Bacillus* and other aerobic endospore-forming bacteria. In: Manual of Clinical Microbiology, Murray PR. (Ed in Chief), ASM Press, Washington DC, 2003, pp. 445–460
3. Mock M, Fouet A. Anthrax. Ann Rev Microbiol 2001;55:647–671
4. Weber DJ, Rutala WA. Risks and prevention of nosocomial transmission of rare zoonotic diseases. Clin Infect Dis 2003;32:446–456
5. Oncu S, Oncu S, Sakarya S. Anthrax – an overview. Med Sci Monit 2003;9:RA276–RA283
6. Centers for Disease Control and Prevention. Summary of notifiable diseases – United States, 2001. Morb Mort Weekly Rep (MMWR) 2003;50:1–97
7. Cieslak TJ, Eitzen EM. Clinical and epidemiologic principles of anthrax. Emerg Infect Dis 1999;5:552–555
8. Inglesby TV, O'Toole T, Henderson DA, et al. Anthrax as a biological weapon, 2002. JAMA 2002;287:2236–2252
9. Spencer RC. *Bacillus anthracis*. J Clin Pathol 2003;56:182–187
10. Centers for Disease Control and Prevention. Biological and chemical terrorism: strategic plan for preparedness and response. Morb Mort Weekly Rep (MMWR) 2000;49(RR-4):1–14
11. Jernigan JA, Stephens DS, Ashford DA, et al. Bioterrorism-related inhalation anthrax: the first 10 cases reported in the United States. Emerg Infect Dis 2001;7:933–944
12. Jernigan DB, Ragunathan PL, Bell BP, et al. Investigation of bioterrorism-related anthrax, United States 2001: epidemiologic findings. Emerg Infect Dis 2002;8:1019–1028
13. Titball RW, Turnball P, Hutson RA. The monitoring and detection of *Bacillus anthracis* in the environment. Soc Appl Bacteriol Symp Ser 1991;20:9S–18S
14. Nicholson WL, Munakata N, Horneck G, Melosh HJ, Setlow P. Resistance of *Bacillus* endospores to extreme terrestrial and extraterrestrial environments. Microbiol Mol Biol Rev 2000;64:548–572
15. Manchee RJ, Broster MG, Melling J, Henstridge RM, Stagg AJ. *Bacillus anthracis* on Gruinlard Island. Nature 1981;294:254–255
16. Manchee RJ, Broster MG, Anderson IS, Henstridge RM, Melling J. Decontamination of *Bacillus anthracis* on Gruinlard Island? Nature 1983;303:239–240
17. Dixon TC, Meselson M, Guillemin J, Hanna PC. (1999) Anthrax. N Engl J Med 1999;341:815–826
18. Swartz MN. Recognition and management of anthrax – an update. N Engl J Med 2001;345:1621–1626
19. Weber DJ, Rutala WA. Recognition and management of anthrax. N Engl J Med 2002;346:944
20. Tutrone WD, Scheinfeld NS, Weinberg JM. Cutaneous anthrax: a concise review. Cutis 2000;69:27–33
21. Celia F. Cutaneous anthrax: an overview. Dermatol Nurs 2002;14:89–92
22. Demirdag K, Ozden M, Saral Y, Kalkan A, Kilic SS, Ozdarendeli A. Cutaneous anthrax in adults: a review of 25 cases in the Eastern Anatolian region of Turkey. Infection 2003;31:327–330
23. Godyn JJ, Siderits R, Dzaman J. Cutaneous anthrax. Arch Pathol Lab Med 2004;128:709–710
24. Shafazand S, Doyle R, Ruoss S, Weinacker A, Raffin TA. Inhalation anthrax. Chest 1999;116:1369–1376
25. Quintiliani Jr. R, Quintiliani R. Inhalation anthrax and bioterrorism. Cur Opin Pulmon Med 2003;9:221–226
26. Cuneo BM. Inhalation anthrax. Respir Care Clin N Am 2004;10:75–82
27. Beatty ME, Ashford DA, Griffin PM, Tauxe RV, Sobel J. Gastrointestinal anthrax. Arch Intern Med 2003;163:2527–2531
28. Meyer ME. Neurologic complications of anthrax. Arch Neurol 2003;60:483–488
29. Lanska DJ. Anthrax meningoencephalitis. Neurol 2002;59:327–334
30. Ascenzi P, Visca P, Ippolito G, Spallarossa A, Bolognesi M, Montecucco C. FEBS Lett 2002;531:384–388
31. Moayeri M, Leppla SH. The role of anthrax toxin in pathogenesis. Curr Opin Microbiol 2004;7:19–24
32. Mourez M. Anthrax toxins. Rev Physiol Biochem Pharmacol 2004;152:135–164
33. Sirsanthana T, Nelson KE, Ezzell JW, Abshire TG. Serological studies of patients with cutaneous and oral-oropharyngeal anthrax from northern Thailand. Am Trop Med Hyg 1988;39:575–581
34. Ichhpujani RL, Rajogopal V, Bhattachary D, et al. An outbreak of human anthrax in Mysore (India). J Commun Dis 2004;36:199–204
35. Kanafani ZA, Ghossain A, Sharara AI, Hatem JM, Kanj SS. Epidemic gastrointestinal anthrax in 1960s Lebanon: clinical manifestations and surgical findings. Emerg Infect Dis 2003;9:520–525
36. Kyriacou DN, Stein AC, Yarnold PR, et al. Clinical predictors of bioterrorism-related inhalational anthrax. Lancet 2004;354:449–452
37. Centers for Disease Control and Prevention. Surveillance for foodborne-disease outbreaks-United States, 1993–1997. Morb Mort Weekly Rep (MMWR) 2000;49(SS-1):1–62
38. Centers for Disease Control and Prevention. Surveillance for foodborne-disease outbreaks-United States, 1998–2002. Morb Mort Weekly Rep (MMWR) 2006;55(SS-10):1–42
39. Dierick K, van Coillie E, Swiecicka I, et al. Fatal family outbreak of *Bacillus cereus*-associated food poisoning. J Clin Microbiol 2005;43:4277–4279
40. Drobniewski FA. *Bacillus cereus* and related species. Clin Microbiol Rev 1993;6:324–338
41. Granum PE, Lund T. *Bacillus cereus* and its food poisoning toxins. FEMS Microbiol Lett 1997;157:223–228
42. Kotiranta A, Lounatmaa K, Haapasalo M. Epidemiology and pathogenesis of *Bacillus cereus* infections. Microbes Infect 2000;2:189–198
43. Gaur AH, Shenep JL. The expanding spectrum of diseases caused by *Bacillus species*. Pediatr Infect Dis J 2001;20:533–534
44. Ehling-Schulz M, Fricher M, Scherer S. *Bacillus cereus*, the causative agent of emetic type of food-borne illness. Mol Nutr Food Res 2004;48:479–487
45. Sliman R, Rehm S, Shlaes DM. Serious infections caused by *Bacillus* species. Medicine 1987;66:218–223
46. Dubouix A, Bonnet E, Alvarez M, et al. *Bacillus cereus* infections in traumatology-orthopaedics department: retrospective investigation and improvement of healthcare practices. J Infect 2005;50:22–30
47. Pillai A, Thomas S, Arora J. *Bacillus cereus*: the forgotten pathogen. Surg Infect 2006;7:305–308
48. Rutala WA, Saviteer SM, Thomann CA, Wilson MB. Plaster-associated *Bacillus cereus* wound infection. Orthopedics 1986;9:575–577
49. Stansfield R, Caudle S. *Bacillus cereus* and orthopaedic surgical wound infection associated with incontinence pads manufactured from virgin wood pulp. J Hosp Infect 1997;37:336–338

50. Hemady R, Zaltas M, Paton B, Foster CS, Baker AS *Bacillus*-induced endophthalmitis: new series of 10 cases and review of the literature. Br J Ophthalmol 1990;74:26–29

51. Reynolds DS, Flynn HW Endophthalmitis after penetrating ocular trauma. Curr Opin Ophthalmol 1997;8:32–38

52. Duch-Samper AM, Chaques-Alepuz V, Menezo JL, Hurtado-Sarrio M. Endophthalmitis following open-glove injuries. Curr Opin Ophthalmol 1998;9:59–65

53. Choudhuri KK, Sharma S, Garg P, Rao GN. Clinical and microbiologic profile of *Bacillus* keratitis. Cornea 2000;19:301–306

54. Das T, Choudhury K, Sharma S, Jaladi S, Nuthethi R. Clinical profile and outcome in *Bacillus* endophthalmitis. Ophthalmology 2001;108:1819–1825

55. Chhabra S, Kunimoto DY, Kazi L, et al. Endophthalmitis after open globe injury: microbiologic spectrum and susceptibilities of isolates. Am J Ophthalmol 2006;142:852–854

56. Gaur AH, Patrick CC, McCullers JA, et al. *Bacillus cereus* bacteremia and meningitis in immunocompromised children. Clin Infect Dis 2001;32:1456–1462

57. Weisse ME, Bass JW, Jarrett RV, Vincent JM. Nonanthrax *Bacillus* infections of the central nervous system. Pediatr Infect Dis J 1991;10:243–246

58. Tokieda K, Morikawa Y, Maeyama K, Mori K, Ikeda K. Clinical manifestations of *Bacillus cereus* meningitis in newborn infants. J Paediatr Child Health 1999;35:582–584

59. Frankard J, Li R, Taccone F, Struelens MJ, Jacobs F, Kentos A. *Bacillus cereus* pneumonia in a patient with acute lymphoblastic leukemia. Eur J Microbiol Infect Dis 2004;23:725–728

60. Steen MK, Bruno-Murtha LA, Chaux G, Lazar H, Bernard S, Sulis C. *Bacillus cereus* endocarditis: report of a case and review. Clin Infect Dis 1992;14:945–946

61. Castedo E, Castro A, Martin P, Roda J, Montero CG. *Bacillus cereus* prosthetic valve endocarditis. Ann Thorac Surg 1999;68:2351–2352

62. Hilliard NJ, Schelonka RL, Waites KB. *Bacillus cereus* bacteremia in a preterm neonate. J Clin Microbiol 2003;41:3441–3444

63. Musa MO, Al Douri MA, Khan S, Shafi T, Al Humaidh A, Al Rasheed AM. Fulminant septicaemic syndrome of *Bacillus cereus*: three case reports. J Infect 1999;39:154–156

64. Zinner SH. Changing epidemiology of infections in patients with neutropenia and cancer: emphasis on Gram-positive and resistant bacteria. Clin Infect Dis 1999;29:490–494

65. Ozkocamen V, Ozcelik T, Ali R, et al. *Bacillus* spp among hospitalized patients with haematological malignancies: clinical features, epidemics and outcomes. J Hosp Infect 2006;64:169–176

66. Clinical and Laboratory Standards Institute. Performance Standards for Antimicrobial Susceptibility Testing; Sixteenth Informational Supplement, 2006. CLSI document M100-S16. Clinical and Laboratory Standards Institute, 940 West Valley Road, Suite 1400, Wayne, PA

67. Mohammed MJ, Marston CK, Popovic T, Weyant RS, Tenover FC. Antimicrobial susceptibility testing of *Bacillus anthracis*: comparison of results obtained by using the National Committee for Clinical Laboratory Standards broth microdilution reference and Etest agar gradient diffusion methods. J Clin Microbiol 2002;40:1902–1907

68. Lightfoot NF, Scott RJD, Turnball PCB. Antimicrobial susceptibility of *Bacillus anthracis*. Salisbury Med Bull 1990;68(suppl):95–98

69. Odendaal MW, Pieterson PM, de Vos V, Botha AD. The antibiotic sensitivity patterns of *Bacillus anthracis* isolated from Kruger National Park. Onderstepoort J Vet Res 1991;58:17–19

70. Doganay M, Aydin N. Antimicrobial susceptibility of *Bacillus anthracis*. Scand J Infect Dis 1991;23:333–335

71. Bryskier A. *Bacillus anthracis* and antibacterial agents. Clin Microbiol Infect 2002;8:467–478

72. Drago L, de Vecchi E, Lombardi A, Nicola L, Valli M, Gismondo MR. Bactericidal activity of levofloxacin, gatifloxacin, penicillin, meropenem and rokitamycin against *Bacillus anthracis* clinical isolates. J Antimicrob Chemother 2002;50:1059–1063

73. Bakici MZ, Eladi N, Bakir M, Bokmetas I, Erandac M, Turan M. Antimicrobial susceptibility of *Bacillus anthracis* in an endemic area. Scand J Infect Dis 2002;34:564–566

74. Cavallo J-D, Ramisse F, Girardet M, Vaissaire J, Mock M, Hernandez E. Antimicrobial susceptibilities of 96 isolates of *Bacillus anthracis* isolated in France between 1994 and 2000. Antimicrob Agents Chemother 2002;46:2307–2309

75. Cooker PR, Smith KL, Hugh-Jones ME. Antimicrobial susceptibilities of diverse *Bacillus anthracis* isolates. Antimicrob Agents Chemother 2002;46:3843–3845

76. Frean J, Klugman KP, Arntzen L, Bukofzer S. Susceptibility of *Bacillus anthracis* to eleven antimicrobial agents including novel fluoroquinolones and a ketolide. J Antimicrob Chemother 2003;52:297–299

77. Jones ME, Goguen J, Critchley IA, et al. Antibiotic susceptibility of isolates of *Bacillus anthracis*, a bacterial pathogen with the potential use in biowarfare. Clin Microbiol Infect 2003;9:984–986

78. Turnbull PCB, Sirianni NM, LeBron CI, et al. MICs of selected antibiotics for *Bacillus anthracis*, *Bacillus cereus*, *Bacillus thuringiensis*, and *Bacillus mycoides* from a range of clinical and environmental sources as determined by Etest. J Antimicrob Chemother 2004;42:3626–3634

79. Athamna A, Massalha M, Athamna M, et al. In vitro susceptibilities of *Bacillus anthracis* to various antibacterial agents and time-kill activity. J Antimicrob Chemother 2004;53:247–251

80. Athamna A, Athamna M, Nura A, et al. Is in vitro antibiotic combination more effective than single-drug therapy against anthrax. Antimicrob Agents Chemother 2005;49:1323–1325

81. Anthamna A, Athamna M, Medlej B, Bast DJ, Rubinstein E. In vitro post-antibiotic effect of fluoroquinolones, macrolides, β-lactams, tetracyclines, vancomycin, clindamycin, linezolid, chloramphenicol, quinupristin–dalfopristin and rifampin on *Bacillus anthracis*. J Antimicrob Chemother 2004;53:609–615

82. Severn M. A fatal case of pulmonary anthrax. Br Med J 1976;1:748

83. Bradaric N, Punda-Polic J. Cutaneous anthrax due to penicillin-resistant *Bacillus anthracis* transmitted by insect bite. Lancet 1992;340:306–307

84. Lalitha MK. Penicillin resistance in *Bacillus anthracis*. Lancet 1997;349:1522

85. Chen Y, Tenover FC, Koekler TM. β-lactamase gene expression in a penicillin-resistant *Bacillus anthracis* strain. Antimicrob Agents Chemother 2004;48:4873–4877

86. Chen Y, Succi J, Tenover FC, Koekler TM. Beta-lactamase genes of the penicillin-susceptible *Bacillus anthracis* Sterne strain. J Bacteriol 2003;185:823–830

87. Materon IC, Queenan AM, Koehler TM, Bush K, Palzkill T. Biochemical characterization of β-lactamases Bla1 and Bla2 from *Bacillus anthracis*. Antimicrob Agents Chemother 2993;47:2040–2042

88. Beharry Z, Chen H, Gadhachanda VR, Buynak JD, Palzkill T. Evaluation of penicillin-based inhibitors of the class A and B β-lactamases from *Bacillus anthracis*. Biochem Biophysical Res Commun 2004;313:541–545

89. Kim HS, Choi EC, Kim BK. A macrolide-lincosamide-streptogramin B resistance determination from *Bacillus anthracis* 590: cloning and expression of ermJ. J Gen Microbiol 1993;139:601–607

90. Choe CH. In vitro development of resistance to ofloxacin and doxycycline in *Bacillus anthracis* Sterne. Antimicrob Agents Chemother 2000;44:1766

91. Brook I, Elliott TB, Pryor II HI, et al. In vitro resistance of *Bacillus anthracis* Sterne to doxycycline, macrolides and quinolones. Int J Antimicrob Agents 2001;18:559–562

92. Athamna A, Athamna M, Abu-Rashed N, Medlej B, Bast DJ, Rubinstein E. Selection of *Bacillus anthracis* isolates resistant to antibiotics. J Antimicrob Chemother 2004;54:424–428

93. Inglesby TV, Henderson DA, Bartlett JG, et al. Anthrax as a biological weapon, 1999. JAMA 2002;281:1735–1745

94. Friedlander AM, Welkos SL, Pitt ML, et al. Postexposure prophylaxis against experimental inhalation anthrax. J Infect Dis 1993;167:1239–1243

95. Centers for Disease Control and Prevention. Update: investigation of bioterrorism-related anthrax and interim guidelines for exposure management and antimicrobial therapy, October 2001. Morb Mort Weekly Rep (MMWR) 2001;50:909–919

96. Centers for Disease Control and Prevention. Update: interim recommendations for antimicrobial prophylaxis for children and breastfeeding mothers and treatment for children with anthrax. Morb Mort Weekly Rep (MMWR) 2001;50:1014–1016

97. Brook I. The prophylaxis and treatment of anthrax. Int J Antimicrob Agents 2002;20:320–325

98. Meselson M, Guillemin J, Langmuir MH-A, Popova I, Yampolskaya ASO. The Sverdlovsk anthrax outbreak of 1979. Science 1994;266:1202–1208

99. Centers for Disease Control and Prevention. Update: investigation of bioterrorism-related anthrax and interim guidelines for clinical evaluation of persons with possible anthrax. Morb Mort Weekly Rep (MMWR) 2001;50:941–948

100. Barlett JG, Inglesby TV, Borio L. Management of anthrax. Clin Infect Dis 2002;35:851–858

101. Brook I, Germana A, Giraldo DE, et al. Clindamycin and quinolone therapy for *Bacillus anthracis* Sterne infection in 60Co-gamma-photon-irradiated and sham-irradiated mice. J Antimicrob Chemother 2005;56:1074–1080

102. Henderson DW, Peacock S, Belton FC. Observations on the prophylaxis of experimental pulmonary anthrax in the monkey. J Hyg 1956;54:28–36

103. Vietri NJ, Purcell BK, Lawler JV, et al. Short-course post-exposure antibiotic prophylaxis combined with vaccination protects against experimental inhalation anthrax. PNAS 2006;103:7813–7816

104. Altboum Z, Gozes Y, Barnea A, Pass A, White M, Kobiler D. Postexposure prophylaxis against anthrax: evaluation of various treatment regiments in intranasally infected guinea pigs. Infect Immun 2002;70:6231–6241

105. Fowler RA, Sanders GD, Bravata DM, et al. Cost-effectiveness of defending against bioterrorism: a comparison of vaccination and antibiotic prophylaxis against anthrax. Ann Intern Med 2005;142:601–610

106. Sejvar JJ, Tenover FC, Stephens DS. Management of anthrax meningitis. Lancet Infect Dis 2005;5:287–295

107. Sever JL, Brenner AI, Gale AD, et al. Safety of anthrax vaccine: an expanded review and evaluation of adverse events reported to the Vaccine Adverse Event Reporting System (VAERS). Pharmacoepidemiol Drug Saf 2004;13:825–840

108. Wells TS, Sato PA, Smith TC, Wang LZ, Reed RJ, Ryan MAK. Military hospitalizations among deployed US service members following anthrax vaccination, 1998–2001. Hum Vaccin 2006;2:54–59

109. Centers for Disease Control and Prevention. Bioterrorism alleging use of anthrax and interim guidelines for management – United States, 1998. Morb Mort Weekly Rep (MMWr) 1999;48:69–74

110. Centers for Disease Control and Prevention. Update: investigation of anthrax-associated with intentional exposure and interim public health guidelines, October 2001. Morb Mort Weekly Rep (MMWR) 2001;50:889–893

111. Centers for Disease Control and Prevention. Updated recommendations for antimicrobial prophylaxis among asymptomatic pregnant women after exposure to *Bacillus anthracis*. Morb Mort Wkly Rep (MMWR) 2001;50:960

112. Centers for Disease Control and Prevention. (2001) Update: investigation of bioterrorism-related anthrax and adverse events from antimicrobial prophylaxis. Morb. Mort Wkly Rep (MMWR) 2001;50:973–976

113. Centers for Disease Control and Prevention. Update: adverse events associated with anthrax prophylaxis among post employees – New Jersey, New York City, and the District of Columbia Metropolitan area, 2001. Morb Mort Weekly Rep (MMWR) 2001;50:1031–1034

114. Centers for Disease Control and Prevention. Update: adverse events associated with anthrax prophylaxis among post employees – New Jersey, New York City, and the District of Columbia Metropolitan area, 2001. Morb Mort Weekly Rep (MMWR) 2001;50:1051–1054

115. Shepard CW, Soriano-Gabarro M, Zell ER, et al. Antimicrobial postexposure prophylaxis for anthrax: adverse events and adherence. Emerg Infect Dis 2002;8:1124–1132

116. Tierney BC, Martin SW, Franzke LH, et al. Serious adverse events among participants in the Centers for Disease Control and Prevention's anthrax vaccine and antimicrobial availability program for persons at risk for bioterrorism-related inhalation anthrax. Clin Infect Dis 2003;37:905–911

117. Martin SW, Tierney BC, Aranas A, et al. An overview of adverse events reported by participants in CDC's anthrax vaccine and antimicrobial availability program. Pharmacoepidemol Drug Saf 2005;14:393–401

118. Jorgensen JH, Hindler JF. New consensus guidelines from the Clinical and Laboratory Standards Institute for antimicrobial susceptibility testing of infrequently isolated or fastidious bacteria. Clin Infect Dis 2007;44:280–286

119. Clinical and Laboratory Standards Institute Methods for Antimicrobial Dilution and Disk Susceptibility Testing of Infrequently Isolated or Fastidious Bacteria; Approved Guideline. CLIS document M45-A, CLIS, 2006, Wayne, PA

120. Andrews JM, Wise R. Susceptibility testing of *Bacillus* species. J Antimicrob Chemother 2002;49:1039–1046

121. Weber DJ, Saviteer SM, Rutala WA, Thomann CA. In vitro susceptibility of *Bacillus* spp. to selected antimicrobial agents. Antimicrob Agents Chemother 1988;32:642–645

122. Turnbull PCB, Sirianni NM, LeBron CI, et al. MICs of selected antibiotics for *Bacillus anthracis, Bacillus cereus, Bacillus thuringiensis*, and *Bacillus mycoides* from a range of clinical and environmental sources as determined by the Etest. J Clin Microbiol 2004;42:3626–3634

123. Banerjee C, Bustamante CI, Wharton R, Talley E, Wade JC. *Bacillus* infections in patients with cancer. Arch Intern Med 1988;148:1769–1774

124. Wong MT, Dolan MJ. Significant infections due to *Bacillus* species following abrasions associated with motor vehicle-related trauma. Clin Infect Dis 1992;15:855–857

125. Krause A, Freeman R, Sisson PR, Murphy OM. Infection with *Bacillus cereus* after close-range gunshot injuries. J Trauma 1996;41:546–548

126. Kunimoto DK, Das T, Sharma S, et al. Microbiologic spectrum and susceptibility of isolates: part II. Posttraumatic endophthalmitis. Am J Ophthalmol 1999;128:242–244

127. Chhabra S, Kunimoto DY, Kazi L, et al. Endophthalmitis after open globe injury: microbiologic spectrum and susceptibilities of isolates. Am J Ophthalmol 2006;142:852–854

128. Handal T, Olsen I, Walker CB, Caugant DA. β-lactamase production and antimicrobial susceptibility of subgingival bacteria from refractory periodontitis. Oral Microbiol Immunol 2004;19:303–308

129. Johnson DM, Biedenbach DJ, Jones RN. Potency and antimicrobial spectrum update for piperacillin/tazobactam (2000): emphasis on its activity against resistant organism populations and generally untested species causing community-acquired respiratory tract infections. Diagn Microbiol Infect Dis 2002;43:49–60

130. Streit JM, Jones RN, Sadar HS. Daptomycin activity and spectrum: a worldwide sample of 6737 clinical Gram-positive organisms. J Antimicrob Chemother 2004;53:669–674

131. Gigantelli JW, Gomez JT, Osato MS. In vitro susceptibilities of ocular *Bacillus cereus* isolates to clindamycin, gentamicin, and vancomycin alone or in combination. Antimicrob Agents Chemother 1991;35:201–202

132. Coonrod JD, Leadley PJ, Eickhoff TC. Antibiotic susceptibility of *Bacillus* species. J Infect Dis 1971;123:102–105

133. Uraz G, Simsek H, Maras Y. Determination of beta-lactamase activities and antibiotic susceptibility of some Bacillus strains causing food poisoning. Drug Metabol Drug Interact 2001;18:69–77

134. Centers for Disease Control and Prevention. Healthcare-Associated Infections. www.cdc.gov/ncidod/dhqp/healthDis.html. Accessed December 27, 2006

135. Spaulding EH. Chemical sterilization of surgical instruments. Surg Gynecol Obstet 1939;69:738–744

136. Weber DJ, Sickbert-Bennett E, Gergen MF, Rutala WA. Efficacy of selected hand hygiene agents used to remove *Bacillus atropheus* (a surrogate of *Bacillus anthracis*) from contaminated hands. JAMA 2003;289:1274–1277

137. Centers for Disease Control and Prevention. Update: cutaneous anthrax in a laboratory worker – Texas, 2002. Morb Mort Weekly Rep (MMWR) 2002;51:482

138. Hseuh P-R, Teng L-J, Yang P-C, Pan H-H, Ho S-W, Luh K-T. Nosocomial pseudoepidemic caused by *Bacillus cereus* traced to contaminated ethyl alcohol from a liquor factory. J Clin Microb 1999;37:2280–2284

139. Brazis AR, Leslie JE, Kabler PW, Woodward RL. The inactivation of spores of *Bacillus globigii* and *Bacillus anthracis* by free available chlorine. Appl Microbiol 1958;6:338–342

140. Lensing HH, Oei HL. Investigations on the sporicidal and fungicidal activity of disinfectants. Zentralbl Bakteriol Mikrobiol Hyg [b] 1985;181:487–495

141. Russell AD. Bacterial resistance to disinfectants: present knowledge and future problems. J Hosp Infect 1998;4(suppl): S57–S68

142. Whitney EAS, Beatty ME, Taylor TH, Weyant R, Sobel J, Arduino MJ, Ashford DA. Inactivation of *Bacillus anthracis* spores. Emerg Infect Dis 2003;9:623–627

Chapter 52
Antibiotic Resistance in *Neisseria*

Margaret C. Bash, Durrie L. McKnew, and John W. Tapsall

1 Introduction

The genus *Neisseria* includes both pathogenic and commensal species. *N. meningitidis* and *N. gonorrhoeae* are obligate human pathogens with no reservoir outside of the human host. *N. lactamica*, *N. sicca*, *N. subflava* (biovars subflava, flava, and perflava), *N. mucosa*, *N. flavescens*, *N. cinerea*, *N. polysaccharea*, and *N. elongata* subspecies *elongata*, *glycolytica*, and *nitroreducens* are human commensal organisms that are rarely associated with disease. Commensal organisms found in animal respiratory tract or oral flora include *N. canis* and *N. weaveri* in dogs, *N. dentrificans* in guinea pigs, *N. macacae* in rhesus monkeys, *N. dentiae* in cows, and *N. iguanae* in iguanid lizards.

While *N. meningitidis* often colonizes the nasopharynx without causing disease, severe and characteristic syndromes are associated with invasion, including sepsis and meningitis. Infection with *N. gonorrhoeae* often presents as cervicitis in women and urethritis in men, but ranges from asymptomatic infections of mucosal surfaces to complicated infections such as pelvic inflammatory disease. In addition, *N. gonorrhoeae* can cause arthritis and other forms of disseminated disease.

Although DNA analysis of *N. gonorrhoeae* and *N. meningitidis* indicates that they are closely related and very similar organisms, vast differences exist in the role that antibiotic resistance plays in disease treatment and prevention. Diversification through genetic exchange is an important aspect of adaptation for both organisms; however, while antibiotic resistance has been a major consideration in control of gonococcal disease almost since the advent of antibiotic use, it has had less dramatic effects on approaches to treating *N. meningitidis* infections.

M.C. Bash (✉)
Center for Biologics Evaluation and Research,
U.S. Food and Drug Administration, Silver Spring, MD, USA
margaret.bash@fda.hhs.gov

2 Neisseria gonorrhoeae

N. gonorrhoeae causes one of the most common communicable diseases in humans. It is a sexually transmitted organism that usually infects mucosal surfaces. Disease presentation is highly variable, and although asymptomatic infections are common, complications of gonococcal infections are particularly burdensome. Substantial evidence now suggests that gonococcal infection is associated with increases in both the acquisition and transmission of human immunodeficiency virus (HIV).

2.1 Overview of Gonococcal Disease

2.1.1 Worldwide Distribution

Gonorrhea is a global disease of tremendous public health importance. The 2001 World Health Organization (WHO) estimate suggests that about 62 million new cases occur each year (1, 2). These estimates are only approximations, because the disease is often under-diagnosed and under-reported, especially in settings where the disease is most prevalent. The incidence of gonorrhea in developed countries, which declined during the 1980s and early 1990s, has steadily increased over the past decade. High rates of gonococcal disease have been maintained in less developed regions.

Gonorrhea has been described as a disease of the disadvantaged. Less developed countries have significantly higher rates of gonorrhea than Western industrialized nations but, in all regions, the most marginalized in social or economic terms have the highest rates of the disease. Incidence rates in regions most affected are often at least ten times higher than those of Western industrialized countries (1, 2). For example, estimates of annual disease rates per 1,000 individuals 15–49 years of age are, for men and women, respectively: 57 and 67 in sub-Saharan Africa,

D.L. Mayers (ed.), *Antimicrobial Drug Resistance*,
DOI 10.1007/978-1-60327-595-8_52, © Humana Press, a part of Springer Science+Business Media, LLC 2009

30 and 31 in South and South-East Asia, and 27 and 29 in Latin America and the Caribbean. In the United Kingdom, where the overall rate of gonorrhea is approximately 40/100,000, exceptionally high disease rates were identified in some populations (3, 4). For example, among males 20–24 years of age in inner London who were of black ethnicity, the incidence rate was 1,685/100,000. Similar rates are present in Australia in indigenous populations (5). In the US, in 2003, as in recent years, the highest rates of gonorrhea were seen among 15- to 19-year-old African-American women (2,947.8 per 100,000), while the rate overall for the US was 116.2 cases per 100,000 population (6). These high rates of gonorrhea currently are either being maintained or are increasing, despite control efforts. A resurgence of gonorrhea in homosexually active men has been noted in many parts of the developed world (7–9) and high rates of disease have been recorded in former Eastern block countries, despite the collapse of mechanisms for case reporting (10).

2.1.2 Clinical Manifestations

Gonococcal disease is defined by the demonstration of *N. gonorrhoeae* in clinical samples. The gonococcus is an organism found only in humans, and is highly adapted to its ecological niche. Most often, it infects mucosal surfaces, causing sexually transmitted urethritis in men and endocervicitis in women. Ano-rectal and pharyngeal infections, which are more difficult to treat, may occur in both sexes and, in neonates, ophthalmic infection is acquired during passage through an infected birth canal. Endocervical, ano-rectal, and pharyngeal infection is commonly asymptomatic, so that clinical presentation is delayed and reservoirs of infection and transmission are established.

The urgent need for control of gonorrhea is amplified by the impact of complications. Extension of mucosal infection may give rise to epididymo-orchitis in men or pelvic inflammatory disease (PID) in women – both of which may result in infertility. Other complications of *N. gonorrhoeae* infections in women include an increased risk of spontaneous abortion, ectopic pregnancy, and chronic pelvic pain. Eye infection may lead to corneal perforation and blindness. Disseminated gonococcal infections (DGI) occur in 0.5–3% of infections, occur four times more frequently in women, and have been associated with strains that are resistant to killing by normal human serum. DGI may present as tenosynovitis, septic arthritis, or even endocarditis and meningitis (11).

In addition, significant amplification of HIV transmission occurs in the presence of gonorrhea, increasing the spread of the virus by up to five times (12). The inflammatory exudate that accompanies gonococcal infection recruits cells that are the target for HIV to the mucosal surfaces, increasing the risk of HIV acquisition. This risk is diminished with effective gonococcal treatment (13, 14). Viral load estimates of HIV in the semen of HIV-infected men with gonorrhea are up to eight times those in HIV-infected men without gonorrhea. The high HIV viral load observed in the presence of gonococcal infection provides an increased inoculum of the virus, and thus a greater transmission risk. Importantly, high viral loads revert to levels as low as those of the uninfected cohort when effective antibiotic treatment is given (13).

2.1.3 Treatment and Control Strategies

It has long been recognized that a comprehensive program aimed at decreasing disease burden, transmissibility, the time a patient remains infected, and the number of sexual contacts, is required for control of gonococcal disease (15). Behavioral change, improved diagnostic capability, adequate surveillance, and enhanced healthcare delivery, including the provision of appropriate antibiotic treatment, all contribute to successful disease control and prevention. The requirement for early and effective treatment is central to this integrated approach. The treatment strategies recommended are for single-dose therapy on first presentation or diagnosis. This treatment should, as a minimum, cure 95% or more of cases. The rationale behind this approach is to achieve compliance rates not possible with multi-dose treatments and to reduce, as quickly as possible, any further disease transmission, as gonococci are no longer viable 12 h after an effective antibiotic treatment (15–17). Adequate treatment of gonorrhea is essential to the overall control of the disease; extensive efforts have been made to define, monitor, and address antimicrobial resistance (AMR) in *N. gonorrhoeae*.

2.2 Antibiotic Resistance in N. gonorrhoeae

N. gonorrhoeae has a well-recognized potential to rapidly develop resistance to antibiotics. The organism's capacity for genetic recombination and phenotypic diversity enhances transmission and evasion of host immune systems, and is essential for survival in the human host (18–20). This propensity for genetic transformation and recombination also results in rapid spread of antibiotic resistance genes that have rendered many treatments ineffective in many parts of the world. This includes the penicillins and early-generation cephalosporins, tetracyclines and, more recently, the quinolone group of antibiotics.

The gonococcus was originally highly susceptible to antibiotics (21). Now, in many parts of the word, only the third-generation cephalosporins, and most notably ceftriaxone, have retained efficacy, and decreased susceptibility to these antibiotics has begun to appear. Widespread resistance to penicillins in gonococci has necessitated demonstration of their efficacy in a given case or setting before their use is considered. A similar picture has developed in many parts of the world for quinolone antibiotics. This means that cheap and effective oral therapy has had to be replaced by expensive and/or injectable agents. In resource-poor settings, effective antibiotics may be unavailable because the cost of the agent precludes its use (22).

In many areas where there are high rates of gonococcal disease, access to antibiotics is by means of the informal health sector. In this environment, adulterated antibiotics, off-patent preparations, and improperly stored antibiotics are all available (22–26). The ready accessibility of these preparations means that inadequate doses may be purchased, with resultant under-dosing. Ironically, unrestricted drug availability leading to over-use and misuse, contributes significantly to the problem of resistance. It is no accident that the WHO Western Pacific Region, where unregulated antibiotics are readily obtainable, has seen the sequential emergence of gonococci with resistance to penicillins, tetracyclines, spectinomycin, and quinolones.

2.2.1 Development and Spread of Antibiotic Resistance in *N. gonorrhoeae*

In general, antibiotic resistance involves reduced access of the antibiotic to the target site or alteration of the target site itself. Access of antibiotics to the target site in gonococci may be limited by reduced permeability of the cell envelope caused by changes in porin proteins, active export of antibiotics from the cell by means of efflux pumps, or destruction of the antibiotic before it can interact with the target. Alteration or deletion of the target site of the antibiotic generally results in a reduction of its affinity for the antibiotic. Genetically, these changes may be mediated by either chromosomal or extra-chromosomal elements (plasmids). Multiple resistance determinants may coexist in a single organism, resulting in increased levels of resistance or, in some cases, resistance to a number of different antibiotics.

In gonococci, chromosomally mediated resistance is generally slow to emerge and disseminate. While genetic transformation, the mechanism of acquisition of these determinants, is common in *N. gonorrhoeae*, clinically relevant resistance requires multiple gene transfers (27). In *N. gonorrhoeae*, plasmid-mediated resistance spreads more rapidly than chromosomally mediated resistance. At present, plasmid-mediated resistance is limited to penicillins and tetracyclines, and is transmitted by means of conjugation. This process requires the presence of a conjugative plasmid to mobilize the resistance plasmid. As not all strains possess conjugative plasmids, the rate of spread may be limited to some extent. However, conjugative plasmids are also transferable during conjugation, so that recipient strains then become donors themselves (27). Different rates of dissemination of extra-chromosomally mediated resistance have thus been observed.

Resistance to Penicillins (Penicillin, Ampicillin, Amoxicillin, Penicillin/β-lactamase Inhibitor Combinations)

The penicillins have been widely used for the treatment of gonorrhea. Originally, *N. gonorrhoeae* was extremely sensitive, and treatment with 150,000 units of penicillin was efficacious in most instances (21). Decreased in vitro susceptibility appeared, and was associated with treatment failure as early as the mid-1950s (28). Increasing the recommended dose of penicillin temporarily alleviated the problem, but levels of resistance rapidly increased and large numbers of treatment failures again occurred, even with high-dose regimens (17). This was an example of stepwise accrual of chromosomal changes over a period of many years. The genetic basis for high-level chromosomally mediated penicillin resistance has only recently been described, and the contributions of mutations in five different genes or loci shown (29).

The targets of β-lactam agents are the penicillin-binding proteins (PBPs), enzymes located in the cell envelope that participate in cell wall peptidoglycan metabolism. Alterations in PBP-2 and PBP-1 decrease their affinity for the penicillins, and thus the susceptibility of the organism (30). PBP-2 is encoded by the *penA* locus (31). Changes in other loci such as *mtr* and *penB* produce additive effects. The *mtr* locus mediates resistance to a wide range of antibiotics, detergents, and dyes through an active efflux system (32, 33). Mutations in the *penB* locus affect the major outer membrane porin protein, which results in reduced permeability of the cell envelope to hydrophilic antibiotics and other compounds (27, 34–36). An additional contribution to resistance by *ponA1* that encodes a mutation in PBP1 has been shown, but only in the presence of *penC* (29). The *penC* mutation has been identified as a mutation in *pilQ* that interferes with the formation of the high molecular weight PilQ secretin complex (37). The combined effect of *penA*, *penB*, *mtr*, *penC*, and *ponA1* is to increase the MIC of penicillin by 120-fold. Gonococci exhibiting these changes are termed chromosomally resistant *N. gonorrhoeae* (CMRNG) (38). The CMRNG phenotype has been associated with strains expressing the P1B allele of the porin that is also the target for serologic typing antibodies, and is found in strains designated serotype IB (historically WII/WIII) (39, 40).

Resistance to penicillin is also mediated by a plasmid-borne, inducible TEM-1 type β-lactamase. This enzyme hydrolyses the β-lactam ring of penicillins, thus inactivating them. In contrast to the slow evolution and incremental increase in resistance associated with chromosomal changes, acquisition of the plasmid confers resistance in a single step. In 1976, penicillinase-producing *N. gonorrhoeae* (PPNG) were detected at the same time in both the UK (41) and the US (42). The first isolates were imported from Africa and the Far East, respectively. Although the same TEM type of β-lactamase was present in both instances, the gene was carried on plasmids of different sizes, which became known as the "African" and "Asian" plasmids. Transmission of resistance by conjugation required the presence of a mobilizing plasmid, which was present in the Asian PPNG when it was first isolated, but was not found in the African strains until 1981 (43). Thus, resistance due to the Asian plasmid disseminated more widely and more quickly. A number of related PPNG carrying plasmids of different sizes have since been described (27). There is evidence that the plasmid was initially acquired from *Haemophilus* species (43–48).

Lactamase production (PPNG) and chromosomal changes (CMRNG) can coexist in the same isolate. Attempts have been made to negate the effects of penicillinase production by combining a β-lactamase inhibitor with a penicillin, e.g. amoxicillin with clavulanic acid. Treatment of gonorrhea with such a combination has met with only limited success (49, 50). Although lactamase inhibitors may neutralize the effect of the hydrolyzing enzyme and leave the penicillin to act on the organism unhindered, if underlying chromosomally mediated mechanisms of resistance are also present, the organism will still be intrinsically resistant (51).

Cephalosporin Antibiotics

Altered susceptibility to cephalosporin antibiotics in gonococci is chromosomally mediated, and is due to the same changes that account for decreased penicillin susceptibility (27, 52). There is cross-resistance between penicillins and early-generation cephalosporins such as cefuroxime (52, 53). However, this is not the case for the later-generation cephalosporins such as ceftriaxone and cefixime. Other β-lactamases (cephalosporinases), which are constitutively expressed by many Gram-negative genera, have not been detected in *Neisseria* sp. Originally, all gonococci were extremely sensitive to ceftriaxone, but a progressive decrease in the in vitro susceptibility of the organism has occurred over time (54), and less-susceptible gonococci have been detected in the Western Pacific region (WHO WPR).

An outbreak of cephamycin-resistant gonorrhea, including treatment failure with aztreonam and cefdinir, has been reported in Japan (55). Subsequent cures of treatment failures were achieved with spectinomycin, cefodizime, and a ceftriaxone/sparfloxacin combination. The resistance to cephamycins, which are used in Japan, is accompanied by decreased susceptibility to ceftriaxone, which is not used in Japan for treatment of gonorrhea. Genetic characterization of strains with decreased susceptibility to cefixime and ceftriaxone have identified mosaic *penA* genes (56, 57), and reports of multidrug-resistant strains with reduced susceptibility to ceftriaxone include mutations in *penA*, *ponA*, *mtrR*, and *penB* (*porB*) (58, 59).

Quinolone Antibiotics

Oral, single-dose fluoroquinolone therapy, such as ciprofloxacin and ofloxacin, has been recommended for the treatment of genital *N. gonorrhoeae* infections since the early 1990s (60). Over the past decade, quinolone-resistant gonococci (QRNG) have been isolated in Asia, Europe, Australia, and North America, threatening the usefulness of quinolone antimicrobials (61, 62). In the WHO Western Pacific Region, for example, data published since 1992 has shown the rapid emergence and spread of quinolone resistance (63). The number of centers identifying quinolone-resistant strains, the number of quinolone-resistant strains in those centers, and the levels of resistance to the quinolones as determined by MICs has escalated dramatically in recent years (64) (Fig. 1).

Fluoroquinolone-resistance has been attributed to point mutations in bacterial genes *gyrA* and *parC*, which code for the target enzymes DNA gyrase and topoisomerase IV, respectively (65). Sequence analysis suggests that multiple mutations in *gyrA* or the combination of *gyrA* and *parC* mutations are generally associated with ciprofloxacin zresistance (Ciprofloxacin MIC ≥ 1 μg/mL), and clinically expressed as treatment failure (65–72). Additionally, porin changes and efflux mechanisms may contribute to resistance (67, 73, 74). Newer quinolones with enhanced ParC activity have been recently released; however, this target site is less important in gonococcal resistance than GyrA, so these agents are unlikely to be effective in areas where high-level resistance to quinolones is well established (66).

Spectinomycin

In *N. gonorrhoeae*, high-level resistance to spectinomycin or to aminoglycosides usually occurs via a single-step chromosomal mutation. The different ribosomal genes involved in spectinomycin and aminoglycoside resistance are

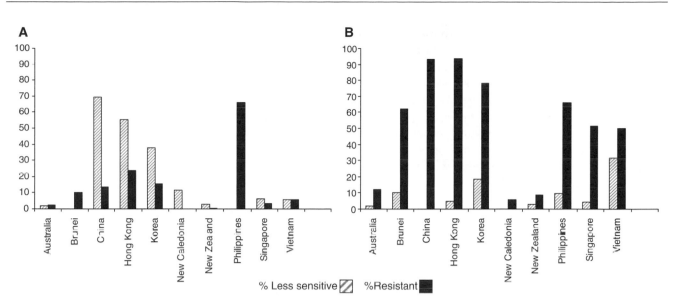

Fig. 1 Percentage of *Neisseria gonorrhoeae* less sensitive and resistant to quinolone antibiotics in ten selected countries in the WHO Western Pacific region in 1996 (**a**) and 2003 (**b**). Less sensitive (*hatched bars*): ciprofloxacin MICs 0.06–0.5 mg/L; resistant (*filled bars*): ciprofloxacin MICs = >1 mg/L

linked (27, 75, 76). Spectinomycin-resistant gonococci appeared in Korea in the 1980s, following widespread use. When spectinomycin treatment was discontinued, antibiotic-resistant strains disappeared. Currently spectinomycin-resistant strains of *N. gonorrhoeae* are uncommonly encountered and, specifically, have not been seen in Korea for many years (63). Apparent treatment failure has been reported where in vitro sensitivity to the antibiotic was demonstrated. This was attributed to failure of the agent to distribute adequately from the site of injection (77), but other mechanisms of resistance may be present.

Tetracyclines

The tetracyclines are generally not recommended for treatment of gonorrhea because they must be administered in multiple doses over several days, resulting in decreased compliance and inadequate dosage. However, they are cheap and therefore widely used, particularly in the informal health sector. Both chromosomal and plasmid-borne tetracycline resistance mechanisms are found in gonococci, the latter being responsible for high-level resistance. Chromosomal resistance is linked to the *mtr* and *penB* alterations, which also reduce susceptibility to the penicillins (27) and a to third locus, tet-2 (31). In *N. gonorrhoeae*, tet-2 has been identified as a single point mutation in the *rpsJ* gene encoding the ribosomal protein S10 (78). The combination of these and other chromosomal mutations result in clinically significant resistance (79). High-level tetracycline resistance in gonococci (TRNG) results from the acquisition of the *tetM* determinant and was first reported in 1986 (80). In *N. gonorrhoeae*, *tetM* exists as two slightly different "Dutch" and "American"

types, located on a self-mobilizing plasmid (81). A study of the molecular epidemiology of the *tetM* genes by PCR suggests that the Dutch type may have originated in the Far East and the American type on the African continent (82). The *tetM* plasmid is widely dispersed in the normal genital tract flora; the mobility of the plasmid and the selective pressure created by the use of tetracyclines to treat other sexually transmitted diseases (STDs) has contributed to the widespread dispersal of the TRNG phenotype (38, 63, 83–86).

Sulfonamide–Trimethoprim Combinations

Sulfamethoxazole and trimethoprim (cotrimoxazole) have been combined in an oral formulation that is used as a multi-dose treatment for gonorrhea. As discussed above for the tetracyclines, the need for multiple doses has implications for the development of resistance due to poor compliance. Trimethoprim is not particularly active against gonococci and is, in fact, used as a selective agent for the growth of gonococci in primary culture plates. This is because of reduced affinity of gonococcal dihydrofolate reductase for trimethoprim. Increased production of dihydrofolate reductase or decreased cell permeability may also contribute to resistance (87). Resistance to the sulfonamides can develop separately (15, 27).

Newer Macrolides

A number of newer macrolides have been made available for treatment of *Chlamydia trachomatis* infection, most notably azithromycin. Chromosomal resistance to erythromycin, an earlier macrolide, was dependent on expression of the *mtr* phenotype (32). Slaney et al. (88) have shown that susceptibility of *N. gonorrhoeae* to azithromycin is also affected by *mtr*. Enhanced resistance to macrolides occurred with mutations in the promoter region of *macAB* that resulted in increased transcription of an additional efflux pump MacA-MacB (89). It is possible that ribosomal mutations may also determine azithromycin resistance in *N. gonorrhoeae* (90). Treatment failures have been reported with low-dose (1 g) azithromycin regimens (91–93).

Aminoglycosides

Aminoglycoside antibiotics, primarily kanamycin and gentamicin, are low-cost injectable agents, sometimes used as first-line treatment. Susceptibility testing suggests that resistance has emerged even though precise definitions of *in vitro* resistance to gentamicin have not been developed (94, 95).

Chloramphenicol/Thiamphenicol

Data on in vitro susceptibility is often lacking, but that which does exist suggests gonococcal resistance to these agents (84, 96).

2.2.2 Laboratory Determination of Resistance

In principle, laboratory methods for susceptibility testing of gonococci are similar to those for other bacteria. However, *N. gonorrhoeae* has specialized growth requirements that have led to the development of tests with numerous variations in methodology.

Agar Dilution (Agar Incorporation) Methods

The agar dilution MIC is the definitive susceptibility test. It is a labor-intensive method and is only performed in specialized laboratories, but it is relatively inexpensive when large numbers of strains are tested in batches. The methods currently in use are not uniform, and different MIC values expressed in mg/L may be obtained in different laboratories (97). MICs are generally accepted to be accurate to plus or minus one doubling dilution.

Disc Diffusion Methods

Disc diffusion susceptibility tests are widely used, and are practical because of low cost and technical simplicity. Their utility and accuracy in assessing gonococcal susceptibility is debated, because the method was initially standardized for rapidly growing organisms, and the slow rate of bacterial growth and increased time of incubation for *N. gonorrhoeae* greatly affect inhibition zone diameters. Attempts have been made to correlate inhibitory zones with MICs in order to develop interpretive criteria. Although not standardized, comparable data can be generated in different laboratories (15, 63, 98).

E-Test

This is a quantitative susceptibility test that uses a strip impregnated with a predefined antibiotic gradient. When performed under reference laboratory conditions, the E-test has compared favorably with the conventional agar dilution MIC. However, the methods were less comparable in a field study in Malawi (94). MICs obtained with this method in reference laboratories tend to be slightly lower than those obtained by conventional agar dilution methods.

Comparability of MIC Data

Many problems exist with comparability of MIC data. Recently, however, it has been suggested that resistance rates obtained by different methods can be compared if certain test parameters are defined, and if internationally agreed-upon controls are used (15, 73). For example, the MIC value (in mg/L) for chromosomal resistance to penicillin is defined as 2 mg/L or more in the USA and Canada, and as 1 mg/L or more in the United Kingdom and Australia. However, qualitative classifications of the strains (i.e. as sensitive or resistant) are the same when the relevant interpretive criteria are applied. The validity of this approach has been demonstrated in the quality assurance aspects of the continuing program of surveillance in the WHO Western Pacific Region (63, 64, 97).

Detection of β-Lactamase (Identification of PPNG)

PPNG express an inducible TEM-type β-lactamase, which is encoded on plasmids. Beta-lactamases can be detected by a number of methods, including a commercially available chromogenic test. The clinical utility of this test may be limited, as resistance to the penicillins is widespread, and CMRNG are not detected by this means. Chromosomally mediated resistance can only be reliably detected in PPNG after strains are cured of plasmids.

Special Test Requirements for Some Antibiotics

Although not generally recommended, co-trimoxazole has been used extensively in some regions to treat gonorrhea, because of its availability and low price. Testing susceptibility to this drug requires that the growth medium be free of substances that interfere with its activity. Azithromycin susceptibility testing is pH-dependent. As CO_2 (needed for the growth of *N. gonorrhoeae*) can alter the pH of the medium, robust controls must be used when assessing the activity of azithromycin.

DNA Probe and Hybridization Techniques for Susceptibility Determination

Chromosomally mediated resistance in *N. gonorrhoeae* is the result of multiple genetic changes, for which there is no simple probe. Probes have been tested that identify known mutations in *gyrA*, *parC*, and *gyrB* genes associated with QRNG (99–101), and those of *penA* and *ponA* that are associated with penicillin resistance (102). Because new mutations that affect levels of resistance are being continually discovered, an alternative approach that uses probes to identify the absence of mutations (wild-type sequence) in resistance-determining regions may be a useful screening strategy for detecting resistance (103). Mutations that may partially reverse resistance, for example suppressed expression of the *mtr* phenotype by the *env* mutation (27), illustrate how complicated identifying phenotypic resistance by molecular methods will be. Identification of resistance markers by DNA testing will add significantly to conventional susceptibility tests only if the ability to reliably and rapidly test non-cultured direct clinical specimens can be developed.

2.3 Clinical Significance of Resistance in N. gonorrhoeae

2.3.1 Epidemiology

The epidemiology of *N. gonorrhoeae* is complex. Although gonococci are generally considered to be non-clonal, outbreaks of antibiotic-resistant gonorrhea have been demonstrated to be caused by strains that are closely related, phenotypically and/or genotypically (79, 104, 105). Studies suggest that the establishment of antibiotic-resistant gonorrhea in a community progresses through several characteristic stages. Initially, resistant isolates are primarily imported and sporadic, with little or no secondary spread. At this stage, resistant isolates are diverse. Sustained local transmission of a resistant strain may develop, establishing endemic transmission. This transition is usually associated with infection of core transmitters, such as commercial sex workers (CSWs) (106), and at this stage, one strain or a few closely

related strains account for a large proportion of resistant isolates. In regions where high rates of resistance have been established for several years, multiple genetically diverse resistant strains can be found.

The spread of QRNG is an interesting example. The emergence of QRNG has been remarkable, particularly in Asia, and since 1999 has accounted for over 50% of Southeast Asian isolates (97, 107). Analysis of variability in mutation patterns and typing characteristics demonstrate worldwide isolate diversity (62, 66, 72, 108, 109), and the initial introduction of QRNG to communities has been characterized by low numbers of diverse strains imported from endemic regions via travelers (110). Rapid increases in the prevalence of QRNG in a community signals the beginning of endemic transmission, which is typically clonal. The pattern of clonal spread of a highly resistant strain establishing high rates of endemic QRNG has been shown in studies conducted in the UK, Australia, Japan, the US, Israel and, more recently, in Sweden (72, 104, 108, 111–114).

2.3.2 Surveillance

Because antibiotic-resistant gonococci arise and spread rapidly and cross national and regional boundaries with ease, data on in vitro susceptibility of prevalent gonococci are needed to establish and maintain effective treatment guidelines (115–118). While in vitro susceptibility data reliably predicts clinical outcome (15), these examinations are generally not performed on an individual basis, and treatment must be provided before results of this testing are available. Therefore an epidemiological approach is utilized, in which the susceptibilities of prevalent gonococci and trends in gonococcal resistance patterns are determined by surveillance systems (15). International travel is an important means of antimicrobial resistance spread, well illustrated by the data on PPNG and QRNG (119, 120). Therefore, to provide effective treatment, it is important to know the origin of an infection, and both local and global patterns of antimicrobial resistance in *N. gonorrhoeae*.

Unfortunately, severe limitations in resources impact the surveillance process. While national schemes have been in existence in developed countries for several decades (121–123), there are few examples of adequate data arising in less developed countries (1). Some regional activity has been implemented, however, and data is progressively being generated, assessed, and validated by international groups (124, 125). An additional limitation to antimicrobial resistance surveillance is the use of nucleic acid-based amplification assays for diagnosis of STDs. A potential disadvantage of these tests is that fewer culture isolates are obtained for susceptibility testing, necessitating new approaches to ensure valid samples of gonococcal isolates for surveillance programs.

Regional Surveillance Data

There are substantial regional differences in rates of antibiotic resistance (1, 121, 122). A number of regional surveillance programs of AMR in GC exist. The Gonococcal Antimicrobial Surveillance Program (GASP) has continuously monitored AMR in GC in the WHO Western Pacific Region since 1992 (63). Similar programs exist in Latin America and South East Asia, but are less developed, and a West African GASP has produced some early data. Attempts are under way to establish a global program of gonococcal susceptibility surveillance (77).

Country-Based Data

There are a number of programs within various countries for surveillance of AMR in gonococci. The Australian Gonococcal Surveillance Program (AGSP) began in 1979 (126), and the US Gonococcal Isolate Surveillance Program (GISP) (127) was established in 1986. Additional country-based programs exist in Canada, the UK (Gonococcal Resistance to Antimicrobials Program – GRASP) (123), Sweden, Denmark, Singapore, China, Hong Kong, Bangladesh, and France, among others. The current data from the AGSP, GISP, and GRASP reveal the loss of utility of penicillins and, increasingly, quinolone antibiotics (121, 128, 129). In Scandinavian surveys, multi-resistant gonococcal infections acquired overseas are prominent. Data from China, Hong Kong, and Bangladesh indicate there are major problems with multiply resistant gonococci in these countries. Individual country-based data have been published periodically from a number of countries in Central and South America, Southern Africa, Central Asia, Europe, and elsewhere, either as intermittent analyses or as one-time studies. In data available from Africa and Latin America, quinolone resistance is not as pronounced as in Asia, but penicillin and tetracycline resistance is at high levels (77).

2.4 Treatment

2.4.1 Management of *N. gonorrhoeae* Infections

In developed countries, the usual practice is to establish an etiological diagnosis in those presenting with symptoms of sexually transmitted infections (STIs). Culture is the usual diagnostic approach, but DNA-based diagnostic techniques have improved case finding, especially asymptomatic cases in high-prevalence populations. In contrast, in many parts of the world where diagnostic facilities are non-existent or rudimentary, treatment algorithms based on syndromic approaches have been developed (130). Treatment is aimed at those infecting agents most likely to be involved in a particular clinical situation. The syndromic approach presumes that clinical symptoms are not only present, but also that they are of sufficient magnitude to induce the patient to seek treatment. However, a considerable proportion of gonococcal infections, particularly in women, produce either no symptoms or else only minimal discomfort (130–132). Such patients fail to present, placing themselves at risk of complications, and serving as a reservoir of infection for others.

Regardless of the level of diagnostic capability, initial treatment is empiric, and the choice of antibiotic used is predetermined by the patterns of antibiotic resistance demonstrated in recently isolated gonococci. Disaggregated local information, as opposed to pooled country-based information, is relevant to tailoring treatment schedules to particular geographic regions. For example, treatment regimens in Sydney were adjusted to account for significant increases in QRNG by substituting ceftriaxone for ciprofloxacin as the recommended therapy in public STD clinics, while penicillins remained suitable for use in remote settings in rural Australia (121). Once resistance to an individual antibiotic in a gonococcal population reaches 5% or more, it is usually removed from recommended treatment schedules (118).

Concomitant infection with other treatable STDs is common. *Chlamydia trachomatis* infection often accompanies gonococcal infection, and can be asymptomatic or produce symptoms similar to those seen with gonorrhea. Based on studies in some populations in which 20–40% of those with gonorrhea were also infected with *C. trachomatis,* it is usual to include anti-chlamydial treatment with initial anti-gonococcal therapy unless co-infection with chlamydia has been specifically excluded (115, 133–135).

Follow-up evaluation of treated patients is standard practice in developed countries. This does not uniformly include a repeat laboratory examination, but cultures should be obtained if symptoms persist or recur, to ensure that the individual patient is cured and, in the case of treatment failure, to determine the reasons for failure (136). It is sometimes difficult to differentiate between failure of antibiotic treatment and reinfection. Comparisons of pre- and post-treatment cultures can sometimes assist in this distinction. It is important to identify treatment failures due to new or spreading forms of resistance, so that control measures can be implemented in a local setting. This practice can also alert practitioners to the existence of novel forms of resistance in the gonococcus. The timing of repeat evaluation needs to be carefully considered. Even if the organism is resistant to an antibiotic or antibiotic combination, symptoms and signs may be temporarily relieved, and recur after cessation of therapy. In this context, anti-chlamydial therapy administered at the same time may have a suppressive, but not curative, effect (91, 137). In less developed settings, access to treatment and clinics is often limited, and follow-up assessments are infrequent.

While the focus here is on antibiotic resistance and treatment strategies, individual case management should include a comprehensive approach to the patient's needs for reproductive health. Counseling, contact tracing, and identification of other possible STDs are all essential to the management of STIs.

2.4.2 Current Antibiotic Recommendations

Optimal practice requires cure of a minimum of 95% of cases by single-dose antibiotic therapy on initial presentation. Ideally, the selected regimen should be low cost, orally administered under direct supervision, and followed by an appropriate clinical review. Due to the propensity for *N. gonorrhoeae* to develop resistance rapidly, any treatment regimen should also be designed and administered so as to prevent emergence of new forms of resistance. Standard protocols that fulfill the above criteria have been developed either for universal application, or else for use in individual countries (115, 116, 118). Recommendations incorporate different requirements for treatment of genital and extra-genital disease (pharyngeal, rectal, and ophthalmic infection), for complicated gonococcal disease, and for the special cases of infections in neonates, children, and during pregnancy. The recommendations are regularly revised to take account of changing susceptibility of gonococci to existing antibiotics, the introduction of new agents or new experience with older agents, the availability of currently used treatments, and the different prevalence of disease in different settings. Updated treatment recommendations for the US are provided by the CDC (http://www.cdc.gov/std/treatment/2006/updated-regimens.htm). Published protocols also include procedures for the prophylaxis of neonatal ophthalmia neonatorum (118, 138, 139). Treatment protocols generally utilize the following antimicrobial agents:

Cephalosporins

Of the antibiotics currently recommended for the treatment of gonorrhea, the third-generation cephalosporins are the most efficacious, and ceftriaxone the most active of these. The original dose recommended was 250 mg, though in some treatment protocols the dose has been reduced to 125 mg. This antibiotic is given by single intramuscular injection, and is suitable for use in all forms of gonococcal disease, including pharyngeal gonorrhea. Intravenous inpatient treatment is usual for disseminated gonococcal infection, including meningitis and endocarditis. Ophthalmic infections of neonates, older infants, and adults also respond to ceftriaxone.

This class of antibiotics can also be administered during pregnancy.

Oral forms of third-generation cephalosporins are also recommended for uncomplicated ano-genital gonorrhea, but their use has been hampered by limited availability in some countries (140). Cefixime is given as a 400 mg single dose. Oral forms of third-generation cephalosporins deliver a lower dose, equivalent to 125 mg of ceftriaxone (115).

Quinolones

Fluoroquinolones, primarily ciprofloxacin or ofloxacin, are widely recommended as standard treatments for gonorrhea in geographic regions where resistance remains low. The standard doses recommended are 500 mg of ciprofloxacin or 400 mg of ofloxacin, given as a single oral dose. Initially, low-dose regimens (e.g. 250 mg doses of ciprofloxacin) were used, but the higher dose recommendation was implemented following reports of treatment failures due to low antibiotic levels. Fluoroquinolone agents given orally are effective for treatment of ano-genital and pharyngeal infection. Fluoroquinolones should not be administered during pregnancy or lactation, or to pre-pubertal children. Parenteral ciprofloxacin or ofloxacin may be used in disseminated and systemic gonococcal infection at doses of 500 mg and 400 mg, respectively, given every 12 h; however, ceftriaxone is preferred for this complication. Earlier-generation non-fluorinated quinolones, which are less efficacious, are not recommended.

Spectinomycin

Spectinomycin is an aminocyclitol compound given by IM injection as a 2 g dose. It is relatively expensive but effective in the treatment of ano-genital infection, but not pharyngeal gonorrhea. Side effects are few. It is usually regarded as a "reserve" agent in the treatment of gonorrhea, for example for those intolerant of cephalosporins or quinolones. It can also be used in pregnant women in standard doses and for disseminated infection, if given twice daily for up to 7 days.

Suboptimal or Obsolete Treatments

Some previously efficacious regimens have become ineffective because of developing resistance, and should only be used if the infecting organism has been clearly demonstrated to be susceptible. Other agents have been used with some success, but only in situations where gonococci have been generally susceptible to all agents. Additionally, inexpensive and readily available treatments continue to be used in some settings, simply because more effective therapy is unaffordable.

Penicillins, including ampicillin and amoxicillin, with or without clavulanate and/or probenecid, were once standard treatments for gonorrhea, but are now rarely used, as a consequence of resistance. The most effective form of administration is a single 3 g oral dose of amoxicillin. Probenecid, 1 g, if given at the same time, will delay renal excretion of the penicillins. Azithromycin is widely used as a treatment for chlamydia as a single 1 g dose. This antibiotic exhibits some anti-gonococcal activity, but treatment failures are unacceptably high, and resistance has appeared during therapy (141). The additive anti-gonococcal effect of azithromycin combined with a specific gonococcal therapy is unquantified, and should not be relied on to effect a cure for gonorrhea (91, 93, 142). Oral tetracyclines like azithromycin are also used as anti-chlamydial agents in conjunction with anti-gonococcal treatments, and also have some anti-gonococcal activity. However, when used for gonorrhea, tetracyclines require multi-dose treatment, and are thus not recommended for compliance as well as other issues. Despite this, the ready availability of tetracyclines and their low-cost results in their continued use in some settings. Some guidelines mention kanamycin (2 g IM) as an alternative treatment where in vitro resistance rates are low. However, data on efficacy and in vitro criteria of resistance are poorly documented (94, 95). Co-trimoxazole (trimethoprim/sulfamethoxazole combination) is a multi-dose oral treatment, and as such is not recommended. Its use should be guided by in vitro data demonstrating susceptibility to the agent. However, considerable technical requirements must be fulfilled before reliable in vitro data can be obtained. Chloramphenicol/thiamphenicol antibiotics are still widely used for the treatment of many diseases in resource-poor settings, even though they are not recommended.

2.4.3 Infection Control Measures

Availability of proper treatment in a community contributes significantly to reductions in both disease and complication rates, including those of enhanced HIV transmission. It has been estimated that effective treatment of 100 women with gonorrhea, 25 of whom were pregnant, would prevent 25 cases of pelvic inflammatory disease (PID), 1 ectopic pregnancy, 6 instances of infertility, and 7 cases of neonatal ophthalmia (15). These estimates have been supported by results of longitudinal studies in Sweden, where a reduction in incidence of PID coincided with a decrease in the incidence of gonorrhea (143–145). It has also been estimated that proper treatment of gonococcal disease in a cohort of 100 high-frequency transmitters of gonorrhea would cumulatively prevent 425 cases of HIV over a period of 10 years (15), and the decreased incidence of new HIV infection observed in a study of improved STD treatment in Mwanza in Tanzania lends support to these projections (130, 146).

The multidisciplinary approach (15) needed for control of antimicrobial resistance in *N. gonorrhoeae* includes rapid and accurate diagnostic testing, ready access to effective antibiotics administered in a setting in which there is an established regulatory framework that oversees drug evaluation and approval, enforcement of prescription-only drug access, reliable drug delivery systems, an informed prescriber base, and laboratory systems with good and evaluable diagnostic standards (147). Prevention measures are also essential, including those aimed at effecting behavioral changes. While control was seemingly achieved in some countries when a concerted effort combining these elements was in place, the reduction in rates has been reversed as "safe sex" practices are seemingly abandoned (7, 148).

Some progress has been made in efforts to control gonococcal antimicrobial resistance: the WHO is developing systems of inexpensive diagnostics to underpin syndromic management algorithms for STIs, effective surveillance systems for AMR in GC have been implemented in settings with few resources at relatively little cost (63), and the WHO is developing easily accessible color-density maps that show the distribution of resistance to agents used for the treatment of gonorrhea by region and country (http://www.who.int/csr/drugresist/infosharing/en/) (Fig. 2). Successful implementation of an aggressive control program in Hawaii indicated that a reversal of resistance trends is possible. Coincident with initiating universal antimicrobial resistance testing, followed by partner identification and treatment of all cases of fluoroquinolone-resistant gonococcal infections, the rate of fluroquinolone resistance in Hawaii was reduced from 19.6% in 2001 to 10.1% in 2002 (149).

Reversal of resistance trends is rare though, and effective measures frequently only succeed in slowing the rate of emerging resistance. Despite its high global incidence and prevalence, its high rate of complications, and the decreasing capacity to treat gonococcal diseases, efforts aimed at the eradication of gonorrhea are minimal, and there is little prospect for diminution of antibiotic-resistant *N. gonorrhoeae* in the near future.

3 Neisseria meningitidis

3.1 Overview of Meningococcal Disease

3.1.1 Epidemiology and Clinical Manifestations

Neisseria meningitidis causes both endemic and epidemic disease worldwide but, as with gonococcal infections, there are significant differences between developed and less developed settings. The clinically significant serogroups, as determined

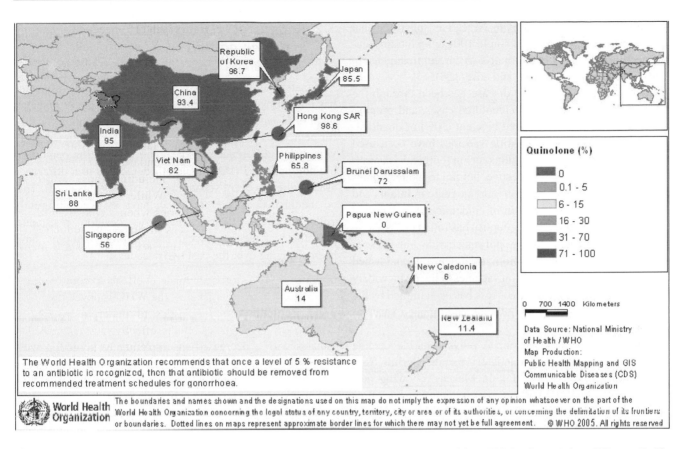

Fig. 2 Quinolone-resistant strains of *N. gonorrhoeae* isolated in countries, area, and territories of the WHO Southeast Asia and Western Pacific Regions (2003)

by their capsular polysaccharides, are groups A, B, C, Y, and W-135. Group A is particularly associated with recurrent epidemics and hyperendemic meningococcal disease in sub-Saharan Africa, often called the "meningitis belt," and parts of Asia. It is estimated that in the 10 years from 1995 to 2004, outbreaks of meningococcal disease in Africa have resulted in about 700,000 cases and 60,000 deaths (150). In Western industrialized countries, infections with serogroup B or C meningococci predominate, and in the US, serogroup Y accounts for over one-third of meningococcal disease cases (151). For endemic disease, the peak incidence is in the very young (less than 4 years), with a predominance of serogroup B infections; a secondary peak occurs in adolescents and young adults, and serogroup C clusters and outbreaks are common in this age group.

Sepsis and meningitis are the most typical presentations of invasive disease, but pneumonia, arthritis, and recurrent bacteremia can occur. Mortality rates vary, and are influenced by many factors, including type of care available, clinical presentation, age of patient, and serogroup. Case-fatality rates in industrialized countries in non-epidemic situations are around 8% (152–154), but are often much higher during epidemics in less-developed countries. Morbidity is substantial, including hearing loss, neurologic sequelae, and

limb loss from auto-amputation. Asymptomatic carriage of the organism in the nasopharynx is common. In a study of healthy individuals observed over 32 months, 18% were found to be carriers at some point (155). Invasive meningococcal disease occurs when the organism penetrates the epithelial surface of the nasopharynx.

3.1.2 Treatment and Control

The first successful treatment of meningococcal disease with sulfonamides was reported in 1937 (156). Penicillin became an effective therapy in the 1940s, followed soon after by chloramphenicol and, most recently, the third-generation cephalosporins (154). Current treatment recommendations for Western industrialized countries are to use high-dose penicillin administered early by the first doctor to see the patient. Cefotaxime, ceftriaxone, and chloramphenicol are alternatives (157). Chemoprophylaxis with rifampin, ceftriaxone, or ciprofloxacin is indicated for close contacts of patients. Effective and cheap antibiotic treatment is difficult to deliver in the meningitis belt, and currently heavy reliance for treatment of individual cases is placed on the use of long-acting chloramphenicol given by intramuscular injection (150). A recent trial in Niger has suggested that ceftriaxone, administered as a single 100 mg/kg intramuscular injection, is a suitable alternative to current treatments in terms of efficacy, ease of use, and cost (158).

Control of meningococcal disease has been through the use of vaccines, treatment of identified cases, and prophylaxis of case contacts. Licensed bivalent (A/C) or quadrivalent (ACYW-135) polysaccharide vaccines have been used in selected "at-risk" populations or in outbreak control. These vaccines are highly effective, but fail to induce immunological memory, and are less immunogenic in infants and young children. In the situation of epidemic meningococcal disease in sub-Saharan Africa, control has relied on "reactive vaccination" programs using polysaccharide vaccines to interrupt outbreaks, and antibiotic treatment for established cases. This approach depends on vaccines being given widely and early, so that their overall success has been limited by the ability to rapidly identify an outbreak and mount a vaccination response (150).

Vaccination with a serogroup A polysaccharide vaccine prior to departure became mandatory for all pilgrims from sub-Saharan Africa to the Hajj in Mecca, following outbreaks of disease attributed to transmission amongst fellow pilgrims. This requirement was later extended to all Hajj pilgrims. The situation in relation to vaccination of pilgrims became more complex after 2000, when widespread disease with serogroup W135 was noted in Hajj pilgrims and their contacts after return to their countries of origin. Vaccination with a polyvalent (A,C, Y, W135) polysaccharide vaccine is now mandatory for Hajj visitors (159).

Development of conjugate vaccines, initially monovalent serogroup C preparations, has seen a marked reduction in disease where universal vaccination programs have been introduced (160). These conjugate vaccines induce T-cell responses and longer-term immunity that can be boosted by repeat vaccination. A booster dose appears to benefit individuals first immunized as infants (161, 162). In 2005, a multivalent conjugate vaccine effective against serogroup A, C, Y, and W135 meningococci was licensed in the USA for use in adolescents and adults. Conjugate vaccines specifically for prevention of epidemic serogroup A disease in Africa are under development (163, 164).

The serogroup B polysaccharide is poorly immunogenic and is chemically identical to material found in the human central nervous system, and therefore non-capsular protein antigens have been studied as vaccine candidates. Serogroup B meningococci are often of diverse subtypes, but individual subtypes may give rise to endemic or hyperendemic disease (165). An outer membrane vesicle (OMV) vaccine, derived from the specific hyperendemic serogroup B strain responsible for the majority of cases of meningococcal disease in New Zealand, has been developed, tested, and implemented as a national immunization program (166–169).

3.2 Antimicrobial Resistance in N. meningitidis

Fortunately, unlike with the gonococcus, antibiotic resistance has not yet had a major impact on clinical disease management of *N. meningitidis* infections. One explanation for this, for penicillins at least, has been provided by Antignac et al, who noted differences in the gene coding for penicillin-binding protein 2 (PBP2) and attributed this to a difference arising after an event separating the two species (170). That is, meningococci and gonococci have evolved differently with regard to their capacity to develop resistance. Nonetheless, meningococcal susceptibility patterns have been changing over the past two decades.

3.2.1 Penicillins

Isolates with a decreased susceptibility to penicillin were first identified in Spain in 1985 (171). Since then, they have been found across much of Europe, North America, Australia, and parts of Africa, although with widely varying rates. Numerous reports show the prevalence of moderately penicillin-susceptible strains is increasing. Spain, in particular, has reported dramatic increases. In a study conducted in 2000, decreased penicillin susceptibility was identified in 55% of the isolates from patients and 39% of those from carriers (172). In this study, decreased susceptibility was more common among disease isolates that were group C (prevalent in Spain in recent years) than in non-group C disease isolates (66% vs. 35%). All stains were fully susceptible to ceftriaxone, cefotaxime, rifampin, and ciprofloxacin, while the majority of strains (89% of clinical strains and 92% of carrier strains) were resistant to sulfadiazine. The association between decreased susceptibility and serogroup C has also been noted elsewhere (173, 174).

In France, reduced susceptibility to penicillin was first reported in 1994. Studies indicate that a large proportion of recently isolated strains have decreased susceptibility to penicillin. A study of 2,167 clinical isolates obtained between 1999 and 2002 found an overall prevalence of 31% (23–39% for each year in the study) (153). In this study, decreased susceptibility was identified most frequently among serogroup C (40%) and W135 (37%) strains. All isolates were fully susceptible to third-generation cephalosporins.

Australia has an active surveillance program for invasive meningococcal isolates. 1,434 clinical isolates from 1994 to 1999 were analyzed for antibiotic susceptibilities. As reported elsewhere, the rates of decreased susceptibility to penicillin have been increasing, from 55% in 1994 to 74% in 1999 (175). Two strains were resistant (MIC 1 mg/L). No link was seen between decreased penicillin susceptibility and disease outcome. Though the treatment regimen was not available for all cases, there was a statistically higher survival rate among those who had penicillin intermediate strains than those who had fully susceptible strains.

The first reported cases in the US of meningococcal disease caused by strains with reduced susceptibility to penicillin are from the early 1990s (176), and the prevalence of such strains has remained low. A surveillance study of cases from 1997 found only 3% of the strains to have reduced susceptibility (177).

Studies from other countries have found quite variable rates of resistance. For example, reduced penicillin susceptibility was present in 3% of isolates reported in a 2003 study from Italy (178), 7% of isolates from a 2001 outbreak in Taiwan (179), 8% in a 2002 study from Scotland (180), 37% of isolates from 2000 to 2001 in Portugal (173), and 43% of strains in a 2002 Turkish study (181).

Resistance to penicillin is due, in part, to development of altered forms of PBP 2, which have decreased affinity for penicillin (170, 172, 182). Mutations in *penA* have been correlated with decreased susceptibility to beta-lactam antibiotics (183). Decreased membrane permeability (184) and efflux (185) may also contribute to resistance. Beta-lactamase production is not an important mechanism of penicillin resistance in meningococci.

3.2.2 Chloramphenicol

Intermediate resistance to chloramphenicol has been identified in France. Recently, 14 out of 2,144 isolates examined had reduced susceptibility to chloramphenicol (153). There have been only two reports of chloramphenicol resistance (186, 187). In the first report, strains were isolated from the CSF of 12 patients, between 1987 and 1996. Of these, 11 were epidemiologically unrelated strains from Vietnam, and one was from France, from a patient with no history of travel to Southeast Asia. While all 12 strains were serogroup B, they were genetically diverse. MICs for these strains were 64 mg/L. Disk-agar dilution tests showed them to also be resistant to sulfonamides and streptomycin, but susceptible to penicillins, cephalosporins, tetracyclines, macrolides, rifampin, and quinolones. The second report is of two isolates, also group B, from Australia, isolated from patients in 1994 and 1997. Chloramphenicol is no longer commonly used in developed nations, and has not been standard therapy for meningococcal meningitis in Vietnam since the 1980s. It is used frequently in topical preparations, especially ophthalmologic preparations, and it remains standard parenteral treatment in many developing countries, particularly in Africa. In both reports, resistance was mediated by a chloramphenicol acetyltransferase, with the gene encoding this enzyme possibly acquired from *Clostridium perfringens*.

Because of widespread use of choramphenicol in Africa, 33 serogroup A strains in the CDC collection were recently examined (188). These strains were obtained between 1963 and 1998 from nine different African countries, and almost 40% were from the time period when chloramphenicol resistance was seen in France and Vietnam. All were fully susceptible, and the *catP* gene encoding chloramphenicol acetyltransferase was not detected. However the small number of isolates studied does not provide complete reassurance in this regard.

3.2.3 *N. Meningitidis* Resistance to Agents Used for Prophylaxis

Resistance of meningococci to sulfonamides was identified in the US as early as 1963, and is now widespread. Although sulfonamides were no longer used for treatment of clinical disease, they were widely prescribed for prophylaxis prior to the identification of resistance (189, 190). Resistance is due to mutations in the gene for dihydropteroate synthase (191).

Resistance to rifampin has also been identified (192, 193). A 1997 study from the CDC found 3 of 97 isolates to be resistant to rifampin (177). A larger study from Australia involving 1,434 isolates obtained over 6 years in the 1990s found only eight isolates resistant to rifampin (MIC 1 mg/L), and one with reduced susceptibility to ciprofloxacin (MIC 0.25 mg/L) (175). A recent study in France found only one out of 2,167 isolates to be resistant to rifampin, and one additional isolate with reduced susceptibility (153). Other studies in Europe found similar patterns (172, 173). A 1996 study in the US showed the development of rifampin resistance during prophylaxis treatment. Oropharyngeal cultures were obtained before and 3 weeks after prophylaxis treatment was instituted in a middle school in Seattle. No secondary cases occurred, but resistance developed in 12% of the isolates, all of which were group B (194). Mutations in the *rpoB* gene as well as changes in membrane permeability account for rifampin resistance (153, 175, 186).

There have been several reports of reduced susceptibility to ciprofloxacin, one a serogroup C strain from a patient with invasive disease in Australia (as noted above), one a group B strain from a carrier in France, and the latest a group B strain isolated from the CSF of a patient in Spain (195, 196). *N. meningitidis* has the ability to develop mutations in the *gyrA* and *parC* genes that are similar to the mutations in QRNG (66, 197).

3.3 Clinical Significance of Resistance in N. meningitidis

A study from the UK looked specifically at the question of a link between reduced susceptibility to penicillin and fatal outcome from meningococcal infection (152). The authors retrospectively looked at over 11,000 cases reported between 1993 and 2000 in England and Wales. During this time period, the frequency of penicillin intermediate strains increased from less than 6% to greater than 18% (12.6% overall), with a higher frequency among serogroups C and W135. The overall case-fatality rate was around 8%, and while there was an association between fatal outcome and specific serogroups and serotypes, there was no link with reduced susceptibility to penicillin. In a Spanish study of isolates from 1988 to 1992, 34% of strains (72 of 213) showed decreased susceptibility to penicillin. Higher morbidity/mortality was associated with these strains, even though penicillin was not used for therapy in all cases (172, 198).

Isolated case reports raise the possibility of treatment failure associated with decreased susceptibility to penicillin. A report from the UK describes an 18-year-old with meningococcal meningitis, who was treated with IV benzylpenicillin and, after an initial clinical response, remained ill after several days. The CSF culture was positive when repeated. After treatment was changed to chloramphenicol, this patient improved rapidly. The *N. meningitidis* isolated from CSF initially and upon repeat had a penicillin MIC of 0.64 (reduced susceptibility). Notably, the dose of penicillin was lower than some use (199). Another report from Argentina also suggests possible treatment failure of penicillin (200).

Prophylaxis failures associated with rifampin resistance have been reported (192, 201). In Israel, three small clusters of disease that occurred in the military were examined. In one, the initial case was rifampicin-sensitive, but two secondary cases occurred among the contacts who had taken rifampicin, and the strains were identified to be rifampicin-resistant. All three strains were group C:NT:P1.2 (193). In the 1997 CDC study, nine contacts of individuals with rifampin-resistant *N. meningitidis* received prophylaxis with rifampin, and none developed disease (177).

3.4 Treatment and Infection Control Recommendations

Penicillin G remains the recommended treatment for invasive meningococcal disease in the US and elsewhere. The dose is 250,000 U/kg per day (up to a maximum of 12 million U/day), divided every 4–6 h. Cefotaxime, ceftriaxone, and ampicillin are acceptable alternatives. Recent data suggest that shorter courses of treatment than the usually accepted 7–10 days of therapy are adequate for management of meningococcal disease (158, 202). Chloramphenicol is recommended for patients with penicillin allergy characterized by anaphylaxis. For disease that may have been acquired in regions of the world where decreased susceptibility to penicillin is common, or resistance has been reported,

cefotaxime, ceftriaxone, or chloramphenicol is recommended. Chemoprophylaxis is recommended for individuals, and for close contacts of individuals with meningococcal disease in whom the risk of developing invasive disease is increased. This includes household contacts, childcare or nursery school contacts during the 7 days prior to disease onset in the index patient, and individuals who have been exposed to the index patient's secretions such as by kissing, or sharing eating utensils, during the 7 days prior to the onset of illness. In addition, healthcare workers who administered mouth-to-mouth resuscitation or those who were unprotected during endotracheal intubation should receive chemoprophylaxis. The patient should also receive prophylaxis to eliminate carriage, unless the infection was treated with ceftriaxone or cefotaxime. Recommended regimens include: rifampin 600 mg (or 10 mg/kg for children over 1 month of age, and 5 mg/kg for infants under 1 month of age) every 12 h for 2 days; ceftriaxone 250 mg intramuscularly as a single dose (125 mg for children less that 15 years of age); or ciprofloxacin 500 mg as a single oral dose.

Secondary cases of meningococcal disease can occur several weeks after onset of disease in an index patient. Therefore, vaccination can be used as an adjunct to chemoprophylaxis if the index case was caused by serogroups A, C, Y, or W-135.

4 Commensal *Neisseria* Species

N. lactamica, *N. sicca*, *N. subflava* (biovars subflava, flava, and perflava), *N. mucosa*, *N. flavescens*, *N. cinerea*, *N. polysaccharea*, and *N. elongata* subspecies *elongata*, *glycolytica*, and *nitroreducens* are human commensal organisms that are rarely associated with disease in a normal host. *N. elongata* subspecies *elongate*, *N. subflava*, and *N. sicca/perflava* have been occasionally associated with infective endocarditis, which occurs on damaged or normal heart valves and in congenital heart disease (203, 204); *N. sicca* and *N. perflava* have been described in pulmonary and disseminated infections in patients with AIDS (205).

Antibodies to *N. lactamica* developed during carriage may provide immunity to meningococcal disease. Interest in *N. lactamica* has thus been focused mainly on the identifying "immunizing" characteristics and the dynamics of carriage of this organism. There are, however, few large studies on antimicrobial resistance in the commensal *Neisseria* sp. derived from these carriage studies.

The commensal *Neisseria* are, by their nature, longer-term inhabitants of the nasopharynx than the more transient, invasive subtypes of *N. meningitidis*. For this reason, they are exposed more often and for a greater duration to resistance pressures arising from use of antimicrobials prescribed for any reason. It is therefore reasonable to suggest that the commensal *Neisseria* may harbor a reservoir of resistance genes available for acquisition by the invasive species. Penicillin-binding proteins, encoded by chromosomal *penA* genes, are the target site for the penicillins. It has been shown that mosaic *penA* genes present in the highly transformable commensal *Neisseria* confer intermediate resistance to penicillin. These resistance genes are then transferred to other commensal *Neisseria*, and also to *N. meningitidis* by recombination (178, 206).

One report (207) of antibiotic resistance in 286 *N. lactamica*, collected in Spain in 1996 and 1998 during studies on meningococcal carriage, demonstrated raised penicillin MICs (0.12–1 mg/L) in all isolates tested. Additionally, about 2% of isolates in this study showed decreased quinolone susceptibility many years before its appearance in pathogenic *N. meningitidis* in that country. In another study, examination of *N. gonorrhoeae* isolates in Japan that had decreased susceptibility to cefixime identified mosaic PBP 2 that had fragments that were identical to the PBP 2 of *N. cinerea* and *N. perflava* (56). Isolates of *N. elongata* subspecies *elongata*, *N. subflava*, and *N. sicca/perflava* found in occasional instances of systemic infection often display resistance or decreased susceptibility to penicillins and other agents. Thus misuse of antibiotics may have profound consequences on the commensal members of this genus in terms of emergence and spread of resistance genes, with subsequent "downstream" effects on both meningococci and gonococci.

References

1. Anonymous. *Global Prevalence and Incidence of Selected Curable Sexually Transmitted Infections: Overview and Estimates.* World Health Organization, Geneva, 15–19, 2001
2. Gerbase AC, Rowley JT, Heymann DH, Berkley SF, Piot P. Global prevalence and incidence estimates of selected curable STDs. Sex Transm Infect 1998; 74 Suppl 1:12–16
3. Lacey CJ, Merrick DW, Bensley DC, Fairley I. Analysis of the sociodemography of gonorrhoea in Leeds, 1989–93. BMJ 1997; 314(7096):1715–1718
4. Low N, Daker-White G, Barlow D, Pozniak AL. Gonorrhoea in inner London: results of a cross sectional study. BMJ 1997; 314(7096):1719–1723
5. Tapsall JW. Perspectives on gonococcal disease in Australia. In: Asche V, ed. *Recent Advances in Microbiology 1999.* The Australian Society for Microbiology, Melbourne, 171–196, 1999
6. Centers for Disease Control and Prevention. *Sexually Transmitted Disease Surveillance, 2003.* U.S. Department of Health and Human Services, CDC, Atlanta, GA, 2004
7. Centers for Disease Control and Prevention. Increases in fluoroquinolone-resistant *Neisseria gonorrhoeae* among men who have sex with men – United States, 2003, and revised recommendations for gonorrhea treatment, 2004. MMWR Morb Mortal Wkly Rep 2004; 53(16):335–338
8. Donovan B, Bodsworth NJ, Rohrsheim R, McNulty A, Tapsall JW. Increasing gonorrhoea reports – not only in London. Lancet 2000; 355(9218):1908
9. Martin IM, Ison CA. Rise in gonorrhoea in London, UK. London Gonococcal Working Group. Lancet 2000; 355(9204):623
10. Waugh MA. Task force for the urgent response to the epidemics of sexually transmitted diseases in eastern Europe and central Asia. Sex Transm Infect 1999; 75(1):72–73
11. Sparling PF, Handsfield HH. *Neisseria gonorrhoeae.* In: Mandell GL, Bennett JE, eds. *Principles and Practice of Infectious Diseases.* Churchill Livingstone, Philadelphia, 2242–2258, 2000
12. Laga M, Manoka A, Kivuvu M, Malele B, Tuliza M, Nzila N et al. Non-ulcerative sexually transmitted diseases as risk factors for HIV-1 transmission in women: results from a cohort study. AIDS 1993; 7(1):95–102
13. Cohen MS, Hoffman IF, Royce RA, Kazembe P, Dyer JR, Daly CC, et al. Reduction of concentration of HIV-1 in semen after treatment of urethritis: implications for prevention of sexual transmission of HIV-1. AIDSCAP Malawi Research Group. Lancet 1997; 349(9069):1868–1873
14. Cohen MS. Sexually transmitted diseases enhance HIV transmission: no longer a hypothesis. Lancet 1998; 351 Suppl 3:5–7
15. Tapsall JW. *Antimicrobial Resistance in Neisseria gonorrhoeae WHO/CDS/CSR/DRS/2001.3.* World Health Organization, Geneva, 2001
16. Haizlip J, Isbey SF, Hamilton HA, Jerse AE, Leone PA, Davis RH et al. Time required for elimination of *Neisseria gonorrhoeae* from the urogenital tract in men with symptomatic urethritis: comparison of oral and intramuscular single-dose therapy. Sex Transm Dis 1995; 22(3):145–148
17. Holmes KK, Johnson DW, Floyd TM. Studies of venereal disease. I. Probenecid-procaine penicillin G combination and tetracycline hydrochloride in the treatment of "penicillin-resistant" gonorrhea in men. JAMA 1967; 202(6):461–473
18. Fussenegger M, Rudel T, Barten R, Ryll R, Meyer TF. Transformation competence and type-4 pilus biogenesis in *Neisseria gonorrhoeae* – a review. Gene 1997; 192(1):125–134
19. Cannon JG, Sparling PF. The genetics of the gonococcus. Annu Rev Microbiol 1984; 38:111–133
20. Hamilton HL, Dillard JP. Natural transformation of *Neisseria gonorrhoeae*: from DNA donation to homologous recombination. Mol Microbiol 2006; 59(2):376–385
21. Reyn A, Korner B, Bentzon MW. Effects of penicillin, streptomycin, and tetracycline on *N. gonorrhoeae* isolated in 1944 and in 1957. Br J Vener Dis 1958; 34(4):227–239
22. Laga M. Epidemiology and control of sexually transmitted diseases in developing countries. Sex Transm Dis 1994; 21 2 Suppl: S45–S50
23. Adu-Sarkodie YA. Antimicrobial self medication in patients attending a sexually transmitted diseases clinic. Int J STD AIDS 1997; 8(7):456–458
24. Abellanosa I, Nichter M. Antibiotic prophylaxis among commercial sex workers in Cebu City, Philippines. Patterns of use and perceptions of efficacy. Sex Transm Dis 1996; 23(5):407–412
25. Taylor RB, Shakoor O, Behrens RH. Drug quality, a contributor to drug resistance? Lancet 1995; 346(8967):122
26. Van der Veen F, Fransen L. Drugs for STD management in developing countries: choice, procurement, cost, and financing. Sex Transm Infect 1998; 74 Suppl 1:S166–S174
27. Johnson SR, Morse SA. Antibiotic resistance in *Neisseria gonorrhoeae*: genetics and mechanisms of resistance. Sex Transm Dis 1988; 15(4):217–224
28. Sparling PF. Antibiotic resistance in *Neisseria gonorrhoeae*. Med Clin North Am 1972; 56(5):1133–1144
29. Ropp PA, Hu M, Olesky M, Nicholas RA. Mutations in ponA, the gene encoding penicillin-binding protein 1, and a novel locus, penC, are required for high-level chromosomally mediated penicillin resistance in *Neisseria gonorrhoeae*. Antimicrob Agents Chemother 2002; 46(3):769–777

30. Dougherty TJ. Involvement of a change in penicillin target and peptidoglycan structure in low-level resistance to beta-lactam antibiotics in *Neisseria gonorrhoeae*. Antimicrob Agents Chemother 1985; 28(1):90–95

31. Sparling PF, Sarubbi FA, Jr, Blackman E. Inheritance of low-level resistance to penicillin, tetracycline, and chloramphenicol in *Neisseria gonorrhoeae*. J Bacteriol 1975; 124(2):740–749

32. Guymon LF, Sparling PF. Altered crystal violet permeability and lytic behavior in antibiotic-resistant and -sensitive mutants of *Neisseria gonorrhoeae*. J Bacteriol 1975; 124(2):757–763

33. Hagman KE, Pan W, Spratt BG, Balthazar JT, Judd RC, Shafer WM. Resistance of *Neisseria gonorrhoeae* to antimicrobial hydrophobic agents is modulated by the mtrRCDE efflux system. Microbiology 1995; 141 (Pt 3):611–622

34. Gill MJ, Simjee S, Al Hattawi K, Robertson BD, Easmon CS, Ison CA. Gonococcal resistance to beta-lactams and tetracycline involves mutation in loop 3 of the porin encoded at the penB locus. Antimicrob Agents Chemother 1998; 42(11):2799–2803

35. Olesky M, Hobbs M, Nicholas RA. Identification and analysis of amino acid mutations in porin IB that mediate intermediate-level resistance to penicillin and tetracycline in *Neisseria gonorrhoeae*. Antimicrob Agents Chemother 2002; 46(9):2811–2820

36. Olesky M, Zhao S, Rosenberg RL, Nicholas RA. Porin-mediated antibiotic resistance in *Neisseria gonorrhoeae*: ion, solute, and antibiotic permeation through PIB proteins with penB mutations. J Bacteriol 2006; 188(7):2300–2308

37. Zhao S, Tobiason DM, Hu M, Seifert HS, Nicholas RA. The penC mutation conferring antibiotic resistance in *Neisseria gonorrhoeae* arises from a mutation in the PilQ secretin that interferes with multimer stability. Mol Microbiol 2005; 57(5):1238–1251

38. Ison CA. Antimicrobial agents and gonorrhoea: therapeutic choice, resistance and susceptibility testing. Genitourin Med 1996; 72(4): 253–257

39. Bygdeman S. Polyclonal and monoclonal antibodies applied to the epidemiology of gonococcal infection. In: Young H, McMillan A, eds. *Immunologic Diagnosis of Sexually Transmitted Diseases*. Marcel Dekker, New York, 117–165, 1988

40. Knapp JS, et al. Nomenclature for the serologic classification of *Neisseria gonorrhoeae*. In: Schoolnik G, Brooks GF, Falkow S, et al. eds. *The Pathogenic Neisseriae*. American Society for Microbiology, Washington DC, 4–5, 1985

41. Phillips I. Beta-lactamase-producing, penicillin-resistant gonococcus. Lancet 1976; 2(7987):656–657

42. Ashford WA, Golash RG, Hemming VG. Penicillinase-producing *Neisseria gonorrhoeae*. Lancet 1976; 2(7987):657–658

43. van Embden JD, van Klingeren B, Dessens-Kroon M, van Wijngaarden LJ. Emergence in the Netherlands of penicillinase-producing gonococci carrying "Africa" plasmid in combination with transfer plasmid. Lancet 1981; 1(8226):938

44. Laufs R, Kaulfers PM, Jahn G, Teschner U. Molecular characterization of a small *Haemophilus influenzae* plasmid specifying beta-lactamase and its relationship to R factors from *Neisseria gonorrhoeae*. J Gen Microbiol 1979; 111(1):223–231

45. van Embden JD, van Klingeren B, Dessens-Kroon M, van Wijngaarden LJ. Penicillinase-producing *Neisseria gonorrhoeae* in the Netherlands: epidemiology and genetic and molecular characterization of their plasmids. Antimicrob Agents Chemother 1980; 18(5):789–797

46. Brunton JL, Clare D, Ehrman N, Meier MA. Evolution of antibiotic resistance plasmids in *Neisseria gonorrhoeae* and *Haemophilus* species. Clin Invest Med 1983; 6(3):221–228

47. Flett F, Humphreys GO, Saunders JR. Intraspecific and intergeneric mobilization of non-conjugative resistance plasmids by a 24.5 megadalton conjugative plasmid of *Neisseria gonorrhoeae*. J Gen Microbiol 1981; 125(1):123–129

48. Roberts M, Elwell LP, Falkow S. Molecular characterization of two beta-lactamase-specifying plasmids isolated from *Neisseria gonorrhoeae*. J Bacteriol 1977; 131(2):557–563

49. Lim KB, Rajan VS, Giam YC, Lui EO, Sng EH, Yeo KL. Two dose augmentin treatment of acute gonorrhoea in men. Br J Vener Dis 1984; 60(3):161–163

50. Lim KB, Thirumoorthy T, Lee CT, Sng EH, Tan T. Three regimens of procaine penicillin G, Augmentin, and probenecid compared for treating acute gonorrhoea in men. Genitourin Med 1986; 62(2):82–85

51. Tapsall JW, Phillips EA, Morris LM. Chromosomally mediated intrinsic resistance to penicillin of penicillinase producing strains of *Neisseria gonorrhoeae* isolated in Sydney: guide to treatment with Augmentin. Genitourin Med 1987; 63(5):305–308

52. Ison CA, Bindayna KM, Woodford N, Gill MJ, Easmon CS. Penicillin and cephalosporin resistance in gonococci. Genitourin Med 1990; 66(5):351–356

53. Rice RJ, Biddle JW, JeanLouis YA, DeWitt WE, Blount JH, Morse SA. Chromosomally mediated resistance in *Neisseria gonorrhoeae* in the United States: results of surveillance and reporting, 1983–1984. J Infect Dis 1986; 153(2):340–345

54. Schwebke JR, Whittington W, Rice RJ, Handsfield HH, Hale J, Holmes KK. Trends in susceptibility of *Neisseria gonorrhoeae* to ceftriaxone from 1985 through 1991. Antimicrob Agents Chemother 1995; 39(4):917–920

55. Muratani T, Akasaka S, Kobayashi T, Yamada Y, Inatomi H, Takahashi K et al. Outbreak of cefozopran (penicillin, oral cephems, and aztreonam)-resistant *Neisseria gonorrhoeae* in Japan. Antimicrob Agents Chemother 2001; 45(12):3603–3606

56. Ito M, Deguchi T, Mizutani KS, Yasuda M, Yokoi S, Ito S et al. Emergence and spread of *Neisseria gonorrhoeae* clinical isolates harboring mosaic-like structure of penicillin-binding protein 2 in Central Japan. Antimicrob Agents Chemother 2005; 49(1):137–143

57. Takahata S, Senju N, Osaki Y, Yoshida T, Ida T. Amino acid substitutions in mosaic penicillin-binding protein 2 associated with reduced susceptibility to cefixime in clinical isolates of *Neisseria gonorrhoeae*. Antimicrob Agents Chemother 2006; 50(11):3638–3645

58. Tanaka M, Nakayama H, Huruya K, Konomi I, Irie S, Kanayama A et al. Analysis of mutations within multiple genes associated with resistance in a clinical isolate of *Neisseria gonorrhoeae* with reduced ceftriaxone susceptibility that shows a multidrug-resistant phenotype. Int J Antimicrob Agents 2006; 27(1):20–26

59. Lindberg R, Fredlund H, Nicholas R, Unemo M. *Neisseria gonorrhoeae* isolates with reduced susceptibility to cefixime and ceftriaxone: association with genetic polymorphisms in penA, mtrR, porB1b, and ponA. Antimicrob Agents Chemother 2007; 51(6):2117–2122

60. Moran JS, Zenilman JM. Therapy for gonococcal infections: options in 1989. Rev Infect Dis 1990; 12 Suppl 6:S633–S644

61. Ghanem KG, Giles JA, Zenilman JM. Fluoroquinolone-resistant *Neisseria gonorrhoeae*: the inevitable epidemic. Infect Dis Clin North Am 2005; 19(2):351–365

62. Dan M. The use of fluoroquinolones in gonorrhoea: the increasing problem of resistance. Expert Opin Pharmacother 2004; 5(4): 829–854

63. Surveillance of antibiotic susceptibility of *Neisseria gonorrhoeae* in the WHO western Pacific region 1992–4. WHO Western Pacific Region Gonococcal Antimicrobial Surveillance Programme. Genitourin Med 1997; 73(5):355–361

64. Surveillance of antibiotic resistance in *Neisseria gonorrhoeae* in the World Health Organization Western Pacific Region, 2003. Commun Dis Intell 2005; 29(1):62–64

65. Belland RJ, Morrison SG, Ison C, Huang WM. *Neisseria gonorrhoeae* acquires mutations in analogous regions of gyrA and

parC in fluoroquinolone-resistant isolates. Mol Microbiol 1994; 14(2):371–380

66. Shultz TR, Tapsall JW, White PA. Correlation of in vitro susceptibilities to newer quinolones of naturally occurring quinolone-resistant *Neisseria gonorrhoeae* strains with changes in GyrA and ParC. Antimicrob Agents Chemother 2001; 45(3):734–738

67. Trees DL, Sandul AL, Whittington WL, Knapp JS. Identification of novel mutation patterns in the parC gene of ciprofloxacin-resistant isolates of *Neisseria gonorrhoeae*. Antimicrob Agents Chemother 1998; 42(8):2103–2105

68. Deguchi T, Saito I, Tanaka M, Sato K, Deguchi K, Yasuda M, et al. Fluoroquinolone treatment failure in gonorrhea. Emergence of a *Neisseria gonorrhoeae* strain with enhanced resistance to fluoroquinolones. Sex Transm Dis 1997; 24(5):247–250

69. Tanaka M, Sagiyama K, Haraoka M, Saika T, Kobayashi I, Naito S. Genotypic evolution in a quinolone-resistant *Neisseria gonorrhoeae* isolate from a patient with clinical failure of levofloxacin treatment. Urol Int 1999; 62(1):64–68

70. Tanaka M, Nakayama H, Haraoka M, Nagafuji T, Saika T, Kobayashi I. Analysis of quinolone resistance mechanisms in a sparfloxacin-resistant clinical isolate of *Neisseria gonorrhoeae*. Sex Transm Dis 1998; 25(9):489–493

71. Tanaka M, Sakuma S, Takahashi K, Nagahuzi T, Saika T, Kobayashi I et al. Analysis of quinolone resistance mechanisms in *Neisseria gonorrhoeae* isolates in vitro. Sex Transm Infect 1998; 74(1):59–62

72. Giles JA, Falconio J, Yuenger JD, Zenilman JM, Dan M, Bash MC. Quinolone resistance-determining region mutations and por type of *Neisseria gonorrhoeae* isolates: resistance surveillance and typing by molecular methodologies. J Infect Dis 2004; 189(11):2085–2093

73. Knapp JS, Fox KK, Trees DL, Whittington WL. Fluoroquinolone resistance in *Neisseria gonorrhoeae*. Emerg Infect Dis 1997; 3(1):33–39

74. Dewi BE, Akira S, Hayashi H, Ba-Thein W. High occurrence of simultaneous mutations in target enzymes and MtrRCDE efflux system in quinolone-resistant *Neisseria gonorrhoeae*. Sex Transm Dis 2004; 31(6):353–359

75. Boslego JW, Tramont EC, Takafuji ET, Diniega BM, Mitchell BS, Small JW et al. Effect of spectinomycin use on the prevalence of spectinomycin-resistant and of penicillinase-producing *Neisseria gonorrhoeae*. N Engl J Med 1987; 317(5):272–278

76. Maness MJ, Foster GC, Sparling PF. Ribosomal resistance to streptomycin and spectinomycin in *Neisseria gonorrhoeae*. J Bacteriol 1974; 120(3):1293–1299

77. Tapsall JW. Antibiotic resistance in *Neisseria gonorrhoeae*. Clin Infect Dis 2005; 41 Suppl 4:S263–S268

78. Hu M, Nandi S, Davies C, Nicholas RA. High-level chromosomally mediated tetracycline resistance in *Neisseria gonorrhoeae* results from a point mutation in the rpsJ gene encoding ribosomal protein S10 in combination with the mtrR and penB resistance determinants. Antimicrob Agents Chemother 2005; 49(10): 4327–4334

79. Faruki H, Kohmescher RN, McKinney WP, Sparling PF. A community-based outbreak of infection with penicillin-resistant *Neisseria gonorrhoeae* not producing penicillinase (chromosomally mediated resistance). N Engl J Med 1985; 313(10):607–611

80. Morse SA, Johnson SR, Biddle JW, Roberts MC. High-level tetracycline resistance in *Neisseria gonorrhoeae* is result of acquisition of streptococcal tetM determinant. Antimicrob Agents Chemother 1986; 30(5):664–670

81. Gascoyne-Binzi DM, Heritage J, Hawkey PM. Nucleotide sequences of the tet(M) genes from the American and Dutch type tetracycline resistance plasmids of *Neisseria gonorrhoeae*. J Antimicrob Chemother 1993; 32(5):667–676

82. Turner A, Gough KR, Leeming JP. Molecular epidemiology of tetM genes in *Neisseria gonorrhoeae*. Sex Transm Infect 1999; 75(1):60–66

83. Ison CA, Dillon JA, Tapsall JW. The epidemiology of global antibiotic resistance among *Neisseria gonorrhoeae* and *Haemophilus ducreyi*. Lancet 1998; 351 Suppl 3:8–11

84. Djajakusumah T, Sudigdoadi S, Meheus A, Van Dyck E. Plasmid patterns and antimicrobial susceptibilities of *Neisseria gonorrhoeae* in Bandung, Indonesia. Trans R Soc Trop Med Hyg 1998; 92(1):105–107

85. West B, Changalucha J, Grosskurth H, Mayaud P, Gabone RM, Ka-Gina G et al. Antimicrobial susceptibility, auxotype and plasmid content of *Neisseria gonorrhoeae* in northern Tanzania: emergence of high level plasmid mediated tetracycline resistance. Genitourin Med 1995; 71(1):9–12

86. Van Dyck E, Crabbe F, Nzila N, Bogaerts J, Munyabikali JP, Ghys P, et al. Increasing resistance of *Neisseria gonorrhoeae* in west and central Africa. Consequence on therapy of gonococcal infection. Sex Transm Dis 1997; 24(1):32–37

87. Ho RI, Lai PH, Corman L, Ho J, Morse SA. Comparison of dihydrofolate reductases from trimethoprim- and sulfonamide-resistant strains of *Neisseria gonorrhoeae*. Sex Transm Dis 1978; 5(2):43–50

88. Slaney L, Chubb H, Ronald A, Brunham R. In-vitro activity of azithromycin, erythromycin, ciprofloxacin and norfloxacin against *Neisseria gonorrhoeae*, Haemophilus ducreyi, and Chlamydia trachomatis. J Antimicrob Chemother 1990; 25 Suppl A:1–5

89. Rouquette-Loughlin CE, Balthazar JT, Shafer WM. Characterization of the MacA-MacB efflux system in *Neisseria gonorrhoeae*. J Antimicrob Chemother 2005; 56(5):856–860

90. Ehret JM, Nims LJ, Judson FN. A clinical isolate of *Neisseria gonorrhoeae* with in vitro resistance to erythromycin and decreased susceptibility to azithromycin. Sex Transm Dis 1996; 23(4):270–272

91. Tapsall JW, Shultz TR, Limnios EA, Donovan B, Lum G, Mulhall BP. Failure of azithromycin therapy in gonorrhea and discorrelation with laboratory test parameters. Sex Transm Dis 1998; 25(10):505–508

92. Steingrimsson O, Olafsson JH, Thorarinsson H, Ryan RW, Johnson RB, Tilton RC. Azithromycin in the treatment of sexually transmitted disease. J Antimicrob Chemother 1990; 25 Suppl A:109–114

93. Young H, Moyes A, McMillan A. Azithromycin and erythromycin resistant *Neisseria gonorrhoeae* following treatment with azithromycin. Int J STD AIDS 1997; 8(5):299–302

94. Daly CC, Hoffman I, Hobbs M, Maida M, Zimba D, Davis R et al. Development of an antimicrobial susceptibility surveillance system for *Neisseria gonorrhoeae* in Malawi: comparison of methods. J Clin Microbiol 1997; 35(11):2985–2988

95. Lkhamsuren E, Shultz TR, Limnios EA, Tapsall JW. The antibiotic susceptibility of *Neisseria gonorrhoeae* isolated in Ulaanbaatar, Mongolia. Sex Transm Infect 2001; 77(3):218–219

96. Bhalla P, Sethi K, Reddy BS, Mathur MD. Antimicrobial susceptibility and plasmid profile of *Neisseria gonorrhoeae* in India (New Delhi). Sex Transm Infect 1998; 74(3):210–212

97. Tapsall JW. Use of a quality assurance scheme in a long-term multicentric study of antibiotic susceptibility of *Neisseria gonorrhoeae*. Genitourin Med 1990; 66(1):8–13

98. Tapsall J, Members of the National Neisseria Network of Australia. Antimicrobial testing and applications in the pathogenic Neisseria. In: Merlino J, ed. *Antimicrobial Susceptibility Testing: Methods and Practices with an Australian Perspective*. Australian Society for Microbiology, Sydney, 175–188, 2005

99. Deguchi T, Yasuda M, Nakano M, Ozeki S, Kanematsu E, Kawada Y et al. Uncommon occurrence of mutations in the gyrB gene associated with quinolone resistance in clinical isolates of *Neisseria gonorrhoeae*. Antimicrob Agents Chemother 1996; 40(10):2437–2438

100. Deguchi T, Yasuda M, Nakano M, Kanematsu E, Ozeki S, Nishino Y et al. Rapid screening of point mutations of the *Neisseria gonorrhoeae* parC gene associated with resistance to quinolones. J Clin Microbiol 1997; 35(4):948–950

101. Deguchi T, Yasuda M, Nakano M, Ozeki S, Ezaki T, Maeda S et al. Rapid detection of point mutations of the *Neisseria gonorrhoeae* gyrA gene associated with decreased susceptibilities to quinolones. J Clin Microbiol 1996; 34(9):2255–2258

102. Vernel-Pauillac F, Merien F. A novel real-time duplex PCR assay for detecting penA and ponA genotypes in *Neisseria gonorrhoeae*: comparison with phenotypes determined by the E-test. Clin Chem 2006; 52(12):2294–2296

103. Giles J, Hardick J, Yuenger J, Dan M, Reich K, Zenilman J. Use of applied biosystems 7900HT sequence detection system and Taqman assay for detection of quinolone-resistant *Neisseria gonorrhoeae*. J Clin Microbiol 2004; 42(7):3281–3283

104. Kilmarx PH, Knapp JS, Xia M, St Louis ME, Neal SW, Sayers D et al. Intercity spread of gonococci with decreased susceptibility to fluoroquinolones: a unique focus in the United States. J Infect Dis 1998; 177(3):677–682

105. van Klingeren B, Ansink-Schipper MC, Dessens-Kroon M, Verheuvel M. Relationship between auxotype, plasmid pattern and susceptibility to antibiotics in penicillinase-producing *Neisseria gonorrhoeae*. J Antimicrob Chemother 1985; 16(2):143–147

106. Rothenberg R, Voigt R. Epidemiologic aspects of control of penicillinase-producing *Neisseria gonorrhoeae*. Sex Transm Dis 1988; 15(4):211–216

107. Increases in fluoroquinolone-resistant *Neisseria gonorrhoeae* – Hawaii and California, 2001. MMWR Morb Mortal Wkly Rep 2002; 51(46):1041–1044

108. Tanaka M, Nakayama H, Haraoka M, Saika T. Antimicrobial resistance of *Neisseria gonorrhoeae* and high prevalence of ciprofloxacin-resistant isolates in Japan, 1993 to 1998. J Clin Microbiol 2000; 38(2):521–525

109. Trees DL, Sandul AL, Neal SW, Higa H, Knapp JS. Molecular epidemiology of *Neisseria gonorrhoeae* exhibiting decreased susceptibility and resistance to ciprofloxacin in Hawaii, 1991–1999. Sex Transm Dis 2001; 28(6):309–314

110. Tapsall JW, Shultz TR, Phillips EA. Characteristics of *Neisseria gonorrhoeae* isolated in Australia showing decreased sensitivity to quinolone antibiotics. Pathology 1992; 24(1):27–31

111. Tapsall JW, Limnios EA, Shultz TR. Continuing evolution of the pattern of quinolone resistance in *Neisseria gonorrhoeae* isolated in Sydney, Australia. Sex Transm Dis 1998; 25(8):415–417

112. Yagupsky P, Schahar A, Peled N, Porat N, Trefler R, Dan M et al. Increasing incidence of gonorrhea in Israel associated with countrywide dissemination of a ciprofloxacin-resistant strain. Eur J Clin Microbiol Infect Dis 2002; 21(5):368–372

113. Palmer HM, Leeming JP, Turner A. Investigation of an outbreak of ciprofloxacin-resistant *Neisseria gonorrhoeae* using a simplified opa-typing method. Epidemiol Infect 2001; 126(2):219–224

114. Unemo M, Sjostrand A, Akhras M, Gharizadeh B, Lindback E, Pourmand N et al. Molecular characterization of *Neisseria gonorrhoeae* identifies transmission and resistance of one ciprofloxacin-resistant strain. APMIS 2007; 115(3):231–241

115. Sexually transmitted diseases treatment guidelines 2002. Centers for Disease Control and Prevention. MMWR Recomm Rep 2002; 51(RR-6):1–78

116. Bignell CJ. BASHH guideline for gonorrhoea. Sex Transm Infect 2004; 80(5):330–331

117. Bignell CJ. European guideline for the management of gonorrhoea. Int J STD AIDS 2001; 12 Suppl 3:27–29

118. World Health Organization. *Guidelines for the Management of Sexually Transmitted Infections*. World Health Organization, Geneva, 2003

119. Backman M, Jacobson K, Ringertz S. The virgin population of *Neisseria gonorrhoeae* in Stockholm has decreased and antimicrobial resistance is increasing. Genitourin Med 1995; 71(4):234–238

120. Marrazzo JM. Sexual tourism: implications for travelers and the destination culture. Infect Dis Clin North Am 2005; 19(1):103–120

121. Annual report of the Australian Gonococcal Surveillance Programme, 2004. Commun Dis Intell 2005; 29(2):137–142

122. Centers for Disease Control and Prevention. *Sexually Transmitted Disease Surveillance, 2002*. U.S. Department of Health and Human Services, CDC, Atlanta, GA, 2003

123. Paine TC, Fenton KA, Herring A, Turner A, Ison C, Martin I et al. GRASP: a new national sentinel surveillance initiative for monitoring gonococcal antimicrobial resistance in England and Wales. Sex Transm Infect 2001; 77(6):398–401

124. Surveillance of antibiotic resistance in *Neisseria gonorrhoeae* in the WHO Western Pacific Region, 2002. Commun Dis Intell 2003; 27(4):488–491

125. Dillon JA, Li H, Sealy J, Ruben M, Prabhakar P. Antimicrobial susceptibility of *Neisseria gonorrhoeae* isolates from three Caribbean countries: Trinidad, Guyana, and St Vincent. Sex Transm Dis 2001; 28(9):508–514

126. Penicillin sensitivity of gonococci in Australia: development of Australian gonococcal surveillance programme. Members of the Australian Gonococcal Surveillance Programme. Br J Vener Dis 1984; 60(4):226–230

127. Gorwitz RJ, Nakashima AK, Moran JS, Knapp JS. Sentinel surveillance for antimicrobial resistance in *Neisseria gonorrhoeae* – United States, 1988–1991. The Gonococcal Isolate Surveillance Project Study Group. MMWR CDC Surveill Summ 1993; 42(3):29–39

128. CDC. *Sexually Transmitted Disease Surveillance 2003 Supplement: Gonococcal Isolate Surveillance Project (GISP) Annual Report – 2003*. U.S. Department of Health and Human Services, Atlanta, GA, 2004

129. GRASP Steering Group. The Gonococccal Resistance to Antimicrobials Surveillance Programme. 2005. London, Health Protection Agency

130. Mayaud P, Hawkes S, Mabey D. Advances in control of sexually transmitted diseases in developing countries. Lancet 1998; 351 Suppl 3:29–32

131. Zenilman JM, Deal CD. Gonorrhoea: epidemiology, control and prevention. In: Stanberry LR, Bernstein DI, eds. *Sexually Transmitted Diseases Vaccines, Prevention and Control*. Academic Press, London, 369–385, 2000

132. Brooks GF, Donegan EA. Uncomplicated gonococcal infection. In: Brooks GF, Donegan GF, eds. *Gonococcal Infection*. Edward Arnold, London, 85–104, 1985

133. Schachter J. Chlamydial infections (second of three parts). N Engl J Med 1978; 298(9):490–495

134. Lyss SB, Kamb ML, Peterman TA, Moran JS, Newman DR, Bolan G et al. Chlamydia trachomatis among patients infected with and treated for *Neisseria gonorrhoeae* in sexually transmitted disease clinics in the United States. Ann Intern Med 2003; 139(3):178–185

135. Miller WC, Zenilman JM. Epidemiology of chlamydial infection, gonorrhea, and trichomoniasis in the United States – 2005. Infect Dis Clin North Am 2005; 19(2):281–296

136. Harry C. The management of uncomplicated adult gonococcal infection: should test of cure still be routine in patients attending genitourinary medicine clinics? Int J STD AIDS 2004; 15(7):453–458

137. Tapsall JW, Limnios EA, Thacker C, Donovan B, Lynch SD, Kirby LJ et al. High-level quinolone resistance in *Neisseria gonorrhoeae*: a report of two cases. Sex Transm Dis 1995; 22(5):310–311

138. Laga M, Plummer FA, Piot P, Datta P, Namaara W, Ndinya-Achola JO, et al. Prophylaxis of gonococcal and chlamydial ophthalmia neonatorum. A comparison of silver nitrate and tetracycline. N Engl J Med 1988; 318(11):653–657

139. Update to CDC's sexually transmitted diseases treatment guidelines, 2006: fluoroquinolones no longer recommended for treatment of gonococcal infections. MMWR Morb Mortal Wkly Rep 2007; 56(14):332–336

140. Discontinuation of cefixime tablets – United States. MMWR Morb Mortal Wkly Rep 2002; 51(46):1052

141. Handsfield HH, Dalu ZA, Martin DH, Douglas JM Jr, Mc Carty JM, Schlossberg D. Multicenter trial of single-dose azithromycin vs. ceftriaxone in the treatment of uncomplicated gonorrhea. Azithromycin Gonorrhea Study Group. Sex Transm Dis 1994; 21(2):107–111

142. Dillon JA, Rubabaza JP, Benzaken AS, Sardinha JC, Li H, Bandeira MG et al. Reduced susceptibility to azithromycin and high percentages of penicillin and tetracycline resistance in *Neisseria gonorrhoeae* isolates from Manaus, Brazil, 1998. Sex Transm Dis 2001; 28(9):521–526

143. Kamwendo F, Forslin L, Bodin L, Danielsson D. Decreasing incidences of gonorrhea- and chlamydia-associated acute pelvic inflammatory disease. A 25-year study from an urban area of central Sweden. Sex Transm Dis 1996; 23(5):384–391

144. Kamwendo F, Forslin L, Bodin L, Danielsson D. Programmes to reduce pelvic inflammatory disease – the Swedish experience. Lancet 1998; 351 Suppl 3:25–28

145. Kamwendo F, Forslin L, Bodin L, Danielsson D. Epidemiology of ectopic pregnancy during a 28 year period and the role of pelvic inflammatory disease. Sex Transm Infect 2000; 76(1):28–32

146. Grosskurth H, Mosha F, Todd J, Mwijarubi E, Klokke A, Senkoro K et al. Impact of improved treatment of sexually transmitted diseases on HIV infection in rural Tanzania: randomised controlled trial. Lancet 1995; 346(8974):530–536

147. Simonsen GS, Tapsall JW, Allegranzi B, Talbot EA, Lazzari S. The antimicrobial resistance containment and surveillance approach – a public health tool. Bull World Health Organ 2004; 82(12):928–934

148. From the Centers for Disease Control and Prevention. Increases in unsafe sex and rectal gonorrhea among men who have sex with men   San Francisco, California, 1994–1997. JAMA 1999; 281(8):696–697

149. Katz AR, Lee MV, Ohye RG, Whiticar PM, Effler PV. Ciprofloxacin resistance in *Neisseria gonorrhoeae*: trends in Hawaii, 1997–2002. Lancet 2003; 362(9382):495

150. Enhanced surveillance of epidemic meningococcal meningitis in Africa: a three-year experience. Wkly Epidemiol Rec 2005; 80(37):313–320

151. Raghunathan PL, Bernhardt SA, Rosenstein NE. Opportunities for control of meningococcal disease in the United States. Annu Rev Med 2004; 55:333–353

152. Trotter CL, Fox AJ, Ramsay ME, Sadler F, Gray SJ, Mallard R et al. Fatal outcome from meningococcal disease – an association with meningococcal phenotype but not with reduced susceptibility to benzylpenicillin. J Med Microbiol 2002; 51(10):855–860

153. Antignac A, Ducos-Galand M, Guiyoule A, Pires R, Alonso JM, Taha MK. *Neisseria meningitidis* strains isolated from invasive infections in France (1999–2002): phenotypes and antibiotic susceptibility patterns. Clin Infect Dis 2003; 37(7):912–920

154. Apicella MA. *Neisseria meningitidis*. In: Mandell GL, Bennett JE, eds. *Principles and Practice of Infectious Diseases*. Churchill Livingstone, Philadelphia, 2228–2241, 2000

155. Greenfield S, Sheehe PR, Feldman HA. Meningococcal carriage in a population of "normal" families. J Infect Dis 1971; 123(1):67–73

156. Schwentker FF, Gelman S, Long PH. Landmark article April 24, 1937. The treatment of meningococci meningitis with sulfanilamide. Preliminary report. By Francis F. Schwentker, Sidney Gelman, and Perrin H. Long. JAMA 1984; 251(6):788–790

157. Meningococcal infections. In: Pickering LK, ed. *Red Book: 2003 Report of the Committee on Infectious Diseases*. American Academy of Pediatrics, Elk Grove Village, 430–436, 2003

158. Nathan N, Borel T, Djibo A, Evans D, Djibo S, Corty JF et al. Ceftriaxone as effective as long-acting chloramphenicol in short-course treatment of meningococcal meningitis during epidemics: a randomised non-inferiority study. Lancet 2005; 366(9482):308–313

159. Aguilera JF, Perrocheau A, Meffre C, Hahne S. Outbreak of serogroup W135 meningococcal disease after the Hajj pilgrimage, Europe, 2000. Emerg Infect Dis 2002; 8(8):761–767

160. Trotter CL, Andrews NJ, Kaczmarski EB, Miller E, Ramsay ME. Effectiveness of meningococcal serogroup C conjugate vaccine 4 years after introduction. Lancet 2004; 364(9431):365–367

161. Auckland C, Gray S, Borrow R, Andrews N, Goldblatt D, Ramsay M et al. Clinical and immunologic risk factors for meningococcal C conjugate vaccine failure in the United Kingdom. J Infect Dis 2006; 194(12):1745–1752

162. De Wals P, Trottier P, Pepin J. Relative efficacy of different immunization schedules for the prevention of serogroup C meningococcal disease: a model-based evaluation. Vaccine 2006; 24(17):3500–3504

163. Frasch CE. Recent developments in *Neisseria meningitidis* group A conjugate vaccines. Expert Opin Biol Ther 2005; 5(2):273–280

164. Kshirsagar N, Mur N, Thatte U, Gogtay N, Viviani S, Preziosi MP, et al. Safety, immunogenicity, and antibody persistence of a new meningococcal group A conjugate vaccine in healthy Indian adults. Vaccine 2007

165. Martin DR, Walker SJ, Baker MG, Lennon DR. New Zealand epidemic of meningococcal disease identified by a strain with phenotype B:4:P1.4. J Infect Dis 1998; 177(2):497–500

166. Thornton V, Lennon D, Rasanathan K, O'hallahan J, Oster P, Stewart J et al. Safety and immunogenicity of New Zealand strain meningococcal serogroup B OMV vaccine in healthy adults: beginning of epidemic control. Vaccine 2005; 24(9):1395–1400

167. Wong S, Lennon D, Jackson C, Stewart J, Reid S, Crengle S et al. New Zealand epidemic strain meningococcal B outer membrane vesicle vaccine in children aged 16–24 months. Pediatr Infect Dis J 2007; 26(4):345–350

168. Oster P, O'Hallahan J, Aaberge I, Tilman S, Ypma E, Martin D. Immunogenicity and safety of a strain-specific MenB OMV vaccine delivered to under 5-year olds in New Zealand. Vaccine 2007; 25(16):3075–3079

169. Ameratunga S, Macmillan A, Stewart J, Scott D, Mulholland K, Crengle S. Evaluating the post-licensure effectiveness of a group B meningococcal vaccine in New Zealand: a multi-faceted strategy. Vaccine 2005; 23(17–18):2231–2234

170. Antignac A, Boneca IG, Rousselle JC, Namane A, Carlier JP, Vazquez JA et al. Correlation between alterations of the penicillin-binding protein 2 and modifications of the peptidoglycan structure in *Neisseria meningitidis* with reduced susceptibility to penicillin G. J Biol Chem 2003; 278(34):31529–31535

171. Saez-Nieto JA, Fontanals D, Garcia DJ, Martinez DAV, Pena P, Morera MA, et al. Isolation of *Neisseria meningitidis* strains with increase of penicillin minimal inhibitory concentrations. Epidemiol Infect 1987; 99(2):463–469

172. Arreaza L, de La FL, Vazquez JA. Antibiotic susceptibility patterns of *Neisseria meningitidis* isolates from patients and asymptomatic carriers. Antimicrob Agents Chemother 2000; 44(6):1705–1707

173. Canica M, Dias R, Nunes B, Carvalho L, Ferreira E. Invasive culture-confirmed *Neisseria meningitidis* in Portugal: evaluation of serogroups in relation to different variables and antimicrobial susceptibility (2000–2001). J Med Microbiol 2004; 53(Pt 9): 921–925

174. Berron S, Vazquez JA. Increase in moderate penicillin resistance and serogroup C in meningococcal strains isolated in Spain. Is there any relationship? Clin Infect Dis 1994; 18(2):161–165

175. Tapsall JW, Shultz T, Limnios E, Munro R, Mercer J, Porritt R et al. Surveillance of antibiotic resistance in invasive isolates of *Neisseria meningitidis* in Australia 1994–1999. Pathology 2001; 33(3):359–361

176. Woods CR, Smith AL, Wasilauskas BL, Campos J, Givner LB. Invasive disease caused by *Neisseria meningitidis* relatively resistant to penicillin in North Carolina. J Infect Dis 1994; 170(2):453–456

177. Rosenstein NE, Stocker SA, Popovic T, Tenover FC, Perkins BA. Antimicrobial resistance of *Neisseria meningitidis* in the United States, 1997. The Active Bacterial Core Surveillance (ABCs) Team. Clin Infect Dis 2000; 30(1):212–213

178. Mastrantonio P, Stefanelli P, Fazio C, Sofia T, Neri A, La Rosa G et al. Serotype distribution, antibiotic susceptibility, and genetic relatedness of *Neisseria meningitidis* strains recently isolated in Italy. Clin Infect Dis 2003; 36(4):422–428

179. Hsueh PR, Teng LJ, Lin TY, Chen KT, Hsu HM, Twu SJ et al. Re-emergence of meningococcal disease in Taiwan: circulation of domestic clones of *Neisseria meningitidis* in the 2001 outbreak. Epidemiol Infect 2004; 132(4):637–645

180. Kyaw MH, Bramley JC, Clark S, Christie P, Jones IG, Campbell H. Prevalence of moderate penicillin resistant invasive *Neisseria meningitidis* infection in Scotland, 1994–9. Epidemiol Infect 2002; 128(2):149–156

181. Punar M, Eraksoy H, Cagatay AA, Ozsut H, Kaygusuz A, Calangu S et al. *Neisseria meningitidis* with decreased susceptibility to penicillin in Istanbul, Turkey. Scand J Infect Dis 2002; 34(1):11–13

182. Saez-Nieto JA, Lujan R, Berron S, Campos J, Vinas M, Fuste C et al. Epidemiology and molecular basis of penicillin-resistant *Neisseria meningitidis* in Spain: a 5-year history (1985–1989). Clin Infect Dis 1992; 14(2):394–402

183. Thulin S, Olcen P, Fredlund H, Unemo M. Total variation in the penA gene of *Neisseria meningitidis*: correlation between susceptibility to beta-lactam antibiotics and penA gene heterogeneity. Antimicrob Agents Chemother 2006; 50(10):3317–3324

184. Orus P, Vinas M. Mechanisms other than penicillin-binding protein-2 alterations may contribute to moderate penicillin resistance in *Neisseria meningitidis*. Int J Antimicrob Agents 2001; 18(2):113–119

185. Rouquette-Loughlin C, Dunham SA, Kuhn M, Balthazar JT, Shafer WM. The NorM efflux pump of *Neisseria gonorrhoeae* and *Neisseria meningitidis* recognizes antimicrobial cationic compounds. J Bacteriol 2003; 185(3):1101–1106

186. Galimand M, Gerbaud G, Guibourdenche M, Riou JY, Courvalin P. High-level chloramphenicol resistance in *Neisseria meningitidis*. N Engl J Med 1998; 339(13):868–874

187. Shultz TR, Tapsall JW, White PA, Ryan CS, Lyras D, Rood JI et al. Chloramphenicol-resistant *Neisseria meningitidis* containing catP isolated in Australia. J Antimicrob Chemother 2003; 52(5):856–859

188. Tondella ML, Rosenstein NE, Mayer LW, Tenover FC, Stocker SA, Reeves MW et al. Lack of evidence for chloramphenicol resist-

ance in *Neisseria meningitidis*, Africa. Emerg Infect Dis 2001; 7(1):163–164

189. Feldman HA. Sulfonamide-resistant meningococci. Annu Rev Med 1967; 18:495–506

190. Millar JW, Siess EE, Feldman HA, Silverman C, Frank P. *In vivo* and *in vitro* resistance to sulfadiazine in strains of *Neisseria meningitidis*. JAMA 1963; 186:139–141

191. Vazquez JA. The resistance of *Neisseria meningitidis* to the antimicrobial agents: an issue still in evolution. Rev Med Microbiol 2001; 12(1):39–45

192. Cooper ER, Ellison RT, III, Smith GS, Blaser MJ, Reller LB, Paisley JW. Rifampin-resistant meningococcal disease in a contact patient given prophylactic rifampin. J Pediatr 1986; 108(1): 93–96

193. Yagupsky P, Ashkenazi S, Block C. Rifampicin-resistant meningococci causing invasive disease and failure of chemoprophylaxis. Lancet 1993; 341(8853):1152–1153

194. Jackson LA, Alexander ER, DeBolt CA, Swenson PD, Boase J, McDowell MG et al. Evaluation of the use of mass chemoprophylaxis during a school outbreak of enzyme type 5 serogroup B meningococcal disease. Pediatr Infect Dis J 1996; 15(11): 992–998

195. Shultz TR, Tapsall JW, White PA, Newton PJ. An invasive isolate of *Neisseria meningitidis* showing decreased susceptibility to quinolones. Antimicrob Agents Chemother 2000; 44(4):1116

196. Alcala B, Salcedo C, de La FL, Arreaza L, Uria MJ, Abad R et al. *Neisseria meningitidis* showing decreased susceptibility to ciprofloxacin: first report in Spain. J Antimicrob Chemother 2004; 53(2):409

197. Shultz TR, White PA, Tapsall JW. In vitro assessment of the further potential for development of fluoroquinolone resistance in *Neisseria meningitidis*. Antimicrob Agents Chemother 2005; 49(5):1753–1760

198. Luaces CC, Garcia Garcia JJ, Roca MJ, Latorre Otin CL. Clinical data in children with meningococcal meningitis in a Spanish hospital. Acta Paediatr 1997; 86(1):26–29

199. Turner PC, Southern KW, Spencer NJ, Pullen H. Treatment failure in meningococcal meningitis. Lancet 1990; 335(8691):732–733

200. Bardi L, Badolati A, Corso A, Rossi MA. [Failure of the treatment with penicillin in a case of *Neisseria meningitidis* meningitis]. Medicina (B Aires) 1994; 54(5 Pt 1):427–430

201. Rainbow J, Cebelinski E, Bartkus J, Glennen A, Boxrud D, Lynfield R. Rifampin-resistant meningococcal disease. Emerg Infect Dis 2005; 11(6):977–979

202. Briggs S, Ellis-Pegler R, Roberts S, Thomas M, Woodhouse A. Short course intravenous benzylpenicillin treatment of adults with meningococcal disease. Intern Med J 2004; 34(7):383–387

203. Brouqui P, Raoult D. Endocarditis due to rare and fastidious bacteria. Clin Microbiol Rev 2001; 14(1):177–207

204. Haddow LJ, Mulgrew C, Ansari A, Miell J, Jackson G, Malnick H et al. *Neisseria elongata* endocarditis: case report and literature review. Clin Microbiol Infect 2003; 9(5):426–430

205. Morla N, Guibourdenche M, Riou JY. *Neisseria* spp. and AIDS. J Clin Microbiol 1992; 30(9):2290–2294

206. Orus P, Vinas M. Transfer of penicillin resistance between Neisseriae in microcosm. Microb Drug Resist 2000; 6(2):99–104

207. Arreaza L, Salcedo C, Alcala B, Vazquez JA. What about antibiotic resistance in Neisseria lactamica?. J Antimicrob Chemother 2002; 49(3):545–547

Chapter 53
Mechanisms of Resistance in *Haemophilus influenzae* and *Moraxella catarrhalis*

Michael R. Jacobs

1 Overview

Haemophilus influenzae and *Moraxella catarrhalis* are found as both respiratory tract commensals and respiratory and invasive pathogens. While it is ideal to tailor chemotherapy to a known pathogen with a known drug susceptibility profile it is often difficult or impractical to isolate the causative agent, and many infections are treated empirically (1). It is therefore important to know the activity of antimicrobial agents against the pathogens associated with diseases being treated empirically and the effect of resistance mechanisms on in vivo activity. Antimicrobial agents should be used rationally, avoiding overuse, tailoring treatment to identified pathogens as much as possible, and basing empiric treatment on the disease being treated and the susceptibility of the predominant pathogens at breakpoints based on pharmacokinetic (PK) and pharmacodynamic (PD) parameters (2). The current status of resistance mechanisms found in *Haemophilus influenzae* and *Moraxella catarrhalis* against the antimicrobial agents recommended for empiric and directed treatment of the diseases caused by these pathogens form the basis of this review.

2 Carriage of *H. influenzae* and *M. catarrhalis*

Many infections, particularly those of the respiratory tract, are superinfections of inflammatory processes, such as viral infections, by bacteria colonizing the nasopharynx and oropharynx. Bacteria normally resident in the mouth and respiratory tract include streptococcal species, especially *Streptococcus pneumoniae*, *H. influenzae*, *M. catarrhalis*,

Neisseria species, various anaerobes, and staphylococcal species. Carriage of *S. pneumoniae*, with 91 serotypes, *H. influenzae*, both encapsulated and nonencapsulated strains, and *M. catarrhalis* changes over time as immunity develops to each strain, and different strains are acquired from other persons (3, 4). Carriage of these species is also influenced by use of protein-conjugated capsular polysaccharide vaccines, *H. influenzae* type b (Hib), and the 7-valent pneumococcal vaccine.

3 Major Diseases Caused by *H. influenzae* and *M. catarrhalis*

The major diseases caused by these pathogens are childhood meningitis and bacteremia, community-acquired pneumonia (CAP) in adults and children, acute otitis media (AOM), acute sinusitis, and acute exacerbations of chronic bronchitis (AECB). Empiric and directed antimicrobial therapy of these diseases will be briefly reviewed to establish the range of antimicrobial agents of clinical importance, and therefore where resistance needs to be considered.

3.1 Meningitis

Whereas Hib vaccination has greatly reduced the incidence of Hib meningitis in countries where it is used, meningitis remains a serious problem in children under 7 years of age in areas where the vaccine is not used (5). The empiric antimicrobial treatment of meningitis recommended by the Infectious Disease Society of America for this age group is vancomycin plus a third-generation cephalosporin such as cefotaxime or ceftriaxone (6). If a Gram stain of cerebrospinal fluid shows Gram-negative bacilli presumptively identified as *H. influenzae*, a third-generation

M.R. Jacobs (✉)
Case Western Reserve University School of Medicine, University Hospitals Case Medical Center, Cleveland, OH, USA
mrj6@cwru.edu

D.L. Mayers (ed.), *Antimicrobial Drug Resistance*,
DOI 10.1007/978-1-60327-595-8_53, © Humana Press, a part of Springer Science+Business Media, LLC 2009

cephalosporin alone is recommended. Alternative therapies for *H. influenzae* include chloramphenicol, cefepime, and meropenem. Once the pathogen has been isolated and identified, and susceptibilities are known, the antibiotic choices can be narrowed or changed if necessary. For β-lactamase-negative *H. influenzae*, ampicillin is recommended as standard therapy, with a third-generation cephalosporin, cefepime, or chloramphenicol as alternate regimens. β-Lactamase-positive *H. influenzae* should be treated with a third-generation cephalosporin, with cefepime or chloramphenicol as alternatives. Meningitis caused by *H. influenzae*, usually untypeable strains, can also occur in patients who have suffered basilar skull fractures. These patients should be treated with the same agents discussed above, with the addition of a fluoroquinolone, either gatifloxacin or moxifloxacin, to the list of alternative agents recommended, for adult patients only.

3.2 Childhood Pneumonia and Bacteremia

In regions where protein-conjugated Hib and pneumococcal capsular polysaccharide vaccines are not used, the most common bacterial causes of childhood pneumonia between 6 months and 5 years of age are *S. pneumoniae*, *H. influenzae* type b, and *M. catarrhalis* (7, 8). *Mycoplasma pneumoniae* and *Chlamydia (Chlamydophilia) pneumoniae* become more common at school age, with *M. pneumoniae* more common in the 5–10-year-old cohort and *C. pneumoniae* more common after age 10 (9, 10). Bacteremia with *S. pneumoniae* and *H. influenzae* type b occurs with or without the presence of pneumonia.

High-dose amoxicillin (90 mg/kg/day), either alone or with the addition of clavulanic acid, is the first-line drug of choice for empiric treatment of outpatients with childhood pneumonia (11). If oral antibiotics are not tolerated, daily intramuscular (IM) ceftriaxone has good coverage for the three major bacterial pathogens (11). In older children with a higher probability of *C. pneumoniae* or *M. pneumoniae*, addition of a macrolide is recommended (10–13). Oral cephalosporins should be avoided because of a lack of coverage for penicillin-resistant pneumococci. Recommended empiric therapy for inpatients includes ceftriaxone or cefotaxime to provide coverage for penicillin-non-susceptible *S. pneumoniae* and β-lactamase-positive *H. influenzae* (11). The addition of azithromycin or erythromycin is recommended to provide coverage for atypical pathogens in older children. Vancomycin should be added for life-threatening pulmonary infections in which *Staphylococcus aureus* is a suspected pathogen, as virulent, community-acquired, methicillin-resistant strains are increasingly being encountered (11). Directed

parenteral therapy for pneumonia due to *H. influenzae* includes ampicillin for β-lactamase-negative strains and ceftriaxone, cefotaxime, or cefuroxime for β-lactamase-positive strains.

3.3 Community-Acquired Pneumonia in Adults

The most common causes of CAP are *S. pneumoniae* (26–60%), *M. pneumoniae* (10–37%), untypeable *H. influenzae* (2–12%), *Legionella pneumophila* (2–6%), *C. pneumoniae* (5–15%), and *M. catarrhalis* (2–3%) (1). Treatment guidelines for management of CAP in immunocompetent adults have been established by the American Thoracic Society and the Infectious Diseases Society of America (14, 15). Recommendations for outpatients with no comorbidities include azithromycin, clarithromycin, and doxycycline if no antibiotic therapy had been administered in the past 3 months; if antibiotic therapy had been administered in the past 3 months, recommendations are levofloxacin, gatifloxacin, gemifloxacin, or moxifloxacin as single agents, or combination macrolide-β-lactam therapy (azithromycin or clarithromycin with amoxicillin (3 g/day) or amoxicillin–clavulanate (4 g/250 mg/day). Recommendations for outpatients with comorbidities include azithromycin, clarithromycin, levofloxacin, gatifloxacin, gemifloxacin, or moxifloxacin if no antibiotic therapy had been administered in the past 3 months; if antibiotic therapy had been administered in the past 3 months, recommendations are levofloxacin, gatifloxacin, gemifloxacin, or moxifloxacin as single agents, or combination macrolide-β-lactam therapy (azithromycin or clarithromycin with amoxicillin–clavulanate (4 g/250 mg/day). Amoxicillin–clavulanate or clindamycin is recommended for suspected aspiration pneumonia. High-dose amoxicillin, high-dose amoxicillin–clavulanate, cefpodoxime, cefprozil, cefuroxime axetil, levofloxacin, gatifloxacin, gemifloxacin, or moxifloxacin is recommended for influenza with bacteral superinfection. Recommendations for inpatients in medical wards include levofloxacin, gatifloxacin, gemifloxacin, or moxifloxacin alone, or azithromycin or clarithromycin plus cefotaxime, ceftriaxone, ampicillin–sulbactam, or ertapenem. Recommendations for patients requiring intensive care are the same plus inclusion of an antipseudomonal agent if infection with *Pseudomonas aeruginosa* is a concern. The guidelines emphasize that the infectious etiology be determined whenever possible and that pathogen-directed therapy be used once the organism has been identified. Virulent, community-acquired, methicillin-resistant *S. aureus* (MRSA) are increasingly being encountered, and the addition of vancomycin or other anti-MRSA agents should also be considered (16).

3.4 Acute Otitis Media

AOM is one of the most common pediatric infections, second only to the common cold in prevalence, occurring most often between 6 months and 3 years of age, especially in children with frequent viral upper respiratory infections (17). The principal bacterial causes of AOM are *S. pneumoniae* (25–50%), untypeable *H. influenzae* (23–67%), and *M. catarrhalis* (12–15%) (18, 19). In the US, introduction of the conjugate pneumococcal vaccine in children has resulted in untypeable, β-lactamase-producing *H. influenzae* and ampicillin-resistant serotype 19A *Streptococcus pneumoniae* becoming more prevalent in patients failing first-line amoxicillin therapy (20–22). Recent guidelines for empiric treatment of AOM include the following (23): Amoxicillin, 80–90 mg/kg/day, is recommended as the first-line agent for less severe disease, with azithromycin or clarithromycin as alternatives for patients with type I penicillin allergy; and cefdinir, cefuroxime axetil, and cefpodoxime as alternatives for patients with non-type I penicillin allergy. Amoxicillin–clavulanate, 90/6.4 mg/kg/day, is recommended as the first-line agent for more severe disease and for patients not responding to treatment after use of amoxicillin for 48–72 h. IM ceftriaxone, 50 mg/kg/day for 1 or 3 days, is recommended for initial therapy of less severe disease for patients with penicillin allergy, and for 3 days for patients not responding to treatment after use of amoxicillin–clavulanate for 48–72 h. In cases of patients with type I penicillin allergy not responding to treatment, clindamycin is recommended for less severe disease, whereas clindamycin and diagnostic tympanocentesis are offered as options for more severe disease (23).

3.5 Acute Sinusitis

Although most cases of acute sinusitis are viral, *S. pneumoniae*, untypeable *H. influenzae*, and *M. catarrhalis* are the predominant pathogens when bacterial superinfection occurs, with *M. catarrhalis* being more common in children (24). Recommended therapy for adults with no recent antibiotic use includes amoxicillin (1.5–4 g/day), amoxicillin-clavulanate (1.75–4 g/250 mg/day), cefpodoxime, cefuroxime, and cefdinir, with these cephalosporins recommended for patients with non-type I penicillin allergy, and trimethoprim–sulfamethoxazole, doxycycline, azithromycin, clarithromycin,

erythromycin, and telithromycin for patients with type I penicillin allergy. Recommendations for patients not responding to therapy after 72 h or that have received antimicrobials in the past 4–6 weeks include gatifloxacin, levofloxacin, moxifloxacin, amoxicillin–clavulanate (4 g/250 mg/day), IM ceftriaxone, and combination therapy (amoxicillin + cefixime; clindamycin + cefixime; amoxicillin + rifampin; clindamycin + rifampin). Recommendations for children are similar to those for adults, except for the following: amoxicillin dose is 90 mg/kg/day; amoxicillin–clavulanate dose is 90/6.4 mg/kg/day; removal of gatifloxacin, levofloxacin, moxifloxacin, doxycycline, and telithromycin as they are not approved for pediatric use; and addition of trimethoprim–sulfamethoxazole as an option for children with type I penicillin allergy that have received antimicrobials in the past 4–6 weeks.

3.6 Acute Exacerbations of Chronic Bronchitis

Acute bacterial exacerbations of chronic bronchitis are predominantly caused by the typical upper respiratory bacteria, untypeable *H. influenzae*, *S. pneumoniae*, and *M. catarrhalis*, which make up 85–95% of cases, with *H. influenzae* usually the most frequent pathogen (25). In addition, *H. parainfluenzae*, *P. aeruginosa*, *S. aureus*, *M. pneumoniae*, *Legionella pneumophila*, and opportunistic Gram-negative organisms are occasionally implicated, with the latter found principally in severe disease. The presence of a new strain of *H. influenzae*, *S. pneumoniae*, or *M. catarrhalis* from the sputum of a patient with chronic bronchitis increases the relative risk of an exacerbation twofold (4).

Recommendations for treatment of AECB are stratified by presence of baseline patient factors (pulmonary function, comorbid illnesses, recurrent exacerbations, chronic steroid use, home oxygen use, and hypercapnia) and severity of the exacerbation. Severity of the exacerbation is based on the presence of increased dyspnea, increased sputum volume, and increased sputum purulence. A "mild" exacerbation is one featuring only one of these three symptoms and does not require antibiotic treatment. "Moderate" or "severe" exacerbations require the presence of any two of the three symptoms and treatment is determined by the severity of baseline patient factors. Recommendations for patients without the baseline risk factors listed above include azithromycin, clarithromycin, telithromycin, doxycycline, cefuroxime axetil, cefpodoxime, and cefdinir. Recommendations for patients with any of the baseline risk factors listed above include amoxicillin–clavulanic acid, levofloxacin, gatifloxacin, gemifloxacin, and moxifloxacin; ciprofloxacin should be considered if *Pseudomonas aeruginosa* is suspected. Patients with worsening clinical status or inadequate response in 72 h should be re-evaluated and have sputum cultures performed (26, 27).

4 Baseline Susceptibility and Development of Resistance

Every bacterial species typically has a baseline, wild-type population with a defined, usually narrow, range of intrinsic susceptibility to antimicrobial agents at the time of introduction of a new antimicrobial drug class (28). This defines the initial spectrum of activity of each antimicrobial agent, and this in turn depends on the dosing regimen and the site of infection. Species can then be studied on the basis of baseline susceptibilities and susceptibilities of strains with decreased susceptibility, should they be present initially or should they develop. Susceptibility breakpoints between susceptibility of baseline, wild-type populations and those of populations with acquired resistance can be used and are referred to as "microbiological breakpoints" (28). Such breakpoints are very useful, but do not necessarily correlate with clinically relevant breakpoints. Unfortunately, many breakpoints in common use for *H. influenzae* are microbiological breakpoints that are of little clinical use, and the current Clinical and Laboratory Standards Institute (CLSI, formerly NCCLS) interpretation guideline for *H. influenzae* states that results of susceptibility testing using breakpoints provided for the oral β-lactam, macrolide, and ketolide agents "are often not useful for the management of individual patients," but "may be appropriate for surveillance or epidemiologic studies" (29).

Clinically relevant susceptibility breakpoints are also typically developed for each agent, enabling isolates to be classified as susceptible, intermediate, or resistant. Such breakpoints should be based on pharmacokinetic and pharmacodymanic (PK/PD) parameters and appropriate clinical studies, and should be the same for all species associated with each clinical syndrome, e.g., pneumonia, meningitis, cystitis, otitis, etc. Many breakpoints were developed before these principles were introduced, and some breakpoints in clinical use have been shown not to be appropriate, particularly for oral agents. This is especially the case for *H. influenzae*, as noted earlier, while CLSI does not have breakpoints for *M. catarrhalis*, although other groups such as the British Society for Antimicrobial Chemotherapy (BSAC) do have these (30). To overcome this problem, breakpoints based on PK/PD parameters and, where available, adequate clinical studies have been developed and will be used in this review to enable meaningful use of the terms clinical susceptibility and clinical resistance (31, 32).

5 Mechanisms of Resistance of *H. influenzae* and *M. catarrhalis*

5.1 β-Lactams

β-Lactams exert an antimicrobial effect by interfering with the formation and maintenance of the peptidoglycan layer of the bacterial cell wall (33, 34). The cross-linking of stem peptides is facilitated by peptidases, which are located on the extracellular surface of the cell membrane (35). β-Lactams exert their antimicrobial effect by irreversibly binding to these peptidases, which are frequently referred to as penicillin-binding proteins (PBPs) (36). Resistance is achieved when genetic alterations result in a PBP that has a reduced affinity for β-lactam antibiotics or when β-lactamases are produced (37–39). β-Lactamases are structurally related to PBPs and have a high affinity for β-lactam antibiotics; the interaction between β-lactams and β-lactamases causes a permanent opening of the β-lactam ring, thereby inactivating the antibiotic (Fig. 1) (34, 40). Unlike the interaction between the antibiotic and PBPs, the interaction between β-lactams and β-lactamases does not result in a covalent bond and the enzyme is free to inactivate other β-lactam molecules.

The predominant mechanism of β-lactam resistance in *H. influenzae* is β-lactamase production, and the genes encoding for β-lactamases in *H. influenzae* are found primarily on plasmids; however, in some cases, these genes are incorporated into the bacterial chromosome (41). Two distinct β-lactamases are produced by strains of *H. influenzae*: TEM-1 and ROB-1, of which, the TEM-1 β-lactamase is more common (42). Three β-lactamases are produced by *M. catarrhalis*: BRO-1, BRO-2, and BRO-3, which are structurally similar to each other, but are distinct from the TEM-1 or ROB-1 β-lactamases (43).

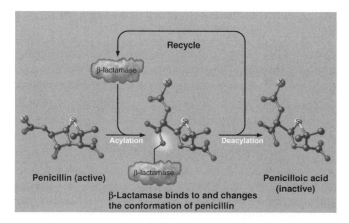

Fig. 1 Antibiotic inactivation of penicillins by β-lactamases of *H. influenzae* and *M. catarrhalis*. Copyright Michael R. Jacobs, used with permission

Resistance via β-lactamase production cannot be overcome by increasing the dose of the β-lactam antibiotic (i.e., the concentration at the site of infection) because the β-lactamase enzyme is regenerated following each interaction with – and subsequent inactivation of – an antibiotic. However, this mechanism of resistance can be overcome by using a combination of a β-lactam antibiotic with a β-lactamase inhibitor (e.g., amoxicillin–clavulanate), or by using β-lactam antibiotics that are stable to the actions of β-lactamases (e.g., ceftriaxone, cefuroxime, cefpodoxime, cefixime, provided the pharmacokinetic properties of the agent are adequate). β-Lactamase inhibitors act as "suicide substrates," forming a covalent bond between the enzyme and the β-lactamase inhibitor, inactivating the enzyme and preventing it from destroying more β-lactam molecules (Fig. 2) (44). β-Lactamase-stable agents evade the action of β-lactamases owing to stereochemical blocking of the attachment site of β-lactamases by the side chains of these agents. Extended-spectrum β-lactamase (ESBL) variants of TEM-1 with increased antibiotic resistance to broad-spectrum β-lactam antibiotics and, in some cases, β-lactamase inhibitors (e.g., clavulanic acid) have appeared in *Enterobacteriaceae*, but have not been detected in clinical isolates of *H. influenzae*, although they have been expressed in cloned strains (45). ESBLs have been reported in two South African isolates of *H. parainfluenzae* that produced a TEM-15 enzyme and had cefotaxime minimum inhibitory concentrations (MICs) of >16 µg/mL (46).

Non-β-lactamase-mediated resistance to β-lactams due to PBP alterations have occurred in *H. influenzae*, both type b and untypeable strains, mediated via changes in PBP3, which is encoded by the *ftsI* gene (38, 47). This PBP is made up of an *N*-terminal hydrophobic region, a central penicillin-binding domain, and a *C*-terminal domain, and the active site of transpeptidase activity is formed by three conserved amino acid motifs, SXXK, SSN, and KTG (Fig. 3). These motifs occur at amino acid positions 326–330,

379–381, and 512–514 in PBP3 of *H. influenzae* (48). Strains with specific mutations in or around these motifs are referred to as β-lactamase-negative ampicillin resistant (BLNAR) or β-lactamase positive amoxicillin-clavulanate resistant (BLPACR) if they are also β-lactamase-positive (47). Strains are further divided into low- and high-level resistant: low-level BLNAR strains have ampicillin MICs of 0.5–4 µg/mL (compared to a modal value 0.12 µg/mL for wild-type strains), and high-level BLNAR strains have ampicillin MIC of 1–16 µg/mL (Fig. 4). Low-level BLNAR and BLPACR strains have N526K or R517H substitutions close to the KTG motif in the *ftsI* gene, while high-level BLNAR and BLPACR strains additionally have S385T or S385T and L389F substitutions close to the SSN motif (Fig. 3) (48–50). Horizontal transfer of the *ftsI* gene in *H. influenzae* has been demonstrated within and between *H. influenzae* and *H. haemolyticus* (51). MICs of all β-lactams are higher against strains with *ftsI* mutations than against wild-type strains, and the clinical significance varies on the basis of the PK/PD breakpoint for each agent (Figs. 4 and 5).

Low-level BLNAR and BLPACR strains are fairly common in many countries, accounting for up to 10% of isolates, while high-level BLNAR and BLPACR strains to date are rare in most areas, accounting for fewer than 1% of isolates (52, 53). However, in Japan low-level BLNAR and BLPACR strains have been reported from 26% of nonmeningeal and 40% of meningeal isolates, while high-level BLNAR and BLPACR strains account for 13% of nonmeningeal and 24% of meningeal isolates (5, 38). Similar findings in nasopharyngeal isolates from Japanese children with AOM have also been reported (37). High-level BLNAR and BLPACR strains have also been reported from Korea and Spain (54, 55).

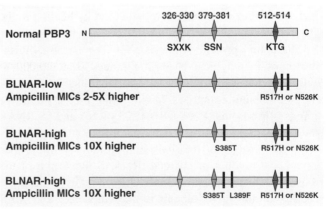

Fig. 3 Primary structures and positions of motifs making up the active transpeptidase sites of PBP3 of *Haemophilus influenzae* and mutations associated with low- and high-level BLNAR strains. Adapted from Ubukata et al. (48), Dabernat et al. (49), and Hasegawa et al. (38). Copyright Michael R. Jacobs, used with permission

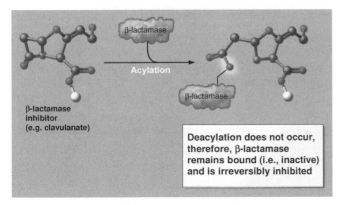

Fig. 2 Irreversible binding of a β-lactamase inhibitor to β-lactamase. Copyright Michael R. Jacobs, used with permission

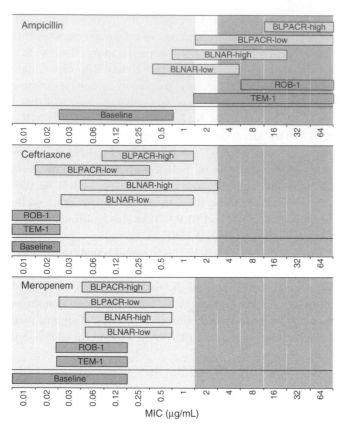

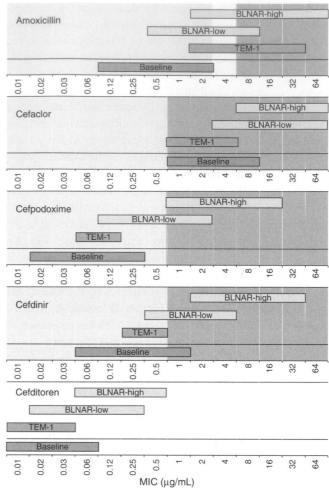

Fig. 4 Correlation between β-lactam resistance mechanisms and susceptibility of *H. influenzae* to ampicillin, ceftriaxone, and meropenem. Background color indicates susceptibility based on PK/PD parameters: Green, susceptible; yellow, intermediate; red, resistant. Adapted from Hasegawa et al. (5) and Sanbongi et al. (50). Copyright Michael R. Jacobs, used with permission

5.2 Protein Synthesis Inhibitors

Several classes of agents inhibit protein systhesis (56). Although these agents are chemically and structurally distinct, they all exert an antimicrobial effect by binding to the 23S component of the 50S subunit of bacterial ribosomes and disrupting protein synthesis (57). The number of 70S ribosomes in a typical bacterium ranges from 20,000 to 70,000, each of which consists of two subunits: 50S and 30S. The 50S subunit comprises 34 ribosomal proteins and two strands of ribosomal RNA (rRNA; 23S RNA and 5S RNA). The rRNA provides structure to the 50S subunit and determines the position of the ribosomal proteins. Tetracyclines prevent the binding of charged tRNA to the A site of the ribosome; chloramphenicol inhibits the peptidyl transferase reaction of the large subunit of the ribosome; and MLS antibiotics, which include macrolides (e.g., erythromycin, clarithromycin), azalides (eg azithromycin,), lincosamides (e.g., clindamycin), ketolides (e.g., telithromycin), and streptogramins, block the ribosome exit tunnel, thereby preventing movement and release of the nascent peptide.

Fig. 5 Correlation between β-lactam resistance mechanisms and susceptibility of *H. influenzae* to amoxicillin, cefaclor, cefpodoxime, cefdinir, and cefditoren. Background color indicates susceptibility based on PK/PD parameters: Green, susceptible; yellow, intermediate; red, resistant. No susceptibility interpretations are available for cefditoren. Adapted from Hasegawa et al. (5) and Sanbongi et al. (50). Copyright Michael R. Jacobs, used with permission

5.3 MLS Agents and Ketolides

Macrolide resistance mechanisms include efflux pumps (either intrinsic or acquired), ribosomal methylase, and alterations in ribosomal proteins and RNA (58, 59). *H. influenzae* is intrinsically resistant to MLS agents and ketolides. This is associated with the presence of an *acr*AB efflux pump homologous to this mechanism in *E. coli*, explaining the limited activity of these agents against most wild-type strains of this pathogen (60–62). Occasional strains of *H. influenzae* lack this efflux pump and have lower MICs than typical wild-type strains, while a few strains have higher MICs associated with mutations in L4 or L22 ribosomal proteins or 23S rRNA (Fig. 6).

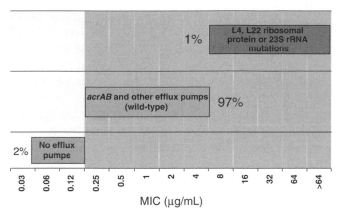

Fig. 6 Correlation between azithromycin MICs and resistance mechanisms of *H. influenzae*. Adapted from Peric et al. (97). Copyright Michael R. Jacobs, used with permission

5.4 Tetracyclines

Tetracyclines exert an antimicrobial effect by binding to the 30S subunit of bacterial ribosomes and preventing tRNA from binding to the A- or P-sites (63). Tetracycline resistance in *H. influenzae* is produced by a cell-membrane-associated efflux mechanism encoded by the *tet*(B) gene, which is usually located on conjugative plasmids (64, 65). The efflux protein encoded by the *tet*(B) gene confers resistance to both tetracycline and minocycline, but not glycylcyclines (65). Tetracycline resistance is often transmitted on conjugative plasmids carrying ampicillin-chloramphenicol-tetracycline-kanamycin resistance genes, which have been described in *H. influenzae* type b isolates in Belgium, Spain, and Cuba (66, 67).

5.5 Quinolones

The quinolones have a broad spectrum of activity and exert an antimicrobial effect by interfering with DNA replication and, subsequently, bacterial reproduction. Two enzymes that are important in the replication process are DNA gyrase and topoisomerase IV, and resistance to quinolones among strains of *H. influenzae* occurs via alterations in the quinolone-resistance-determining region (QRDR) of these genes (68, 69). These alterations can occur via spontaneous mutations or via the acquisition of DNA from other bacteria. The newer quinolones are potent against *H. influenzae*, and the prevalence of resistance among clinical strains is low (39). However, spontaneous quinolone-resistant mutants are readily selected in vitro by exposure to quinolones, and this has resulted in development of considerable resistance to this drug class in other species (70, 71). Quinolone-resistant

isolates of *H. influenzae* have been shown to have high mutation frequencies (72).

5.6 Chloramphenicol

Chloramphenicol resistance in *H. influenzae* is usually associated with plasmid-mediated production of chloramphenicol acetyltransferase (CAT) encoded by the *cat* gene, with occasional strains having a penetration barrier (73, 74). The *cat* gene is carried on conjugative plasmids ranging in molecular weight from 34 to 46×10^6, and these plasmids often carry genes encoding for resistance to tetracycline and ampicillin as well. These conjugative plasmids can also be incorporated into the chromosome (75). The CAT enzyme produced resembles the Type-II CATs produced by enterobacteria. Resistance associated with a permeability barrier is due to the loss of an outer membrane protein (73).

5.7 Folic Acid Metabolism Inhibitors

Trimethoprim and sulfamethoxazole (used alone or in combination) exert an antimicrobial effect by interfering with cellular metabolism and replication by sequentially blocking the production of tetrahydrofolate. During normal cellular metabolism, dihydrofolate is reduced to tetrahydrofolate by the enzyme dihydrofolate reductase (DHFR) (76). Tetrahydrofolate is an important cofactor in many cellular reactions, supplying single carbon moieties for the production of thymidylate, purine nucleotides, methionine, serine, glycine, and other compounds (77). Inhibiting the production of tetrahydrofolate causes the bacterial cells to die because the lack of thymine prevents DNA replication (78). Trimethoprim is a substrate analog of dihydrofolate and blocks the reduction of dihydrofolate to tetrahydrofolate by DHFR, whereas sulfamethoxazole is a substrate analog of *para*-aminobenzoic acid, which is involved in the production of dihydropteroate, a precursor compound of dihydrofolate, blocking the enzyme dihydropteroate synthetase (DHPS) (Fig. 7) (76). Thus, the use of these compounds in combination limits the production of dihydrofolate and prevents the conversion from dihydrofolate to tetrahydrofolate. Both compounds, trimethoprim and sulfamethoxazole, selectively inhibit bacterial metabolism with little toxicity to humans because humans do not synthesize folic acid; rather, the necessary levels of folic acid are obtained from dietary sources.

Resistance to trimethoprim occurs via alteration in the affinity between trimethoprim and DHFR. The decreased affinity is the result of altered genes that encode for DHFR, which often are carried on plasmids or transposons and

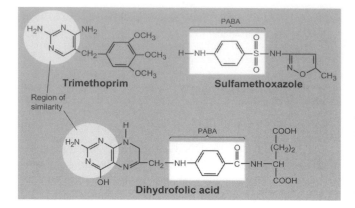

Fig. 7 Mechanism of action of trimethoprim and sulfonamides by mimicry of dihydrofolic acid components, blocking the enzymes involved in conversion of PABA to dihydrofolic acid, and dihydrofolic acid to tetrahydropholic acid, the active form of the enzyme. Regions of similarity of trimethoprim and sulfamethoxazole with dihydrofolic acid are highlighted. Copyright Michael R. Jacobs, used with permission

probably originated from closely related bacteria. Studies have shown that substitutions in the amino acid sequence of DHFR result in resistance to trimethoprim without affecting the affinity of the natural substrates (79–81). Resistance to trimethoprim–sulfamethoxazole among strains of *H. influenzae* is common and is caused by an increase in the production of DHFR with altered affinity for trimethoprim (82). Resistance to trimethoprim–sulfamethoxazole also has been noted among strains of *M. catarrhalis*, which is intrinsically resistant to trimethoprim (83–86).

Resistance of *H. influenzae* to sulfonamides is associated with two mechanisms (87). The first is mediated via the *sul2* gene, a common mediator of acquired sulfonamide resistance in enteric bacteria, which encodes for drug-resistant forms of DHPS. The second is mediated via the mutations in the chromosomal gene encoding DHPS, *folP*, associated with insertion of a 15-bp segment together with other missense mutations.

6 History of Geographical Spread

Bacterial antibiotic resistance results from antibiotic pressure and natural selection and can be spread either through clonal expansion or horizontal transfer, usually through plasmids, phage vectors, or natural transformation systems. The key antimicrobial class to which resistance in *H. influenzae* and *M. catarrhalis* has developed has been the β-lactams, predominantly owing to β-lactamase production.

6.1 Haemophilus influenzae

Cases of ampicillin treatment failure in *H. influenzae* meningitis were first reported in 1973 (88) and confirmed in 1974

(89, 90), at which time β-lactamase production was identified as the mediating cause (91). These cases were dispersed throughout the US, England, and New Zealand. By the late 1970s, ampicillin resistance in *H. influenzae* in the UK was already reported to be at 6.2%, 92% of which was β-lactamase mediated (92). In the early 1980s, BLNAR strains of *H. influenzae* began to be isolated in the US, UK, New Zealand, and Japan (92–94). BLNAR and BLPACR strains are now common in Japan, Korea, and Spain (5, 50, 54, 55). β-Lactamase production among strains of *H. influenzae* has generally increased throughout the past two decades (95). During the early 1980s, the proportion of strains that produced β-lactamases in the US was approximately 10–15%, whereas more recent surveillance studies have demonstrated a prevalence of up to 30%. Prevalence of β-lactamase production in various countries varies from 4.2% in Russia to 29.6% in the US (Fig. 8) (96).

The activity of macrolides against *H. influenzae* has remained essentially unchanged throughout the past 30 years, although a few hyper-resistant strains have developed (5, 50, 54, 55 31, 97). Resistance to tetracyclines and chloramphenicol has developed, associated with plasmids carrying ampicillin-chloramphenicol-tetracycline-kanamycin resistance genes, as noted earlier, predominantly in type b isolates (98). Resistance to quinolones among clinical isolates of *H. influenzae* is also rare; however, surveillance studies have identified a few clinical strains with increased quinolone MICs, and an outbreak of a highly resistant clone was recently detected in a long-term care facility (31, 96, 99). Twelve of 457 isolates (2.6%) of *H. influenzae* isolated in Hokkaido prefecture, Japan, during 2002–2004 were quinolone resistant, with resistant isolates found only in patients over 58 years of age (100). In contrast, resistance to trimethoprim–sulfamethoxazole has increased over the past two decades, with resistance varying from a low of 8.5% in Belgium to a high of 55.2% in Kenya in a recent study (Fig. 8) (96).

6.2 Moraxella catarrhalis

β-Lactamase production among strains of *M. catarrhalis* also is prevalent. β-Lactamase-mediated resistance first appeared in the late 1970s and is now present in at least 90% of worldwide isolates. Walker and Levy, working from a 10-year Veterans Administration hospital collection of *M. catarrhalis* isolates, examined the genetic changes that accompanied the transition from less than 30% to greater than 95% of isolates being β-lactamase-positive in that comparatively brief period (101). From a recent surveillance study, it was noted that nearly 100% of strains of *M. catarrhalis* produce β-lactamases (96). Amoxicillin-clavulanate is active against *M. catarrhalis*, with MICs of 0.12–0.25 μg/mL. β-Lactamase-stable cepha-

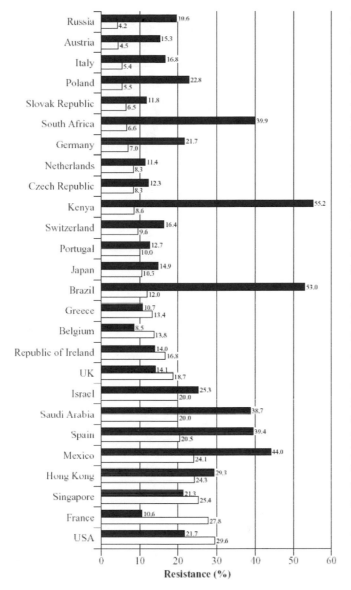

Fig. 8 Prevalence of trimethoprim–sulfamethoxazole resistance (MIC ≥ 1 μg/mL) (*filled square*) and β-lactamase production (*open square*) in *H. influenzae*, Alexander Project 1998–2000. Reproduced with permission from Jacobs et al. (96)

losporins, macrolides, and fluoroquinolones all are active against most strains of *M. catarrhalis*.

7 Clinical Significance

Significant advances have recently been made in understanding the relationships between in vitro susceptibility and in vivo response to infection on the basis of PK/PD correlations. In the absence of human studies or to complement limited human data, susceptibility breakpoints can be established on the basis of animal models and pharmacokinetic parameters. Clinically relevant susceptibility breakpoints

can then be derived by applying these PK/PD parameters to standard dosing regimens. For nonmeningeal infections, breakpoints can be derived from non-protein-bound plasma drug levels present for 25–50% of the dosing interval for time-dependent agents such as β-lactams, and from AUC:MIC ratios exceeding 30 for concentration-dependent agents such as most non-β-lactam agents. These principles have repeatedly been validated in animal models and in bacteriologic outcome studies of AOM, AECB, and sinusitis (2, 32, 102–105). Breakpoints for agents recommended for use against *H. influenzae* and *M. catarrhalis* on the basis of PK/PD parameters, as well as current CLSI and BSAC breakpoints, are shown in Table 1. While PK/PD and BSAC breakpoints are very similar, many CLSI breakpoints for *H. influenzae* are considerably higher and generally represent microbiological rather than clinical breakpoints as discussed earlier. Susceptibility of worldwide isolates of *H. influenzae* and *M. catarrhalis* to agents recommended for treatment of diseases due to these pathogens is shown in Table 2, with regional differences in susceptibility of *H. influenzae* in Table 3.

The relationships between MIC distributions and susceptibility breakpoints are important, as they determine the clinical activity of agents. MICs of clinically useful agents should be below PK/PD breakpoints, and the greater the difference between MICs and breakpoints, the greater the likelihood that the agent will be successful in clinical use. It is therefore important to examine MIC distributions in relation to breakpoints, and several patterns are found with *H. influenzae* (Figs. 9 and 10) (24, 31, 38, 47, 48, 96, 106, 107):

- A unimodal MIC distribution with modal MIC value fourfold (i.e., two doubling dilutions) or more below the breakpoint. This is the case with cefuroxime (parenteral), amoxicillin-clavulanate, cefixime, cefpodoxime, and the quinolones. These agents are therefore highly active against *H. influenzae* and are most suitable for empiric use.
- A unimodal MIC distribution with breakpoint within the MIC distribution, as seen with cefuroxime (oral), cefdinir, cefprozil, and doxycycline. These are agents with limited clinical activity and their use should be limited to circumstances where other more suitable agents cannot be used.
- A unimodal MIC distribution with breakpoint below the MIC distribution, as seen with cefaclor, erythromycin, azithromycin, clarithromycin, and telithromycin. These agents have intrinsic resistance due to pharmacokinetic limitations and have essentially no clinically useful activity against *H. influenzae*.
- A bimodal MIC distribution with a clearly defined susceptible population below the breakpoint and a clearly defined resistant population, typically with defined resistance mechanisms. This is the case with the ampicillin- and amoxicillin-resistant populations associated with β-lactamase production, tetracycline-resistant population

Table 1 Breakpoints (µg/mL) used to determine susceptible (S), intermediate (I) and resistant (R) categories, based on PK/PD, BSAC and CLSI interpretative breakpoints (29, 30, 95, 96, 103). No CLSI breakpoints are available for *M. catarrhalis*. PK/PD breakpoints are applicable to both species

Antimicrobial	PK/PD breakpoints		H. influenzae BSAC breakpoints			M. catarrhalis BSAC breakpoints			H. influenzae CLSI breakpoints		
	S	R	S	I	R	S	I	R	S	I	R
Parenteral agents											
Ampicillin	≤2	≥4	≤1	–	≥2	≤1	–	≥2	≤1	2	≥4[a]
Ampicillin–sulbactam	≤2	≥4	–	–	–	–	–	–	≤2	–	≥2
Piperacillin–tazobactam	≤8	≥16	–	–	–	–	–	–	≤1	–	≥2
Cefuroxime sodium	≤4	≥4	≤1	–	≥2	≤1	–	≥2	≤4	8	≥16
Cefotaxime	≤2	≥4	≤1	–	≥2	–	–	–	≤2	–	–
Ceftriaxone	≤2	≥4	≤1	–	≥2	–	–	–	≤2	–	–
Cefepime	≤4	≥8	–	–	–	–	–	–	≤2	–	–
Ceftazidime	≤8	≥16	≤2	–	≥4	–	–	–	≤2	–	–
Meropenem	≤4	≥8	≤4	–	≥8	–	–	–	≤0.5	–	–
Imipenem	≤4	≥8	≤4	–	≥8	–	–	–	≤4	–	–
Ertapenem	≤1	≥2	≤2	–	≥4	≤2	–	≥4	≤0.5	–	–
Parenteral and oral agents											
Erythromycin	≤0.25	≥0.5	≤0.5	1–8	≥16	≤0.5	–	≥1	–	–	–
Clarithromycin	≤0.25	≥0.5	≤0.5	1–16	≥32	≤0.5	–	≥1	≤8	16	≥32
Azithromycin	≤0.12	≥0.25	≤0.25	0.5–4	≥8	–	–	–	≤4	–	–
Doxycycline	≤0.25	≥0.5	–	–	–	–	–	–	–	–	–
Trimethoprim–sulfamethoxazole[d]	≤0.5/9.5	≥1/19	≤1.6/30.4	–	≥32./60.8	≤1.6/30.4	–	≥32./60.8	≤0.5/9.5	1/19–2/38	≥4/76
Ciprofloxacin	≤1	≥2	≤0.5	–	≥1	≤0.5	–	≥1	≤1	–	–
Ofloxacin	≤2	≥4	≤0.5	–	≥1	≤0.5	–	≥1	≤2	–	–
Gemifloxacin	≤0.25	≥0.5	≤0.25	–	≥0.5	≤0.25	–	≥0.5	–	–	–
Levofloxacin	≤2	≥4	≤1	–	≥2	≤1	–	≥2	≤2	–	–
Gatifloxacin	≤1	≥2	≤1	–	≥2	≤1	–	≥2	≤1	–	–
Moxifloxacin	≤1	≥2	≤0.5	–	≥1	≤0.5	–	≥1	≤1	–	–
Rifampin	ND	ND	–	–	–	–	–	–	≤1	2	≥4
Chloramphenicol	≤2	≥4	≤2	–	≥4	≤2	–	≥4	≤2	4	≥8
Oral agents											
Amoxicillin (1.5 g/day; 45 mg/k/day)	≤2	≥4	≤1	–	≥2	–	–	–	–	–	–
Amoxicillin (3–4 g/day; 90 mg/kg/day)	≤4[b]	≥8[b]	–	–	–	–	–	–	–	–	–
Amoxicillin–clavulanate (1.5 g/250 mg/day; 45/6.4 mg/kg/day)	≤2[b]	≥4[b]	≤1	–	≥2	≤1	–	≥2	≤4	–	≥8[c]
Amoxicillin–clavulanate (4 g/6.4 mg/day; 45 mg/kg/day)	≤4[b]	≥8[b]	–	–	–	–	–	–	–	–	–
Cefaclor	≤0.5	≥1	≤1	–	≥2	≤1	–	≥2	≤8	16	≥32
Cefuroxime axetil	≤1	≥2	≤1	–	≥2	≤1	–	≥2	≤4	8	≥16
Cefixime	≤1	≥2	–	–	–	–	–	–	≤1	–	–
Cefprozil	≤1	≥2	–	–	–	–	–	–	≤8	16	≥32
Cefdinir	≤0.5	≥1	–	–	–	–	–	–	≤1	–	–
Cefpodoxime	≤0.5	≥1	–	–	–	–	–	–	≤2	–	–
Telithromycin	≤0.5[e]	≥1[e]	≤0.5	1–2	≥4	≤0.5	–	≥1	≤4	8	≥16
Tetracycline	≤2[f]	≥4[f]	≤1	–	≥2	≤1	–	≥2	≤2	4	≥8

ND not defined; *CLSI* Clinical and Laboratory Standards Institute; *BSAC* British Society for Antimicrobial Chemotherapy –, no breakpoint available

[a]CLSI breakpoint used to define β-lactamase-negative ampicillin resistant (BLNAR) isolates. CLSI states that BLNAR strains of *H. influenzae* should be considered resistant to amoxicillin–clavulanate, ampicillin–sulbactam, cefaclor, cefamandole, cefetamet, cefonicid, cefprozil, cefuroxime, lorocarbef, and piperacillin–tazobactam despite apparent in vitro susceptibility of some BLNAR strains to these agents (29)

[b]Breakpoints are expressed as amoxicillin component; testing was performed using a 2:1 ratio of amoxicillin:clavulanic acid

[c]Breakpoint used to define β-lactamase positive amoxicillin–clavulanate resistant (BLPACR) isolates

[d]Breakpoints are expressed as trimethoprim component; testing was performed using a 1:19 ratio of trimethoprim:sulfamethoxazole

[e]Limited information is currently available to determine PK/PD breakpoints

[f]Microbiological breakpoint used in absence of PK/PD studies

Table 2 Susceptibility of worldwide isolates of *H. influenzae* ($N = 8523$) and *M. catarrhalis* ($N - 874$) to 23 antimicrobials and MIC_{50}'s and MIC_{90}'s. Alexander Project 1998–2000

	H. influenzae					*M. catarrhalis*		
	MIC_{50}	MIC_{90}	PK/PD	CLSI		MIC_{50}	MIC_{90}	PK/PD
Antimicrobial	(µg/mL)	(µg/mL)	S (%)	S (%)	R (%)	(µg/mL)	(µg/mL)	S (%)
Ampicillin	0.25	>16	NA	81.9	17.0	8	16	NA
Amoxicillin	0.5	>16	81.6	83.2	16.8	8	16	22.7
Amoxicillin–clavulanate, lower dose	0.5	1	98.1	99.6	0.4	≤0.12	0.25	100
Amoxicillin–clavulanate, higher dose	0.5	1	99.6	NA	NA	≤0.12	0.25	100
Cefaclor	4	16	1.4	89.7	3.6	2	4	10.9
Cefuroxime axetil	1	2	83.6	98.1	0.7	1	2	61.9
Cefixime	0.03	0.06	99.8	99.8	NA	0.12	0.5	100
Ceftriaxone	≤0.004	0.008	100	100	NA	0.12	1	97.4
Cefprozil	2	8	22.3	92.5	2.6	4	8	16.0
Cefdinir	0.25	0.5	92.0	97.6	NA	0.25	0.5	100
Erythromycin	4	8	<0.5	NA	NA	≤0.5	≤0.5	99.7[a]
Clarithromycin	8	16	<0.3	79.6	0.9	≤0.5	≤0.5	99.9[a]
Azithromycin	1	2	<1.2	99.5	NA	0.06	0.12	99.3
Chloramphenicol	0.5	1	98.1	97.9	1.9	0.5	0.5	100
Doxycycline	0.5	1	28.9	NA	NA	0.12	0.25	95.8
Trimethoprim-sulfamethoxazole	0.12	>4	78.3	78.3	17.0	0.25	1	72.0
Ciprofloxacin	0.015	0.03	99.9	99.9	NA	0.03	0.06	99.9
Ofloxacin	0.03	0.06	99.9	99.9	NA	0.12	0.12	99.8
Gemifloxacin	0.004	0.015	99.9	NA	NA	0.008	0.015	99.8
Levofloxacin	0.015	0.015	99.9	99.9	NA	0.03	0.06	>99.5
Gatifloxacin	0.008	0.015	99.9	99.9	NA	0.03	0.03	100
Moxifloxacin	0.015	0.03	99.8	99.8	NA	0.06	0.06	100

Adapted from Jacobs et al. (96); *NA* not available

[a]For *M. catarrhalis*, the percentage susceptibility to erythromycin and clarithromycin was based on the lowest concentration tested (0.5 µg/mL) instead of at the breakpoints of 0.25 (µg/mL)

Table 3 Regional differences in susceptibility (%) of *H. influenzae* to antimicrobials based on PK/PD breakpoints (refer to Table 1 for breakpoints). Alexander Project 1998–2000

Region/country	N	Ampicillin	Ampicillin, β-lactamase negative	Amoxicillin	Amoxicillin, β-lactamase negative	Amoxicillin-clavulanate, lower dose	Amoxicillin-clavulanate, higher dose	Cefaclor	Cefuroxime axetil	Cefixime	Ceftriaxone	Cefprozil	Cefdinir	Chloramphenicol	Doxycycline	Trimethoprim-sulfamethoxazole	Ofloxacin
Africa	361	91.4	98.2	90.6	97.3	97.5	100	0.8	80.1	99.4	100	19.7	93.5	96.1	26.6	57.6	100
E. Europe	1393	93.6	99.8	93.6	99.8	99.7	100	0.5	88.0	99.9	99.9	26.4	95.4	99.3	26.5	82.1	100
W. Europe	3064	85.5	99.1	85.7	99.3	99.1	99.9	0.2	87.4	100	100	22.4	93.5	98.7	35.1	83.5	100
Hong Kong	379	74.9	99.0	72.3	95.5	96.0	99.5	0.5	73.4	100	100	8.4	87.3	90.8	16.4	70.7	99.7
Japan	457	81.0	90.5	80.1	89.5	87.1	94.5	0.4	53.8	96.7	100	9.2	66.2	95.4	18.4	85.1	99.8
Saudi Arabia	225	79.1	98.9	78.2	97.8	98.2	100	0.0	80.0	100	100	9.8	88.8	92.0	16.9	61.3	100
Brazil	183	88.5	100	89.1	100	100	100	9.3	95.6	100	100	60.7	100	94.5	49.7	47.0	100
Mexico	191	75.4	99.3	75.4	99.3	99.5	100	5.2	88.0	99.5	100	30.4	94.0	99.5	45.5	56.0	100
USA	2073	69.7	98.8	69.2	98.2	98.5	99.8	3.2	83.5	100	100	23.4	93.9	99.7	23.6	78.3	99.8
All isolates	8523	81.9	98.6	81.6	98.2	98.1	99.6	1.4	83.6	99.8	100	22.3	92.0	98.1	28.9	78.3	99.9

Adapted from Jacobs et al. (96)

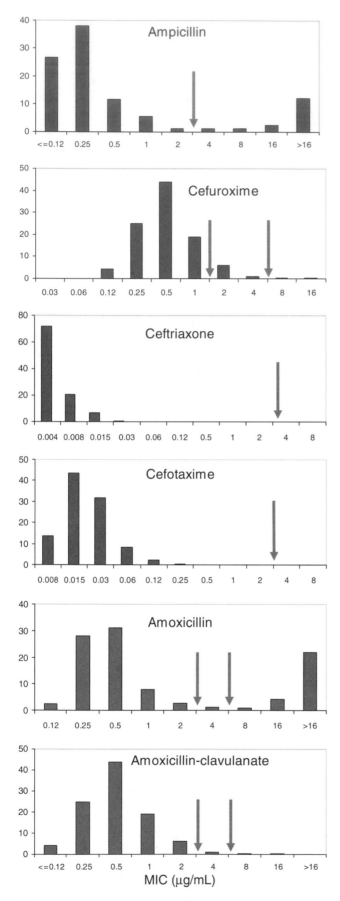
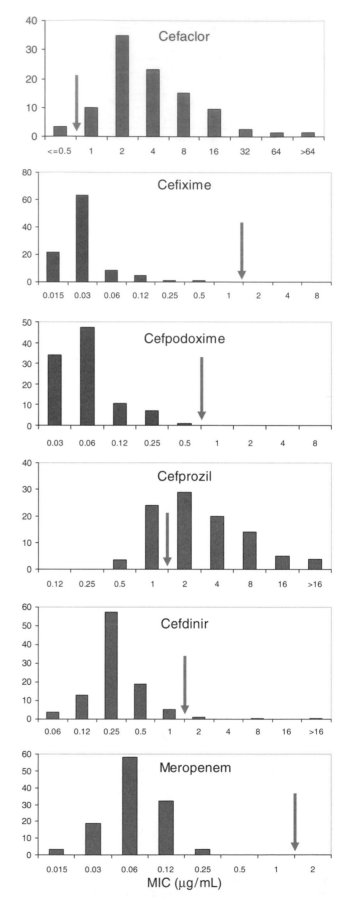

Fig. 9 MIC distributions of selected β-lactam antimicrobial agents for *H. influenzae*. Arrows indicate PK/PD breakpoints. The two arrows shown for amoxicillin and amoxicillin-clavulanate indicate breakpoints applicable to lower (*left*) and higher (*right*) dosing regimens. The two arrows shown for cefuroxime indicate breakpoints applicable to oral (*left*) and parenteral (*right*) dosing regimens. Data adapted from literature or the data bases used to generate these publications (24, 31, 38, 48, 96, 106, 107). Copyright Michael R. Jacobs, used with permission

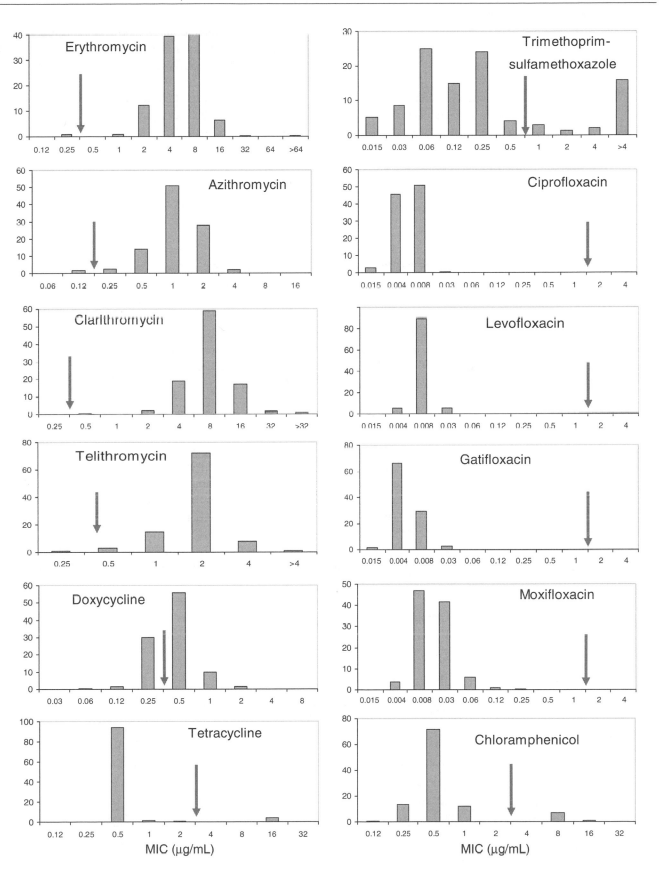

Fig. 10 MIC distributions of selected non-β-lactam antimicrobial agents for *H. influenzae*. Arrows indicate PK/PD breakpoints. Data adapted from literature or the data bases used to generate these publications (24, 31, 38, 48, 96, 106, 107). Copyright Michael R. Jacobs, used with permission.

associated with *tetB* gene, trimethoprim-sulfamethox-azole-resistant population associated with mutations in DHFR and DHPS, and chloramphenicol-resistant population associated with *cat* gene. These agents are suitable for directed use against *H. influenzae*, and for empiric use where resistance is low, or the consequences of treatment failure are minor, although drug toxicity also needs to be considered.

Comparison of these PK/PD based susceptibility interpretations with current recommendations for treatment of diseases associated with *H. influenzae* reveal the following:

• *Meningitis*. Current empiric therapy recommendations, vancomycin plus a third-generation cephalosporin such as cefotaxime or ceftriaxone, or a third-generation cephalosporin alone if Gram stain enables presumptive pathogen identification as *H. influenzae*, are still valid except in areas where high-level BLNAR and BLPACR strains are prevalent and Hib is not in use, such as Japan, where treatment failures with cefotaxime or ceftriaxone monotherapy have been encountered (5). Suggested therapy for areas where high-level BLNAR and BLPACR strains occur is cefotaxime or ceftriaxone plus meropenem based on no additional loss of affinity of meropenem for PBP3 between low and high BLNAR strains (Table 4 and Fig. 4) (5, 50). Alternative therapies recommended for *H. influenzae*: chloramphenicol, cefepime, and meropenem, appear to be valid except in areas where chloramphenicol-resistant strains or high-level BLNAR and BLPACR strains are prevalent. Gatifloxacin and moxifloxacin are also recommended as alternative agents for adults, and these are also valid options, as virtually all *H. influenzae* are currently susceptible, although gatifloxacin is no longer available in many countries. Use of quinolones in children should also be considered if other options are contraindicated. Development of susceptibility breakpoints for *H. influenzae* applicable to meningitis would be very worthwhile.

• *Childhood pneumonia and bacteremia*. Current empiric and directed treatment recommendations are valid except for areas where BLNAR and BLPACR strains are prevalent, where the efficacy of oral amoxicillin and amoxicillin-clavulanate against high-level BLNAR strains may be compromised. The efficacy of parenteral cephalosporins and meropenem may also be compromised, but MICs of high-level BLNAR strains are currently below PK/PD breakpoints (Tables 4 and 5, and Fig. 4) (5, 50).

• *CAP in adults*. Recommendations of azithromycin, clarithromycin, or doxycycline for outpatients with no comorbidities, and of azithromycin or clarithromycin for outpatients with comorbidities if no antibiotic therapy had been administered in the past 3 months, are problematic as these agents have little, if any, clinical activity against *H. influenzae*, and the activity of these agents against macrolide-resistant pneumococci is also a concern (108). The remaining recommendations for CAP are valid except for areas where BLNAR and BLPACR *H. influenzae* are found as discussed earlier, in which case respiratory quinolones and meropenem are suitable agents.

• *AOM*. Current recommendations are valid with the exception again of areas where BLNAR and BLPACR *H. influenzae* are found, where MIC_{90}'s of amoxicillin, cefaclor, cefpodoxime, and cefdinir against high-level BLNAR and BLPACR strains are above PK/PD breakpoints (Table 5). The MIC_{90} of cefditoren against high-level BLNAR strains is 0.25 µg/mL; however, the PK/PD breakpoint for this agent has not been established, but is likely to be lower than the MIC_{90} value (109, 110). Cefixime may have clinically useful activity against high-level BLNAR strains, but additional information is needed, and use of quinolones should be considered (21, 109, 111).

• *Acute sinusitis*. As is the case for AOM, current recommendations for sinusitis are valid with the exception of areas where BLNAR and BLPACR *H. influenzae* are found.

Table 4 MIC_{50}/MIC_{90} values of 621 meningeal isolates of *H. influenzae* type b, Japan 2000–2004, based on β-lactam resistance mechanisms

	MIC_{50}/MIC_{90} values (µg/mL) for isolates based on resistance mechanism					
	None (N = 155, 25%)	TEM-1[a] (N = 68, 11%)	Low-level BLNAR[b] (N = 189, 30%)	High-level BLNAR[c] (N = 138, 22%)	Low-level BLPACR[d] (N = 59, 10%)	High-level BLPACR[e] (N = 12, 2%)
Ampicillin	0.25/0.5	8/16	1/2	2/4	16/32	32/64
Cefotaxime	0.016/0.03	0.016/0.03	0.06/0.125	0.5/1	0.06/0.125	0.5/1
Ceftriaxone	0.004/0.008	0.004/0.008	0.016/0.03	0.125/0.25	0.016/0.03	0.125/0.25
Meropenem	0.03/0.06	0.06/0.06	0.125/0.25	0.125/0.25	0.125/0.25	0.125/0.25

Adapted from Hasegawa et al. (5)
[a]TEM-1, TEM-1 β-lactamase gene present
[b]N256K or R517H substitution in *ftsI* gene
[c]S385T substitution with either N256K or R517H substitution in *ftsI* gene
[d]TEM-1 β-lactamase gene and N256K or R517H substitution in *ftsI* gene
[e]TEM-1 β-lactamase gene and S385T substitution with either N256K or R517H substitution in *ftsI* gene

Table 5 MIC$_{50}$/MIC$_{90}$ values of 296 Japanese and 100 US respiratory isolates of untypeable respiratory isolates of *H. influenzae*, 1999, based on β-lactam resistance mechanisms

	None		TEM-1[a]		ROB-1[b]		Low-level BLNAR[c]		High-level BLNAR[d]	
Country	Japan	US	Japan	US	Japan	US	Japan	US	Japan	US
N (%)	163 (55%)	45 (46%)	9 (3%)	26 (26%)	–[e]	10 (10%)	78 (26%)	13 (13%)	39 (13%)	–
Ampicillin	0.25/0.5	0.25/.025	4/32	8/32	–	16/64	1/2	1/1	2/8	–
Amoxicillin	0.5/0.5	0.5/0.5	4/32	8/32	–	16/64	2/4	2/8	4/16	–
Piperacillin	0.016/0.06	0.016/0.03	1/32	4/32	–	16/64	0.03/0.06	0.03/0.125	0.06/0.25	–
Cefotaxime	0.016/0.03	0.016/0.03	0.016/0.03	0.016/0.016	–	0.008/0.016	0.06/0.25	0.06/0.06	0.5/1	–
Ceftriaxone	0.004/0.008	0.004/0.008	0.004/0.008	0.004/0.004	–	0.004/0.008	0.016/0.03	0.016/0.03	0.125/0.25	–
Cefaclor	2/8	2/8	2/4	2/4	–	16/64	16/64	16/64	32/64	–
Cefpodoxime	0.06/0.125	0.06/0.125	0.06/0.125	0.06/0.06	–	0.06/0.06	0.25/1	0.25/0.5	2/8	–
Cefdinir	0.5/0.5	0.25/0.5	0.25/0.5	0.25/0.5	–	0.25/0.25	1/4	0.5/1	8/16	–
Cefditoren	0.016/0.03	0.016/0.03	0.016/0.06	0.008/0.016	–	0.016/0.016	0.03/0.125	0.03/0.03	0.25/0.25	–
Meropenem	0.06/0.125	0.06/0.06	0.06/0.125	0.06/0.06	–	0.06/0.06	0.125/0.5	0.12/0.25	0.25/0.5	–

Adapted from Hasegawa et al. (38)
[a]TEM-1, TEM-1 β-lactamase gene present
[b]ROB-1, ROB-1 β-lactamase gene present
[c]N256K or R517H substitution in *ftsI* gene
[d]S385T substitution with either N256K or R517H substitution in *ftsI* gene
[e]–, not applicable

- *AECB.* Recommendations for patients with baseline risk factors, amoxicillin–clavulanate and respiratory quinolones, are valid as *H. influenzae* is the predominant pathogen and these agents are active on the basis of PK/PD breakpoints. However, of the agents recommended for patients without baseline risk factors, azithromycin, clarithromycin, telithromycin, doxycycline, cefuroxime axetil, cefpodoxime, and cefdinir, only cefpodoxime is active against *H. influenzae* on the basis of PK/PD breakpoints. The rationale for these latter recommendations of agents that will not be effective for the patient group with a high probability of spontaneous resolution is unclear.

consists of cation-supplemented Mueller–Hinton broth supplemented with 5 mg of yeast extract per mL, 15 μg of NAD per mL, and 15 μg of hematin per mL (29, 112). The medium specified by BSAC is Isosensitest agar or broth supplemented with 5% horse blood (lysed for the broth formulation) and 20 μg of NAD per mL (30). Results obtained with these two methods and other variations are comparable (113, 114). Media containing hematin should be fresh, as hematin tends to precipitate out of solution on storage (113). *M. catarrhalis* can be tested with Mueller–Hinton broth or agar, or with media used to test *H. influenzae* (96). BSAC recommends Isosensitest agar supplemented with 5% horse blood (30).

8 Laboratory Determination of Susceptibility

8.1 MIC Determination

Susceptibility testing of *H. influenzae* by MIC determination has been well standardized, with CLSI, BSAC, and other methods generally providing comparable results (29, 30). The main requirements for testing are to ensure that concentrations of hematin, hemoglobin, blood or other iron source, and NAD adequately support growth, that the inoculum size is correct, and that appropriate quality control strains are included in each test batch. The medium specified by CLSI is Haemophilus Test Medium (HTM), which

8.2 Disk Diffusion Testing

CLSI and BSAC both show interpretative disk diffusion criteria for a number of agents against *Haemophilus* species (29, 30). However, most MIC distributions are unimodal, and testing of these agents is best performed by MIC determination rather than disk diffusion. Agents showing bimodal MIC distributions, such as ampicillin, amoxicillin, tetracycline, chloramphenicol, and trimethoprim-sulfamethoxazole, are the most suitable for testing by disk diffusion. BSAC also has disk diffusion interpretations for *M. catarrhalis* (30). A major limitation of disk diffusion testing is that interpretative criteria for many agents are based on microbiological rather than PK/PK breakpoints, so their clinical relevance is limited.

8.3 Gradient Diffusion (E-test)

This method has been widely used and is generally comparable to standard MIC methods for testing *H. influenzae* (115). MICs of macrolides, ketolides, and quinolones are generally twofold higher by E-test with incubation in a 5–10% CO_2 atmosphere, so this needs to be considered when interpreting and comparing results (116, 117). The accuracy of E-test for differentiation of BLNAR and BLPACR strains from baseline strains has not been adequately established (47).

8.4 β-Lactamase Detection

This is best determined by the chromogenic cephalosporin method using nitrocefin, which is converted from a yellow to a pink compound when hydrolized by β-lactamases, or other comparable agents (118).

9 Infection Control Measures

Prior to the introduction of the Hib vaccine, *H. influenzae* type b was the most common cause of bacterial meningitis in children between the ages of 2 months and 5 years. Prevention, through widespread use of the Hib vaccine, has been highly effective. In areas where the vaccine is unavailable or in unvaccinated children, *H. influenzae* type b meningitis remains a childhood threat (119). The disease remains communicable as long as the organism is present in the nasopharynx and until 24–48 h after beginning effective antibiotic treatment. Contacts, particularly those under 6 years of age, should receive prophylactic treatment with rifampin (20 mg/kg in children and 600 mg in adults, once daily, by mouth for 4 days) (120).

Prevention of AOM due to untypeable *H. influenzae* using a novel vaccine containing polysaccharides from 11 *S. pneumoniae* serotypes each conjugated to *H. influenzae*-derived protein D has been demonstrated (121). In addition to protection against pneumococcal AOM, efficacy of this vaccine was also shown by a 35.5% reduction in episodes of AOM caused by non-typeable *H. influenzae*.

10 Conclusions

H. influenzae and *M. catarrhalis* are major pathogens associated with common respiratory tract infections, and *H. influenzae* type b is an invasive pathogen of unimmunized children. Treatment of these infections is limited by both intrinsic and acquired resistance, and mechanisms of resistance continue to evolve in these pathogens. Application of PK/PD principles to these pathogens is essential to understanding the clinical relationship between in vitro susceptibility and in vivo response. Judicious use of antimicrobial agents is the key to preserving the activity of these agents and to prevent further development of resistance.

References

1. Bartlett JG, Dowell SF, Mandell LA, File Jr TM, Musher DM, Fine MJ. Practice guidelines for the management of community-acquired pneumonia in adults. Infectious Diseases Society of America. Clin Infect Dis 2000; 31:347–382
2. Jacobs MR. Anti-infective pharmacodynamics – maximizing efficacy, minimizing toxicity. Drug Discovery Today 2004; 1:505–512
3. Coles CL, Kanungo R, Rahmathullah L, et al. Pneumococcal nasopharyngeal colonization in young South Indian infants. Pediatr Infect Dis J 2001; 20:289–295
4. Sethi S, Evans N, Grant BJ, Murphy TF. New strains of bacteria and exacerbations of chronic obstructive pulmonary disease. N Engl J Med 2002; 347:465–471
5. Hasegawa K, Kobayashi R, Takada E, et al. High prevalence of type b {beta}-lactamase-non-producing ampicillin-resistant *Haemophilus influenzae* in meningitis: the situation in Japan where Hib vaccine has not been introduced. J Antimicrob Chemother 2006; 57:1077–1082
6. Tunkel AR, Hartman BJ, Kaplan SL, et al. Practice guidelines for the management of bacterial meningitis. Clin Infect Dis 2004; 39:1267–1284
7. Juven T, Mertsola J, Waris M, et al. Etiology of community-acquired pneumonia in 254 hospitalized children. Pediatr Infect Dis J 2000; 19:293–298
8. McCracken GH, Jr. Etiology and treatment of pneumonia. Pediatr Infect Dis J 2000; 19:373–377
9. Heiskanen-Kosma T, Korppi M, Jokinen C, et al. Etiology of childhood pneumonia: serologic results of a prospective, population-based study. Pediatr Infect Dis J 1998; 17:986–991
10. McIntosh K. Community-acquired pneumonia in children. N Engl J Med 2002; 346:429–437
11. Bradley JS. Management of community-acquired pediatric pneumonia in an era of increasing antibiotic resistance and conjugate vaccines. Pediatr Infect Dis J 2002; 21:592–598; discussion 613–614
12. Block S, Hedrick J, Hammerschlag MR, Cassell GH, Craft JC. *Mycoplasma pneumoniae* and *Chlamydia pneumoniae* in pediatric community-acquired pneumonia: comparative efficacy and safety of clarithromycin vs. erythromycin ethylsuccinate. Pediatr Infect Dis J 1995; 14:471–477
13. McMillan JA. *Chlamydia pneumoniae* revisited. Pediatr Infect Dis J 1998; 17:1046–1047
14. Mandell LA, Bartlett JG, Dowell SF, File TM, Jr, Musher DM, Whitney C. Update of practice guidelines for the management of community-acquired pneumonia in immunocompetent adults. Clin Infect Dis 2003; 37:1405–1433
15. Niederman MS, Mandell LA, Anzueto A, et al. Guidelines for the management of adults with community-acquired pneumonia. Diagnosis, assessment of severity, antimicrobial therapy, and prevention. Am J Respir Crit Care Med 2001; 163:1730–1754

16. Stevens DL. The role of vancomycin in the treatment paradigm. Clin Infect Dis 2006; 42 Suppl 1:S51–5S7

17. Daly KA. Epidemiology of otitis media. Otolaryngol Clin North Am 1991; 24:775–786

18. Dagan R, Leibovitz E. Bacterial eradication in the treatment of otitis media. Lancet Infect Dis 2002; 2:593–604

19. Dowell SF, Butler JC, Giebink GS, et al. Acute otitis media: management and surveillance in an era of pneumococcal resistance – a report from the drug-resistant *Streptococcus pneumoniae* Therapeutic Working Group. Pediatr Infect Dis J 1999; 18:1–9

20. Casey JR, Pichichero ME. Changes in frequency and pathogens causing acute otitis media in 1995–2003. Pediatr Infect Dis J 2004; 23:824–828

21. Pichichero ME, Casey JR. Emergence of a multiresistant serotype 19A pneumococcal strain not included in the 7-valent conjugate vaccine as an otopathogen in children. JAMA 2007; 298:1772–1778

22. Pelton SI, Huot H, Finkelstein JA, et al. Emergence of 19A as virulent and multidrug resistant pneumococcus in Massachusetts following universal immunization of infants with pneumococcal conjugate vaccine. Pediatr Infect Dis J 2007; 26:468–472

23. American Academy of Pediatrics and American Academy of Family Physicians Clinical Practice Guideline. Diagnosis and management of acute otitis media. Pediatrics 2004; 113:1451–1465

24. Anon JB, Jacobs MR, Poole MD, et al. Antimicrobial treatment guidelines for acute bacterial rhinosinusitis. Otolaryngol Head Neck Surg 2004; 130:1–45

25. Sethi S. Infectious exacerbations of chronic bronchitis: diagnosis and management. J Antimicrob Chemother 1999; 43 Suppl A:97–105

26. Sethi S, Murphy TF. Acute exacerbations of chronic bronchitis: new developments concerning microbiology and pathophysiology – impact on approaches to risk stratification and therapy. Infect Dis Clin North Am 2004; 18:861–882, ix

27. Balter MS, La Forge J, Low DE, Mandell L, Grossman RF. Canadian guidelines for the management of acute exacerbations of chronic bronchitis. Can Respir J 2003; 10 Suppl B:3B–32B

28. Turnidge J, Kahlmeter G, Kronvall G. Statistical characterisation of bacterial wild-type MIC value distributions and the determination of epidemiological cut-off values. Clin Microbiol Infect 2006; 12:418–425

29. Clinical and Laboratory Standards Institute. *Performance Standards for Antimicrobial Susceptibility Testing*, Sixteenth Informational Supplement. M100-S16. CLSI, Wayne, PA 2006

30. BSAC. *BSAC Methods for Antimicrobial Susceptibility Testing*, Version 5, January 2006. http://www.bsac.org.uk/_db/_documents/version_5_.pdf 2006

31. Jacobs MR, Bajaksouzian S, Windau A, et al. Susceptibility of *Streptococcus pneumoniae*, *Haemophilus influenzae*, and *Moraxella catarrhalis* to 17 oral antimicrobial agents based on pharmacodynamic parameters: 1998–2001 U S Surveillance Study. Clin Lab Med 2004; 24:503–530

32. Andes D, Anon J, Jacobs MR, Craig WA. Application of pharmacokinetics and pharmacodynamics to antimicrobial therapy of respiratory tract infections. Clin Lab Med 2004; 24:477–502

33. Chambers HF. Penicillin-binding protein-mediated resistance in pneumococci and staphylococci. J Infect Dis 1999; 179 Suppl 2:S353–359

34. Massova I, Mobashery S. Structural and mechanistic aspects of evolution of beta-lactamases and penicillin-binding proteins. Curr Pharm Des 1999; 5:929–937

35. Ghuysen JM. Molecular structures of penicillin-binding proteins and beta-lactamases. Trends Microbiol 1994; 2:372–380

36. Blumberg PM, Strominger JL. Interaction of penicillin with the bacterial cell: penicillin-binding proteins and penicillin-sensitive enzymes. Bacteriol Rev 1974; 38:291–335

37. Hotomi M, Sakai KF, Billal DS, Shimada J, Suzumoto M, Yamanaka N. Antimicrobial resistance in *Haemophilus influenzae* isolated from the nasopharynx among Japanese children with acute otitis media. Acta Otolaryngol 2006; 126:130–137

38. Hasegawa K, Yamamoto K, Chiba N, et al. Diversity of ampicillin-resistance genes in *Haemophilus influenzae* in Japan and the United States. Microb Drug Resist 2003; 9:39–46

39. Jacobs MR. Worldwide trends in antimicrobial resistance among common respiratory tract pathogens in children. Pediatr Infect Dis J 2003; 22:S109–S119

40. Massova I, Mobashery S. Kinship and diversification of bacterial penicillin-binding proteins and beta-lactamases. Antimicrob Agents Chemother 1998; 42:1–17

41. Jordens JZ, Slack MP. *Haemophilus influenzae*: then and now. Eur J Clin Microbiol Infect Dis 1995; 14:935–948

42. Rubin LG, Medeiros AA, Yolken RH, Moxon ER. Ampicillin treatment failure of apparently beta-lactamase-negative *Haemophilus influenzae* type b meningitis due to novel beta-lactamase. Lancet 1981; 2:1008–1010

43. Wallace RJ, Jr., Steingrube VA, Nash DR, et al. BRO beta-lactamases of *Branhamella catarrhalis* and *Moraxella* subgenus Moraxella, including evidence for chromosomal beta lactamase transfer by conjugation in *B. catarrhalis*, *M. nonliquefaciens*, and *M. lacunata*. Antimicrob Agents Chemother 1989; 33: 1845–1854

44. Bush K. Beta-lactamase inhibitors from laboratory to clinic. Clin Microbiol Rev 1988; 1:109–123

45. Bozdogan B, Tristram S, Appelbaum PC. Combination of altered PBPs and expression of cloned extended-spectrum beta-lactamases confers cefotaxime resistance in *Haemophilus influenzae*. J Antimicrob Chemother 2006; 57:747–749

46. Pitout M, MacDonald K, Musgrave H, et al. Characterization of extended spectrum beta-lactamase (ESBL) activity in *Haemophilus influenzae*. In: *Program and Abstracts of the 42nd Interscience Conference on Antimicrobials and Chemotherapy*, San Diego, CA. American Society for Microbiology, Washington, DC, USA. Abstract C2–C645, p. 96, 2002

47. Tristram S, Jacobs MR, Appelbaum PC. Antimicrobial resistance in *Haemophilus influenzae*. Clin Microbiol Rev 2007; 20:368–389

48. Ubukata K, Shibasaki Y, Yamamoto K, et al. Association of amino acid substitutions in penicillin-binding protein 3 with beta-lactam resistance in beta-lactamase-negative ampicillin-resistant *Haemophilus influenzae*. Antimicrob Agents Chemother 2001; 45:1693–1699

49. Dabernat H, Delmas C, Seguy M, et al. Diversity of beta-lactam resistance-conferring amino acid substitutions in penicillin-binding protein 3 of *Haemophilus influenzae*. Antimicrob Agents Chemother 2002; 46:2208–2218

50. Sanbongi Y, Suzuki T, Osaki Y, Senju N, Ida T, Ubukata K. Molecular evolution of beta-lactam-resistant *Haemophilus influenzae*: 9-year surveillance of penicillin-binding protein 3 mutations in isolates from Japan. Antimicrob Agents Chemother 2006; 50:2487–2492

51. Takahata S, Ida T, Senju N, et al. Horizontal gene transfer of ftsI, encoding penicillin-binding protein 3, in *Haemophilus influenzae*. Antimicrob Agents Chemother 2007; 51:1589–1595

52. Fluit AC, Florijn A, Verhoef J, Milatovic D. Susceptibility of European beta-lactamase-positive and -negative *Haemophilus influenzae* isolates from the periods 1997/1998 and 2002/2003. J Antimicrob Chemother 2005; 56:133–138

53. Dabernat H, Seguy M, Faucon G, Delmas C. Epidemiology of *Haemophilus influenzae* strains identified in 2001 in France, and assessment of their susceptibility to beta-lactams. Med Mal Infect 2004; 34:97–101

54. Kim IS, Ki CS, Kim S, et al. Diversity of ampicillin resistance genes and antimicrobial susceptibility patterns in *Haemophilus*

influenzae strains isolated in Korea. Antimicrob Agents Chemother 2007; 51:453–460

55. Garcia-Cobos S, Campos J, Lazaro E, et al. Ampicillin-resistant non-beta-lactamase-producing *Haemophilus influenzae* in Spain: recent emergence of clonal isolates with increased resistance to cefotaxime and cefixime. Antimicrob Agents Chemother 2007; 51:2564–2573

56. Ng WL, Kazmierczak KM, Robertson GT, Gilmour R, Winkler ME. Transcriptional regulation and signature patterns revealed by microarray analyses of *Streptococcus pneumoniae* R6 challenged with sublethal concentrations of translation inhibitors. J Bacteriol 2003; 185:359–370

57. Vazquez D, Monro RE. Effects of some inhibitors of protein synthesis on the binding of aminoacyl tRNA to ribosomal subunits. Biochim Biophys Acta 1967; 142:155–173

58. Tait-Kamradt A, Davies T, Cronan M, Jacobs MR, Appelbaum PC, Sutcliffe J. Mutations in 23S rRNA and ribosomal protein L4 account for resistance in pneumococcal strains selected in vitro by macrolide passage. Antimicrob Agents Chemother 2000; 44:2118–2125

59. Tait-Kamradt A, Davies T, Appelbaum PC, et al. Two new mechanisms of macrolide resistance in clinical strains of *Streptococcus pneumoniae* from Eastern Europe and North America. Antimicrob Agents Chemother 2000; 44:3395–3401

60. Sanchez L, Leranoz S, Puig M, Loren JG, Nikaido H, Vinas M. Molecular basis of antimicrobial resistance in non-typable *Haemophilus influenzae*. Microbiologia 1997; 13:309–314

61. Sanchez L, Pan W, Vinas M, Nikaido H. The acrAB homolog of *Haemophilus influenzae* codes for a functional multidrug efflux pump. J Bacteriol 1997; 179:6855–6857

62. Bogdanovich T, Bozdogan B, Appelbaum PC. Effect of efflux on telithromycin and macrolide susceptibility in *Haemophilus influenzae*. Antimicrob Agents Chemother 2006; 50:893–898

63. Chopra I, Hawkey PM, Hinton M. Tetracyclines, molecular and clinical aspects. J Antimicrob Chemother 1992; 29:245–277

64. Marshall B, Roberts M, Smith A, Levy SB. Homogeneity of transferable tetracycline-resistance determinants in *Haemophilus* species. J Infect Dis 1984; 149:1028–1029

65. Chopra I, Roberts M. Tetracycline antibiotics: mode of action, applications, molecular biology, and epidemiology of bacterial resistance. Microbiol Mol Biol Rev 2001; 65:232–260

66. Campos J, Chanyangam M, deGroot R, Smith AL, Tenover FC, Reig R. Genetic relatedness of antibiotic resistance determinants in multiply resistant *Hemophilus influenzae*. J Infect Dis 1989; 160:810–817

67. Levy J, Verhaegen G, De Mol P, Couturier M, Dekegel D, Butzler JP. Molecular characterization of resistance plasmids in epidemiologically unrelated strains of multiresistant *Haemophilus influenzae*. J Infect Dis 1993; 168:177–187

68. Wang JC. DNA topoisomerases. Annu Rev Biochem 1985; 54:665–697

69. Pan XS, Fisher LM. DNA gyrase and topoisomerase IV are dual targets of clinafloxacin action in *Streptococcus pneumoniae*. Antimicrob Agents Chemother 1998; 42:2810–2816

70. Davies TA, Kelly LM, Hoellman DB, et al. Activities and postantibiotic effects of gemifloxacin compared to those of 11 other agents against *Haemophilus influenzae* and *Moraxella catarrhalis*. Antimicrob Agents Chemother 2000; 44:633–639

71. Davies TA, Kelly LM, Pankuch GA, Credito KL, Jacobs MR, Appelbaum PC. Antipneumococcal activities of gemifloxacin compared to those of nine other agents. Antimicrob Agents Chemother 2000; 44:304–310

72. Perez-Vazquez M, Roman F, Garcia-Cobos S, Campos J. Fluoroquinolone resistance in *Haemophilus influenzae* is associated with hypermutability. Antimicrob Agents Chemother 2007; 51:1566–1569

73. Burns JL, Mendelman PM, Levy J, Stull TL, Smith AL. A permeability barrier as a mechanism of chloramphenicol resistance in *Haemophilus influenzae*. Antimicrob Agents Chemother 1985; 27:46–54

74. Roberts MC, Swenson CD, Owens LM, Smith AL. Characterization of chloramphenicol-resistant *Haemophilus influenzae*. Antimicrob Agents Chemother 1980; 18:610–615

75. Powell M, Livermore DM. Mechanisms of chloramphenicol resistance in *Haemophilus influenzae* in the United Kingdom. J Med Microbiol 1988; 27:89–93

76. Burchall JJ, Hitchings GH. Inhibitor binding analysis of dihydrofolate reductases from various species. Mol Pharmacol 1965; 1:126–136

77. Hartman PG. Molecular aspects and mechanism of action of dihydrofolate reductase inhibitors. J Chemother 1993; 5:369–376

78. Then R, Angehrn P. Nature of the bacterial action of sulfonamides and trimethoprim, alone and in combination. J Infect Dis 1973; 128:Suppl:498–501

79. Adrian PV, Klugman KP. Mutations in the dihydrofolate reductase gene of trimethoprim-resistant isolates of *Streptococcus pneumoniae*. Antimicrob Agents Chemother 1997; 41:2406–2413

80. Maskell JP, Sefton AM, Hall LM. Multiple mutations modulate the function of dihydrofolate reductase in trimethoprim-resistant *Streptococcus pneumoniae*. Antimicrob Agents Chemother 2001; 45:1104–1108

81. Pikis A, Donkersloot JA, Rodriguez WJ, Keith JM. A conservative amino acid mutation in the chromosome-encoded dihydrofolate reductase confers trimethoprim resistance in *Streptococcus pneumoniae*. J Infect Dis 1998; 178:700–706

82. de Groot R, Chaffin DO, Kuehn M, Smith AL. Trimethoprim resistance in *Haemophilus influenzae* is due to altered dihydrofolate reductase(s). Biochem J 1991; 274 (Pt 3):657–662

83. Then RL. Neisseriaceae, a group of bacteria with dihydrofolate reductases, moderately susceptible to trimethoprim. Zentralbl Bakteriol [Orig A] 1979; 245:450–458

84. Burman LG. The antimicrobial activities of trimethoprim and sulfonamides. Scand J Infect Dis 1986; 18:3–13

85. Wallace RJ, Jr, Nash DR, Steingrube VA. Antibiotic susceptibilities and drug resistance in *Moraxella (Branhamella) catarrhalis*. Am J Med 1990; 88:46S–50S

86. Eliopoulos GM, Wennersten CB. In vitro activity of trimethoprim alone compared with trimethoprim–sulfamethoxazole and other antimicrobials against bacterial species associated with upper respiratory tract infections. Diagn Microbiol Infect Dis 1997; 29:33–38

87. Enne VI, King A, Livermore DM, Hall LM. Sulfonamide resistance in *Haemophilus influenzae* mediated by acquisition of sul2 or a short insertion in chromosomal folP. Antimicrob Agents Chemother 2002; 46:1934–1939

88. Bower BD. Ampicillin 'failure' in *H. influenzae* meningitis. Dev Med Child Neurol 1973; 15:813–814

89. Khan W, Ross S, Rodriguez W, Controni G, Saz AK. *Haemophilus influenzae* type B resistant to ampicillin. A report of two cases. JAMA 1974; 229:298–301

90. Tomeh MO, Starr SE, McGowan JE, Jr, Terry PM, Nahmias AJ. Ampicillin-resistant *Haemophilus influenzae* type B infection. JAMA 1974; 229:295–297

91. Farrar WE, Jr., O'Dell NM. Beta-lactamase activity in ampicillin-resistant *Haemophilus influenzae*. Antimicrob Agents Chemother 1974; 6:625–629

92. Philpott-Howard J, Williams JD. Increase in antibiotic resistance in *Haemophilus influenzae* in the United Kingdom since 1977: report of study group. Br Med J (Clin Res Ed) 1982; 284:1597–1599

93. Markowitz SM. Isolation of an ampicillin-resistant, non-beta-lactamase-producing strain of *Haemophilus influenzae*. Antimicrob Agents Chemother 1980; 17:80–83

94. Mendelman PM, Chaffin DO, Stull TL, Rubens CE, Mack KD, Smith AL. Characterization of non-beta-lactamase-mediated ampicillin resistance in *Haemophilus influenzae*. Antimicrob Agents Chemother 1984; 26:235–244

95. Jacobs MR, Bajaksouzian S, Zilles A, Lin G, Pankuch GA, Appelbaum PC. Susceptibilities of *Streptococcus pneumoniae* and *Haemophilus influenzae* to 10 oral antimicrobial agents based on pharmacodynamic parameters: 1997 U.S. Surveillance study. Antimicrob Agents Chemother 1999; 43:1901–1908

96. Jacobs MR, Felmingham D, Appelbaum PC, Gruneberg RN. The Alexander Project 1998–2000: susceptibility of pathogens isolated from community-acquired respiratory tract infection to commonly used antimicrobial agents. J Antimicrob Chemother 2003; 52:229–246

97. Peric M, Bozdogan B, Jacobs MR, Appelbaum PC. Effects of an efflux mechanism and ribosomal mutations on macrolide susceptibility of *Haemophilus influenzae* clinical isolates. Antimicrob Agents Chemother 2003; 47:1017–1022

98. Tamargo I, Fuentes K, Llop A, Oteo J, Campos J. High levels of multiple antibiotic resistance among 938 *Haemophilus influenzae* type b meningitis isolates from Cuba (1990–2002). J Antimicrob Chemother 2003; 52:695–698

99. Nazir J, Urban C, Mariano N, et al. Quinolone-resistant *Haemophilus influenzae* in a long-term care facility: clinical and molecular epidemiology. Clin Infect Dis 2004; 38:1564–1569

100. Yokota SI, Ohkoshi Y, Sato K, Fujii N. Emergence of fluoroquinolone-resistant *Haemophilus influenzae* strains among elderly patients but not in children. J Clin Microbiol 2007

101. Walker ES, Levy F. Genetic trends in a population evolving antibiotic resistance. Evol Int J Org Evol 2001; 55:1110–1122

102. Jacobs M. Optimisation of antimicrobial therapy using pharmacokinetic and pharmacodynamic parameters. Clin Microbiol Infect 2001; 7:589–596

103. Craig WA. Basic pharmacodynamics of antibacterials with clinical applications to the use of beta-lactams, glycopeptides, and linezolid. Infect Dis Clin North Am 2003; 17:479–501

104. Craig WA. Pharmacokinetic/pharmacodynamic parameters: rationale for antibacterial dosing of mice and men. Clin Infect Dis 1998; 26:1–10; quiz 11–12

105. Ambrose PG, Anon JB, Owen JS, et al. Use of pharmacodynamic end points in the evaluation of gatifloxacin for the treatment of acute maxillary sinusitis. Clin Infect Dis 2004; 38:1513–1520

106. Hasegawa K, Chiba N, Kobayashi R, et al. Rapidly increasing prevalence of beta-lactamase-nonproducing, ampicillin-resistant *Haemophilus influenzae* type b in patients with meningitis. Antimicrob Agents Chemother 2004; 48:1509–1514

107. Kooth LM, Jacobs MR, Good CE, et al. Comparative in vitro activity of a pharmacokinetically enhanced oral formulation of amoxicillin/clavulanic acid (2000/125 mg twice daily) against 9172 respiratory isolates collected worldwide in 2000. Int J Infect Dis 2004; 8:362–373

108. Jacobs MR. In vivo veritas: in vitro macrolide resistance in systemic *Streptococcus pneumoniae* infections does result in clinical failure. Clin Infect Dis 2002; 35:565–569

109. Nakamura T, Takahashi H. Antibacterial activity of oral cephems against various clinically isolated strains and evaluation of efficacy based on the pharmacokinetics/pharmacodynamics theory. Jpn J Antibiot 2004; 57:465–474

110. Liu P, Rand KH, Obermann B, Derendorf H. Pharmacokinetic-pharmacodynamic modelling of antibacterial activity of cefpodoxime and cefixime in *in vitro* kinetic models. Int J Antimicrob Agents 2005; 25:120–129

111. Schaad UB. Fluoroquinolone antibiotics in infants and children. Infect Dis Clin North Am 2005; 19:617–628

112. Clinical and Laboratory Standards Institute. *M7-A7 Methods for Dilution Antimicrobial Susceptibility Tests for Bacteria That Grow Aerobically*; Approved Standard, 7th edn. CLSI, Wayne, PA 2006

113. Jacobs MR, Bajaksouzian S, Windau A, et al. Effects of various test media on the activities of 21 antimicrobial agents against *Haemophilus influenzae*. J Clin Microbiol 2002; 40: 3269–3276

114. Reynolds R, Shackcloth J, Felmingham D, MacGowan A. Comparison of BSAC agar dilution and NCCLS broth microdilution MIC methods for in vitro susceptibility testing of *Streptococcus pneumoniae*, *Haemophilus influenzae* and *Moraxella catarrhalis*: the BSAC Respiratory Resistance Surveillance Programme. J Antimicrob Chemother 2003; 52:925–930

115. Fuchs PC, Barry AL, Brown SD. Influence of variations in test methods on susceptibility of *Haemophilus influenzae* to ampicillin, azithromycin, clarithromycin, and telithromycin. J Clin Microbiol 2001; 39:43–46

116. Bouchillon SK, Johnson JL, Hoban DJ, Stevens TM, Johnson BM Impact of carbon dioxide on the susceptibility of key respiratory tract pathogens to telithromycin and azithromycin. J Antimicrob Chemother 2005; 56:224–227

117. Perez-Vazquez M, Roman F, Varela MC, Canton R, Campos J. Activities of 13 quinolones by three susceptibility testing methods against a collection of *Haemophilus influenzae* isolates with different levels of susceptibility to ciprofloxacin: evidence for cross-resistance. J Antimicrob Chemother 2003; 51: 147–151

118. Sutton LD, Biedenbach DJ, Yen A, Jones RN. Development, characterization, and initial evaluations of S1. A new chromogenic cephalosporin for beta-lactamase detection. Diagn Microbiol Infect Dis 1995; 21:1–8

119. Yogev R, Guzman-Cottrill J. Bacterial meningitis in children: critical review of current concepts. Drugs 2005; 65:1097–1112

120. American Academy of Pediatrics. *Haemophilus influenzae* infections. In: Pickering LK, editor. *Red Book: 2003 Report of the Committee on Infectious Diseases*, 26th edn. Elk Grove Village, IL: American Academy of Pediatrics; 2003, 293–301

121. Prymula R, Peeters P, Chrobok V, et al. Pneumococcal capsular polysaccharides conjugated to protein D for prevention of acute otitis media caused by both *Streptococcus pneumoniae* and nontypable *Haemophilus influenzae*: a randomised double-blind efficacy study. Lancet 2006; 367:740–748

Chapter 54
Enterobacteriaceae

David L. Paterson

1 Overview of Resistance Trends

Approximately 50% of *Escherichia coli* isolates are resistant to ampicillin (1). This resistance is mediated by narrow-spectrum β-lactamases such as TEM-1 (2). The addition of β-lactamase inhibitors, such as clavulanic acid, can protect penicillins from hydrolysis from TEM-1. Thus, rates of resistance of *E. coli* to amoxicillin/clavulanate are only approximately 5% (2, 3). When all Enterobacteriaceae are considered, almost one-quarter of isolates are resistant to amoxicillin/clavulanate (3). This is likely due to production of β-lactamases, by organisms such as *Enterobacter cloacae*, that are not inhibited by commonly used β-lactamase inhibitors.

The third-generation cephalosporins were developed, in part, because of the advent of narrow-spectrum β-lactamases such as TEM-1. In the United States, the Centers for Disease Control and Prevention coordinate the National Nosocomial Infections Surveillance (NNIS) System. As of the time of writing (January 2008), the most recent report by NNIS or the National Healthcare Safety Network (NHSN) comprised the 2003 data. In 2003, 20.6% of all *K. pneumoniae* isolates from patients in intensive-care units (ICUs) in the United States were nonsusceptible to third-generation cephalosporins (4). This represented a 47% increase compared to resistance rates for 1998–2002. Nonsusceptibility to third-generation cephalosporins was also observed in 31.1% of *Enterobacter* species and 5.8% of *E. coli* isolated from patients in ICUs that year. Those rates were approximately the same as for 1998–2002. International studies report even higher rates of nonsusceptible *K. pneumoniae* in hospitals and particularly in ICU settings (5).

Neither NNIS nor NHSN has provided data on resistance of the Enterobacteriaceae to antibiotic classes other than third-generation cephalosporins. In a recently published report describing susceptibility of more than 20,000 *E. coli* isolates from a variety of medical centers in North America, Latin America, and Europe from 1999 to 2004, 5% of isolates had an ESBL phenotype. Resistance rates to non-β-lactam antibiotics were 12.5% for ciprofloxacin, 24.4% for trimethoprim/sulfamethoxazole, and 5.8% for gentamicin (3). Undoubtedly, there are geographic differences in these rates of resistance. Different populations within certain areas are also likely to have different rates of resistance. For example, in a study of bacterial isolates from women in Spain with uncomplicated cystitis, women greater than 65 years of age had a 29% rate of *E. coli* resistance to ciprofloxacin, while younger women had a rate of ciprofloxacin resistance of just 13% (6).

Across the various species of Enterobacteriaceae, approximately 10% of isolates are resistant to ciprofloxacin (3). On the basis of previous trends, however, these rates are likely to rise. Rates are highest in indole-positive Proteae (18.3% resistant), *P. mirabilis* (13.9% resistant), *E. coli* (12.5% resistant), and *E. aerogenes* (12.5% resistant). Interestingly, rates of ciprofloxacin resistance in *Salmonella* spp. are just 0.1% (3). However, approximately 10% of *Salmonella* strains are nalidixic-acid resistant (7). Among nalidixic-acid-resistant *Salmonella* isolates, ciprofloxacin MICs are 8- to 32-fold higher than "wild-type" strains, despite the ciprofloxacin MIC not entering the resistant range (7). An increased failure rate is observed when ciprofloxacin is used to treat infections with nalidixic-acid-resistant Salmonella (8).

Rates of aminoglycoside resistance worldwide in Enterobacteriaceae are approximately 8% (3). Rates of gentamicin resistance are highest in *K. pneumoniae* (14.6% resistant), most likely reflecting presence of genes encoding aminoglycoside-modifying enzymes on plasmids harboring genes encoding ESBLs. Methylation of 16S ribosomal RNA is emerging as a mechanism of resistance of Enterobacteriaceae to the aminoglycosides (9). However, this mechanism likely accounts for just a small percentage of aminoglycoside-resistant isolates at the present time. Methylation of 16S ribosomal RNA leads to resistance not just to gentamicin and tobramycin but also to amikacin (9).

D.L. Paterson (✉)
Professor of Medicine, University of Queensland,
Centre for Clinical Research, Royal Brisbane
and Women's Hospital, Brisbane, QLD, Australia
david.antibiotics@gmail.com

D.L. Mayers (ed.), *Antimicrobial Drug Resistance*,
DOI 10.1007/978-1-60327-595-8_54, © Humana Press, a part of Springer Science+Business Media, LLC 2009

Least commonly, the Enterobacteriaceae are resistant to carbapenems. In most hospitals, fewer than 5% of isolates of the Enterobacteriaceae are resistant to carbapenem. However, in recent years, there have been pockets of increased resistance to this antibiotic class (10, 11). Acquired resistance to tigecycline and polymyxins is extremely uncommon. However, some species (for example, *Proteus* spp. in the case of tigecycline) may be intrinsically resistant (12, 13).

2 ESBL-Producing Enterobacteriaceae

2.1 General Issues and Nomenclature

Infections caused by ESBL-producing Enterobacteriaceae are of serious concern in the current environment. Some ESBLs represent enzymes that have evolved from narrow-spectrum β-lactamases such as TEM-1, TEM-2, and SHV-1. The CTX-M type ESBLs appear to be derived from chromosomally encoded β-lactamases produced by *Kluyvera* spp (2). ESBLs can hydrolyze most cephalosporins and penicillins. However, ESBLs are typically not active against cephamycins (e.g., cefotetan, cefoxitin, or cefmetazole) or carbapenems (doripenem, imipenem, ertapenem, and meropenem) and can generally be inhibited by β-lactamase inhibitors, such as clavulanate, sulbactam, or tazobactam. Unlike most ESBLs that have been found in *E. coli*, *K. pneumoniae*, and other Enterobacteriaceae, OXA-type ESBLs have been found mainly in *Pseudomonas aeruginosa* and only rarely in Enterobacteriaceae (14).

ESBLs should be distinguished from other β-lactamases capable of hydrolyzing extended-spectrum cephalosporins and penicillins. Examples include AmpC-type β-lactamases and carbapenemases. Carbapenemases may be further grouped as either metallo-β-lactamases (class B) or serine carbapenemases (classes A and D). Like ESBLs, AmpC β-lactamases hydrolyze third-generation or expanded-spectrum cephalosporins, but unlike ESBLs, they are also active against cephamycins and are resistant to inhibition by clavulanate or other β-lactamase inhibitors (15, 16). Carbapenemases have broader-range activity, inactivating carbapenems as well as expanded-spectrum cephalosporins (15, 17).

2.2 In Vitro Susceptibility Profiles and Clinical Outcomes

Rates of resistance of ESBL-producing Enterobacteriaceae to the cephalosporins can be misleading. In general, a much greater proportion of Enterobacteriaceae are genotypically defined as ESBL producers than would be suggested by examining resistance rates to third-generation cephalosporins defined by Clinical and Laboratory Standards Institute (CLSI) criteria (18). This has clinical relevance. In a study of patients with ESBL-producing *K. pneumoniae* bacteremia, 54% of patients receiving treatment with a susceptible cephalosporin, as determined by CLSI criteria, experienced clinical failure (18). These results are consistent with those from a variety of observational studies, which show rates of clinical failure of >90%, approximately 67%, and <30% with cephalosporin minimal inhibitory concentrations (MICs) of 8, 4, and ≤2 μg/mL, respectively, when third-generation cephalosporins are used to treat ESBL producers (19, 20). The 2007 CLSI guidelines recommend that laboratories report ESBL-producing isolates as resistant to all penicillins, cephalosporins, and aztreonam irrespective of the in vitro tests results (21).

2.3 Treatment of ESBL Producers

The presence of ESBL-producing Enterobacteriaceae complicates therapy, especially since these organisms are often multidrug resistant. When isolates from a patient indicate an ESBL-producing organism, the first thing to consider is whether the patient has a true infection versus colonization. Patients with positive isolates from urine or perhaps the respiratory tract may be only colonized, and, clearly, there is no indication for treatment in those situations. Assuming the patient has a serious infection due to ESBL-producing Enterobacteriaceae, the choice of empiric therapy is made difficult by the likelihood of multidrug resistance and the fact that there are no data from large, randomized, controlled trials designed to compare one antibiotic therapy with another for infections caused by ESBL-producing organisms. Moreover, for a variety of reasons, it is unlikely that such a study will ever be performed. Nonetheless, data from a number of studies strongly point to carbapenems as the drugs of choice for empiric treatment of serious infections involving ESBL-producing Enterobacteriaceae.

Subgroup analysis from a randomized, evaluator-blind trial comparing cefepime with imipenem in patients with nosocomial pneumonia showed that 100% of patients (10 out of 10) receiving imipenem for pneumonia caused by an ESBL producer experienced a positive clinical response compared with only 69% of patients (9 out of 13) treated with cefepime (22). Similarly, a prospective, observational, international study of patients with *K. pneumonia* bacteremia reported an all-cause 14-day mortality rate of 3.7% (1 out of 27) with use of a carbapenem alone, compared with rates of 36.3% and 44.% with quinolone and non-carbapenem β-lactam monotherapy, respectively (20). For patients infected with ESBL-producing *K. pneumoniae*, the corresponding 14-day mortality rates were 4.8% (2 out of 42) among patients receiving carbapenem monotherapy or combination therapy and 27.6% (8 out of 29) among those receiving treatment with a non-carbapenem antibiotic.

While TEM- and SHV-type ESBLs do not effectively hydrolyze cephamycins (such as cefoxitin or cefotetan), Enterobacteriaceae may exhibit resistance to those agents because of plasmid-mediated expression (23) or overexpression (24) of AmpC β-lactamases. Additionally, resistance to β-lactam/β-lactamase inhibitor combinations (such as piperacillin/tazobactam) may occur owing to the coexistence of AmpC-type β-lactamases and ESBLs. The development of porin-deficient mutants may also contribute to resistance to cephamycins and β-lactam/β-lactamase inhibitor combinations (25). Such occurrences are not infrequent and argue against the use of cephamycins or β-lactamase/β-lactamase inhibitor combinations in patients with serious infections due to ESBL-producing Enterobacteriaceae. As mentioned earlier, the CLSI recommends that isolates found to be ESBL producing be considered resistant to all penicillins, all cephalosporins, and aztreonam.

Similarly, quinolones, aminoglycosides, and trimethoprim–sulfamethoxazole (TMP/SMX) are generally not appropriate initial therapeutic choices for serious infections caused by ESBL-producing Enterobacteriaceae because ESBL producers are often resistant to these drugs as well (26–28). Moreover, multidrug resistance among ESBL-producing *K. pneumoniae* and *E. coli* species appears to be increasing (28). With quinolones, even in the presence of apparent susceptibility, there may be a substantial failure rate. In the international study discussed earlier, 36.4% of patients who received treatment with a quinolone for bacteria caused by ESBL-producing *K. pneumoniae* died within 14 days (20). Quinolone resistance in Enterobacteriaceae is described in greater detail below.

2.4 Community-Acquired ESBLs

ESBL-producing Enterobacteriaceae are prevalent in the hospital setting, and there is now evidence that they are emerging and spreading in the community as well (29). Most cases of ESBL-producing organisms in the community have been reported internationally, although reports from the United States are emerging (30). Most commonly, the cases of community-acquired ESBL producers involve urinary tract infections (UTIs), although gastrointestinal infections in the community may also be important. A population-based laboratory surveillance study of ESBL-producing *E. coli* infections in the Calgary Health Region of Canada reported

that 71% of patients had community-onset disease (31). The study did not address whether the ESBL-producing *E. coli* were necessarily acquired in the community, but the data do speak to the high prevalence of infections associated with ESBL-producing species in the community (29). The most common ESBL type in *E. coli* isolated from patients with community-onset infections are of the CTX-M type (30, 31). This contrasts with the general preponderance of TEM- and SHV-type ESBLs in isolates from hospitalized patients with *K. pneumoniae* or *E. coli* infections both in the United States and worldwide.

The typical clinical picture for community-associated infection involving ESBLs is UTI (sometimes associated with bacteremia) due to CTX-M-producing *E. coli*, with elderly women being most commonly affected. Isolates are resistant to typical first-line agents for UTI, such as ciprofloxacin, TMP/SMX, gentamicin, and ceftriaxone. So there is now the very real risk that treatment of community-acquired infections with *E. coli* may be compromised because of multidrug resistance. Data for January 1998 through June 2004 from the US-based Intensive Care Antimicrobial Resistance Epidemiology (ICARE) project indicated that only 0.6% of *E. coli* isolates and 1.8% of *K. pneumoniae* isolates from so-called outpatient areas were nonsusceptible to third-generation cephalosporins (4). At present, the existence of community-associated ESBL-producing Enterobacteriaceae appears to be very limited in the United States. Nonetheless, the healthcare community needs to be aware of the potential problem that community-acquired ESBL producers may present in the United States in the future, especially given what has been observed in the United Kingdom and Canada.

ESBL-producing pathogens may also be involved in gastrointestinal infections acquired in the community. Bacterial species that have been reported to produce ESBLs leading to drug-resistant gastroenteritis include *Salmonella* species, *Shigella*, and Shiga toxin-producing *E. coli* (32–38). The possible emergence and spread of *Salmonella* strains resistant to antibiotics commonly used as treatment are of concern because those infections can be invasive. Outside the United States, TEM-, SHV-, and CTX-M-type ESBLs, as well as AmpC β-lactamases, have been identified in infection-causing *Salmonella* (32, 33, 39). Within the United States, the mechanism of *Salmonella* resistance to third-generation cephalosporins has been linked to production of AmpC β-lactamases (40–42). In particular, resistance has been associated with the plasmid-mediated AmpC β-lactamase known as CMY-2. *Salmonella* strains resistant to third-generation cephalosporins are of concern because (1) ceftriaxone and, secondarily, quinolones are the drugs of choice for invasive salmonella disease and (2) quinolones are not indicated for use in children. Fortunately, ceftriaxone-resistant *Salmonella* are currently rare in the

United States, but they represent an area that bears further watching.

3 Antibiotic Resistance in *Enterobacter* Species

Enterobacter species are significant causes of nosocomial infection and are intrinsically resistant to aminopenicillins, cefazolin, and cefoxitin owing to production of constitutive chromosomal AmpC β-lactamases (43). Moreover, β-lactam exposure is capable of inducing expression of AmpC *beta*-lactamases in *Enterobacter* species – with consequent resistance to third-generation cephalosporins. Furthermore, mutations can result in permanent hyperproduction and persistent resistance. Treatment of *Enterobacter* infections with third-generation cephalosporins may select for mutant strains associated with hyperproduction of AmpC β-lactamase. The prevalence of *Enterobacter* species resistant to third-generation cephalosporins has increased since the introduction and common use of these antibiotics. For example, in one study, resistance to third-generation cephalosporins emerged in approximately 20% of patients during treatment for *Enterobacter* bacteremia (44). Multidrug-resistant *Enterobacter* species in initial positive blood cultures were significantly more prevalent (*P* <0.001) among patients who had previously received third-generation cephalosporins than among patients who had previously received other antibiotic treatments, and they were associated with higher mortality rates (44).

Third-generation cephalosporins should be avoided as treatment for serious infection with *Enterobacter* species because their use in such situations results in selection of derepressed mutants which hyperproduce AmpC. In contrast, cefepime is comparatively stable to AmpC β-lactamases and therefore has been regarded as a suitable option for treatment of *Enterobacter* infections (43). However, ESBL-producing *Enterobacter* species, particularly *E. cloacae*, have been identified in the United States (45–47), Europe (48), and Asia (49–51). SHV-type ESBLs may have elevated cefepime MICs and compromise the activity of the antibiotic (52).

4 Emerging Quinolone and Carbapenem Resistance

4.1 Quinolone Resistance

Quinolones are used widely for the treatment of serious *E. coli* UTIs and may also be used to treat other infections caused by other members of the Enterobacteriaceae family

(53, 54). Hence, quinolone resistance in Enterobacteriaceae may lead to treatment failures and is a significant concern, as is the recent emergence of plasmid-mediated resistance to quinolones. According to the 2004 NNIS report, means of 7.3% and 8.2% of *E. coli* isolates from U.S. patients in both ICUs and non-ICU areas of hospitals, respectively, and a mean of 3.6% from U.S. outpatients exhibited quinolone resistance (4). Higher rates of quinolone resistance may be found in ESBL-producing strains of *E. coli* and *K. pneumoniae*. For example, 55.8% of infections in the University of Pennsylvania Health System caused by ESBL-producing *E. coli* or *K. pneumoniae* were fluoroquinolone resistant (26). In Shanghai, China, 86.1% of ESBL-producing *E. coli* and 45.6% of ESBL-producing *K. pneumoniae* were reported to be resistant to levofloxacin (55). Prior receipt of a quinolone has been shown to be an independent risk factor for quinolone resistance (26).

Quinolone resistance in Enterobacteriaceae is usually due to alterations in target enzymes (DNA gyrase and/ or topoisomerase IV) or to impaired access to the target enzymes, occurring either because of changes in porin expression or because of efflux mechanisms (56). Both these principal means of resistance are caused by chromosomal mutations. More recently, plasmid-mediated quinolone resistance has emerged in *K. pneumoniae* and *E. coli*. The first case of plasmid-mediated resistance to quinolones in *K. pneumoniae* was reported in the United States in 1998 and was from a strain isolated at the University of Alabama in 1994 (57). The plasmid, pMG252, confers multidrug resistance and was shown to greatly increase quinolone resistance when transferred to strains of *K. pneumoniae* deficient in outer-membrane porins. The gene associated with that resistance has been designated *qnr*. Quinolone resistance associated with *qnr*-containing plasmids has now emerged in *E. coli* and *K. pneumoniae* strains (58–60). A recent study in the United States reported that 11.1% of *K. pneumoniae* strains from six states exhibited plasmid-mediated quinolone resistance associated with the *qnr* gene, although none of the *E. coli* strains examined contained *qnr* (61). Some of the strains contained the original pMG252 plasmid, but *qnr* was carried on different plasmids for others. The mechanism of quinolone resistance associated with *qnr*-containing plasmids appears to involve inhibition of quinolone binding with DNA gyrase (62). Another mechanism of quinolone resistance in Enterobacteriaceae is encoded by a variant of the gene encoding the aminoglycoside acetyltransferase AAC(6′)-lb (63).

The emergence of this new plasmid-mediated mechanism of quinolone resistance is particularly worrisome because it provides a mechanism for the rapid development and spread of quinolone and multidrug resistance to important members of the Enterobacteriaceae family.

4.2 Carbapenem Resistance

As mentioned earlier, carbapenems are currently considered to be the preferred agents for treatment of serious infections caused by ESBL-producing Enterobacteriaceae. Carbapenems are highly stable to β-lactamase hydrolysis, and porin penetration is facilitated by their general size and structure. Their susceptibility for most strains of Enterobacteriaceae makes them generally useful as treatment for multidrug-resistant organisms. Carbapenem resistance is currently rare among Enterobacteriaceae, but some worrisome signs have appeared in recent years.

The expression of AmpC or class A (TEM or SHV type) ESBLs plus loss of outer-membrane proteins has been associated with carbapenem resistance in *K. pneumoniae* (64–69). Resistance to carbapenems has also been reported in *K. pneumoniae* producing class B β-lactamases (metallo-β-lactamases) in various countries, including Brazil (70), Greece (71), China (72), and Singapore (73). A metallo-β-lactamase-producing strain of *E. cloacae* with reduced susceptibility to carbapenems has been observed in Greece (74). Standard susceptibility testing may categorize metallo-β-lactamase-producing Enterobacteriaceae as susceptible to carbapenems, but an inoculum effect has been observed, suggesting that the susceptibility testing may falsely predict the susceptibility of particular Enterobacteriaceae to carbapenems in the clinical environment (74, 75).

In the United States, carbapenem resistance has been observed in strains of *K. pneumoniae*–producing class A carbapenemases – KPC-1, KPC-2, or KPC-3 (10, 76–82). These enzymes are apparently obtained via plasmid conjugation and are capable of hydrolyzing and inactivating the carbapenems. KPC-producing strains have generally been shown to exhibit multidrug resistance that includes piperacillin/tazobactam, third- and fourth-generation cephalosporins, fluoroquinolones, and aminoglycosides, as well as carbapenems (82). KPC-1 expression itself was apparently associated with moderate- to high-level carbapenem resistance (76), while loss of outer-membrane proteins appeared to be a required cofactor for high-level resistance in KPC-2- and KPC-3-producing strains (77, 79). In 96 isolates obtained from ten New York hospitals, more than 80% of the KPC-producing organisms belonged to a single ribotype (82). This is worrisome because it suggests that these isolates are not being selected by antibiotic use but, rather, are being passed from person to person as a result of breakdown in infection control. As with metallo-β-lactamase-producing Enterobacteriaceae, susceptibility testing may falsely indicate the clinical susceptibility of KPC-producing *K. pneumoniae* due to an inoculum effect (10, 80, 81). In vitro testing suggests that tigecycline and polymyxins may exhibit the most consistent activity against KPC-producing strains of *K. pneumoniae*, but this has yet to be demonstrated clinically (82). KPC-producing strains of

Enterobacter (81) and *Salmonella* species (83) have also been identified in the United States.

Hence, strains of clinically important *Enterobacteriaceae* have now emerged with broader multidrug resistance than has ever before been observed. As the list of antibiotics with potential activity against those strains continues to shrink, measures that prevent and slow the spread of multidrug-resistant *Enterobacteriaceae* strains throughout the world need to be put in action.

5 Conclusions

Enterobacteriaceae are significant causes of serious infections, and many of the most important members of this family are becoming increasingly resistant to currently available antibiotics. It is a troubling trend and one that requires vigilance and intensified measures to control the further spread of resistance by these important Gram-negative pathogens. It should be emphasized that improvements in infection control and antibiotic management are necessary if the steady rise in ESBL-producing Enterobacteriaceae and in other forms of resistance in these species is to be slowed or stopped. The widespread use of third-generation cephalosporins as the driving force behind the emergence of ESBL-producing organisms has been shown in many studies. Quinolones seem to have replaced third-generation cephalosporins as "workhorse therapy" in some hospitals, yet their overuse, particularly in light of plasmid-mediated quinolone resistance in Enterobacteriaceae, may be of concern.

Infection control is a key aspect in restriction of the emergence and spread of resistant Enterobacteriaceae. With regard to ESBL and KPC producers, there is ample evidence of person-to-person spread. Combining reductions in third-generation cephalosporin use with traditional infection control measures – such as the use of gloves, gowns, and hand hygiene in the care of colonized or infected patients – has been reported to control the hospital spread of multidrug-resistant *K. pneumoniae*. What is not yet well elucidated is the relationship between antibiotic-resistant Enterobacteriaceae in farm animals and resistance in humans. This is an important area to be explored in the next decade.

References

1. Gobernado M, Valdes L, Alos JI, Garcia-Rey C, Dal-Re R, Garcia-de-Lomas J. Antimicrobial susceptibility of clinical *Escherichia coli* isolates from uncomplicated cystitis in women over a 1-year period in Spain. Rev Esp Quimioter 2007;20:68–76
2. Paterson DL, Bonomo RA. Extended-spectrum beta-lactamases: a clinical update. Clin Microbiol Rev 2005;18:657–686
3. Sader HS, Fritsche TR, Jones RN. In vitro activity of garenoxacin tested against a worldwide collection of ciprofloxacin-susceptible

and ciprofloxacin-resistant Enterobacteriaceae strains (1999–2004). Diagn Microbiol Infect Dis 2007;58:27–32

4. National Nosocomial Infections Surveillance (NNIS) System Report, data summary from January 1992 through June 2004, issued October 2004. Am J Infect Control 2004;32:470–485

5. Paterson DL, Ko WC, Von Gottberg A, et al. International prospective study of *Klebsiella pneumoniae* bacteremia: implications of extended-spectrum beta-lactamase production in nosocomial Infections. Ann Intern Med 2004;140:26–32

6. Gobernado M, Valdes L, Alos JI, Garcia-Rey C, Dal-Re R, Garcia-de-Lomas J. Quinolone resistance in female outpatient urinary tract isolates of Escherichia coli: age-related differences. Rev Esp Quimioter 2007;20:206–210

7. Biedenbach DJ, Toleman M, Walsh TR, Jones RN. Analysis of *Salmonella* spp. with resistance to extended-spectrum cephalosporins and fluoroquinolones isolated in North America and Latin America: report from the SENTRY Antimicrobial Surveillance Program (1997–2004). Diagn Microbiol Infect Dis 2006; 54:13–21

8. Crump JA, Barrett TJ, Nelson JT, Angulo FJ. Reevaluating fluoroquinolone breakpoints for *Salmonella enterica* serotype Typhi and for non-Typhi salmonellae. Clin Infect Dis 2003;37:75–81

9. Doi Y, Arakawa Y. 16S ribosomal RNA methylation: emerging resistance mechanism against aminoglycosides. Clin Infect Dis 2007;45:88–94

10. Bratu S, Mooty M, Nichani S, et al. Emergence of KPC-possessing *Klebsiella pneumoniae* in Brooklyn, New York: epidemiology and recommendations for detection. Antimicrob Agents Chemother 2005;49:3018–3020

11. Nordmann P, Poirel L. Emerging carbapenemases in Gram-negative aerobes. Clin Microbiol Infect 2002;8:321–331

12. Livermore DM. Tigecycline: what is it, and where should it be used? J Antimicrob Chemother 2005;56:611–614

13. Li J, Nation RL, Turnidge JD, et al. Colistin: the re-emerging antibiotic for multidrug-resistant Gram-negative bacterial infections. Lancet Infect Dis 2006;6:589–601

14. Bradford PA. Extended-spectrum beta-lactamases in the 21st century: characterization, epidemiology, and detection of this important resistance threat. Clin Microbiol Rev 2001;14:933–951

15. Jacoby GA, Munoz-Price LS. The new beta-lactamases. N Engl J Med 2005;352:380–391

16. Rupp ME, Fey PD. Extended spectrum beta-lactamase (ESBL)-producing Enterobacteriaceae: considerations for diagnosis, prevention and drug treatment. Drugs 2003;63:353–365

17. Walsh TR, Toleman MA, Poirel L, Nordmann P. Metallo-beta-lactamases: the quiet before the storm? Clin Microbiol Rev 2005;18:306–325

18. Paterson DL, Ko WC, Von Gottberg A, et al. Outcome of cephalosporin treatment for serious infections due to apparently susceptible organisms producing extended-spectrum beta-lactamases: implications for the clinical microbiology laboratory. J Clin Microbiol 2001;39:2206–2212

19. Wong-Beringer A, Hindler J, Loeloff M, et al. Molecular correlation for the treatment outcomes in bloodstream infections caused by *Escherichia coli* and *Klebsiella pneumoniae* with reduced susceptibility to ceftazidime. Clin Infect Dis 2002;34:135–146

20. Paterson DL, Ko WC, Von Gottberg A, et al. Antibiotic therapy for *Klebsiella pneumoniae* bacteremia: implications of production of extended-spectrum beta-lactamases. Clin Infect Dis 2004;39:31–37

21. Peleg AY, Paterson DL. Modifying antibiotic prescribing in primary care. Clin Infect Dis 2006;42:1231–1233

22. Zanetti G, Bally F, Greub G, et al. Cefepime versus imipenem-cilastatin for treatment of nosocomial pneumonia in intensive care unit patients: a multicenter, evaluator-blind, prospective, randomized study. Antimicrob Agents Chemother 2003;47: 3442–3447

23. Alvarez M, Tran JH, Chow N, Jacoby GA. Epidemiology of conjugative plasmid-mediated AmpC beta-lactamases in the United States. Antimicrob Agents Chemother 2004;48:533–537

24. Tracz DM, Boyd DA, Bryden L, et al. Increase in ampC promoter strength due to mutations and deletion of the attenuator in a clinical isolate of cefoxitin-resistant *Escherichia coli* as determined by RT-PCR. J Antimicrob Chemother 2005;55:768–772

25. Martinez-Martinez L, Hernandez-Alles S, Alberti S, Tomas JM, Benedi VJ, Jacoby GA. In vivo selection of porin-deficient mutants of *Klebsiella pneumoniae* with increased resistance to cefoxitin and expanded-spectrum-cephalosporins. Antimicrob Agents Chemother 1996;40:342–348

26. Lautenbach E, Strom BL, Bilker WB, Patel JB, Edelstein PH, Fishman NO. Epidemiological investigation of fluoroquinolone resistance in infections due to extended-spectrum beta-lactamase-producing *Escherichia coli* and *Klebsiella pneumoniae*. Clin Infect Dis 2001;33:1288–1294

27. DiPersio JR, Deshpande LM, Biedenbach DJ, Toleman MA, Walsh TR, Jones RN. Evolution and dissemination of extended-spectrum beta-lactamase-producing *Klebsiella pneumoniae*: epidemiology and molecular report from the SENTRY Antimicrobial Surveillance Program (1997–2003). Diagn Microbiol Infect Dis 2005;51:1–7

28. Hyle EP, Lipworth AD, Zaoutis TE, et al. Risk factors for increasing multidrug resistance among extended-spectrum beta-lactamase-producing *Escherichia coli* and *Klebsiella* species. Clin Infect Dis 2005;40:1317–1324

29. Pitout JD, Nordmann P, Laupland KB, Poirel L. Emergence of Enterobacteriaceae producing extended-spectrum {beta}-lactamases (ESBLs) in the community. J Antimicrob Chemother 2005

30. Rodriguez-Bano J, Paterson DL. A change in the epidemiology of infections due to extended-spectrum beta-lactamase-producing organisms. Clin Infect Dis 2006;42:935–937

31. Pitout JD, Hanson ND, Church DL, Laupland KB. Population-based laboratory surveillance for *Escherichia coli*-producing extended-spectrum beta-lactamases: importance of community isolates with blaCTX-M genes. Clin Infect Dis 2004;38: 1736–1741

32. Munday CJ, Whitehead GM, Todd NJ, Campbell M, Hawkey PM. Predominance and genetic diversity of community- and hospital-acquired CTX-M extended-spectrum beta-lactamases in York, UK. J Antimicrob Chemother 2004;54:628–633

33. Kruger T, Szabo D, Keddy KH, et al. Infections with nontyphoidal *Salmonella* species producing TEM-63 or a novel TEM enzyme, TEM-131, in South Africa. Antimicrob Agents Chemother 2004;48:4263–4270

34. Ishii Y, Kimura S, Alba J, et al. Extended-spectrum beta-lactamase-producing Shiga toxin gene (Stx1)-positive *Escherichia coli* O26:H11: a new concern. J Clin Microbiol 2005;43:1072–1075

35. Kim S, Kim J, Kang Y, Park Y, Lee B. Occurrence of extended-spectrum beta-lactamases in members of the genus *Shigella* in the Republic of Korea. J Clin Microbiol 2004;42:5264–5269

36. Petroni A, Corso A, Melano R, et al. Plasmidic extended-spectrum beta-lactamases in *Vibrio cholerae* O1 El Tor isolates in Argentina. Antimicrob Agents Chemother 2002;46:1462–1468

37. Radice M, Gonzealez C, Power P, Vidal MC, Gutkind G. Third-generation cephalosporin resistance in *Shigella sonnei*, Argentina. Emerg Infect Dis 2001;7:442–443

38. Vignoli R, Varela G, Mota MI, et al. Enteropathogenic *Escherichia coli* strains carrying genes encoding the PER-2 and TEM-116 extended-spectrum beta-lactamases isolated from children with diarrhea in Uruguay. J Clin Microbiol 2005;43:2940–2943

39. Li WC, Huang FY, Liu CP, et al. Ceftriaxone resistance of nontyphoidal *Salmonella enterica* isolates in Northern Taiwan attributable

to production of CTX-M-14 and CMY-2 {beta}-lactamases. J Clin Microbiol 2005;43:3237–3243

40. Carattoli A, Tosini F, Giles WP, et al. Characterization of plasmids carrying CMY-2 from expanded-spectrum cephalosporin-resistant *Salmonella* strains isolated in the United States between 1996 and 1998. Antimicrob Agents Chemother 2002;46: 1269–1272

41. Dunne EF, Fey PD, Kludt P, et al. Emergence of domestically acquired ceftriaxone-resistant *Salmonella* infections associated with AmpC beta-lactamase. JAMA 2000;284:3151–3156

42. Fey PD, Safranek TJ, Rupp ME, et al. Ceftriaxone-resistant salmonella infection acquired by a child from cattle. N Engl J Med 2000;342:1242–1249

43. Bouza E, Cercenado E. *Klebsiella* and *Enterobacter*: antibiotic resistance and treatment implications. Semin Respir Infect 2002;17:215–230

44. Chow JW, Fine MJ, Shlaes DM, et al. Enterobacter bacteremia: clinical features and emergence of antibiotic resistance during therapy. Ann Intern Med 1991;115:585–590

45. Levison ME, Mailapur YV, Pradhan SK, et al. Regional occurrence of plasmid-mediated SHV-7, an extended-spectrum beta-lactamase, in *Enterobacter cloacae* in Philadelphia Teaching Hospitals. Clin Infect Dis 2002;35:1551–1554

46. Sanders CC, Ehrhardt AF, Moland ES, Thomson KS, Zimmer B, Roe DE. BetalasEN: microdilution panel for identifying beta-lactamases present in isolates of Enterobacteriaccae. J Clin Microbiol 2002;40:123–127

47. D'Agata E, Venkataraman L, DeGirolami P, Weigel L, Samore M, Tenover F. The molecular and clinical epidemiology of enterobacteriaceae-producing extended-spectrum beta-lactamase in a tertiary care hospital. J Infect 1998;36:279–285

48. Tzelepi E, Giakkoupi P, Sofianou D, Loukova V, Kemeroglou A, Tsakris A. Detection of extended-spectrum beta-lactamases in clinical isolates of *Enterobacter cloacae* and *Enterobacter aerogenes*. J Clin Microbiol 2000;38:542–546

49. Park YJ, Park SY, Oh EJ, et al. Occurrence of extended-spectrum beta-lactamases among chromosomal AmpC-producing *Enterobacter cloacae*, *Citrobacter freundii*, and *Serratia marcescens* in Korea and investigation of screening criteria. Diagn Microbiol Infect Dis 2005;51:265–269

50. Jiang X, Ni Y, Jiang Y, et al. Outbreak of infection caused by *Enterobacter cloacae* producing the novel VEB-3 beta-lactamase in China. J Clin Microbiol 2005;43:826–831

51. Pai H, Hong JY, Byeon JH, Kim YK, Lee HJ. High prevalence of extended-spectrum beta-lactamase-producing strains among blood isolates of *Enterobacter* spp. collected in a tertiary hospital during an 8-year period and their antimicrobial susceptibility patterns. Antimicrob Agents Chemother 2004;48:3159–3161

52. Szabo D, Bonomo RA, Silveira F, et al. SHV-type extended-spectrum beta-lactamase production is associated with reduced cefepime susceptibility in *Enterobacter cloacae*. J Clin Microbiol 2005;43:5058–5064

53. Carson C, Naber KG. Role of fluoroquinolones in the treatment of serious bacterial urinary tract infections. Drugs 2004;64: 1359–1373

54. Hooper DC. Clinical applications of quinolones. Biochim Biophys Acta 1998;1400:45–61

55. Xiong Z, Zhu D, Wang F, Zhang Y, Okamoto R, Inoue M. Investigation of extended-spectrum beta-lactamase in *Klebsiellae pneumoniae* and *Escherichia coli* from China. Diagn Microbiol Infect Dis 2002;44:195–200

56. Hooper DC. Mechanisms of fluoroquinolone resistance. Drug Resist Updat 1999;2:38–55

57. Martinez-Martinez L, Pascual A, Jacoby GA. Quinolone resistance from a transferable plasmid. Lancet 1998;351:797–799

58. Wang M, Tran JH, Jacoby GA, Zhang Y, Wang F, Hooper DC. Plasmid-mediated quinolone resistance in clinical isolates of

Escherichia coli from Shanghai, China. Antimicrob Agents Chemother 2003;47:2242–2248

59. Mammeri H, Van De Loo M, Poirel L, Martinez-Martinez L, Nordmann P. Emergence of plasmid-mediated quinolone resistance in *Escherichia coli* in Europe. Antimicrob Agents Chemother 2005; 49:71–76

60. Rodriguez-Martinez JM, Pascual A, Garcia I, Martinez-Martinez L. Detection of the plasmid-mediated quinolone resistance determinant qnr among clinical isolates of *Klebsiella pneumoniae* producing AmpC-type beta-lactamase. J Antimicrob Chemother 2003;52:703–706

61. Wang M, Sahm DF, Jacoby GA, Hooper DC. Emerging plasmid-mediated quinolone resistance associated with the qnr gene in *Klebsiella pneumoniae* clinical isolates in the United States. Antimicrob Agents Chemother 2004;48:1295–1299

62. Tran JH, Jacoby GA. Mechanism of plasmid-mediated quinolone resistance. Proc Natl Acad Sci U S A 2002;99:5638–5642

63. Robicsek A, Strahilevitz J, Jacoby GA, et al. Fluoroquinolone-modifying enzyme: a new adaptation of a common aminoglycoside acetyltransferase. Nat Med 2006;12:83–88

64. Bornet C, Davin-Regli A, Bosi C, Pages JM, Bollet C. Imipenem resistance of enterobacter acrogenes mediated by outer membrane permeability. J Clin Microbiol 2000;38:1048–1052

65. de Champs C, Henquell C, Guelon D, Sirot D, Gazuy N, Sirot J. Clinical and bacteriological study of nosocomial infections due to *Enterobacter aerogenes* resistant to imipenem. J Clin Microbiol 1993;31:123–127

66. Chow JW, Shlaes DM. Imipenem resistance associated with the loss of a 40 kDa outer membrane protein in *Enterobacter aerogenes*. J Antimicrob Chemother 1991;28:499–504

67. Poirel L, Heritier C, Tolun V, Nordmann P. Emergence of oxacillinase-mediated resistance to imipenem in *Klebsiella pneumoniae*. Antimicrob Agents Chemother 2004;48:15–22

68. Martinez-Martinez L, Pascual A, Hernandez-Alles S, et al. Roles of beta-lactamases and porins in activities of carbapenems and cephalosporins against *Klebsiella pneumoniae*. Antimicrob Agents Chemother 1999;43:1669–1673

69. Bradford PA, Urban C, Mariano N, Projan SJ, Rahal JJ, Bush K. Imipenem resistance in *Klebsiella pneumoniae* is associated with the combination of ACT-1, a plasmid-mediated AmpC beta-lactamase, and the foss of an outer membrane protein. Antimicrob Agents Chemother 1997;41:563–569

70. Lincopan N, McCulloch JA, Reinert C, Cassettari VC, Gales AC, Mamizuka EM. First isolation of metallo-beta-lactamase-producing multiresistant *Klebsiella pneumoniae* from a patient in Brazil. J Clin Microbiol 2005;43:516–519

71. Giakkoupi P, Xanthaki A, Kanelopoulou M, et al. VIM-1 Metallo-beta-lactamase-producing *Klebsiella pneumoniae* strains in Greek hospitals. J Clin Microbiol 2003;41:3893–3896

72. Yan JJ, Ko WC, Tsai SH, Wu HM, Wu JJ. Outbreak of infection with multidrug-resistant *Klebsiella pneumoniae* carrying bla(IMP-8) in a university medical center in Taiwan. J Clin Microbiol 2001;39:4433–4439

73. Koh TH, Sng LH, Babini GS, Woodford N, Livermore DM, Hall LM. Carbapenem-resistant *Klebsiella pnuemoniae* in Singapore producing IMP-1 beta-lactamase and lacking an outer membrane protein. Antimicrob Agents Chemother 2001;45: 1939–1940

74. Galani I, Souli M, Chryssouli Z, Orlandou K, Giamarellou H. Characterization of a new integron containing bla(VIM-1) and aac(6″)-IIc in an *Enterobacter cloacae* clinical isolate from Greece. J Antimicrob Chemother 2005;55:634–638

75. Giakkoupi P, Tzouvelekis LS, Daikos GL, et al. Discrepancies and interpretation problems in susceptibility testing of VIM-1-producing *Klebsiella pneumoniae* isolates. J Clin Microbiol 2005;43:494–496

76. Yigit H, Queenan AM, Anderson GJ, et al. Novel carbapenem-hydrolyzing beta-lactamase, KPC-1, from a carbapenem-resistant strain of *Klebsiella pneumoniae*. Antimicrob Agents Chemother 2001;45:1151–1161

77. Smith Moland E, Hanson ND, Herrera VL, et al. Plasmid-mediated, carbapenem-hydrolysing beta-lactamase, KPC-2, in *Klebsiella pneumoniae* isolates. J Antimicrob Chemother 2003;51: 711–714

78. Bradford PA, Bratu S, Urban C, et al. Emergence of carbapenem-resistant *Klebsiella* species possessing the class A carbapenem-hydrolyzing KPC-2 and inhibitor-resistant TEM-30 beta-lactamases in New York City. Clin Infect Dis 2004;39:55–60

79. Woodford N, Tierno PM, Jr, Young K, et al. Outbreak of *Klebsiella pneumoniae* producing a new carbapenem-hydrolyzing class A beta-lactamase, KPC-3, in a New York Medical Center. Antimicrob Agents Chemother 2004;48:4793–4799

80. Bratu S, Landman D, Haag R, et al. Rapid spread of carbapenem-resistant *Klebsiella pneumoniae* in New York City: a new threat to our antibiotic armamentarium. Arch Intern Med 2005;165: 1430–1435

81. Bratu S, Landman D, Alam M, Tolentino E, Quale J. Detection of KPC carbapenem-hydrolyzing enzymes in *Enterobacter* spp. from Brooklyn, New York. Antimicrob Agents Chemother 2005;49:776–778

82. Bratu S, Tolaney P, Karumudi U, et al. Carbapenemase-producing *Klebsiella pneumoniae* in Brooklyn, NY: molecular epidemiology and in vitro activity of polymyxin B and other agents. J Antimicrob Chemother 2005;56:128–132

83. Miriagou V, Tzouvelekis LS, Rossiter S, Tzelepi E, Angulo FJ, Whichard JM. Imipenem resistance in a *Salmonella* clinical strain due to plasmid-mediated class A carbapenemase KPC-2. Antimicrob Agents Chemother 2003;47:1297–1300

Chapter 55
Pseudomonas aeruginosa

David L. Paterson and Baek-Nam Kim

1 Microbiology

P. aeruginosa is a Gram-negative bacillus that is typically 1–3 μm in length. The organism is typically a strict aerobe. It grows on many solid media and can grow at both 37 and 42°. Most strains have a characteristic grapelike odor. It does not ferment carbohydrates. It is positive in the indophenol oxidase test, and is Simmon's citrate positive, L-arginine dehydrolase positive, L-lysine decarboxylase negative, and L-ornithine decarboxylase negative (1).

2 Habitats of *P. aeruginosa*

P. aeruginosa is typically found in moist environments and can be found in water and soil as well as on fruits, vegetables, and flowers (1). Hence, groups at high risk of serious infections with *P. aeruginosa* (for example, those who are neutropenic) are advised not to consume fruits and uncooked vegetables (2). Other examples of moist environments that can be colonized with *P. aeruginosa* include swimming pools, hot tubs, contact-lens solutions, illicit injectable drugs, and the inner soles of sneakers (1). In the hospital environment, aqueous solutions used in medical care (for example, irrigation fluids, eye drops, dialysis fluids, and even soaps and disinfectants) may also become contaminated with the organism (3). *P. aeruginosa* may also be found in the aerators and traps of sinks, in respiratory therapy equipment, on inadequately cleaned bronchoscopes (4), and on showerheads. This has potential infection control implications (Table 1).

P. aeruginosa is rarely found as part of the microbial flora of healthy individuals (2). In the rare circumstance that colonization of healthy individuals occurs, the sites of colonization include the gastrointestinal tract and moist body sites such as the throat, nasal mucosa, axillary skin, and perineum. In hospitalized patients, the most likely site of colonization is the respiratory tract. Patients with long-term urinary tract catheterization may also have urinary tract colonization. Occasionally, hospitalized patients have gastrointestinal tract colonization with *P. aeruginosa*.

3 Pulmonary Infections with *P. aeruginosa*

P. aeruginosa may cause acute pneumonia or may be a chronic colonizer of the lungs. *P. aeruginosa* is consistently identified as the most commonly isolated pathogen causing ventilator-associated pneumonia (VAP) (5). Typically, patients with VAP due to *P. aeruginosa* have had a prolonged duration of mechanical ventilation and have received antibiotics for other infections. It must be remembered that ventilated patients with *P. aeruginosa* in their respiratory secretions may merely have respiratory tract colonization. Clinical assessment (for example, by way of use of the clinical pulmonary infection score) or assessment of quantitative culture of bronchoalveolar lavage may be used to differentiate patients with true VAP from those with respiratory tract colonization (6).

The organism is increasingly recognized as an important etiology of healthcare-associated pneumonia (HCAP) (7). This entity encompasses patients presenting to hospital with pneumonia, but who (1) have come from a nursing home, rehabilitation hospital, or other long-term nursing care facility; (2) have been hospitalized in the preceding 12 months; (3) receive outpatient dialysis or infusion therapy necessitating regular visits to a hospital-based clinic; or (4) have an immunocompromised state (7). In a single-center review of patients with culture positive HCAP, *P. aeruginosa* was responsible for 25.5% of cases (7). In contrast, *P. aeruginosa* is a rare cause of true community-acquired pneumonia.

D.L. Paterson (✉)
Professor of Medicine, University of Queensland,
Centre for Clinical Research, Royal Brisbane
and Women's Hospital, Brisbane, QLD, Australia
david.antibiotics@gmail.com

D.L. Mayers (ed.), *Antimicrobial Drug Resistance*,
DOI 10.1007/978-1-60327-595-8_55, © Humana Press, a part of Springer Science+Business Media, LLC 2009

Table 1 Infection control and multiresistant *P. aeruginosa*

It should not be assumed that multiresistant *P. aeruginosa* purely arises de novo from antibiotic use

Molecular epidemiologic investigations may be useful to delineate whether strains are clonally related

Inadequately cleaned bronchoscopes and other environmental sources have been described

Patient-to-patient transmission via the hands of healthcare workers is possible

P. aeruginosa is well known as a cause of chronic infection of the lungs and airways in patients with cystic fibrosis. Patients with cystic fibrosis, an autosomal recessive genetic disorder, have chronic cough with episodes of deterioration in respiratory status. *P. aeruginosa*, along with *Staphylococcus aureus*, is responsible for most respiratory infections in patients with cystic fibrosis. Patients with bronchiectasis may also have chronic colonization with *P. aeruginosa*, punctuated by exacerbations of respiratory infection.

4 Bloodstream Infections with *P. aeruginosa*

Patients with neutropenia (typically as a result of chemotherapy) are classically regarded as at high risk of pseudomonal bacteremia. However, the proportion of neutropenic patients who develop *P. aeruginosa* bacteremia in the current era appears quite low. Others at risk of bloodstream infection with *P. aeruginosa* include those undergoing procedures or with known infections of the hepatobiliary system, those with VAP, those with extensive burns, and patients with urinary tract colonization with the organism. Patients with pseudomonal bacteremia are typically febrile and hypotensive. In some patients, distinctive skin lesions, known as ecthyma gangrenosum, occur in conjunction with *P. aeruginosa* bloodstream infection.

5 Other Serious Infections with *P. aeruginosa*

A proportion of cases of post-neurosurgical meningitis are due to *P. aeruginosa*. However, the organism is distinctly unusual as a cause of community-acquired meningitis. *P. aeruginosa* may cause a rapidly progressive keratitis, which can lead to a loss of vision in the affected eye. Occasionally, *P. aeruginosa* may cause significant bone and joint infections. This may be secondary to bacteremia. Alternatively, the organism may enter bone from infection at a contiguous site or be inoculated directly into bone (for example, from puncture wounds through the rubber soles of sneakers). *P. aeruginosa* is the classic cause of malignant otitis externa, whereby extension of ear infection occurs to cartilage of the ear, the middle ear, and eventually temporal bone. This condition is most typically seen in elderly diabetics. Finally, *P. aeruginosa* is a rare cause of infective endocarditis.

6 Less Serious Infections with *P. aeruginosa*

P. aeruginosa is the classic cause of "swimmer's ear" – otitis externa due to pseudomonal infection of moist, macerated skin of the external ear canal. The organism is also typically the cause of "whirlpool folliculitis" – folliculitis related to exposure to water colonized with *P. aeruginosa*.

7 Mechanisms of Resistance of *P. aeruginosa* to Antimicrobial Agents

P. aeruginosa is intrinsically resistant to a multitude of antibiotics presumably as a result of impermeability of the outer membrane combined with active efflux pumps (8). Thus, commonly used antibiotics such as ampicillin, ceftriaxone, cefotaxime, and tigecycline do not have clinically useful activity against the organism. Additionally, *P. aeruginosa* has a chromosomally encoded AmpC β-lactamase which, when hyperproduced is able to hydrolyze penicillins and cephalosporins (with the exception of cefepime) (9). This β-lactamase is not inhibited by β-lactamase inhibitors such as clavulanic acid. Furthermore, some antibiotics and some β-lactamase inhibitors are able to induce expression of the AmpC β-lactamase. This may have relevance in antibiotic choice for serious *P. aeruginosa* infections. Potentially, for example, clavulanate may induce production of the AmpC β-lactamase, which, in turn, may inactivate ticarcillin (10). It is noteworthy that tazobactam does not induce production of the AmpC β-lactamase, so piperacillin/tazobactam is not subject to this risk (10).

Genes encoding a broad range of β-lactamases may be acquired by *P. aeruginosa*. These include the OXA and PSE type β-lactamases. Most noteworthy, however, are the metallo-β-lactamases (MBLs). Although still quite rare in many geographic areas, these β-lactamases may confer resistance to all β-lactam antibiotics (except aztreonam) and are not inhibited by commercially available β-lactamase inhibitors. Thus, widely used antipseudomonal antibiotics such as piperacillin, ceftazidime, cefepime, imipenem, and meropenem may all be inactivated by this type of β-lactamase.

Furthermore, the genes encoding MBLs are often linked to genes encoding resistance to other antibiotic classes (11). It is important to note that MBLs have been described in the United States (12–19).

Another type of carbapenem-hydrolyzing β-lactamase is the KPC type (20). These β-lactamases, although more common in Enterobacteriaceae such as *Klebsiella pneumoniae*, have been found in *P. aeruginosa* (20). Extended-spectrum β-lactamases (ESBLs) are actually quite rare in *P. aeruginosa* (9). These β-lactamases inactivate penicillins and most cephalosporins but are inhibited by currently available β-lactamase inhibitors (21). With few exceptions, the ESBLs do not hydrolyze carbapenems. In certain geographic areas, the PER and GES β-lactamases have been produced by "outbreak" strains of *P. aeruginosa* (9).

Even with the advent of carbapenem-hydrolyzing β-lactamases (MBLs and KPC), the most common mechanism of resistance of *P. aeruginosa* to carbapenems is mutational loss of an outer-membrane protein, known as OprD or the D2 porin (22). Loss of OprD causes reduced susceptibility to both imipenem and meropenem, with the effect being substantially more pronounced with imipenem. Loss of OprD does not confer resistance to other antibiotic classes. The MexXY-OprN efflux pump system may be coregulated with OprD (23). Upregulation of the MexAB-OprM efflux pump system may lead to a decrease in meropenem susceptibility, with imipenem susceptibility usually not being affected (22). It is noteworthy that upregulated efflux pumps in *P. aeruginosa* may lead to resistance to multiple antibiotic classes, including the fluoroquinolones, penicillins, cephalosporins, and aminoglycosides.

Resistance of *P. aeruginosa* to aminoglycosides may be due to outer-membrane impermeability, upregulated efflux pumps, and enzymatic modification of the antibiotics themselves (9). Additionally, a new mechanism of resistance, 16S ribosomal RNA methylation, has been described in *P. aeruginosa* (24). This mechanism leads to high-level resistance to gentamicin, tobramycin, and amikacin (25). Resistance of *P. aeruginosa* to fluoroquinolones may also be due to outer-membrane impermeability or upregulated efflux pumps. Additionally, mutations of target enzymes for the quinolones (topoisomerases II and IV, encoded by gyrA and parC, respectively) are an important mechanism of quinolone resistance (9).

8 Epidemiology of Infections Due to Multidrug Resistant *P. aeruginosa*

Multidrug resistance in *P. aeruginosa* (resistance to more than one of the key antipseudomonal drug classes) has been variably defined. Panresistance implies resistance to *all* of the antibiotics recommended for the empiric treatment of

ventilator-associated pneumonia due to Gram-negative pathogens – cefepime, ceftazidime, imipenem, meropenem, piperacillin/tazobactam, ciprofloxacin, and levofloxacin (2). Extreme drug resistance (XDR) in *P. aeruginosa* implies resistance to all these antibiotics plus aminoglycosides and colistin/polymyxin B (26, 27). In other words, XDR strains are not susceptible to any commercially available antibiotic.

There is evidence that multidrug-resistant strains of *P. aeruginosa* appear to emerge in association with certain antibiotic choices and to have the potential for patient-to-patient spread. Carbapenem resistance emerges in approximately 25% patients with *P. aeruginosa* treated with this antibiotic class (28–32). However, typically resistance is to carbapenems only and not to multiple classes. The preponderance of data suggests that fluoroquinolones may be the class most likely to select for resistance of *P. aeruginosa* to multiple classes (33–36). A case–control study conducted in France assessed patients infected with *P. aeruginosa* isolates that were resistant to piperacillin, ceftazidime, imipenem, and ciprofloxacin and compared the antibiotic histories of these patients with patients from the same intensive care unit (ICU) who did not have *P. aeruginosa* infection and whose length of stay in ICU was at least as long as the infected patients (36). Prolonged therapy with ciprofloxacin was found to be the only risk factor for infection with multidrug-resistant *P. aeruginosa* (36). Similar findings were made in studies in Italy and Brazil (34, 37). In an assessment in New York City, hospitals with the highest rates of resistance to imipenem, fluoroquinolones, and piperacillin/tazobactam were those that had highest rates of use of fluoroquinolones (35).

Early studies of panresistance in *P. aeruginosa* showed little evidence of clonality among these strains (38). However, subsequent studies have shown that these strains can be responsible for outbreaks of infection, especially in ICUs (34, 39–41). Bratu and colleagues performed ribotyping on 195 imipenem-resistant *P. aeruginosa* isolates and found that two strains (present in at least eight hospitals in Brooklyn) accounted for 40% of all isolates (35). It is not clear whether transmission occurred via the hands of healthcare workers or from common environmental sources. Both have potential to be implicated.

8.1 Treatment of Serious Infections with *P. aeruginosa*

As mentioned earlier, the antibiotic armamentarium active against *P. aeruginosa* is intrinsically limited by virtue of the organism's impermeable outer membrane coupled with active efflux pumps. Thus, only some cephalosporins (ceftazidime and cefepime), some carbapenems (imipenem, meropenem, and doripenem), some fluoroquinolones (ciprofloxacin and levofloxacin), some penicillins (piperacillin

Table 2 Optimizing therapy against *P. aeruginosa*

Combination therapy may be needed empirically, but it has no proven role in definitive therapy
Piperacillin/tazobactam can be dosed as 4 h infusions (50)
Cefepime should be dosed at 2 g every 8 h and extended infusions considered[a] (52)
Carbapenems can be dosed as extended infusions (51)
Aminoglycosides should not be used as monotherapy, but when used can be given as large, infrequent doses[a] (56)
Ciprofloxacin can be dosed at 400 mg every 8 h[a] (55)

[a] Modifications required for patients with abnormal renal function

and ticarcillin), aminoglycosides, aztreonam, and polymyxins have potentially useful activity against *P. aeruginosa*. Acquired or mutational mechanisms of resistance have limited all these antibiotics.

There are two fundamental questions in addressing treatment of serious infections with *P. aeruginosa*. The first is whether combination therapy should be used. The second is whether dosing of individual antipseudomonal antibiotics can be optimized. These are summarized in Table 2.

8.1.1 Combination Therapy for *P. aeruginosa*

Combination therapy for serious infections with *P. aeruginosa* has long been practiced, but recent evidence questions its utility. Rationale for use of combination therapy includes in vitro synergy between certain antibiotics, prevention of emergence of resistance, and improved clinical outcome. In vitro, the susceptibility testing of combinations of antibiotics – especially, β-lactam antibiotics plus aminoglycosides – may show synergy when these combinations are used. However, in vitro synergy has never been shown conclusively to result in a clinical advantage. Furthermore, in vitro testing for synergy is fraught with difficulties in performance, standardization, and interpretation (42).

Much of the support for combination therapy emanated from a prospective observational study of 200 patients with *P. aeruginosa* bloodstream infection (43). Mortality in those patients receiving combination therapy (27%) was significantly lower than in those receiving monotherapy (47%). It should be noted that most patients receiving monotherapy received aminoglycosides; the most commonly used combinations were piperacillin or ticarcillin combined with gentamicin or tobramycin (43). Few patients received cephalosporins, aztreonam, carbapenems, or fluoroquinolones, so the relevance of this study to current practice is debatable. Furthermore, other observational studies have shown no benefit from the use of combination therapy (44, 45), and a meta-analysis of randomized controlled trials showed no benefit of combination therapy (46, 47).

Having questioned the value of routine combination therapy for *P. aeruginosa* infections, it may, however, be reasonable to use combination therapy empirically when *P. aeruginosa* is suspected. In most ICUs, fewer than 90% *P. aeruginosa* strains are susceptible to any particular antipseudomonal β-lactam. Therefore, combination therapy may be necessary empirically to ensure that empiric therapy is microbiologically adequate (that is, able to cover the vast majority of strains that a patient may potentially be infected by). How is an appropriate empiric combination chosen? Mizuta and colleagues have discussed the role of "combination antibiogram" to address this question (48). A combination antibiogram provides information on the percentage of isolates susceptible to a particular antibiotic if the isolate is resistant to a core antipseudomonal antibiotic. For example, Bhat and colleagues showed that of *P. aeruginosa* isolates resistant to cefepime in their institution 19.5% were resistant to amikacin, 100% were resistant to aztreonam, 82.9% were resistant to ciprofloxacin, 43.9% were resistant to gentamicin, 87.8% were resistant to levofloxacin, and 39.0% were resistant to tobramycin (49). Therefore, for example, combinations of cefepime and amikacin would be much more likely to improve the adequacy of initial empiric antibiotic therapy than a combination of cefepime and a fluoroquinolone.

8.1.2 Optimizing Therapy Aimed at *P. aeruginosa*

Once the decision regarding choice of antibiotic regimen has been made, it is necessary to ensure that the dose, frequency of administration, and duration of infusion are optimized. The product information of each antibiotic mentioned thus far gives some guidance as to appropriate dosage regimens. There are some exceptions to this statement: for example, dosage regimens for patients receiving continuous renal replacement are typically absent from approved product information. Furthermore, there are some lines of evidence to suggest that some adjustment of dosage regimens in patients with all degrees of renal function may optimize pharmacodynamic parameters and could potentially result in superior clinical outcome (50, 51). It should be emphasized that, at present, most of this data does not come from randomized, controlled trials.

Lodise and colleagues have examined the impact of a novel dosing regimen of piperacillin/tazobactam on outcome (50). They compared clinical outcomes of patients who received the antibiotic dosed at 3.375 g infused over 30 min every 4–6 h (conventional dosing) with those who received the antibiotic dosed at 3.375 g infused over 4 h every 8 h (extended-infusion dosing). Among patients with APACHE-2 scores of 17 or more, infected with *P. aeruginosa*, 14-day mortality was significantly lower in those treated with the extended-infusion strategy than those given conventional dosing (12.2% vs. 31.6%; $p = 0.04$). This data does not come from a randomized controlled trial but provides provocative evidence to suggest that dosing of piperacillin/tazobactam should be altered in seriously ill patients with suspected *P. aeruginosa* infections.

United States Food and Drug Administration (U.S. FDA) approved product information for cefepime suggests a range of possible doses from 0.5 g every 12 h to 2 g every 8 h. It is likely that dosing at the lower end of this range is inappropriate for patients with serious infections with organisms that may have cefepime minimal inhibitory concentrations (MICs) in the higher part of the susceptible range. *P. aeruginosa* strains may have cefepime MICs of 8 µg/mL and yet be reported by laboratories using Clinical and Laboratory Standards Institute (CLSI) breakpoints as cefepime susceptible. A recent analysis of 204 patients with bloodstream infection with Gram-negative bacteria primarily treated with cefepime showed that patients with an organism with a cefepime MIC of 8 µg/mL had a 28-day mortality rate of 56.3% compared to 24.1% for those with a cefepime MIC less than 8 µg/mL (52). Specifically with regards to the 28-day mortality in those patients with *P. aeruginosa* bloodstream infection, 66.7% (8/12) died with a cefepime MIC of 8 µg/mL compared to 20.8% (5/24 died) with a cefepime MIC of ≤4 µg/mL (52). Pharmacodynamic assessments using Monte Carlo simulation suggest that dosing regimens of 1–2 g administered over 30 min every 12 h have a low probability of "target attainment" when the cefepime MIC is 8 µg/mL (52). Again this data does not come from a randomized trial, but would suggest that cefepime should be administered empirically at 2 g every 8 h or as a prolonged infusion in order to adequately treat *P. aeruginosa* which may have cefepime MICs as high as 8 µg/mL.

The antipseudomonal carbapenems (imipenem, meropenem, and doripenem) share with antipseudomonal penicillins the pharmacodynamic characteristic that best predicts antimicrobial activity. That is, the percentage of time during the dosing interval during which the serum concentration exceeds the MIC predicts antimicrobial activity. Monte Carlo simulation predicts that extending the infusion duration of meropenem from 30 min to 3 h increases the probability of bactericidal target attainment (53, 54). In a nonrandomized assessment, Lorente and colleagues assessed outcomes of patients with ventilator-associated pneumonia given meropenem either by continuous infusion (1 g over 360 min every 6 h) or by 30-min infusions (1 g over 30 min every 6 h) (51). The group receiving meropenem by continuous infusion had a superior clinical cure rate than those receiving the 30-min infusions (90.5% cure rate vs. 59.6%, *p* <0.001). It is important to note that extended infusions of meropenem or imipenem are not approved by any regulatory agency. An extended infusion of doripenem is currently under review by the FDA.

For serious infections with *P. aeruginosa*, ciprofloxacin could potentially be dosed at 400 mg every 8 h instead of 400 mg every 12 h (28, 55). Aminoglycosides, even when in combination therapy, should be given in large, infrequent doses when aimed against *P. aeruginosa* (56). Tobramycin or gentamicin at 5–7 mg/kg/day and amikacin at 15–20 mg/kg/day are recommended. In some situations, colistin or polymyxin B needs to be used in treatment of *P. aeruginosa* infections. Unfortunately, the optimal dosage regimen of the polymyxins is unknown at the present time (57). Tigecycline has no role in the therapy of *P. aeruginosa* infections.

9 Conclusions

P. aeruginosa is likely to remain a formidable pathogen for many years to come. Unfortunately, discovery of new antibiotics with antipseudomonal activity has waned, which means that many patients are likely to have multiresistant, untreatable infections in the future. This underscores the need for strategies to prevent infections with *P. aeruginosa*, particularly those with resistance to multiple antibiotics.

References

1. Kiska DL, Gilligan PH. *Pseudomonas*. In: Murray PR, Baron EJ, Jorgensen JH, Pfaller MA and Yolken RH, eds. Manual of Clinical Microbiology, 8th ed, Vol. 1. Washington, DC: American Society for Microbiology Press, 2003:719–728
2. Paterson DL. The epidemiological profile of infections with multidrug-resistant *Pseudomonas aeruginosa* and *Acinetobacter* species. Clin Infect Dis 2006;43 Suppl 2:S43–S48
3. Morrison AJ, Jr, Wenzel RP. Epidemiology of infections due to *Pseudomonas aeruginosa*. Rev Infect Dis 1984;6 Suppl 3: S627–S642
4. Srinivasan A, Wolfenden LL, Song X, et al. An outbreak of *Pseudomonas aeruginosa* infections associated with flexible bronchoscopes. N Engl J Med 2003;348:221–227
5. Chastre J, Fagon JY. Ventilator-associated pneumonia. Am J Respir Crit Care Med 2002;165:867–903
6. Chastre J, Luyt CE, Combes A and Trouillet JL. Use of quantitative cultures and reduced duration of antibiotic regimens for patients with ventilator-associated pneumonia to decrease resistance in the intensive care unit. Clin Infect Dis 2006;43 Suppl 2:S75–S81
7. Micek ST, Kollef KE, Reichley RM, Roubinian N and Kollef MH. Health care-associated pneumonia and community-acquired pneumonia: a single-center experience. Antimicrob Agents Chemother 2007;51:3568–3573
8. Livermore DM. Of Pseudomonas, porins, pumps and carbapenems. J Antimicrob Chemother 2001;47:247–250
9. Bonomo RA, Szabo D. Mechanisms of multidrug resistance in Acinetobacter species and Pseudomonas aeruginosa. Clin Infect Dis 2006;43 Suppl 2:S49–56
10. Lister PD, Gardner VM and Sanders CC. Clavulanate induces expression of the *Pseudomonas aeruginosa* AmpC cephalosporinase at physiologically relevant concentrations and antagonizes the antibacterial activity of ticarcillin. Antimicrob Agents Chemother 1999;43:882–889
11. Doi Y, de Oliveira Garcia D, Adams J and Paterson DL. Coproduction of novel 16S rRNA methylase RmtD and

metallo-beta-lactamase SPM-1 in a panresistant *Pseudomonas aeruginosa* isolate from Brazil. Antimicrob Agents Chemother 2007;51:852–856

12. Lolans K, Queenan AM, Bush K, Sahud A and Quinn JP. First nosocomial outbreak of *Pseudomonas aeruginosa* producing an integron-borne metallo-beta-lactamase (VIM-2) in the United States. Antimicrob Agents Chemother 2005;49:3538–3540

13. Naumovski L, Quinn JP, Miyashiro D, et al. Outbreak of ceftazidime resistance due to a novel extended-spectrum beta-lactamase in isolates from cancer patients. Antimicrob Agents Chemother 1992;36:1991–1996

14. Queenan AM, Shang W, Schreckenberger P, Lolans K, Bush K and Quinn J. SME-3, a novel member of the *Serratia marcescens* SME family of carbapenem-hydrolyzing beta-lactamases. Antimicrob Agents Chemother 2006;50:3485–3487

15. Queenan AM, Torres-Viera C, Gold HS, et al. SME-type carbapenem-hydrolyzing class A beta-lactamases from geographically diverse Serratia marcescens strains. Antimicrob Agents Chemother 2000;44:3035–3039

16. Quinn JP, Miyashiro D, Sahm D, Flamm R and Bush K. Novel plasmid-mediated beta-lactamase (TEM-10) conferring selective resistance to ceftazidime and aztreonam in clinical isolates of *Klebsiella pneumoniae*. Antimicrob Agents Chemother 1989;33:1451–1456

17. Rasmussen BA, Bradford PA, Quinn JP, Wiener J, Weinstein RA and Bush K. Genetically diverse ceftazidime-resistant isolates from a single center: biochemical and genetic characterization of TEM-10 beta-lactamases encoded by different nucleotide sequences. Antimicrob Agents Chemother 1993;37:1989–1992

18. Wiener J, Quinn JP, Bradford PA, et al. Multiple antibiotic-resistant *Klebsiella* and *Escherichia coli* in nursing homes. JAMA 1999;281:517–523

19. Wong-Beringer A, Hindler J, Loeloff M, et al. Molecular correlation for the treatment outcomes in bloodstream infections caused by *Escherichia coli* and *Klebsiella pneumoniae* with reduced susceptibility to ceftazidime. Clin Infect Dis 2002;34:135–146

20. Villegas MV, Lolans K, Correa A, Kattan JN, Lopez JA and Quinn JP. First identification of *Pseudomonas aeruginosa* isolates producing a KPC-type carbapenem-hydrolyzing beta-lactamase. Antimicrob Agents Chemother 2007;51:1553–1555

21. Paterson DL, Bonomo RA. Extended-spectrum beta-lactamases: a clinical update. Clin Microbiol Rev 2005;18:657–686

22. Livermore DM. Multiple mechanisms of antimicrobial resistance in *Pseudomonas aeruginosa*: our worst nightmare? Clin Infect Dis 2002;34:634–640

23. Ochs MM, McCusker MP, Bains M and Hancock RE. Negative regulation of the *Pseudomonas aeruginosa* outer membrane porin OprD selective for imipenem and basic amino acids. Antimicrob Agents Chemother 1999;43:1085–1090

24. Doi Y, Arakawa Y. 16S ribosomal RNA methylation: emerging resistance mechanism against aminoglycosides. Clin Infect Dis 2007;45:88–94

25. Doi Y, Ghilardi AC, Adams J, de Oliveira Garcia D and Paterson DL. High prevalence of metallo-beta-lactamase and 16S rRNA methylase coproduction among imipenem-resistant *Pseudomonas aeruginosa* isolates in Brazil. Antimicrob Agents Chemother 2007;51:3388–3390

26. Paterson DL, Doi Y. A step closer to extreme drug resistance (XDR) in gram-negative bacilli. Clin Infect Dis 2007;45:1179–1181

27. Paterson DL, Lipman J. Returning to the pre-antibiotic era in the critically ill: the XDR problem. Crit Care Med 2007;35:1789–1791

28. Fink MP, Snydman DR, Niederman MS, et al. Treatment of severe pneumonia in hospitalized patients: results of a multicenter, randomized, double-blind trial comparing intravenous ciprofloxacin with imipenem–cilastatin. The Severe Pneumonia Study Group. Antimicrob Agents Chemother 1994;38:547–557

29. Carmeli Y, Troillet N, Eliopoulos GM and Samore MH. Emergence of antibiotic-resistant *Pseudomonas aeruginosa*: comparison of risks associated with different antipseudomonal agents. Antimicrob Agents Chemother 1999;43:1379–1382

30. Cometta A, Baumgartner JD, Lew D, et al. Prospective randomized comparison of imipenem monotherapy with imipenem plus netilmicin for treatment of severe infections in nonneutropenic patients. Antimicrob Agents Chemother 1994;38:1309–1313

31. Jaccard C, Troillet N, Harbarth S, et al. Prospective randomized comparison of imipenem–cilastatin and piperacillin–tazobactam in nosocomial pneumonia or peritonitis. Antimicrob Agents Chemother 1998;42:2966–2972

32. Zanetti G, Bally F, Greub G, et al. Cefepime versus imipenem–cilastatin for treatment of nosocomial pneumonia in intensive care unit patients: a multicenter, evaluator-blind, prospective, randomized study. Antimicrob Agents Chemother 2003;47:3442–3447

33. Defez C, Fabbro-Peray P, Bouziges N, et al. Risk factors for multidrug-resistant *Pseudomonas aeruginosa* nosocomial infection. J Hosp Infect 2004;57:209–216

34. Nouer SA, Nucci M, de-Oliveira MP, Pellegrino FL and Moreira BM. Risk factors for acquisition of multidrug-resistant *Pseudomonas aeruginosa* producing SPM metallo-beta-lactamase. Antimicrob Agents Chemother 2005;49:3663–3667

35. Bratu S, Quale J, Cebular S, Heddurshetti R and Landman D. Multidrug-resistant *Pseudomonas aeruginosa* in Brooklyn, New York: molecular epidemiology and in vitro activity of polymyxin B. Eur J Clin Microbiol Infect Dis 2005;24:196–201

36. Paramythiotou E, Lucet JC, Timsit JF, et al. Acquisition of multidrug-resistant *Pseudomonas aeruginosa* in patients in intensive care units: role of antibiotics with antipseudomonal activity. Clin Infect Dis 2004;38:670–677

37. Tacconelli E, Tumbarello M, Bertagnolio S, et al. Multidrug-resistant *Pseudomonas aeruginosa* bloodstream infections: analysis of trends in prevalence and epidemiology. Emerg Infect Dis 2002;8:220–221

38. Harris A, Torres-Viera C, Venkataraman L, DeGirolami P, Samore M and Carmeli Y. Epidemiology and clinical outcomes of patients with multiresistant *Pseudomonas aeruginosa*. Clin Infect Dis 1999;28:1128–1133

39. Crespo MP, Woodford N, Sinclair A, et al. Outbreak of carbapenem-resistant *Pseudomonas aeruginosa* producing VIM-8, a novel metallo-beta-lactamase, in a tertiary care center in Cali, Colombia. J Clin Microbiol 2004;42:5094–5101

40. Tsakris A, Pournaras S, Woodford N, et al. Outbreak of infections caused by *Pseudomonas aeruginosa* producing VIM-1 carbapenemase in Greece. J Clin Microbiol 2000;38:1290–1292

41. Deplano A, Denis O, Poirel L, et al. Molecular characterization of an epidemic clone of panantibiotic-resistant *Pseudomonas aeruginosa*. J Clin Microbiol 2005;43:1198–1204

42. Hsieh MH, Yu CM, Yu VL and Chow JW. Synergy assessed by checkerboard. A critical analysis. Diagn Microbiol Infect Dis 1993;16:343–349

43. Hilf M, Yu VL, Sharp J, Zuravleff JJ, Korvick JA and Muder RR. Antibiotic therapy for *Pseudomonas aeruginosa* bacteremia: outcome correlations in a prospective study of 200 patients. Am J Med 1989;87:540–546

44. Leibovici L, Paul M, Poznanski O, et al. Monotherapy versus beta-lactam-aminoglycoside combination treatment for gram-negative bacteremia: a prospective, observational study. Antimicrob Agents Chemother 1997;41:1127–1133

45. Vidal F, Mensa J, Almela M, et al. Epidemiology and outcome of *Pseudomonas aeruginosa* bacteremia, with special emphasis on the influence of antibiotic treatment. Analysis of 189 episodes. Arch Intern Med 1996;156:2121–2126

46. Paul M, Benuri-Silbiger I, Soares-Weiser K and Leibovici L. Beta lactam monotherapy versus beta lactam-aminoglycoside combination

therapy for sepsis in immunocompetent patients: systematic review and meta-analysis of randomised trials. BMJ 2004;328:668

47. Paul M, Leibovici L. Combination antibiotic therapy for *Pseudomonas aeruginosa* bacteraemia. Lancet Infect Dis 2005;5: 192–193; discussion 193–194

48. Mizuta M, Linkin DR, Nachamkin I, et al. Identification of optimal combinations for empirical dual antimicrobial therapy of *Pseudomonas aeruginosa* infection: potential role of a combination antibiogram. Infect Control Hosp Epidemiol 2006;27: 413–415

49. Bhat S, Fujitani S, Potoski BA, et al. Pseudomonas aeruginosa infections in the Intensive Care Unit: can the adequacy of empirical beta-lactam antibiotic therapy be improved? Int J Antimicrob Agents 2007;30:458–462

50. Lodise TP, Jr, Lomaestro B and Drusano GL. Piperacillin-tazobactam for *Pseudomonas aeruginosa* infection: clinical implications of an extended-infusion dosing strategy. Clin Infect Dis 2007;44:357–363

51. Lorente L, Lorenzo L, Martin MM, Jimenez A and Mora ML. Meropenem by continuous versus intermittent infusion in ventilator-associated pneumonia due to gram-negative bacilli. Ann Pharmacother 2006;40:219–223

52. Bhat SV, Peleg AY, Lodise TP, Jr, et al. Failure of current cefepime breakpoints to predict clinical outcomes of bacteremia caused by gram-negative organisms. Antimicrob Agents Chemother 2007;51:4390–4395

53. Capitano B, Nicolau DP, Potoski BA, et al. Meropenem administered as a prolonged infusion to treat serious gram-negative central nervous system infections. Pharmacotherapy 2004;24: 803–807

54. Li C, Du X, Kuti JL and Nicolau DP. Clinical pharmacodynamics of meropenem in patients with lower respiratory tract infections. Antimicrob Agents Chemother 2007;51:1725–1730

55. Yang JC, Tsuji BT and Forrest A. Optimizing use of quinolones in the critically ill. Semin Respir Crit Care Med 2007;28:586–595

56. Rea RS, Capitano B. Optimizing use of aminoglycosides in the critically ill. Semin Respir Crit Care Med 2007;28:596–603

57. Li J, Nation RL, Turnidge JD, et al. Colistin: the re-emerging antibiotic for multidrug-resistant Gram-negative bacterial infections. Lancet Infect Dis 2006;6:589–601

Chapter 56
Acinetobacter

David L. Paterson and Anton Y. Peleg

1 Overview

Acinetobacter spp. are Gram-negative coccobacilli. Like organisms such as *Pseudomonas aeruginosa* they are non-fermentative and thus can be readily differentiated by the clinical microbiology laboratory from the Enterobacteriaceae. The most important genomospecies is *Acinetobacter calcoaceticus-baumannii* complex. *Acinetobacter* spp. can actually be a normal inhabitant of the human skin (1) – and may occasionally be a contaminant of blood cultures. In a recent survey, 17% of healthy American soldiers in Texas had skin colonization with *Acinetobacter* (2). Throat carriage may occur in up to 10% of people outside hospital, especially in those with excessive alcohol consumption. It should be noted that such surveys are limited in their geographical scope (3). *Acinetobacter* nares colonization was not found in healthy U.S. soldiers (4). Typically, *Acinetobacter* spp. are considered to be nonpathogenic to healthy individuals (5). Hospitalized patients, and those with extensive healthcare contact, may have cutaneous, respiratory and gastrointestinal colonization with the organism. This patient population is also that which is at greatest risk of true infection due to the organisms.

Acinetobacter spp. are ubiquitous in the environment both outside the hospital and within it. Villegas and Hartstein have published a comprehensive review of hospital outbreaks with *Acinetobacter* spp. (6). This provides examples of locations in the hospital environment where *Acinetobacter* has been found. Examples of contaminated fluids have included ventilator tubing, suction catheters, humidifiers, distilled water, urine collection jugs, intravenous nutrition, multidose medications, potable water, moist articles of bedding and inadequately sterilized reusable arterial pressure transducers (7).

A recent example of moist site contamination associated with an outbreak of multiple resistant *Acinetobacter* spp. was that occurring during pulsatile lavage wound treatment, a high pressure irrigation treatment used to debride wounds (8). Contamination of the hospital environment with *Acinetobacter* spp. is apparently quite frequent (9), and since the organism can survive in dry conditions for a prolonged period of time (10), it is not surprising that even dry parts of the hospital environment may be potential reservoirs of infection (11). Survival on hospital bed rails for up to 9 days after the discharge of an infected patient has been described (12). Survival of *Acinetobacter* spp. on hospital computer keyboards is also possible and may be unsuspected (13).

Given the propensity for prolonged hospital contamination it is not surprising that outbreaks of hospital-acquired *Acinetobacter* infections are frequent. Compounding this is the ability for the organism to acquire genetic elements encoding mechanisms of antibiotic resistance. Although the organism is typically considered to be of low pathogenicity, it is of great importance as a cause of multiresistant infection in compromised patients such as those in intensive care units (ICUs) and burns units.

2 History of Geographical Spread

Hospital-acquired infections caused by *Acinetobacter* have now been reported worldwide (14). In a recent review of *Acinetobacter* outbreaks from 1977 to 2000, a stepwise trend in the reporting of outbreaks with increasingly resistant organisms was noted (6). Initial reports, mostly through the 1980s, focused on aminoglycoside resistance. This was soon followed by a larger number of outbreaks reporting resistance to multiple antibiotic classes (multidrug resistant), including third- and fourth-generation cephalosporins, quinolones and aminoglycosides (6). As a result, carbapenems became the agents of choice for serious *Acinetobacter* infections, inevitably leading to the most recent outbreaks involving carbapenem-resistant organisms (6, 15, 16). Some organisms

D.L. Paterson (✉)
Professor of Medicine, University of Queensland, Centre for Clinical Research, Royal Brisbane and Women's Hospital, Brisbane, QLD, Australia
david.antibiotics@gmail.com

D.L. Mayers (ed.), *Antimicrobial Drug Resistance*,
DOI 10.1007/978-1-60327-595-8_56, © Humana Press, a part of Springer Science+Business Media, LLC 2009

have become "panresistant" (17). This term implies resistance to all representatives of all of the following antibiotic classes: cephalosporins, carbapenem, beta-lactam/beta-lactamase inhibitors and fluoroquinolones. The only available options to treat such organisms are aminoglycosides (typically amikacin), tigecycline and polymyxins (colistin and polymyxin B).

Panresistant *Acinetobacter* isolates have been reported from every inhabited continent. In the United States, early reports were from New York City (18). However, these resistant pathogens have now been detected in major medical centers nationwide. In Europe, virtually all nations have been affected, with the Mediterranean countries and ICUs in the larger cities elsewhere being particularly hard hit. Although contemporaneous data is lacking, rates of panresistant *Acinetobacter* in South America, Asia and South Africa appear to be as high as any other nation in the world. Some cases of panresistant *Acinetobacter* in Australia have arisen in patients transferred from Asian ICUs, such as that which occurred in the aftermath of the Bali terrorist bombing (17).

3 Epidemiology

Infections with *Acinetobacter* spp. tend to occur most frequently in ICUs and in highly specialized units within the hospital, such as burns units. Molecular epidemiologic studies frequently show evidence of clonal outbreaks of infection. The vector for the spread of infection may be healthcare workers with poor hand hygiene. However, as noted above, the organism can persist for a prolonged period of time in the hospital environment and thus contamination from hospital equipment is quite possible.

Numerous studies have assessed antibiotic risk factors for infections with multiply resistant *Acinetobacter* spp., although few have studied risk factors for panresistance. Exposure to any antibiotic active against Gram-negative bacteria has been related to isolation of multiply resistant *Acinetobacter* organisms (19), but three classes of antibiotics have been most frequently implicated. Third-generation cephalosporin use has been implicated in numerous case-control studies (20–22). Additionally, Landman, Quale and colleagues found that an aggregate usage of cephalosporins plus aztreonam, but not other antibiotic classes, was associated with multiply resistant (including carbapenem resistant) *Acinetobacter* isolates (23). Others have found that carbapenems have been risk factors for carbapenem resistant, multiply resistant *Acinetobacter* isolates (24). Finally, fluoroquinolone use has been also associated with emergence of multiply resistant *Acinetobacter* isolates (25).

4 Clinical Significance

The growth of *Acinetobacter* spp. from clinical specimens frequently represents colonization rather than true infection. The isolation of *Acinetobacter* from respiratory specimens is a particular issue because while the organism may cause pneumonia, it may equally well represent respiratory tract colonization. Quantitative cultures of bronchoalveolar lavage may be useful in differentiating ventilator-associated pneumonia from respiratory tract colonization (26). Positive blood cultures with *Acinetobacter* from hospitalized patients usually represent true bloodstream infections, but as noted above, the organism may be a part of normal skin flora (2) and therefore may contaminate blood cultures. *Acinetobacter* is rarely a cause of intra-abdominal infections, and when doing so is usually present in mixed growth in patients with prolonged hospitalization and multiple previous operations (27). *Acinetobacter* may occasionally cause urinary tract infections or postneurosurgical meningitis (28).

5 Laboratory Diagnosis of Resistance

The *ampC Acinetobacter* derived cephalosporinase, bla_{ADC}, is present in almost all *Acinetobacter* isolates. ADC is regarded as the major intrinsic cephalosporinase of *A. baumannii* and confers resistance to ceftazidime and cefotaxime (29, 30). Some ADC-producing *Acinetobacter* isolates are susceptible to both extended spectrum cephalosporins as well as the other antibiotics tested. This susceptibility may result from a lack or diminished expression of this resistance determinant. OXA-69 is also characteristically produced by *A. baumannii* isolates although its contribution to clinically important resistance is uncertain (31). *Acinetobacter* may acquire genes encoding other beta-lactamases. The most important clinically are the carbapenemases. Typically these are OXA type beta-lactamases (such as OXA-23) and metallo-beta-lactamases (such as those of the IMP, VIM, GIM or SPM types) (32). Metallo-beta-lactamases may be suspected in carbapenem resistant isolates by using a test comparing imipenem with imipenem combined with EDTA (33). TEM-1 and occasionally ESBL-type beta-lactamases may be produced by *Acinetobacter* isolates, although their presence is usually overshadowed by other resistance mechanisms. There are no recommendations for detecting ESBLs in nonfermentative organisms such as *Acinetobacter*.

Fluoroquinolone resistance in *Acinetobacter* spp. is typically due to point mutations in the quinolone resistance determining region (QRDRs) of DNA gyrase genes. Most frequently these are point mutations at Ser83 in *gyr*A or Ser80 in *par*C leading to a change in the amino acid sequence of QRDR and therefore quinolone resistance (30). Upregulated efflux pumps may also contribute to fluoroquinolone resistance in *Acinetobacter*. Newer quinolone resistance mechanisms such as the presence of the qnr do not appear to be common in *Acinetobacter*. It is not typically easy for clinical microbiology laboratories to differentiate these mechanisms of quinolone resistance.

Aminoglycoside resistance in *Acinetobacter* spp. is typically due to the presence of aminoglycoside modifying enzymes, although the upregulated efflux pumps may also contribute. It is not certain if 16S rRNA methylases are prevalent in *Acinetobacter* spp. (34). Amikacin resistant isolates typically produce *aphA6* 3′-aminoglycoside phosphotransferase type VI enzyme (30). Mechanisms of resistance to gentamicin or tobramycin include the adenylyltransferases, such as *aadA1* and *aadB*, and the acetyltransferases such as *aacC1* and *aacC2* (30, 35).

Tigecycline susceptibility should be sought in all panresistant isolates in which the antibiotic is being considered for use. Typically MIC based methods (such as use of the E-test) are used. Tigecycline resistance in *Acinetobacter* may be due to the upregulated efflux pumps of the AdeABC type (36).

6   Treatment Alternatives

Treatment options for serious infections with *Acinetobacter* include ampicillin/sulbactam, piperacillin/tazobactam, ceftazidime, cefepime, imipenem, meropenem, tigecycline, polymyxins, fluoroquinolones and aminoglycosides. The choice of the particular agent for any given infection depends on local susceptibility patterns and an individual's allergies and renal function. A number of specific points are worthy of mention. Ampicillin/sulbactam appears to have greater activity than other beta-lactam/beta-lactamase inhibitor combinations (such as amoxicillin/clavulanate, piperacillin/tazobactam or ticarcillin/clavulanate). This is by virtue of antibacterial activity mediated by sulbactam which has high affinity for the penicillin-binding proteins of *Acinetobacter* spp. (37). With regard to carbapenems, imipenem, meropenem and doripenem have activity against *Acinetobacter* spp. whereas ertapenem lacks such activity and should not be used to treat this organism.

Tigecycline, a new, semisynthetic glycylcycline has provided hope for the treatment of infections caused by certain resistant Gram-negative organisms, including *A. baumannii*. As with other tetracycline derivatives, tigecycline inhibits the 30S ribosomal subunit, but its unique feature is its ability to evade the major determinants of tetracycline resistance, active efflux and ribosomal protection. Thus, tigecycline has a broad spectrum of in-vitro activity, including susceptible and multi-drug resistant Gram-positive and -negative organisms, as well as, anaerobes and atypical organisms. The U.S.

Food and Drug Administration (FDA) indicates that a tigecycline minimal inhibitory concentration of ≤2 μg/mL is considered susceptible for Enterobacteriaceae, but no interpretive criteria are yet available for non-fermentative bacteria such as *Acinetobacter* spp. Pharmacokinetic studies indicate that tigecycline, given in the regimen validated in clinical trials (100-mg loading dose followed by 50 mg every 12-h), achieves a mean (±SD) maximum serum steady-state concentration of 0.63 (±0.28) μg/mL in hospitalized patients (38). Others have reported similar levels (39). Serum concentrations up to 2.8 μg/mL have been described from healthy subjects after a 300 mg dose but such dosing is limited by troublesome nausea and vomiting, and greatly exceeds current recommendations. With regard to *Acinetobacter* spp., the majority of studies have demonstrated an MIC_{90} of 2 μg/mL. A study involving 12 Spanish medical centers demonstrated an MIC_{90} of 8 μg/mL from 64 *A. baumannii* isolates (40), whereas a study from the United Kingdom showed approximately 50% of isolates had an MIC of 1 μg/mL or more (41). Since *Acinetobacter* isolates may have a tigecyline MIC exceeding the peak achievable blood level, the drug should be used with great caution in treating *Acinetobacter* bloodstream infection (39). Tigecycline may have greater utility in treating pneumonia due to *Acinetobacter* spp. since the antibiotic tends to accumulate in pulmonary tissue.

Colistin (polymyxin E) and polymyxin B have been available for over 50 years. Their use was abandoned in the early 1980s as a consequence of unacceptable rates of nephrotoxicity compared to newer antimicrobial options. However, the use of polymyxins have undergone a necessary revival as a result of the dearth of agents available for treating highly resistant Gram-negative bacilli, including *Acinetobacter* (42). Unfortunately the optimal dosing regimen of colistin is unknown, because its pharmacokinetics were never studied completely when the drug was developed. This is of particular concern in seriously ill patients such as those with acute renal failure on renal replacement therapy. Nevertheless, reasonable outcomes have been reported when colistin is used for multiply resistant *Acinetobacter* infections. Furthermore, recent studies suggest that toxicity may not be as profound as was observed in the early decades of its use. A combination therapy of colistin plus rifampicin has shown favorable results in preliminary studies and may provide a more effective option for management of these challenging infections (42). Nebulized colistin has also been investigated but studies of this treatment modality are small. We would only recommend such therapy in combination with an active systemic agent. The numerous uncertainties of colistin dosing and potential usefulness in combination therapy should act as a stimulus for further research. Of concern, and in keeping with the behavior of this organism, rates of resistance to colistin have recently been reported as high as 58% in multidrug-resistant *Acinetobacter* in Israel, although a larger study of 2,621 *Acinetobacter* isolates from four major geographic regions found rates of resistance of less than 5% (43). Li and colleagues have recently demonstrated heteroresistance to colistin in an *Acinetobacter* isolate (44).

Acinetobacter isolates resistant to both tigecycline and polymyxins, as well as cephalosporins, carbapenem, beta-lactam/beta-lactamase inhibitors and fluoroquinolones, have recently been referred to as "XDR" – possessing extreme drug resistance (45). Unfortunately, there are no novel antibiotic classes in an advanced stage of clinical development in active against such strains. The specter of increasing numbers of XDR *Acinetobacter* isolates in the coming decade is therefore quite likely.

7 Infection Control Measures

Villegas and Hartstein (6) in their review of *Acinetobacter* infections clearly demonstrated the propensity for outbreaks of multiresistant infections that were to occur. Only one or two strain types were found in the majority of more than 20 outbreaks assessed which used pulsed field gel electrophoresis or PCR-based typing tests to assess clonality (6). In Brooklyn, New York City, two strain types accounted for more than 80% of carbapenem resistant isolates. Among six panresistant isolates, three separate ribotypes were identified (18). This clearly demonstrates the importance of infection control interventions in response to outbreaks of multiply resistant *Acinetobacter* infections.

The following infection control interventions are appropriate in regard to *Acinetobacter* outbreaks: (1) molecular epidemiologic investigations to determine if a clonal outbreak strain is present; (2) environmental cultures to determine if a common environmental source is present. If such a source is found it should be removed from the patient care setting; (3) enhanced isolation procedures, aimed at optimizing contact isolation. This implies improvement in hand hygiene and the usage of gloves and gowns when dealing with colonized patients or their environment; (4) antibiotic management processes to ensure that "at-risk" antibiotics are not being used excessively. A number of investigators have demonstrated that interventions such as these can be effective in the control of *Acinetobacter* infections (46).

References

1. Seifert H, Dijkshoorn L, Gerner-Smidt P, Pelzer N, Tjernberg I, Vaneechoutte M. Distribution of *Acinetobacter* species on human skin: comparison of phenotypic and genotypic identification methods. *J Clin Microbiol.* 1997;35(11):2819–2825

2. Griffith ME, Ceremuga JM, Ellis MW, Guymon CH, Hospenthal DR, Murray CK. Acinetobacter skin colonization of US Army Soldiers. *Infect Control Hosp Epidemiol.* 2006;27(7):659–661
3. Anstey NM, Currie BJ, Hassell M, Palmer D, Dwyer B, Seifert H. Community-acquired bacteremic *Acinetobacter pneumonia* in tropical Australia is caused by diverse strains of *Acinetobacter baumannii*, with carriage in the throat in at-risk groups. *J Clin Microbiol.* 2002;40(2):685–686
4. Griffith ME, Ellis MW, Murray CK. Acinetobacter nares colonization of healthy US soldiers. *Infect Control Hosp Epidemiol.* 2006;27(7):787–788
5. Schreckenberger PCea. *Acinetobacter, Achromobacter, Chryseobacterium, Moraxella* and other non-fermentative Gram negative rods. In: Murray PR, ed. *Manual of Clinical Microbiology,* 8th edn, Washington, DC: ASM Press; 2003
6. Villegas MV, Hartstein AI. Acinetobacter outbreaks, 1977–2000. *Infect Control Hosp Epidemiol.* 2003;24(4):284–295
7. Villegas MV, Kattan JN, Correa A, et al. Dissemination of *Acinetobacter baumannii* clones with OXA-23 carbapenemase in Colombian Hospitals. *Antimicrob Agents Chemother.* 2007;51(6):2001–2004
8. Maragakis LL, Cosgrove SE, Song X, et al. An outbreak of multidrug-resistant *Acinetobacter baumannii* associated with pulsatile lavage wound treatment. *JAMA.* 2004;292(24):3006–3011
9. Denton M, Wilcox MH, Parnell P, et al. Role of environmental cleaning in controlling an outbreak of *Acinetobacter baumannii* on a neurosurgical intensive care unit. *J Hosp Infect.* 2004;56(2):106–110
10. Jawad A, Seifert H, Snelling AM, Heritage J, Hawkey PM. Survival of *Acinetobacter baumannii* on dry surfaces: comparison of outbreak and sporadic isolates. *J Clin Microbiol.* 1998;36(7):1938–1941
11. Bureau-Chalot F, Drieux L, Pierrat-Solans C, Forte D, de Champs C, Bajolet O. Blood pressure cuffs as potential reservoirs of extended-spectrum beta-lactamase VEB-1-producing isolates of *Acinetobacter baumannii. J Hosp Infect.* 2004;58(1):91–92
12. Catalano M, Quelle LS, Jeric PE, Di Martino A, Maimone SM. Survival of *Acinetobacter baumannii* on bed rails during an outbreak and during sporadic cases. *J Hosp Infect.* 1999;42(1):27–35
13. Neely AN, Maley MP, Warden GD. Computer keyboards as reservoirs for *Acinetobacter baumannii* in a burn hospital. *Clin Infect Dis.* 1999;29(5):1358–1360
14. Navon-Venezia S, Ben-Ami R, Carmeli Y. Update on *Pseudomonas aeruginosa* and *Acinetobacter baumannii* infections in the healthcare setting. *Curr Opin Infect Dis.* 2005;18(4):306–313
15. Go ES, Urban C, Burns J, et al. Clinical and molecular epidemiology of acinetobacter infections sensitive only to polymyxin B and sulbactam. *Lancet.* 1994;344(8933):1329–1332
16. Peleg AY, Franklin C, Bell JM, Spelman DW. Emergence of carbapenem resistance in *Acinetobacter baumannii* recovered from blood cultures in Australia. *Infect Control Hosp Epidemiol.* 2006;27(7):759–761
17. Paterson DL. The epidemiological profile of infections with multidrug-resistant *Pseudomonas aeruginosa* and *Acinetobacter* species. *Clin Infect Dis.* 2006;43 Suppl 2:S43–S48
18. Quale J, Bratu S, Landman D, Heddurshetti R. Molecular epidemiology and mechanisms of carbapenem resistance in *Acinetobacter baumannii* endemic in New York City. *Clin Infect Dis.* 2003;37(2):214–220
19. Maslow JN, Glaze T, Adams P, Lataillade M. Concurrent outbreak of multidrug-resistant and susceptible subclones of *Acinetobacter baumannii* affecting different wards of a single hospital. *Infect Control Hosp Epidemiol.* 2005;26(1):69–75
20. Husni RN, Goldstein LS, Arroliga AC, et al. Risk factors for an outbreak of multi-drug-resistant Acinetobacter nosocomial pneumonia among intubated patients. *Chest.* 1999;115(5):1378–1382

21. Scerpella EG, Wanger AR, Armitige L, Anderlini P, Ericsson CD. Nosocomial outbreak caused by a multiresistant clone of *Acinetobacter baumannii*: results of the case-control and molecular epidemiologic investigations. *Infect Control Hosp Epidemiol.* 1995;16(2):92–97

22. Carbonne A, Naas T, Blanckaert K, et al. Investigation of a nosocomial outbreak of extended-spectrum beta-lactamase VEB-1-producing isolates of *Acinetobacter baumannii* in a hospital setting. *J Hosp Infect.* 2005;60(1):14–18

23. Landman D, Quale JM, Mayorga D, et al. Citywide clonal outbreak of multiresistant *Acinetobacter baumannii* and Pseudomonas aeruginosa in Brooklyn, NY: the preantibiotic era has returned. *Arch Intern Med.* 2002;162(13):1515–1520

24. Corbella X, Montero A, Pujol M, et al. Emergence and rapid spread of carbapenem resistance during a large and sustained hospital outbreak of multiresistant *Acinetobacter baumannii. J Clin Microbiol.* 2000;38(11):4086–4095

25. Villers D, Espaze E, Coste-Burel M, et al. Nosocomial *Acinetobacter baumannii* infections: microbiological and clinical epidemiology. *Ann Intern Med.* 1998;129(3):182–189

26. Fagon JY, Chastre J, Wolff M, et al. Invasive and noninvasive strategies for management of suspected ventilator-associated pneumonia. A randomized trial. *Ann Intern Med.* 2000;132(8):621–630

27. Paterson DL, Rossi F, Baquero F, et al. In vitro susceptibilities of aerobic and facultative Gram-negative bacilli isolated from patients with intra-abdominal infections worldwide: the 2003 Study for Monitoring Antimicrobial Resistance Trends (SMART). *J Antimicrob Chemother.* 2005;55(6):965–973

28. Paramythiotou E, Karakitsos D, Aggelopoulou H, Sioutos P, Samonis G, Karabinis A. Post-surgical meningitis due to multiresistant *Acinetobacter baumannii.* Effective treatment with intravenous and/or intraventricular colistin and therapeutic dilemmas. *Med Mal Infect.* 2007;37(2):124–125

29. Hujer KM, Hamza NS, Hujer AM, et al. Identification of a new allelic variant of the *Acinetobacter baumannii* cephalosporinase, ADC-7 beta-lactamase: defining a unique family of class C enzymes. *Antimicrob Agents Chemother.* 2005;49(7):2941–2948

30. Hujer KM, Hujer AM, Hulten EA, et al. Analysis of antibiotic resistance genes in multidrug-resistant Acinetobacter sp. isolates from military and civilian patients treated at the Walter Reed Army Medical Center. *Antimicrob Agents Chemother.* 2006;50(12):4114–4123

31. Heritier C, Poirel L, Fournier PE, Claverie JM, Raoult D, Nordmann P. Characterization of the naturally occurring oxacillinase of *Acinetobacter baumannii. Antimicrob Agents Chemother.* 2005;49(10):4174–4179

32. Walsh TR, Toleman MA, Poirel L, Nordmann P. Metallo-beta-lactamases: the quiet before the storm? *Clin Microbiol Rev.* 2005;18(2):306–325

33. Franklin C, Liolios L, Peleg AY. Phenotypic detection of carbapenem-susceptible metallo-beta-lactamase-producing gram-negative bacilli in the clinical laboratory. *J Clin Microbiol.* 2006;44(9):3139–3144

34. Doi Y, de Oliveira Garcia D, Adams J, Paterson DL. Coproduction of novel 16S rRNA methylase RmtD and metallo-beta-lactamase SPM-1 in a panresistant Pseudomonas aeruginosa isolate from Brazil. Antimicrob Agents Chemother. 2007;51(3):852–856

35. Doi Y, Wachino J, Yamane K, et al. Spread of novel aminoglycoside resistance gene aac(6)-Iad among Acinetobacter clinical isolates in Japan. Antimicrob Agents Chemother. 2004;48(6):2075–2080

36. Ruzin A, Keeney D, Bradford PA. AdeABC multidrug efflux pump is associated with decreased susceptibility to tigecycline in Acinetobacter calcoaceticus–Acinetobacter baumannii complex. J Antimicrob Chemother. 2007;59:1001–1004

37. Bonomo RA, Szabo D. Mechanisms of multidrug resistance in Acinetobacter species and Pseudomonas aeruginosa. Clin Infect Dis. 2006;43 Suppl 2:S49–S56

38. Owen J, Darling I, Troy S, Cirincione B. Noncompartmental pharmacokinetics of tigecycline in patients with complicated skin and skin structure infections [abstract A-11]. In: Program and abstracts of the 44th Interscience Conference on Antimicrobial Agents and Chemotherapy (Washington DC), Washington, DC: American Society for Microbiology; 2004:2

39. Peleg AY, Potoski BA, Rea R, et al. Acinetobacter baumannii bloodstream infection while receiving tigecycline: a cautionary report. J Antimicrob Chemother. 2007;59(1):128–131

40. Betriu C, Rodriguez-Avial I, Sanchez BA, Gomez M, Alvarez J, Picazo JJ. In vitro activities of tigecycline (GAR-936) against recently isolated clinical bacteria in Spain. Antimicrob Agents Chemother. 2002;46(3):892–895

41. Henwood CJ, Gatward T, Warner M, et al. Antibiotic resistance among clinical isolates of Acinetobacter in the UK, and in vitro evaluation of tigecycline (GAR-936). J Antimicrob Chemother. 2002;49(3):479–487

42. Li J, Nation RL, Turnidge JD, et al. Colistin: the re-emerging antibiotic for multidrug-resistant Gram-negative bacterial infections. Lancet Infect Dis. 2006;6(9):589–601

43. Peleg AY, Paterson DL. Multidrug-resistant Acinetobacter: a threat to the antibiotic era. Intern Med J. 2006;36(8):479–482

44. Li J, Rayner CR, Nation RL, et al. Heteroresistance to colistin in multidrug-resistant Acinetobacter baumannii. Antimicrob Agents Chemother. 2006;50(9):2946–2950

45. Paterson DL, Lipman J. The end of the antibiotic era. The XDR problem. Crit Care Med. 2007;35:1789–1791

46. Chan PC, Huang LM, Lin HC, et al. Control of an outbreak of pan-drug-resistant Acinetobacter baumannii colonization and infection in a neonatal intensive care unit. Infect Control Hosp Epidemiol. 2007;28(4):423–429

Chapter 57
Antimicrobial Resistance of *Shigella* spp., Typhoid *Salmonella* and Nontyphoid *Salmonella*

Herbert L. DuPont

1 Introduction

At the end of the nineteenth century, the two great forms of dysentery were identified: sporadically occurring amoebic dysentery (amoebiasis) and bacillary dysentery (shigellosis) that tended to produce outbreaks of diarrheal disease. Since first identified, *Shigella* spp. have been shown to be important causes of mortality worldwide and for epidemic strains of *S. dysenteriae* type 1 (Shiga bacillus) major causes of mortality in tropical endemic regions.

Enteric or typhoid fever is a striking syndrome of fever with abdominal symptoms and signs associated with bacteremic salmonellosis. If untreated, typhoid fever may progress to life-threatening complications in the second week of illness, including perforated intestine and intestinal hemorrhage. The major causes of enteric fever are *Salmonella* Typhi and or *S*. Paratyphi.

Nontyphoid strains of *Salmonella* are important causes of self-limiting food-borne gastroenteritis with antimicrobial therapy directed to the subset of cases at extremes of age, when illness is complicated by presence of fever and systemic toxicity or when persons also have underlying medical conditions that predispose to systemic or bacteremic infection and associated complications.

For nontyphoid *Salmonella* strains, animals serve as the major microbial reservoir where use of antibiotics in animals facilitates the emergence of a relatively stable form of antibacterial resistance. The widespread use of antibacterial drugs in human medicine is more relevant for emergence of antibacterial resistance among the bacterial enteropathogens showing a human reservoir, including *Shigella* and typhoid *Salmonella*. In these cases, self-medication and purchase of antibacterial drugs without a prescription are commonly practiced in many areas of the developing world. In industrialized regions, antibiotic use for viral infections and other conditions for which antibiotics are not indicated contributes to rising rates of resistance.

This review looks at the current state of antibacterial resistance among shigellae and salmonellae and focuses on current guidelines of antimicrobial therapy in the setting of growing resistance.

2 Importance of *Shigella* and *Salmonella*

2.1 *Shigella*

The annual number of *Shigella* diarrhea and dysentery cases has been estimated to be 165 million leading to approximately one million deaths in the developing world (1). *S. dysenteriae* 1 (the Shiga bacillus) characteristically has a more severe outcome and can produce widespread and severe epidemics. In the US it is estimated that we have approximately 500,000 cases of shigellosis each year (2). *Shigella* strains continue to be important causes of travelers' diarrhea in international visitors and military populations (3, 4). Shigellosis is uniquely pathogenic among bacterial pathogens resulting in common person-to-person spread because of low dose required for illness (5). Strains of *Shigella* should be suspected as a potential etiologic agent in patients with sporadically occurring dysentery where many stools of small volume are passed that contain gross blood and mucus. The illness tends to be clinically striking and may persist for a week or longer if untreated.

2.2 *Typhoid Salmonella*

It is estimated that there are up to 16–33 million cases of typhoid fever per year in the world resulting in more than 600,000 deaths (6, 7). The infectious dose of typhoid

H.L. DuPont (✉)
University of Texas – Houston School of Public Health,
St. Luke's Episcopal Hospital and Baylor College of Medicine,
Houston, TX, USA
hdupont@sleh.com

D.L. Mayers (ed.), *Antimicrobial Drug Resistance*,
DOI 10.1007/978-1-60327-595-8_57, © Humana Press, a part of Springer Science+Business Media, LLC 2009

Salmonella is moderately high (8), explaining the lack of person-to-person spread and the need for a food or water vehicle for disease transmission. Typhoid fever is particularly endemic in the Indian subcontinent, Southeast Asia, Africa and South America. The disease is striking and patients with typhoid fever often present themselves to medical centers for evaluation. It is one of the most important febrile conditions among international travelers to endemic areas. Blood cultures should always be obtained in travelers with fever following return from endemic tropical regions to evaluate for the presence of typhoid fever.

2.3 Nontyphoid Salmonella

Nontyphoid salmonellosis causes approximately 1.4 million cases of food-borne disease in the US leading to an estimated 16,000 hospitalizations and nearly 600 deaths (2). A surprisingly high incidence of the organism is seen in young infants less than 1 year of age which appears to be related to a reduced number of organisms needed for development of gastroenteritis in this age group plus household exposure to the organism from common in-home cross contamination.

3 Patterns of Susceptibility of *Shigella* spp. by Geography

The first antibiotic shown to be effective in shortening the course of shigellosis was ampicillin (9). In children with severe shigellosis, orally absorbable ampicillin was shown to be superior to orally administered nonabsorbable neomycin, with both drugs showing similar levels of in vitro susceptibility. This study provided indirect evidence that drug absorption was required for mucosally invasive shigellosis. With the subsequent widespread use of ampicillin for therapy of bacterial diarrhea in the 1970s and 1980s, ampicillin resistance occurred widely (10), leading to the search for other drugs to treat this severe form of diarrhea and dysentery. Nelson et al. (11) demonstrated that trimethoprim–sulfamethoxazole (TMP/SMX) was active in vitro and showed that the drug shortened clinical shigellosis in infected children. Soon after this study in pediatric shigellosis, adults with endemic shigellosis were shown to have improvement in their clinical disease by administration of the drug (12), and our group showed that TMP/SMX was active in shortening the duration of travelers' diarrhea due to strains of *Shigella* during short-term stay in Mexico (13). During the 1980s, TMP/SMX remained active against isolated strains of *Shigella* in the US, Europe, Latin America and Asia (10), while in the 1990s identified enteric bacterial pathogens

including strains of *Shigella* began to lose their susceptibility to TMP/SMX with rates of resistance reaching 50–94% throughout the world. In the US we initially found TMP/SMX resistance among persons returning from international travel after visiting these regions and showing resistance (14).

One of the first drugs to be used successfully to treat TMP/SMX-resistant shigellosis was nalidixic acid, a quinolone available in pediatric suspension form and with in vitro activity against enteric bacterial pathogens (14). The drug possessed a potential for quinolone toxicity in children, limiting its widespread use. Mecillinam (pivamdinicillin) was further evaluated and found to have value in the treatment of shigellosis in Bangladesh (15) for susceptible and more resistant forms of *Shigella*. Resistance to nalidixic acid became common, particularly in strains of *S. dysenteriae* 1 (16). This emergence of resistance was presumably due to widespread use of nalidixic acid. With the availability of the newer fluoroquinolones, beginning with norfloxacin and followed by ciprofloxacin and levofloxacin, the outcome of treatment of shigellosis in adults was immediately improved.

In the US, nalidixic acid resistance has occurred in approximately 1% of tested strains with a high percent of the nalidixic acid-resistant strains found also to be resistant to fluoroquinolones (17). In recent years, nalidixic acid resistance has reached very high levels for *S. flexneri* and *S. dysenteriae* strains in Asia, and these strains typically show resistance to fluoroquinolones as well (18, 19). A clonal epidemic of an antimicrobial-susceptible strain of *S. dysenteriae* 2 has been seen in Bangladesh (20).

Antimicrobial susceptibility of strains of *Shigella* has been related to general use of antimicrobials in the population, as well as to the species of pathogen causing illness. *S. flexneri* showed greater resistance to common drugs than *S. sonnei* (21), and *S. dysenteriae* 1 showed the highest degree of resistance compared with other serotypes (14). Over a period of time in endemic areas such as Bangladesh, nalidixic acid resistance has become clinically important so that the drug is no longer helpful in the management of Shiga dysentery (14).

In Table 1 we have provided a world region summary of antimicrobial susceptibility data for isolated *Shigella* strains in various published studies.

4 Enteric Fever Due to Strains of *Salmonella* Typhi and *S.* Paratyphoid

Since the 1940s, typhoid fever has been managed in the developing world with choloramphenicol. The drug was inexpensive and effective in shortening the course of illness. In the 1970s, choloramphenicol resistance among typhoid *Salmonella* strains emerged in the Indian subcontinent and in

Table 1 Changing susceptibility of *Shigella* spp. to various antibiotics from the 1970s–1980s to the 1990s–2000 in various regions of the World

Region	Amp	TMP/SMX	Nalidixic acid	Quinolone	Azithromycin	References
U.S.	18→63	0→59	Low→0.3	Low→5	?	(10, 17, 71, 72)
Europe, Middle East	18→73	6→70	Low→0	Low→5	?	(10, 72–77)
Latin America	15→90	0→90	?	0→5	Low→<5	(78–81)
Asia	10→90	10→90[a]	Low→<1–90[a]	0→55[a]	Low→0	(14, 19, 21, 82–86)
Africa	37→90	6→90	Low→10[a]	Low→5	?	(87–89)
Worldwide(≥3 countries)	50→90	10→90	?	0→5	Low→0	(78, 81)

Values are expressed in percentages

[a]Antimicrobial resistance is currently highest for strains of *S. dysenteriae* 1 with high rates also seen in strains of *S. flexneri* and low rates for *S. sonnei* isolates

Mexico (22), leading to the successful evaluation of other antimicrobial agents, including ampicillin and then trimethoprim–sulfamethoxazole for therapy of typhoid fever (23). Beginning with the 1980s, multi-drug-resistant strains of typhoid *Salmonella* emerged in Asia and Europe. The plasmid-encoded resistance identified was directed not only to chloramphenicol but also to ampicillin and trimethoprim–sulfamethoxazole, thereby complicating the therapy and leading to increased mortality (24). Worldwide occurrence of resistance to chloramphenicol, ampicillin and trimethoprim–sulfamethoxazole in *Salmonella* Typhi has continued to increase.

Nalidixic acid resistance among enteric *S*. Typhi strains was shown to be an important predictor of intermediate resistance to the fluoroquinolones and indicated the need to administer higher doses of fluoroquinolones for successful treatment (25). Fluoroquinolone resistance has been documented among isolated strains of typhoid *Salmonella* (26, 27), although it has not yet become important or widespread (25, 28). Most fluoroquinolone-resistant *S* Typhi strains have been shown to have point mutations in the genes encoding DNA gyrase or DNA topoimerase IV enzymes located within their chromosomes (29). Fluoroquinolones act on *GyrA* and at higher concentrations on *ParC*, with point mutations leading to reduced susceptibility to ofloxacin, ciprofloxacin and gatifloxacin (30).

In the US, where most cases of typhoid fever occur secondarily to international travel, particularly to the Indian subcontinent, multi-drug resistance rates have gone from <1 to >10% (31, 32). In Europe, multi-resistance became even more common in recent years, with nearly one-third of isolates showing reduced fluoroquinolone susceptibility, thus indicating a need for higher doses for treatment with this class of drugs (33). In some areas with an increasing resistance of *S*. Typhi strains to fluoroquinolones, a concomitant decrease in resistance to choloramphenicol has been found (34), which could influence future treatment recommendations in developing countries where the cost differential between fluoroquinolones and chloramphenicol is great. In a study carried out in Nepal, multi-resistant and extended-spectrum beta-lactamase-producing enteric fever strains were more commonly classified in the laboratory as Paratyphi A than Typhi (35). A study of Paratyphi isolates from India also demonstrated nalidixic acid resistance and a reduced susceptibility to ciprofloxacin (36). Susceptibility testing of isolated typhoid and paratyphoid *Salmonella* is important in managing enteric fever in patients to identify the optimal therapy and to prevent delayed recovery and treatment failures.

5 Gastroenteritis Due to Nontyphoid *Salmonella*

During the 1970s and 1980s, strains of nontyphoid *Salmonella* were shown to have variable susceptibility to ampicillin, tetracycline and TMP/SMX (10). In more recent years, resistance to ampicillin, TMP/SMX, chloramphenicol, aminoglycosides, chloramphenicol and sulfonamides has become widespread throughout the world, related at least in part to the potential of these bacterial pathogens for horizontal transfer of resistance mediated by plasmids, transposons or integron cassettes. There is evidence for the nontyphoid *Salmonella* that dissemination of multi-drug resistance is secondary to both local antimicrobial use with local selection of resistant strains as well as by more widespread dissemination of resistant clones of *Salmonella* amplified within livestock and other animal populations (37–39). Resistant *Salmonella* enterica serovars isolated from different institutions may show the same genetic lineage, thus supporting the concept of clonal spread (40).

Non*Salmonella* enterica pathogens, including *Shigella*, typhoid *Salmonella* and *Campylobacter jejuni*, characteristically develop polyclonal resistance in response to local antibiotic use patterns. The occurrence of an important clonal spread of nontyphoid *Salmonella* strains has facilitated widespread distribution of antimicrobial resistance, resembling the problem of methicillin-resistant *Staphylococcus aureus*, which has spread within the community from a hospital reservoir. For the study of clonal spread of nontyphoid *Salmonella,* multiple genetic typing procedures may be needed for epidemiologic study, as a single gene characterization may give an incomplete epidemiologic picture (41). Although less important from a public health standpoint, multiclonal spread can also occur for *Salmonella* enterica strains (42).

Rates of fluoroquinolone resistance among strains of nontyphoid *Salmonella* were shown to increase from 1995 to 1999 in travelers returning to the US. Ciprofloxacin resistance increased from 4 to 24% for various travel destinations, while for those returning from Thailand, the increase was even greater, with increase in resistance rates from 6 to 50% (43).

Retail meat can be shown to harbor antibacterial-resistant strains of *Salmonella,* supporting current recommendations that national surveillance for antimicrobial-resistant *Salmonella* should include the monitoring of retail foods and that restrictions for use of antibiotics important in human medicine should be imposed for all food animals (44). Removing the selective influence of fluoroquinolones in animal populations is an important public health effort in the US and needs to be extended to additional areas of the world beyond the European Union (45). Resistant *Salmonella* enterica serovars may be isolated from poultry (46), and shell eggs have been found to harbor resistant *Salmonella*, including strains resistant to nalidixic acid, with the resistance pattern showing serotype-dependence (47).

Of the many serotypes of *Salmonella,* serovar Typhimurium is the most resistant to antibacterial drugs. Multi-drug-resistant definitive type (DT) 104 *S.* Typhimurium has emerged worldwide and has appeared in the US. DT 104 strains are responsible for about one-third of infections in the US. They are characteristically resistant to ampicillin, chloramphenicol, tetracycline, streptomycin, sulfamethoxazole and kanamycin (48). Bacteriophage typing can identify various DT 104 types belonging to multiple serotypes but with a similar mechanism of integron gene resistance that may confer resistance to aminoglycosides, trimethoprim and β-lactam drugs (44). *Salmonella* phage type DT104 harbors a genomic island called *Salmonella* genomic island 1 (SGI-1) containing an antibiotic gene cluster conferring multi-drug resistance (49). The CDC-sponsored FoodNet program demonstrated that human acquisition of DT 104 in the US was related to prior receipt of an antimicrobial agent during the 4 weeks preceding illness onset (48).

Between 1998 and 2002 multi-drug-resistant *Salmonella* Newport emerged as an important public health problem in the United States (50). This strain is particularly important because it is not only resistant to the drugs seen with DT 104 strains, but it is resistant to the third-generation cephalosporin, ceftriaxone, which is the treatment of choice for systemic pediatric salmonellosis. This resistance in *S.* Newport has been attributed to plasmid-mediated AmpC (CMY-2) β-lactamase (51). Resistance in these strains appears to be encouraged by the use of antibacterial drugs in livestock with resultant spread to humans (50, 52). The spread from bovine sources to humans may also be facilitated by human use of antibacterial drugs (53). Currently *S.* Newport is the third most common *Salmonella* serotype in the US, having increased in incidence fivefold from 1998 to 2001 (50).

When compared with susceptible strains, multi-drug-resistant strains of *Salmonella* are more likely to produce severe infection and mortality (54) and to lead to hospitalization (55). There is evidence that antimicrobial-resistant *Salmonella* are not only able to resist the effect of antibiotics to which they show low susceptibility, but they may be more virulent than susceptible strains, causing more prolonged and more severe illness than their antibiotic-susceptible counterparts (56). Comorbid conditions of the host may affect susceptibility to salmonellosis and influence the outcome. In one study in Ethiopia, the *Salmonella* isolates from patients with HIV infection showed greater resistance to antimicrobials than those from HIV-negative controls (57). It will be important to monitor the incidence of antimicrobial-resistant *Salmonella* in human populations as well as the food supply to help predict the evolution of antimicrobial resistance in human infections (58, 59).

6 Current Therapeutic Recommendations

In Table 2, recommendations for therapy of the various bacterial enteric infections considered herein are summarized.

6.1 Shigella

The fluoroquinolones have become the mainstay of therapy for adult patients with shigellosis. Most cases should be treated with antibacterial drugs for three full days, although for many persons with milder forms of shigellosis caused by species other than *S. dysenteriae* type 1, single-dose treatment may be effective (60, 61). A single-dose therapy with azithromycin appears to be effective in treating many forms of shigellosis (62). Azithromycin or one of the third-generation cephalosporins should currently be considered the drug of choice for treatment of pediatric shigellosis. Strains of *S. sonnei* resistant to third-generation cephalosporins have been encountered (63). While azithromycin is an important form of therapy for shigellosis, there may be challenges with the interpretation of in vitro susceptibility testing of *Shigella* isolates using E-test and disk diffusion (64).

Table 2   Recommended therapy of shigellosis and salmonellosis based on current susceptibility patterns

Condition	Children		Adults	
Shigellosis	Azithromycin[b]	10 mg/kg/d	Norfloxacin (NF) or ciprofloxacin (CF) or levofloxacin (LF) or azithromycin (AZ)	NF 400 mg bid, CF 500 mg bid or LV 500 qd for 3 d or AZ 1,000 mg in a single dose
Typhoid fever	Ceftriaxone	50 mg/kg/d in two IV doses/d for 7–10 days	CF, LF or other fluoroquinolone (FQ) or azithromycin (AZ)	FQ given in full doses for 7–10 days AZ 500 mg qd for 7 days
Salmonellosis (afebrile, non-toxic in health host)	Fluid therapy and observation		Fluid therapy and observation	
Salmonellosis (febrile, toxic or in special host[a])	Treat for bacteremia as typhoid fever or with azithromycin (AZ) for cephalosporin-resistant strains	See above for ceftriaxone dosing, AZ 10 mg/kg/d in single daily dose for 7 days	Treat for bacteremia as typhoid fever[c]	

[a]Extremes of age (<3 months, >65 years of age), sickle cell anemia, inflammatory bowel disease, hemodialysis, receiving systemic corticosteroids or anti-cancer or anti-immunity drugs, AIDS (for AIDS or immunocompromised continue therapy for at least 2 weeks)
[b]Ciprofloxacin can be safely given for 3 days to older children although not approved for bacterial diarrhea
[c]Immunocompromised patients may need prolonged treatment

One concern in the therapy of Shiga dysentery due to *S. dysenteriae* 1 is the development of hemolytic uremic syndrome (HUS), an association which has been reported (65). The importance of antimicrobial therapy to the development of HUS in Shiga dysentery was studied by Bennish and coworkers (66), who found in one small study that treatment of Shiga bacillus dysentery did not predispose to HUS and stools in treated subjects showed a reduction of Shiga toxin.

6.2 Typhoid Fever

Although it has been the drug of choice for three decades, choloramphenicol, has been used more sparingly in recent years due to the emergence of resistance, high relapse rate and failure to eradicate intestinal carriage of the organism (8). Resistance to chloramphenicol, ampicillin and TMP/SMX has been seen worldwide for strains of *Salmonella* Typhi. Fluoroquinolones remain active in vitro, render high concentrations in bile and macrophages and can also be given for shorter courses. For adults in regions where they are not prohibitively expensive, the fluoroquinolones represent the current treatment of choice (28, 32). The recommended duration of fluoroquinolone use in adults with typhoid fever is 7–10 days and the drug should be given orally as soon as oral medications can be taken. Ceftriaxone (1–2 g per day) for 7–10 days is effective in adults with typhoid fever and the third-generation cephalosporins represent the treatment of choice for pediatric typhoid fever (67). Oral cefixime and oral azithromycin remain alternatives for strains resistant to other drugs (68).

6.3 Nontyphoid Salmonellosis

Over the years multi-drug-resistant strains of nontyphoid *Salmonella* have emerged, confounding the therapy of human infections. Fortunately, most cases of nontyphoid salmonellosis produce just mild-to-moderate self-limiting gastroenteritis. In a subset of patients, bacteremia or other systemic infection including meningitis may occur, which explains that nearly 600 deaths in the US each year is associated with intestinal salmonellosis. Conditions in which *Salmonella* bacteremia and systemic infection should be suspected, and where antimicrobial therapy should be initiated empirically, include patients with *Salmonella* gastroenteritis in the following patient groups: (1) extremes of age (<3 months and >65 years of age); (2) undergoing regular hemodialysis; (3) receiving high-dose steroid treatment; (4) presence of AIDS or cancer or receipt of anti-cancer drugs that alter immunocompetence; and (5) presence of inflammatory bowel disease or sickle cell disease. In these cases antibiotics are given for 7–10 days to treat bacteremic disease rather than a localized enteric infection. In immuno-compromised persons with cancer or AIDS and possible systemic salmonellosis, the antibiotics are given for at least 2 weeks, and some need therapy even longer. The antimicrobials given to patients with known or possible bacteremic disease do not shorten nonsystemic intestinal disease and may encourage the emergence of resistant forms with transient shedding (69) without decreasing post-diarrhea shedding of *Salmonella* (70).

The treatment of choice for therapy of systemic nontyphoid *Salmonella* infection in adults is a fluoroquinolone, given orally when it can be taken by that route. The fluoroquinolones remain active against strains of *Salmonella* encountered in the US (58). For children, parenteral third-generation cephalosporins should ordinarily be used for systemic salmonellosis. With the occurrence of cephalosporin-resistant nontyphoid *Salmonella* from animal populations, new treatments are needed for children.

Since most nontyphoid *Salmonella* strains now are multi-drug-resistant, in vitro susceptibility testing should routinely be performed with isolated strains, so that initial empiric therapy can be altered if indicated by susceptibility results.

References

1. Kotloff KL, Winickoff JP, Ivanoff B, et al. Global burden of *Shigella* infections: implications for vaccine development and implementation of control strategies. *Bull World Health Organ.* 1999;77(8):651–666
2. Mead PS, Slutsker L, Dietz V, et al. Food-related illness and death in the United States. *Emerg Infect Dis.* 1999;5(5):607–625
3. Jiang ZD, Lowe B, Verenkar MP, et al. Prevalence of enteric pathogens among international travelers with diarrhea acquired in Kenya (Mombasa), India (Goa), or Jamaica (Montego Bay). *J Infect Dis.* 2002;185(4):497–502
4. Thornton SA, Sherman SS, Farkas T, Zhong W, Torres P, Jiang X. Gastroenteritis in US marines during operation Iraqi freedom. *Clin Infect Dis.* 2005;40(4):519–525
5. DuPont HL, Levine MM, Hornick RB, Formal SB. Inoculum size in shigellosis and implications for expected mode of transmission. *J Infect Dis.* 1989;159(6):1126–1128
6. World Health Organization. The World Health report 1996 – fighting disease, fostering development. *World Health Forum.* 1997;18(1):1–8
7. Edelman R, Levine MM. Summary of an international workshop on typhoid fever. *Rev Infect Dis.* 1986;8(3):329–349
8. Hornick RB, Greisman SE, Woodward TE, DuPont HL, Dawkins AT, Snyder MJ. Typhoid fever: pathogenesis and immunologic control. *N Engl J Med.* 1970;283(13):686–691
9. Haltalin KC, Nelson JD, Hinton LV, Kusmiesz HT, Sladoje M. Comparison of orally absorbable and nonabsorbable antibiotics in shigellosis. A double-blind study with ampicillin and neomycin. *J Pediatr.* 1968;72(5):708–720
10. Murray BE. Resistance of *Shigella*, *Salmonella*, and other selected enteric pathogens to antimicrobial agents. *Rev Infect Dis.* 1986;8 Suppl 2:S172–S181
11. Nelson JD, Kusmiesz H, Jackson LH, Woodman E. Trimethoprim–sulfamethoxazole therapy for shigellosis. *JAMA.* 1976;235(12):1239–1243
12. Barada FA, Jr, Guerrant RL. Sulfamethoxazole–trimethoprim versus ampicillin in treatment of acute invasive diarrhea in adults. *Antimicrob Agents Chemother.* 1980;17(6):961–964
13. DuPont HL, Reves RR, Galindo E, Sullivan PS, Wood LV, Mendiola JG. Treatment of travelers' diarrhea with trimethoprim/sulfamethoxazole and with trimethoprim alone. *N Engl J Med.* 1982;307(14):841–844
14. Bennish ML, Salam MA, Hossain MA, et al. Antimicrobial resistance of Shigella isolates in Bangladesh, 1983–1990: increasing frequency of strains multiply resistant to ampicillin, trimethoprim–sulfamethoxazole, and nalidixic acid. *Clin Infect Dis.* 1992;14(5):1055–1060
15. Salam MA, Dhar U, Khan WA, Bennish ML. Randomised comparison of ciprofloxacin suspension and pivmecillinam for childhood shigellosis. *Lancet.* 1998;352(9127):522–527
16. Munshi MH, Sack DA, Haider K, Ahmed ZU, Rahaman MM, Morshed MG. Plasmid-mediated resistance to nalidixic acid in Shigella dysenteriae type 1. *Lancet.* 1987;2(8556):419–421
17. Sivapalasingam S, Nelson JM, Joyce K, Hoekstra M, Angulo FJ, Mintz ED. High prevalence of antimicrobial resistance among *Shigella* isolates in the United States tested by the National Antimicrobial Resistance Monitoring System from 1999 to 2002. *Antimicrob Agents Chemother.* 2006;50(1):49–54
18. Talukder KA, Khajanchi BK, Islam MA, et al. Genetic relatedness of ciprofloxacin-resistant *Shigella dysenteriae* type 1 strains isolated in south Asia. *J Antimicrob Chemother.* 2004;54(4):730–734
19. Taneja N. Changing epidemiology of shigellosis and emergence of ciprofloxacin-resistant Shigellae in India. *J Clin Microbiol.* 2007;45(2):678–679
20. Talukder KA, Khajanchi BK, Islam MA, et al. The emerging strains of *Shigella dysenteriae* type 2 in Bangladesh are clonal. *Epidemiol Infect.* 2006;134(6):1249–1256
21. Hoge CW, Gambel JM, Srijan A, Pitarangsi C, Echeverria P. Trends in antibiotic resistance among diarrheal pathogens isolated in Thailand over 15 years. *Clin Infect Dis.* 1998;26(2):341–345
22. Paniker CK, Vimala KN. Transferable chloramphenicol resistance in *Salmonella typhi*. *Nature.* 1972;239(5367):109–110
23. Snyder MJ, Gonzalez O, Palomino C, et al. Comparative efficacy of chloramphenicol, ampicillin, and co-trimoxazole in the treatment of typhoid fever. *Lancet.* 1976;2(7996):1155–1157
24. Rowe B, Ward LR, Threlfall EJ. Multidrug-resistant *Salmonella typhi*: a worldwide epidemic. *Clin Infect Dis.* 1997;24 Suppl 1:S106–S109
25. Wain J, Hoa NT, Chinh NT, et al. Quinolone-resistant *Salmonella typhi* in Vietnam: molecular basis of resistance and clinical response to treatment. *Clin Infect Dis.* 1997;25(6):1404–1410
26. Joshi S, Amarnath SK. Fluoroquinolone resistance in *Salmonella typhi* and *S. paratyphi* A in Bangalore, India. *Trans R Soc Trop Med Hyg.* 2007;101(3):308–310
27. Saha SK, Darmstadt GL, Baqui AH, et al. Molecular basis of resistance displayed by highly ciprofloxacin-resistant *Salmonella enterica* serovar Typhi in Bangladesh. *J Clin Microbiol.* 2006;44(10):3811–3813
28. Parry CM, Ho VA, Phuong le T, et al. Randomized controlled comparison of ofloxacin, azithromycin, and an ofloxacin–azithromycin combination for treatment of multidrug-resistant and nalidixic acid-resistant typhoid fever. *Antimicrob Agents Chemother.* 2007;51(3):819–825
29. Hirose K, Hashimoto A, Tamura K, et al. DNA sequence analysis of DNA gyrase and DNA topoisomerase IV quinolone resistance-determining regions of *Salmonella enterica* serovar Typhi and serovar Paratyphi A. *Antimicrob Agents Chemother.* 2002;46(10):3249–3252
30. Turner AK, Nair S, Wain J. The acquisition of full fluoroquinolone resistance in Salmonella Typhi by accumulation of point mutations in the topoisomerase targets. *J Antimicrob Chemother.* 2006;58(4):733–740
31. Ackers ML, Puhr ND, Tauxe RV, Mintz ED. Laboratory-based surveillance of Salmonella serotype Typhi infections in the United States: antimicrobial resistance on the rise. *JAMA.* 2000;283(20):2668–2673
32. Mermin JH, Townes JM, Gerber M, Dolan N, Mintz ED, Tauxe RV. Typhoid fever in the United States, 1985–1994: changing risks of international travel and increasing antimicrobial resistance. *Arch Intern Med.* 1998;158(6):633–638
33. Threlfall EJ, Fisher IS, Berghold C, et al. Trends in antimicrobial drug resistance in *Salmonella enterica* serotypes Typhi and

Paratyphi A isolated in Europe, 1999–2001. *Int J Antimicrob Agents.* 2003;22(5):487–491

34. Gautam V, Gupta NK, Chaudhary U, Arora DR. Sensitivity pattern of Salmonella serotypes in Northern India. *Braz J Infect Dis.* 2002;6(6):281–287

35. Pokharel BM, Koirala J, Dahal RK, Mishra SK, Khadga PK, Tuladhar NR. Multidrug-resistant and extended-spectrum beta-lactamase (ESBL)-producing *Salmonella enterica* (serotypes Typhi and Paratyphi A) from blood isolates in Nepal: surveillance of resistance and a search for newer alternatives. *Int J Infect Dis.* 2006;10(6):434–438

36. Mandal S, Mandal MD, Pal NK. Antibiotic resistance of Salmonella enterica serovar Paratyphi A in India: emerging and reemerging problem. *J Postgrad Med.* 2006;52(3):163–166

37. Heurtin-Le Corre C, Donnio PY, Perrin M, Travert MF, Avril JL. Increasing incidence and comparison of nalidixic acid-resistant *Salmonella enterica* subsp. enterica serotype typhimurium isolates from humans and animals. *J Clin Microbiol.* 1999;37(1):266–269

38. Malorny B, Schroeter A, Bunge C, Hoog B, Steinbeck A, Helmuth R. Evaluation of molecular typing methods for *Salmonella enterica* serovar Typhimurium DT104 isolated in Germany from healthy pigs. *Vet Res.* 2001;32(2):119–129

39. Prager R, Liesegang A, Rabsch W, et al. Clonal relationship of *Salmonella enterica* serovar typhimurium phage type DT104 in Germany and Austria. *Zentralbl Bakteriol.* 1999;289(4):399–414

40. Fonseca EL, Mykytczuk OL, Asensi MD, et al. Clonality and antimicrobial resistance gene profiles of multidrug-resistant *Salmonella enterica* serovar infantis isolates from four public hospitals in Rio de Janeiro, Brazil. *J Clin Microbiol.* 2006;44(8):2767–2772

41. Liebana E, Garcia-Migura L, Clouting C, et al. Multiple genetic typing of *Salmonella enterica* serotype typhimurium isolates of different phage types (DT104, U302, DT204b, and DT49) from animals and humans in England, Wales, and Northern Ireland. *J Clin Microbiol.* 2002;40(12):4450–4456

42. Ghilardi AC, Tavechio AT, Fernandes SA. Antimicrobial susceptibility, phage types, and pulse types of *Salmonella typhimurium*, in Sao Paulo, Brazil. *Mem Inst Oswaldo Cruz.* 2006;101(3):281–286

43. Hakanen A, Kotilainen P, Huovinen P, Helenius H, Siitonen A. Reduced fluoroquinolone susceptibility in *Salmonella enterica* serotypes in travelers returning from Southeast Asia. *Emerg Infect Dis.* 2001;7(6):996–1003

44. White DG, Zhao S, Sudler R, et al. The isolation of antibiotic-resistant salmonella from retail ground meats. *N Engl J Med.* 2001;345(16):1147–1154

45. Bager F, Helmuth R. Epidemiology of resistance to quinolones in Salmonella. *Vet Res.* 2001;32(3–4):285–290

46. Shahada F, Chuma T, Tobata T, Okamoto K, Sueyoshi M, Takase K. Molecular epidemiology of antimicrobial resistance among *Salmonella enterica* serovar Infantis from poultry in Kagoshima, Japan. *Int J Antimicrob Agents.* 2006;28(4):302–307

47. Musgrove MT, Jones DR, Northcutt JK, et al. Antimicrobial resistance in *Salmonella* and *Escherichia coli* isolated from commercial shell eggs. *Poult Sci.* 2006;85(9):1665–1669

48. Glynn MK, Bopp C, Dewitt W, Dabney P, Mokhtar M, Angulo FJ. Emergence of multidrug-resistant *Salmonella enterica* serotype typhimurium DT104 infections in the United States. *N Engl J Med.* 1998;338(19):1333–1338

49. Quinn T, O'Mahony R, Baird AW, Drudy D, Whyte P, Fanning S. Multi-drug resistance in *Salmonella enterica*: efflux mechanisms and their relationships with the development of chromosomal resistance gene clusters. *Curr Drug Targets.* 2006;7(7):849–860

50. Gupta A, Fontana J, Crowe C, et al. Emergence of multidrug-resistant *Salmonella enterica* serotype Newport infections resistant to expanded-spectrum cephalosporins in the United States. *J Infect Dis.* 2003;188(11):1707–1716

51. Dunne EF, Fey PD, Kludt P, et al. Emergence of domestically acquired ceftriaxone-resistant *Salmonella* infections associated with AmpC beta-lactamase. *JAMA.* 2000;284(24):3151–3156

52. Spika JS, Waterman SH, Hoo GW, et al. Chloramphenicol-resistant Salmonella newport traced through hamburger to dairy farms. A major persisting source of human salmonellosis in California. *N Engl J Med.* 1987;316(10):565–570

53. Varma JK, Marcus R, Stenzel SA, et al. Highly resistant Salmonella Newport-MDRAmpC transmitted through the domestic US food supply: a FoodNet case-control study of sporadic Salmonella Newport infections, 2002–2003. *J Infect Dis.* 2006;194(2):222–230

54. Helms M, Vastrup P, Gerner-Smidt P, Molbak K. Excess mortality associated with antimicrobial drug-resistant *Salmonella typhimurium*. *Emerg Infect Dis.* 2002;8(5):490–495

55. Martin LJ, Fyfe M, Dore K, et al. Increased burden of illness associated with antimicrobial-resistant *Salmonella enterica* serotype typhimurium infections. *J Infect Dis.* 2004;189(3):377–384

56. Travers K, Barza M. Morbidity of infections caused by antimicrobial-resistant bacteria. *Clin Infect Dis.* 2002;34 Suppl 3:S131–S134

57. Wolday D, Erge W. Antimicrobial sensitivity pattern of Salmonella: comparison of isolates from HIV-infected and HIV-uninfected patients. *Trop Doct.* 1998;28(3):139–141

58. Herikstad H, Hayes P, Mokhtar M, Fracaro ML, Threlfall EJ, Angulo FJ. Emerging quinolone-resistant Salmonella in the United States. *Emerg Infect Dis.* 1997;3(3):371–372

59. Kiessling CR, Cutting JH, Loftis M, Kiessling WM, Datta AR, Sofos JN. Antimicrobial resistance of food-related Salmonella isolates, 1999–2000. *J Food Prot.* 2002;65(4):603–608

60. Bassily S, Hyams KC, el-Masry NA, et al. Short-course norfloxacin and trimethoprim-sulfamethoxazole treatment of shigellosis and salmonellosis in Egypt. *Am J Trop Med Hyg.* 1994;51(2):219–223

61. Bennish ML, Salam MA, Khan WA, Khan AM. Treatment of shigellosis: III. Comparison of one- or two-dose ciprofloxacin with standard 5-day therapy. A randomized, blinded trial. *Ann Intern Med.* 1992;117(9):727–734

62. Shanks GD, Smoak BL, Aleman GM, et al. Single dose of azithromycin or three-day course of ciprofloxacin as therapy for epidemic dysentery in Kenya. Acute Dysentery Study Group. *Clin Infect Dis.* 1999;29(4):942–943

63. Huang IF, Chiu CH, Wang MH, Wu CY, Hsieh KS, Chiou CC. Outbreak of dysentery associated with ceftriaxone-resistant Shigella sonnei: First report of plasmid-mediated CMY-2-type AmpC beta-lactamase resistance in S. sonnei. *J Clin Microbiol.* 2005;43(6):2608–2612

64. Jain SK, Gupta A, Glanz B, Dick J, Siberry GK. Antimicrobial-resistant *Shigella sonnei*: limited antimicrobial treatment options for children and challenges of interpreting in vitro azithromycin susceptibility. *Pediatr Infect Dis J.* 2005;24(6):494–497

65. Taneja N, Lyngdoh VW, Sharma M. Haemolytic uraemic syndrome due to ciprofloxacin-resistant *Shigella dysenteriae* serotype 1. *J Med Microbiol.* 2005;54(Pt 10):997–998

66. Bennish ML, Khan WA, Begum M, et al. Low risk of hemolytic uremic syndrome after early effective antimicrobial therapy for *Shigella dysenteriae* type 1 infection in Bangladesh. *Clin Infect Dis.* 2006;42(3):356–362

67. Girgis NI, Sultan Y, Hammad O, Farid Z. Comparison of the efficacy, safety and cost of cefixime, ceftriaxone and aztreonam in the treatment of multidrug-resistant *Salmonella typhi* septicemia in children. *Pediatr Infect Dis J.* 1995;14(7):603–605

68. Girgis NI, Tribble DR, Sultan Y, Farid Z. Short course chemotherapy with cefixime in children with multidrug-resistant *Salmonella typhi* septicaemia. *J Trop Pediatr.* 1995;41(6):364–365

69. Neill MA, Opal SM, Heelan J, et al. Failure of ciprofloxacin to eradicate convalescent fecal excretion after acute salmonellosis: experience during an outbreak in health care workers. *Ann Intern Med.* 1991;114(3):195–199

70. Sirinavin S, Thavornnunth J, Sakchainanont B, Bangtrakulnonth A, Chongthawonsatid S, Junumporn S. Norfloxacin and azithromycin for treatment of nontyphoidal salmonella carriers. *Clin Infect Dis.* 2003;37(5):685–691

71. Outbreaks of multidrug-resistant *Shigella sonnei* gastroenteritis associated with day care centers – Kansas, Kentucky, and Missouri, 2005. *MMWR Morb Mortal Wkly Rep.* 2006;55(39):1068–1071

72. Replogle ML, Fleming DW, Cieslak PR. Emergence of antimicrobial-resistant shigellosis in Oregon. *Clin Infect Dis.* 2000;30(3):515–519

73. Ashkenazi S, Levy I, Kazaronovski V, Samra Z. Growing antimicrobial resistance of *Shigella* isolates. *J Antimicrob Chemother.* 2003;51(2):427–429

74. Aysev AD, Guriz H. Drug resistance of *Shigella* strains isolated in Ankara, Turkey, 1993–1996. *Scand J Infect Dis.* 1998;30(4):351–353

75. Mates A, Eyny D, Philo S. Antimicrobial resistance trends in *Shigella* serogroups isolated in Israel, 1990–1995. *Eur J Clin Microbiol Infect Dis.* 2000;19(2):108–111

76. Ozmert EN, Gokturk B, Yurdakok K, Yalcin SS, Gur D. *Shigella* antibiotic resistance in central Turkey: comparison of the years 1987–1994 and 1995–2002. *J Pediatr Gastroenterol Nutr.* 2005;40(3):359–362

77. Vasilev V, Japheth R, Yishai R, Andorn N. Antimicrobial resistance of *Shigella flexneri* serotypes in Israel during a period of three years: 2000–2002. *Epidemiol Infect.* 2004;132(6):1049–1054

78. Carlson JR, Thornton SA, DuPont HL, West AH, Mathewson JJ. Comparative in vitro activities of ten antimicrobial agents against bacterial enteropathogens. *Antimicrob Agents Chemother.* 1983;24(4):509–513

79. Flores A, Araque M, Vizcaya L. Multiresistant *Shigella* species isolated from pediatric patients with acute diarrheal disease. *Am J Med Sci.* 1998;316(6):379–384

80. Fulla N, Prado V, Duran C, Lagos R, Levine MM. Surveillance for antimicrobial resistance profiles among *Shigella* species isolated from a semirural community in the northern administrative area of santiago, Chile. *Am J Trop Med Hyg.* 2005;72(6):851–854

81. Gomi H, Jiang ZD, Adachi JA, et al. In vitro antimicrobial susceptibility testing of bacterial enteropathogens causing traveler's diarrhea in four geographic regions. *Antimicrob Agents Chemother.* 2001;45(1):212–216

82. Isenbarger DW, Hoge CW, Srijan A, et al. Comparative antibiotic resistance of diarrheal pathogens from Vietnam and Thailand, 1996–1999. *Emerg Infect Dis.* 2002;8(2):175–180

83. Jahan Y, Hossain A. Multiple drug-resistant *Shigella dysenteriae* type 1 in Rajbari district, Bangladesh. *J Diarrhoeal Dis Res.* 1997;15(1):17–20

84. MoezArdalan K, Zali MR, Dallal MM, Hemami MR, Salmanzadeh-Ahrabi S. Prevalence and pattern of antimicrobial resistance of *Shigella* species among patients with acute diarrhoea in Karaj, Tehran, Iran. *J Health Popul Nutr.* 2003;21(2):96–102

85. Tjaniadi P, Lesmana M, Subekti D, et al. Antimicrobial resistance of bacterial pathogens associated with diarrheal patients in Indonesia. *Am J Trop Med Hyg.* 2003;68(6):666–670

86. Pazhani GP, Ramamurthy T, Mitra U, Bhattacharya SK, Niyogi SK. Species diversity and antimicrobial resistance of *Shigella* spp. isolated between 2001 and 2004 from hospitalized children with diarrhoea in Kolkata (Calcutta), India. *Epidemiol Infect.* 2005;133(6):1089–1095

87. Ahmed SF, Riddle MS, Wierzba TF, et al. Epidemiology and genetic characterization of *Shigella flexneri* strains isolated from three paediatric populations in Egypt (2000–2004). *Epidemiol Infect.* 2006;134(6):1237–1248

88. Iwalokun BA, Gbenle GO, Smith SI, Ogunledun A, Akinsinde KA, Omonigbehin EA. Epidemiology of shigellosis in Lagos, Nigeria: trends in antimicrobial resistance. *J Health Popul Nutr.* 2001;19(3):183–190

89. Shapiro RL, Kumar L, Phillips-Howard P, et al. Antimicrobial-resistant bacterial diarrhea in rural western Kenya. *J Infect Dis.* 2001;183(11):1701–1704

Chapter 58
Antimicrobial Resistance in Vibrios

Michael L. Bennish, Wasif A. Khan, and Debasish Saha

1 Introduction

This chapter addresses antimicrobial resistance in a genus – *Vibrio* – that results in two distinct clinical syndromes. One is profound diarrheal disease – cholera – caused by *Vibrio cholerae* O1 or O139. The other is often the fatal wound infection and sepsis caused by a variety of halophilic (salt-loving) vibrios (1) – with *V. vulnificus* and *V. parahaemolyticus* perhaps being the most commonly occurring species (2–4) but including infections with *V. alginolyticus* (5), *V. harveyi, V. fluvialis,* and others (6).

V. cholerae serogroups in addition to *V. cholerae* O1 and O139 have been associated with diarrhea (7, 8), as have other *Vibrio* species, including *V. parahaemolyticus* (9) and *V. mimicus* (10). Lacking the genetic endowment to produce cholera toxin (11), these other vibrios rarely cause diarrhea severe enough to require antimicrobial therapy and will not be discussed in this chapter.

The primary reservoir for all vibrios is marine or estuarine waters – primarily in tropical and subtropical areas, but occasionally in temperate regions as well (12). The pathogenesis and epidemiology, however, of the two clinical syndromes caused by vibrios – cholera or wound infection and sepsis – differ substantially, and affect how antimicrobials are used and the development of resistance to antimicrobial use.

Cholera caused by infection with *V. cholerae* O1 or O139 results from ingestion of contaminated water or food, and infection is confined to the intestinal lumen. Hundreds of thousands of persons are reported infected worldwide annually (13). The actual number is likely to be in the millions, as many countries, including those with endemic cholera, do not report cases to the World Health Organization (13). Both the endemic disease and epidemics, which can affect tens or hundreds of thousands of persons in nonendemic areas (particularly

refugee camps), occur (14). Infections are almost entirely confined to poor countries lacking basic hygiene, sanitation, and access to potable water. Infections occur in all ages, but in endemic areas disproportionately affect the young (15, 16).

Because of the large numbers of persons infected, numerous randomized controlled trials have been conducted since the 1960s on the utility and choice of antimicrobial agents for therapy, providing a solid evidence base for determining therapy (17–25). The large number of infected persons has also provided extensive information on resistance patterns, usually obtained as part of systematic surveys or at large research centers devoted to the study of enteric infections (26–41).

Because most infections occur in isolated areas of the poorest developing countries, without access to basic diagnostic microbiologic facilities, most facilities that provide care to patients with cholera are not able to isolate the infecting organism or determine antimicrobial susceptibility. In any case, antimicrobial treatment is required early in the course of illness if it is to be useful. Cholera is a disease that strikes rapidly (patients can purge a volume of water equal to their body weight in 24 h). By the time the organism is isolated and susceptibility patterns determined, the patient will be either dead or better.

In contrast, vibrio infections causing wound infections or sepsis result from ingestion of contaminated seafood, or inoculation through skin by injury while in contaminated waters, or while handling seafood (42–45); are locally and systemically invasive (2, 3, 45); occur sporadically and in relatively small numbers (44–46); and disproportionately infect the elderly and the immunocompromised, especially those with cirrhosis (4, 44, 45, 47). Infections are most commonly reported from rich and medium-income countries, perhaps because ascertainment is difficult in poor countries. There have been no randomized trials defining best antimicrobial therapy, and reports on patterns of resistance are based upon small numbers of clinical isolates or surveys of environmental isolates (6, 48–53). Patients are most likely to be cared for in hospital settings where definitive microbiologic diagnoses and ascertainment of antimicrobial resistance can be done (3).

This chapter will discuss each of the two clinical syndromes – cholera and wound infection and sepsis – in turn.

M. Bennish (✉)
Department of Population, Family and Reproductive Health, Bloomberg School of Public Health, Johns Hopkins University, Baltimore, MD Mpilonhle, Mtubatuba, South Africa
mbennish@jhsph.edu

D.L. Mayers (ed.), *Antimicrobial Drug Resistance,*
DOI 10.1007/978-1-60327-595-8_58, © Humana Press, a part of Springer Science+Business Media, LLC 2009

2 Cholera Caused by *V. cholerae* O1 or O139

2.1 *Geographic Spread and Epidemiology of Resistance*

Tetracycline was the first antimicrobial agent systematically evaluated for the treatment of cholera (23–25) and it soon established itself as the drug of choice for treating this disease. For the first two decades of its use – until the late 1970s – reported resistance to tetracycline was rare. Resistance to other agents used for cholera treatment – including ampicillin, chloramphenicol, and trimethoprim–sulfamethoxazole – was also infrequent. In a report on 1,109 isolates of *V. cholerae* O1 obtained from patients in the Philippines in 1969, only 11 (1.0%) demonstrated resistance to drugs then in use for treatment (54). In a report of 1,156 strains from Asia, Africa, and Europe reported on in 1976, only 27 (2.7%) were resistant to one of the drugs tested – tetracycline, ampicillin, chloramphenicol, or a sulfa agent – all drugs then used to treat cholera (55).

By the end of the 1970s, however, plasmid-mediated multiple-drug-resistance to tetracycline, ampicillin, chloramphenicol, and trimethoprim–sulfamethoxazole was being commonly reported from *V. cholerae* O1 strains isolated in Asia and Africa (56–58). Since then, multiple-antimicrobial resistance has been a characteristic feature of *V. cholerae* O1 from Africa (33, 36, 59–61), Asia (18–20, 28–31, 35, 39–41, 62–77), Europe (38, 78), and South and Central America (Table 1) (79–81).

V. cholerae O139 was a new serogroup of *V. cholerae* first identified in 1992 when it caused large epidemics of cholera in Bangladesh and subsequently in other Asian countries (82). This was the first non-O1 serogroup of *V. cholerae* to produce cholera toxin and to cause epidemic cholera. The epidemic strain evolved from a *V. cholerae* El Tor O1 strain that had acquired the O139 antigen-encoding genes following horizontal gene transfer from a donor strain and recombination with the El Tor O1 chromosome (83, 84). The O139 epidemic strain also differed from endemic O1 strains by its resistance to trimethoprim, sulfamethoxazole, streptomycin, and furazolidone. Resistance to the first three of these antibiotics was conferred by the presence in initial isolates of *V. cholerae* O139 of a novel transmissible genetic element – termed a "constin" for an acronym of its properties: conjugative, self-transmissible, and integrating (85, 86).

Resistance in both *V. cholerae* O1 and O139 is not easily predictable for a number of reasons. In endemic areas, especially in south Asia, there may be multiple clones of either *V. cholerae* O1 or O139 circulating simultaneously, and these different clones may have differing antimicrobial susceptibilities (63, 66, 87–89). In nonendemic areas, outbreaks usually result from introduction of a single strain of *V. cholerae* O1 or O139 (90), and most initial infections will be due to organisms with identical antimicrobial resistance profiles (90). Over time, however, these epidemic strains may acquire antimicrobial resistance. Isolates obtained from patients later in the epidemic may have differing antimicrobial resistance patterns when compared to initial isolates (27, 36, 61, 76, 91).

Antimicrobial resistance in *V. cholerae* O1 and O139 is encoded by a number of mobile genetic elements – plasmids (36, 57, 59, 61, 70, 71, 78, 92), integrons (27, 34, 78, 91–95), and constins (85, 86, 93–96) – that can be acquired from other *V. cholerae*, including non-O1 or O139 serogroups that are in the aquatic environment where *V. cholerae* O1 and O139 reside, and from other Gram-negative bacteria in the gut (79). These mobile elements are not stable (86). With changing antimicrobial pressure and other ecological changes, resistance can be acquired and resistant strains quickly propagate, or resistance genes can be lost and susceptibility reestablished. Such ecological pressure also enhances the selection of isolates with chromosomal mutational changes in antimicrobial gene targets or antimicrobial efflux pump mechanisms (97, 98) – such as the recent emergence of *V. cholerae* O1 isolates with diminished susceptibility, and clinical resistance, to the fluoroquinolones (19, 31, 67, 68, 73, 99).

Acquisition and loss of resistance genes have been clearly illustrated by recent experience with *V. cholerae* O139 infections in Asia. After the initial epidemics of cholera caused by this new serogroup of *V. cholerae* in the first half of the 1990s, this pathogen largely disappeared as a cause of diarrhea. When infections reappeared in the latter part of the decade, the organism had lost its resistance to trimethoprim–sulfamethoxazole, one of its original defining characteristics (28, 63, 100–102). This was due to the antibiotic resistance gene cluster in the SXT-related constin having been deleted (86). Paradoxically, the clones of *V. cholerae* O1 that emerged after the *V. cholerae* O139 epidemic had subsided (*V. cholerae* O1 as a cause of cholera virtually disappeared during the height of the O139 epidemic in the Indian subcontinent) were resistant to trimethoprim–sulfamethoxazole as a result of acquisition of the trimethoprim–sulfamethoxazole (SXT) constin encoding resistance to trimethoprim–sulfamethoxazole (86). Multidrug-resistant isolates of *V. cholerae* O1 containing the SXT element have also been identified in Africa (27).

What is the current status of antimicrobial resistance in *V. cholerae* O1 and O139? Making broad generalizations is difficult. Resistance patterns vary geographically because circulating strains in any area are likely to have evolved from parent strains that may have been the source of the initial epidemics, either acquiring or losing resistance genotypes.

Table 1 Reports of susceptibility of *V. cholerae* O1 to antimicrobial agents

Author and reference	Country	Years isolates obtained	Number of isolates tested	Percent of isolates resistant									
				AMP	AZM	CHL	CIP	DOX	ERY	FUR	NAL	SXT	TET
Israil et al. (38)	Romania	1995	116	–	–	3	–	0	–	100	97	100	2
Yamamoto et al. (37)	India	1985–1990	67	–	–	99	–	–	–	99	–	99	0
	Bangladesh	1994	30	–	–	83	–	–	–	97	–	100	43
	Peru	1991	52	–	–	0	–	–	–	0	–	2	0
Sheikh et al. (39)	Pakistan	1996	54	–	–	29	–	–	56	–	2	96	91
Mwansa et al. (36)	Zambia	1990	163	–	–	13	–	–	–	–	–	–	2
		1990–1991	121	–	–	39	–	–	–	–	–	–	3
		1991–1992	263	–	–	78	–	70	0	–	–	97	95
		1992–1993	26	–	–	–	–	–	–	–	–	–	93
		1994–1997	39	–	–	64	–	–	0	–	–	92	77
		1998–2002	50	–	–	0	–	–	2	–	–	100	24
		2003[a]	125	100	–	a	–	–	a	–	–	100	0
		2004[a]	150	100	–	a	–	–	a	–	–	100	0
Campos et al. (79)	Brazil	1991–1999	92	93	–	0	2	–	–	40	0	0	79
Olukoya et al. (59)	Nigeria	1992	86	58	–	9	0	–	0	–	–	–	41
Mukhopadhyay et al. (64)	India	1992	27	33	–	15	0	–	–	96	07	37	11
		1993	20	25	–	30	0	–	–	85	05	80	10
		1994	22	82	–	64	0	–	–	100	96	100	9
Garg et al. (30)	India	1997	73	100	–	19	19	–	–	100	94	98	–
Dhar et al. (29)	Bangladesh	1993–1994	110	–	–	–	0	1	1	73	–	95	42
Srifuenfung et al. (77)	Thailand	1994–2001	290	8	–	–	0	–	–	–	–	1	16
Das et al. (28)	India	2000	150	–	–	0	–	–	–	98	100	98	0
Dubon et al. (80)	Honduras	1997	11	36	–	27	27	75	9	–	0	27	27
Urassa et al. (33)	Tanzania	1999	87	54	–	53	0	–	54	–	81	97	41
Sundaram et al. (74)	India	1997–2001	321	–	–	0	0	–	–	–	–	97	0
Zachariah et al. (60)	Malawi	1999–2000	32		–	47	3	28	50	94	19	91	–
Mishra et al. (40)	India	2003	198	85	–	–	62	–	–	–	–	–	68
Sabeena et al. (75)	India	2000	25	52	–	16	16	–	–	100	92	88	08
Saha (20)[b]	Bangladesh	2001–02	141	–	–	0	0	0	0	100	–	99	0
Saha et al. (19)[b]	Bangladesh	2002–04	168	–	0	0	0	0	0	100	–	100	0
Sur et al. (16)[c]	India	2003–04	77	–	33	–	18	10	91	92	–	79	01
ICDDR,B Dhaka Hospital Surveillance System – unpublished data	Bangladesh	2006	618	–	–	–	0	41	99	100	–	99	41

Abbreviation for antimicrobial agents: *AMP* ampicillin; *AZM* azithromycin; *CHL* chloramphenicol; *CIP* ciprofloxacin; *DOX* doxycycline; *ERY* erythromycin; *FUR* furazolidone; *NAL* nalidixic acid, *SXT* trimethoprim–sulfamethoxazole; *TET*, tetracycline

All studies included in the table used the agar disc-diffusion method to determine susceptibility, with the exception of Yamamoto et al. (37), which used broth dilution MIC testing

[a]Isolates were reported to show reduced susceptibility to chloramphenicol and erythromycin during these 2 years

[b]Strains were susceptible to ciprofloxacin when tested by disc-diffusion method, but the MIC values were increased for these strains when compared to strains isolated in earlier years, and clinical response to ciprofloxacin was poor

[c]Strains that tested as having intermediate susceptibility were reported as resistant

This results in a great variety of resistance phenotypes in areas where cholera is endemic or epidemic.

Making the tracking and reporting of resistance more difficult, there is no easily available and up-to-date source tracking resistance patterns. As can be ascertained from Table 1, summarizing global resistance patterns in *V. cholerae* O1, or Table 2, summarizing resistance to O139 requires for the most part relying on literature reporting on findings, which even at the time of publication are likely to be – because of time required for data collation, manuscript writing, and the publication process – 2 or more years old. In addition, reports are likely to be weighted to reporting resistance, which is presumably more publication worthy, than reporting the absence of resistance, thus providing a skewed picture of actual resistance patterns. The Weekly Epidemiologic Record published by the World Health Organization is the one publication that regularly contains updates on cholera outbreaks as part of its "Outbreak News" feature, but these reports most often do not contain information on antimicrobial susceptibility patterns (Table 2).

Despite the increased awareness in recent years of the problem of resistance, there is no available online source where resistance patterns for tropical infections such as *V. cholerae* can be reported and the results obtained in a timely fashion. Such a resource would greatly enhance management of cholera in remote areas, where healthcare providers are now more likely to have access to the Internet than to published reports on antimicrobial resistance. Susceptibility profiles determined in reference hospitals in national capitals, or as part of outbreak investigations by international teams, rarely filter down to healthcare staff at the district level.

With the above as a caveat, the current picture of resistance in *V. cholerae* O1, the major current cause of cholera, is disconcerting (Table 1). Multidrug-resistant *V. cholerae* O1 is now commonplace in most areas where cholera is endemic.

This situation is nowhere more evident than at the International Centre for Diarrhoeal Disease Research, Bangladesh (ICDDR, B) Hospital in Dhaka, Bangladesh, which cares for more than 30,000 patients with cholera caused by *V. cholerae* O1 annually (*V. cholerae* O139 has again disappeared as a cause of cholera in Bangladesh). During 2006, most isolates of *V. cholerae* O1 were commonly resistant or had diminished susceptibility to all the antimicrobial agents that have been shown in clinical trials to be effective in the treatment of cholera (103). Virtually all isolates at the ICDDR,B in 2006 were resistant by disc-diffusion testing to trimethoprim–sulfamethoxazole and furazolidone, barely half were susceptible to tetracycline and its congener doxycycline, only 5% were fully susceptible to erythromycin and its congener azithromycin, and virtually all isolates had diminished susceptibility and clinical resistance to the fluoroquinolones (Fig. 1) (103, 104).

Table 2 Reports of susceptibility of *V. cholerae* O139 to antimicrobial agents

Authors and reference	Country	Years isolates obtained	Number of isolates tested	Percentage of isolates resistant									
				AMP	AZM	CHL	CIP	DOX	ERY	FUR	NAL	SXT	TET
Yamamoto et al. (37)	Bangladesh, India, Thailand	1992–1993	167	–	–	96	–	–	–	95	–	96	0
Garg et al. (30)	India	1997	71	100	–	3	01	–	–	100	7	–	1
Dhar et al. (29)	Bangladesh	1993–1994	132	–	–	–	0	0	0	07	–	97	100
Sheikh et al. (39)	Pakistan	1994	112	–	–	35	–	–	75	–	01	99	01
Mukhopadhyay et al. (64)	India	1994	17	71	–	29	0	–	–	100	0	100	0
Srifuenfung et al. (77)	Thailand	1994–2001	240	01	–	–	0	–	–	–	–	0	71
Das et al. (28)	India	2000	150	–	–	0	–	–	–	93	100	3	0
Sundaram et al. (74)	India	1997–2001	479	–	–	0	0	–	–	–	–	49	0
Saha et al. (20)	Bangladesh	2001–2002	21	–	–	0	0	0	0	–	–	0	0
Saha et al. (19)	Bangladesh	2002–2004	14	–	0	–	0	0	0	0	–	0	0

Abbreviation for antimicrobial agents: *AMP* ampicillin; *AZM* azithromycin; *CHL* chloramphenicol; *CIP* ciprofloxacin; *DOX* doxycycline; *ERY* erythromycin; *FUR* furazolidone; *NAL* nalidixic acid; *SXT* trimethoprim–sulfamethoxazole; *TET* tetracycline

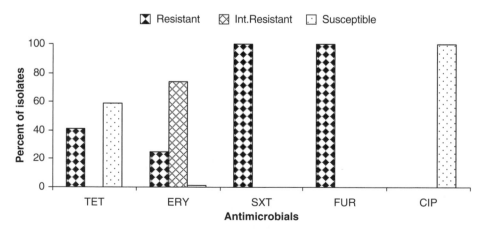

Fig. 1 Antimicrobial susceptibility of 683 *V. cholerae* O1 isolates from the ICDDR,B Dhaka Diarrhea Treatment Centre, in 2006. Antimicrobial susceptibility testing was done by the disc diffusion method. Key to antimicrobial agents: *TET* tetracycline; *ERY* erythromycin; *SXT* trimethoprim–sulfamethoxazole; *FUR* furazolidone; *CIP* ciprofloxacin. Although all isolates were susceptible to ciprofloxacin when tested by the disc-diffusion method, testing of selected isolates by broth dilution showed a 125-fold increase in minimum inhibitory concentration from previous years (from 0.002 μg/mL in 1996 to 0.250 μg/mL in 2006), and infected patients did not respond clinically to treatment with ciprofloxacin. Intermediate susceptibility to erythromycin was defined as a zone size of 14–22 mm

Virtually all *V. cholerae* O1 isolates at the ICDDR,B appear to be susceptible to fluoroquinolones when tested by either the disc-diffusion method (zone of inhibition >21 mm) or the minimum inhibitory concentration method (MICs below the threshold level of <1 μg/mL that is used for defining resistance) (104). From 1994 to 2006, however, the MIC (90) to ciprofloxacin of *V. cholerae* O1 increased from 0.012 to 0.250 μg/mL (19, 104). At the same time, the MIC (90) for nalidixic acid increased from 32 to ≥256 μg/mL. Isolates resistant to nalidixic acid by disc-diffusion had a median ciprofloxacin MIC of 0.190 μg/mL compared to 0.002 μg/mL for nalidixic acid-susceptible isolates. Importantly, the rate of clinical success of single-dose ciprofloxacin treatment of patients infected with nalidixic acid-resistant isolates was only 18%, compared to 94% for the treatment of patients with nalidixic acid-susceptible isolates (104). Clearly, as with *Salmonella* (105) and *Neisseria gonorrheae* (106), applying the in vivo breakpoints for determining susceptibility of Enterobacteriaceae to the fluoroquinolones does not predict in vivo response to these agents during cholera.

Resistance is not fixed. With diminished antimicrobial pressure there is hope that susceptible isolates may again establish themselves. In addition to the example of loss of resistance genotypes in *V. cholerae* O139, the experience at the ICDDR,B is that resistance to tetracycline can vary quickly over time. Resistance rates among *V. cholerae* O1 reached over 80% in the early 1990s, disappeared by the latter part of that decade, only to return in 2004, and then greatly diminish in early 2007 (103).

The picture is not entirely grim. Reports from some areas suggest that most strains of *V. cholerae* O1 remain susceptible to commonly used agents. Of 77 *V. cholerae* O1 isolates from Kolkata, India, in 2003 and 2004, all but 1 remained susceptible to tetracycline (16). These isolates are, however, from a period before tetracycline resistance in *V. cholerae* O1 reemerged in the neighboring megalopolis of Durban, and the susceptibility pattern in Kolkata may also have changed since this study was reported. In Jakarta, Indonesia, more than 90% of *V. cholerae* O1 isolates from 2001 to 2003 remained susceptible to the first-line agents tetracycline, trimethoprim–sulfamethoxazole, and the fluoroquinolones (15). In Vietnam, *V. cholerae* O1 multidrug resistance was common in surveys in 1995 and 2000, but had become susceptible to all agents tested in 2002 – a change associated with the loss of the class I integron and the SXT constin that *V. cholerae* O1 strains had earlier contained (34).

2.2 Clinical Significance

Fortunately, antimicrobial use in cholera is adjunctive therapy, rather than essential for cure. Because *V. cholerae* O1 and O139 are noninvasive and self-limited infections, the infectious process is in itself not lethal – i.e., there are no infection-induced inflammatory changes leading to cell death, tissue destruction, and organ dysfunction. The lethal consequence of *V. cholerae* O1 and O139 are related to cholera toxin production. The latter elicits in the small bowel the voluminous secretory diarrhea that is characteristic of the disease. Replacement of fluids – either orally (for patients with mild or moderate disease), or both orally and intravenously (for patients with severe cholera) – is lifesaving (107).

Antimicrobials can, however, reduce the volume of diarrhea by half to two-thirds, and duration of diarrhea by half (20, 107, 108). Without antimicrobial therapy, patients severely ill with cholera will purge approximately 750 mL/kg body weight after presenting for care; with effective antimicrobial therapy it is reduced to 250 mL/kg body weight (20, 24, 25, 108). In a 50 kg person, a 500 mL/kg difference amounts to 25 L during the course of their stay for treatment. The duration of diarrhea is reduced from a mean of slightly less than 4 days to slightly less than 2 days.

The reduction in fluid losses and the consequent reduction in fluid replacement needs have important consequences for management of patients. In inexperienced hands, management of fluid volume replacement in severely dehydrated cholera patients can be problematic, with healthcare providers often not giving sufficient fluids, resulting in unnecessary mortality. In experienced hands, mortality in cholera should be 0.2% or less (41). Cholera mortality, overall, however, remain 10–20 times higher than that (13), and during epidemics can reach almost 50%, as it did during a large outbreak of multiple-drug-resistant *V. cholerae* O1 infection in Rwandan refugee camps (14). Inexperienced or overwhelmed staff has difficulty judging the magnitude of fluid replacement required, most often underestimating the volume needed. Operational constraints – too many patients, too few staff, very few, if any, trained staff, lack of supplies – are also major impediments to successful treatment of patients with cholera. These problems are exacerbated by the fact that cholera is most common where capacity is most limited. By reducing fluid requirements and duration of illness, effective antimicrobial therapy can greatly reduce the logistic constraints of treating patients with severe cholera. In the end, effective antimicrobial therapy reduces not only the cost of treatment, but can substantially affect mortality.

Treatment of cholera is empiric. In cholera-endemic areas, or during cholera outbreaks, any adult with severe watery diarrhea is assumed to have cholera (107). Standard therapy is replacement of fluids – orally if the patient is not vomiting excessively and has none to some dehydration according to WHO criteria, or intravenously if the patient is severely dehydrated or has a high rate of purging (>5 mL/kg body weight/h) (109). All patients with dehydration or a high purging rate should also be treated with an antimicrobial, with the choice of agent guided by pre-existing knowledge of the susceptibility pattern of circulating strains (109).

2.3 Laboratory Diagnosis of Resistance

Laboratory diagnosis of resistance in individual patients for the purposes of selecting an antimicrobial agent is not useful. The benefit of antimicrobial treatment is evinced when treatment is provided early in the course of illness, rather than after the 48–72 h required for isolation and susceptibility testing of the infecting strain of *V. cholerae* O1 and O139. The choice of antibiotic for treatment must be based on knowledge of the pattern of resistance of circulating strains. Susceptibility testing is used therefore for monitoring the resistance profile of circulating strains as part of surveillance of endemic or epidemic disease.

Disc-diffusion testing on agar plates is the most commonly used means of determining susceptibility (110, 111). Disc-diffusion testing has the advantage of simplicity, low cost, and reproducibility, all crucial concerns when conducting antimicrobial susceptibility testing in the impoverished settings where cholera occurs. These settings often lack even the most basic diagnostic capacity, and field laboratories usually have to be established during epidemics so that isolation and susceptibility testing can be conducted. These conditions preclude the use of more sophisticated automated systems, no matter how reliable they might be in other settings (112).

There are limitations to the use of the disc-diffusion method. Clinical and Laboratory Standards Institute (CLSI, formerly National Committee for Clinical Laboratory Standards, NCCLS) interpretive standards have been established for testing of *V. cholerae* only for ampicillin, chloramphenicol, sulfonamides, tetracycline, and trimethoprim–sulfamethoxazole (110). Disc-diffusion testing of doxycycline susceptibility does not accurately predict clinical response. Patients infected with *V. cholerae* strains that test susceptible to doxycycline but resistant to tetracycline will not respond to doxycycline administration (17). Therefore tetracycline susceptibility testing, rather than doxycycline susceptibility testing, should be used when doxycycline is being considered for treatment of *V. cholerae* O1 or O139 infections. Neither disc-diffusion nor broth-dilution susceptibility standards have been established for testing of erythromycin or azithromycin. It is important, therefore, to determine clinical response when these agents are used. The latter is easier said than done, as systematic evaluation of clinical response is often deficient during the tumult and chaos surrounding a cholera epidemic, or even in endemic settings where cholera is treated.

Disc-diffusion breakpoints for ciprofloxacin, furazolidone, and nalidixic acid have not been established, and the breakpoints used for Enterobacteriaceae are commonly used instead when interpreting *V. cholerae* O1 or O139 susceptibility to these agents (110). Tentative zone diameter breakpoints have been proposed: ≥18 mm for furazolidone, ≥19 mm for nalidixic acid, and ≥21 mm for ciprofloxacin (110). The latter proposed breakpoint does not, however, correlate with clinical response. Patients infected with *V. cholerae* O1 strains that were susceptible to ciprofloxacin using the proposed ciprofloxacin susceptibility breakpoint, but that had ciprofloxacin MICs of 0.250 μg/mL when determined using the E-test, did not respond to ciprofloxacin treatment (19). Thus ciprofloxacin disc-diffusion results cannot be used for determining susceptibility in *V. cholerae* O1 and O139.

Because fluoroquinolones are an important option for treatment of cholera and other enteric infections, it is important to have some method of determining susceptibility in the absence of disc-diffusion testing. One option is to use nalidixic acid susceptibilities – and consider all isolates resistant to nalidixic acid in disc-diffusion testing clinically resistant to the fluoroquinolones (104). Another option is to use the E-test to determine MICs.

The E-test, though more expensive than disc-diffusion testing, has the same advantages as disc-diffusion testing of simplicity and reliability for use in the developing-country settings. Strains with an MIC to ciprofloxacin of ≥0.250 μg/mL should be considered clinically resistant (19); strains with an MIC ≤0.025 μg/mL, though resistant to nalidixic acid by the disc-diffusion method, will have at least an intermediate clinical response to ciprofloxacin (20, 104); strains with a ciprofloxacin E-test MIC of ≤0.002 μg/mL will be susceptible to nalidixic acid by disc-diffusion testing, and will be fully responsive to ciprofloxacin therapy.

Although disc-diffusion standards for erythromycin or azithromycin susceptibility have not been established, strains with an E-test MIC of ≤0.750 μg/mL of erythromycin or an azithromycin E-test MIC of ≤0.125 μg/mL have been shown to be clinically responsive to these agents (18, 19).

A common problem with medical care in countries where cholera is endemic is the lack of access to current information on susceptibility patterns. Libraries and journals are often not available in remote regions – or even in capital cities. The Internet could potentially lessen the problem of access, but cost – of both Internet access and journals – remains a problem. CLSI updates are costly, as are journal subscriptions.

2.4 Treatment Alternatives

In situations where almost half of all *V. cholerae* isolates are resistant to all antimicrobial agents known to be effective in the treatment of cholera, as has recently been the case in Bangladesh, alternatives for empiric therapy are limited.

One nonrandomized study suggested that the use of tetracycline has some efficacy even in patients whose isolates are resistant in vitro (113). Although single-dose ciprofloxacin was ineffective in the treatment of *V. cholerae* O1 infections with an increased MIC to ciprofloxacin (19), retrospective observations suggest that multiple-dose therapy might be effective (104). Both observations need evaluation in randomized, controlled trials.

Rifaximin is an older, nonabsorbable antimicrobial agent that has drawn interest as a treatment for enteric infections (114, 115). *V. cholerae* are in vitro susceptible to concentrations achievable in the gut lumen (32). Initial clinical studies, however, have not been promising. The pipeline of new antimicrobials that might be used for treatment of multiply resistant *V. cholerae* infections is sparse (116). A drug to be useful in cholera must be active in vitro, attain high concentrations in the gut lumen, be orally administered, and be inexpensive. No antimicrobial agent currently under evaluation meets those criteria – even if the cost is not considered.

A novel, and potentially more promising approach to treatment is inhibition of virulence gene expression during infection (117, 118). A small molecule (termed virstatin by its discoverers) has been identified that inhibits a transcriptional regulator governing expression of two virulence factors – cholera toxin and toxin-coregulated pilus – essential in the pathogenesis of clinical cholera. Virstatin has been shown to be effective in a mouse model of cholera, but has not yet been tested in humans (117).

2.5 Infection Control Measures

The most effective means of avoiding the problem of antimicrobial resistance in *V. cholerae* is to prevent cholera by the provision of potable water and improved santiation (119). Unfortunately, most parts of the of the world still lack access to clean water – something that should be considered a basic human right (120). Efforts for the provision of potable water from central systems have proved problematic in the rural areas of developing countries. There have been substantial efforts to dig tube wells, but maintenance and unintended consequences (high levels of arsenic in some tube wells in the Indian subcontinent) have been proven to be stumbling blocks to these programs (121). Even within confined geographic areas, arsenic contamination of aquifers is not consistent, however, and efforts have been made to identify sites were tube wells can be safely placed.

An alternative, or supplemental, solution for the provision of potable water has been efforts to sterilize water after it is collected but before it is ingested. These efforts have included using locally available materials – such as the cloth that is used for making saris – to filter out the copepods and other marine life that carry *V. cholerae* (122). Other methods include the use of narrow-mouth (to prevent continued contamination) water containers to which chlorine is added (123), or use of ceramic water filters (124). All such methods recognize that centralized systems to provide potable water remain a distant aspiration for most of the world's population, especially those living in rural areas, and that methods for providing safe drinking water have to be inexpensive (for instance boiling water is too expensive for most persons lacking clean water) and adapted to poor, rural conditions.

An alterative to provision of clean water for prevention is provision of cholera vaccine (13). There are two killed vaccines that are currently licensed in at least some countries. Current WHO recommendations are that these vaccines may be of use during emergency and refugee situations at high risk of cholera outbreaks. Their utility and routine use in endemic situations are still being debated (13).

3 Disease Caused by Vibrios Other than *V. cholerae* O1 or O139

3.1 Geographic Spread and Epidemiology of Resistance

Summarizing resistance patterns for *V. vulnificus* and other non-cholera *Vibrio* species causing invasive disease is complicated by their relatively rarity of isolation from humans, the equal rarity of reports in the literature on susceptibility, the scarcity of reports on mechanisms of resistance, the diversity of geographic sites in which they can be isolated, the absence for the most part of human-to-human spread and therefore the absence of a single strain causing multiple infections, and the absence until recently of standardized methods for susceptibility testing.

Ecologic studies suggest that there are a diverse array of non-cholera vibrios in the aquatic environment, with differing antimicrobial resistance patterns, that may cause infection (125). Reports on antimicrobial susceptibility that do exist in the literature often incorporate environmental isolates as well as human isolates. Many reports on susceptibility date from the 1970s and 1980s when the taxonomy of the non-cholera *Vibrio* species was first being established, and their relevance to current susceptibility patterns is uncertain (1, 6, 52, 126, 127).

More recent reports on *V. vulnificus*, the most common of the non-cholera vibrios causing invasive disease, suggest that *V. vulnificus* is susceptible to the fluoroquinolones

(2, 48–50, 53, 128, 129), cefotaxime and other third-generation cephalosporins (2, 49, 50, 53, 129, 130), trimethoprim–sulfamethoxazole (50, 53, 128), tetracycline or minocycline (2, 49, 50, 53, 129, 130), and imipenem (2, 50). Resistance to ampicillin was noted at the time these species were first characterized (1, 6, 52, 128), and resistance or intermediate susceptibility (MIC ≥1 μg/mL) remains common, as it does to first- or second-generation cephalosporins (2, 50, 53, 129, 130). The addition of clavulanate to ampicillin or amoxicillin reduces the MIC of strains that are frankly resistant to the β-lactam, but only to an MIC (90) of 4 μg/mL (50). Gentamicin has also shown at best intermediate activity against *V. vulnificus*, with a reported MIC (50) of 2 μg/mL MIC (90) of 4 μg/mL in two studies (2, 49), and MIC values double that in an earlier study (128).

Studies have also reported on the susceptibility of *V. alginolyticus,* and for the most part the pattern of resistance is similar to that reported for *V. vulnificus* (50, 53, 127). Reports on other tissue-invasive *Vibrio* species are even scarcer.

3.2 Clinical Significance

There are no controlled studies of antimicrobial therapy for tissue-invasive vibrios. Choice of therapy, therefore, is based upon relatively small series of patients, and extrapolated from in vitro or animal studies (2, 43, 48, 49, 126, 130). Unlike *V. cholerae* O1, where resistance is now widespread, the many drug classes that remain active against most of the halophilic (non-cholera) vibrios potentially offer multiple options for therapy.

Because patients with invasive disease caused by non-cholera vibrios are often immunocompromised, and the disease can be fulminate (illness onset within 36 h of exposure, 50% or higher fatality rate in most series), antimicrobial therapy must be started when infection is first suspected on the basis of clinical presentation and epidemiologic profile, and then adjusted on the basis of subsequent laboratory findings. Drug regimens suggested on the basis of in vitro and animal studies include ciprofloxacin and cefotaxime (49), single-agent treatment with tetracycline (126), single-agent fluoroquinolone therapy (48), and a combination of cefotaxime and minocycline, which was synergistic in vitro (131, 132).

In recent years, the largest series of patients reported in the literature has come from Taiwan. In general, the approach has been to treat with two drugs that are known to have good in vitro activity against non-cholera vibrios. A recent series reporting on 93 patients who received a variety of antimicrobial regimens suggested that the lowest fatality rate was achieved with a combination of a third-generation cephalosporin and tetracycline or a congener; patients treated with a first- or second-generation cephalosporin and an aminogly-coside did noticeably worse (3). These studies, like all uncontrolled retrospective studies, are subject to the limitations inherent to studies – selection of treatment regimens by severity of illness, changing antimicrobial regimens over time, and differences in provider care.

3.3 Laboratory Diagnosis of Resistance

Guidelines for susceptibility testing of non-cholera *Vibrio* species have only recently been established (133). The absence of such guidelines reflected the relative rarity of the isolation of these organisms from patients, thus resulting in a scarcity of information on the clinical and bacteriologic response to antimicrobial agents. The latter is a critical element for establishing breakpoints.

Both broth-dilution MIC and disc-diffusion testing are now considered appropriate and acceptable for determining susceptibility of these organisms, using standard media (cation-adjusted Mueller–Hinton broth or Mueller–Hinton agar, respectively). The recommended disc-diffusion breakpoints and the control organisms to use are derived from, and are the same as, for the more commonly isolated Enterobacteriaceae (133). The use of derived breakpoints for these "orphan" organisms recognizes that because of their infrequent isolation it was not possible to adhere to all the rigorous requirements for establishing breakpoints, especially correlation of the breakpoints with clinical response (133). The full guidelines for susceptibility testing of infrequently isolated bacteria, including non-cholera vibrios, can by found in CLSI standard M45-A (134).

3.4 Treatment Alternatives

Surgical treatment (incision and drainage, debridement of necrotic tissue, fasciotomies, or amputations) when required is an important adjunct to antimicrobial therapy (2, 3, 42, 43). Other crucial supportive measures include maintenance of blood pressure (septic shock is a common manifestation of infection, especially in immunocompromised hosts) and measures to control disseminated intravascular coagulation. But unlike the non-invasive disease caused by *V. cholerae* O1 or O139, antimicrobial therapy is essential for survival (Table 3).

3.5 Infection Control Measures

Patients with liver disease are at high risk for *V. vulnificus* septicemia. Raw seafood, especially oysters, is the most common vehicle of transmission (51). Efforts should be

Table 3 Options for antimicrobial treatment of cholera in adults and children

Drug	Dose	Adult dose	Pediatric dose
Ampicillin	Multiple	Not evaluated	12.5 mg/kg body weight every 6 h for 3 days (137)
	Single	Not evaluated	Not evaluated
Azithromycin	Multiple	Not evaluated	Not evaluated
	Single	1 g (19)	20 mg/kg body weight (18)
Ciprofloxacin	Multiple	500 mg every 24 h for 3 days (138, 139)	Not evaluated
	Single	1 g (17)	20 mg/kg body weight (20)
Doxycycline	Multiple	100 mg twice (q 12 h) on day 1, then 100 mg once on days 2–4 (22)	2 mg/kg body weight twice (q 12 h) on day 1, then 2 mg/kg body weight once on days 2–4 (22)
	Single	300 mg (21)	4 mg/kg body weight (22)
Erythromycin	Multiple	500 mg every 6 h for 3 days (138)	12.5 mg/kg body weight every 6 h for 3 days (140)
	Single	Not evaluated	Not evaluated
Tetracycline	Multiple	500 mg every 6 h for 3 days (138)	12.5 mg/kg body weight every 6 h for 3 days (137)
	Single	1 g (141)	Not evaluated
Trimethoprim–sulfamethoxazole	Multiple	160 mg of trimethoprim – 800 mg of sulfamethoxazole every 12 h for 3 days (142)	10 mg/kg trimethoprim – 50 mg/kg sulfamethoxazole per kg body weight every 12 h × 3 days (140)
	Single	Not evaluated	Not evaluated

Resistance to all of the listed agents is common. Selection of an agent for treatment of cholera depends on knowing the contemporaneous susceptibility pattern of *V. cholerae* in the locale where the infection occurred

made to warn all persons who are at high risk of disease to avoid eating raw or undercooked seafood. Posted warnings in restaurants or seafood shops are often not noticed by those at risk, either because they are not conspicuous, or they are in a language that is not understood by the person at risk (English language signs for high-risk Hispanic persons with liver disease in the US, for instance) (135). In at least one report from Japan, many healthcare providers in endemic areas were also unaware of the risk to persons with hepatic disease from eating raw or undercooked seafood (136). Other precautions include the use of gloves for all persons handling seafood commercially.

References

1. Hollis DG, Weaver RE, Baker CN, Thornsberry C. Halophilic Vibrio species isolated from blood cultures. J Clin Microbiol 1976;3:425–431
2. Chiang SR, Chuang YC. *Vibrio vulnificus* infection: clinical manifestations, pathogenesis, and antimicrobial therapy. J Microbiol Immunol Infect 2003;36:81–88
3. Liu JW, Lee IK, Tang HJ, Ko WC, Lee HC, Liu YC, Hsueh PR, Chuang YC. Prognostic factors and antibiotics in *Vibrio vulnificus* septicemia. Arch Intern Med 2006;166:2117–2123
4. Hally RJ, Rubin RA, Fraimow HS, Hoffman-Terry ML. Fatal *Vibrio parahemolyticus* septicemia in a patient with cirrhosis. A case report and review of the literature. Dig Dis Sci 1995;40:1257–1260
5. Schmidt U, Chmel H, Cobbs C. *Vibrio alginolyticus* infections in humans. J Clin Microbiol 1979;10:666–668
6. French GL, Woo ML, Hui YW, Chan KY. Antimicrobial susceptibilities of halophilic vibrios. J Antimicrob Chemother 1989;24:183–194
7. Jesudason MV, Lalitha MK, Koshi G. Non 01 *Vibrio cholerae* in intestinal and extra intestinal infections in Vellore, S. India. Indian J Pathol Microbiol 1991;34:26–29
8. Lesmana M, Subekti DS, Tjaniadi P, Simanjuntak CH, Punjabi NH, Campbell JR, Oyofo BA. Spectrum of vibrio species associated with acute diarrhea in North Jakarta, Indonesia. Diagn Microbiol Infect Dis 2002;43:91–97
9. Fuenzalida L, Hernandez C, Toro J, Rioseco ML, Romero J, Espejo RT. *Vibrio parahaemolyticus* in shellfish and clinical samples during two large epidemics of diarrhoea in southern Chile. Environ Microbiol 2006;8:675–683
10. Ananthan S, Dhamodaran S. Toxigenicity & drug sensitivity of *Vibrio mimicus* isolated from patients with diarrhoea. Indian J Med Res 1996;104:336–341
11. Makino K, Oshima K, Kurokawa K, Yokoyama K, Uda T, Tagomori K, Iijima Y, Najima M, Nakano M, Yamashita A, Kubota Y, Kimura S, Yasunaga T, Honda T, Shinagawa H, Hattori M, Iida T. Genome sequence of *Vibrio parahaemolyticus*: a pathogenic mechanism distinct from that of *V. cholerae*. Lancet 2003;361:743–749
12. Back E, Ljunggren A, Smith H, Jr. Non-cholera Vibrios in Sweden. Lancet 1974;1:723–724
13. Cholera 2005. Wkly Epidemiol Rec 2006;81:297–307
14. Siddique AK, Salam A, Islam MS, Akram K, Majumdar RN, Zaman K, Fronczak N, Laston S. Why treatment centres failed to prevent cholera deaths among Rwandan refugees in Goma, Zaire. Lancet 1995;345:359–361
15. Agtini MD, Soeharno R, Lesmana M, Punjabi NH, Simanjuntak C, Wangsasaputra F, Nurdin D, Pulungsih SP, Rofiq A, Santoso H, Pujarwoto H, Sjahrurachman A, Sudarmono P, von Seidlein L, Deen JL, Ali M, Lee H, Kim DR, Han O, Park JK, Suwandono A, Ingerani, Oyofo BA, Campbell JR, Beecham HJ, Corwin AL, Clemens JD. The burden of diarrhoea, shigellosis, and cholera in North Jakarta, Indonesia: findings from 24 months surveillance. BMC Infect Dis 2005;5:89
16. Sur D, Deen JL, Manna B, Niyogi SK, Deb AK, Kanungo S, Sarkar BL, Kim DR, Danovaro-Holliday MC, Holliday K, Gupta VK, Ali M, von Seidlein L, Clemens JD, Bhattacharya SK. The burden of cholera in the slums of Kolkata, India: data from a prospective, community based study. Arch Dis Child 2005;90:1175–1181
17. Khan WA, Bennish ML, Seas C, Khan EH, Ronan A, Dhar U, Busch W, Salam MA. Randomised controlled comparison of single-dose ciprofloxacin and doxycycline for cholera caused by *Vibrio cholerae* 01 or 0139. Lancet 1996;348:296–300

18. Khan WA, Saha D, Rahman A, Salam MA, Bogaerts J, Bennish ML. Comparison of single-dose azithromycin and 12-dose, 3-day erythromycin for childhood cholera: a randomised, double-blind trial. Lancet 2002;360:1722–1727

19. Saha D, Karim MM, Khan WA, Ahmed S, Salam MA, Bennish ML. Single-dose azithromycin for the treatment of cholera in adults. N Engl J Med 2006;354:2452–2462

20. Saha D, Khan WA, Karim MM, Chowdhury HR, Salam MA, Bennish ML. Single-dose ciprofloxacin versus 12-dose erythromycin for childhood cholera: a randomised controlled trial. Lancet 2005;366:1085–1093

21. Alam AN, Alam NH, Ahmed T, Sack DA. Randomised double blind trial of single dose doxycycline for treating cholera in adults. BMJ 1990;300:1619–1621

22. Sack DA, Islam S, Rabbani H, Islam A. Single-dose doxycycline for cholera. Antimicrob Agents Chemother 1978;14:462–464

23. Greenough WB, III, Gordon RS, Jr, Rosenberg IS, Davies BI, Benenson AS. Tetracycline in the treatment of cholera. Lancet 1964;41:355–357

24. Lindenbaum J, Greenough WB, Islam MR. Antibiotic therapy of cholera in children. Bull World Health Organ 1967;37:529–538

25. Lindenbaum J, Greenough WB, Islam MR. Antibiotic therapy of cholera. Bull World Health Organ 1967;36:871–883

26. Aidara A, Koblavi S, Boye CS, Raphenon G, Gassama A, Grimont F, Grimont PA. Phenotypic and genotypic characterization of Vibrio cholerae isolates from a recent cholera outbreak in Senegal: comparison with isolates from Guinea-Bissau. Am J Trop Med Hyg 1998;58:163–167

27. Dalsgaard A, Forslund A, Sandvang D, Arntzen L, Keddy K. Vibrio cholerae O1 outbreak isolates in Mozambique and South Africa in 1998 are multiple-drug resistant, contain the SXT element and the aadA2 gene located on class 1 integrons. J Antimicrob Chemother 2001;48:827–838

28. Das S, Gupta S. Diversity of Vibrio cholerae strains isolated in Delhi, India, during 1992–2000. J Health Popul Nutr 2005;23:44–51

29. Dhar U, Bennish ML, Khan WA, Seas C, Huq Khan E, Albert MJ, Abdus Salam M. Clinical features, antimicrobial susceptibility and toxin production in Vibrio cholerae O139 infection: comparison with V. cholerae O1 infection. Trans R Soc Trop Med Hyg 1996;90:402–405

30. Garg P, Chakraborty S, Basu I, Datta S, Rajendran K, Bhattacharya T, Yamasaki S, Bhattacharya SK, Takeda Y, Nair GB, Ramamurthy T. Expanding multiple antibiotic resistance among clinical strains of Vibrio cholerae isolated from 1992–7 in Calcutta, India. Epidemiol Infect 2000;124:393–399

31. Garg P, Sinha S, Chakraborty R, Bhattacharya SK, Nair GB, Ramamurthy T, Takeda Y. Emergence of fluoroquinolone-resistant strains of Vibrio cholerae O1 biotype El Tor among hospitalized patients with cholera in Calcutta, India. Antimicrob Agents Chemother 2001;45:1605–1606

32. Scrascia M, Forcillo M, Maimone F, Pazzani C. Susceptibility to rifaximin of Vibrio cholerae strains from different geographical areas. J Antimicrob Chemother 2003;52:303–305

33. Urassa WK, Mhando YB, Mhalu FS, Mjonga SJ. Antimicrobial susceptibility pattern of Vibrio cholerae O1 strains during two cholera outbreaks in Dar es Salaam, Tanzania. East Afr Med J 2000;77:350–353

34. Ehara M, Nguyen BM, Nguyen DT, Toma C, Higa N, Iwanaga M. Drug susceptibility and its genetic basis in epidemic Vibrio cholerae O1 in Vietnam. Epidemiol Infect 2004;132:595–600

35. Mohanty S, Kapil A, Das BK. Seasonality and antimicrobial resistance pattern of Vibrio cholerae in a tertiary care hospital of North India. Trop Doct 2004;34:249–251

36. Mwansa JC, Mwaba J, Lukwesa C, Bhuiyan NA, Ansaruzamman M, Ramamurthy T, Alam M, Balakrish Nair G. Multiply antibiotic-resistant Vibrio cholerae O1 biotype El Tor strains emerge during cholera outbreaks in Zambia. Epidemiol Infect 2006:1–7

37. Yamamoto T, Nair GB, Albert MJ, Parodi CC, Takeda Y. Survey of in vitro susceptibilities of Vibrio cholerae O1 and O139 to antimicrobial agents. Antimicrob Agents Chemother 1995;39:241–244

38. Israil A, Nacescu N, Cedru CL, Ciufecu C, Damian M. Changes in Vibrio cholerae O1 strains isolated in Romania during 1977–95. Epidemiol Infect 1998;121:253–258

39. Sheikh A, Khan A, Malik T, Fisher-Hoch SP. Cholera in a developing megacity; Karachi, Pakistan. Epidemiol Infect 1997;119: 287–292

40. Mishra M, Mohammed F, Akulwar SL, Katkar VJ, Tankhiwale NS, Powar RM. Re-emergence of El Tor Vibrio in outbreak of cholera in & around Nagpur. Indian J Med Res 2004;120:478–480

41. Ryan ET, Dhar U, Khan WA, Salam MA, Faruque AS, Fuchs GJ, Calderwood SB, Bennish ML. Mortality, morbidity, and microbiology of endemic cholera among hospitalized patients in Dhaka, Bangladesh. Am J Trop Med Hyg 2000;63:12–20

42. Ulusarac O, Carter E. Varied clinical presentations of Vibrio vulnificus infections: a report of four unusual cases and review of the literature. South Med J 2004;97:163–168

43. Chuang YC, Yuan CY, Liu CY, Lan CK, Huang AH. Vibrio vulnificus infection in Taiwan: report of 28 cases and review of clinical manifestations and treatment. Clin Infect Dis 1992;15:271–276

44. Shapiro RL, Altekruse S, Hutwagner L, Bishop R, Hammond R, Wilson S, Ray B, Thompson S, Tauxe RV, Griffin PM. The role of Gulf Coast oysters harvested in warmer months in Vibrio vulnificus infections in the United States, 1988–1996. Vibrio Working Group. J Infect Dis 1998;178:752–759

45. Klontz KC, Lieb S, Schreiber M, Janowski HT, Baldy LM, Gunn RA. Syndromes of Vibrio vulnificus infections. Clinical and epidemiologic features in Florida cases, 1981–1987. Ann Intern Med 1988;109:318–323

46. Hoge CW, Watsky D, Peeler RN, Libonati JP, Israel E, Morris JG, Jr. Epidemiology and spectrum of Vibrio infections in a Chesapeake Bay community. J Infect Dis 1989;160:985–993

47. Oliver JD. Wound infections caused by Vibrio vulnificus and other marine bacteria. Epidemiol Infect 2005;133:383–391

48. Tang HJ, Chang MC, Ko WC, Huang KY, Lee CL, Chuang YC. In vitro and in vivo activities of newer fluoroquinolones against Vibrio vulnificus. Antimicrob Agents Chemother 2002;46:3580–3584

49. Kim DM, Lym Y, Jang SJ, Han H, Kim YG, Chung CH, Hong SP. In vitro efficacy of the combination of ciprofloxacin and cefotaxime against Vibrio vulnificus. Antimicrob Agents Chemother 2005;49:3489–3491

50. Zanetti S, Spanu T, Deriu A, Romano L, Sechi LA, Fadda G. In vitro susceptibility of Vibrio spp. isolated from the environment. Int J Antimicrob Agents 2001;17:407–409

51. Vibrio vulnificus infections associated with eating raw oysters – Los Angeles, 1996. MMWR Morb Mortal Wkly Rep 1996;45:621–624

52. Joseph SW, DeBell RM, Brown WP. In vitro response to chloramphenicol, tetracycline, ampicillin, gentamicin, and beta-lactamase production by halophilic Vibrios from human and environmental sources. Antimicrob Agents Chemother 1978;13:244–248

53. Ottaviani D, Bacchiocchi I, Masini L, Leoni F, Carraturo A, Giammarioli M, Sbaraglia G. Antimicrobial susceptibility of potentially pathogenic halophilic vibrios isolated from seafood. Int J Antimicrob Agents 2001;18:135–140

54. Kobari K, Takakura I, Nakatomi M, Sogame S, Uylangco C. Antibiotic-resistant strains of El Tor vibrio in the Philippines and the use of furalazine for chemotherapy. Bull World Health Organ 1970;43:365–371

55. O'Grady F, Lewis MJ, Pearson NJ. Global surveillance of antibiotic sensitivity of Vibrio cholerae. Bull World Health Organ 1976;54:181–185

56. Glass RI, Huq I, Alim AR, Yunus M. Emergence of multiply antibiotic-resistant Vibrio cholerae in Bangladesh. J Infect Dis 1980;142:939–942

57. Glass RI, Huq MI, Lee JV, Threlfall EJ, Khan MR, Alim AR, Rowe B, Gross RJ. Plasmid-borne multiple drug resistance in *Vibrio cholerae* serogroup O1, biotype El Tor: evidence for a point-source outbreak in Bangladesh. J Infect Dis 1983;147:204–209

58. Towner KJ, Pearson NJ, Mhalu FS, O'Grady F. Resistance to anti-microbial agents of *Vibrio cholerae* El Tor strains isolated during the fourth cholera epidemic in the United Republic of Tanzania. Bull World Health Organ 1980;58:747–751

59. Olukoya DK, Ogunjimi AA, Abaelu AM. Plasmid profiles and antimicrobial susceptibility patterns of *Vibrio cholerae* O1 strain isolated during a recent outbreak in Nigeria. J Diarrhoeal Dis Res 1995;13:118–121

60. Zachariah R, Harries AD, Arendt V, Nchingula D, Chimtulo F, Courteille O, Kirpach P. Characteristics of a cholera outbreak, patterns of *Vibrio cholerae* and antibiotic susceptibility testing in rural Malawi. Trans R Soc Trop Med Hyg 2002;96:39–40

61. Finch MJ, Morris JG, Jr, Kaviti J, Kagwanja W, Levine MM. Epidemiology of antimicrobial resistant cholera in Kenya and East Africa. Am J Trop Med Hyg 1988;39:484–490

62. Khan WA, Dhar U, Begum M, Salam MA, Bardhan PK, Mahalanabis D. Antimicrobial treatment of adults with cholera due to *Vibrio cholerae* 0139 (synonym Bengal). Drugs 1995;49 Suppl 2:460–462

63. Basu A, Garg P, Datta S, Chakraborty S, Bhattacharya T, Khan A, Ramamurthy S, Bhattacharya SK, Yamasaki S, Takeda Y, Nair GB. *Vibrio cholerae* O139 in Calcutta, 1992–1998: incidence, antibiograms, and genotypes. Emerg Infect Dis 2000;6:139–147

64. Mukhopadhyay AK, Garg S, Nair GB, Kar S, Ghosh RK, Pajni S, Ghosh A, Shimada T, Takeda T, Takeda Y. Biotype traits and antibiotic susceptibility of *Vibrio cholerae* serogroup O1 before, during and after the emergence of the O139 serogroup. Epidemiol Infect 1995;115:427–434

65. Niyogi SK, Sengupta PG, Bhattacharya SK, Garg S, Mukhapadhayay AK, Nair GB. Emergence of furazolidone and cotrimoxazole resistant *Vibrio cholerae* 01 in eastern India. J Infect 1995;30:265–266

66. Ramamurthy T, Rajendran K, Garg P, Shimada T, Basu A, Chowdhury NR, Nandy RK, Yamasaki S, Bhattacharya SK, Takeda Y, Nair GB. Cluster-analysis & patterns of dissemination of multidrug resistance among clinical strains of *Vibrio cholerae* in Calcutta, India. Indian J Med Res 2000;112:78–85

67. Jesudason MV, Balaji V, Thomson CJ. Quinolone susceptibility of *Vibrio cholerae* O1 & O139 isolates from Vellore. Indian J Med Res 2002;116:96–98

68. Jesudason MV, Saaya R. Resistance of *Vibrio cholerae* O1 to nalidixic acid. Indian J Med Res 1997;105:153–154

69. Dalsgaard A, Forslund A, Bodhidatta L, Serichantalergs O, Pitarangsi C, Pang L, Shimada T, Echeverria P. A high proportion of *Vibrio cholerae* strains isolated from children with diarrhoea in Bangkok, Thailand are multiple antibiotic resistant and belong to heterogenous non-O1, non-O139 O-serotypes. Epidemiol Infect 1999;122:217–226

70. Tabtieng R, Wattanasri S, Echeverria P, Seriwatana J, Bodhidatta L, Chatkaeomorakot A, Rowe B. An epidemic of *Vibrio cholerae* el tor Inaba resistant to several antibiotics with a conjugative group C plasmid coding for type II dihydrofolate reductase in Thailand. Am J Trop Med Hyg 1989;41:680–686

71. Yamamoto T, Nair GB, Takeda Y. Emergence of tetracycline resistance due to a multiple drug resistance plasmid in *Vibrio cholerae* O139. FEMS Immunol Med Microbiol 1995;11:131–136

72. Bhattacharya MK, Ghosh S, Mukhopadhyay AK, Deb A, Bhattacharya SK. Outbreak of cholera caused by *Vibrio cholerae* 01 intermediately resistant to norfloxacin at Malda, West Bengal. J Indian Med Assoc 2000;98:389–390

73. Mukhopadhyay AK, Basu I, Bhattacharya SK, Bhattacharya MK, Nair GB. Emergence of fluoroquinolone resistance in strains of *Vibrio cholerae* isolated from hospitalized patients with acute diarrhea in Calcutta, India. Antimicrob Agents Chemother 1998;42:206–207

74. Sundaram SP, Revathi J, Sarkar BL, Bhattacharya SK. Bacteriological profile of cholera in Tamil Nadu (1980–2001). Indian J Med Res 2002;116:258–263

75. Sabeena F, Thirivikramji G, Radhakutty G, Indu P, Singh DV. In vitro susceptibility of *Vibrio cholerae* O1 biotype El Tor strains associated with an outbreak of cholera in Kerala, Southern India. J Antimicrob Chemother 2001;47:361–362

76. Radu S, Vincent M, Apun K, Abdul-Rahim R, Benjamin PG, Yuherman, Rusul G. Molecular characterization of *Vibrio cholerae* O1 outbreak strains in Miri, Sarawak (Malaysia). Acta Trop 2002;83:169–176

77. Srifuenfung S, Komolpis P, Yungyuen T, Techachaiwiwat W, Tribuddharat C. Prevalence of Vibrio species isolated from fecal specimens of patients with diarrhea in Siriraj Hospital during 1994–2001. J Infect Dis Antimicrob Agents 2004;21:83–88

78. Falbo V, Carattoli A, Tosini F, Pezzella C, Dionisi AM, Luzzi I. Antibiotic resistance conferred by a conjugative plasmid and a class I integron in *Vibrio cholerae* O1 El Tor strains isolated in Albania and Italy. Antimicrob Agents Chemother 1999;43:693–696

79. Campos LC, Zahner V, Avelar KE, Alves RM, Pereira DS, Vital BJ, Freitas FS, Salles CA, Karaolis DK. Genetic diversity and antibiotic resistance of clinical and environmental *Vibrio cholerae* suggests that many serogroups are reservoirs of resistance. Epidemiol Infect 2004;132:985–992

80. Dubon JM, Palmer CJ, Ager AL, Shor-Posner G, Baum MK. Emergence of multiple drug-resistant *Vibrio cholerae* O1 in San Pedro Sula, Honduras. Lancet 1997;349:924

81. Weber JT, Mintz ED, Canizares R, Semiglia A, Gomez I, Sempertegui R, Davila A, Greene KD, Puhr ND, Cameron DN, et al. Epidemic cholera in Ecuador: multidrug-resistance and transmission by water and seafood. Epidemiol Infect 1994;112:1–11

82. Large epidemic of cholera-like disease in Bangladesh caused by *Vibrio cholerae* O139 synonym Bengal. Cholera Working Group, International Centre for Diarrhoeal Diseases Research, Bangladesh. Lancet 1993;342:387–390

83. Waldor MK, Mekalanos JJ. Emergence of a new cholera pandemic: molecular analysis of virulence determinants in *Vibrio cholerae* O139 and development of a live vaccine prototype. J Infect Dis 1994;170:278–283

84. Waldor MK, Mekalanos JJ. *Vibrio cholerae* O139 specific gene sequences. Lancet 1994;343:1366

85. Waldor MK, Tschape H, Mekalanos JJ. A new type of conjugative transposon encodes resistance to sulfamethoxazole, trimethoprim, and streptomycin in *Vibrio cholerae* O139. J Bacteriol 1996;178:4157–4165

86. Hochhut B, Lotfi Y, Mazel D, Faruque SM, Woodgate R, Waldor MK. Molecular analysis of antibiotic resistance gene clusters in *Vibrio cholerae* O139 and O1 SXT constins. Antimicrob Agents Chemother 2001;45:2991–3000

87. Faruque SM, Abdul Alim AR, Rahman MM, Siddique AK, Sack RB, Albert MJ. Clonal relationships among classical *Vibrio cholerae* O1 strains isolated between 1961 and 1992 in Bangladesh. J Clin Microbiol 1993;31:2513–2516

88. Faruque SM, Ahmed KM, Abdul Alim AR, Qadri F, Siddique AK, Albert MJ. Emergence of a new clone of toxigenic *Vibrio cholerae* O1 biotype El Tor displacing V. cholerae O139 Bengal in Bangladesh. J Clin Microbiol 1997;35:624–630

89. Faruque SM, Saha MN, Asadulghani, Sack DA, Sack RB, Takeda Y, Nair GB. The O139 serogroup of *Vibrio cholerae* comprises diverse clones of epidemic and nonepidemic strains derived from multiple V. cholerae O1 or non-O1 progenitors. J Infect Dis 2000;182:1161–1168

90. Scrascia M, Maimone F, Mohamud KA, Materu SF, Grimont F, Grimont PA, Pazzani C. Clonal relationship among *Vibrio cholerae* O1 El Tor strains causing the largest cholera epidemic in Kenya in the late 1990s. J Clin Microbiol 2006;44:3401–3404

91. Dalsgaard A, Forslund A, Tam NV, Vinh DX, Cam PD. Cholera in Vietnam: changes in genotypes and emergence of class I integrons containing aminoglycoside resistance gene cassettes in *Vibrio cholerae* O1 strains isolated from 1979 to 1996. J Clin Microbiol 1999;37:734–741

92. Ceccarelli D, Salvia AM, Sami J, Cappuccinelli P, Colombo MM. New cluster of plasmid-located class 1 integrons in *Vibrio cholerae* O1 and a dfrA15 cassette-containing integron in *Vibrio parahaemolyticus* isolated in Angola. Antimicrob Agents Chemother 2006;50:2493–2499

93. Vora GJ, Meador CE, Bird MM, Bopp CA, Andreadis JD, Stenger DA. Microarray-based detection of genetic heterogeneity, antimicrobial resistance, and the viable but nonculturable state in human pathogenic *Vibrio* spp. Proc Natl Acad Sci U S A 2005;102:19109–19114

94. Iwanaga M, Toma C, Miyazato T, Insisiengmay S, Nakasone N, Ehara M. Antibiotic resistance conferred by a class I integron and SXT constin in *Vibrio cholerae* O1 strains isolated in Laos. Antimicrob Agents Chemother 2004;48:2364–2369

95. Amita, Chowdhury SR, Thungapathra M, Ramamurthy T, Nair GB, Ghosh A. Class I integrons and SXT elements in El Tor strains isolated before and after 1992 *Vibrio cholerae* O139 outbreak, Calcutta, India. Emerg Infect Dis 2003;9:500–502

96. Toma C, Nakasone N, Song T, Iwanaga M. *Vibrio cholerae* SXT element, Laos. Emerg Infect Dis 2005;11:346–347

97. Baranwal S, Dey K, Ramamurthy T, Nair GB, Kundu M. Role of active efflux in association with target gene mutations in fluoroquinolone resistance in clinical isolates of *Vibrio cholerae*. Antimicrob Agents Chemother 2002;46:2676–2678

98. Colmer JA, Fralick JA, Hamood AN. Isolation and characterization of a putative multidrug resistance pump from *Vibrio cholerae*. Mol Microbiol 1998;27:63–72

99. Krishna BV, Patil AB, Chandrasekhar MR. Fluoroquinolone-resistant *Vibrio cholerae* isolated during a cholera outbreak in India. Trans R Soc Trop Med Hyg 2006;100:224–226

100. Albert MJ, Bhuiyan NA, Talukder KA, Faruque AS, Nahar S, Faruque SM, Ansaruzzaman M, Rahman M. Phenotypic and genotypic changes in *Vibrio cholerae* O139 Bengal. J Clin Microbiol 1997;35:2588–2592

101. Faruque SM, Chowdhury N, Kamruzzaman M, Ahmad QS, Faruque AS, Salam MA, Ramamurthy T, Nair GB, Weintraub A, Sack DA. Reemergence of epidemic *Vibrio cholerae* O139, Bangladesh. Emerg Infect Dis 2003;9:1116–1122

102. Jabeen K, Hasan R. Re-emergence of *Vibrio cholerae* O139 in Pakistan: report from a tertiary care hospital. J Pak Med Assoc 2003;53:335–338

103. Saha D, Khan WA, Ahmed S, Faruque ASG, Salam MA, Bennish ML. Resurgent, multiresistant *V. cholerae* O1 in Bangladesh. In: 46th Interscience Conference on Antimicrobial Agents and Chemotherapy. San Francisco, CA, USA; 2006

104. Khan WA, Saha D, Ahmed S, Salam MA, Bennish ML. Identification and treatment of *V. cholerae* O1 with diminished susceptibility to ciprofloxacin. In: 46th Interscience Conference on Antimicrobial Agents and Chemotherapy. San Francisco, CA, USA; 2006

105. Crump JA, Barrett TJ, Nelson JT, Angulo FJ. Reevaluating fluoroquinolone breakpoints for *Salmonella enterica* serotype Typhi and for non-Typhi salmonellae. Clin Infect Dis 2003;37:75–81

106. Knapp JS, Hale JA, Neal SW, Wintersheid K, Rice RJ, Whittington WL. Proposed criteria for interpretation of susceptibilities of strains of *Neisseria gonorrhoeae* to ciprofloxacin, ofloxacin, enoxacin, lomefloxacin, and norfloxacin. Antimicrob Agents Chemother 1995;39:2442–2445

107. Bennish ML. Cholera: pathophysiology, clinical features, and treatment. In: Wachsmuth IK, Blake PA, Olsvik O, eds. *Vibrio cholerae* and Cholera Molecular to Global Perspectives. Washington, DC: ASM Press; 1994:229–256

108. Karchmer AW, Curlin GT, Huq MI, Hirschhorn N. Furazolidone in paediatric cholera. Bull World Health Organ 1970;43:373–378

109. World Health Organization. The Treatment of Diarrhoea: A Manual for Physicians and Other Senior Health Workers. http://www.who.int/child-adolescent-health/New_Publications/CHILD_HEALTH/ISBN_92_4_159318_0.pdf (accessed 1 February 2007); 2005

110. Centers for Disease Control and Prevention Atlanta Georgia. Laboratory Methods for the Diagnosis of Epidemic Dysentery and Cholera; 1999

111. Bacterial agents of enteric diseases of public health concern: *Salmonella* serotype typhi, *Shigella*, *Vibrio cholerae*. In: Manual for the Laboratory Identification and Antimicrobial Susceptibility Testing of Bacterial Pathogens of Public Health Importance in the Developing World. Geneva: World Health Organization 2003;103–162

112. Sciortino CV, Johnson JA, Hamad A. Vitek system antimicrobial susceptibility testing of O1, O139, and non-O1 *Vibrio cholerae*. J Clin Microbiol 1996;34:897–900

113. Khan AM, von Gierke U, Hossain MS, Fuchs GJ. Tetracycline in the treatment of cholera caused by *Vibrio cholerae* O1 resistant to the drug in vitro. J Health Popul Nutr 2003;21:76–78

114. Jiang ZD, Ke S, Palazzini E, Riopel L, Dupont H. In vitro activity and fecal concentration of rifaximin after oral administration. Antimicrob Agents Chemother 2000;44:2205–2206

115. DuPont HL, Jiang ZD, Ericsson CD, Adachi JA, Mathewson JJ, DuPont MW, Palazzini E, Riopel LM, Ashley D, Martinez-Sandoval F. Rifaximin versus ciprofloxacin for the treatment of traveler's diarrhea: a randomized, double-blind clinical trial. Clin Infect Dis 2001;33:1807–1815

116. Wenzel RP. The antibiotic pipeline – challenges, costs, and values. N Engl J Med 2004;351:523–526

117. Hung DT, Shakhnovich EA, Pierson E, Mekalanos JJ. Small-molecule inhibitor of *Vibrio cholerae* virulence and intestinal colonization. Science 2005;310:670–674

118. Waldor MK. Disarming pathogens – a new approach for antibiotic development. N Engl J Med 2006;354:296–297

119. Guerrant RL. Cholera – still teaching hard lessons. N Engl J Med 2006;354:2500–2502

120. MacDonald R. Access to clean water in rural Africa is inadequate. BMJ 2005;331:70

121. Mukherjee A, Sengupta MK, Hossain MA, Ahamed S, Das B, Nayak B, Lodh D, Rahman MM, Chakraborti D. Arsenic contamination in groundwater: a global perspective with emphasis on the Asian scenario. J Health Popul Nutr 2006;24:142–163

122. Colwell RR, Huq A, Islam MS, Aziz KMA, Yunus M, Khan NH, Mahmud A, Sack RB, Nair GB, Chakraborty J, Sack DA, Russek-Cohen E. Reduction of cholera in Bangladeshi villages by simple filtration. Proc Natl Acad Sci U S A 2003;100:1051–1055

123. Quick RE, Venczel LV, Gonzalez O, Mintz ED, Highsmith AK, Espada A, Damiani E, Bean NH, De Hannover EH, Tauxe RV. Narrow-mouthed water storage vessels and in situ chlorination in a Bolivian community: a simple method to improve drinking water quality. Am J Trop Med Hyg 1996;54:511–516

124. Clasen TF, Brown J, Collin S, Suntura O, Cairncross S. Reducing diarrhea through the use of household-based ceramic water filters: a randomized, controlled trial in rural Bolivia. Am J Trop Med Hyg 2004;70:651–657

125. Radu S, Elhadi N, Hassan Z, Rusul G, Lihan S, Fifadara N, Yuherman, Purwati E. Characterization of *Vibrio vulnificus* isolated from cockles (*Anadara granosa*): antimicrobial resistance,

plasmid profiles and random amplification of polymorphic DNA analysis. FEMS Microbiol Lett 1998;165:139–143

126. Bowdre JH, Hull JH, Cocchetto DM. Antibiotic efficacy against *Vibrio vulnificus* in the mouse: superiority of tetracycline. J Pharmacol Exp Ther 1983;225:595–598

127. Molitoris E, Joseph SW, Krichevsky MI, Sindhuhardja W, Colwell RR. Characterization and distribution of *Vibrio alginolyticus* and *Vibrio parahaemolyticus* isolated in Indonesia. Appl Environ Microbiol 1985;50:1388–1394

128. Morris JG, Jr, Tenney JH, Drusano GL. In vitro susceptibility of pathogenic Vibrio species to norfloxacin and six other antimicrobial agents. Antimicrob Agents Chemother 1985;28:442–445

129. Su BA, Tang HJ, Wang YY, Liu YC, Ko WC, Liu CY, Chuang YC. In vitro antimicrobial effect of cefazolin and cefotaxime combined with minocycline against *Vibrio cholerae* non-O1 non-O139. J Microbiol Immunol Infect 2005;38:425–429

130. do Nascimento SM, dos Fernandes Vieira RH, Theophilo GN, Dos Prazeres Rodrigues D, Vieira GH. *Vibrio vulnificus* as a health hazard for shrimp consumers. Rev Inst Med Trop Sao Paulo 2001;43:263–266

131. Chuang YC, Liu JW, Ko WC, Lin KY, Wu JJ, Huang KY. In vitro synergism between cefotaxime and minocycline against *Vibrio vulnificus*. Antimicrob Agents Chemother 1997;41:2214–2217

132. Chuang YC, Ko WC, Wang ST, Liu JW, Kuo CF, Wu JJ, Huang KY. Minocycline and cefotaxime in the treatment of experimental murine *Vibrio vulnificus* infection. Antimicrob Agents Chemother 1998;42:1319–1322

133. Jorgensen JH, Hindler JF. New consensus guidelines from the Clinical and Laboratory Standards Institute for antimicrobial susceptibility testing of infrequently isolated or fastidious bacteria. Clin Infect Dis 2007;44:280–286

134. Clinical and Laboratory Standards Institute. Methods for antimicrobial dilution and disk susceptibility testing of infrequently isolated or fastidious bacteria. Approved standard M45-A. Wayne, PA: Clinical and Laboratory Standards Institute; 2006

135. Mouzin E, Mascola L, Tormey MP, Dassey DE. Prevention of *Vibrio vulnificus* infections. Assessment of regulatory educational strategies. JAMA 1997;278:576–578

136. Osaka K, Komatsuzaki M, Takahashi H, Sakano S, Okabe N. *Vibrio vulnificus* septicaemia in Japan: an estimated number of infections and physicians' knowledge of the syndrome. Epidemiol Infect 2004;132:993–996

137. Roy SK, Islam A, Ali R, Islam KE, Khan RA, Ara SH, Saifuddin NM, Fuchs GJ. A randomized clinical trial to compare the efficacy of erythromycin, ampicillin and tetracycline for the treatment of cholera in children. Trans R Soc Trop Med Hyg 1998;92:460–462

138. Khan WA, Begum M, Salam MA, Bardhan PK, Islam MR, Mahalanabis D. Comparative trial of five antimicrobial compounds in the treatment of cholera in adults. Trans R Soc Trop Med Hyg 1995;89:103–106

139. Gotuzzo E, Seas C, Echevarria J, Carrillo C, Mostorino R, Ruiz R. Ciprofloxacin for the treatment of cholera: a randomized, double-blind, controlled clinical trial of a single daily dose in Peruvian adults. Clin Infect Dis 1995;20:1485–1490

140. Kabir I, Khan WA, Haider R, Mitra AK, Alam AN. Erythromycin and trimethoprim–sulphamethoxazole in the treatment of cholera in children. J Diarrhoeal Dis Res 1996;14:243–247

141. Islam MR. Single dose tetracycline in cholera. Gut 1987;28:1029–1032

142. Grados P, Bravo N, Battilana C. Comparative effectiveness of cotrimoxazole and tetracycline in the treatment of cholera. Bull Pan Am Health Organ 1996;30:36–42

Chapter 59
Antimicrobial Resistance in *Helicobacter* and *Campylobacter*

Patrick F. McDermott, Joanne L. Simala-Grant, and Diane E. Taylor

1 Introduction

Helicobacter and *Campylobacter* are Gram-negative spiral flagellated bacteria that inhabit and cause diseases of the gastrointestinal tract. Despite early microscopic observations of "*Vibrio*-like" organisms in blood, stool and gastric contents, the role of these two genera in infectious disease was established only recently. *Campylobacter* was first generally accepted as an important fecal pathogen in the 1970s, when improvements in culture methods made it feasible to study the role of *Campylobacter* systematically in diarrheal disease (1). Today, it is recognized as one of the leading causes of foodborne gastroenteritis in the United States and worldwide, with *Campylobacter jejuni* and *Campylobacter coli* being the most commonly isolated species. It is also the most common antecedent microbial infection of Guillain–Barré syndrome (2). *Campylobacter* are enteric commensals in several animal hosts, which include various avian and mammalian species from which most infections are thought to originate. *Helicobacter* is a common microbial constituent of the mammalian gastric mucosa. Despite the fact that they commonly persist in the human stomach asymptomatically, infection by *Helicobacter pylori* is the most important risk factor for peptic ulcers and gastric cancers (3). The relatively recent realization of the importance of *Campylobacter* and *Helicobacter* in human illness has sparked intensive research over the past 20 years into the epidemiology, microbiology, and treatment of diseases caused by these organisms.

2 *Helicobacter pylori*

Infection with *Helicobacter pylori* causes gastritis and increases one's risk for the development of gastric and duodenal ulcers, mucosal-associated lymphoid tissue lymphoma, and gastric cancer (3, 4). Approximately 80% of adults in developing countries are infected with *H. pylori*, whereas fewer than 40% are infected in industrialized countries (5). Poor socio-economic status has been postulated as a risk factor for infection (5). Although the method of transmission of *H. pylori* is unknown, oral-oral or fecal-oral is the most probable route of transmission and occurs primarily in early childhood (5). Although most consider family members, and particularly mothers (6), to play an important role in infection, consensus has not yet been reached (5, 7, 8). There is very little evidence for existence of viable *H. pylori* outside the human host.

The standard eradication therapy in patients with these disease symptoms normally involves triple therapy, consisting of two antibiotics, most often clarithromycin (Cla) and amoxicillin (Amx), and a proton pump inhibitor (9, 10). Primary therapy is successful in 60–85% of patients (11). Antibiotic resistance of *H. pylori* is an important cause of treatment failure (12–14), and varies widely by geographic region and among subpopulations within a region. As a result, alternative treatment regimens may include a bismuth compound, metronidazole (Mtz), tetracycline (Tc), rifamycin derivatives (15–17), or, more rarely, fluoroquinolones (FQs) (18, 19), the penem β-lactam antibiotic, faropenem (20), or nitrofurans (21, 22). Sequential therapy with multiple antimicrobials is also being examined (9).

Rates of *H. pylori* reinfection are lower in industrialized than developing countries, with averages of 3.4% and 8.7%, respectively, however reinfection rates vary from 0 to 100% per year (7). In those countries where reinfection rates are high, repeated treatment and concomitant antibiotic resistance is likely to result in increasing resistance among *H. pylori* over time. Some cases of reinfection may be mistaken for relapse due to incomplete eradication of the

P.F. McDermott (✉)
Director, Division of Animal and Foor Microbiology,
Office of Research, Center for Veterinary Medicine,
U.S. Food and Drug Administration, Laurel, MD, USA
Patrick.McDermott@fda.hhs.gov

D.L. Mayers (ed.), *Antimicrobial Drug Resistance*,
DOI 10.1007/978-1-60327-595-8_59, © Humana Press, a part of Springer Science+Business Media, LLC 2009

organism (7). It is difficult to differentiate relapse from rein-fection, since some individuals may harbor genotypically different strains of *H. pylori* simultaneously (23, 24). In addition, one could be reinfected by the same strain from the same source. It has been observed that recurrence is more common within 1 year of the eradication therapy when less efficacious antimicrobials are given or less sensitive diagnostic methods are used to determine eradication (7).

The "gold standard" for *H. pylori* diagnosis is histopathology of gastric biopsy specimens. Other diagnostic methods include the non-invasive urea breath test (25), serology, or stool antigen tests (26). A number of molecular diagnostic techniques are also being examined for diagnosis of *H. pylori* infection, including fluorescence in situ hybridization of gastric biopsy specimens (27, 28), real-time polymerase chain reaction (PCR) of gastric biopsy and stool specimens (29), and restriction fragment length polymorphism (RFLP) PCR using gastric biopsy and stool specimens (30).

2.1 In Vitro Antimicrobial Susceptibility Testing and Interpretive Criteria for H. pylori

The Clinical and Laboratory Standards Institute (CLSI) (formerly NCCLS) recognizes only the agar dilution susceptibility testing method for *H. pylori*. This method requires a cell suspension equivalent to a 2.0 McFarland standard, Mueller-Hinton plates containing 5% aged (>2 months) sheep blood, and incubation for 72 h in a microaerobic atmosphere at $35°C ± 2°C$. *H. pylori* ATCC 43504 is the quality control (QC) strain. Currently, there are QC ranges for Amx, Cla, Mtz, telithromycin, and Tc, but interpretive criteria are established only for Cla (resistant breakpoint $\geq 1 \mu g/mL$) (31). While it is reproducible, this method is labor intensive and not amenable to regular testing of small numbers of clinical isolates. There is a need for a more rapid and affordable method for routine laboratory use.

A variety of other methods have been examined for their suitability for testing antimicrobial susceptibility of *H. pylori*. These include disk diffusion (32), the Epsilometer testing method (Etest, AB BIODISK, Solna, Sweden) (33, 34), and broth dilution (35). Disk diffusion is generally not considered a good choice for slow-growing organisms such as *H. pylori*, since the antibiotic gradient decays over time (13, 36). It has been suggested that if young cultures of *H. pylori* are used, disk diffusion plates can be read within 31 h (37). This method has not yet been validated in multi-laboratory studies.

While the Etest is relatively expensive in comparison to other methods of susceptibility testing, it is much simpler than agar dilution, and thus is often preferred in clinical settings. Several studies have evaluated the Etest relative to the agar dilution reference method for testing *H. pylori*, often with conflicting results. Because the majority of these studies did not assay the CLSI-established quality control organism with the comparator method, they are often difficult to interpret. Regardless, these studies suggest that, in general, the Etest correlates well with agar dilution when testing Amx and Cla, but is less reliable for Mtz (38–43) and rifampicin (44), for which the Etest generates higher MIC values. Even when using the agar dilution, Mtz susceptibility testing results, while stable for the QC organism, are more variable among clinical isolates than are the results for other agents. The reasons for this appear to be due in part to heteroresistant subpopulations (45) or infection by multiple strains (23).

Numerous reports describe heterogeneous susceptibility in *H. pylori* cultures when grown both from a single colony from a single gastric biopsy (23, 45–48) or from multiple biopsies (22–38% show heteroresistance) from the same patient (17, 24, 49). The potential for patients to be infected simultaneously by more than one strain, or a strain with heteroresistant subpopulations, can compromise the predictive value of in vitro susceptibility testing, thereby limiting the success of eradication. Table 1 lists suggested breakpoints for the most commonly used antimicrobial agents used in the treatment of *H. pylori*-induced gastritis.

Traditional methods of susceptibility testing require prior isolation and identification of *H. pylori*. Because the isolation of *H. pylori* from a biopsy may take several days, empiric therapy is often initiated long before antibiotic susceptibility results are available. To circumvent this problem, rapid molecular methods have been developed recently to help guide therapy based on the presence of

Table 1 Interpretive breakpoints for *Helicobacter pylori*

Antimicrobial	MIC breakpoint (µg/mL)		
	S	I	R
Amoxicillin	≤0.5	NA	≥1
Ciprofloxacin	≤0.5	NA	≥1
Clarithromycin	≤0.5	NA	≥1
Furazolidone	≤1	NA	≥2
Levofloxacin	≤0.5	NA	≥1
Metronidazole	≤1	2–4	≥8
Moxifloxacin	≤0.5	NA	≥1
Nitrofurantoin	≤1	NA	≥2
Rifampin	≤2	NA	≥4
Tetracycline	≤1	2–8	≥16
Tinidazole	≤1	2–4	≥8

NA not applicable; *S, I, R* susceptible, intermediate, resistant specific resistance determinants. Rapid tests have been investigated for detecting resistance to FQs (50), Cla (27–29, 47, 51–59), and Tc (59–62) using DNA from gastric juice, gastric biopsy, or stool specimens. The results from this type of testing can be obtained on the same day as endoscopy, even in the presence of contaminating organisms. Comparisons are beginning to be made between traditional antibiotic susceptibility testing methods and emerging molecular diagnostic techniques (27–29, 47, 51, 53, 56). While similar approaches have been taken with other slow-growing bacteria, the value of this approach for reliably guiding *H. pylori* antimicrobial therapy must be correlated with clinical success.

2.2 Clinical Significance of Resistance

Despite the inherent difficulty in clearing the gastric mucosa of antibiotic-susceptible *Helicobacter*, antimicrobial resistance in *H. pylori* may also be a critical factor in therapeutic failure. While some studies report similar eradication rates for patients infected with resistant and susceptible strains (63–67), it is generally agreed that resistance to Amx (68), Cla (69–77), and Mtz (49, 71, 73, 74, 76, 78–81) correlates with reduced eradication success rates. Since susceptibility testing of *H. pylori* is rare, the selection of appropriate therapy is therefore usually based on local susceptibility patterns for *H. pylori*.

2.3 Resistance to Specific Antimicrobials

Below we consider the mechanisms of resistance to specific antimicrobials used to treat illness caused by *H. pylori*. Because initial attempts at eradication therapy can frequently fail, we will discuss resistance and antimicrobial use in the context of primary, secondary, and rescue therapies.

2.3.1 β-Lactam Resistance

β-lactams interfere with cell wall biosynthesis, resulting in lysis of replicating cells (82). Resistance to Amx, the only β-lactam commonly used to treat *H. pylori* infections (13), is generally rare (17, 33, 83), although there have been reports of Amx resistance in 11% to 72% of clinical isolates (14, 23, 84, 85). Amx resistance has been linked to mutations within penicillin-binding protein 1A (86–90) that reduce the binding of Amx to this target, and also to decreased membrane permeability for Amx (87, 88, 90). Amx-resistant *H. pylori* have also shown resistance to other β-lactams (87), and in one study showed cross-resistance to chloramphenicol and Tc (88).

2.3.2 Fluoroquinolone Resistance

The FQ family of antibiotics includes, among others, ciprofloxacin (Cip), pefloxacin, norfloxacin, trovafloxacin, moxifloxacin, and levofloxacin (91). They act through inhibitions of the DNA gyrase and topoisomerase IV enzymes in DNA synthesis (92). FQs are not generally used for primary eradication of *H. pylori*, but may be used in rescue treatment regimens when other antibiotics fail (18, 93, 94). Resistance to FQs may be acquired rapidly (95), and thus the use of this group of agents for the treatment of *H. pylori* should be used with caution. In addition, FQs are not recommended for use in children (34). Resistance of *H. pylori* isolates to FQs has been reported to vary from 0 to 33% (34, 96) from primary treatments, and 9–24% from secondary treatments (33, 97, 98).

Cip resistance (Cip^R) in *H. pylori* is due primarily to various mutations in the quinolone resistance-determining region (QRDR) of *gyrA*, the gene that encodes the A subunit of DNA gyrase (34, 95, 96, 99–101). In Cip$_R$ *H. pylori* isolates, several types of base substitutions, usually resulting in a single amino acid change at Asp91 in the QRDR of *gyrA*, were associated with increased MICs of Cip from <0.25 to 4 to 16 μg/mL, with cross-resistance to other FQs (34, 96, 99, 100). Acquisition of a second mutation in the QRDR at Asn87 resulted in higher FQ resistance (99). A real-time PCR technique has been developed to detect mutations in *gyrA* associated with FQ resistance (50). So far, this technique has been optimized only for use with a select number of *gyrA* mutations using DNA isolated from culture, but it should be possible to modify the technique for use with gastric biopsy, gastric fluids, or stool specimens.

2.3.3 Macrolide Resistance

Cla is a macrolide that binds to the 50S subunit of bacterial ribosomes and interferes with protein synthesis by inhibiting the elongation of peptide chains (102). This antibiotic is frequently used as one component of *H. pylori* eradication therapy (21), whereas the macrolides roxithromycin and josamycin (91) are less commonly used. Primary macrolide resistance in *H. pylori* varies between 0 and 46% (24, 27, 29, 32, 34, 46, 55, 64, 71, 83, 103), while secondary resistance varies from 29 to 100% (17, 33, 83, 103, 104). It has been suggested that Cla resistance may be lost in vivo when there is no selection pressure (105, 106), but it is possible that a heterogeneous Cla-resistant *H. pylori* population is maintained and that resistant bacteria will reappear if selection pressure is once again applied.

Point mutations in the 23S rRNA gene have been associated with increased Cla MICs (100, 106–109), and cross-resistance to all other macrolides and lincosamides, with varying resistance to streptogramins (107, 110). The most common point mutations are substitutions of adenine (A) with guanine (G) at either of two nucleotides (corresponding to positions 2,058 and 2,059 using *Escherichia coli* coordinates) within domain IV of the peptidyl transferase loop of 23S rRNA (106). The positions of the two nucleotides were demonstrated to be 2,142 and 2,143 in *H. pylori* coordinates, based on the determination of the transcription start site of *H. pylori* 23S rRNA (109). Other much less common mutations observed in the 23S rRNA include A2115G, G2141A, A2142C, A2142T, 2142G (MIC > 256 mg/mL) (108), A2144G (111), A2144T (no effect on MIC and no evidence as to importance) (103), T2182C (MIC 1 to ≥64 μg/mL) (55, 112–114), C2195T (55), A2215G, T2717C (0.5–1 μg/mL) (115), T2727C, G2224A, C2245T, T2289C and T2717C (MIC !μg/mL) (108). Controversy remains as to the clinical importance of these mutations to Cla resistance, but one study has shown that A2143G mutations in the 23SrRNA significantly hinder eradication (116).

A number of molecular diagnostic methods have been developed to identify Cla resistance determinants in *H. pylori*. These include a DNA microarray (59), double gradient-denaturing gel electrophoresis (47), PCR-based denaturing high pressure liquid chromatography (55), 3′-mismatched reverse primer PCR (52), PCR single-strand conformation polymorphism (75), PCR-oligonucleotide ligation (58), DNA enzyme immunoassay (54), line-probe (57, 117), real-time PCR (29, 51, 53, 116, 118), and fluorescent in situ hybridization (27, 28, 56) assays.

2.3.4 Nitrofuran Resistance

The nitrofurans include nifuratel, furazolidone, and nitrofurantoin. Nitrofurans function through multiple mechanisms by binding to a variety of proteins. While none of these agents is commonly used in primary eradication of *H. pylori,* they may be used when primary treatment fails (22, 119). The susceptibility of *H. pylori* to these antibiotics is not commonly measured; however, resistance to nitrofurans has been found in 1.5 to 4% of primary isolates (24, 84, 120, 121). In other bacteria, resistance is associated with reduced nitrofuran reductase (122). As yet, no studies have been published on the mechanisms of resistance to nitrofurans in *H. pylori*.

2.3.5 Nitroimidazole Resistance

Nitroimidazoles include such compounds as Mtz and tinidazole. Mtz is a pro-drug that is reduced to a hydroxylamine derivative that damages DNA and appears to cause cell death by nicking DNA (123). Nitroimidazoles in general, and Mtz in particular, were among the first groups of antibiotics to be used for the treatment of *H. pylori* (13). Resistance to Mtz is widespread, and may be as high as 82% (32, 46, 64, 71, 83), whereas secondary resistance rates range from 14 to 100% (17, 33, 78, 103, 104).

Resistance in bacteria to nitroimidazole compounds appear to be due to an inability to reduce the pro-drug (13). Goodwin et al. (124) convincingly demonstrated that mutations in *rdxA*, which encodes an oxygen-insensitive NADPH nitroreductase, resulted in Mtz^R. Mutations in *rdxA* were confirmed by others to correlate with Mtz^R in *H. pylori* (100, 125–130). Later, Kwon et al. (88) and Jeong et al. (131) independently demonstrated that *frxA*, which codes for an NAD(P)H-flavin oxidoreductase, a paralog of RdxA, can also be involved in Mtz^R. They showed that inactivation of *rdxA* alone resulted in moderate Mtz^R (MIC 16–32 μg/mL), whereas single mutations in both *rdxA* and *frxA* conferred higher-level resistance (MIC > 64 μg/mL). There is still a controversy as to the roles of *rdxA* and *frxA* in Mtz^R, as other groups have not found the same correlation between mutations within *rdxA* and *frxA* and Mtz MIC (132, 133). As a result, it has been suggested that other genes may play a role in Mtz^R. Mutations in *recA* (134), and *fdxB* (encoding a ferredoxin-like protein) (135), repression of pyruvate oxidoreductase (POR) and α-ketoglutarate oxidoreductase (136), decreased transcription of *rdxA* and *for* (ferrodoxin oxidoreductase) and possibly *por* and *fdxB* all have been implicated in Mtz^R in *H. pylori* (137). Therefore, diverse mutations in *H. pylori* may result in Mtz^R.

2.3.6 Rifamycin Resistance

Resistance of *H. pylori* to rifamycin and its derivatives results from the inability of these compounds to bind to the β-subunit of RNA polymerase, which is encoded by *rpoB* (44, 100, 138, 139). Rifamycins are rarely used for treatment of *H. pylori*, but rifaximin and rifabutin have been examined for use in rescue therapies (15). At present, rifampin resistance has been reported very infrequently in *H. pylori* (17, 34, 97, 139).

2.3.7 Tetracycline Resistance

Tc inhibits protein synthesis by binding reversibly to the 16S rRNA in the 30S ribosomal subunits, blocking the binding of aminoacyl-tRNA, and thus stalling the synthesis of the growing peptide chains (140, 141). Tetracycline resistance (Tc^R) is not very common in *H. pylori* (33, 46, 60, 61, 64, 142, 143), with primary resistance rates ranging from 5 to 56% (14, 24, 32, 84, 120, 143). Tc is often used in secondary therapies (144).

In *H. pylori*, mutations in both copies of the16S rRNA genes, ^{965}AGA^{967} to ^{965}TTC^{967} (*Escherichia coli* numbering), was determined to be solely responsible for high-level Tc^R (61, 145, 146). Single and double mutations at nucleotides 965–967 result in lower levels of Tc^R (85, 147). Decreased binding of Tc to *E. coli* ribosomes with nucleotide substitutions in positions 965 to 967 of the 16S rRNA has been demonstrated (148). Molecular diagnostic assays have been developed to identify mutations in the 16S rRNA leading to Tc^R. These include a microelectronic chip array using stool specimens (59), real-time PCR on DNA from gastric biopsies (60, 61), and PCR-RFLP using DNA from cultured bacteria (62).

Other studies have suggested that additional gene products and DNA mutations may play roles in Tc^R (147). One study showed 16S rRNA mutations in only 54% of Tc-resistant *H. pylori* isolates, while the remainder showed decreased Tc uptake (85). A role for efflux was demonstrated by Li et al, who showed that inactivation of a Tc efflux homologue abrogated inducible Tc^R (149).

While Tc-susceptible isolates of *H. pylori* show modal MICs of 0.5 µg/mL, Tc-resistant isolates show a range of MICs from 32 to $\geq$ 258 µg/mL (150). The reason for the wide range in Tc MICs has not yet been clearly explained. A mixture of susceptible wild-type and Tc-resistant mutant ribosomes may account for intermediate levels of Tc^R in some cases (146). It is possible that the interaction of Tc with ribosomes containing 16S rRNA that is modified by mutations leads to unstable interactions; and these may influence the MIC values, perhaps depending on growth medium or other variables. Site-directed mutagenesis in *H. pylori* using limited (seven) substitutions within the triplet mutation suggested that single- and double-base-pair mutations mediate only low-level Tc^R (MIC 1–2 µg/mL) and also decrease growth rates in the presence of Tc (145). This study thus offers a possible explanation for the prevalence of the ^{965}TTC^{967} mutation observed in clinical Tc^R isolates of *H. pylori*.

Further studies are necessary to understand exactly how the mutations found in the Tc^R *H. pylori* are selected in vivo, why such a wide variation in MICs is possible in *H. pylori* isolates which contain similar 16S rRNA mutations, and the possible importance of genes other than the 16S rRNA mutation which may contribute to Tc^R.

3 *Campylobacter jejuni/coli*

The majority of *Campylobacter* enteritis cases are sporadic in nature, occurring in individuals, households, or small groups. In infected humans, the most usual illness is a gastroenteritis that is indistinguishable from that caused by other enteric bacterial pathogens such as *Salmonella* and *Shigella*. Most studies to determine risk factors have identified consumption of contaminated food, milk, or untreated water. It is presumed that these sources of infection are the result of contamination from animal waste. *Campylobacter* colonize a wide variety of wild and domestic mammalian and avian species. Among food animals, *C. jejuni* is most often isolated from chickens and cattle, while *C. coli* is more common in pigs and turkeys. Although the organisms can be transmitted directly to humans from farm animals (151) and pets (152–155), undercooked or mishandled fresh poultry meat appears to be the most important source of infection (156–162). Therefore, interventions have focused on reducing the prevalence of *Campylobacter*-positive poultry flocks destined for human consumption or the freezing of meats derived from birds colonized by *Campylobacter* (156).

Depending on the host factors, inoculum size, and strain virulence, symptoms follow 1–7 days after ingesting the organism. In the only reported study with human volunteers (163), the infectious dose for some strains was as low as 500 organisms. Symptoms usually consist of diarrhea (with or without blood), severe abdominal pain and fever; headache, myalgia, and nausea are also common. Extra-intestinal infections include cholecystitis, pancreatitis, hepatitis, bacteremia, and peritonitis (164). Gastritis symptoms usually resolve within 3–7 days, and primary treatment consists of fluid and electrolyte replacement. As with other types of bacterial gastroenteritis, campylobacteriosis is usually self-limiting. Antimicrobial chemotherapy may be necessary only in cases of severe, relapsing, or invasive illness.

A number of different laboratory approaches have been examined for isolating *Campylobacter* on primary culture medium. Most clinical laboratories employ selective culture methods optimized for the recovery of *C. jejuni* and *C. coli*, which requires incubation in a microaerobic atmosphere (5% O_2, 10% CO_2, and 85% N_2). Selective enrichment includes growth at 42°C and use of a medium containing one or more antimicrobial agents (usually cefoperazone) to inhibit competing enteric flora. Using this approach, Gram-stained smears showing small curved or spiral bacilli from typical *Campylobacter* colonies is a very reliable presumptive diagnosis. Additional methods may be employed to confirm the identification and to determine the species.

Treatment with erythromycin is effective if given early in the course of infection (165), and is currently considered the drug of choice for treating culture-confirmed cases of campylobacteriosis (166). Because symptoms are indistinguishable from salmonellosis, a FQ is often given pending (or in the absence of) culture results, and it is the treatment of choice for traveler's diarrhea (167). In some countries, Tc, doxycycline, and azithromycin have been used as alternative therapeutics, but resistance to these agents has been documented.

Gentamicin, clindamycin, tigecycline, and meropenem all show potent in vitro activity, and may prove valuable for treating infections.

3.1 In Vitro Antimicrobial Susceptibility Testing and Interpretive Criteria

The relatively recent recognition of *Campylobacter* as a common cause of diarrhea, the self-limiting nature of most infections, and the fastidious growth requirements of the organism all contributed to the delay in developing a standardized in vitro susceptibility testing method for members of this genus. A broth microdilution susceptibility testing method for *Campylobacter* was recently established along with quality control ranges for 14 antimicrobial agents (168). The method requires testing in Mueller-Hinton broth supplemented with 2–5% lysed horse blood and incubation in a humid atmosphere of 10% CO_2 and 5% O_2. Testing can be done at either 36–37°C for 48h or 42°C for 24h, the latter applying only to thermotolerant species (169). It is important that testing be done using a well-controlled gas mixture and constant temperature, since not all isolates will grow at incubation temperatures of 35°C or 43°C and not all commercially available gas-generating systems produce consistent results (168).

Other methods have been used to measure antimicrobial susceptibility. Disk diffusion testing is an attractive method because of its convenience and low cost. Some researchers have reported consistent results for certain drugs obtained by disk diffusion within a single laboratory (170). However, when tested in a multi-laboratory format, there has been a lack of intra- and inter-laboratory reproducibility, which was greater for certain antimicrobial agents (P.F. McDermott, unpublished results). This problem was ascribed to the peculiar growth characteristic of *Campylobacter* and to variations in commercially prepared media. This resulted in widely different interpretations of zone sizes for the same strain/antimicrobial combinations, depending on the angle and intensity of the light source. Until growth conditions are identified that eliminate ambiguity in zone endpoint determinations, and QC ranges have been established for this testing method, disk diffusion should not be used for testing *Campylobacter*. A variation on the standard disk diffusion susceptibility testing is the use of disks to screen for resistance. This approach uses the lack of a zone of inhibition as an indicator of resistance. This method works very well to predict resistant to Cip (5-µg disks) and erythromycin (15-µg disks) (171, 172), the drugs of choice for treating *Campylobacter* infections (172). Another widely used method for antimicrobial susceptibility testing of *Campylobacter* is the Etest method (173–175). This technique is convenient, and has the advantage of providing MIC values over a wide range (15 log$_2$

dilutions). Using incubation at 36°C, it has been observed that, for many agents, the Etest endpoints fall one or more dilutions above or below those observed using agar dilution (174, 176). The two methods compare favorably for some drugs, with a reported overall agreement between Etest and agar dilution ranging from 62% (174) to 83% (177).

The interpretation of antimicrobial susceptibility testing results for *Campylobacter* isolates is hindered by the lack of validated breakpoints for any antimicrobial agent. Establishing interpretive criteria requires clinical outcome studies, data on population MIC distributions, and information on the pharmacokinetic/pharmacodynamic properties at the site of infection. Because controlled clinical studies are lacking, breakpoints used at different institutions may differ considerably. The CLSI recently (June, 2006) used a population MIC distribution to set tentative MIC breakpoints for resistance to Cip (MIC ≥ 4µg/mL), erythromycin (MIC ≥ 32µg/mL), doxycycline (MIC ≥ 8µg/mL), and Tc (MIC ≥ 16µg/mL) (172). Similar approaches have been taken by other consensus standards organizations such as the British Society for Antimicrobial Chemotherapy (BSAC) and the Comite de L'Antibiogramme de la Societe Francaise de Microbiologie (SFM) (http://www.sfm.asso.fr/), among others. The BSAC has proposed resistance breakpoints of ≥2µg/mL for erythromycin and ≥4µg/mL for Cip (178), whereas the SFM has proposed ≥8µg/mL for erythromycin and ≥4µg/mL for Cip (179).

For other agents, population MIC distributions can be used to suggest interpretive breakpoints. Table 2 shows suggested *Campylobacter* MIC breakpoints, inferred from MIC distributions generated using broth microdilution testing of more than 850 human and retail meat isolates. CLSI proposed breakpoints also are indicated. These breakpoints were used in the NARMS program beginning in 2004, as reference points for monitoring purposes. They should be considered with caution as guidelines to anti-infective therapy until supporting clinical outcome data are available.

Table 2 Suggested interpretive breakpoints for *Campylobacter*

Antibiotic	MIC breakpoint (µg/mL)		
	S	I	R
Azithromycin	≤2	4	≥8
Ciprofloxacin[a]	≤1	2	≥4
Clindamycin	≤2	4	≥8
Doxycycline[a]	≤2	4	≥8
Erythromycin[a]	≤8	16	≥32
Gentamicin	≤2	4	≥8
Telithromycin	≤4	8	≥16
Tetracycline[a]	≤4	8	≥16

S, I, R susceptible, intermediate, resistant
[a] Indicates CLSI established interpretive criteria

3.2 Clinical Significance of Resistance

As has been reported for *Salmonella* (180), there is evidence that antimicrobial resistance causes adverse health outcomes in patients with *Campylobacter* infections. The first report by Smith et al. (181) calculated that, among subjects treated with a quinolone, the median duration of diarrhea was 7 days if the causative strain was susceptible, versus 10 days if it was resistant. Engberg et al. (182) also observed a longer duration of illness in patients with a quinolone-resistant *C. jejuni* infection (median 13.2 days), compared to patients infected with a susceptible strain (median 10.3, $p = 0.01$). Based on the analysis of 3,471 patients with *Campylobacter* infections, quinolone resistance was associated with a sixfold increased risk of invasive illness or death within 30 days of infection (183). Comparing infections caused by quinolone-resistant and -susceptible strains, a Center for Disease Control study estimated a 2-day increase in duration of diarrhea caused by resistant strains (9 vs. 7 days) (184). Importantly, this difference was greater among subjects who did not take antidiarrheal medications or antimicrobial agents (12 vs. 6 days).

The biological mechanisms of protracted illness from resistant strains, even in the absence of antimicrobial therapy, are not clear. Using competitive growth experiments in a chicken animal model, Luo et al. observed that quinolone-resistant *C. jejuni* isolates (with targeted *gyrA* mutations), repeatedly out-competed isogenic susceptible strains in the animal gut (185). Whether a competitive growth/colonization advantage reflects increased resistance to immune eradication is not known, nor is it clear how the underlying DNA gyrase mutations confer this selective advantage. It is interesting that antimicrobial-resistant *Helicobacter* strains appear to have enhanced invasiveness in tissue culture models (186). Regardless of the potential biological relationships between virulence and antimicrobial resistance in *Campylobacter*, the clinical evidence suggests a greater health burden due to infections caused by resistant strains.

3.3 Resistance to Specific Antimicrobials

The known genetic elements underlying *Campylobacter* resistance include the common chromosomal and plasmid-borne mechanisms present in other bacteria, namely, target-site modification, structural gene mutation, enzymatic inactivation, and energy-dependent drug efflux. Resistance to the major antimicrobial drug classes is presented below.

3.3.1 Macrolides

Macrolides are considered a primary treatment for *Campylobacter* infections. As noted above, macrolides are bacterio-static agents that inhibit peptide chain elongation by binding to the 50S subunit of the bacterial ribosome (102). Resistance is uncommon in *C. jejuni* from the U.S., with approximately 1% of human isolates showing erythromycin MICs $\geq 8\,\mu g/mL$ (187); however, higher rates have been reported in other countries (188). Resistance to macrolides (and other antimicrobials) is usually higher in *C. coli*, where resistance to erythromycin resistance ranges from 4 to 6% in the U.S (187) and up to 14% in other regions (189). Among strains isolated from animals, resistance is generally higher in isolates from swine and poultry production environments (189), where macrolides are used routinely.

In *C. jejuni* and *C. coli*, macrolide resistance is caused by target-site mutations and efflux. The only example of an extra-chromosomal macrolide resistance determinant in *Campylobacter* is a plasmid-encoded rRNA methylase (*erm*), which has been found only in *C. rectus* to date (190).

As in other bacteria, macrolide resistance results from target-site mutations in two positions of domain V (peptidyl transferase region) of the 23S rRNA genes. *Campylobacter* contains three copies of the rRNA gene; evidence suggests that at least two copies must be mutated to cause resistance (191). It is worth mentioning that ribosomal gene mutations are present only in isolates with erythromycin MICs $\geq 32\,\mu g/mL$ (192), supporting the use of $32\,\mu g/mL$ as an MIC breakpoint denoting resistance. Nucleotide changes at positions A2074 and A2075 are most common, corresponding in *E. coli* to positions 2,058 and 2,059 (193). An A2075G transition is the most frequent mutation observed in clinical strains (191, 194–196). It is usually present in all three copies of the 23S rRNA gene (191), and can confer high MICs ($>128\,\mu g/mL$). In vitro transformation experiments demonstrated that these mutations are readily transferred and stably incorporated into the chromosomes of susceptible recipient *C. jejuni* and *C. coli* strains (191, 197). While ribosomal mutations in *Campylobacter* can confer cross-resistance to tylosin, azithromycin, and Cla. Erythromycin MICs are identical to those of Cla; therefore, erythromycin can be used as a surrogate for this compound. While ribosomal mutations imparting erythromycin resistance also impact susceptibility to tylosin and azithromycin, the MICs to the latter drugs are not equivalent to those of erythromycin (198).

It is known that efflux plays a role both in baseline erythromycin susceptibility levels and in elevated MICs conferring clinical resistance (192, 199). The first report of a multidrug efflux system in *Campylobacter* was made by Charvalos et al. (200) using *C. jejuni* mutants selected on pefloxacin and on cefotaxime. The MDR phenotype included β-lactams, quinolones, chloramphenicol, and Tc, in addition to macrolides, but the genes were not identified. In resistant clinical isolates, studies by Lin et al. (201). and by Pumbwe and Piddock (202) identified an efflux system encoded by the *cmeABC* locus. CmeB is related to multidrug transporters of the resistance nodulation and cell division (RND) superfamily, which includes AcrB in *E. coli* and MexB in *Pseudomonas*. This pump extrudes a variety of structurally unrelated antimicrobials, as well as detergents and dyes, and is widespread in *C. jejuni* and *C. coli* (203). *cmeABC* also confers resistance to bile, and is consequently required for intestinal colonization in chickens (204). Activity of CmeB is down-regulated by CmeR (205), but no transcriptional activators have been identified to date. Inactivation of *cme* yielded a 4- to 16-fold reduction in erythromycin MICs in wild-type susceptible strains (201, 206). Overexpression of *cmeB* also confers resistance to ampicillin, chloramphenicol, and Tc. A second macrolide efflux phenotype was revealed by exposure to the efflux pump inhibitor Phe-Arg-ß-naphthylamide (PAßN). This compound increased erythromycin susceptibility to wild-type levels in intermediately-susceptible strains, and to a lesser degree in resistant strains. Furthermore, it made a wild-type isolate hyper-susceptible (199). Further characterization of this phenotype confirmed that this pump was independent of *cmeB* (207). Ge et al. examined ten putative *Campylobacter* efflux pumps, including CmeB and CmeF, which were identified based on sequence homology. Using site-directed mutagenesis, they found that only *cmeB* influenced susceptibility to chloramphenicol, erythromycin, nalidixic acid, and Tc (208).

3.3.2 Quinolones

In contrast to the relatively stable low incidence of macrolide resistance, FQ-resistant *C. jejuni* has emerged in many regions over the past two decades (187, 193, 209–211). This rise has been attributed in part to the use of FQs (sarafloxacin and enrofloxacin) in poultry medicine. Endtz et al. reported that the emergence of FQ resistance in human *C. jejuni* infections in the Netherlands coincided with the approval of enrofloxacin in poultry in 1987 (210). In Minnesota from 1992 to 1998, the number of quinolone-resistant infections increased from 1.3 to 10.2%. In only 2 years after approval of the poultry FQ sarafloxacin in 1995, Cip[R] among *Campylobacter* in Minnesota had doubled. Part of this increase was attributed to the acquisition of resistant strains from poultry meats (181). In a study examining *C. jejuni* infections among patients treated at Philadelphia-area hospitals, Nachamkin et al. reported Cip[R] rising from 8.3% in 1996 to 40.5% in 2001 (212). Among human *Campylobacter* isolates submitted to the CDC, Cip[R] rose from 0% in 1989–1990 (209) to 21% in 2002 (187). In 2004, NARMS data showed that 15.5% of *Campylobacter* isolated from retail chicken breast samples were resistant to Cip (213). The associations of Cip[R] *Campylobacter* in humans to selection in the poultry production environment prompted the Food and Drug Administration to withdraw approval of FQs in poultry (214).

Cip[R] in *Campylobacter* results from a single topoisomerase mutation in *gyrA*, similar to that seen in *H. pylori*; but unlike *Salmonella* and *E. coli*, in which two mutations are required for clinical levels of ciprofloxacin resistance (215). The sufficiency of a single mutation in *Campylobacter gyrA* does not appear to be the case for all FQs. A study by Ruiz et al. (216) showed that moxifloxacin resistance required double topoisomerase mutations (Ile86, Asn90), suggesting that the efficacy of this newer FQ may be less subject to compromise by *gyrA* mutation. For Cip, however, the most common mutation associated with high-level MICs (≥32 μg/mL) is a substitution of Ile at Thr86 (217–220). Mutations at Asp90 and Ala70 (185, 217) impart intermediate levels of Cip resistance (MICs 1–4 μg/mL). A small number of *Campylobacter* that show resistance to nalidixic acid but not to Cip have been reported. This phenotype has been associated with a Thr86Ala substitution in *gyrA* (221). Other *gyrA* mutations have been detected, but their respective contributions to quinolone resistance have not been measured (222). No changes in GyrB have been associated with FQ resistance, and *C. jejuni* lacks the *parC* gene encoding topoisomerase IV (223). The requirement of only a single base change for high-level Cip MICs may help explain the rapid evolution of Cip[R] in *Campylobacter* from animals (224, 225) and humans (226) exposed to FQs, as well as the widespread occurrence of Cip[R] in retail raw meats (213) and human clinical isolates (187).

Multidrug efflux pumps, including CmeB, contribute to baseline levels of FQ susceptibility in *Campylobacter*. Wild type susceptible isolates of *Campylobacter* display higher Cip MICs (0.125–0.5 μg/mL) than do wild type strains of other Gram-negative enterics such as *E. coli* and *Salmonella* (MIC, 0.015–0.06 μg/mL). This intrinsic resistance appears to result from the constitutive expression of *cmeB* (201, 202). Inactivation of *cmeB* by site-directed mutagenesis lowered Cip MICs in susceptible isolates to levels in the range for *E. coli* and *Salmonella* (201, 202). Similarly, in resistant strains (also containing *gyrA* mutations), inactivation of the *cmeABC* operon reduced Cip MICs near to that of wild-type isolates (227). These findings show that, as with macrolide resistance (198), *cmeB* functions cooperatively in isolates with target-site mutations to maintain acquired high-level FQ MICs in *Campylobacter*. Expression of *cmeB*, and perhaps of *cmeF* as well as of other uncharacterized loci (206), likely also contribute to acquired quinolone/multidrug resistance.

3.3.3 Tetracycline

Tc is considered as a second-line treatment for *Campylobacter*. It is used mainly in developing regions due to its low cost and low toxicity. Resistance to Tc has risen in many countries, making this class of antimicrobials less attractive for therapy. In Canada, Tc^R has increased from 7 to 9% in 1980–1981 (228) to 43–68% in 1998–2001 (229), with more recent resistant strains also showing even higher MIC values (230). In the U.S. from 1997 to 2002, Tc^R ranged from 38 to 48% (187). In some countries, the proportion of resistant isolates is much higher (231, 232).

While efflux plays a role (208), Tc^R is mainly due to ribosomal protection mediated by the *tet(O)* gene product (233). Tet(O) confers resistance by allosterically displacing Tc from its primary binding site on the ribosome (234, 235). The *tet(O)* gene is widespread in *Campylobacter* worldwide, and is also present in various Gram-positive species. Alleles of *tet(O)* in *C. jejuni* usually impart MIC levels of Tc ranging from 32 to 128 μg/mL, but mutations in *tet(O)* can lead to MICs as high as 512 μg/mL (230).

The *tet(O)* gene is usually plasmid-borne (236), but may be located on the chromosome (237). Two large self-transmissible Tc^R plasmids have been sequenced (238), one from *C. jejuni* and one from *C. coli*, isolated on separate continents about 20 years apart. Both plasmids had mosaic sequence structures, with gene signatures suggesting origins in various commensal and pathogenic bacteria, including *H. pylori*. Remarkably, the two plasmids were 94.3% identical at the DNA sequence level, and are widespread in plasmid-containing Tc-resistant *Campylobacter* isolates. Other plasmid vehicles, ranging in size up to 100 kb, also carry Tc^R determinants (236).

3.3.4 Aminoglycosides

The genetic determinants that cause aminoglycoside resistance are well characterized in several bacteria. In *Campylobacter*, kanamycin resistance is due to the presence of the *aphA-3* gene (239), usually located on large plasmids (40 to >100 kb) that often carry *tet(O)* as well (240). Integrons also have been identified in *Campylobacter* (241, 242), which in one report were found to be common (16.4%) in isolates from different sources, and to contain the aminoglycoside-modifying enzyme encoded by *aadA2* (243). Spectinomycin/streptomycin resistance due to adenylyltranferases encoded by *aadA* and *aadE* has been associated with plasmids from human clinical isolates (244). Resistance to the aminoglycoside streptothricin has been linked to the *sat4* gene product in animal and clinical isolates from Europe (245). In isolates recovered from a poultry production house, integrons carrying the *aacA-4* gene were detected in strains resistant to tobramycin and gentamicin (241). It is not known if this mechanism is present in human clinical isolates. Gentamicin has been recommended for the treatment of campylobacteriosis, particularly in patients with systemic infection (164).

Resistance to gentamicin is rare in *Campylobacter*, and has not been characterized at the genetic level.

3.3.5 Other Resistances

Most *Campylobacter* strains are resistant to β-lactam antimicrobials, with over 80% of *C. jejuni* carrying β-lactamases (246). *C. jejuni* are resistant to cefamandole, cefoxitin, and cefoperazone. Most isolates also are resistant to cephalothin and cefazolin, and resistance is variable for cefotaxime, moxalactam, piperacillin, and ticarcillin (247). The most active β-lactam agents include ampicillin, amoxicillin, cefpirome, and imipenem (246). Meropenem also shows good activity against *Campylobacter* (248), and has been recommended as a treatment option (249, 250).

Campylobacter are generally resistant to trimethoprim and sulfonamides, through mechanisms common to other bacteria. Trimethoprim resistance in *C. jejuni* is due to the chromosomal presence of acquired trimethoprim resistance-associated dihydrofolate reductase gene cassettes (*dfr1*, *dfr9*) (251). Sulfonamide resistance in *Campylobacter*, as in other bacteria, results from mutations in dihydropteroate synthase (252). Chloramphenicol resistance is rare in *Campylobacter*, and results from acetylase activity encoded by *cat* genes (253).

References

1. Skirrow MB. *Campylobacter* enteritis: a "new" disease. Br Med J 1977; 2(6078):9–11
2. Nachamkin I, Allos BM, Ho T. *Campylobacter* species and Guillain–Barre syndrome. Clin Microbiol Rev 1998; 11(3):555–567
3. Cave D. Transmission and epidemiology of *Helicobacter pylori*. Am J Med 1996; 100(5A):12S–17S
4. Montalban C, Manzanal A, Boixeda D, Redondo C, Alvarez I, Calleja J et al. *Helicobacter pylori* eradication for the treatment of low-grade gastric MALT lymphoma: follow-up together with sequential molecular studies. Ann Oncol 1997; 8 Suppl:37–39
5. Perez-Perez GI, Rothenbacher D, Brenner H. Epidemiology of *Helicobacter pylori* infection. Helicobacter 2004; 9 Suppl 1:1–6
6. Weyermann M, Adler G, Brenner H, Rothenbacher D. The mother as source of *Helicobacter pylori* infection. Epidemiol 2006; 17:1–3
7. Gisbert JP. The recurrence of *Helicobacter pylori* infection: incidence and variables influencing it. A critical review. Am J Gastroenterol 2005; 100:2083–2099
8. Konno M, Fujii N, Yokota S, Sato K, Takajashi M, Sato K et al. Five-year follow-up study of mother-to-child transmission of *Helicobacter pylori* infection detected by a random amplified polymorphic DNA fingerprinting method. J Clin Microbiol 2005; 43:2246–2250
9. Calvet X. *Helicobacter pylori* infection: treatment options. Digestion 2006; 73 Suppl 1:119–128
10. Hunt RH, Fallone CA, Thomson AB. Canadian *Helicobacter pylori* Consensus Conference update: infections in adults. Canadian *Helicobacter* Study Group. Can J Gastroenterol 1999; 13(3):213–217

11. Graham DY. Therapy of *Helicobacter pylori*: current status and issues. Gastroenterol 2000; 118:S2-S8

12. Bytzer P, O'Morain C. Treatment of *Helicobacter pylori*. Helicobacter 2005; 10 Suppl 1:40–46

13. Megraud F. Resistance of *Helicobacter pylori* to antibiotics and its impact on treatment options. Drug Res Updates 2001; 4:178–186

14. Realdi G, Dore MP, Piana AAA, Carta MLC, et al. Pretreatment antibiotic resistance in *Helicobacter pylori* infection: results of three randomized controlled studies. Helicobacter 1999; 4:106–112

15. Bock H, Koop H, Lehn N, Heep M. Rifabutin-based triple therapy after failure of *Helicobacter pylori* eradication treatment. J Clin Gastroenterol 2000; 31:222–225

16. Gasbarrini A, Gasbarrini G, Pelosini I. Eradication of *Helicobacter pylori*: are rifaximin-based regimens effective. Digestion 2006; 73 Suppl 1:129–135

17. Toracchio S, Capodicasa S, Soraja DB, Cellini L, Marzio L. Rifabutin based triple therapy for eradication of *H. pylori* primary and secondary resistant to tinidazole and clarithromycin. Dig Liver Dis 2005; 37:33–38

18. Gisbert JP, Castro-Fernandez M, Bermejo F, Perez-Aisa A, Ducons J, Fernandez-Bermejo M et al. Third-line rescue therapy with levofloxacin after two *H. pylori* treatment failures. Am J Gastroenterol 2006; 101(2):243–247

19. Matsumoto Y, Miki I, Aoyama N, Shirasaka D, Wantanabe Y, Morita Y et al. Levofloxacin versus metronidazole-based rescue therapy for *H. pylori* infection in Japan. Dig Liver Dis 2005; 37:821–825

20. Togawa J, Inamori M, Furisawa N, Takahashi H, Yoneda M, Kawamura H et al. Efficacy of a triple therapy with rabeprazole, amoxicillin, and faropenem as a second-line treatment after failure of initial *Helicobacter pylori* eradication therapy. Hepatogastroenterology 2005; 52:645–648

21. Gisbert JP, Pajares JM. *Helicobacter pylori* "rescue" therapy after failure of two eradication treatments. Helicobacter 2005; 10(5):363–372

22. Nijevitch AA, Shcherbakov PL, Sataev VU, Khasanov RSh, Khashash RA, Tuygunov MM. *Helicobacter pylori* eradication in childhood after failure of initial treatment: advantage of quadruple therapy with nifuratel to furazolidone. Aliment Pharmacol Ther 2005; 22:881–887

23. Dore MP, Osato MS, Kwon DH, Graham DY, Wl-Zaatari FAK. Demonstration of unexpected antibiotic resistance of genotypically identical *Helicobacter pylori* isolates. Clin Infect Dis 1998; 27:84–89

24. Kim JJ, Kim JG, Kwon DH. Mixed-infection of antibiotic susceptible and resistant *Helicobacter pylori* isolates in a single patient and underestimation of antimicrobial susceptibility testing. Helicobacter 2003; 8:202–206

25. Gisbert JP, Pajares JM. 13C-urea breath test in the management of *Helicobacter pylori* infection. Dig Liver Dis 2005; 37:899–906

26. Gisbert JP, Parjares JM. Diagnosis of *Helicobacter pylori* infection by stool antigen determination: a systematic review. Am J Gastroenterol 2001; 96:2829–2838

27. Can F, Yilmaz Z, Demirbilek M, Bilezikci B, Kunefeci G, Atac FB et al. Diagnosis of *Helicobacter pylori* infection and determination of clarithromycin resistance by fluorescence *in situ* hybridization from formalin-fixed, paraffin-embedded gastric biopsy specimens. Can J Microbiol 2005; 51:569–573

28. Russmann H, Kempf CAJ, Koletzko S, Heesemann J, Autenrieth IB. Comparison of fluorescent *in situ* hybridization and conventional culturing for detection of *Helicobacter pylori* in gastric biopsy specimens. J Clin Microbiol 2001; 39:304–308

29. Schabereiter-Gurtner C, Hirschl AM, Dragosics B, Hufnagl P, Puz S, Kovach Z et al. Novel real-time PCR assay for detection of *Helicobacter pylori* infection and simultaneous clarithromycin susceptibility testing of stool and biopsy specimens. J Clin Microbiol 2004; 42:4512–4518

30. Rimbara E, Noguchi N, Yamaguchi T, Narui K, Kawai T, Sasatsu M. Development of a highly sensitive method for detection of clarithromycin-resistant *Helicobacter pylori* from human feces. Curr Microbiol 2005; 51:1–5

31. CLSI. Clinical and Laboratory Standards Institute/NCCLS. *Performance Standards for Antimicrobial Susceptibility Testing; Fifteenth Informational Supplement.* CLSI/NCCLS document M100-S15. 940 West Valley Road, Suite 1400, Wayne, PA 19087–1898 USA: Clinical and Laboratory Standards Institute, 2005

32. Falsafi T, Mobasheri F, Nariman F, Najafi M. Susceptibilities to different antibiotics of *Helicobacter pylori* strains isolated from patients at the pediatric medical center of Tehran, Iran. J Clin Microbiol 2004; 42:387–389

33. Branca G, Spanu R, Cammarota G, Schito AM, Gasbarrini A, Gasbarrini GB, et al. High levels of dual resistance to clarithromycin and metronidazole and *in vitro* activity of levofloxacin against *Helicobacter pylori* isolates from patients after failure of therapy. Int J Antimicrob Agents 2004; 433–438

34. Fujimura S, Kato S, Kawamura T, Watanabe A. *In vitro* activity of rifampicin against *Helicobacter pylori* isolated from children and adults. J Antimicrob Chemother 2002; 49:541–543

35. Osato MS, Reddy R, Graham DY. Metronidazole and clarithromycin resistance amongst *Helicobacter pylori* isolates from a large metropolitan hospital in the United States. Int J Antimicrob Agents 1999; 12(4):341–347

36. Solnick JV. Editorial response: antibiotic resistance in *Helicobacter pylori*. Clin Infect Dis 1998; 27:90–92

37. Henriksen TH, Brorson O, Schoyen R, Thoresen T, Lia A. A simple method for determining metronidazole resistance of *Helicobacter pylori*. J Clin Microbiol 1997; 35:1424–1426

38. Cederbrant G, Kahlmeter G, Ljungh A. The E test for antimicrobial susceptibility testing of *Helicobacter pylori*. J Antimicrob Chemother 1993; 31:65–71

39. DeCross AJ, Marshall BJ, McCallum RW, Hoffman SR, Barrett LJ, Guerrant RL. Metronidazole susceptibility testing for *Helicobacter pylori*: comparison of disk, broth, and agar dilution methods and their clinical relevance. J Clin Microbiol 1993; 31(8):1971–1974

40. Glupczynski Y, Labbe M, Hansen W, Crokaert F, Yourassowsky E. Evaluation of the E test for quantitative antimicrobial susceptibility testing of *Helicobacter pylori*. J Clin Microbiol 1991; 29:2072–2075

41. Hirschl AM, Hirschl MM, Rotter ML. Comparison of three methods for the determination of the sensitivity of *Helicobacter pylori* to metronidazole. J Antimicrob Chemother 1993; 32:45–49

42. Megraud F, Lehn N, Lind T, Bayerdorffer E, O'Morain C, Spiller R et al. Antimicrobial susceptibility testing of *Helicobacter pylori* in a large multicenter trial: the MACH 2 study. Antimicrob Agents Chemother 1999; 43(11):2747–2752

43. Piccolomini R, Di Bonaventura G, Catamo G, Carbone F, Neri M. Comparative evaluation of the E test, agar dilution, and broth microdilution for testing susceptibilities of *Helicobacter pylori* strains to 20 antimicrobial agents. J Clin Microbiol 1997; 35(7):1842–1846

44. Heep M, Beck D, Bayerdorffer E, Lehn N. Rifampin and rifabutin resistance mechanism in *Helicobacter pylori*. Antimicrob Agents Chemother 1999; 43:1497–1499

45. van der Wouden EJ, Jong AD, Thijs JC, Kleibeuker JH, vanZwet AA. Subpopulations of *Helicobacter pylori* are responsible for discrepancies in the outcome of nitroimidazole susceptibility testing. Antimicrob Agents Chemother 1999; 43:1484–1486

46. Raymond J, Nguyen B, Bergeret M, Dupont C, Kalach N. Heterogeneous susceptibility to metronidazole and clarithromycin of *Helicobacter pylori* isolates from a single biopsy in adults is confirmed in children. Int J Antimicrob Agents 2005; 26:272–278

47. Scarpellini P, Carrera P, Cavallero A, Cernuschi M, Mezzi G, Testoni PA et al. Direct detection of *Helicobacter pylori* mutations associated with macrolide resistance in gastric biopsy material

taken from human immunodeficiency virus-infected subjects. J Clin Microbiol 2002; 40:2234–2237

48. Weel JFL, vanderHulst RWM, Gerrits Y, Tytgat GNJ, vander-Ende A, Dankert J. Heterogeneity in susceptibility to metronidazole among *Helicobacter pylori* isolates from patients with gastritis or peptic ulcer disease. J Clin Microbiol 1996; 34:2158–2162

49. Jorgensen M, Daskalopoulos G, Warburton V, Mitchell HM, Hazell SL. Multiple strain colonization and metronidazole resistance in *Helicobacter pylori*-infected patients: identification from sequential and multiple biopsy specimens. J Infect Dis 1996; 174:631–635

50. Glocker E, Kist M. Rapid detection of point mutations in the *gyrA* gene of *Helicobacter pylori* conferring resistance to ciprofloxacin by a fluorescence resonance energy transfer based real-time PCR approach. J Clin Microbiol 2004; 42:2241–2246

51. Chisholm SA, Owen RJ, Teare EL, Saverymuttu S. PCR-based diagnosis of *Helicobacter pylori* infection and real-time determination of clarithromycin resistance directly from human gastric biopsy samples. J Clin Microbiol 2001; 39:1217–220

52. Elviss NC, Lawson AJ, Owen RJ. Application of 3′-mismatched reverse primer PCR compared with real-time PCR and PCR-RFLP for the rapid detection of 23S rDNA mutations associated with clarithromycin resistance in *Helicobacter pylori*. Int J Antimicrob Agents 2004; 23:349–355

53. Lascols C, Lamarque D, Costa JM, Copie-Bergman C, Glaumec JML, Deforges L et al. Fast and accurate quantitative detection of *Helicobacter pylori* and identification of clarithromycin resistance mutations in *H. pylori* isolates from gastric biopsy specimens by real-time PCR. J Clin Microbiol 2003; 41:4573–4577

54. Marais A, Monteiro L, Occhialini A, Pina M, Lamouliatte H, Megraud F. Direct detection of *Helicobacter pylori* resistance to macrolides by a polymerase chain reaction/DNA enzyme immunoassay in gastric biopsy specimens. Gut 1999; 44:463–467

55. Posteraro P, Branca G, Sanguinetti M, Ranno S, Cammarota G, Rahimi S et al. Rapid detection of clarithromycin resistance in *Helicobacter pylori* using a PCR-based denaturing HPLC assay. J Antimicrob Chemother 2006; 57(1):71–78

56. Russmann H, Adler K, Haai R, Gebert B, Koletzko S, heesemann J. Rapid and accurate determination of genotypic clarithromycin resistance in cultured *Helicobacter pylori* by fluorescent *in situ* hybridization. J Clin Microbiol 2001; 39:4142–4144

57. Ryan KA, Doorn LV, Moran AP, Glennon M, Smith T, Maher M. Evaluation of clarithromycin resistance and *cagA* and *vacA* genotyping of *Helicobacter pylori* strains from the west of Ireland using line probe assays. J Clin Microbiol 2001; 39:1978–1980

58. Stone GG, Shortridge D, Versalovic J, Beyer J, Flamm RK, Graham DY et al. A PCR-oligonucleotide ligation assay to determine the prevalence of 23S rRNA gene mutations in clarithromycin-resistant *Helicobacter pylori*. Antimicrob Agents Chemother 1997; 41:712–714

59. Xing JZ, Clarke C, Zhu L, Gabos S. Development of a microelectronic chip array for high throughput genotyping of *Helicobacter* species and screening for antimicrobial resistance. J Biomol Screen 2005; 10:235–245

60. Glocker E, Berning M, Gerrits MM, Kusters JG, Kist M. Real-time PCR screening for 16S rRNA mutations associated with resistance to tetracycline in *Helicobacter pylori*. Antimicrob Agents Chemother 2005; 49:3166–3170

61. Lawson AJ, Elviss NC, Owen RJ. Real-time PCR detection and frequency of 16S rDNA mutations associated with resistance and reduced susceptibility to tetracycline in *Helicobacter pylori* from England and Wales. J Antimicrob Chemother 2005; 56:282–286

62. Ribeiro ML, Gerrits MM, Benvengo YH, Berning M, Godoy AP, Kuipers EJ et al. Detection of high-level tetracycline resistance in clinical isolates of *Helicobacter pylori* using PCR-RFLP. FEMS Immunol Med Microbiol 2004; 40(1):57–61

63. Murakami K, Sato R, Okimoto T, Nasu M, Fujioka T, Kodama M et al. Efficacy of triple therapy comprising rabeprazole, amoxicillin, and metronidazole for second-line *Helicobacter pylori* eradication in Japan, and the influence of metronidazole resistance. Aliment Pharmacol Ther 2003; 17:119–123

64. Wheeldon TU, Granstrom M, Hoang TTH, Phuncarg DC, Nilsson LE, Sorberg M. The importance of the level of metronidazole resistance for the success of *Helicobacter pylori* eradication. Aliment Pharmacol Ther 2004; 19:1315–1321

65. Gomollon F, Sicilia B, Ducons JA, Sierra E, Revillo MJ, Ferrero M. Third line treatment for *Helicobacter pylori*: a prospective, culture-guided study in peptic ulcer patients. Aliment Pharmacol Ther 2001; 15:1543–1547

66. Miwa H, Nagahara A, Kurosawa A, Ohkusa T, Ohkura R, Hojo M et al. Is antimicrobial susceptibility testing necessary before second-line treatment for *Helicobacter pylori*?. Aliment Pharmacol Ther 2003; 17:1545–1551

67. Neri M, Milano A, Laterza F, DiBonaventura G, Piccolomini R, Caldarella MP et al. Role of antibiotic sensitivity testing before first-line *Helicobacter pylori* eradication treatments. Aliment Pharmacol Ther 2003; 18:821–827

68. Dore MP, Piana A, Carta M, Atzei A, Are BM, Mura I et al. Amoxycillin resistance is one reason for failure of amoxycillin–omeprazole treatment of *Helicobacter pylori* infection. Aliment Pharmacol Ther 1998; 12:635–639

69. Broutet N, Tchamgoue S, Pereira E, Lamouliatte H, Salamon R, Megraud F. Risk factors for failure of *Helicobacter pylori* therapy-results of an individual data analysis of 2751 patients. 2003; 17:99–109

70. Ducons JA, Santolaria S, Guirao R, Ferrero M, Montoro M, Gomollon F. Impact of clarithromycin resistance on the effectiveness of a regime for *Helicobacter pylori*: a prospective study of 1 week lansoprazole, amoxicillin and clarithromycin in active peptic ulcer. Aliment Pharmacol Ther 1999; 13:775–780

71. Faber J, Ber-Meir M, Rudensky B, Schlesinger Y, Rachman E, Benenson S et al. Treatment regimes for *Helicobacter pylori* infection in children: is in vitro susceptibility testing helpful? J Pediatr Gastroenterol Nutr 2005; 40:571–574

72. Furuta T, Shirai N, Xiao F, El-Omar EM, Rabkin CS, Sugimura H et al. Polymorphism of interleukin-1β affects the eradication rates of *Helicobacter pylori* by triple therapy. Clin Gastroenterol Hepatol 2004; 2:22–30

73. Kawabata H, Habu Y, Tomioka H, Kutsumi H, Kobayashi M, Oyasu K et al. Effect of different proton pump inhibitors, differences in CYP2C19 genotype and antibiotic resistance on the eradication rate of *Helicobacter pylori* infection by a 1-week regimen of proton pump inhibitor, amoxicillin and clarithromycin. Aliment Pharmacol Ther 2003; 17:259–264

74. Koivisto TT, Rautelin HI, Voutilainen ME, Heikkinen MT, Koskenpato JP, Farkkila MA. First-line eradication therapy for *Helicobacter pylori* in primary health care based on antibiotic resistance: results of three eradication regimens. Aliment Pharmacol Ther 2005; 21:773–782

75. Masuda H, Hiyama T, Yoshihara M, Tanaka S, Haruma K, Chayama K. Characteristics and trends of clarithromycin-resistant *Helicobacter pylori* isolates in Japan over a decade. Pathobiology 2004; 71:159–163

76. Megraud F. *H. pylori* antibiotic resistance: prevalence, importance and advances in testing. Gut 2004; 53:1374–1384

77. Tankovic J, Lamarque D, Lascols C, Soussy CJ, Delchier JC. Clarithromycin resistance of *Helicobacter pylori* has a major impact on the efficacy of the omeprazole-amoxicillin-clarithromycin therapy. Pathol Biol 2001; 49:528–533

78. Adamek RJ, Suerbaum S, Pfaffenbach B, Opferkuch W. Primary and acquired *Helicobacter pylori* resistance to clarithromycin, metronidazole, and amoxicillin – influence on treatment outcome. Am Coll Gastroenterol 1998; 93:386–389

79. Buckley MJM, Xia H, Hyde DM, Keane CT, O'Morain COO. Metronidazole resistance reduces efficacy of triple therapy and leads to secondary clarithromycin resistance. Dig Dis Sci 1997; 42:2111–2115

80. Houben MH, Beek DVD, Hensen EF, Craen AJ, Rauws EA, Tytget GN. A systematic review of *Helicobacter pylori* eradication therapy-the impact of antimicrobial resistance on eradication rates. Aliment Pharmacol Ther 1999; 13:2131–2140

81. Noach LA, Langenberg WL, Bertola MA, Dankert J, Tytgat GNJ. Impact of metronidazole resistance on the eradication of *Helicobacter pylori*. Scand J Infect Dis 1994; 26:321–327

82. Ghuysen JM. Serine β-lactamases and penicillin-binding proteins. Annu Rev Microbiol 1991; 45:37–67

83. Boyanova L, Nikolov R, Lazarova E, Gergova G, Katsarov N, Kamburov V et al. Antibacterial resistance in *Helicobacter pylori* strains from Bulgarian children and adult patients over 9 years. J Med Microbiol 2006; 55:65–68

84. Mendonca S, Ecclissato C, Sartori MS, Godoy AP, Guerzoni RA, Degger M et al. Prevalence of *Helicobacter pylori* resistance to metronidazole, clarithromycin, amoxicillin, tetracycline, and furazolidone in Brazil. Helicobacter 2000; 5(2):79–83

85. Wu JY, Kim JJ, Reddy R, Wang WM, Graham DY, Kwon DH. Tetracycline-resistant clinical *Helicobacter pylori* isolates with and without mutations in 16S rRNA-encoding genes. Antimicrob Agents Chemother 2005; 49:578–583

86. DeLoney CR, Schiller NL. Characterization of an *in vitro*-selected amoxicillin-resistant strain of *Helicobacter pylori*. Antimicrob Agents Chemother 2000; 44:3368–3373

87. Gerrits MM, Schuijffel D, vanZwet AA, Kuipers EJ, Vandenbroucke-Grauls CM, Kusters JG. Alterations in penicillin-binding protein 1A confer resistance to beta-lactam antibiotics in *Helicobacter pylori*. Antimicrob Agents Chemother 2002; 46:2229–2233

88. Kwon DH, Dore MP, Kim JJ, Kato M, Lee M, Wu JY et al. High-level β-lactam resistance associated with acquired multidrug resistance in *Helicobacter pylori*. Antimicrob Agents Chemother 2003; 47:2169–2178

89. Okamoto T, Yoshiyama H, Nakazawa T, Park ID, Chang MW, Yanai H et al. A change in PBP1 is involved in amoxicillin resistance of clinical isolates of *Helicobacter pylori*. J Antimicrob Chemother 2002; 60:849–856

90. Paul R, Postius S, Melchers K, Schafer KP. Mutations in *Helicobacter pylori* genes *rdxA* and *pbp1* cause resistance against metronidazole and amoxicillin. Antimicrob Agents Chemother 2001; 45:962–965

91. Candelli M, Nista EC, Carloni E, Pignataro G, Zocco MA, Cazzato A et al. Treatment of *H. pylori* infection: a review. Curr Med Chem 2005; 12:375–384

92. Vila J. Fluoroquinolone resistance. In: Vila J, editor. Frontiers in Antimicrobial Resistance: A Tribute to Stuart B. Levy. Washington, DC: ASM Press, 2005: 41–52

93. Cheon JH, Kim N, Lee DH, Kim JM, Kim JS, JUng HC et al. Efficacy of moxifloxacin-based triple therapy as second-line treatment for *Helicobacter pylori* infection. Helicobacter 2006; 11(1):46–51

94. Gatta L, Zullo A, Perna F, Ricci CVDF, Tampieri A et al. A 10 day levofloxacin-based triple therapy in patients who have failed two eradication courses. Aliment Pharmacol Ther 2005; 22:45–49

95. Moore RA, Beckthold B, Wong S, Kureishi A, Bryan LE. Nucleotide sequence of the *gyrA* gene and characterization of ciprofloxacin-resistant mutants of *Helicobacter pylori*. Antimicrob Agents Chemother 1995; 39:107–111

96. Kim JM, Kim JS, JUng HC, Kim N, Kim T, Song IS. Distribution of antibiotic MICs for *Helicobacter pylori* strains over a 16-year period in patients from Seoul, South Korea. Antimicrob Agents Chemother 2004; 48:4843–4847

97. Heep M, Kist M, Strobel S, Beck D, Lehn N. Secondary resistance among 554 isolates of *Helicobacter pylori* after failure of therapy. Eur J Clin Microbiol Infect Dis 2000; 19:538–541

98. Yahav J, Shmuely H, Niv Y, Bechor J, Samra Z. *In vitro* activity of levofloxacin against *Helicobacter pylori* isolates from patients after treatment failure. Diagnost Microbiol Infect Dis 2006; 55:81–83

99. Tankovic J, Lascols C, Sculo Q, Petit J, Soussy C. Single and double mutations in *gyrA* but not in *gyrB* are associated with low- and high-level fluoroquinolone resistance in *Helicobacter pylori*. Antimicrob Agents Chemother 2003; 47:3942–3944

100. Wang G, Wilson TJ, Jiang Q, Taylor DE. Spontaneous mutations that confer antibiotic resistance in *Helicobacter pylori*. Antimicrob Agents Chemother 2001; 45(3):727–733

101. Yoshida HM, Bogaki M, Nakamura M, Nakamura S. Quinolone resistance-determining region in the DNA gyrase *gyrA* gene of *Escherichia coli*. Antimicrob Agents Chemother 1990; 34:1271–1272

102. Weisblum B. Erythromycin resistance by ribosome modification. Antimicrob Agents Chemother 1995; 39(3):577–585

103. Toracchio S, Aceto GM, Mariani-Constantini R, Battista P, Marzio L. Identification of a novel mutation affecting domain V of the 23S rRNA gene in *Helicobacter pylori*. Helicobacter 2004; 9:396–399

104. Masaoka T, Suzuki H, Kurabayashi K, Kamiya AG, Ishii H. Second-line treatment of *Helicobacter pylori* infection after dilution agar methods and PCR-RFLP analysis. Aliment Pharmacol Ther 2004; 20 Suppl. 1:68–73

105. Bjorkholm B, Sjolund M, Falk PG, Berg OG, Engstrand L, Andersson DI. Mutation frequency and biological cost of antibiotic resistance in *Helicobacter pylori*. PNAS 2001; 98: 14607–14612

106. Versalovic J, Shortridge D, Kibler K, Griffy MV, Beyer J, Flamm RK et al. Mutations in 23S rRNA are associated with clarithromycin resistance in *Helicobacter pylori*. Antimicrob Agents Chemother 1996; 40(2):477–480

107. Occhialini A, Urdaci M, Doucet-Populaire F, Bebear CM, Lamouliatte H, Megraud F. Macrolide resistance in *Helicobacter pylori*: rapid detection of point mutations and assays of macrolide binding to ribosomes. Antimicrob Agents Chemother 1997; 41(12):2724–2728

108. Soltermann A, Perren A, Schmid S, Eigenmann F, Guller R, Weber KB et al. Assessment of *Helicobacter pylori* clarithromycin resistance mutations in archival gastric biopsy samples. Swiss Med Wkly 2005; 135:327–332

109. Taylor DE, Ge Z, Purych D, Lo T, Hiratsuka K. Cloning and sequence analysis of two copies of a 23S rRNA gene from *Helicobacter pylori* and association of clarithromycin resistance with 23S rRNA mutations. Antimicrob Agents Chemother 1997; 41(12):2621–2628

110. Wang G, Taylor DE. Site-specific mutations in the 23S rRNA gene of *Helicobacter pylori* confer two types of resistance to macrolide-lincosamide-streptogramin B antibiotics. Antimicrob Agents Chemother 1998; 42(8):1952–1958

111. Kaneko F, Suzuki H, Hasegawa N, Kurabayshi K, Saito H, Otani S et al. High prevalence rate of *Helicobacter pylori* resistance to clarithromycin during long-term multiple antibiotic therapy for chronic respiratory disease caused by nontuberculous mycobacteria. Aliment Pharmacol Ther 2004; 20 Suppl 1:62–67

112. Burucoa C, Landron C, Garnier M, Fauchere JL. T2182C mutation is not associated with clarithromycin resistance in *Helicobacter pylori*. Antimicrob Agents Chemother 2005; 49: 868–870

113. Khan R, Rahman M. Authors reply. Antimicrob Agents Chemother 2005; 49:868–870

114. Kim KS, Kang JO, Eun CS, Han DS, Choi TY. Mutations in the 23S rRNA gene of *Helicobacter pylori* associated with clarithromycin resistance. J Korean Med Sci 2002; 17:599–603

115. Fontana C, Favaro M, Minelli S, Criscuolo AA, Pietroiusti A, Galante A et al. New site of modification of 23S rRNA associated with clarithromycin resistance of *Helicobacter pylori* clinical isolates. Antimicrob Agents Chemother 2002; 46: 3765–3769

116. DeFrancesco V, Margiotta M, Zullo A, Hassan C, Triani L, Burattini O et al. Clarithromycin-resistant genotypes and eradication of *Helicobacter pylori*. Ann Intern Med 2006; 144: 94–100

117. vanDoorn LJ, Debets-Ossenkopp YJ, Marais A, Sanna R, Megraud F, Kusters JG et al. Rapid detection, by PCR and reverse hybridzation, of mutations in the 23S rRNA gene, associated with macrolide resistance. Antimicrob Agents Chemother 1999; 43:1779–1782

118. DeFrancesco V, Margiotta M, Zullo A, Hassan C, Valles N, Burattini O et al. Primary clarithromycin resistance in Italy assessed on *Helicobacter pylori* DNA sequences by TaqMan real-time polymerase chain reaction. Aliment Pharmacol Ther 2006; 23: 429–435

119. Eisig JN, Silva FM, Rodriguez TN, Hashimoto CL, Barbuti RC. A furazolidone-based quadruple therapy for *Helicobacter pylori* retreatment in patients with peptic ulcer disease. Clin 2005; 60:485–488

120. Kim JJ, Reddy R, Lee M, Kim JG, El-Zaatari FAK, Osato MS et al. Analysis of metronidazole, clarithromycin and tetracycline resistance of *Helicobacter pylori* isolates from Korea. J Antimicrob Chemother 2001; 47:459–461

121. Kwon DH, Lee M, Kim JJ, Kim JG, El Zaatari FAK, Osato MS et al. Furazolidone- and nitrofurantoin resistant *Helicobacter pylori*: prevalence and role of genes involved in metronidazole resistance. Antimicrob Agents Chemother 2001; 45:306–308

122. Breeze AS, Obaseiki-Ebor EE. Nitrofuran reductase activity in nitrofurantoin-resistant strains of *Escherichia coli* K12: some with chromosomally determined resistance and others carrying R-plasmids. J Antimicrob Chemother 1983; 12(6):543–547

123. Edwards DI. Nitroimidazole drugs-action and resistance mechanisms. I. Mechanisms of action. J Antimicrob Chemother 1993; 31:19–20

124. Goodwin A, Kersulyte D, Sisson G, Veldhuyzen van Zanten SJ, Berg DE, Hoffman PS. Metronidazole resistance in *Helicobacter pylori* is due to null mutations in a gene (*rdxA*) that encodes an oxygen-insensitive NADPH nitroreductase. Mol Microbiol 1998; 28(2):383–393

125. Debets-Ossenkopp YJ, Pot RG, vanWesterloo DJ, Goodwin A, Vandenbroucke-Grauls CM, Berg DE et al. Insertion of mini-IS605 and deletion of adjacent sequences in the nitroreductase (*rdxA*) gene cause metronidazole resistance in *Helicobacter pylori* NCTC11637. Antimicrob Agents Chemother 1999; 43:57–62

126. Jenks PJ, Ferrero RL, Labigne A. The role of the *rdxA* gene in the evolution of metronidazole resistance in *Helicobacter pylori*. J Antimicrob Chemother 1999; 43:753–758

127. Kwon DH, Pena JA, Osato MS, Fox JG, Graham DY, Versalovic J. Frameshift mutations in *rdxA* and metronidazole resistance in North American *Helicobacter pylori* isolates. J Antimicrob Chemother 2000; 46:793–796

128. Latham SR, Labigne A, Jenks PJ. Production of the RdxA protein in metronidazole-susceptible and -resistant isolates of *Helicobacter pylori* cultured from treated mice. J Antimicrobial Chemother 2002; 49:675–678

129. Tankovic J, Lamarque D, Delchier JC, Soussy CJ, Labigne A, Jenks PJ. Frequent association between alteration of the *rdxA* gene and metronidazole resistance in French and North African

isolates of *Helicobacter pylori*. Antimicrob Agents Chemother 2000; 44:608–613

130. Yang YJ, Wu JJ, Sheu BS, Kao AW, Huang AH. The *rdxA* gene plays a more major role than *frxA* gene mutation in high-level metronidazole resistance of *Helicobacter pylori* in Taiwan. Helicobacter 2004; 9(5):400–407

131. Jeong JY, Mukhopadhyay AK, Dailidiene D, Wang Y, Velapatino B, Gilman RH et al. Sequential inactivation of *rdxA* (HP0954) and *frxA* (HP0642) nitroreductase genes causes moderate and high-level metronidazole resistance in *Helicobacter pylori*. J Bacteriol 2000; 182:5082–5090

132. Aldana LP, Kato M, Kondo T, Nakagawa S, Zheng R, Sugiyama T et al. In vitro induction of resistance to metronidazole, and analysis of mutations in *rdxA* and *frxA* genes from *Helicobacter pylori* isolates. J Infect Chemother 2005; 11:59–63

133. Mendz GL, Megraud F. Is the molecular basis of metronidazole resistance in microaerophilic organisms understood? Trends Microbiol 2002; 10:370–375

134. Chang KC, Ho SW, Yang JC, Wang JT. Isolation of a genetic locus associated with metronidazole resistance in *Helicobacter pylori*. Biochem Biophys Res Commun 1997; 236(3):785–788

135. Kwon DH, Zaatari FAE, Kato M, Osato MS, Reddy R, Yamaoka Y et al. Analysis of *rdxA* and involvement of additional genes encoding NAD(P)H flavin oxidoreductase (FrxA) and ferredoxin-like protein (FdxB) in metronidazole resistance of *Helicobacter pylori*. Antimicrob Agents Chemother 2000; 44:2133–2142

136. Hoffman PS, Goodwin A, Johnsen J, Magee K, Zanten SJVV. Metabolic activities of metronidazole-sensitive and -resistant strains of *Helicobacter pylori*: repression of pyruvate oxidoreductase and expression of isocitrate lyase activity correlate with resistance. J Bacteriol 1996; 178:4822–4829

137. Kwon DH, Osato MS, Graham DY, El-Zaatari FAK. Quantitative RT-PCR analysis of multiple gene encoding putative metronidazole nitroreductases from *Helicobacter pylori*. Int J Antimicrob Agents 2000; 15:31–36

138. Heep M, Odenbreit S, Beck D, Decker J, Prohaska E, Rieger U et al. Mutations at four distinct regions of the *rpoB* gene can reduce the susceptibility of *Helicobacter pylori* to rifamycins. Antimicrob Agents Chemother 2000; 44:1713–1715

139. Heep M, Rieger U, Beck D, Lehn N. Mutations in the beginning of the *rpoB* gene can induce resistance to rifamycins in both *Helicobacter pylori* and *Mycobacterium tuberculosis*. Antimicrob Agents Chemother 2000; 44:1075–1077

140. Brodersen DE, Clemons WM, Jr, Carter AP, Morgan-Warren RJ, Wimberly BT, Ramakrishnan V. The structural basis for the action of the antibiotics tetracycline, pactamycin, and hygromycin B on the 30S ribosomal subunit. Cell 2000; 103(7):1143–1154

141. Pioletti M, Schlunzen F, Harms J, Zarivach R, Gluhmann M, Avila H et al. Crystal structures of complexes of the small ribosomal subunit with tetracycline, edeine and IF3. EMBO J 2001; 20(8):1829–1839

142. Boyanova L, Gergova G, Koumanova R, Jelev C, Lazarova E, Mitov I et al. Risk factors for primary *Helicobacter pylori* resistance in Bulgarian children. J Med Microbiol 2004; 53: 911–914

143. Hao Q, Li Y, Zhang ZJ, Liu Y, Gao H. New mutation points in 23S rRNA gene associated with *Helicobacter pylori* resistance to clarithromycin in northeast China. World J Gastroenterol 2004; 10:1075–1077

144. McLoughlin R, O'Morain C. Effectiveness of antiinfectives. Chemother 2005; 51:243–246

145. Gerrits MM, Berning M, van Vliet AH, Kuipers EJ, Kusters JG. Effects of 16S rRNA gene mutations on tetracycline resistance in *Helicobacter pylori*. Antimicrob Agents Chemother 2003; 47(9):2984–2986

146. Trieber CA, Taylor DE. Mutations in the 16S rRNA genes of *Helicobacter pylori* mediate resistance to tetracycline. J Bacteriol 2002; 184:2131–2140

147. Dailidiene D, Bertoli MT, Miciuleviciene J, Mukhopadhyay AK, Dailide G, Pascasio MA et al. Emergence of tetracycline resistance in *Helicobacter pylori*: multiple mutational changes in 16S ribosomal DNA and other genetic loci. Antimicrob Agents Chemother 2002; 46(12):3940–3946

148. Nonaka L, Connell SR, Taylor DE. 16S rRNA mutations that confer tetracycline resistance in *Helicobacter pylori* decrease drug binding in *Escherichia coli* ribosomes. J Bacteriol 2005; 187(11):3708–3712

149. Li Y, Dannelly K. Inactivation of the putative tetracycline resistance gene HP1165 in *Helicobacter pylori* led to loss of inducible tetracycline resistance. Arch Microbiol 2006; 185(4): 255–262

150. Midolo PD, Korman MG, Turnidge JD, Lambert JR. *Helicobacter pylori* resistance to tetracycline. Lancet 1996; 347(9009): 1194–1195

151. Potter RC, Kaneene JB, Hall WN. Risk factors for sporadic *Campylobacter jejuni* infections in rural Michigan: a prospective case-control study. Am J Public Health 2003; 93(12): 2118–2123

152. Workman SN, Mathison GE, Lavoie MC. Pet dogs and chicken meat as reservoirs of *Campylobacter* spp. in Barbados. J Clin Microbiol 2005; 43(6):2642–2650

153. Hald B, Pedersen K, Waino M, Jorgensen JC, Madsen M. Longitudinal study of the excretion patterns of thermophilic *Campylobacter* spp. in young pet dogs in Denmark. J Clin Microbiol 2004; 42(5):2003–2012

154. Damborg P, Olsen KE, Moller NE, Guardabassi L. Occurrence of *Campylobacter jejuni* in pets living with human patients infected with *C. jejuni*. J Clin Microbiol 2004; 42(3):1363–1364

155. Tenkate TD, Stafford RJ. Risk factors for *Campylobacter* infection in infants and young children: a matched case-control study. Epidemiol Infect 2001; 127(3):399–404

156. Wingstrand A, Neimann J, Engberg J, Nielsen EM, Gerner-Smidt P, Wegener HC et al. Fresh chicken as main risk factor for campylobacteriosis, Denmark. Emerg.Infect.Dis. 12, 280–284. 2006

157. Friedman CR, Neimann J, Wegener HC, Tauxe RV. Epidemiology of *Campylobacter jejuni* infections in the United States and other industrialized nations. In: Nachamkin I, Blaser MJ, editors. Campylobacter. Washington, DC: American Society for Microbiology, 2000: 130

158. Harris NV, Weiss NS, Nolan CM. The role of poultry and meats in the etiology of *Campylobacter jejuni/coli* enteritis. Am J Public Health 1986; 76(4):407–11

159. Friedman CR, Hoekstra RM, Samuel M, Marcus R, Bender J, Shiferaw B et al. Risk factors for sporadic *Campylobacter* infection in the United States: a case-control study in FoodNet sites. Clin Infect Dis 2004; 38 Suppl 3:S285–S296

160. Eberhart-Phillips J, Walker N, Garrett N, Bell D, Sinclair D, Rainger W et al. Campylobacteriosis in New Zealand: results of a case-control study. J Epidemiol Community Health 1997; 51(6):686–691

161. Kapperud G, Skjerve E, Bean NH, Ostroff SM, Lassen J. Risk factors for sporadic *Campylobacter* infections: results of a case-control study in southeastern Norway. J Clin Microbiol 1992; 30(12):3117–3121

162. Kapperud G, Espeland G, Wahl E, Walde A, Herikstad H, Gustavsen S et al. Factors associated with increased and decreased risk of *Campylobacter* infection: a prospective case-control study in Norway. Am J Epidemiol 2003; 158(3):234–242

163. Black RE, Levine MM, Clements ML, Hughes TP, Blaser MJ. Experimental *Campylobacter jejuni* infection in humans. J Infect Dis 1988; 157(3):472–479

164. Skirrow MB, Blaser MJ. *Campylobacter jejuni*. In: Blaser MJ, Smith PD, Ravdin JI, Greenberg HB, Guerrant RL, editors. Infections of the Gastrointestinal Tract. Baltimore, MD: Lippincott Williams and Wilkins, 2002: 719–739

165. Williams MD, Schorling JB, Barrett LJ, Dudley SM, Orgel I, Koch WC et al. Early treatment of *Campylobacter jejuni* enteritis. Antimicrob Agents Chemother 1989; 33(2):248–250

166. Anonymous. The Sanford Guide to Antimicrobial Therapy. 3rd ed. Hyde Park, VT: Antimicrobial Therapy, Inc., 2003

167. Guerrant RL, Van Gilder T, Steiner TS, Thielman NM, Slutsker L, Tauxe RV et al. Practice guidelines for the management of infectious diarrhea. Clin Infect Dis 2001; 32(3):331–351

168. McDermott PF, Bodeis-Jones SM, Fritsche TR, Jones RN, Walker RD. Broth microdilution susceptibility testing of *Campylobacter jejuni* and the determination of quality control ranges for fourteen antimicrobial agents. J Clin Microbiol 2005; 43(12):6136–6138

169. McDermott PF, Bodeis SM, Aarestrup FM, Brown S, Traczewski M, Fedorka-Cray P et al. Development of a standardized susceptibility test for *Campylobacter* with quality-control ranges for ciprofloxacin, doxycycline, erythromycin, gentamicin, and meropenem. Microb Drug Resist 2004; 10(2):124–131

170. Gaudreau C, Gilbert H. Comparison of disc diffusion and agar dilution methods for antibiotic susceptibility testing of *Campylobacter jejuni* subsp. *jejuni* and *Campylobacter coli*. J Antimicrob Chemother 1997; 39(6):707–712

171. McDermott PF, Bodeis-Jones SM, Nachamkin I. The Use of Disk Diffusion to Screen for Antimicrobial Resistance in *Campylobacter*. Abstracts of the 12th International Workshop of *Campylobacter, Helicobacter* and Related Organisms. Aarhus, Denmark. 2003

172. CLSI. Clinical and Laboratory Standards Institute (CLSI). *Methods for Antimicrobial Dilution and Disk Susceptibility Testing of Infrequently – Isolated or Fastidious Bacteria; Proposed Guideline*. CLSI document M45-P (ISBN 1–56238–000–0). Wayne, Pennsylvania 19087–1898 USA, 2005: Clinical and Laboratory Standards Institute, 940 West Valley Road, Suite 1400, 2006

173. Engberg J, Andersen S, Skov R, Aarestrup FM, Gerner-Smidt P. Comparison of two agar dilution methods and three agar diffusion methods, including the Etest, for antibiotic susceptibility testing of thermophilic *Campylobacter* species. Clin Microbiol Infect 1999; 5(9):580–584

174. Ge B, Bodeis S, Walker RD, White DG, Zhao S, McDermott PF et al. Comparison of the Etest and agar dilution for *in vitro* antimicrobial susceptibility testing of *Campylobacter*. J Antimicrob Chemother 2002; 50(4):487–494

175. Oncul O, Zarakolu P, Oncul O, Gur D. Antimicrobial susceptibility testing of *Campylobacter jejuni*: a comparison between Etest and agar dilution method. Diagn Microbiol Infect Dis 2003; 45(1):69–71

176. Valdivieso-Garcia A, Imgrund R, Deckert A, Varughese B, Harris K, Bunimov N, et al. Cost analysis and antimicrobial susceptibility testing comparing the Etest and the agar dilution method in *Campylobacter* spp Abstracts of the Annual Meeting of the American Society for Microbiology, May 2003, Washington, DC. 2003

177. Huang MB, Baker CN, Banerjee S, Tenover FC. Accuracy of the E test for determining antimicrobial susceptibilities of staphylococci, enterococci, *Campylobacter jejuni*, and gram-negative bacteria resistant to antimicrobial agents. J Clin Microbiol 1992; 30(12):3243–3248

178. King A. Recommendations for susceptibility tests on fastidious organisms and those requiring special handling. J Antimicrob Chemother 2001; 48 Suppl 1:77–80

179. Anonymous. Comite de l'Antibiogramme de la Societe Francaise de Microbiologie report 2003. Int J Antimicrob Agents 2003; 21(4):364–391

180. Molbak K. Human health consequences of antimicrobial drug-resistant *Salmonella* and other foodborne pathogens. Clin Infect Dis 2005; 41(11):1613–1620

181. Smith KE, Besser JM, Hedberg CW, Leano FT, Bender JB, Wicklund JH et al. Quinolone-resistant *Campylobacter jejuni* infections in Minnesota, 1992–1998. Investigation Team. N Engl J Med 1999; 340(20):1525–32

182. Engberg J, Neimann J, Nielsen EM, Aerestrup FM, Fussing V. Quinolone-resistant *Campylobacter* infections: risk factors and clinical consequences. Emerg Infect Dis 2004; 10(6): 1056–1063

183. Helms M, Simonsen J, Olsen KE, Molbak K. Adverse health events associated with antimicrobial drug resistance in *Campylobacter* species: a registry-based cohort study. J Infect Dis 2005; 191(7):1050–1055

184. Nelson JM, Smith KE, Vugia DJ, Rabatsky-Ehr T, Segler SD, Kassenborg HD et al. Prolonged diarrhea due to cipro floxacin-resistant *Campylobacter* infection. J Infect Dis 2004; 190(6):1150–1157

185. Luo N, Pereira S, Sahin O, Lin J, Huang S, Michel L et al. Enhanced *in vivo* fitness of fluoroquinolone-resistant *Campylobacter jejuni* in the absence of antibiotic selection pressure. Proc Natl Acad Sci U S A 2005; 102(3):541–546

186. Lai CH, Kuo CH, Chen PY, Poon SK, Chang CS, Wang WC. Association of antibiotic resistance and higher internalization activity in resistant *Helicobacter pylori* isolates. J Antimicrob Chemother 2006; 57(3):466–471

187. CDC. 2003 National Antimicrobial Resistance Monitoring System (NARMS) For Enteric Bacteria. Available at: http://www.cdc.gov/ncidod/dbmd/narms/. NARMS. 2006

188. Rao D, Rao JR, Crothers E, McMullan R, McDowell D, McMahon A et al. Increased erythromycin resistance in clinical *Campylobacter* in Northern Ireland an update. J Antimicrob Chemother 2005

189. Aarestrup FM, Nielsen EM, Madsen M, Engberg J. Antimicrobial susceptibility patterns of thermophilic *Campylobacter* spp. from humans, pigs, cattle, and broilers in Denmark. Antimicrob Agents Chemother 1997; 41(10):2244–2250

190. Roe DE, Weinberg A, Roberts MC. Mobile rRNA methylase genes in *Campylobacter* (*Wolinella*) *rectus*. J Antimicrob Chemother 1995; 36(4):738–740

191. Gibreel A, Kos VN, Keelan M, Trieber CA, Levesque S, Michaud S et al. Macrolide resistance in *Campylobacter jejuni* and *Campylobacter coli*: molecular mechanism and stability of the resistance phenotype. Antimicrob Agents Chemother 2005; 49(7):2753–2759

192. Payot S, Avrain L, Magras C, Praud K, Cloeckaert A, Chaslus-Dancla E. Relative contribution of target gene mutation and efflux to fluoroquinolone and erythromycin resistance, in French poultry and pig isolates of *Campylobacter coli*. Int J Antimicrob Agents 2004; 23(5):468–472

193. Engberg J, Aarestrup FM, Taylor DE, Gerner-Smidt P, Nachamkin I. Quinolone and macrolide resistance in *Campylobacter jejuni* and *C. coli*: resistance mechanisms and trends in human isolates. Emerg Infect Dis 2001; 7(1):24–34

194. Vacher S, Menard A, Bernard E, Santos A, Megraud F. Detection of mutations associated with macrolide resistance in thermophilic *Campylobacter* spp. by real-time PCR. Microb Drug Resist 2005; 11(1):40–47

195. Niwa H, Chuma T, Okamoto K, Itoh K. Simultaneous detection of mutations associated with resistance to macrolides and quinolones in *Campylobacter jejuni* and *C. coli* using a PCR-line probe assay. Int J Antimicrob Agents 2003; 22(4): 374–379

196. Niwa H, Chuma T, Okamoto K, Itoh K. Rapid detection of mutations associated with resistance to erythromycin in *Campylobacter*

197. *jejuni/coli* by PCR and line probe assay. Int J Antimicrob Agents 2001; 18(4):359–364

197. Kim JS, Carver DK, Kathariou S. Natural transformation-mediated transfer of erythromycin resistance in *Campylobacter coli* strains from turkeys and swine. Appl Environ Microbiol 2006; 72(2):1316–1321

198. Cagliero C, Mouline C, Payot S, Cloeckaert A. Involvement of the CmeABC efflux pump in the macrolide resistance of *Campylobacter coli*. J Antimicrob Chemother 2005; 56(5):948–950

199. Mamelli L, Amoros JP, Pages JM, Bolla JM. A phenylalanine-arginine beta-naphthylamide sensitive multidrug efflux pump involved in intrinsic and acquired resistance of *Campylobacter* to macrolides. Int J Antimicrob Agents 2003; 22(3):237–241

200. Charvalos E, Tselentis Y, Hamzehpour MM, Kohler T, Pechere JC. Evidence for an efflux pump in multidrug-resistant *Campylobacter jejuni*. Antimicrob Agents Chemother 1995; 39(9):2019–2022

201. Lin J, Michel LO, Zhang Q. CmeABC functions as a multidrug efflux system in *Campylobacter jejuni*. Antimicrob Agents Chemother 2002; 46(7):2124–2131

202. Pumbwe L, Piddock LJ. Identification and molecular characterisation of CmeB, a *Campylobacter jejuni* multidrug efflux pump. FEMS Microbiol Lett 2002; 206(2):185–189

203. Corcoran D, Quinn T, Cotter L, O'Halloran F, Fanning S. Characterization of a *cmeABC* operon in a quinolone-resistant *Campylobacter coli* isolate of Irish origin. Microb Drug Resist 2005; 11(4):303–308

204. Lin J, Sahin O, Michel LO, Zhang Q. Critical role of multidrug efflux pump CmeABC in bile resistance and *in vivo* colonization of *Campylobacter jejuni*. Infect Immun 2003; 71(8): 4250–4259

205. Lin J, Akiba M, Sahin O, Zhang Q. CmeR functions as a transcriptional repressor for the multidrug efflux pump CmeABC in *Campylobacter jejuni*. Antimicrob Agents Chemother 2005; 49(3):1067–1075

206. Pumbwe L, Randall LP, Woodward MJ, Piddock LJ. Expression of the efflux pump genes *cmeB*, *cmeF* and the porin gene *porA* in multiple-antibiotic-resistant *Campylobacter jejuni*. J Antimicrob Chemother 2004; 54(2):341–347

207. Mamelli L, Prouzet-Mauleon V, Pages JM, Megraud F, Bolla JM. Molecular basis of macrolide resistance in *Campylobacter*: role of efflux pumps and target mutations. J Antimicrob Chemother 2005; 56(3):491–497

208. Ge B, McDermott PF, White DG, Meng J. Role of efflux pumps and topoisomerase mutations in fluoroquinolone resistance in *Campylobacter jejuni* and *Campylobacter coli*. Antimicrob Agents Chemother 2005; 49(8):3347–3354

209. Gupta A, Nelson JM, Barrett TJ, Tauxe RV, Rossiter SP, Friedman CR et al. Antimicrobial resistance among *Campylobacter* strains, United States, 1997–2001. Emerg Infect Dis 2004; 10(6):1102–1109

210. Endtz HP, Ruijs GJ, van Klingeren B, Jansen WH, van der Reyden T, Mouton RP. Quinolone resistance in *Campylobacter* isolated from man and poultry following the introduction of fluoroquinolones in veterinary medicine. J Antimicrob Chemother 1991; 27(2):199–208

211. DANMAP. DANMAP 2004 – Use of antimicrobial agents and occurrence of antimicrobial resistance in bacteria from food animals, foods and humans in Denmark. ISSN 1600–2032. 40–41. 2005

212. Nachamkin I, Ung H, Li M. Increasing fluoroquinolone resistance in *Campylobacter jejuni*, Pennsylvania, USA, 1982–2001. Emerg Infect Dis 2002; 8(12):1501–1503

213. FDA. National Antimicrobial Resistance Monitoring System for Enteric Bacteria (NARMS): NARMS Retail Meat Annual Report, 2003. Rockville, MD: U.S. Department of Health and Human Services, FDA. 2004

214. Federal Register, 65. 64954 (Oct 31, 2000).

215. Piddock LJ. Mechanisms of fluoroquinolone resistance: an update 1994–1998. Drugs 1999; 58 Suppl 2:11–18

216. Ruiz J, Moreno A, Jimenez de Anta MT, Vila J. A double mutation in the *gyrA* gene is necessary to produce high levels of resistance to moxifloxacin in *Campylobacter spp.* clinical isolates. Int J Antimicrob Agents 2005; 25(6):542–545

217. Wang Y, Huang WM, Taylor DE. Cloning and nucleotide sequence of the *Campylobacter jejuni gyrA* gene and characterization of quinolone resistance mutations. Antimicrob Agents Chemother 1993; 37(3):457–463

218. Alonso R, Mateo E, Girbau C, Churruca E, Martinez I, Fernandez-Astorga A. PCR-restriction fragment length polymorphism assay for detection of *gyrA* mutations associated with fluoroquinolone resistance in *Campylobacter coli*. Antimicrob Agents Chemother 2004; 48(12):4886–4888

219. Beckmann L, Muller M, Luber P, Schrader C, Bartelt E, Klein G. Analysis of *gyrA* mutations in quinolone-resistant and -susceptible *Campylobacter jejuni* isolates from retail poultry and human clinical isolates by non-radioactive single-strand conformation polymorphism analysis and DNA sequencing. J Appl Microbiol 2004; 96(5):1040–1047

220. Hakanen AJ, Lehtopolku M, Siitonen A, Huovinen P, Kotilainen P. Multidrug resistance in *Campylobacter jejuni* strains collected from Finnish patients during 1995–2000. J Antimicrob Chemother 2003; 52(6):1035–1039

221. Jesse TW, Englen MD, Pittenger-Alley LG, Fedorka-Cray PJ. Two distinct mutations in *gyrA* lead to ciprofloxacin and nalidixic acid resistance in *Campylobacter coli* and *Campylobacter jejuni* isolated from chickens and beef cattle. J Appl Microbiol 2006; 100(4):682–688

222. Ge B, White DG, McDermott PF, Girard W, Zhao S, Hubert S et al. Antimicrobial-resistant *Campylobacter* species from retail raw meats. Appl Environ Microbiol 2003; 69(5): 3005–3007

223. Parkhill J, Wren BW, Mungall K, Ketley JM, Churcher C, Basham D et al. The genome sequence of the food-borne pathogen *Campylobacter jejuni* reveals hypervariable sequences. Nature 2000; 403(6770):665–668

224. McDermott PF, Bodeis SM, English LL, White DG, Walker RD, Zhao S et al. Ciprofloxacin resistance in *Campylobacter jejuni* evolves rapidly in chickens treated with fluoroquinolones. J Infect Dis 2002; 185(6):837–840

225. van Boven M, Veldman KT, de Jong MC, Mevius DJ. Rapid selection of quinolone resistance in *Campylobacter jejuni* but not in *Escherichia coli* in individually housed broilers. J Antimicrob Chemother 2003; 52(4):719–723

226. Wretlind B, Stromberg A, Ostlund L, Sjogren E, Kaijser B. Rapid emergence of quinolone resistance in *Campylobacter jejuni* in patients treated with norfloxacin. Scand J Infect Dis 1992; 24(5):685–686

227. Luo N, Sahin O, Lin J, Michel LO, Zhang Q. In vivo selection of *Campylobacter* isolates with high levels of fluoroquinolone resistance associated with *gyrA* mutations and the function of the CmeABC efflux pump. Antimicrob Agents Chemother 2003; 47(1):390–394

228. Gaudreau C, Gilbert H. Antimicrobial resistance of clinical strains of *Campylobacter jejuni* subsp. *jejuni* isolated from 1985 to 1997 in Quebec, Canada. Antimicrob Agents Chemother 1998; 42(8):2106–2108

229. Gaudreau C, Gilbert H. Antimicrobial resistance of *Campylobacter jejuni* subsp. *jejuni* strains isolated from humans in 1998 to 2001 in Montreal, Canada. Antimicrob Agents Chemother 2003; 47(6):2027–2029

230. Gibreel A, Tracz DM, Nonaka L, Ngo TM, Connell SR, Taylor DE. Incidence of antibiotic resistance in *Campylobacter jejuni* isolated in Alberta, Canada, from 1999 to 2002, with special reference to *tet(O)*-mediated tetracycline resistance. Antimicrob Agents Chemother 2004; 48(9):3442–3450

231. Schwartz D, Goossens H, Levy J, Butzler JP, Goldhar J. Plasmid profiles and antimicrobial susceptibility of *Campylobacter jejuni* isolated from Israeli children with diarrhea. Zentralbl Bakteriol 1993; 279(3):368–376

232. Li CC, Chiu CH, Wu JL, Huang YC, Lin TY. Antimicrobial susceptibilities of *Campylobacter jejuni* and *coli* by using E-test in Taiwan. Scand J Infect Dis 1998; 30(1):39–42

233. Manavathu EK, Hiratsuka K, Taylor DE. Nucleotide sequence analysis and expression of a tetracycline-resistance gene from *Campylobacter jejuni*. Gene 1988; 62(1):17–26

234. Trieber CA, Burkhardt N, Nierhaus KH, Taylor DE. Ribosomal protection from tetracycline mediated by Tet(O): Tet(O) interaction with ribosomes is GTP-dependent. Biol Chem 1998; 379(7):847–855

235. Spahn CM, Blaha G, Agrawal RK, Penczek P, Grassucci RA, Trieber CA et al. Localization of the ribosomal protection protein Tet(O) on the ribosome and the mechanism of tetracycline resistance. Mol Cell 2001; 7(5):1037–1045

236. Tenover FC, Williams S, Gordon KP, Nolan C, Plorde JJ. Survey of plasmids and resistance factors in *Campylobacter jejuni* and *Campylobacter coli*. Antimicrob Agents Chemother 1985; 27(1):37–41

237. Pratt A, Korolik V. Tetracycline resistance of Australian *Campylobacter jejuni* and *Campylobacter coli* isolates. J Antimicrob Chemother 2005

238. Batchelor RA, Pearson BM, Friis LM, Guerry P, Wells JM. Nucleotide sequences and comparison of two large conjugative plasmids from different *Campylobacter* species. Microbiology 2004; 150(Pt 10):3507–3517

239. Lambert T, Gerbaud G, Trieu-Cuot P, Courvalin P. Structural relationship between the genes encoding 3″-aminoglycoside phosphotransferases in *Campylobacter* and in gram-positive cocci. Ann Inst Pasteur Microbiol 1985; 136B(2):135–150

240. Gibreel A, Skold O, Taylor DE. Characterization of plasmid-mediated *aphA-3* kanamycin resistance in *Campylobacter jejuni*. Microb Drug Resist 2004; 10(2):98–105

241. Lee MD, Sanchez S, Zimmer M, Idris U, Berrang ME, McDermott PF. Class 1 integron-associated tobramycin-gentamicin resistance in *Campylobacter jejuni* isolated from the broiler chicken house environment. Antimicrob Agents Chemother 2002; 46(11):3660–3664

242. Lucey B, Crowley D, Moloney P, Cryan B, Daly M, O'Halloran F et al. Integronlike structures in *Campylobacter* spp. of human and animal origin. Emerg Infect Dis 2000; 6(1):50–55

243. O'Halloran F, Lucey B, Cryan B, Buckley T, Fanning S. Molecular characterization of class 1 integrons from Irish thermophilic *Campylobacter* spp. J Antimicrob Chemother 2004; 53(6):952–957

244. Pinto-Alphandary H, Mabilat C, Courvalin P. Emergence of aminoglycoside resistance genes *aadA* and *aadE* in the genus *Campylobacter*. Antimicrob Agents Chemother 1990; 34(6):1294–1296

245. Jacob J, Evers S, Bischoff K, Carlier C, Courvalin P. Characterization of the *sat4* gene encoding a streptothricin acetyltransferase in *Campylobacter coli* BE/G4. FEMS Microbiol Lett 1994; 120(1–2):13–17

246. Tajada P, Gomez-Graces JL, Alos JI, Balas D, Cogollos R. Antimicrobial susceptibilities of *Campylobacter jejuni* and *Campylobacter coli* to 12 beta-lactam agents and combinations with beta-lactamase inhibitors. Antimicrob Agents Chemother 1996; 40(8):1924–1925

247. Lachance N, Gaudreau C, Lamothe F, Lariviere LA. Role of the beta-lactamase of *Campylobacter jejuni* in resistance to beta-lactam agents. Antimicrob Agents Chemother 1991; 35(5):813–818

248. Kwon SY, Cho DH, Lee SY, Lee K, Chong Y. Antimicrobial susceptibility of *Campylobacter fetus* subsp. *fetus* isolated from blood and synovial fluid. Yonsei Med J 1994; 35(3): 314–319

249. Monselise A, Blickstein D, Ostfeld I, Segal R, Weinberger M. A case of cellulitis complicating *Campylobacter jejuni* subspecies jejuni bacteremia and review of the literature. Eur J Clin Microbiol Infect Dis 2004; 23(9):718–721

250. Burch KL, Saeed K, Sails AD, Wright PA. Successful treatment by meropenem of *Campylobacter jejuni* meningitis in a chronic alcoholic following neurosurgery. J Infect 1999; 39(3):241–243

251. Gibreel A, Skold O. An integron cassette carrying *dfr1* with 90-bp repeat sequences located on the chromosome of trimethoprim-resistant isolates of *Campylobacter jejuni*. Microb Drug Resist 2000; 6(2):91–98

252. Gibreel A, Skold O. Sulfonamide resistance in clinical isolates of *Campylobacter jejuni*: mutational changes in the chromosomal dihydropteroate synthase. Antimicrob Agents Chemother 1999; 43(9):2156–2160

253. Wang Y, Taylor DE. Chloramphenicol resistance in *Campylobacter coli*: nucleotide sequence, expression, and cloning vector construction. Gene 1990; 94(1):23–28

Chapter 60
Pertussis (Whooping Cough)

Michael A. Saubolle

1 Overview and Bacteriology

Bronchitis, an inflammatory process involving the lower respiratory tract, presents in very differing forms (acute and chronic). Each form requires a different management approach. *Bordetella* spp., *Mycoplasma pneumoniae*, and *Chlamydophila pneumoniae* have been implicated as significant bacterial etiologies of acute bronchitis, while other usual bacteria have not been commonly associated with this syndrome in otherwise healthy patients (1, 2). *Bordetella* spp. are commonly associated with clinical presentations characterized by prolonged, persistent, coughing which often tends to be paroxysmal. Such presentations have been referred to as pertussis or whooping cough.

The genus *Bordetella* is presently known to be comprised of at least eight species (*Bordetella pertussis*, *Bordetella parapertussis*, *Bordetella bronchiseptica*, *Bordetella avium*, *Bordetella hinzii*, *Bordetella holmesii*, *Bordetella trematum*, and *Bordetella petrii* (recently described)) of fastidious Gram-negative coccobacilli. The most common clinical etiology in human cases of pertussis is *B. pertussis*, with *B. parapertussis* causing only occasional cases. *Bordetella bronchiseptica*, *B. holmesii*, *B. hinzii*, and *B. trematum* are rarely isolated from human cases (See Table 1) (3–5). On rare occasions, one may find *B. pertussis* and *B. parapertussis* co-infecting the same patient (6, 7).

The clinically important *Bordetella spp.* produce a number and variety of adhesins (filamentous hemagglutinins (FHA) and fimbriae (FIM)) as well as autotransporters (a surface protein:pertactin (PRN); an outer membrane protein:Vag8; and a secreted protein:tracheal colonization factor (TcfA)) (4). These help the organisms attach to respiratory cilia. The organisms also express several toxins, including pertussis toxin (PT), adenylate cyclase (CyaA),

type III secretion, dermonecrotic toxin (DNT), and tracheal cytotoxin (TCT). These toxins help disrupt the architecture of the epithelial lining of the respiratory tract and provide protection to the organisms from the immune system (Table 1) (4). Together, these biologically active products are responsible for the organisms' ability to colonize and survive in the respiratory tract, to cause the clinical features of pertussis, and to induce immunity in the host.

2 History of Geographic Spread

Pertussis was first noted in the literature in the fifteenth century, seemingly being first recognized as originating in France in 1414 (4). The first large epidemic was reported in Paris in 1578. In 1679, Sydenham introduced the term "pertussis," meaning "violent cough," for the syndrome. The first *Bordetella pertussis* isolate was recovered in 1906 by Bordet and Gengou, with the other three species associated with human disease being isolated in the first decade of the twentieth century (*B. bronchiseptica*), in the 1930s (*B. parapertussis*), and in the 1980s and 1990s (*B. holmesii*) (4).

Pertussis was recognized as a severe global problem with most countries having epidemic and endemic forms of the disease. Prior to the introduction of vaccines, almost every child contracted the disease. The worldwide introduction of whole-cell vaccines from the 1940s to the 1960s dramatically decreased its effect on morbidity and mortality, with infections reduced by as much as 80 to >90%.

Even with availability of vaccine, pertussis remains a major contributor to morbidity and mortality worldwide, causing the reporting of an estimated 5 million infections and 60,000 deaths each year (7). However, because of high variability in the success of vaccination programs, outside estimates attribute as many as 48.5 million cases and almost 295,000 deaths to pertussis (4, 8). Sharp increases in the incidence in pertussis cases is seen every 3–5 years worldwide, but the rate seems to be increasing since the 1980s.

M.A. Saubolle (✉)
Department of Clinical Pathology, Banner Good Samaritan Medical Center, Phoenix, AZ, USA
mike.saubolle@bannerhealth.com

D.L. Mayers (ed.), *Antimicrobial Drug Resistance*,
DOI 10.1007/978-1-60327-595-8_60, © Humana Press, a part of Springer Science+Business Media, LLC 2009

Table 1 Bacteriology of *Bordetella spp.* pathogenic to humans

Species pathogenic to humans	*Bordetella pertussis* (common), *Bordetella parapertussis$_{hu}$* (infrequent), *Bordetella bronchiseptica* (rare), *Bordetella holmesii* (rare), *Bordetella hinzii* (very rare), *Bordetella trematum* (very rare)
Cellular morphology	Gram-negative coccobacilli
Overall pathogenic properties (primarily in *B. pertussis*)	Adhesin: filamentous hemagglutinins, fimbriae
	Autotransporters: pertactin, VagB, BrkA, SphB1
	Toxins: pertussis toxin, adenylate cyclase, type 3 secretion, dermonecrotic toxin, tracheal cytotoxin
	Lipopolysaccharides: *wlb* locus, *wbm* locus, PagP
Reservoirs	*B. pertussis*: humans only
	B. parapertussis: human strain in humans only
	B. bronchiseptica: many mammal species and rarely humans, especially in dogs and swine, but primary reservoir unknown
	B. holmesii: occurs in humans, but epidemiology presently unknown
	B. hinzii: poultry; rarely associated with humans
	B. trematum: rarely associated with nonrespiratory infections in humans

Adapted from (4, 5)

The incidence of pertussis in the United States between 1922 and 1940 (prior to the vaccine) was approximately 150/100,000 population. After the introduction of the vaccine, the incidence decreased to 1/100,000 by the 1980s. It has since re-emerged in the United States (as in the rest of the world), with the number of cases steadily increasing from only 1,010 in 1976 to 9,771 in 2002, 11,000 in 2003, and 25,827 in 2004 (9). The incidence is rising as well in countries like France, Finland, other northern European countries, and Canada, which have very strong pediatric vaccination programs. The most recent increases throughout the world are attributable to the increasing number of cases in adolescents and adults (4, 5, 7, 10, 11).

3 Epidemiology

Whooping cough or pertussis is highly contagious and its primary etiology, *B. pertussis*, has a predilection for humans and has no other known reservoir (4). *Bordetella bronchiseptica*, *B. parapertussis*, and *B. holmesii* do have other animal reservoirs, although little is known about *B. holmesii*. *Bordetella bronchiseptica* infects a wide range

of other hosts while in humans it is primarily associated with the immunocompromised patients (e.g. AIDS). A strain of *B. parapertussis* has adapted to humans (*B. parapertussis$_{hu}$*) and now has no other environmental reservoirs, but causes milder disease. Recently, *B. holmesii* has been associated with human disease, being isolated from bacteremic young adults and from some sputum specimens. Little is known of its epidemiology. Even more recently, *B. hinzii* and *B. trematum* have been reported in association with some rare cases of respiratory and nonrespiratory disease in humans (5).

The number of cases in adolescents and adults has increased significantly (5, 7, 10). Reasons for this dramatic increase are unclear, but may include an increase in prevalence of circulating *B. pertussis* in the general population and transmission of infection from adults to infants. Possible reasons given for this increase have been a waning immunity, changes in the vaccine and in the organism, better diagnostic capability and greater awareness. Revaccination of older children and adults with pertussis vaccine had been contraindicated until just recently because of the vaccine's side effects; yet, immunity wanes in about 5–10 years post-initial administration of vaccine. Thus, adolescents and adults are considered to be a significant reservoir for pertussis. Patients are most contagious in the catarrhal phase of disease and especially within the first 3 weeks of onset of cough (9). Secondary attack rates can exceed 80 percent in the susceptible population.

4 Clinical Significance

Traditionally, pertussis has been considered a childhood illness. But recently, an increasing numbers of infections have been associated with adolescent and adult populations (12). Clinical presentations of pertussis are vastly different between the younger and older groups and often may not be recognized by clinicians in the latter.

After an incubation period of 7–10 days (range: 5–21 days), classic symptoms of pertussis in infants include an insidious catarrhal stage lasting approximately 1–2 weeks. The catarrhal stage is indistinguishable from other common upper respiratory ailments characterized by nasal congestion, mild sore throat, and mild, dry cough; with either no or minimally elevated fever being present. The first stage is followed by a paroxysmal stage lasting from 1 to 6–10 weeks. In this stage, the cough worsens from intermittent to paroxysmal, characterized by succession of coughing without inspiration between coughs, and ending in an inspiratory "whoop". The frequent episodes of convulsive coughing and inspiratory whoop are commonly followed by post-cough emesis. The symptoms in older children and adults may be more atypical (especially in previously vaccinated individuals) and are usually milder. In these older patients, paroxysmal coughing may still be prolonged (often lasting for 1–6 weeks), but the whooping is present only in 20–40% of cases and may not be as characteristic as in the younger children and infants. Post-tussive emesis is frequently missing in adults. Leukocytosis ($50,000/mm^3$ WBCs with absolute lymphocyte counts greater than $10,000/mm^3$) is commonly present in classical pertussis, but may be diminished or absent in atypical cases as well as in the older adolescent and adult patients. Finally, the paroxysmal stage is followed by a gradual and protracted convalescent stage which can stretch from 2 to 4 weeks to several months. Coughing and the toll of the illness wanes as convalescence continues, although nonparoxysmal coughing can continue throughout the course. New viral infection during this period can cause recurrence of symptoms (4, 9).

Severe pertussis, with its paroxysmal coughing can have many complications, including sleep deprivation, pneumothorax, rib fracture, rectal prolapse, subdural hematoma, subconjunctival hemorrhage, and neurologic complications. Secondary bacterial pneumonias and otitis media can further complicate the scenario. Complications are greatest in the susceptible infants of less than 1 year of age.

The differential diagnoses include viral infection, bacterial infection, tuberculosis, and exacerbation of chronic bronchitis, as well as noninfectious causes such as asthma, presence of a foreign object, postnasal drip, gastrointestinal reflux, and malignancy.

5 Laboratory Diagnosis

To some degree, the severity of symptoms of pertussis may be lessened and its period of communicability shortened by its rapid diagnosis and institution of appropriate therapy (6). Antimicrobial therapy is especially useful in patients with symptoms of less than 3–4 weeks duration. Direct specimen evaluation by direct fluorescent antibody (DFA) detection or nucleic acid amplification testing (NAAT) methods such as PCR, culture, and serologic methods are all available to help make the diagnosis of pertussis.

Pertussis is a notifiable disease. Laboratories need to review the specific reporting requirements of each local state health authority in order to comply.

5.1 Specimen Collection and Transport

Preferred specimens include aspirates or swabbed specimens taken from the posterior nasopharynx. In culture, nasopharyngeal aspirates (NP) have slightly better recovery yields then NP swabbed specimens, but in many clinical situations are harder to obtain. Specimens should contain ciliated epithelial cells with which Bordetella are associated. Cotton-tipped swabs are not acceptable for culture studies since they contain fatty acids toxic to Bordetella. Flexible dacron, rayon or calcium-alginate swabs should be used in collecting swab specimens for culture. Dacron or rayon swabs should be used for molecular studies as calcium alginate swabs may inhibit NAAT (5). Specimens from the throat and anterior nares are not acceptable because of the decreased yield from those sites. However, throat swabs may be adequate for NAAT studies (4, 5).

Specimens should be processed as rapidly as possible since Bordetella spp. are susceptible to drying (5). If not processed immediately, the specimens for culture should be placed in transport medium. Regan-Lowe (RL) enrichment medium containing cephalexin (substitution of methicillin for cephalexin may increase isolation of B. holmesii), defibrinated horse blood, and semisolid (half strength) charcoal agar, together with nonenrichment media such as Casamino acids made of 1% acid-hydrolyzed casein and Amies charcoal medium are now commercially available. Transport media may maintain adequate viability for less than 24 h; however specimens should be processed within a day of collection. Transport at 4°C maintains better viability than at ambient room temperature (4, 5).

Fine, flexible wire, Dacron- or rayon-tipped swabs should be used for collection of nasopharyngeal secretions for NAAT studies. Calcium alginate swabs should not be used.

After collecting the specimen, the swab tip should be agitated vigorously while immersed in 0.4 mL of 0.9% saline in a tube or vial. The swab may then be discarded, and the container sealed for transport (4).

5.2 Direct Detection

Bordetella spp. do not stain well by routine methods and are difficult to be viewed and recognized in direct specimen preparations. However, they can be rapidly detected by commercially available monoclonal or polyclonal DFA or by NAAT studies.

Direct fluorescent antibody detection. Both, monoclonal and polyclonal antibodies are commercially available for the detection of either or both B. pertussis and B. parapertussis on the same slide or separately. DFA testing lacks sensitivity (30–71%) and also often has been shown to lack specificity (4, 5). It should only be performed in conjunction with culture or NAAT studies and the results of DFA should be considered presumptive and correlated to clinical considerations as well as to results of other laboratory findings.

Direct NAAT. Molecular-based NAAT studies such as PCR have been described using a number of gene targets, including the *B. pertussis* toxin gene (*cyaA*) or its S1 promoter (specific for *B. pertussis*), the adenylate cyclase gene, and insertion sequence elements such as IS481 (for *B. pertussis* and *B holmesii*) and IS1001 (for *B. parapertussis* and *B. holmesii*). PCR increases diagnostic yields significantly and results show a high level of agreement with serologic studies (4, 13). PCR has a higher recovery rate than culture in patients who present with atypical disease manifestations (e.g. older patients or those with a history of vaccination) and can continue to detect organisms for longer periods of time than culture during pertussis, even after initiation of therapy. Sensitivities of PCR as well as culture decrease with evolution of the disease process.

Methods for PCR have not been standardized and require verification and validation against culture and clinical data in individual laboratories. False-positive results can occur because of contamination in the laboratory or during specimen collection (4, 6). False-negative results can also occur because of inhibitory substances in respiratory secretions. Both problems can be minimized by taking appropriate quality-control steps in the processing and testing of specimens.

Molecular-based NAAT studies for pertussis are presently recommended as adjunct tests to cultures and isolation of the etiologic agent is still recommended by the Centers for Disease Control (CDC). However, real-time PCR technology now allows rapid screening for *B. pertussis*, with the capability for same-day results and may replace the far less sensitive DFA or even culture in the future.

5.3 Culture

Culture is recommended by the CDC as isolates are available for in vitro susceptibility testing and molecular typing when clinically or epidemiologically necessitated (6). Culture may not be as sensitive as serologic or NAAT studies and least useful in the diagnosis of pertussis in the older child and adult, especially if previously vaccinated. Culture still remains an important tool in the diagnosis of pertussis. Successful isolation of *Bordetella* is influenced by a number of factors, including patients' clinical presentation and age, as well as the previous vaccination and antimicrobial therapy.

Specimens can be inoculated onto RL media and /or Bordet–Gengou (BG) agar (potato infusion with 10% glycerol and 20% sheep blood) both with and without cephalexin added (40 mcg/mL). The cephalexin-containing selective plates may inhibit a small percent of *Bordetella* spp. and should not be used alone (5).

Culture plates should be incubated at 35 °C for 7 days in a humidified atmosphere in ambient air; CO_2 should not be used. In some instances, longer incubation may be required. *B. pertussis* can be recognized as "mercury droplets" (because of their mercury-silver color) after 3–4 days incubation. *B. parapertussis* can normally be recognized within 2–3 days (5).

5.4 In Vitro Antimicrobial Susceptibility Testing

Therapy of active pertussis and prophylaxis of close contacts is considered to minimize transmission (6). However, clinical resistance of *B. pertussis* to the macrolides was first reported in 1995 (14). This resistance seems to have arisen because of a mutation of the erythromycin binding site in the 23S rRNA gene (15). At least eleven isolates of highly erythromycin-resistant *B. pertussis* have been documented to date (5). Nonetheless, routine antimicrobial susceptibility testing is not recommended because of the rarity of resistant isolates (6, 9). Clinical cases, which do not respond to appropriate therapy, can be screened by in vitro susceptibility studies.

In vitro susceptibility studies have been described and evaluated, but not yet been standardized (16). Screening methods for resistance of clinical isolates in laboratories include disk diffusion and the E-test (AB Biodisk, Solna, Sweden) using RL agar without cephalexin (14, 16). Resistant strains tested had no zone of inhibition around the erythromycin disk and E-test MICs >256 mcg/mL, whereas susceptible strains were characterized by zones of 43–46 mm and a modal MIC of 0.12 mcg/mL, respectively. A known susceptible strain of *B. pertussis* should be run concurrently with the isolate being screened for comparative purposes. Isolates indicated as resistant by screen should be immediately submitted to the local health departments for confirmation and epidemiologic evaluation.

5.5 Serology

Assays available for serological evaluations of *B. pertussis* infection include the EIA, CF, immunoblotting, agglutination, indirect hemagglutination, and toxin neutralization (5). EIA is the most commonly used. IgA, IgG, and IgM can be measured against a number of *Bordetella* antigens. However, a fourfold rise in IgG against the pertussis toxin (PT) is considered the most specific serodiagnostic indicator of *B. pertussis* infection.

Serodiagnostic strategy for pertussis also depends on the vaccination status and age of the patient (5). Although serologic studies have been shown to be useful in some clinical situations, they have neither been FDA-approved, nor adequately standardized; they are difficult to interpret and should not be routinely relied upon for diagnosis and confirmation of pertussis (5, 6). The CDC recommends that cases that are culture and PCR-negative, but serologically positive and fit the clinical definition of pertussis, be considered as "probable" cases. Individual laboratories that require more information on serologic diagnosis in specific cases should consult their local state health departments for guidance.

6 Alternative Treatments

Erythromycin has traditionally been the antimicrobial of choice for therapy and postexposure prophylaxis of pertussis (6). The newer macrolides, clarithromycin and azithromycin, have been shown to be as effective as erythromycin and seem to be better tolerated because of fewer adverse side effects (9). These newer agents may have a better patient compliance. Trimethoprim–sulfamethoxazole is recommended for patients intolerant of the macrolides or in the cases of B. pertussis resistance to macrolides (9, 14). In general, antimicrobials active against B. pertussis are also active against B. parapertussis (5).

Other antimicrobial agents such as penicillins, cephalosporins, tetracyclines, chloramphenicol, and the fluoroquinolones are not normally recommended for use in pertussis. None of these have been shown to be clinically effective (9). Their pharmacokinetic and pharmacodynamic properties may not be adequate against Bordetella in the respiratory tract; their minimal inhibitory concentrations may be unacceptably high, or they may have potentially adverse side effects (9).

A set of recent recommendations unanimously approved by the CDC, the American Academy of Pediatrics (AAP), the American Academy of Family Physicians (AAFP), and the Health Care Infection Control Practices Advisory Committee for the therapy and prophylaxis of pertussis have been recently published by the CDC (9). The macrolides erythromycin, clarithromycin, and azithromycin are the recommended agents of choice for treatment of pertussis in patients of 1 month of age or older. However, it must be noted that the U.S. Food and Drug Administration (FDA) has not approved any of the macrolides for use in children under the age of 6 months, and overall data in that age group is limited. Trimethoprim–sulfamethoxazole remains the recommended alternative to macrolides in patients 2 months of age or older. It should be used in situations in which the patient is intolerant to macrolides, the Bordetella isolate is resistant to the macrolides (which is found on very rare occasions), or the patient is not responding to the primary agent (macrolide of choice). The final choice of a prescribed antimicrobial agent should take into account not only an agent's effectiveness, but also its tolerability, ease of patient compliance with its dosing regimen, and overall cost. A more detailed overview of the CDC recommendations is outlined in Table 2.

Table 2 Centers for Disease Control guidelines for the use of antimicrobial agents for the treatment and postexposure prophylaxis of pertussis [a]

Patient age group	Guideline
Infant's age <1 month	Azithromycin: 10 mg/kg/day for 5 days
	Clarithromycin: not recommended
	Erythromycin: not recommended, but if it is the only available choice, then 40–50 mg/kg/day in four divided doses/day for 14 days [b]
	Trimethoprim–sulfamethoxazole: contraindicated
Infants' and children' age ≥ 1 month	Azithromycin
	<6 months: 10 mg/kg/day for 5 days
	≥6 months: 10 mg/kg/day (up to 500 mg maximum/day) on day 1, then 5 mg/kg/day (up to 250 mg maximum/day) for a full 5-day course
	Clarithromycin: 15 mg/kg/day (up to a 1 g maximum/day) in two divided doses/day for 7 days
	Erythromycin: 40–50 mg/kg/day (up to a 2 g maximum/day) in four divided doses/day for 14 days
	Trimethoprim–sulfamethoxazole (only for patients ≥2 months [c]): trimethoprim 8 mg/kg/day, sulfamethoxazole 40 mg/kg/day in two divided doses/day for 14 days
Adults	Azithromycin: 500 mg on day 1, then 250 mg/day for days 2 through 5
	Clarithromycin: 1 g/day in two divided doses/day for 7 days
	Erythromycin: 2 g/day in four divided doses/day for 14 days
	Trimethoprim–sulfamethoxazole: trimethoprim 320 mg/day, sulfamethoxazole 1,600 mg/day in two divided doses/day for 14 days

[a] Adapted from (9)

[b] Has been associated with infantile hypertrophic pyloric stenosis (IHPS)

[c] Should not be used in patients of less than 2 months of age, pregnant women, or nursing mothers because of potential kernicterus in infants

7 Infection Control and Prevention Measures

Pertussis is a highly contagious disease with an approximate 80% secondary attack rate in susceptible patients. Transmission from person to person occurs via aerosolized droplets released during forceful expulsion (coughing, sneezing) or via exposure by direct contact of susceptible persons with excretions from acutely infected patients. In 80–90% of cases, untreated symptomatic patients may clear Bordetella spp. spontaneously from their respiratory tract in approximately 3–4 weeks after onset of symptoms; symptomatic infants may continue to shed for over 6 weeks. Thus, strong vaccination programs of children, adolescents, and adults, together with infection control programs minimizing exposure of persons at high risk of contracting the disease, will help prevent pertussis. Patients, suspected of presenting with suspected or diagnosed pertussis, should be placed in droplet precautions. Early antimicrobic therapy of diagnosed symptomatic cases and timely postexposure prophylaxis of close contacts is also paramount in controlling the disease in the community (Table 2). Close contact includes exposure to symptomatic patients in the form of (a) face-to-face exposure within close quarters (3 feet); (b) direct contact with upper respiratory secretions; and (c) sharing a confined space for more than an hour. Prophylaxis should be given to exposed health care workers to help abrogate nosocomial outbreaks. Prophylaxis regimens are of the same dosage and time course as therapeutic regimens.

Childhood vaccination programs have been recommended since the mid-1940s and are a very effective means to control pertussis in the general public. In fact, in many countries full-scale vaccination programs brought the number of cases of pertussis close to zero. Unfortunately, cessation of such programs in some countries resulted in an almost immediate resurgence of the disease in young children, indicating a previously unrecognized reservoir. It is now thought that asymptomatic adult or adolescent family members may be a major source of Bordetella for infants at risk (7, 17).

The childhood vaccine is normally given to children in five doses of a formulation of acellular pertussis in combination with diphtheria and tetanus toxoid (DTaP). The recommended schedule of vaccination remains at 2, 4, and 6 months, then again at 15–18 months, and followed by a final dose at 4–6 years. Vaccine- and natural disease-induced immunity does not last life-long and begins to decrease within 5–10 years of a vaccine dose. Thus, adolescents and adults are at the risk of having symptomatic disease or carrying the organisms thereby remaining as reservoirs of Bordetella. DTaP has potentially severe side effects in age groups past childhood and cannot be used as a booster of immunity in adolescents and adults (9).

Two new vaccines were cleared in 2005 by the U. S. Food and Drug Administration for safer use in the older population. These are tetanus and reduced diphtheria toxoid and acellular pertussis adsorbed (Tdap) formulations (BOOSTRIX^R, GlaxoSmithkline Biologicals, Rixensart, Belgium, and ADACEL, Sanofi Pasteur, Toronto, Canada). Tdap is recommended as a single dose for both adolescents and adults (9).

With increasing prevalence of pertussis in the community, there have been reports of nosocomial transmission of cases from health care workers who had acquired it in either the community or health care facility settings. It was suggested that such nosocomial outbreaks are substantially disruptive to facilities and an economic burden on medical institutions. A model has been described which predicted that a vaccination program using the new vaccines for health care workers would be cost-effective, with substantial savings to health care facilities in abrogating outbreaks (18).

Additional infection control practices should include standard precautions together with droplet precautions on patients admitted to the health care facility with a potential diagnosis of pertussis. The precautions should be in effect for 5 days after the initiation of effective therapy or 3 weeks after the onset of symptoms if the patient remains untreated. In day care or school facilities, infected children should be kept at home for the same time frame as health care givers under the two scenarios presented above.

8 Summary

Pertussis continues to be a problem in public health and outbreaks will probably continue to occur, despite the introduction of newer vaccines for adolescence and adults.

Diagnosis is often hampered by the limitations of the available methods including culture, NAAT, and serologies. Use of multiple methods, paired up at certain temporal junctions of the progression of the disease may be most efficacious at the arrival of a diagnosis of pertussis. Thus, within 2 weeks of symptoms, use of a combination of culture and NAAT may have the best ability to detect the organisms whereas NAAT alone may be most useful on specimens collected after the first 2 weeks of illness (19).

References

1. Sethi, S. (1999) Etiology and management of infections in chronic obstructive pulmonary disease. Clin. Pulmon. Med. 6, 327–332
2. Wadowsky, R. M., Castilla, E. A., Laus, S., et al. (2002) Evaluation of Chlamydia pneumoniae and Mycoplasma pneumoniae as etiologic agents of persistent cough in adolescents and adults. J. Clin. Microbiol. 40, 637–640
3. Heininger, U., Klemens, S., Schmitt-Grohe, S., Lorenz, C., Rost, R., Christenson, P. D., Uberall, M., and Cherry, J. D. (1994) Clinical characteristics of illness caused by Bordetella parapertussis compared with illness caused by Bordetella pertussis. Pediatr. Infect. Dis. J. 13, 306–309
4. Mattoo, S. and Cherry, J. D. (2005) Molecular pathogenesis, epidemiology, and clinical manifestations of respiratory infections due to Bordetella pertussis and other Bordetella subspecies. Clin. Microbiol. Rev. 18, 326–382
5. Loeffelholze, M. J. and Sandin, G. N. (2007) Bordetella. In: Manual of Clinical Microbiology, 9th ed. Murray, P. R., Baron, E. J., Jorgensen, J. H., Landry, M. L., and Pfaller, M. A., eds., ASM Press, Washington, DC, pp. 803–814
6. Bisgard, K., Pascual, F. B., Tiwari, T., and Murphy, T. V. (2002) VPD Surveillance Manual, 3rd ed., Chapter 8, Pertussis, pp 8–17. At www.cdc.gov/nip/publications/sur-manual/Chpt08_pertussis.pdf, CDC, Atlanta, GA
7. Bisgard, K. M., Pascual, F. B., Ehresmann, K. R., Rebmann, C. A., Gabel, J., Schauer, S. L., and Lett, S. M. (2004). Infant pertussis: who was the source? Pediatr. Infect. Dis. J. 23, 985–989
8. Crowcroft, N.S., Stein, C., Duclos, P., and Birmingham, M. (2003) How best to estimate the global burden of pertussis? Lancet Infect. Dis. 3, 413–418

9. Tiwari, T., Murphy, T. V., and Moran, J. (2005). Recommended antimicrobial agents for the treatment and postexposure prophylaxis of pertussis: 2005 CDC guidelines. MMWR 54(RR14), 1–23

10. Guris, D., Strebel, P. M., Bardenheier, B., Brennan, M., Tachdjian, R., Finch, E., Wharton, M., and Livengood, J. R. (1999) Changing epidemiology of Pertussis in the United States: increasing reported incidence among adolescents and adults, 1990–1996. Clin. Infect. Dis. 28, 1230–1237

11. Hardwick, T. W., Cassiday, P., Weyant, R. S., Bisgard, K. M., and Sanden, G. N. (2006) Changes in predominance and diversity of genomic subtypes of *Bordetella pertussis* in the United States, 1935 to 1999. Emerg. Infect. Dis. 8, 1–12

12. Guiso, N. (2005) Is Bordetella pertussis changing? ASM News 71, 230–234

13. Fry, N. K., Tzivia, O., Li, Y. T., McNiff, A., Doshi, N., Maple, P. A., Crowcroft, N. S., Miller, E., George, R. C., and Harrison, T. G. (2004) Laboratory diagnosis of pertussis infections: the role of PCR and serology. J. Med. Microbiol. 53, 519–525

14. Lewis, K., Saubolle, M. A., Tenover, F. C., Rudinsky, M. F., Barbour, S. D., and Cherry, J. D. (1995) Pertussis caused by an erythromycin-resistant strain of Bordetella pertussis. Pediatr. Infect. Dis. J. 14, 388–391

15. Bartkus, J. M., Juni, B. A., Ehresmann, K., Miller, C. A., Sandan, G. N., Cassiday, P. K., Saubolle, M., Lee, B., Long, J., Harrison, A. R. Jr., and Besser, J. M. (2003) Identification of a mutation associated with erythromycin resistance in *Bordetella pertussis*: implication for surveillance of antimicrobial resistance. J. Clin. Microbiol. 41, 1167–1172

16. Hill, B. C., Baker, C. N., and Tenover, F. (2000) A simplified method for testing *Bordetella pertussis* for resistance to erythromycin and other antimicrobial agents. J. Clin. Microbiol. 38, 1151–1155

17. Heininger, U., Cherry, J. D., and Stehr, K. (2004) Serologic response and antibody-titer decay in adults with pertussis. Clin. Infect. Dis. 38, 591–594

18. Calugar, A., Ortega-Sanchez, I. R., Tiwari, T., Oakes, L., Jahre, J. A., and Murphy, T. V. (2006) Nosocomial pertussis: costs of an outbreak and benefits of vaccinating health care workers. Clin. Infect. Dis. 42, 981–988

19. Sotir, M. J., Cappozo, D. L., Warshauer, D. M., Schmidt, C. E., Monson, T. A., Berg, J. L., Zastrow, J. A., Gabor, G. W., and Davis, J. P. (2007) Evaluation of polymerase chain reaction and culture for diagnosis of pertussis in the control of a county wide outbreak focused among adolescence and adults. Clin. Infect. Dis. 44, 1216–1219

Chapter 61
Antibiotic Resistance of Anaerobic Bacteria

Itzhak Brook

1 Infections Caused by Anaerobic Bacteria

Infections caused by anaerobic bacteria are common, and may be serious and life-threatening. Anaerobes are the predominant components of the bacterial flora of normal human skin and mucous membranes (1), and are therefore a common cause of bacterial infections of endogenous origin. Because of their fastidious nature, these organisms are difficult to isolate from infectious sites and are often overlooked. Failure to direct therapy against these organisms often leads to clinical failures. Their isolation requires appropriate methods of collection, transportation, and cultivation of specimens (2–4). Anaerobic infections can occur in all body sites, including the central nervous system, head and neck, chest, abdomen, pelvis, skin, and soft tissues. Treatment of anaerobic bacterial infection is complicated by the slow growth of these organisms, which makes diagnosis in the laboratory only possible after several days, by the often polymicrobial nature of the infection and by the growing resistance of anaerobic bacteria to antimicrobial agents.

The inadequate isolation, identification, and subsequent performance of susceptibility testing of anaerobes from an infected site can prevent the detection of antimicrobial resistance and the correlation of resistance with clinical outcome (1, 2). Correlation of the results of in vitro susceptibility and clinical and bacteriological response is not always possible. This discrepancy occurs because of a variety of reasons: Individuals may improve without antimicrobial or surgical therapy and others can get better because of adequate drainage. In some instances of polymicrobial infection, eradication of the aerobic component may be adequate, although it is well established that it is important to eliminate the aerobic pathogens as well. In most cases, infections vary in duration, severity and extent; and failure can occur because of lack of needed surgical drainage; hence the response depends on individual patients status such as underlying condition, age and nutritional status; and the antimicrobial may not be effective because of enzymatic inactivation or a low Eh or pH at the infection site, or low levels at the site of infection; and because of variations or imperfections in the susceptibility testing.

Microbiological quantitation of all of the infecting flora is important; it is not necessary to eliminate all of the infecting organisms because reduction in counts or modification of the metabolism of certain isolates alone may be sufficient to achieve a good clinical response. Synergy between two or more infecting organisms, which is a common event in anaerobic infections, may confuse the clinical picture.

A correlation between the antibiotic susceptibility of anaerobes and poor clinical outcome have been reported in several retrospective studies (5, 6). A prospective study of *Bacteroides* bacteremia reported the adverse clinical outcomes in 128 individuals who received an antibiotic to which the organism was not susceptible (7). The clinical outcome was correlated with results of in vitro susceptibility testing of *Bacteroides* isolates recovered from blood and/or other sites, and was determined with by the use of three end points: mortality at 30 days, clinical response (cure vs. failure), and microbiological response (eradication vs. persistence). The mortality rate among those who received inactive therapy (45%) was higher than among patients who received active therapy (16%; $P = 04$). Clinical failure (82%) and microbiological persistence (42%) were higher for those who received inactive therapy than for patients who received active therapy (22 and 12%, respectively; $P = 0.0002$ and 0.06, respectively). In vitro activity of agents directed at *Bacteroides* spp. reliably predicts outcome (specificity 97%, and positive predictive value 82%). The authors conclude that the antimicrobial susceptibility testing may be indicated for patients whose blood specimens yield *Bacteroides* spp. (7). All these observations enhanced the recommendation that susceptibility testing of anaerobic bacteria should be performed in selected cases (8, 9).

I. Brook (✉)
Department of Pediatrics, Georgetown University School of Medicine, Washington, DC, USA
ib6@georgetown.edu

D.L. Mayers (ed.), *Antimicrobial Drug Resistance*,
DOI 10.1007/978-1-60327-595-8_61, © Humana Press, a part of Springer Science+Business Media, LLC 2009

These findings emphasize that it is important, to perform susceptibility testing to isolates recovered from sterile body sites, those that are isolated in pure culture or those that are clinically important and have variable or unique susceptibility (Table 1). Screening of anaerobic Gram-negative bacteria (AGNB) isolates (particularly *Prevotella*, *Bacteroides* and *Fusobacterium* spp.) for beta-lactamase (BL) activity is also helpful. However, occasionally resistance to beta-lactam antibiotics is through other mechanisms. Recent standardization of testing methods by the NCCLS allows for comparison of resistance trends among various laboratories (8, 9). Organisms that should be considered for individual isolate testing include highly virulent pathogens for which susceptibility cannot be predicted, such as *Bacteroides*, *Prevotella*, *Fusobacterium*, and *Clostridium* spp., *Bilophila wadsworthia*, and *Sutterella wadworthensis* (8, 9).

The routine susceptibility testing of all anaerobic isolates is extremely time-consuming and in many cases unnecessary. Therefore, susceptibility testing should be limited to selected anaerobic isolates. Antibiotics tested should include penicillin, a broad-spectrum penicillin, a penicillin plus a BL inhibitor, clindamycin, chloramphenicol, cefoxitin, a third-generation cephalosporin, metronidazole, a carbapenem (e.g., imipenem), tigecycline, and an extended-spectrum quinolone.

The antimicrobial resistance among anaerobes has consistently increased in the past three decades and the susceptibility of anaerobic bacteria to antimicrobial agents has become less predictable. The most commonly isolated antibiotic-resistant anaerobe is the *Bacteroides fragilis* group. Resistance to several antimicrobial agents by *B. fragilis* group and other AGNB has increased over the past decade (8, 9). Antimicrobial resistance has also increased among other anaerobes such as *Clostridium* spp. that were previously very susceptible to antibiotics. This increase made the choice of appropriate empirical therapy more difficult. Even though resistance patterns have been monitored through national and local surveys, susceptibility testing of anaerobic bacteria at individual hospitals is rarely done.

Table 1 Anaerobic infections for which susceptibility testing is indicated

1. Serious or life-threatening infections (e.g., brain abscess, bacteremia, or endocarditis)
2. Infections that failed to respond to empiric therapy
3. Infections that relapsed after initially responding to empiric therapy
4. Infections where an antimicrobial will have a special role in the patient's outcome
5. When an empirical decision is difficult because of absence of precedent
6. When there are few susceptibility data available on a bacterial species
7. When the isolate(s) is often resistant to antimicrobial
8. When the patients require prolonged therapy (e.g., septic arthritis, osteomyelitis, undrained abscess, or infection of a graft or a prosthesis)

2 Susceptibility Patterns of Anaerobic Bacteria

The increase in antibiotic resistance among anaerobes generated extensive studies of the mechanisms of resistance and resistance-gene transfer. These investigations brought about more insight into the causes of the rapid development of resistance. The observed resistance patterns to different antibiotics vary among the different groups of organisms as variations in the mechanisms of resistance exist.

AGNB which are among the most important anaerobic pathogens recovered from infectious sites also possess the broadest spectrum of recognized resistances to antimicrobials. Their resistance and its transfer mechanisms were extensively investigated.

Studies that monitor the development of antimicrobial resistance in specific organisms are routinely conducted in many countries. The antimicrobial agents that are studied include those that have been extensively used to treat anaerobic infections (beta-lactams, clindamycin, metronidazole, and chloramphenicol), as well as newer agents.

B. fragilis group as well as many other AGNB and *Fusobacterium* spp. are resistant to the penicillins and the ureidopenicillin (i.e., piperacillin) through the production of BL. However, the addition of a BL inhibitor enables penicillins to overcome this mechanism of resistance. Cefoxitin, a second-generation cephalosporin formerly very active against anaerobes, has lost potency in most recent surveys. The carbapenems are the most effective beta-lactam agents.

Metronidazole as well as clindamycin are active against the *B. fragilis* group. However, although resistance to clindamycin of up to 25% has been noted in localized areas such as southern Europe, Japan, and some regions of the USA (10–12). Penicillins are still effective against other anaerobes including *Clostridium* and *Propionibacterium* spp., and most *Fusobacterium* spp. Resistance to metronidazole has been observed in a few strains of *Clostridium perfringens*, and is common in *Propionibacterium* spp. (12).

As a guide to the efficacy of a available antibiotics effective against anaerobic bacteria, the susceptibility results from the Wadsworth Anaerobic Laboratory at Los Angeles are presented in Tables 2 and 3 (13).

3 Susceptibility Testing and Their Interpretation

There are currently three susceptibility testing methods for anaerobic bacteria that provide reproducible results that correlate with a reference standard: the agar dilution, the broth micro dilution, and the E-test (AB Biodisk) (8, 14). At

Table 2 Susceptibility of Gram-negative anaerobic bacteria (13)

Anaerobe	% Susceptible to[a]						
	<50	50–69	70–84	85–95		>95	
B. fragilis	PEN[b] CIP FLE LOM AZM ERY ROX TET	CFP CTX CAZ SPX	MOX CRO CLR	CTT ZOX CLI MIN	PIP AMC SAM CPS TZP TIM	FOX BIA IPM MEM CHL CLX	SIT LUZ OFX TVZ MND
Other *B. fragilis* group[c]	PEN CTX CAZ CRO CIP FLE LOM AZM ERY ROX	CFP CTT MOX OFX SPX	LVX CLR CLI	AMC PIP FOX ZOX	SAM CPS TZP TIM BIA	IPM MEM CHL CLX	SIT TVA MND MIN
Other *Bacteroides* spp.	FLE LOM	CIP TET	PEN MOX OFX SPX AZM	CTT CAZ CRO CLR ERY ROX MIN	PIP AMC SAM TIM CFP CPS	CTX FOX ZOX BIA IPM CHL	CLX SIT LVX TVA MND CLI
Prevotella spp.	FLE LOM	TET	CIP OFX SPX MIN	CRO AZM CLR ERY ROX	PIP AMC SAM TZP TIM FOX	ZOX BIA IPM MEM CHL	CLX SIT TVA MND CLI
Porphyromonas spp.	FLE LOM	TET		CIP CLR CLI ERY ROX	PIP AMC FOX ZOX CRO BIA	IPM MEM CHL CLX SIT	SPX TVA MND AZM MIN
F. nucleatum	FLE LOM CLR ERY ROX			CIP AZM	PIP AMC TZP TIM FOX ZOX CRO	BIA IPM MEM CHL CLX SIT LVX	OFX SPX TVA CLI MND MIN TET
F. mariqferum and *F. varium*	FLE LOM AZM CLR ERY ROX	CIP SPX TEM	CLI TET	AMC ZOX CRO	PIP TZP TIM FOX BIA	IPM MEM CHL CLX	SIT TVA MND MIN
Other *Fusobacterium* spp.	FLE LOM CLR ERY ROX		CAZ MOX CIP SPX AZM	PIP AMC TIM CPS CTX	PEN SAM TZP FOX BIA	IPM MEM CHL CLX SIT	MND CLI MIN TET

(continued)

Table 2 (continued)

Anaerobe	% Susceptible to[a]				
	<50	50–69	70–84	85–95	>95
				CTT	
				ZOX	
				CRO	

[a]The order of listing of drugs within percent susceptible categories is not significant. *AMC* amoxicillin/clavulanate; *AZM* azithromycin; *BIA* biapenem; *CAZ* ceftazidime; *CFP* cefoperazone; *CHL* chloramphenicol; *CIP* ciprofloxacin; *CLI* clindamycin; *CLR* clarithromycin; *CLX* clinafloxacin; *CPS* cefoperazone/sulbactam; *CRO* ceftriaxone; *CTT* cefotetan; *CTX* cefotaxime; *ERY* etythromycin; *FLE* fleroxacin; *FOX* cefoxitin; *IPM* imipenem; *LOM* lomefloxacin; *LVX* levofloxacin; *MEM* meropenem; *MIN* minocycline; *MND* metronidazole; *MOX* moxalactam; *OFX* ofloxacin; *PEN* penicillin; *PIP* piperacillin; *ROX* roxithromycin; *SAM* ampicillin/sulbactam; *SIT* sitafloxacin; *SPX* sparfloxacin; *TEM* temafloxacin; *TET* tetracycline; *TIM* ticarcillin/clavulanate; *TVA* trovafloxacin; *TZP* piperacillin/tazobactam; *ZOX* ceftizoxime
[b]NCCLS approved breakpoint is 4 µg/mL. However, the breakpoint should probably be lowered to 1 µg/mL, which will considerably lower the values for % susceptible. For example, at 1 µg/mL, no strains of the *B. fragilis* group were susceptible
[c]Excluding *B. fragilis*

present there are no automated methods. The NCCLS currently recommends that for surveillance purposes to monitor for resistance trends, the agar dilution method is used to test at least 100 anaerobic isolates per year at individual hospitals. The agar dilution method is reproducible, labor-intensive, and allows for batch testing of up to 30 anaerobic isolates at one time against a single antibiotic.

The broth micro dilution panel is a convenient, user-friendly method that determines susceptibilities of a single anaerobic isolate to several antibiotics at the same time. This panel provides results that correlate well with those of the agar dilution standard for anaerobes that grow well in broth supplemented with NCCLS-recommended *Brucella* blood agar. Both methods are equivalent for determining antimicrobial susceptibilities of *B. fragilis* group isolates, but the NCCLS does not recommend the broth micro dilution for non-bacteroides anaerobes unless the laboratory validates their results against the agar dilution standard.

The E-test (AB Biodisk) is a simple user-friendly, gradient method that delivers accurate results. However, the limitation of this test is that each test strip is only for a single isolate. Both the broth micro dilution, and the E-test methods are adequate for testing individual isolates and can provide guidance in selection of therapy on the basis of positive culture results.

The susceptibility results are considered when antibiotic treatment is chosen. The results are expressed as the minimal inhibitory concentration (MIC) or by providing degrees of susceptibility as sensitive (S), intermediate (I), and resistant (R). These sensitivity breakpoints are established by the NCCLS and the US Food and Drug Administration (FDA). The MIC value obtained by any of the methods does not represent an absolute number because the accurate MIC is actually between the obtained MIC and the next-lower or -higher test concentration. Also a twofold difference on successive testing is allowed in all dilution-based susceptibility methods (8). The phenotypic interpretation of the results of the MIC tests as sensitive, intermediate, and resistant are based on the MIC distribution of the bacterial population, the antibiotic pharmacokinetics and pharmacodynamics, and the verification of antibiotic efficacy in clinical studies. The dosages of antibiotics administered for infections caused by anaerobic organisms whose MICs are at or near the S or I breakpoints, should be maximal to overcome their lower penetration and instability at the site of most infections (8).

4 Resistance Mechanisms of Anaerobic Bacteria

Antimicrobial susceptibility tests results may depend on the methods and media used, the study size (single vs. numerous hospitals), the geographic location, and the antibiotic utilization. Whenever the susceptibility of an individual isolate is not available, the most clinically relevant antibiotic susceptibility information can be provided by longitudinal surveys that use the same methodology over time.

4.1 Clindamycin Resistance

Clindamycin has been used for the treatment of anaerobic bacterial infection since the 1960s. Antibiotic resistance to clindamycin among anaerobes has gradually increased over the past 25 years. The national anaerobe survey in the USA reported frequencies of resistance among anaerobes in the *B. fragilis* group to be 3% in 1987, with increases to 16, 26, and 43% in 1996, 2000, and 2003 respectively (15–18). Resistance at some locations reached 44% (19). Results derived from one medical center can not predict those at other centers as resistance to clindamycin in individual sites varies. Surveillance of local resistance is therefore essential

Table 3 Susceptibility of Gram-positive anaerobic bacteria (13)

Anaerobe	Susceptible to[a]						
	<50	50–69	70–84	85–95	>95		
Peptosreptococcus spp.	LOM	FLE	CIP	LVX	PEN	CTT	MEM
		TET	OFX	CLI	PIP	FOX	CHL
		ROX	AZM	MIN	AMC	CAZ	CLX
			CLR		SAM	ZOX	SIT
			ERY		TZP	CRO	SPX
					TIM	BIA	TVA
					CFP	IPM	MND
					CPS		
C. difficile[b]	FOX	CLI		CRO	AMP	TZP	CLX
	ZOX	MIN		BIA	PIP	TIM	SIT
	CIP	TET		CHL	TIC	CTT	TVA
	FLE	AZM			AMC	IPM	MND
	LOM	CLR			SAM	MEM	
	SPX	ERY					
		ROX					
C. ramosum	CIP	SPX	FOX	AMP	AMC	ZOX	SIT
	FLE	MIN		PIP	TZP	IPM	MND
	LOM	TET		SAM	TIM	CLX	
	AZM			CHL			
	CLR			TVA			
	ERY			CLI			
	ROX						
C. perfringens		TET	MIN	LOM	AMP	ZOX	SPX
				CLI	PIP	BIA	TVA
					TIC	IPM	MND
					SAM	CHL	AZM
					AMC	CIP	CLR
					TZP	CLX	ERY
					TIM	SIT	ROX
					CTT	FLE	
Other *Clostridium* spp.	CAZ	CFP	LVX	MOX	AMX	TIC	CLX
	FLE	CTX	OFX		AMP	SAM	SIT
	LOM	FOX	SPX		CAR	AMC	TVA
		ZOX	CLI		PEN	BIA	MND
		CRO	TET		PIP	IPM	MIN
		CIP				CHL	
		AZM					
		CLR					
		ERY					
		ROX					
Nonspore-forming Gram-positive rod	FLE	CIP	CFP	CTT	PEN	FTX	CLI
	LOM	OFX	MOX	FOX	PIP	ZOX	CLX
		MND	SPX	CRO	AMC	BIA	SIT
			TET	CPS	SAM	IPM	LVX
				TVA	TZP	MEM	MIN
				AZM	TIM	CHL	
				CLR			
				ERY			
				ROX			

[a]The order of listing of drugs within percent susceptible categories is not significant. According to the NCCLS-approved breakpoints (M11-A3), using the intermediate category as susceptible. *AMP* ampicillin; *AMX* amoxicillin; *TIC* ticarcillin. See Table 2 footnote for other antimicrobial agents

[b]Breakpoint is used only as a reference point. *C. difficile* is primarily of interest in relation to antimicrobial-induced pseudomembranous colitis. These data must be interpreted in the context of level of drug achieved in the colon and impact of agent on indigenous colonic flora

in assessing the utility of clindamycin as a therapeutic agent at a certain location. Even though longitudinal survey data on non-bacteroides organisms is limited, resistance to clindamycin among *Prevotella*, *Fusobacterium*, *Porphyromonas*, and *Peptostreptococcus* spp. is generally much lower and is often less than 10% (20). The anaerobe most resistant to clindamycin is *Clostridium difficile* with up to 67% of isolates resistant (21).

Clindamycin resistance can develop due to three mechanisms: inactivation of the drug, altered permeability, and changed ribosomal target site (22, 23). Several genetic clindamycin-resistance determinants were identified in the *B. fragilis* group (*ermF*, *ermG*, and *ermS*), *C. perfringens* (*ermQ* and *ermP*), *C. difficile* (*ermZ*, *ermB*, and *ermBZ*), and *Porphyromonas*, *Prevotella*, *Peptostreptococcus*, and *Eubacterium* spp. (*ermF*) (24). These determinants were located on the chromosome, plasmids, or transposons and were transferable by conjugation for both *B. fragilis* and *C. difficile*. Similar to that in staphylococci, resistance is mediated by a macrolide-lincosamide-streptogramin type 23S RNA methylase at one of the two adenine residues (25, 26). This methylation prevents binding of clindamycin to the ribosomes and makes them resistant. The same mechanism of resistance was detected in *Bacteroides* spp. Ribosomes isolated from a clindamycin resistance *Bacteroides vulgatus* strain, induced with either clindamycin or erythromycin, showed decreased susceptibility to clindamycin compared with ribosomes isolated from a clindamycin-susceptible strain or a strain with clindamycin resistance that was not induced (25, 27). These findings showed that resistance to clindamycin is at the ribosomal level and probably occurs via methylation of the rRNA.

Three different, but closely related (over 95% homology), MLS resistance genes were cloned from various *Bacteroides* strains. These genes exist within a transposon or on a conjugal element: *ermF* is encoded on *Tn4351*, *ermFS* is encoded on *Tn4551*, and *ermFU* is encoded on a *B. vulgatus* conjugal element (28–30). In addition to being very homologous with each other, their encoded proteins have sequence identities that are very similar to those of the MLS resistance genes from Gram-positive organisms (28–30). Most clindamycin-resistant *Bacteroides* contain an *erm* gene related to one of the three above-mentioned genes. The genes generally encode high-level resistance and are driven by strong promoters. However, not all clindamycin-resistant *Bacteroides* contain DNA sequences that crosshybridize with the *ermF* gene (31–33), suggesting that another unrelated MLS resistance gene or another mechanism of resistance also exists.

Clindamycin resistance can be inducible as well as constitutive. That conjugal transfer of clindamycin resistance is plasmid-mediated with a frequent cotransfer of tetracycline resistance, was first reported in 1979 (34–36). These plasmids are mostly self-transmissible and vary in size from 14.6 kilobases (kb) (pBFTM 10) to 41 kb (pIP411 and pBF4) (35) to −82 kb (pBI136) (37). Studies with the plasmids pBFTM I O and pBF4 demonstrated that these clindamycin resistance genes are carried on transposons *Tn4400* and *Tn4351*, respectively (38, 39). Resistance to clindamycin can also be chromosomally encoded. Chromosomal resistance to clindamycin has also been linked with resistance to tetracycline; and the clindamycin resistance gene was found to exist within the tetracycline resistance transfer element (39–41).

With the rapid increase in the prevalence of clindamycin resistance, especially among the *B. fragilis* group, this agent is no longer considered to be a first-line agent for anaerobic infections due to these organisms (42). Clindamycin can still be considered when treating AGNB with known susceptibilities or other mixed infections that do not harbor or are not likely to harbor these bacteria, such as oral and upper respiratory tract infections or aspiration pneumonia.

4.2 Beta-lactam Resistance

Beta-lactam agents are important for the treatment of infections involving anaerobes, although significant resistance to some of them has also been noted. The *B. fragilis* group have the highest prevalence of resistance to beta-lactams among anaerobes. Almost all (>97%) of *B. fragilis* group isolates are resistant to penicillin G. In contrast, the cephamycins cefoxitin and cefotetan have much better activity, although the prevalence of resistance among *B. fragilis* group has increased. During 1987–2000, resistance to cefoxitin was observed in 8–14% of *B. fragilis* group (15, 17). Significant variations were seen among individual medical centers, with resistance of 22% of isolates at one site (15).

Cefotetan is as active as cefoxitin against *B. fragilis*, but is much less effective against other members of the *B. fragilis* group with resistance rates of 30–87%, depending on the species. This high prevalence of resistance resulted in recent recommendations against the use of both cephamycins as empirical therapy for intra-abdominal infections (42). However, these agents can still be used when susceptible testing shows them to be active. Piperacillin resistance has also increased from <10% in 1980 to 25% in recent studies, with significant variability among the *B. fragilis* group (15, 24), which is why it is not currently recommended for empirical therapy for intra-abdominal infections.

The most active beta-lactam agents against anaerobic bacteria are the carbapenems (imipenem, meropenem, and ertapenem) with worldwide resistance of <0.2% of *B. fragilis* group isolates (15, 20, 43), and the combinations of a beta-lactam agent with a BL inhibitor (ampicillin/sulbactam, ticarcillin/clavulanate, and piperacillin/tazobactam) were less than 4%

of *B. fragilis* group strains and were resistant, in 2003 (18). When organisms are resistant to penicillins through the production of BL, the addition of a BL inhibitor usually makes them effective against these isolates. However, strains of non-BL-resistant *Bacteroides distasonis* frequently have higher MICs for all inhibitor combinations.

Resistance to beta-lactam agents among non-bacteroides anaerobes is variable but is generally lower than the *B. fragilis* group. Because non-bacteroides anaerobes are more difficult to isolate and identify, the frequency of their susceptibility testing is very low. However, in one multicenter study 83% of *Prevotella* isolates were resistant to penicillin G, whereas resistance was much lower for species of *Porphyromonas* (21%), *Fusobacterium* (9%), and *Peptostreptococcus* (6%) (20). Isolates from all these genera were completely susceptible to cefoxitin, beta-lactam/BL inhibitor combinations, and carbapenems, except for *Peptostreptococcus* isolates (4% were resistant to ampicillin/sulbactam) and *Porphyromonas* (5% were resistant to cefoxitin) (20).

Resistance to beta-lactam antibiotics is mediated by one of three resistance mechanisms: inactivating enzymes (BL); reduced-affinity penicillin-binding proteins; or decreased antimicrobial permeability. The production of BLs is the most common mechanism and mediates the most diverse mechanisms of resistance.

4.2.1 Production of beta-Lactamase

BL hydrolyzes the cyclic amide bond of the penicillin or cephalosporin nucleus, causing its inactivation. There are a variety of BLs which are produced by different organisms. These enzymes can be exoenzymes, inducible or constitutive; and genetically they can be of either chromosomal or plasmid origin (44). There are different classifications of the enzymes. A classification based on amino-acid sequence was created by Ambler (45), and a classification based upon substrate of inhibition profiles, molecular weight, and isoelective points was proposed by Richmond and Sykes (46).

Most *B. fragilis* groups produce constitutive BLs that are primarily cephalosporinases (47, 48). Pigmented *Prevotella* and *Porphyromonas*, *Prevotella bivia*, *Prevotella disiens*, and *Fusobacterium nucleatum* produce primarily penicillinases (49).

Over 97% of *Bacteroides* isolates in the USA (45, 46) and 76% in Great Britain (47, 48) produce BLs. Of the non-*fragilis* 65% produce BLs (49). Most enzymes produced by *Bacteroides* are constitutive and are chromosomally mediated. They include enzymes with serine at the active site as well as metalloenzymes that require an active site with Zn^{2+}.

Other anaerobes that are capable of producing BL include *Clostridium butyricum* (50, 51), *Clostridium clostridioforme* (52), *Clostridium ramosum* (53), *Prevotella*,

Porphyromonas (54), and *Fusobacterium* spp. (54, 55). Although only rare strains of Clostridium can produce BLs, *Prevotella*, *Porphyromonas*, and *Fusobacterium* spp. produce these enzymes more often (71, 30, and 41% respectively) (46, 55). Enzymes produced by clostridia are usually inducible except the one produced by *C. ramosum* which is plasmid-mediated TEM-1 enzyme (53).

Acidic isoelectric points are present in most enzymes produced by the anaerobes. Most of the *B. fragilis* group enzymes are group 2e cephalosporinases (56, 57) which can be inhibited by BL inhibitors, making *Bacteroides* strains susceptible to the combinations of a beta-lactam agent with a BL inhibitor. Cefoxitin-hydrolyzing proteins that are encoded by *cepA* and *cfxA* that are less common, were found in the *B. fragilis* group (58).

Sequencing of several of these enzymes illustrated that they belong to the molecular class A serine cephalosporinases (58 60), that are of a smaller molecular size than the inducible group 1 (molecular class C) cephalosporinases from Gram-negative bacteria. Only a single strain of *Bacteroides intermedius* produced a group 1 cephalosporinase not inhibited by clavulanic acid (61).

An uncharacterized cefoxitin-hydrolyzing enzyme, which may belong to the group 2e, was detected in several members of the *B. fragilis* group (62, 63). Although HPLC revealed that the group 2e (class A) CfxA beta-lactamase from *Bacteroides vulgatus* degraded cefoxitin slowly in overnight cultures, the hydrolysis was not detected in standard spectrophotometric assays (60). It is possible that the slow enzymatic hydrolysis is coupled with decreased permeability as the organisms were clinically resistant to cefoxitin.

Fusobacteria and clostridia produce BLs that are usually inhibited by clavulanic acid. However, exceptions among some *Clostridium* spp. were reported (52, 64). These organisms produce at least three groups of enzymes, although not all substrates have been tested with all enzymes.

BLs produced by fusobacteria and *C. butyricum* are inhibited by clavulanic acid, whereas the BL from *C. clostridioforme* was not inhibited by any BL inhibitors (52). This suggests that these enzymes belong to molecular class D BLs, which are the group 2d cloxacillin-hydrolyzing enzymes.

Anaerobes that produce zinc metallo-BLs are potentially the most capable of producing clinical resistance to beta-lactam agents in *B. fragilis* group. These enzymes, encoded by the *ccrA* or *cfiA* genes, readily hydrolyze the carbapenems imipenem, meropenem, and ertapenem, as well as all beta-lactam agents that are active against anaerobes except the monobactam agents (62, 63). These BLs are not inactivated by current BL inhibitors. Although these enzymes are generally chromosomally mediated, a plasmid-mediated metallo-BL has been reported in Japan (65). Even though this resistance mechanism was first reported in 1986 in *B. fragilis* (66), it remains relatively rare. As many as 4% of *Bacteroides* spp. actually carry the *ccrA* or *cfiA* genes, the proteins are not usually expressed at a high-enough level to classify the strains as resistant (<0.8%) (67). However, high-level expression of this enzyme can happen following in vitro selection with imipenem (68). These imipenem-resistant strains contain insertion sequences, that are mobile genetic elements with divergent promoters inserted immediately upstream of the *ccrA* or *cfiA* genes, causing an increased expression of the enzymes leading to resistance (69, 70). These laboratory observations were supported by the findings of an imipenem-resistant clinical isolate that also contained this arrangement of insertion sequence and promoter gene (68). For patients who are infected with these resistant strains, treatment with antibiotics other than beta-lactams may be required.

The rate of recovery of anaerobic beta-lactamase-producing bacteria (BLPB) in clinical infections and their clinical and therapeutic implications have been extensively investigated and are presented later in this chapter (See Section 6.0).

4.2.2 Penicillin Binding Proteins

Penicillin binding to the PBPs determines whether a beta-lactam antimicrobial will be effective. Maintaining PBPs, function in the final stage of cell wall synthesis is essential for bacterial growth. beta-Lactams work by successfully competing for binding to the active site of the essential PBP, thus causing cell death. Three to five PBPs can be found in *Bacteroides* strains: a PBP 1 complex with one to three different enzymes, PBP 2, and PBP 3. These PBPs are most likely similar to the high-molecular-weight PBPs present in aerobic Gram-negative bacteria. It may be possible that other low molecular-weight PBPs also exist, but the number of these proteins vary among strains, and are probably not essential for bacterial growth (71).

Alteration in PBP are not major mechanisms of resistance in anaerobes as the binding of most beta-lactam agents to PBP 1 complex and PBP 2 is adequate. An exception are the monobactams (i.e., aztreonam) that are not active against *B. fragilis* because they do not have good affinity for their PBPs (72). Decreased affinity of cephalosporins for PBP 3 was demonstrated in *B. fragilis* G-232 recovered in Japan (73). Cefoxitin resistance in some *Bacteroides* strains has also been attributed to decreased binding to the PBP 1 complex or the PBP 2 (74, 75). This resistance was also inducable in vitro (76).

4.2.3 Permeability

Increased BL production was associated with decreased permeability in Gram-negative bacteria. Permeability factors can vary among strains of *B. fragilis* (66, 77, 78), and in certain *B. fragilis* strains, resistance was associated with

both reduced permeability and BL production (78). Cefoxitin resistance correlated with a decrease in outer-membrane permeability and the loss of an outer-membrane protein with a molecular size of 49–50 kid (75).

Studies of pore-forming proteins of *Bacteroides*, *Porphyromonas*, and *Fusobacterium* spp. identified and cloned outer-membrane proteins from these AGNB. The absence of at least one outer-membrane protein was associated in some strains with resistance to ampicillin/sulbactam (79).

Selective pressure similar to that observed for many aerobic species most likely also plays a role in the development and selection of resistance to beta-lactams. Although the prevalence of resistance of anaerobes to beta-lactams has increased, several of these antibiotics are still clinically useful. However, their utilization should be determined according to the local resistance patterns or the susceptibility of individual isolates.

4.3 Metronidazole (5-Nitroimidazoles) Resistance

Metronidazole resistance is common among Gram-positive anaerobic bacteria, and includes most isolates of *Propionibacterium acnes* and *Actinomyces* spp., some strains of lactobacilli and *Peptostreptococcus* spp. (43). Resistance of Gram-negative anaerobes to metronidazole is unusual. Although resistant strains of *B. fragilis* (MICs >16 μg/mL) were reported in European countries (80, 81), these were not found in the USA.

Metronidazole is the first of the 5-nitroimidazole that was used clinically since 1960. Other 5-nitroimidazoles include tinidazole, and ornidazole. A metronidazole resistant isolate of *B. fragilis* was first recovered in 1978 from a patient who had received prolonged therapy (82). Even though the rates of metronidazole resistance remain very low (<1%) (10, 83–91), and the drug remains very effective as treatment of bacteroides infections, metronidazole-resistant *Bacteroides* isolates were subsequently isolated from patients who had not received metronidazole therapy (92–94). It was postulated that in mixed infection metronidazole can be inactivated by another bacteria such *E. faecalis* thus protecting *B. fragilis* (95).

The 5-nitroimidazoles must be reduced to form the active antibacterial agent which is stable only under anaerobic conditions because it is rapidly reversed in the presence of oxygen (96, 97). The development of resistance to metronidazole generally occurs with the simultaneously decrease in nitroreductase activity and reduction of uptake of the drug (96, 97).

A decrease in the pyruvate ferredoxin oxidoreductase activity that is combined with a compensatory increase in the lactate dehydrogenate activity results in a decrease in the reducing state of the cell (96, 97). Although the ease with which this change in enzyme activities can occur within a cell is unknown, the phenotype in a metronidazole-resistant isolate has been identified (98).

Two genes, *nimA* and *nimB*, that can confer moderate- to high-level nitroimidazole resistance were identified in strains with high MICs of metronidazole (i.e., >4 μg/mL) (99). *nim* genes encode a nitroimidazole reductase, which reduces 4- or 5-nitroimidazole to 4- or 5-aminoimidazole thus preventing the formation of toxic nitroso residues that are required for the agents' activity (100). Six related chromosomal or plasmid-based *nim* genes (*nim A–F*) were found in *Bacteroides* spp. (99). Elements of insertion sequence, that are identical or similar to those present in imipenem-resistant strains, are also located upstream of the *nim* genes, and possibly increase their expression (101). Evaluation of metronidazole-resistant *B. fragilis* isolates revealed that all harbored DNA sequences hybridized with either an *nimA* or *nimB* DNA probe, while none of the metronidazole-susceptible isolates contained DNA sequences that cross-hybridized with an *nimA* or *nimB* DNA probe (102). The DNA sequence of the *nimA* and *nimB* genes is −73% similar, and may represent two classes of genes that generate resistance through the same mechanism (99). The mechanism of resistance has not been elucidated, but drug uptake studies showed that neither the active efflux nor reduced drug penetration was involved (99).

Both the *nimA* and *nimB* genes were present in the chromosome and various plasmids (103, 104). The plasmids containing these gene were not self-transmissible, but were mobilized by other conjugal elements or were acquired by transformation (105). The transcriptional start information for both the genes is provided by an insertion sequence (IS) element integrated 12–14 bases upstream from the protein-coding region. For the *nimA* gene, this element is *IS1168* (104) and a closely related IS element delivers the transcriptional start information for the *nimB* gene (99). The *IS1168* is almost similar to an IS element, *IS1186*, that has been identified to provide transcriptional initiation signals for the *Bacteroides* metallo BL gene (99, 106). The mechanisms for resistance among non-bacteroides strains was not studied.

Because only few anaerobic isolates are resistant to metronidazole, this agent is still the mainstay for combination treatment of mixed aerobic-anaerobic infections. However, the presence of transferable resistance determinants may bring about the development of resistance in the future (107).

4.4 Fluoroquinolones Resistance

Fluoroquinolones (FQ) were not considered to be active agents against anaerobic bacteria because they are bacteriostatic under anaerobic conditions (108, 109). However, three broad-spectrum FQ that are effective against *Bacteroides* spp. and most other anaerobic species (temafloxacin, trovafloxacin, and moxifloxacin), were approved by the FDA for treatment of infections caused by anaerobic bacteria. Temafloxacin was used for a short time in the early 1990s and was withdrawn because of toxicity. The use of trovafloxacin that was approved in 1997 was severely curtailed also because of toxicity. Resistance to trovafloxacin was noted in 3–8% of *B. fragilis* group in 1994–1996, before the introduction of the drug, and it rose to 13% in 1997, and 15% in 1998, when the drug was launched and reached 25% in 2001 (17, 110). This pattern of increase in resistance may be due to the effect of the use of other older FQ. A similar pattern of increase in *Bacteroides* resistance was also noted with moxifloxacin (110).

Several concurrent resistance mechanisms to the FQ are employed by anaerobes. The FQ inhibit the DNA gyrase and topoisomerase IV, both of which are essential for aerobic and facultative anaerobic bacterial DNA replication. So is the case in aerobic bacteria resistance in *B. fragilis* developed by mutations in the gyrase (*gyrA*) and topoisomerase IV (*parC*) genes and by increased expression of efflux pump. Cloning of both *gyrA* and *gyrB* from *B. fragilis* genome, using stepwise selection with levofloxacin, generated a mutation at residue Ser-82-Phe of GyrA which corresponded to Ser-83-Phe of the FQ resistance-determining region (QRDR) of *gyrA*, in *Escherichia coli* (111). Three mutants with high MICs of levofloxacin had the identical Ser-82-Phe substitutions and cross-resistance to other FQ was also noted.

The oral administration of clinafloxacin to healthy volunteers induced mutations leading to substitutions in the QRDR region which was selected for in vitro resistance against ciprofloxacin, trovafloxacin and other FQ (112, 113). At least one efflux pump mediated resistance to both fluorinated and nonfluorinated quinolones which was recently identified in *B. fragilis* (114, 115). These observations illustrate the potential for developing of resistance among anaerobes to quinolones that are currently at the earlier stages of development. The possible emergence of a combination of mutations QRDR region in one of the and the other in the efflux pumps threatens the long-term efficacy of all quinolones.

4.5 Aminoglycosides Resistance

Anaerobic bacteria are resistant to all aminoglycosides because they do not reach their target site in these bacteria. Of interest is the anaerobe that do not inactivate aminiglycosides and that in a cell-free system both streptomycin and gentamicin are able to bind and inhibit protein synthesis in both *B. fragilis* and *C. perfringens* ribosomes (116).

The uptake of aminoglycosides involves a two-step process: an energy-independent and an energy-dependent one. The energy necessary for the energy-driven phase of drug uptake is obtained from an oxygen- or nitrogen-dependent electron transport system. Strictly anaerobes do not possess this electron transport system and are therefore incapable of importing aminoglycosides (115, 117). This is supported by the fact that aminoglycosides were not accumulated inside either *B. fragilis* or *C. perfringens* (114).

4.6 Chloramphenicol Resistance

Chloramphenicol is active against most anaerobes and no resistance has been noted in any surveys (84, 85, 89, 91). However, clinical failures using this agent have been reported (118). The absence of resistance can be explained by the rare clinical utilization of this agent.

Bacteroides spp. harbor two unique classes of chloramphenicol resistance genes that convey resistance through drug inactivation, either by nitroreduction at the *p*-nitro group on the benzene ring (119) or by acetylation (120, 121). In the case of acetylation, the resistance is transferable and associated with the transfer of a 39.5-kb plasmid, pRYC3373 (120).

4.7 Tetracycline Resistance

The rate of tetracycline resistance among *Bacteroides*, is greater than 80–90% (91, 122). Because of the high rate of resistance, most surveys of antimicrobial resistance do not include a tetracycline and it is currently no longer considered as an effective first-line agent for the empirical treatment of *Bacteriodes* infections. Susceptibility testing is therefore required for the use of these agents for the treatment of such infections.

The mechanism of tetracycline resistance in *Bacteroides* spp. is through modification or protection of the target site. The *tetQ* gene encodes a protein that makes the ribosomal protein synthesis resistant to the inhibitory effects of tetracyclines (33, 123, 124). The DNA sequences of several *Bacteroides tetQ* genes have been determined (123, 124). The TetQ is 40% homologous with TetM and TetO proteins and may represent a new class of ribosomal protection proteins (123, 124).

DNA cross-hybridization studies revealed that a *tetQ* or *tetQ*-related gene are present in most tetracycline-resistant *Bacteroides* isolates (33). However, other mechanisms (such as tetracycline efflux) or other classes of ribosomal protection proteins may also contribute to tetracycline resistance because some tetracycline-resistant isolates do not contain *tetQ* DNA sequences. Support for this possibility is provided by the identification of a tetM-related determinant in some tetracycline-resistant isolates of *Bacteroides ureolyticus* (125).

C. perfringens possesses two tetracycline resistance genes— the *tetA(P)* and *tetB(P)* genes that create an operon that encodes two unrelated proteins which conveys resistance by two unique mechanisms (126). The *tetA(P)* gene generates a tetracycline efflux pump, and the *tetB(P)* creates a protein generating ribosomal resistance (126).

Bacteroides spp. can harbor two additional genes that are related to tetracycline resistance but may not contribute to clinical resistance. The oxidation of tetracycline is brought about by the product of the *tetX* gene that is active only under aerobic conditions (127–129). Another gene encodes a protein that produces tetracycline efflux in *Bacteroides* but is unable to produce tetracycline resistance in *E. coli* (130, 131).

The *tetQ* gene that mediated tetracycline resistance is inducible (123, 132) and transferable (34, 133). The mechanism of transfer of tetracycline resistance is by conjugation mediated by the tetracycline resistance transfer element (132, 134, 135). The frequency of transfer is usually very low except when the organisms are preexposed to tetracycline (83–85). The transfer is controlled by a prokaryotic two-component regulatory system (132, 135). The two regulatory genes, *rteA* and *rteB*, are present in the *tetQ* operon downstream from the *tetQ* gene (135), and their expression is facilitated by the presence of tetracycline.

RteA, the cytoplasmic membrane protein component of the system is encoded by the *rteA* gene, and the RteB is encoded by the *rteB* gene (135). RteB participates in the transfer and mobilization of the tetracycline resistance transfer element. An additional gene, *rteC*, that produces RteC, can play a role in the self-transfer of tetracycline resistance (132).

RteA and RteB also regulate the transfer of unlinked chromosomal elements termed nonreplicating *Bacteroides* units (NBUs) (33, 136, 137). Even though most NBUs do not harbor an identifiable phenotype, a cefoxitin-hydrolyzing, BL gene (*cfxA* [55]) can be located on an NBU (138). The transfer of the cefoxitin=hydrolyzing, BL is facilitated by pretreatment with tetracycline (138, 139).

The transfer elements of tetracycline resistance are chromosomally located and are similar to the conjugal transposon *Tn916* in *Enterococcus faecalis* (33, 140–142). Their size is large (70–80 kbp) (134), and they often contain other resistance genes (e.g., *ermF*) (40).

5 Transfer of Antibiotic Resistance

Anaerobic bacteria are capable of acquiring and disseminating by conjugation a variety of mobile DNA transfer factors, many of which harbor antibiotic resistance genes. These organisms are the main component of the normal human gastrointestinal flora, which contribute to polymicrobial infections including abscesses, and can survive in hypoxic/anoxic environments. All these environments can provide conditions for the rapid dissemination of antibiotic resistance determinants.

The transfer of resistance genes has been observed in the *B. fragilis* group and in *Prevotella*, *Clostridium*, and *Fusobacterium* spp. (24). Bacterial conjugation, which is the dominant mechanism in the *Bacteroides*, is the most common transmission method of antibiotic resistance genes in anaerobes. The resistance genes are situated in DNA transfer factors that contain sometimes mobile transposons, plasmids, and chromosomal elements (143, 144). These elements can be small harboring only the genes needed for initiation of DNA transfer. The actual transfer of the DNA from one cell to another cell requires a mating connector bridge that is encoded by much larger transferable conjugative transposons (143). Two sets of biochemical processes are needed for successful horizontal transmission of the transmissible DNA. One process forms a DNA protein complex (called the relaxosome), comprising a transfer factor-encoded mobilization protein that is assembled on the origin of transfer (*oriT*), and results in the formation of a single-stranded nick that creates the transferred molecule. The nicked DNA is then unwound and is transmitted from the donor to the recipient cell. This process occurs during conjugation alongside with the restoration to the double-stranded form in both cells. One to three mobilization proteins are required for adequate relaxosome formation in *Bacteroides* spp. with mobilization proteins specific for their cognate *oriT*s.

The second process needed for transfer is the formation of the mating or conjugal apparatus. This apparatus is a proteinaceous structure that spans the donor and recipient cell membranes and facilitates the transfer of DNA and has not been well-characterized among the anaerobes. It is believed to be encoded by the transfer region of conjugative transposons. Genes that possibly encode this apparatus have been found on a conjugative transposon called cTnDOT (145), and the formation of a pilus-like cell-surface appendage is required for the conjugation (146).

Members of the *B. fragilis* group that resist tetracycline are likely to harbor conjugative transposons. CTnDOT, which is the most thoroughly investigated conjugative transposon, contains a tetracycline resistance determinant and genes whose by-products are involved in the formation of the mating bridge (147).

Anaerobic conjugative transposons are mobile genetic elements that are also called Tet elements. The name entails their ability to harbor a tetracycline-resistance gene that confers ribosomal protection (148). These elements encode the conjugative transfer apparatus that assembles at the interface of donor and recipient cells and forms the physical conduit through which DNA containing antibiotic resistance genes is transferred from cell to cell (145, 146). Exposure of the bacteria to a low, sub-inhibitory concentration of tetracycline seems to upregulate the expression of transfer apparatus proteins in *Bacteroides* spp. (131). This exposure increases the conjugative transfer frequency of the intracellular Tet element and the other co-resident mobile (149). Multiple unrelated transfer factors that may carry different antibiotic resistance genes can therefore be transferred during conjugation. This may result in the rapid rise in stable antibiotic resistance among the different bacterial genera of anaerobic bacteria (150). A conjugative transposon named CTnGERM1 that carries an erythromycin resistance gene and was previously identified only in Gram-positive bacteria was also found in *Bacteroides* spp. (151). Based on hybridization and DNA sequence analyses, it is assumed that Gram-positive bacteria are likely to be the origin of this transposon. This phenomena of transposon transfer can be demonstrated in the laboratory, where resistance determinants can be efficiently transferred by conjugation within *Bacteroides* spp. and from *Bacteroides* spp. to *E. coli* and other unrelated bacteria.

Animal bacterial flora may also be a source of resistant anaerobic bacteria as transfer factors can also be transmitted from ruminal animals to humans (152). Human colonic bacterial flora may acquire resistance determinants from animal sources. The extensive use of antibiotic in livestock has generated an increase in the spread of resistant determinants among ruminal gut flora, many of which may also be acquired by humans.

6 The Role of beta-Lactamase-Producing-Bacteria in Mixed Infections

Penicillins have been the agents of choice for the therapy of a variety of anaerobic infections at different anatomical locations. However, within the last 50 years, an increased resistance to these drugs has been observed especially in AGNB (*Bacteroides fragilis* group, Pigmented *Prevotella* and *Porphyromonas*, *Prevotella bivia*, and *Prevotella disiens*) and *Fusobacterium* spp.) (2, 3, 153).

BLPB may have an important clinical role in infections. Not only can these organisms cause the infection, they may have an indirect effect through their ability to produce the BLs. BLPB may not only survive penicillin therapy but also may protect other penicillin-susceptible bacteria from penicillins by releasing the free enzyme into their environment (154).

Anaerobic BLPB were isolated in a variety of mixed infections. These include respiratory tract, skin, soft tissue, and surgical infections and other infections. The clinical in vitro and in vivo evidence supporting the role of these organisms in the increased failure rate of penicillin in eradication of these infections and the implication of that increased rate on the management of infections is discussed below.

6.1 Mixed Infections Involving Anaerobic BLPB

Anaerobic BLPB can be isolated from a variety of infections in adults and children, sometimes as the only isolates and sometimes mixed with other flora (Table 4). Table 5 summarizes our experience in the recovery of these organisms from skin and soft tissue infections (156–165), upper respiratory tract (166–178), lower respiratory tract (179–188), obstetric and gynecologic (183), intraabdominal (183–185), and miscellaneous infections (186–188).

The rate of isolation of these organisms varies in each infection entity (Table 5) (189). BLPB were present in 288 (44%) of 648 patients with *skin and soft tissue infections*, 75% harbored aerobic and 36% had anaerobic BLPB. The infections in which BLPB were most frequently recovered were vulvovaginal abscesses (80% of patients), perirectal and buttock abscesses (79%), decubitus ulcers (64%), human bites (61%) and abscesses of the neck (58%). The predominant BLPB were *S. aureus* (68% of patients with BLPB) and the *B. fragilis* group (26% of patients with BLPB).

BLPB were found in 262 (51%) of 514 patients with *upper respiratory tract infection* (URTI); 72% had aerobic BLPB and 57% had anaerobic. The infections in which these organisms were most frequently recovered were adenoiditis (83% of patients), tonsillitis in adults (82%) and children (74%), and retropharyngeal abscess (71%). The predominant BLPB were *S. aureus* (49% of patients with BLPB), Pigmented *Prevotella* and *Porphyromonas* (28% of patients with BLPB) and the *B. fragilis* group (20% of patients with BLPB).

BLPB were isolated in 81 (59%) of 137 children with *pulmonary infections*; 75% had aerobic BLPB, and 53% had anaerobic BLPB. The largest number of patients with BLPB was found in patients with cystic fibrosis (83% of patients), followed by pneumonia in intubated patients (78%) and lung abscesses (70%). The predominant BLPB was *B. fragilis* group (36% of patients with BLPB), *S. aureus* (35% of patients with BLPB), pigmented *Prevotella* and *Porphyromonas* spp. (16% of patients with BLPB), *P. aeruginosa* (14% of patients with BLPB), *K. pneumoniae* (11% of patients with BLPB), and *E. coli* (10% of patients with BLPB).

BLPB were recovered in 104 (92%) of 113 patients with *surgical infections*; 5% of the patients had aerobic BLPB and 98% had anaerobic BLPB (Table 3). The most predominant BLPB was the *B. fragilis* group (98% of patients with BLPB).

BLPB were recovered in 16 (28%) of 57 patients with *miscellaneous infections*, which included periapical and intracranial abscesses and anaerobic osteomyelitis; 25% had aerobic BLPB and 80% had anaerobic BLPB. The rate of recovery of BLPB was not significantly different in these infections. The most frequently recovered BLPB were pigmented *Prevotella* and *Porphyromonas* spp. (37% of patients with BLPB), *S. aureus* and *B. fragilis* groups (25% each of patients with BLPB).

Pelvic inflammatory disease (PID) is a polymicrobial infection (190) involving in most cases numerous isolates, including *N. gonorrhoeae*, *Chlamydia trachomatis*, *Enterobacteriaceae*, and AGNB (*B. fragilis*, *P. bivius*, and *P. disiens*). All of the above organisms (except for *C. trachomatis*) are capable of producing BL. In a summary of 36 studies published from 1973 to 1985, Eschenbach found BLPB in 1,483 (22%) of 6,637 specimens obtained from obstetric

Table 4 Infections involving beta-lactamase-producing bacteria (BLPB)

Infections	Predominant BLPB
Respiratory tract	
Acute sinusitis and otitis	*H. influenzae, M. catarrhalis*
Chronic sinusitis and otitis	*S. aureus*, anaerobic Gram-negative bacilli
Tonsillitis	*S. aureus*, anaerobic Gram-negative bacilli
Bronchitis, pneumonia	*H. influenzae, M. catarrhalis, L. pneumophila*
Aspiration pneumonia, lung abscesses	*S. aureus*, anaerobic Gram-negative bacilli, *Enterobacteriaceae*
Skin and soft tissue	
Abscesses, wounds, and burns in the oral areas, paronychia, bites	*S. aureus*, pigmented *Prevotella* and *Porphyromonas*
Abscesses, wounds, and burns in the rectal area	*E. coli, B. fragilis* group, *P. aeruginosa*
Abscesses, wounds, and burns in the trunk and extremities	*S. aureus, P. aeruginosa*
Obstetric and gynecologic	
Vaginitis, endometritis, salpingitis, pelvic inflammatory disease	*N. gonorrhoeae, E. coli, Prevotella* spp.
Intraabdominal	
Peritonitis, chronic cholangitis, abscesses	*E. coli, B. fragilis* group
Miscellaneous	
Periapical and dental abscesses	Pigmented *Prevotella* and *Porphyromonas*
Intracranial abscesses	*S. aureus*, anaerobic Gram-negative bacilli
Osteomyelitis	*S. aureus*, anaerobic Gram-negative bacilli

Anaerobic Gram-negative bacilli = *Bacteroides, Prevotella,* and *Porphyromonas*

Table 5 Recovery rate of anaerobic BLPB from various sites (155)

Infection	No. patients with BLPB/total no. patients (%)	Total no. of BLPB	Pigmented Prevotella and Porphyromonas spp.	P. oralis	P. oris-buccae	B. fragilis group	Bacteroides and other anaerobic Gram-negative bacilli
Skin/subcutaneous	288/648 (44%)	332	19/87[a]	2/9	2/3	75/75	8/63
	Percentage of patients[b]		7	1	0.6	26	3
Upper respiratory Tract	262/514 (51%)	344	73/191	19/45	2/14	52/52	3/98
	Percentage of patients		28	7	1	20	1
Pulmonary	81/137 (59%)	104	13/59	0/1	1/9	29/29	0/11
	Percentage of patients		16	0	1	36	0
Surgical	104/113 (92%)	113	0/26			102/102	5/23
	Percentage of patients		0			98	5
Other infections	16/57 (28%)	17	6/24	2/7		4/4	1/10
	Percentage of patients		37	12		25	6
All patients	744/1,469 (51%)	910	111/387	23/62	5/26	262/262	17/205
	Percentage of patients		15	3	1	35	2

[a]Number of strains producing beta-lactamase/total number of strains
[b]Number of patients with the specific BLPB/total number of patients with BLPB

and gynecologic infections (190). The predominant BLPB were *Enterobacteriaceae*, *S. aureus*, *B. fragilis* group and pigmented *Prevotella* and *Porphyromonas* spp. The increase in the failure rate of penicillin in eradicating these infections is an indirect proof of their importance (191–193).

We have recovered 2,052 isolates from 736 patients with obstetrical and gynecological infections (193). Of these isolates, 355 (17%) were BLPB, 211 (59%) were anaerobes, and 144 (41%) were aerobes and facultative. These BLPB were recovered from 276 (37%) of all 736 patients. The most frequently recovered BLPB were *Bacteroides* spp. Among them *B. fragilis* group accounted for 129 (36%) of all 355 BLPB. Ninety-nine percent of *B. fragilis* group were BLPB. Others were *P. bivia* (49 of 151 isolates, or 32%, were BLPB), *P. disiens* (6 of 17, or 35%), and *P. melaninogenica* (23 of 110, or 21%). *S. aureus* was the second most common BLPB isolated in 21% of patients.

6.2 Production of BL by AGNB in Clinical Infections

B. fragilis group has been known to be capable of producing BL. These organisms are the predominant anaerobic Gram-negative bacilli present in intra-abdominal infections (184) and anaerobic bacteremias (194). Within the last decade, however, other AGNB previously not recognized as capable of producing BL have acquired this ability. These include the pigmented *Prevotella* and *Porphyromonas* (*P. intermedia*, *P. melaninogenica*, *Porphyromonas asacchanolytica* and *Porphyromonas gingivalis*), *Prevottela oralis* and *Prevotella oris-buccae* (all are the most common AGNB in respiratory tract infections), and *Prevottela disiens* and *Prevotella bivia*

(the most prominent AGNB in pelvic and other obstetrical and gynecological infections) (191).

All 262 isolates of *B. fragilis* group that we recovered from our patients produced BL (Table 4). These isolates accounted for 29% of the BLPB and were isolated in 35% of the patients with BLPB. *B. fragilis* was recovered in 98% of patients with BLPB with surgical infections, in 36% of those with pulmonary infections, in 26% of those with skin and soft tissue infections, and in 20% of those with URTI.

One hundred and eleven of 387 (29%) pigmented *Prevotella* and *Porphyromonas* spp., which accounted for 12% of BLPB, were isolated in 15% of the patients with BLPB. The highest frequency of recovery of BL-producing pigmented *Prevotella* and *Porphyromonas* spp. isolates was found in URTI (38% of all pigmented *Prevotella* and *Porphyromonas* spp. isolates); the isolates were recovered in 28% of patients with URTI, mostly in those with recurrent tonsillitis and chronic OM. In pulmonary infections 22% of the pigmented *Prevotella* and *Porphyromonas* spp. isolates produced BL, and they were isolated in 16% of the patients. Although 22% of the isolates of the pigmented *Prevotella* and *Porphyromonas* spp. produced BL in skin and soft tissue infections, these organisms were isolated only in 7% of patients with these infections, mostly in those that were in close proximity or originated from the oral cavity.

Although 37% of isolates of *P. oralis* produced BL, they were isolated in 3% of the patients. Smaller percentages of *P. oris-buccae* and other AGNB were also detected. Their distribution among the infectious processes was similar to the distribution of pigmented *Prevotella* and *Porphyromonas* spp.

Penicillin resistance through production of BL is increasingly seen in the genus *Fusobacterium*. This is most commonly seen in *F. nucleatum*, but also in other members of the genus such as in *Fusobacterium varium* and *Fusobacterium mortiferum* (195, 196). Since *Fusobacterium* spp. is predominant in oral infection, it is not surprising that their presence was associated with failure of the therapy of respiratory infections (197).

6.3 Evidence for Indirect Pathogenicity of Anaerobic BLPB

The production of the enzyme BL is an important mechanism of indirect pathogenicity of aerobic and anaerobic bacteria that is especially apparent in polymicrobial infection. Not only are the organisms that produce the enzyme protected from the activity of penicillins, but other penicillin-susceptible organisms can also be shielded. This protection can occur when the enzyme BL is secreted into the infected tissues or abscess fluid in sufficient quantities to break the penicillin's beta-lactam ring before it can kill the susceptible bacteria (198–202) (Fig. 1).

Clinical and laboratory studies will be described that provide support for this hypothesis.

6.3.1 In Vivo and In Vitro Studies

Animal studies demonstrated the ability of the enzyme BL to influence polymicrobial infections. Hackman and Wilkins showed that penicillin-resistant strains of *B. fragilis*, pigmented *Prevotella* and *Porphyromonas* spp., and *P. oralis* protected a penicillin-sensitive *Fusobacterium necrophorum* from penicillin therapy in mice (203) Brook et al. (198–202), using a subcutaneous abscess model in mice, demonstrated protection of group A beta-hemolytic streptococci (GABHS) from penicillin by *B. fragilis* and *P. melaninogenica*. Clindamycin or the combination of penicillin and clavulanic acid (a BL inhibitor), which are active against both GABHS and AGNB, were effective in eradicating the infection. Similarly, BL-producing facultative

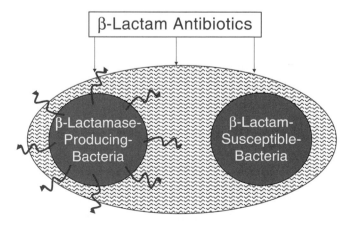

Fig. 1 Protection of penicillin-susceptible bacteria from penicillin by beta-lactamase-producing bacteria

bacteria protected a penicillin-susceptible *P. melaninogenica* from penicillin (199). O'Keefe et al. (204) demonstrated inactivation of penicillin-G in an experimental *B. fragilis* infection model in the rabbit peritoneum.

In vitro studies have also demonstrated this phenomenon. A 200-fold increase in resistance of GABHS to penicillin was observed when it was inoculated with *S. aureus* (200). An increase in resistance was also noted when GABHS was grown with *Haemophilus parainfluenzae* (201). When mixed with cultures of *B. fragilis* the resistance of GABHS to penicillin increased 8,500-fold (202).

6.3.2 BL in Clinical Infections

Several studies demonstrate the activity of the enzyme BL produced by anaerobic bacteria in polymicrobial infections. De Louvois and Hurley (205) demonstrated degradation of penicillin, ampicillin, and cephaloridine by purulent exudates obtained from 4 of 22 patients with abscesses. Studies by Masuda and Tomioka (206) demonstrated BL activity in empyema fluid. Most infections were polymicrobial and involved both *K. pneumoniae* and *P. aeruginosa*.

The presence of the enzyme BL in clinical specimens was also reported. Bryant et al. (207) detected strong enzyme activity in 4 of 11 pus specimens obtained from 12 patients with polymicrobial intraabdominal abscess or polymicrobial empyema.

We measured BL activity in 40 (55%) of 109 abscesses (183). One hundred BLPB were recovered in 88 (77%) specimens. These included all 28 isolates of *B. fragilis*, 18 of 30 pigmented *Prevotella* and *Porphyromonas* spp., 42 of 43 *S. aureus*, and 11 of 14 *E. coli*.

We detected the presence of BL activity in 46 of 88 (55%) ear aspirates that contained BLPB (183). We were also able to find BL activity in ear aspirates of 30 of 38 (79%) children with chronic otitis media (208), in 17 of 19 (89%) ear aspirates of children with acute otitis media who failed amoxicillin (AMX) therapy (209), and in 12 sinus aspirates (three acute and nine chronic infection) of the 14 aspirates that contained BLPB. The predominant BLPBs in acute sinusitis were *H. influenzae*, and *M. catarrhalis*; those in chronic sinusitis were *S. aureus*, *Prevotella* spp., *Fusobacterium* spp., and *B. fragilis* (Table 6) (210).

A study investigated the monthly changes in the rate of recovery of aerobic and anaerobic penicillin-resistant bacteria in the oropharynx of children (211). Each month during 1993, 30 children who presented with URTI were studied. The maximal total number of aerobic and anaerobic BLPB and number of patients with BLPB was in April (60% of patients) and the lowest was in September (13%). A gradual increase of BLPB and penicillin-resistant *S. pneumoniae* occurred from September to April, and a slow decline took place from April to August. These changes correlated directly with the intake of beta-lactam antibiotics. The study

Table 6 beta-Lactamase detected in four patients with chronic sinusitis aspirates (210)

beta-Lactamase detected in chronic sinusitis aspirates

	Patient no.			
Organism	1	2	3	4
Staphylococcus aureus (BL+)		+		+
Streptococcus pneumoniae	+			
Peptostreptococcus spp.	+			+
Propionibacterium acnes	+			
Fusobacterium spp. (BL+)		+		+
Fusobacterium spp. (BL−)		+		+
Prevotella spp. (BL+)			+	
Prevotella spp. (BL−)	+	+	+	
Bacteroides fragilis group (BL+)	+			+
beta-Lactamase activity in plus	+	+	+	+

BL+ = beta-Lactamase-producing bacteria

was reported over the following year with similar results. The crowding and the increased use of antibiotics that are more common in the winter might have also contributed to the spread of BLPB. Monitoring the local seasonal variation in the rate of BLPB may be helpful in the empiric choice of antimicrobials. Judicious use of antimicrobials may control the increase of BLPB.

6.3.3 Clinical Studies Illustrating Failure of Penicillins Due to Anaerobic BLPB

The recovery of penicillin-susceptible bacteria mixed with BLPB in patients who have failed to respond to penicillin or cephalosporin therapy suggests the ability of BLPB to protect a penicillin-susceptible or cephalosporin-susceptible organism from the activity of those drugs.

Selection of BLPB following antimicrobial therapy may account for many of the clinical failures after penicillin therapy. Heimdahl et al. described five adults with clinical failures after penicillin therapy associated with the isolation of anaerobic BLPB (212). In a study of 185 children with orofacial and respiratory infections who failed to respond to penicillin, BLPB were recovered in 75 (40%) (213). The predominant BLPB were *S. aureus*, pigmented *Prevotella* and *Porphyromonas* spp., *B. fragilis* group, and *P. oralis*.

Increased failure rate of penicillins in the therapy of PID has also been noticed and these agents are no longer recommended for this infection. Treatment failure has been noticed in as many as 33% of patients (151) and increased frequency of abscess formation has been observed (214). Therapy with penicillin, either alone or with an aminoglycoside or tetracycline, failed in 15–25% of cases (192). This increased failure rate may be due to the increased resistance to penicillin of anaerobic Gram-negative bacilli and *N. gonorrhoeae* as well as that of the *Enterobacteriaceae* involved in PID.

The URTI in which the phenomenon of indirect pathogenicity was most thoroughly studied is recurrent tonsillitis due to GABHS. Penicillin was considered the drug of choice for the therapy of this infection. However, the frequently reported inability of penicillin to eradicate GABHS is of concern. GABHS persists in the pharynx despite treatment with intramuscular penicillin in 21% of the patients after the first course of therapy and in 83% of the remainder of the patients after retreatment (215). Two randomized, single-blind, trials illustrated that either oral penicillin V or intramuscular penicillin failed to eradicate GABHS in pharyngitis in 35% children treated with oral penicillin V and 37% of intramuscular penicillin (216).

Various theories have been offered to explain this penicillin failure. One theory is that repeated penicillin administration results in a shift in the oral microflora with selection of BL-producing strains of *Haemophillus* spp., *S. aureus*, *M. catarrhalis*, and anaerobic Gram-negative bacilli (200, 201, 212, 212, 217, 218). It is possible that these BLPB can protect the GABHS from penicillin by inactivation of the antibiotic.

Clinical evidence supporting the ability of a BLPB to protect a penicillin-susceptible pathogen was reported in numerous studies (200, 201, 219).

The role of anaerobic BLPB in persistence of GABHS was suggested by Brook et al. (175, 176) who studied core tonsillar cultures recovered from children and young adults suffering from recurrent tonsillitis. One or two strains of aerobic and/or anaerobic BLPB were recovered in over 3/4 of the tonsils. The anaerobic BLPB included strains of *B. fragilis* group, pigmented *Prevotella* and *Porphyromonas* spp. and *P. oralis*, while the aerobic bacteria were *S. aureus*, *Haemophilus* spp., and *M. catarrhalis*. This observation was confirmed by Reilly et al. (220), Chagollan et al. (221), and Tuner and Nord (222). Assays of the free enzyme in the tissues demonstrated its presence in 33 of 39 (85%) tonsils that harbored BLPB, while the enzyme was not detected in any of the 11 tonsils without BLPB (223).

Tuner and Nord (223) and Brook and Gober (224) have demonstrated the rapid emergence of aerobic and anaerobic BLPB following penicillin therapy. Tuner and Nord (223) studied the emergence of BLPB in the oropharynx of ten healthy volunteers treated with penicillin for 10 days. A significant increase in the number of beta-lactamase producing strains of *Bacteroides* spp. *F. nucleatum* and *S. aureus* was observed. BL activity in saliva increased significantly in parallel to the increase of BLPB.

Brook and Gober isolated BLPB in 3 of 21 (14%) children prior to penicillin therapy, and in 10 of 21 (48%) following one course of penicillin (224). These organisms were also isolated from household contacts of children repeatedly treated with penicillin, suggesting their possible transfer within a family. The organisms were members of the pigmented *Prevotella* and *Porphyromonas* spp., *S. aureus*, *M. catarrhalis*, and *H. influenzae*. In a study of 26 children who received

7 days' therapy with penicillin, prior to therapy 11% harbored BLPB in their oropharyngeal flora (225). This increased to 45% at the conclusion of therapy, and the incidence was still 27% 3 months later. These data suggest that it is easy to induce BL production in the upper respiratory tract. Following penicillin therapy, these patients became colonized with BLPB.

Certain groups of children are at greater risk for developing penicillin-resistant flora. The daily administration of AMX chemoprophylaxis selected for colonization with aerobic and anaerobic BLPB in all 20 children was studied by Brook and Gober (226).

An association has been noted between the presence of BLPB even prior to therapy of acute GABHS tonsillitis and the outcome of 10-day oral penicillin therapy (227). Of 98 children with acute GABHS tonsillitis, 36 failed to respond to therapy (Table 7). Prior to therapy, 18 isolates of BLPB were detected in 16 (26%) of those cured and following therapy 30 such organisms were recovered in 19 (31%) of these children. In contrast, prior to therapy, 40 BLPB were recovered from 25 (69%) of the children who failed, and following therapy, 62 such organisms were found in 31 (86%) of the children in that group.

Roos et al. (228) observed high levels of BL in saliva reflecting colonization with numerous BLPB. These investigators also demonstrated that patients with recurrent GABHS tonsillitis had detectable amounts of BL in their saliva compared to patients with tonsillitis that did not recur.

6.4 Therapeutic Implications of Indirect Pathogenicity

The presence of BLPB in mixed infection warrants administration of drugs that will be effective in eradication of BLPB as well as the other pathogens. The high failure rate of penicillin therapy associated with the recovery of BLPB in a growing number of cases of mixed aerobic-anaerobic infections highlights the importance of this therapeutic approach (211, 212).

One infection in which this therapeutic approach has been successful is recurrent tonsillitis (215, 229–242). Antimicrobial agents active against BLPB as well as GABHS were effective in the eradication of this infection. Studies demonstrated the superiority of lincomycin (229–232),

clindamycin (233–238), amoxicillin-clavulanate (242), and penicillin plus rifampin (239, 240), over penicillin alone. The superiority of these drugs compared to penicillin is due to their efficacy against GABHS, S. aureus as well as anaerobic Gram-negative bacilli.

Over 83% of the adenoids in children with chronic adenotonsillitis are colonized with aerobic and anaerobic BLPB (243). The existence of BLPB within the adenoid's core may explain the persistence of many pathogens including S. pneumoniae where they may be shielded from the activity of penicillins. The effect on the adenoid bacterial flora of 10-day therapy with either AMX, AMX-C (244), or clindamycin (245) prior to adenoidectomy for recurrent OM was recently studied. The total number of isolates and bacteria per gram of tissue were lower in those treated with any of the antibiotics. However, the number of potential pathogens and BLPB was lower in those treated with AMX-C (244) and clindamycin 9238) as compared to amoxicillin and controls (P < 0.001).

A similar study evaluated the effects of AMX-C and AMX therapy on the nasopharyngeal flora of 50 children with acute otitis media (246). After therapy, 16 (64%) of the 25 patients treated with AMX and 23 (92%) of the 25 patients treated with AMX-C were considered clinically cured. A significant reduction in the number of both aerobic and anaerobic isolates occurred after therapy in those treated with either agent. The number of all isolates recovered after therapy in those treated with AMX-C was significantly lower (60 isolates) than in those treated with AMX (133 isolates, P < 0.001). The recovery of known aerobic pathogens (e.g., S. pneumoniae, S. aureus, GABHS, Haemophilus spp., and M. catarrhalis) and penicillin-resistant bacteria after therapy was lower in the AMX-C group than in the AMX group (P < 0.005).

The superiority of AMX-C and clindamycin over AMX in eradicating penicillin-susceptible pathogens such as S. pneumoniae and GABHS may be due to their activity against aerobic and anaerobic BLPB. The elimination of both potential pathogenic and non-pathogenic BLPB may be beneficial, as these organisms might "shield" penicillin susceptible pathogens from penicillins. This phenomenon might explain the survival of penicillin-susceptible bacteria such as S. pneumoniae in children treated with AMX.

Table 7 beta-Lactamase-producing organisms isolated from tonsillar cultures of 98 children with group A streptococci (GABHS) tonsillitis (227)

| | Prior to penicillin therapy | | Following 10 days of penicillin therapy | |
	Group A (62 patients)	Group B (36 patients)	Group A (62 patients)	Group B (36 patients)
Aerobic and facultative	6	20	11	30
Anaerobic	12	20	19	32
Total	18	40	30	62

Two studies compared the efficacy of clindamycin to penicillin in the therapy of lung abscesses (247, 248). Clindamycin was superior to penicillin in treating the infection. The superiority of clindamycin over penicillin was postulated to be due to its ability to eradicate the BL-producing anaerobic Gram-negative bacilli present in lung abscess.

Antimicrobials effective against anaerobic BLPB (ticarcillin-clavulanate or clindamycin) were superior to an antibiotic without such coverage (ceftriaxone) in the therapy of aspiration or tracheostomy-associated pneumonia in children (93% vs. 46%, $p < .05$) (249).

7 Antimicrobial Therapy of Anaerobic Infections

The recovery from an anaerobic infection depends on prompt and proper management. The principles of managing anaerobic infections include neutralizing bacterial toxins, preventing bacterial proliferation by changing the environment and hampering bacterial spread into healthy tissues.

Toxin neutralization by specific antitoxins may be employed, especially in infections caused by *Clostridium* spp. (tetanus and botulism). Controlling the environment is achieved by debriding of necrotic tissue, draining the pus, improving circulation, alleviating the obstruction and increasing the tissue oxygenation. In many cases surgical therapy is the most important and sometimes the only form of treatment required, whereas in others it is an adjunct to a pharmacologic approach. Without drainage the infection may persist despite antimicrobial therapy and serious complications can develop. The primary role of antimicrobials is in limiting the local and systemic spread of the organism.

7.1 Antimicrobial Therapy

Appropriate management of mixed aerobic and anaerobic infections requires the administration of antimicrobials effective against both components (Tables 8–11). A number of factors should be considered when choosing appropriate antimicrobial agents. They should have efficacy against all target organisms, induce little or no resistance, achieve sufficient levels in the infected site, and have minimal toxicity and maximum stability.

Antimicrobials often fail to cure the infection. Among the reasons for this are the development of bacterial resistance, achievement of insufficient tissue levels, incompatible drug interaction, and the development of an abscess. The abscess environment is detrimental to many antibiotics. The abscess capsule interferes with the penetration of drugs, and the low pH and the presence of binding proteins or inactivating enzymes (i.e., BL) may impair their activity. The low pH and the anaerobic environment within the abscess are especially unfavorable for the aminoglycosides and quinolones. However, an acidic pH, high osmolarity, and an anaerobic environment can also develop in the absence of an abscess.

When choosing antimicrobials for the therapy of mixed infections, their aerobic and anaerobic antibacterial spectrum (Tables 8 and 10) and their availability in oral or parenteral form should be considered. Some antimicrobials have a limited range of activity. For example, metronidazole is active only against anaerobes and therefore cannot be administered as a single agent for the therapy of mixed infections. Others (i.e., carbapenems) have wide spectra of activity against aerobes and anaerobes.

The selection of antimicrobials is simplified when reliable culture results are available. However, this may be difficult to achieve in anaerobic infections because

Table 8 Susceptibility of anaerobic bacteria present in URTI and head and neck infections to antimicrobial agents

Bacteria	Penicillin	A penicillin and a beta-Lactamase inhibitor	Ureido- and carboxy-penicillin	Cefoxitin	Chloramphenicol	Clindamycin	Macrolides	Metronidazole	Carbapenem
Peptostreptococcus spp.	4	4	3	3	3	3	2–3	2	3
Fusobacterium spp.	3–4	3–4	3	3	3	2–3	1	3	3
B. fragilis group	1	4	2–3	3	3	3–4	1–2	4	4
Prevotella and *Porphyromonas* spp.	1–3	4	2–3	3	3	3–4	2–3	4	4
Clostridium perfringens	4	4	3	3	3	3	3	3	3
Clostridium spp.	3	3	3	2–3	3	2	2	3	3
Actinomyces spp.	4	4	3	3	3	3	3	1	3

Degrees of activity: 1 = minimal; 2 = moderate; 3 = good; 4 = excellent

Table 9 Antimicrobial drugs of choice for anaerobic bacteria

	First	Alternate
Peptostreptococcus spp.	Penicillin	Clindamycin, chloramphenicol, cephalosporins
Clostridium spp.	Penicillin	Metronidazole, chloramphenicol, cefoxitin, clindamycin
Clostridium difficile	Vancomycin	Metronidazole, bacitracin
Gram-negative bacilli[a] (BL−)	Penicillin	Metronidazole, clindamycin, chloramphenicol
Gram-negative bacilli[a] (BL+)	Metronidazole, imipenem, a penicillin and beta-lactamase inhibitor, clindamycin	Cefoxitin, chloramphenicol, piperacillin

BL = beta-Lactamal

[a]*B. fragilis* group; *Prevotella* spp., *Porphyromonas* spp., *Fusobacterium* spp.

Table 10 Antimicrobial agents effective against mixed infection[a]

Antimicrobial agent	Anaerobic bacteria		Aerobic bacteria	
	beta-Lactamase-producing bacteroides	Other anaerobes	Gram-positive cocci	Enterobacteriaceae
Penicillin[b]	0	+ + +	+	0
Chloramphenicol[b]	+ + +	+ + +	+	+
Cephalothin	0	+	+ +	+/−
Cefoxitin	+ +	+ + +	+ +	+ +
Imipenem/meropenem, doripenem	+ + +	+ + +	+ + +	+ + +
Clindamycin[b]	+ + +	+ + +	+ + +	0
Ticarcillin	+	+ + +	+	+ +
Amoxicillin + clavulanic acid[b]	+ + +	+ + +	+ +	+ +
Piperacillin + tazobactam	+ + +	+ + +	+ +	+ +
Metronidazole[b]	+ + +	+ + +	0	0
Moxifloxacin[b]	+ +	+ +	+ +	+ + +
Tigecycline	++	+++	+++	++

[a]Degrees of activity: 0 to + + +

[b]Available also in oral form

of problems in obtaining appropriate specimens. Many patients are treated empirically on the basis of suspected, rather than established, pathogens. Fortunately, the types of organisms involved in many anaerobic infections and their antimicrobial susceptibility patterns tend to be predictable. However, the pattern of resistance to antimicrobials may vary in a particular hospital and resistance to antimicrobial agents may emerge while a patient is receiving therapy. Although identification of the infecting organisms and their antimicrobial susceptibility may be needed for selection of optimal therapy, the clinical setting and Gram-stain preparation of the specimen may indicate the types of anaerobes present in the infection as well as the nature of the infectious process.

Apart from susceptibility patterns, other factors influencing the choice of antimicrobial therapy include the pharmacologic characteristics of the various drugs, their toxicity, their effect on the normal flora and bactericidal activity.

7.2 Antimicrobial Agents (Tables 8–11)

Some classes of agents have poor activity against anaerobic bacteria. These include the aminoglycosides, the monobactams

and the older quinolones. Antimicrobials suitable for use in anaerobic infections are discussed in more detail below.

7.2.1 Penicillins

Penicillin G is still the drug of choice against most non-BLPB. These include anaerobic streptococci, *Clostridium* spp., nonsporulating anaerobic bacilli, and non-beta-lactamase-producing Gram-negative anaerobic rods (250). However, in addition to the *B. fragilis* group, which is known to resist the drug, many other AGNB are showing increased resistance. These include *Fusobacterium* spp., pigmented *Prevotella* and *Porphyromonas* spp. (prevalent in orofacial infections), *Prevotella bivia* and *Prevotella disiens* (common in obstetric and gynecologic infections), and *Bilophila wadsworthia* and *Bacteroides splanchinus*. Resistance to penicillin of some *Clostridium* spp. (*C. ramosum, C. clostridioforme,* and *C. butyricum*) through production of BL was also noted (46, 49).

The utilization of combinations of BL inhibitors (e.g., clavulanic acid, sulbactam, tazobactam) plus a beta-lactam antibiotic (ampicillin, amoxicillin, ticarcillin, or piperacillin) can overcome this resistance and its sequella of shielding non-BLPB. However, if other mechanisms of resistance emerge,

Table 11 Antimicrobial recommended for the therapy of site specific anaerobic infections

	Surgical		
	Prophylaxis	Parenteral	Oral
Intracranial	1. Penicillin	1. Metronidazole[a]	1. Metronidazole[a]
	2. Vancomycin	2. Chloramphenicol	2. Chloramphenicol
Dental	1. Penicillin	1. Clindamycin	1. Clindamycin, amoxicillin + CA
	2. Erythromycin	2. Metronidazole[a], chloramphenicol	2. Metronidazole[a], chloramphenicol
Upper respiratory tract	1. Cefoxitin	1. Clindamycin	1. Clindamycin, amoxicillin + CA
	2. Clindamycin	2. Chloramphenicol, metronidazole[a]	2. Chloramphenicol, metronidazole[b]
Pulmonary	NA	1. Clindamycin[b]	1. Clindamycin[c]
		2. Chloramphenicol, ticarcillin + CA, ampicillin + SU[d], imipenem, meropenem, doripenem	2. Chloramphenicol, metronidazole[b], amoxicillin + CA
Abdominal	1. Cefoxitin	1. Clindamycin[e], cefoxitin[e], metronidazole[e]	1. Clindamycin[c], metronidazole[c]
	2. Clindamycin[e]	2. Imipenem, meropenem, doripenem, ticarcillin + CA	2. Chloramphenicol, amoxacillin + CA
Pelvic	1. Cefoxitin	1. Cefoxitin[d], clindamycin[e]	1. Clindamycin[d]
	2. Doxycycline	2. Ticarcillin + CA[d], ampicillin + SU[d], metronidazole[d]	2. Amoxicillin + CA[d], metronidazole[d]
Skin	1. Cefazolin[f]	1. Clindamycin, cefoxitin	1. Clindamycin, amoxicillin + CA
	2. Vancomycin	2. Metronidazole[a] + methicillin	2. Metronidazole[b]
Bone and joint	1. Cefazolin[f]	1. Clindamycin, imipenem, meropenem	1. Clindamycin
	2. Vancomycin	2. Chloramphenicol, metronidazole[a], ticarcillin + CA	2. Chloramphenicol, metronidazole[a]
Bacteremia with BLPB	NA	1. Imipenem, meropenem, doripenem, metronidazole	1. Clindamycin, metronidazole
		2. Cefoxitin, ticarcillin + CA	2. Chloramphenicol, amoxacillin + CA
Bacteremia with non-BLPB	NA	1. Penicillin	1. Penicillin
		2. Clindamycin, metronidazole, cefoxitin	2. Metronidazole, chloramphenicol, clindamycin

1 – drug(s) of choice; 2 = alternative drugs

NA not applicable; *CA* clavulanic acid; *SU* sulbactam; *BLPB* beta-lactamase-producing bacteria

[a]Plus penicillin

[b]Plus a macrolide (i.e. erythromycin)

[c]Plus a quinolone (only in adults)

[d]Plus doxycycline

[e]Plus aminoglycoside

[f]In location proximal to the rectal and oral areas use cefoxitin

blockage of the enzyme BL will not prevent resistance. Other mechanisms of resistance include alteration in the porin canal and changes in the penicillin-binding protein.

The semisynthetic penicillins, carbenicillin, ticarcillin, piperacillin, and mezlocillin are generally administered in large quantities to achieve high serum concentrations. These drugs have good activity against Enterobacteriaceae and most anaerobes in these concentrations. However, they are not absolutely resistant to BL produced by AGNB.

7.2.2 Cephalosporins

The efficacy of cephalosporins varies against *Bacteroides* spp. (250). The activity of the first-generation cephalosporins against anaerobes is similar to that of penicillin G, although on a weight basis they are less active. Most strains of the *B. fragilis* group and many *Prevotella* and *Porphyromonas* spp. are resistant by virtue of cephalosporinase production. The second-generation cephalosporin cefoxitin is relatively resistant to this enzyme and is the most effective cephalosporin against the *B. fragilis* group and is often used for the therapy and prophylaxis of mixed infections. However, growing number of *B. fragilis* group may be resistant, reflecting hospital use pattern. Cefoxitin is relatively inactive against most species of *Clostridium* (including *C. difficile*); *C. perfringens* is an exception. The second-generation cephalosporins, cefotetan and cefmetazole, have a longer half-life than cefoxitin, which are as effective as cefoxitin against *B. fragilis*, but have poor efficacy against other members of the *B. fragilis* group (i.e., *B. thetaiotaomicron*). Third-generation cephalosporins have inferior activity against *Bacteroides* spp.

7.2.3 Carbapenems (Imipenem, Meropenem, Doripenem, Ertapenem)

All carbapenems have excellent activity against a broad spectrum of aerobic bacteria and anaerobic bacteria, including beta-lactamase-producing *Bacteroides* spp., Enterobacteriaceae and *Pseudomonas* spp. Resistance of the *B. fragilis* group is very rare (<1%). Ertapenem has similar efficacy, but is not active against *Pseudomonas* spp. and *Acinetobacter* spp. (251).

7.2.4 Chloramphenicol

Chloramphenicol has excellent in vitro activity against most anaerobic bacteria, resistance is rare and it penetrates well into the cerebro-spinal fluid (CSF). It is also effective against many Enterobacteriaceae and aerobic Gram-positive cocci. The toxicity of chloramphenicol, the rare but fatal aplastic anemia and the dose-dependent leukopenia limit its use.

7.2.5 Clindamycin and Lincomycin

Clindamycin and lincomycin are effective against anaerobes and have good activity against aerobic Gram-positive cocci (250). Clindamycin has the broader coverage against anaerobes, including BL-producing *Bacteroides* spp. Resistance of *B. fragilis* group is 5–10%, and some *Clostridium* spp. other than *C. perfringens* are resistant. Antibiotic-associated colitis caused by *C. difficile* was first described after clindamycin therapy. However, colitis has been associated with many other antimicrobial agents, including penicillins and cephalosporins.

7.2.6 Metronidazole

Metronidazole has excellent activity limited to anaerobes. Microaerophilic streptococci, *Propionibacterium acnes,* and *Actinomyces* spp. are often resistant (43). It penetrates well into the CSF, Concern was raised about the carcinogenic and mutagenic effects of this drug; however, these effects were shown only in one species of mice and were never substantiated in other animals or humans (2, 3).

7.2.7 Macrolides (Erythromycin, Azithromycin, Clarithromycin)

Macrolides have moderate-to-good in vitro activity against anaerobes other than *B. fragilis* group and fusobacteria. They are active against *Prevotella* and *Porphyromonas* spp., microaerophilic and anaerobic streptococci, Gram-positive

nonspore-forming anaerobic bacilli and certain clostridia such as *C. perfringens*. They have poor or inconsistent activity against AGNB.

7.2.8 Glycopeptides (Vancomycin, Teicoplanin)

The glycopeptides are effective against all Gram-positive anaerobes (including *C. difficile*), but are inactive against AGNB.

7.2.9 Tetracyclines (Tetracycline, Doxycycline, Minocycline)

Resistance to tetracycline has increased. The newer tetracycline analogs (doxycycline and minocycline) are more active than tetracycline. Because of significant resistance to these drugs, they can be used if the organisms are susceptible or in less severe infections in which a therapeutic trial is feasible.

7.2.10 Glycylcyclines

Tigecycline is the first antibiotic of this class approved by the FDA. It is indicated for the empiric monotherapy of a variety of complicated intraabdominal and complicated skin and skin structure infections. Glycylcyclines are tetracycline antibiotics containing a glycylamido moiety attached to the 9- position of a tetracycline ring; tigecycline is a direct analog of minocycline with a 9-glycylamide moiety. It has activity against both Gram-negative and Gram-positive bacteria, anaerobes, and certain drug-resistant pathogens. It is active against *Streptococcus anginosus* group (includes *S. anginosus, S. intermedius,* and *S. constellatus*), *B. fragilis, B. thetaiotaomicron, Bacteroides uniformis, Bacteroides vulgatus, C. perfringens,* and *Peptostreptococcus micros.*

7.2.11 Floroquinolones

Quinolones with low activity against anaerobes include ciprofloxacin, ofloxacin, levofloxacin, fleroxacin, pefloxacin, enoxacin, and lomefloxacin. Compounds with intermediate antianaerobic activity include sparfloxacin and grepafloxacin. Trovafloxacin, gatifloxacin, and moxifloxacin yield low MICs against most groups of anaerobes. FQ with the greatest in vitro activity against anaerobes include clinafloxacin and sitafloxacin (253). The use of the quoinolones is restricted in growing children and pregnancy because of their possible adverse effects on the cartilage.

7.2.12 Other Agents

Bacitracin is active against pigmented *Prevotella* and *Porphyromonas* spp. but is inactive against *B. fragilis* and *F. nucleatum* (2). Quinupristin/dalfopristin is active against *Clostridium perfringens*, *Lactobacillus* spp. and *Peptostreptococcus*. Linezolid is active against *Fusobacterium*, *Porphyromonas*, *Prevotella*, and *Peptostreptococci* spp. Minimal clinical experience has been gained, however, in the treatment of anaerobic bacteria using these agents.

7.3 Choice of Antimicrobial Agents

The available parenteral antimicrobials in most infections (Tables 8–11) are clindamycin, metronidazole, chloramphenicol, cefoxitin, a penicillin (i.e., ticarcillin, ampicillin, piperacillin) and a BL inhibitor (i.e., clavulanic acid, sulbactam, tazobactam), and a carbapenem (i.e., imipenem, meropenem, ertapenem). An agent effective against Gram-negative enteric bacilli (i.e., aminoglycoside) or an antipseudomonal cephalosporin (i.e., cefepime) are generally added to clindamycin, metronidazole and, occasionally, cefoxitin when treating intra-abdominal infections to provide coverage for these bacteria. Penicillin can be added to metronidazole in the therapy of intracranial, pulmonary, and dental infections to cover for microaerophilic streptococci, and *Actinomyces*. A macrolide (i.e., erythromycin) is added to metronidazole in upper respiratory infections to treat *S. aureus* and aerobic streptococci. Penicillin is added to clindamycin to supplement its coverage against *Peptostreptococcus* spp. and other Gram-positive anaerobic organisms.

Doxycycline is added to most regimens in the treatment of pelvic infections for chlamydia and mycoplasma. Penicillin is still the drug of choice for bacteremia caused by non-BLPB. However, other agents should be used for the therapy of bacteremia caused by BLPB.

Because the duration of therapy for anaerobic infections, which are often chronic, is generally longer than for infections caused by aerobic and facultative anaerobes, oral therapy is often substituted for parenteral therapy. The agents available for oral therapy are limited and include clindamycin, amoxicillin plus clavulanic acid, chloramphenicol, and metronidazole.

Clinical judgment, personal experience, safety, and patient compliance should direct the physician in the choice of the appropriate antimicrobial agents. The length of therapy generally ranges between 2 and 4 weeks, but should be individualized depending on the response. In some cases, such as lung abscesses, treatment may be required for as long as 6–8 weeks, but can often be shortened with proper surgical drainage.

References

1. Hentges DJ. The anaerobic microflora of the human body. *Clin Infect Dis* 1993; 164:S175–80.
2. Finegold SM. Anaerobic infections in humans: an overview. *Anaerobe* 1995; 1:3–9.
3. Brook I. Pediatric anaerobic infection: diagnosis and management, 3rd ed. New York: Marcel Dekker, 2002.
4. Summanen P, Baron EJ, Ciron DM, et al. Wadsworth anaerobic bacteriology manual, 5th ed. Belmont, CA: Star Publishing, 1993.
5. Snydman DR, Cuchural GJ Jr., McDermott L, Gill M. Correlation of various in vitro testing methods with clinical outcomes in patients with *Bacteroides fragilis* group infections treated with cefoxitin: a retrospective analysis. *Antimicrob Agents Chemother* 1992; 36:540–4.
6. Finegold SR. National Committee for Clinical Laboratory Standards Working Group on Anaerobic Susceptibility Testing. Susceptibility testing of anaerobic bacteria. *J Clin Microbiol* 1988; 26:1253–6.
7. Nguyen MH, Yu VL, Morris AJ, et al. Antimicrobial resistance and clinical outcome of *Bacteroides* bacteremia: findings of a multicenter prospective observational trial. *Clin Infect Dis* 2000; 30:870–6.
8. NCCLS. Methods for antimicrobial susceptibility testing of anaerobic bacteria, 6th ed. Villanova, PA: NCCLS, 2004. Document no. M11-A6.
9. Citron DM, Hecht DW. Susceptibility test methods: anaerobic bacteria. In: Murray PR, Baron EJ, Jorgensen JH, Pfaller MA, Yolken RH, eds. Manual of clinical microbiology, 8th ed. Washington, DC: American Society for Microbiology Press, 2003, pp. 1141–8.
10. Betriu C, Cabronero C, Gomez M, Picazo JJ. Changes in the susceptibility of *Bacteroides fragilis* group organisms to various antimicrobial agents 1979–1989. *Eur J Clin Microbiol Infect Dis* 1992; 11:352–6.
11. Watanabe K, Ueno K, Kato N, et al. In vitro susceptibility of clinical isolates of *Bacteroides fragilis* and *Bacteroides thetaiotaomicron* in Japan. *Eur J Clin Microbiol Infect Dis* 1992; 11:1069–73.
12. Tuner K, Nord CE. Antibiotic susceptibility of anaerobic bacteria in Europe. *Clin Infect Dis* 1993; 16(suppl 4):S387–9.
13. Wexler HM, Finegold SM. Current susceptibility patterns of anaerobic bacteria. *Yonsei Med J* 1998; 39:495–501.
14. NCCLS. Methods for antimicrobial susceptibility testing of anaerobic bacteria, 4th ed. Villanova, PA: NCCLS, 1997. Document no. M11-A4.
15. Snydman DR, Jacobus NV, McDermott LA, et al. National survey on the susceptibility of *Bacteroides fragilis* group: report and analysis of trends for 1997–2000. *Clin Infect Dis* 2002; 35:S126–34.
16. Cornick NA, Cuchural GJ Jr., Snydman DR, et al. The antimicrobial susceptibility patterns of the *Bacteroides fragilis* group in the United States, 1987. *J Antimicrob Chemother* 1990; 25:1011–9.
17. Snydman DR, Jacobus NV, McDermott LA, et al. Multicenter study of in vitro susceptibility of the *Bacteroides fragilis* group, 1995 to 1996, with comparison of resistance trends from 1990 to 1996. *Antimicrob Agents Chemother* 1999; 43:2417–22.
18. Jacobus NV, Mc Dernott LA, Golan Y, et al. US survey on the susceptibility of the *B. fragilis* group, report: 2002–2003. Abstract of the 7th Biennial Congress of the Anaerobe Society of the Americas. Annapolis, MD, July 19–21, 2004 (# PII-18).
19. Hecht DW, Osmolski JR, O'Keefe JP. Variation in the susceptibility of *Bacteroides fragilis* group isolates from six Chicago hospitals. *Clin Infect Dis* 1993; 16(Suppl 4):S357–60.
20. Aldridge KE, Ashcraft D, Cambre K, Pierson CL, Jenkins SG, Rosenblatt JE. Multicenter survey of the changing in vitro antimicrobial susceptibilities of clinical isolates of *Bacteroides fragilis* group, *Prevotella*, *Fusobacterium*, *Porphyromonas*, and

Peptostreptococcus species. *Antimicrob Agents Chemother* 2001; 45:1238–43.

21. Drummond LJ, McCoubrey J, Smith DG, Starr JM, Poxton IR. Changes in sensitivity patterns to selected antibiotics in *Clostridium difficile* in geriatric in-patients over an 18-month period. *J Med Microbiol* 2003; 52:259–63.

22. Leclercq R, Courvalin P. Bacterial resistance to macrolide, lincosamide, and streptogramin antibiotics by target modification. *Antimicrob Agents Chemother* 1991; 35:1267–72.

23. Leclercq R, Courvalin P. Intrinsic and unusual resistance to macrolide, lincosamide, and streptogramin antibiotics in bacteria. *Antimicrob Agents Chemother* 1991; 35:1273–6.

24. Hecht DW, Vedantam G. Anaerobe resistance among anaerobes: what now? *Anaerobe* 1999; 5:421–9.

25. Jimenez-Diaz A, Reig M, Baquero F, Ballesta JP. Antibiotic sensitivity of ribosomes from wild-type and clindamycin resistant *Bacteroides vulgatus* strains. *J Antimicrob Chemother* 1992; 30:295–301.

26. Lai CJ, Weisblum B. Altered methylation of ribosomal RNA in an erythromycin-resistant strain of *Staphylococcus aureus*. *Proc Natl Acad Sci U S A* 1971; 68:856–60.

27. Reig M, Fernandez MC, Ballesta JPG, Baquero F. Inducible expression of ribosomal clindamycin resistance in *Bacteroides vulgatus*. *Antimicrob Agents Chemother* 1992; 36:639–42.

28. Rasmussen JL, Odelson DA, Macrina FL. Complete nucleotide sequence and transcription of *ermF*, a macrolide-lincosamide-streptogramin B resistance determinant from *Bacteroides fragilis*. *J Bacteriol* 1986; 168:523–33.

29. Smith CJ. Nucleotide sequence analysis of Tn4551: use of *ermFS* operon fusions to detect promoter activity in *Bacteroides fragilis*. *J Bacteriol* 1987; 169:4589–96.

30. Halula MC, Manning S, Macrina FL. Nucleotide sequence of *ermFU*, a macrolide-lincosamide-streptogramin (MLS) resistance gene encoding an RNA methylase from the conjugal element of *Bacteroides fragilis* V503. *Nucleic Acids Res* 1991; 19:3453.

31. Marsh PK, Malamy MH, Shimell MJ, Tally FP. Sequence homology of clindamycin resistance determinants in clinical isolates of *Bacteroides* spp. *Antimicrob Agents Chemother* 1983; 23:726–30.

32. Callihan DR, Young FE, Clark VL. Presence of two unique genes encoding macrolide-lincosamide-streptogramin resistance in members of the *Bacteroides fragilis* group as determined by DNA–DNA homology. *J Antimicrob Chemother* 1984; 14:329–38.

33. Fletcher HM, Macrina FL. Molecular survey of clindamycin and tetracycline resistance determinants in *Bacteroides* species. *Antimicrob Agents Chemother* 1991; 35:2415–8.

34. Privitera G, Dublanchet A, Sebald M. Transfer of multiple antibiotic resistance between subspecies of *Bacteroides fragilis*. *J Infect Dis* 1979; 139:97–101.

35. Welch RA, Jones KR, Macrina FL. Transferable lincosamide-macrolide resistance in *Bacteroides*. *Plasmid*. 1979; 2:261–8.

36. Tally FP, Snydman DR, Gorbach SL, Malamy MH. Plasmid-mediated, transferable resistance to clindamycin and erythromycin in *Bacteroides fragilis*. *J. Infect. Dis.* 1979; 139:83–8.

37. Smith CJ, Macrina FL. Large transmissible clindamycin resistance plasmid in *Bacteroides ovatus*. *J Bacteriol* 1984; 158:739–41.

38. Robillard NJ, Tally FP, Malamy MH. *Tn4400*, a compound transposon isolated from *Bacteroides fragilis*, functions in *Escherichia coli*. *J Bacteriol* 1985; 164:1248–55.

39. Shoemaker NB, Guthrie EP, Salyers AA, Gardner JF. Evidence that the clindamycin-erythromycin resistance gene of *Bacteroides* plasmid pBF4 is on a transposable element. *J Bacteriol* 1985; 162:626–32.

40. Shoemaker NB, Barber BD, Salyers AA. Cloning and characterization of a *Bacteroides* conjugal tetracycline-erythromycin resistance element by using a shuttle cosmid vector. *J Bacteriol* 1989; 171:1294–302.

41. Mays TD, Smith CJ, Welch RA, Delfini C, Macrina FL. Novel antibiotic resistance transfer in *Bacteroides*. *Antimicrob Agents Chemother* 1982; 21:110–8.

42. Solomkin JS, Mazuski JE, Baron EJ, et al. Guidelines for the selection of anti-infective agents for complicated intra-abdominal infections. *Clin Infect Dis* 2003; 37:997–1005.

43. Goldstein EJ, Citron DM, Vreni MC, Warren Y, Tyrrell KL. Comparative in vitro activities of ertapenem (MK-0826) against 1001 anaerobes isolated from human intra-abdominal infections. *Antimicrob Agents Chemother* 2000; 44:2389–94.

44. Bush K. beta-Lactamases of increasing clinical importance. *Curr Pharm Des* 1999; 5:839–45.

45. Ambler RP. The structure of beta-lactamases. *Philos Trans R Soc Lond (Biol)* 1980; 289:321–31.

46. Richmond MH, Sykes RB. The beta-lactamases of Gram-negative bacteria and their possible physiological role. *Adv Microb Physiol* 1973; 9:31–88.

47. Mastrantonio P, Cardines R, Spigaglia P. Oligonucleotide probes for detection of cephalosporinases among Bacteroides strains. *Antimicrob Agents Chemother* 1996; 40:1014–6.

48. Edwards R, Greenwood D. An investigation of beta-lactamases from clinical isolates of *Bacteroides* species. *J Med Microbiol* 1992; 36:89–95.

49. Appelbaum PC, Spangler SK, Jacobs MR. beta-Lactamase production and susceptibilities to amoxicillin, amoxicillin-clavulanate, ticarcillin, ticarcillin-clavulanate, cefoxitin, imipenem and metronidazole of 320 *non-Bacteroides fragilis* Bacteroides isolates and 129 fusobacteria from 28 U.S. centers. *Antimicrob Agents Chemother* 1990; 34:1546–50.

50. Nord CE. Mechanisms of beta-lactam resistance in anaerobic bacteria. *Rev Infect Dis* 1986; 8(suppl 5):S543–8.

51. Hart CA, Barr K, Makin T, Brown P, Cooke RWI. Characteristics of a beta-lactamase produced by *Clostridium butyricum*. *J Antimicrob Chemother* 1982; 10:31–5.

52. Appelbaum PC, Spangler SK, Pankuch GA, et al. Characterization of a beta-lactamase from *Clostridium clostridioforme*. *J Antimicrob Chemother* 1994; 33:33–40.

53. Matthew M. Plasmid-mediated beta-lactamases of Gram-negative bacteria: properties and distribution. *J Antimicrob Chemother* 1979; 5:349–58.

54. Appelbaum PC, Spangler SK, Jacobs MR. Evaluation of two methods for rapid testing for beta-lactamase production in *Bacteroides* and *Fusobacterium*. *Eur J Clin Microbiol Infect Dis* 1990; 9:47–50.

55. Tuner K, Lennart L, Nord CE. Purification and properties of a novel beta-lactamase from *Fusobacterium nucleatum*. *Antimicrob Agents Chemother* 1985; 27:943–7.

56. Appelbaum PC, Philippon A, Jacobs MR, Spangler SK, Gutmann L. Characterization of beta-lactamases from non-*Bacteroides fragilis* group Bacteroides spp. belonging to seven species and their role in beta-lactam resistance. *Antimicrob Agents Chemother* 1990; 34:2169–76.

57. Giraud-Morin C, Madinier I, Fosse T. Sequence analysis of cfxA2-like β-lactamases in *Prevotella* species. *J Antimicrob Chemother* 2003; 51:1293–6.

58. Rogers MB, Parker AC, Smith CJ. Cloning and characterization of the endogenous cephalosporinase gene, *cepA*, from *Bacteroides fragilis* reveals a new subgroup of Ambler class A beta-lactamases. *Antimicrob Agents Chemother* 1993; 37:2391–400.

59. Smith CJ, Bennett TK, Parker AC. Molecular and genetic analysis of the *Bacteroides uniformis* cephalosporinase gene *cblA*, encoding the species-specific beta-lactamase. *Antimicrob Agents Chemother* 1994; 38:1711–5.

60. Parker AC, Smith CJ. Genetic and biochemical analysis of a novel Ambler class A beta-lactamase responsible for cefoxitin resistance in *Bacteroides* species. *Antimicrob Agents Chemother* 1993; 37:1028–36.

61. Tajima M, Sawa K, Watanabe K, Ueno K. The beta-lactamase of genus *Bacteroides*. *J Antibiot (Tokyo)* 1983; 36:423–8.
62. Rasmussen BA, Bush K, Tally FP. Antimicrobial resistance in *Bacteroides*. *Clin Infect Dis* 1993; 16(suppl 4):S390–400.
63. Yang Y, Rasmussen BA, Bush K. Biochemical characterization of the metallo-beta-lactamase CcrA from *Bacteroides fragilis* TAL3636. *Antimicrob Agents Chemother* 1992; 36:1155–7.
64. Rasmussen BA, Bush K, Tally FP. Antimicrobial resistance in anaerobes. *Clin Infect Dis* 1997; 24(Suppl 1):S110–20.
65. Bandoh K, Watanabe K, Muto Y, Tanaka Y, Kato N, Ueno K. Conjugal transfer of imipenem resistance in *Bacteroides fragilis*. *J Antibiot (Tokyo)* 1992; 45:542–7.
66. Cuchural GJ Jr., Malamy MH, Tally FP. beta-Lactamase-mediated imipenem resistance in *Bacteroides fragilis*. *Antimicrob Agents Chemother* 1986; 30:645–8.
67. Podglajen I, Breuil J, Casin I, Collatz E. Genotypic identification of two groups within the species *Bacteroides fragilis* by ribotyping and by analysis of PCR-generated fragment patterns and insertion sequence content. *J Bacteriol* 1995; 177:5270–5.
68. Podglajen I, Breuil J, Bordon F, Gutmann L, Collatz E. A silent carbapenemase gene in strains of *Bacteroides fragilis* can be expressed after a one step mutation. *FEMS Microbiol Lett* 1992, 70:21–9.
69. Podglajen I, Breuil J, Collatz E. Insertion of a novel DNA sequence, 1S1186, upstream of the silent carbapenemase gene *cfiA*, promotes expression of carbapenem resistance in clinical isolates of *Bacteroides fragilis*. *Mol Microbiol* 1994; 12:105–14.
70. Edwards R, Read PN. Expression of the carbapenemase gene (*cfiA*) in *Bacteroides fragilis*. *J Antimicrob Chemother* 2000; 46:1009–12.
71. Piddock LJV, Wise R. Properties of the penicillin-binding proteins of four species of the genus *Bacteroides*. *Antimicrob Agents Chemother* 1986; 29:825–32.
72. Georgopapadakou NH, Smith SA, Sykes RB. Mode of action of azthreonam. *Antimicrob Agents Chemother* 1982; 21:950–6.
73. Yotsuji A, Mitsuyama J, Hori R, et al. Mechanism of action of cephalosporins and resistance caused by decreased affinity for penicillin-binding proteins in *Bacteroides fragilis*. *Antimicrob Agents Chemother* 1988; 32:1848–53.
74. Wexler HM, Halebian S. Alterations to the penicillin-binding proteins in the *Bacteroides fragilis* group: a mechanism for non-beta-lactamase mediated cefoxitin resistance. *J Antimicrob Chemother* 1990; 26:7–20.
75. Piddock LJV, Wise R. Cefoxitin resistance in *Bacteroides* species: evidence indicating two mechanisms causing decreased susceptibility. *J Antimicrob Chemother* 1987; 19:161–70.
76. Fang H, Edlund C, Nord CE, Hedberg M. Selection of cefoxitin-resistant *Bacteroides thetaiotaomicron* mutants and mechanisms involved in b-lactam resistance. *Clin Infect Dis* 2002; 35:S47–53.
77. Hurlbut S, Cuchural GJ, Tally FP. Imipenem resistance in *Bacteroides distasonis* mediated by a novel beta-lactamase. *Antimicrob Agents Chemother* 1990; 34:117–20.
78. Rasmussen BA, Yang Y, Jacobus N, Bush K. Contribution of enzymatic properties, cell permeability, and enzyme expression to microbiological activities of beta-lactams in three *Bacteroides fragilis* isolates that harbor a metallo-beta-lactamase gene. *Antimicrob Agents Chemother* 1994; 38:2116–20.
79. Wexler HM. Outer-membrane pore-forming proteins in gram-negative anaerobic bacteria. *Clin Infect Dis* 2002; 35:S65–71.
80. Breuil J, Dublanchet A, Truffaut N, Sebald M. Transferable 5-nitroimidazole resistance in the *Bacteroides fragilis* group. *Plasmid* 1989; 21:151–4.
81. Urban E, Soki J, Brazier JS, Nagy E, Duerden BI. Prevalence and characterization of *nim* genes of *Bacteroides* sp. isolated in Hungary. *Anaerobe* 2002; 8:175–79.
82. Ingham HR, Eaton S, Venables CW, Adams PC. *Bacteroides fragilis* resistant to metronidazole after long-term therapy [letter]. *Lancet* 1978; 1:214.
83. Dubreuil L, Breuil J, Dublanchet A, Sedallian A. Survey of the susceptibility patterns of Bacteroides fragilis group strains in France from 1977 to 1992. *Eur J Clin Microbiol Infect Dis* 1992; 11:1094–9.
84. Chen SCA, Gottlieb T, Palmer JM, Morris G, Gilbert GL. Antimicrobial susceptibility of anaerobic bacteria in Australia. *J Antimicrob Chemother* 1992; 30:811–20.
85. Bourgault A-M, Lamothe F, Hoban DJ, et al. Survey of Bacteroides fragilis group susceptibility patterns in Canada. *Antimicrob Agents Chemother* 1992; 36:343–7.
86. Horn R, Lavallee J, Robson HG. Susceptibilities of members of the Bacteroides fragilis group to 11 antimicrobial agents. *Antimicrob Agents Chemother* 1992; 36:2051–3.
87. Suata K, Watanabe K, Ueno K, Homma M. Antimicrobial susceptibility patterns and resistance transferability among Bacteroides fragilis group isolates from patients with appendicitis in Bali, Indonesia. *Clin Infect Dis* 1993; 16:561–6.
88. Hill GB, Ayers OM, Everett BQ. Susceptibilities of anaerobic Gramnegative bacilli to thirteen antimicrobials and beta-lactamase inhibitor combinations. *J Antimicrob Chemother* 1991; 28:855–67.
89. Cuchural GJ Jr., Snydman DR, McDermott L, et al. Antimicrobial susceptibility patterns of the Bacteroides fragilis group in the United States, 1989. *Clin Ther* 1992; 14:122–36.
90. Aldridge KE, Gelfand M, Reller LB, et al. A five-year multicenter study of the susceptibility of the Bacteroides fragilis group isolates to cephalosporins, cephamycins, penicillins, clindamycin, and metronidazole in the United States. *Diagn Microbiol Infect Dis* 1994; 18:235–41.
91. Phillips I, King A, Nord CE, Hoffstedt B. Antibiotic sensitivity of the *Bacteroides fragilis* group in Europe. European Study Group. *Eur J Clin Microbiol Infect Dis* 1992; 11:292–304.
92. Lamothe F, Fijalkowski C, Malouin F, Bourgault A-M, Delorme L. *Bacteroides fragilis* resistant to both metronidazole and imipenem [letter]. *J Antimicrob Chemother* 1986; 18:642–3.
93. Brogan O, Garnett PA, Brown R. *Bacteroides fragilis* resistant to metronidazole, clindamycin and cefoxitin [letter]. *J Antimicrob Chemother* 1989; 23:660–2.
94. Rotimi VO, Duerden BI, Ede V, MacKinnon AE. Metronidazole-resistant *Bacteroides* from untreated patient. *Lancet*, 1979; 1(8120):833.
95. Nagy E, Foldes J. Inactivation of metronidazole by *Enterococcus faecalis* chromosomal determinant coding for 5-nitroimidazole resistance. *FEMS Microbiol Lett* 1992; 95:1–6.
96. Edwards DI. Nitroimidazole drugs-action and resistance mechanisms. I. Mechanisms of action. *J Antimicrob Chemother* 1993; 1:9–20.
97. Edwards DI. Nitroimidazole drugs-action and resistance mechanisms. II. Mechanisms of resistance. *J Antimicrob Chemother* 1993; 31:201–10.
98. Narikawa S, Suzuki T, Yamamoto M, Nakamura M. Lactate dehydrogenase activity as a cause of metronidazole resistance in *Bacteroides* of a tetracycline resistance determinant related to *tetM*. *J Antimicrob Chemother* 1991; 27:721–31.
99. Haggoud A, Reysset G, Azeddoug H, Sebald M. Nucleotide sequence analysis of two 5-nitroimidazole resistance determinants from *Bacteroides* strains and of a new insertion sequence upstream of the two genes. *Antimicrob Agents Chemother* 1994; 38:1047–51.
100. Carlier JP, Sellier N, Rager MN, Reysset G. Metabolism of a 5-nitroimidazole in susceptible and resistant isogenic strains of *Bacteroides fragilis*. *Antimicrob Agents Chemother* 1997; 41:1495–9.
101. Trinh S, Haggoud A, Reysset G, Sebald M. Plasmids pIP419 and pIP421 from *Bacteroides*: 5-nitroimidazole resistance genes and their upstream insertion sequence elements. *Microbiology* 1995; 141:927–35.
102. Reysset G, Haggoud A, Sebald M. Genetics of resistance of *Bacteroides* species to 5-nitroimidazole. *Clin Infect Dis* 1993; 16(suppl 4):S401–3.

103. Haggoud A, Reysset G, Sebald M. Cloning of a *Bacteroides fragilis* chromosomal determinant coding for 5-nitroimidazole resistance. *FEMS Microbiol Lett* 1992; 95:1–6.

104. Reysset G, Haggoud A, Su W-J, Sebald M. Genetic and molecular analysis of pIP417 and pIP419: *Bacteroides* plasmids encoding 5-nitroimidazole resistance. *Plasmid* 1992; 27:181–90.

105. Breuil J, Dublanchet A, Truffaut N, Sebald M. Transferable 5-nitroimidazole resistance in the *Bacteroides fragilis* group. *Plasmid* 1989; 21:151–4.

106. Podglajen L, Breuil J, Collatz E. Insertion of a novel DNA sequence, *IS1186*, upstream of the silent carbapenemase gene, *cfiA*, promotes expression of carbapenem resistance in clinical isolates of *Bacteroides fragilis*. *Mol Microbiol* 1994; 12:105–14.

107. Brazier JS, Stubbs SL, Duerden BI. Metronidazole resistance among clinical isolates belonging to the *Bacteroides fragilis* group: time to be concerned? *J Antimicrob Chemother* 1999; 44:580–1.

108. Lewin CS, Morrissey I, Smith JT. Role of oxygen in the bactericidal action of the 4-quinolones. *Rev Infect Dis* 1989; 11 (suppl 5): S913–4.

109. Lewin CS, Morrissey I, Smith JT. The mode of action of quinolones: the paradox in activity of low and high concentrations and activity in the anaerobic environment. *Eur J Clin Microbiol Infect Dis* 1991; 10:240–8.

110. Golan Y, McDermott LA, Jacobus NV, et al. Emergence of fluoroquinolone resistance among *Bacteroides* species. *J Antimicrob Chemother* 2003; 52:208–13.

111. Onodera Y, Sato K. Molecular cloning of the *gyrA* and *gyrB* genes of *Bacteroides fragilis* encoding DNA gyrase. *Antimicrob Agents Chemother* 1999; 43:2423–9.

112. Bachoual R, Dubreuil L, Soussy CJ, Tankovic J. Roles of *gyrA* mutations in resistance of clinical isolates and in vitro mutants of *Bacteroides fragilis* to the new fluoroquinolone trovafloxacin. *Antimicrob Agents Chemother* 2000; 44:1842–5.

113. Oh H, El Amin N, Davies T, Appelbaum PC, Edlund C. *gyrA* mutations associated with quinolone resistance in *Bacteroides fragilis* group strains. *Antimicrob Agents Chemother* 2001; 45: 1977–81.

114. Oh H, Hedberg M, Edlund C. Efflux-mediated fluoroquinolone resistance in the *Bacteroides fragilis* group. *Anaerobe* 2002; 8: 277–82.

115. Ricci V, Piddock L. Accumulation of garenoxacin by *Bacteroides fragilis* compared with that of five fluoroquinolones. *J Antimicrob Chemother* 2003; 52:605–9.

116. Bryan LE, Kowand SK, Van Den Elzen HM. Mechanism of aminoglycoside antibiotic resistance in anaerobic bacteria: *Clostridium perfringens* and *Bacteroides fragilis*. *Antimicrob Agents Chemother* 1979; 15:7–13.

117. Bryan LE, Van Den Elzen HM. Streptomycin accumulation in susceptible and resistant strains of *Escherichia coli* and *Pseudomonas aeruginosa*. *Antimicrob Agents Chemother* 1976; 9:928–38.

118. Salzer W, Pegram PS Jr., McCall CE. Clinical evaluation of moxalactam: evidence of decreased efficacy in gram-positive aerobic infections. *Antimicrob Agents Chemother* 1983; 23: 65–70.

119. Onderdonk AB, Kasper DL, Mansheim BJ, Louie TJ, Gorbach SL, Bartlett JG. Experimental animal models for anaerobic infections. *Rev Infect Dis* 1979; 1:291–301.

120. Britz ML, Wilkinson RG. Chloramphenicol acetyltransferase of *Bacteroi des fragilis*. *Antimicrob Agents Chemother* 1978; 14: 105–11.

121. Martinez-Suarez JV, Baquero F, Reig M, Perez-Diaz JC. Transferable plasmid-linked chloramphenicol acetyltrans-

ferase conferring highlevel resistance in *Bacteroides uniformis*. *Antimicrob Agents Chemother* 1985; 28:113–7.

122. Martinez-Suarez JV, Baquero F. Molecular and ecological aspects of antibiotic resistance in the *Bacteroides fragilis* group. *Microbiolgia SEM* 1987; 3:149–62.

123. Nikolich MP, Shoemaker NB, Salyers AA. A *Bacteroides* tetracycline resistance gene represents a new class of ribosome protection tetracycline resistance. *Antimicrob Agents Chemother* 1992; 36:1005–12.

124. Lepine G, Lacroix J-M, Walker CB, Progulske-Fox A. Sequencing of a *tet(Q)* gene isolated from *Bacteroides fragilis* 1126. *Antimicrob Agents Chemother* 1993; 37:2037–41.

125. de Barbeyrac B, Dutilh B, Quentin C, Renaudin H, Bebear C. Susceptibility of *Bacteroides ureolyticus* to antimicrobial agents and identification of a tetracycline resistance determinant related to tetM. *J Antimicrob Chemother* 1991; 27:721–31.

126. Sloan J, McMurry LM, Lyras D, Levy SB, Rood JI. The *Clostridium perfringens* TetP determinant comprises two overlapping genes: *tetA(P)*, which mediates active tetracycline efflux, and *tetB(P)*, which is related to the ribosomal protection family of tetracycline-resistance determinants. *Mol Microbiol* 1994; 11:403–15.

127. Speer BS, Bedzyk L, Salyers AA. Evidence that a novel tetracycline resistance gene found on two *Bacteroides* transposons encodes an NADP-requiring oxidoreductase. *J Bacteriol* 1991; 173:176–83.

128. Speer BS, Salyers AA. Novel aerobic tetracycline resistance gene that chemically modifies tetracycline. *J Bacteriol* 1989; 171:148–53.

129. Speer BS, Salyers AA. Characterization of a novel tetracycline resistance that functions only in aerobically grown *Escherichia coli*. *J Bacteriol* 1988; 170:1423–9.

130. Park BH, Hendricks M, Malamy MH, Tally FP, Levy SB. Cryptic tetracycline resistance determinant (class F) from *Bacteroides fragilis* mediates resistance in *Escherichia coli* by actively reducing tetracycline accumulation. *Antimicrob Agents Chemother* 1987; 31:1739–43.

131. Speer BS, Salyers AA. A tetracycline efflux gene on *Bacteroides* transposon *Tn4400* does not contribute to tetracycline resistance. *J Bacteriol* 1990; 172:292–8.

132. Stevens AM, Shoemaker NB, Li L-Y, Salyers AA. Tetracycline regulation of genes on *Bacteroides* conjugative transposons. *J Bacteriol* 1993; 175:6134–41.

133. Privitera G, Sebald M, Fayolle F. Common regulatory mechanism of expression and conjugative ability of a tetracycline resistance plasmid in *Bacteroides fragilis*. *Nature* 1979; 278:657–9.

134. Bedzyk LA, Shoemaker NB, Young KE, Salyers AA. Insertion and excision of *Bacteroides* conjugative chromosomal elements. *J Bacteriol* 1992; 174:166–72.

135. Stevens AM, Sanders JM, Shoemaker NB, Salyers AA. Genes involved in production of plasmidlike forms by a *Bacteroides* conjugal chromosomal element share amino acid homology with two-component regulatory systems. *J Bacteriol* 1992; 174:2935–42.

136. Privitera G, Fayolle F, Sebald M. Resistance to tetracycline, erythromycin, and clindamycin in the *Bacteroides fragilis* group: inducible versus constitutive tetracycline resistance. *Antimicrob Agents Chemother* 1981; 20:314–20.

137. Shoemaker NB, Wang G-R, Stevens AM, Salyers AA. Excision, transfer, and integration of NBUI, a mobilizable site-selective insertion element. *J Bacteriol* 1993; 175:6578–87.

138. Li L-Y, Shoemaker NB, Salyers AA. Characterization of the mobilization region of a *Bacteroides* insertion element (NBU1) that is excised and transferred by *Bacteroides* conjugative transposons. *J Bacteriol* 1993; 175:6588–98.

139 Smith CJ, Parker AC. Identification of a circular intermediate in the transfer and transposition of *Tn4555*, a mobilizable transposon from *Bacteroides* spp. *J Bacteriol* 1993; 175:2682–91.

140. Rashtchian A, Dubes GR, Booth SJ. Tetracycline-inducible transfer of tetracycline resistance in *Bacteroides fragilis* in the absence of detectable plasmid DNA. *J Bacteriol* 1982; 150:141–7.

141. Smith CJ, Welch RA, Macrina FL. Two independent conjugal transfer systems operating in *Bacteroides fragilis* V479-1. *J Bacteriol* 1982; 151:281–7.

142. Franke AF, Clewell DB. Evidence for a chromosome borne resistance transposon *(Tn916)* in *Streptococcus faecalis* that is capable of "conjugal" transfer in the absence of a conjugative plasmid. *J Bacteriol* 1981; 145:494–502.

143. Whittle G, Shoemaker NB, Salyers AA. The role of *Bacteroides* conjugative transposons in the dissemination of antibiotic resistance genes. *Cell Mol Life Sci* 2002; 59; 2044–54.

144. Smith CJ, Tribble GD, Bayley DP. Genetic elements of *Bacteroides* species: a moving story. *Plasmid* 1998; 40:12–29.

145. Whittle G, Hund BD, Shoemaker NB, Salyers AA. Characterization of the 13-kilobase *ermF* region of the *Bacteroides* conjugative transposon CTnDOT. *Appl Environ Microbiol* 2001; 67:3488–95.

146. Vedantam G, Hecht DW. Isolation and characterization of BTF-37: chromosomal DNA captured from *Bacteroides fragilis* that confers self-transferability and expresses a pilus-like structure in *Bacteroides* spp. and *Escherichia coli*. *J Bacteriol* 2002; 184:728–38.

147. Bonheyo GT, Hund BD, Shoemaker NB, Salyers AA. Transfer region of a *Bacteroides* conjugative transposon contains regulatory as well as structural genes. *Plasmid* 2001; 46:202–9.

148. Salyers AA, Shoemaker NB, Li LY, Stevens AM. Conjugative transposons: an unusual and diverse set of integrated gene transfer elements. *Microbiol Rev* 1995; 59:579–90.

149. Valentine PJ, Shoemaker NB, Salyers AA. Mobilization of *Bacteroides* plasmids by *Bacteroides* conjugal elements. *J Bacteriol* 1988; 170:1319–24.

150. Shoemaker NB, Vlamakis H, Hayes K, Salyers AA. Evidence for extensive resistance gene transfer among *Bacteroides* spp. and among *Bacteroides* and other genera in the human colon. *Appl Environ Microbiol* 2001; 67:561–8.

151. Wang Y, Wang GR, Shelby A, Shoemaker NB, Salyers AA. A newly discovered *Bacteroides* conjugative transposon, CTnGERM1, contains genes also found in Gram-positive bacteria. *Appl Environ Microbiol* 2003; 69:4595–603.

152. Nikolich MP, Hong G, Shoemaker NB, Salyers AA. Evidence for natural horizontal transfer of *tetQ* between bacteria that normally colonize humans and bacteria that normally colonize livestock. *Appl Environ Microbiol* 1994; 60:3255–60.

153. Brook I, Calhoun L, Yocum P. beta-Lactamase-producing isolates of *Bacteroides* species from children. *Antimicrob Agents Chemother* 1980; 18:264–6.

154. Brook I. The role of beta-lactamase-producing bacteria in the persistence of streptococcal tonsillar infection. *Rev Infect Dis* 1984; 6:601–7.

155. Brook I. Recovery of beta-lactamase producing bacteria in pediatric patients. *Can J Microbiol* 1987; 33:888.

156. Brook I. Microbiology of abscesses of head and neck in children. *Ann Otol Rhinol Laryngol* 1987; 96:429–33.

157. Brook I, Finegold SM. Aerobic and anaerobic bacteriology of cutaneous abscesses in children. *Pediatrics* 1981; 67:891–5.

158. Brook I, Martin WJ. Aerobic and anaerobic bacteriology of perirectal abscess in children. *Pediatrics* 1980; 66:282–4.

159. Brook I, Anderson KD, Controni G, Rodriguez WJ. Aerobic and anaerobic bacteriology of pilonidal cyst abscess in children. *Am J Dis Child* 1980; 134:629–30.

160. Brook I. Aerobic and anaerobic bacteriology of cervical adenitis in children. *Clin Pediatr* 1980; 19:693–6.

161. Brook I, Randolph J. Aerobic and anaerobic flora of burns in children. *J Trauma* 1981; 21:313–18.

162. Brook I. Bacteriology of paronychia in children. *Am J Surg* 1981; 141:703–5.

163. Brook I. Anaerobic and aerobic bacteriology of decubitus ulcers in children. *Am Surg* 1980; 6:624–6.

164. Brook I. Microbiology of human and animal bites in children. *Pediatr Infect Dis J* 1987; 6:29–32.

165. Brook I. Bacteriology of neonatal omphalitis. *J Infect* 1982; 5:127–31.

166. Brook I. Aerobic and anaerobic bacterial isolates of acute conjunctivitis in children: a prospective study. *Arch Ophthalmol* 1980; 98:833–5.

167. Brook I, Finegold SM. Bacteriology of chronic otitis media. *JAMA* 1979; 241:487–8.

168. Brook I. Microbiology of chronic otitis media with perforation in children. *Am J Dis Child* 1980; 130:564–6.

169. Brook I. Prevalence of beta-lactamase-producing bacteria in chronic suppurative otitis media. *Am J Dis Child* 1985; 139:280–4.

170. Brook I, Yocum P, Shah K, Feldman B, Epstein S. The aerobic and anaerobic bacteriology of serous otitis media. *Am J Otolaryngol* 1983; 4:389–92.

171. Brook I. Aerobic and anaerobic bacteriology of cholesteatoma. *Laryngoscope* 1981; 91:250–3.

172. Brook I. Aerobic and anaerobic bacteriology of chronic mastoiditis in children. *Am J Dis Child* 1981; 135.478–9.

173. Brook I. Bacteriological features of chronic sinusitis in children. *JAMA* 1981; 246:567–9.

174. Brook I. Aerobic and anaerobic bacteriology of adenoids in children: comparison between patients with chronic adenotonsillitis and adenoid hypertrophy. *Laryngoscope* 1981; 91:377–82.

175. Brook I, Yocum P, Friedman EM. Aerobic and anaerobic flora recovered from tonsils of children with recurrent tonsillitis. *Ann Otol Rhinol Laryngol* 1981; 90:261–3.

176. Brook I, Yocum P. Bacteriology of chronic tonsillitis in young adults. *Arch Otolaryngol* 1984; 110:803–5.

177. Brook I. Aerobic and anaerobic bacteriology of peritonsillar abscess in children. *Acta Paediatr Scand* 1981; 70:831–5.

178. Brook I. Microbiology of retropharyngeal abscesses in children. *Am J Dis Child* 1987; 141:202–3.

179. Brook I, Finegold SM. Bacteriology of aspiration pneumonia in children. *Pediatrics* 1980; 65:1115–20.

180. Brook I, Finegold SM. The bacteriology and therapy of lung abscess in children. *J Pediatr* 1979; 94:10–4.

181. Brook I. Bacterial colonization, trachitis, tracheobronchitis and pneumonia following tracheostomy and long-term intubation in pediatric patients. *Chest* 1979; 70:420–24.

182. Brook I, Fink R. Transtracheal aspiration in pulmonary infection in children with cystic fibrosis. *Eur J Respir Dis* 1983; 64:51–7.

183. Brook I. Presence of beta-lactamase-producing bacteria and beta-lactamase activity in abscesses. *Am J Clin Pathol* 1986; 86:97–101.

184. Brook I. Bacterial studies of peritoneal cavity and postoperative surgical wound drainage following perforated appendix in children. *Ann Surg* 1980; 192:208–12.

185. Brook I, Altman RP. The significance of anaerobic bacteria in biliary tract infections following hepatic porto-enterostomy for biliary atresia. *Surgery* 1984; 95:281–3.

186. Brook I, Grimm S, Kielich RB. Bacteriology of acute periapical abscess in children. *J Endodon* 1981; 7:378–80.

187. Brook I. Aerobic and anaerobic bacteriology of intracranial abscesses. *Pediatr Neurol* 1992; 8:210–4.

188. Brook I. Anaerobic osteomyelitis in children. *Pediatr Infect Dis J* 1986; 5:550–6.

189. Brook I. Recovery of anaerobic bacteria from clinical specimens in 12 years at two military hospitals. *J Clin Microbiol* 1988; 26:1181–8.

190. Eschenbach DA. A review of the role of beta-lactamase producing bacteria in obstetric-gynecologic infection. *Am J Obstet Gynecol* 1987; 156:495–503.

191. Martens MG, Faro S, Maccato M, Hammill HA, Riddle G. Prevalence of beta-lactamase enzyme production in bacteria isolated from women with postpartum endometritis. *J Reprod Med* 1993; 38:795–8.

192. Quentin R, Lansac J. Pelvic inflammatory disease: medical treatment. *Eur J Obstet Gynecol Reprod Biol* 2000; 92:189–92.

193. Brook I, Frazier EH, Thomas RL. Aerobic and anaerobic microbiologic factors and recovery of beta-lactamase producing bacteria from obstetric and gynecologic infection. *Surg Gynecol Obstet* 1991; 172:138–44.

194. Brook I. Anaerobic bacterial bacteremia: 12-year experience in two military hospitals. *J Infect Dis* 1989; 160:1071–5.

195. Brook I. Infections caused by beta-lactamase-producing *Fusobacterium* spp. in children. *Pediatr Infect Dis J* 1993; 12: 532–3.

196. Kononen E, Kanervo A, Salminen K, Jousimies-Somer H. beta-Lactamase production and antimicrobial susceptibility of oral heterogenous *Fusobacterium nucleatum* populations in young children. *Antimicrob Agents Chemother* 1999; 43:1270–3.

197. Goldstein EJ, Summanen PH, Citron DM, Rosove MH, Finegold SM. Fatal sepsis due to a beta-lactamase-producing strain of *Fusobacterium nucleatum* subspecies polymorphum. *Clin Infect Dis* 1995; 20:797–800.

198. Brook I, Pazzaglia G, Coolbaugh JC, Walker RI. *In vivo* protection of group A beta-hemolytic streptococci by beta-lactamase producing *Bacteroides* species. *J Antimicrob Chemother* 1983; 12:599–606.

199. Brook I, Pazzaglia G, Coolbaugh JC, Walker RI. *In vivo* protection of penicillin susceptible *Bacteroides melaninogenicus* from penicillin by facultative bacteria which produce beta-lactamase. *Can J Microbiol* 1984; 30:98–104.

200. Simon HM, Sakai W. Staphylococcal anatagosim to penicillin group therapy of hemolytic streptococcal pharyngeal infection: effect of oxacillin. *Pediatrics* 1963; 31:463–9.

201. Scheifele DW, Fussell SJ. Frequency of ampicillin resistant *Haemophilus parainfluenzae* in children. *J Infect Dis* 1981; 143:495–8.

202. Brook I, Yocum P. *In vitro* protection of group A beta-hemolytic streptococci from penicillin and cephalothin by *Bacteroides fragilis*. *Chemotherapy* 1983; 29:18–23.

203. Hackman AS, Wilkins TD. *In vivo* protection of *Fusobacterium necrophorum* from penicillin by *Bacteroides fragilis*. *Antimicrob Agents Chemother* 1975; 7:698–703.

204. O'Keefe JP, Tally FP, Barza M, Gorbach SL. Inactivation of penicillin-G during experimental infection with *Bacteroides fragilis*. *J Infect Dis* 1978; 137:437–42.

205. De Louvois J, Hurley R. Inactivation of penicillin by purulent exudates. *Br Med J* 1977; 2:998–1000.

206. Masuda G, Tomioka S. Possible beta-lactamase activities detectable in infective clinical specimens. *J Antibiot (Tokyo)* 1977; 30:1093–7.

207. Bryant RE, Rashad AL, Mazza JA, Hammond D. beta-Lactamase activity in human plus. *J Infect Dis* 1980; 142:594–601.

208. Brook I. Quantitative cultures and beta-lactamase activity in chronic suppurative otitis media. *Ann Otol Rhinol Laryngol* 1989; 98:293–7.

209. Brook I, Yocum P. Bacteriology and beta-lactamase activity in ear aspirates of acute otitis media that failed amoxicillin therapy. *Pediatr Infect Dis J* 1995; 14:805–8.

210. Brook I, Yocum P, Frazier EH. Bacteriology and beta-lactamase activity in acute and chronic maxillary sinusitis. *Arch Otolaryngol Head Neck Surg* 1996; 122:418–22.

211. Brook I, Gober AE. Monthly changes in the rate of recovery of penicillin-resistant organisms from children. *Pediatr Infect Dis J* 1997; 16:255–7.

212. Heimdahl A, Von Konow L, Nord CE. Isolations of beta-lactamase-producing *Bacteroides* strains associated with clinical failures with penicillin treatment of human orofacial infections. *Arch Oral Biol* 1980; 25:288–92.

213. Brook I. beta-Lactamase-producing bacteria recovered after clinical failures with various penicillin therapy. *Arch Otolaryngol* 1984; 110:228–31.

214. Ross J. Pelvic inflammatory disease. *BMJ* 2001; 322:658–9.

215. Smith TD, Huskins WC, Kim KS, Kaplan EL. Efficacy of beta-lactamase-resistant penicillin and influence of penicillin tolerance in eradicating streptococci from the pharynx after failure of penicillin therapy for group A streptococcal pharyngitis. *J Pediatr* 1987; 110:777–82.

216. Kaplan EL, Johnson DR. Unexplained reduced microbiological efficacy of intramuscular benzathine penicillin G and of oral penicillin V in eradication of group A streptococci from children with acute pharyngitis. *Pediatrics* 2001; 108:1180–6.

217. Campos J, Roman F, Perez-Vazquez M, Oteo J, Aracil B, Cercenado E. Spanish Study Group for *Haemophilus influenzae* Type E. Infections due to *Haemophilus influenzae* serotype E: microbiological, clinical, and epidemiological features. *Clin Infect Dis* 2003; 37:841–5.

218. Jacobs MR. Worldwide trends in antimicrobial resistance among common respiratory tract pathogens in children. *Pediatr Infect Dis J* 2003; 22(8 Suppl):S109–19.

219. Kovatch AL, Wald ER, Michaels RH. beta-Lactamase-producing *Branhamella catarrhalis* causing otitis media in children. *J Pediatr* 1983; 102:260–3.

220. Reilly S, Timmis P, Beeden AG, Willis AT. Possible role of the anaerobe in tonsillitis. *J Clin Pathol* 1981; 34:542–7.

221. Chagollan JR, Macias JR, Gil JS. Flora indigena de las amigalas. *Invest Med Int* 1984; 11:36–43.

222. Tuner K, Nord CE. beta-Lactamase-producing microorganisms in recurrent tonsillitis. *Scand J Infect Dis Suppl* 1983; 39:83–5.

223. Tuner K, Nord CE. Emergence of beta-lactamase producing microorganisms in the tonsils during penicillin treatment. *Eur J Clin Microbiol* 1986; 5:399–404.

224. Brook I, Gober AE. Emergence of beta-lactamase-producing aerobic and anaerobic bacteria in the oropharynx of children following penicillin chemotherapy. *Clin Pediatr* 1984; 23:338–41.

225. Brook I. Emergence and persistence of beta-lactamase-producing bacteria in the oropharynx following penicillin treatment. *Arch Otolaryngol Head Neck Surg* 1988; 114:667–70.

226. Brook I, Gober AE. Prophylaxis with amoxicillin or sulfisoxazole for otitis media: effect on the recovery of penicillin-resistant bacteria from children. *Clin Infect Dis* 1996; 22:143–5.

227. Brook I. Role of beta-lactamase-producing bacteria in penicillin failure to eradicate group A streptococci. *Pediatr Infect Dis J* 1985; 4:491–5.

228. Roos K, Grahn E, Holn SE. Evaluation of beta-lactamase activity and microbial interference in treatment failures of acute streptococcal tonsillitis. *Scand J Infect Dis* 1986; 18:313–8.

229. Breese BB, Disney FA, Talpey WB. beta-Hemolytic streptococcal illness: comparison of lincomycin, ampicillin and potassium penicillin-G in treatment. *Am J Dis Child* 1966; 112:21–7.

230. Breese BB, Disney FA, Talpey, WB, et al. beta-Hemolytic streptococcal infection: comparison of penicillin and lincomycin in the treatment of recurrent infections or the carrier state. *Am J Dis Child* 1969; 117:147–52.

231. Randolph MF, DeHaan RM. A comparison of lincomycin and penicillin in the treatment of group A streptococcal infections: speculation on the "L" forms as a mechanism of recurrence. *Del Med J* 1969; 41:51–62.

232. Howie VM, Plousard JH. Treatment of group A streptococcal pharyngitis in children: comparison of lincomycin and penicillin G given orally and benzathine penicillin G given intramuscularly. *Am J Dis Child* 1971; 121:477.

233. Randolph MF, Redys JJ, Hibbard EW. Streptococcal pharyngitis III. Streptococcal recurrence rates following therapy with penicillin or with clindamycin (7-chlorlincomycin). *Del Med J* 1970; 42:87–92.

234. Stillerman M, Isenberg HD, Facklan RR. Streptococcal pharyngitis therapy: comparison of clindamycin palmitate and potassium phenoxymethyl penicillin. *Antimicrob Agents Chemother* 1973; 4:516–20.

235. Massell BF. Prophylaxis of streptococcal infection and rheumatic fever: a comparison of orally administered clindamycin and penicillin. *JAMA* 1979; 241:1589–94.

236. Brook I, Leyva F. The treatment of the carrier state of group A beta-hemolytic streptococci with clindamycin. *Chemotherapy* 1981; 27:360–7.

237. Brook I, Hirokawa R. Treatment of patients with recurrent tonsillitis due to group A beta-hemolytic streptococci: a prospective randomized study comparing penicillin, erythromycin and clindamycin. *Clin Pediatr* 1985; 24:331–6.

238. Orrling A, Stjernquist-Desatnik A, Schalen C. Clindamycin in recurrent group A streptococcal pharyngotonsillitis – an alternative to tonsillectomy? *Acta Otolaryngol* 1997; 117:618–22.

239. Chaudhary S, Bilinsky SA, Hennessy JL, Soler SM, Wallace SF, Schacht CM, Bisno AL. Penicillin V and rifampin for the treatment of group A streptococcal pharyngitis: a randomized trial of 10 days penicillin vs 10 days penicillin with rifampin during the final 4 days of therapy. *J Pediatr* 1985; 106:481–6.

240. Tanz RR, Shulman ST, Barthel MJ, Willert C, Yogev R. Penicillin plus rifampin eradicate pharayngeal carrier of group A streptococci. *J Pediatr* 1985; 106:876–80.

241. Tanz RR, Poncher JR, Corydon KE, Kabat K, Yogev R, Shulman ST. Clindamycin treatment of chronic pharyngeal carriage of group A streptococci. *J Pediatr* 1991; 119:123–8.

242. Brook I. Treatment of patients with acute recurrent tonsillitis due to group A beta-haemolytic streptococci: a prospective randomized study comparing penicillin and amoxycillin/clavulanate potassium. *J Antimicrob Chemother* 1989; 24:227–33.

243. Brook I, Shah K, Jackson W. Microbiology of healthy and diseased adenoids. *Laryngoscope* 2000; 110:994–9.

244. Brook I, Shah K. Effect of amoxycillin with or without clavulanate on adenoid bacterial flora. *J Antimicrob Chemother* 2001; 48:269–73.

245. Brook I, Shah K. Effect of amoxycillin or clindamycin on the adenoids bacterial flora. *Otolaryngol Head Neck Surg* 2003; 129:5–10.

246. Brook I, Gober AE. Effect of amoxicillin and co-amoxiclav on the aerobic and anaerobic nasopharyngeal flora. *J Antimicrob Chemother* 2002; 49:689–92.

247. Levison ME, Mangura CT, Lorber B, Abrutyn E, Pesanti EL, Levy RS, MacGregor RR, Schwartz AR. Clindamycin compared with penicillin for the treatment of anaerobic lung abscess. *Ann Intern Med* 1983; 98:466–71.

248. Gudiol F, Manresa F, Pallares R, Dorca J, Rufi G, Boada J, Ariza X, Casanova A, Viladrich PF. Clindamycin vs penicillin for anaerobic lung infections. High rate of penicillin failures associated with penicillin-resistant *Bacteroides melaninogenicus*. *Arch Intern Med* 1990; 150:2525–9.

249. Brook I. Treatment of aspiration or tracheostomy-associated pneumonia in neurologically impaired children: effect of antimicrobials effective against anaerobic bacteria. *Int J Pediatr Otorhinolaryngol* 1996; 35:171–7.

250. Sutter VL, Finegold SM. Susceptibility of anaerobic bacteria to 23 antimicrobial agents. *Antimicrob Agents Chemother* 1976; 10:736–52.

251. Hoellman DB, Kelly LM, Credito K, Anthony L, Ednie LM, Jacobs MR, Appelbaum PC. In vitro antianaerobic activity of ertapenem (MK-0826) compared to seven other compounds. *Antimicrob Agents Chemother* 2002; 46:220–4.

252. Goldstein EJ, Citron DM, Merriam CV, Warren YA, Tyrrell KL, Fernandez HT. Comparative in vitro susceptibilities of 396 unusual anaerobic strains to tigecycline and eight other antimicrobial agents. *Antimicrob Agents Chemother* 2006; 50:3507–13.

253. Goldstein EJ. Possible role for the new fluoroquinolones (levofloxacin, grepafloxacin, trovafloxacin, clinafloxacin, sparfloxacin, and DU-6859a) in the treatment of anaerobic infections: review of current information on efficacy and safety. *Clin Infect Dis* 1996; 23:S25–30.

Chapter 62
Mycobacteria: Tuberculosis

Francis A. Drobniewski and Yanina Balabanova

1 Overview

There were 9 million new tuberculosis (TB) cases (and approximately 2 million TB deaths) in 2004, of which 3.9 million (62/100,000) were highly infectious, i.e. the bacteria of the *Mycobacterium tuberculosis* complex, which cause TB, and could be seen in preparations of expectorated sputum under the microscope ("pulmonary sputum smear-positive" cases). Patients with infectious tuberculosis (pulmonary and laryngeal) are the main sources of transmission of the disease and therefore they are the key targets in the international effort to combat tuberculosis in the world. Their timely diagnosis and prompt treatment has two purposes: cure which is of individual benefit to the patient and by rendering infectious cases non-infectious, reduction in the spread of further infection. Non-pulmonary cases are usually not infectious to others. Of the new cases of TB detected in 2005, at least 741,000 cases were in adults co-infected with the human immuno-deficiency virus (HIV) (1).

The targets proposed by the World Health Organisation several years ago to detect, by 2005, 70% of new sputum smear-positive cases and to successfully treat 85% of these cases, have not been achieved. The global case detection rate was 53% (globally) in 2004 (although very variable across different countries), and reached approximately 60% in 2005, falling short of the 70% target. Treatment success was 82% (approaching the 85% target) in the 2003 cohort of 1.7 million patients (1).

The Stop TB Partnership (the umbrella coalition of the main international agencies and non-governmental organisations) endorsed additional targets of halving the 1990 prevalence and deaths rates by 2015. Implementation of the new Global Plan for TB is expected to reverse the rise in incidence globally by 2015, as specified in the Millennium Development Goals (MDG), and to halve the 1990 prevalence and death rates globally and in most regions by 2015, although this is not expected to occur in Africa (mainly due to the frequency of co-infection with HIV) and in the former Soviet Union countries (due to the level of drug resistance and particularly multiple drug resistant TB) (2–6).

Drug resistance is often divided into two different types. Acquired drug resistance (or drug resistance among previously treated cases) develops in a patient who has received or is currently receiving treatment due to interruptions in therapy or an inadequate therapeutic regimen. Primary drug resistance is a resistance in newly diagnosed TB cases, who have previously not received anti-TB treatment, i.e. they have been infected with a resistant strain of bacteria. Multidrug resistance (MDR), i.e. resistance to at least isoniazid and rifampin – the two most powerful anti-TB drugs – is the most problematic form of resistance. The global rate of drug resistant tuberculosis is not known with certainty but modelling studies have suggested, for example, that there are almost half a million cases of multi-drug resistant tuberculosis (MDRTB) occurring each year. High MDRTB rates are often used as a marker of contemporary weaknesses in the TB programme as they reflect problems with TB treatment and active transmission of resistant cases.

2 Epidemiology

The real extent of drug resistance, and particularly MDRTB, is unknown. In part this uncertainty has been due to methodological problems including the absence of longitudinal studies to detect trends, the failure to differentiate primary and acquired drug resistance in studies, the selection bias of many surveys and the absence of high quality laboratory culture facilities (4, 7). Nevertheless, there are now clear recommendations for standardising drug resistance surveillance (8).

F.A. Drobniewski (✉)
Professor, Institute of Cell and Molecular Sciences, Barts and the London School of Medicine, Queen Mary College, London, UK
f.drobniewski@qmul.ac.uk

D.L. Mayers (ed.), *Antimicrobial Drug Resistance*,
DOI 10.1007/978-1-60327-595-8_62, © Humana Press, a part of Springer Science+Business Media, LLC 2009

For the last 12 years, the WHO and International Union Against Tuberculosis and Lung Disease (IUATLD), underpinned by a global international network of Supranational Reference Laboratories have been systematically mapping the extent of drug resistance, including MDRTB, and reporting their findings in three key reports which have demonstrated the existence of drug resistance and MDRTB in every corner of the globe (4, 9, 10). There remain sizeable gaps in our understanding of the distribution of cases globally, as detailed systematic determinations of temporal trends remain limited, and our comprehension of the magnitude of the global burden of disease due to MDRTB is therefore uncertain. Currently over two-thirds of the countries and half of the 22 WHO-defined "high TB burden countries" have not reported adequate drug resistance data. These gaps not withstanding, estimates of the global burden have been made; in 2004, an estimated 424,203 (95% CI, 376,019–620,061) MDRTB cases occurred, or 4.3% (95% CI, 3.8–6.1%) of all new and previously treated TB cases. National and regional studies also indicate that drug resistance has been increasing in recent years (1, 4, 11). However, the distribution of drug resistant TB varies greatly across the world. Most North American Western and Central European countries do not have a significant problem with drug resistance in newly diagnosed cases, reporting approximately 5–10% isoniazid resistance and 1–2% MDRTB (1, 4, 12–14).

Cities within North America and Europe such as New York and London have suffered disproportionately in the incidence and prevalence of drug resistance and particularly MDRTB cases. New York in a long campaign turned the tide against MDRTB in a successful but costly rejuvenation of the TB control system including improvements in diagnosis, case management, clinical and public health infrastructure including improved staffing and outreach provision and modifications in public health law to improve patient adherence (15, 16). The need for continued effort and vigilance is reinforced by a recent study of trends drawn from a comparison of four surveys in New York in 1991, 1994, 1997, and 2003. These demonstrated that the percentage of prevalent cases with resistance to any antituberculosis drug decreased from 33.5% in 1991 to 23.8% in 1994 and to 21.5% in 1997 ($P < 0.001$, by test for trend); cases of MDRTB also decreased significantly, from 19% in 1991 to 6.8% in 1997 ($P < 0.001$, by test for trend). Among incident cases in the four surveys, the decrease in resistance to any antituberculosis drugs was not statistically significant; however, the decrease in MDRTB (from 9% in 1991 to 2.8% in 2003) was statistically significant ($P = 0.002$, by test for trend). However, in 2003, there was an increase of 23% in incident cases of MDRTB in previously treated patients with pulmonary tuberculosis not born in the United States (17).

The situation is very different in China, India, and the Russian Federation – these three countries account for almost two-thirds (62%), or 261,362 (95% CI 180,779–414,749), of MDRTB cases (18).

The highest rates of MDRTB in the world have been reported from Eastern Europe, particularly from the Baltic region (19–22) and countries of the former Soviet Union including Russia (23). Unfortunately only a limited number of internationally validated drug resistance surveys (DRS) have been conducted in very few parts of Russia and these demonstrated extremely high rates of MDRTB of approximately 10–20% in new patients and of approximately 40% in re-treatment cases (2, 5, 6, 24–33).

Interestingly, in some parts of Russia, for example in Oriel, MDRTB was seen in only 3% of new cases but 92% of patients had had no previous TB treatment and none were HIV positive, differing from other regions of Russia (34).

These figures support the need for the expansion and provision of better diagnostic systems to detect MDRTB and have appropriate treatment services even in middle to low resource settings reflecting the change in WHO policy in recent years (see also "Economic value of treating MDRTB").

Attempts have been made to determine whether the results of detailed (but more costly) special DRS surveys are in agreement with routinely collected systematic data obtained from National Tuberculosis Programmes (NTP). In this first analysis MDRTB prevalence rates among new TB patients were calculated from both routine and survey data from more than 100 countries. The comparison supported the view that the Global DRS Project provided more reliable epidemiological data than that obtained from routine surveillance (and indeed the MDRTB figure quoted earlier relies heavily on these surveys). When comparing countries the MDRTB prevalence rates were more variable in the routinely collected data, and the absolute prevalence rates calculated from the two sources did not agree closely. They were also poorly correlated in general, though there was a clear association between surveys and routine surveillance for European countries. If the routinely collected data are to be used for assessing MDRTB burden and trends, they must be unbiased, and drug susceptibility testing (DST) must follow recommended laboratory procedures. In European countries, DST is offered to a large proportion of TB patients, which probably reduces selection bias and explains the relatively strong association between measures of MDRTB prevalence for countries in the European Region from the DRS project and surveillance (4). A summary of the global prevalence of any drug resistance and MDRTB in new cases from 1994 until 2002 drawn from the special surveys is given in Figs. 1 and 2 respectively.

There is little systematic data on second-line drug resistance regionally or nationally (most data has been based on studies from a single or a small number of institutions) with

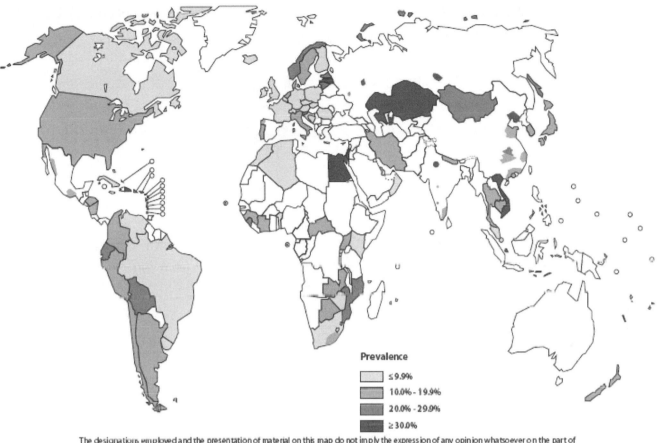

Prevalence

☐	≤9.9%
☐	10.0% - 19.9%
☐	20.0% - 29.9%
■	≥30.0%

The designations employed and the presentation of material on this map do not imply the expression of any opinion whatsoever on the part of
the World Health Organization concerning the legal status of any country, territory, city or area of its authorities, or concerning the delimitation
of its frontiers or boundaries. Dashed lines represent approximate border lines for which there may not be full agreement

Fig. 1 Global prevalence in any drug resistance in new TB cases 1994–2002 (4)

most studies based in Eastern Europe where the majority of MDRTB cases have been found.

Indicative data is presented for systematic first and second-line drug resistance in MDRTB cases in a study of 17 European countries from 2003 to 2005 (where the ex-Soviet Baltic states of Latvia and Estonia accounted for 66% of reported MDRTB cases) and in Samara, a comparable region of the Russian Federation (Table 1) (23).

3 Laboratory Diagnosis of Resistance

3.1 First-Line Drugs Susceptibility Testing

3.1.1 Conventional Methods

Drug susceptibility testing is recommended for all new cases for first-line drugs with specimens taken before initiating treatment and if the patient continues to be culture positive after 2–3 months and if there is a history of prior TB treatment (a major risk factor for drug resistance). Individual circumstances may dictate additional testing. Accuracy is more important than speed and DST results should come from a small number of well-equipped, experienced laboratories that participate and perform well in an international DST quality control scheme. The WHO Supranational Laboratory Quality Control Network offers the greatest global coverage assessing participating laboratories in their ability to identify isoniazid, rifampin, ethambutol and streptomycin resistance correctly (4).

The absolute concentration, resistance ratio, and proportion methods can all give accurate results provided they are carefully quality controlled and standardised (4, 36, 37). As a minimum, laboratories supplying DST data to clinicians, government, and the WHO, and for surveys or surveillance, should correctly identify resistance to isoniazid and rifampin in over 90% of quality control samples in two out of the last three quality control rounds of the WHO scheme.

The early identification of mycobacterial growth as *M. tuberculosis* complex (principally *M. tuberculosis* and *M. bovis*) and the identification of rifampin resistance should be the first priority as rifampin resistance invalidates standard 6-month short-course chemotherapy and is a useful marker

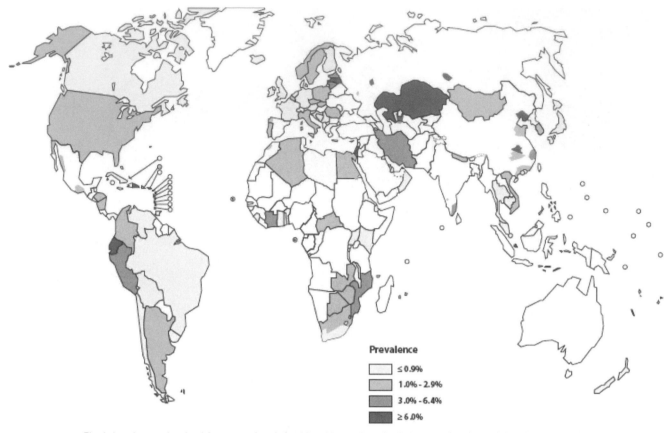

Prevalence

≤ 0.9%

1.0% - 2.9%

3.0% - 6.4%

≥ 6.0%

The designations employed and the presentation of material on this map do not imply the expression of any opinion whatsoever on the part of the World Health Organization concerning the legal status of any country, territory, city or area of its authorities, or concerning the delimitation of its frontiers or boundaries. Dashed lines represent approximate border lines for which there may not be full agreement

Fig. 2 Prevalence of MDR among new cases 1994–2002 (4)

Table 1 Comparative data on drug resistance from Latvia and Estonia (*n* = 800), Samara Region, Russia and other countries in Europe (*n* = 246)

Drug	Estonia and Latvia		Other countries[a]		Samara, Russia	
	No resistant	% resistant	No resistant	% resistant	No resistant	% resistant
Streptomycin	773	97	142	58	281	49
Ethambutol	641	80	105	43	161	28
Pyrazinamide	441	55	82	33	23	9
Kanamycin	425	53	26	11	–	–
Capreomycin	249	31	11	4	–	–
Ethionamide	234	29	42	17	–	–
PAS	172	22	55	22	–	–
Ofloxacin	124	16	10	4	–	–
Ciprofloxacin	–	–	11	4	3/69	5
Amikacin	34	4	25	10	5/69	8
Cycloserine	11	1	20	8	1/69	2
Rifabutin	–	–	106	43	60/68	88
Clofazamine	–	–	–	–	2/68	3
Doxycycline	–	–	–	–	5/68	8

Adapted from (19, 23, 26, 35)

[a]Countries involved: Belgium, Croatia, Cyprus, Czech Republic, Denmark, Finland, Ireland, Israel, Netherlands, Norway, Romania, Slovenia, Spain, Sweden, Switzerland

in most countries for MDRTB. Laboratories should aim to identify isolates as *M. tuberculosis* complex and perform rifampin resistance in 90% of isolates within 1–2 working days (38). This is challenging but technologically feasible (39–55).

Laboratories should also aim to identify *M. tuberculosis* and rifampin resistance in over 90% of cases from smear-positive sputum directly where resources are available for this (this will require an investment in appropriate infrastructure, staffing, and the implementation of new methodological techniques).

3.1.2 Other Methods

Rapid Non-radiometric Automated Culture Methods

Rapid non-radiometric automated culture methods used for the rapid culture of mycobacteria are being used for drug resistance analysis. Studies when these systems were applied to determine isoniazid and rifampin resistance as well as other first-line drugs have been published (56–65).

Their use is likely to increase but mainly in large reference centres due to their higher cost when compared with solid culture-based methods. All of them are based on a modification of the proportion method. Most studies have utilised indirect assays (i.e. you culture the bacteria first) with greatest success for isoniazid and rifampin resistance measurement. Smear positive material, however, can be analysed in direct assays on solid media and may be almost as fast as indirect assays and are cheaper. Capital costs are high and laboratory containment facilities must be of the highest order.

The TB programme must be in a position to send specimens rapidly to the laboratory and act quickly on results; for example a recent study in Peru demonstrated that the total turnaround time from sputum production to diagnosis of MDRTB and subsequent modification of treatment to a more appropriate one, took 5 months, almost twice as long as the bacteriological procedures per se (66).

Molecular Assays

Novel molecular assays offer several potential advantages including faster turnaround times and minimal, or possibly no prior culture for MDRTB analysis.

Many of the key gene mutations conferring resistance have been identified permitting the development of in-house and commercial molecular assays (39–52, 67–84).

Considerable problems remain in the clinical development of assays. The majority are more costly than current methods, the exact proportion of resistant to susceptible organisms producing resistance clinically is unclear and the presence of common gene mutations is not always associated with drug resistance (i.e. silent mutations). Nevertheless for drugs such as rifampin and isoniazid the mutations associated with resistance are now well known and studies have demonstrated their value in the context of centralised national and regional services (22, 43, 53, 79, 85, 86). They may be of particular value in countries with high rates of MDRTB. Nevertheless, although the choice of drugs for therapy can be partially determined using molecular systems but usually require culture-based methods. Another remaining problem is the timely transport of specimens to a laboratory and use of these assays in TB programmes. Further operational research is needed to develop methods which can identify TB, rifampin, and isoniazid resistance in all sputum specimens directly with the same sensitivity as the best bacterial culture methods but within 1–2 working days.

3.2 Second-Line Susceptibility Testing

For patients with proven MDRTB or who are genuinely unable to tolerate first-line therapy, second-line drug therapy should be instituted which will require accurate and ideally rapid determination of susceptibility to second-line drugs (87). It appears that the earlier WHO guidelines on second-line DST analysis (87) may have been premature as a subsequent multicentre analysis concluded that the results obtained from different second-line DST methods were not comparable (88, 89) but until recently there had been no comparative analyses between the MGIT 960 system and solid media-based methods such as the resistance ratio or proportion methods; these have now been completed (65, 90). There was good correlation for most, but for not all, second-line drugs between the solid medium-based resistance ratio and proportion methods and the MGIT 960 system.

Other methods have explored the use of early bactericidal assays (EBA) as surrogates for the above methods with some success (91–93).

Measuring resistance to second-line drugs is complex and for many drugs lacks standardisation. Most countries have few MDRTB cases and maintaining the technical expertise needed for accurate assessment is difficult. Commercial companies may be reluctant to facilitate standard measurement by providing the pure drug reagents needed, tempting some incorrectly, to use pharmaceutical preparations in drug testing. This is particularly important where different drugs within a class are being used for treatment, e.g. it would be negligent to utilise rifabutin to treat rifampin without accurate drug susceptibility testing for example, and similarly for amikacin in strains resistant to streptomycin. International quality assurance programmes for second-line drug testing are being developed (38, 94).

In many countries, however, laboratory diagnosis of drug resistance and MDRTB is of poor quality and this coupled with intermittent drug supply or the supply of poor quality first- and second-line drugs compromises the success of individual therapy as well as the TB programme as a whole. Standardised second-line treatment programmes based on surveys or individualised treatment will produce higher treatment cure rates than no therapy or first-line drug therapy alone although treatment must be prolonged. Although individualised treatment strategies will produce the highest cure rates, this will be dependent on the continuous availability of appropriate drugs and the adherence of the patient to the regimen. It is the responsibility of the laboratory in consultation with the clinician to determine the spectrum of drugs to be tested within the laboratory rather than the other way round.

4 Clinical Significance and Treatment

4.1 Drug Sensitive Tuberculosis

Treatment of drug sensitive TB is highly effective and is based on a standardised strategy proved over several decades in international clinical trials; a treatment regimen includes a combination of drugs administered for a defined period, usually 6–9 months depending on the form of TB and history of anti-TB treatment in the past. Modern treatment regimens include four so-called first-line drugs (isoniazid, rifampin, pyrazinamide, ethambutol or streptomycin (95–98)) and treatment is divided into a 2-month intensive phase using three or four of the first-line drugs followed by a continuation phase usually with isoniazid and rifampin for a total of 6 months (sometimes 9 months, or 12 months for TB meningitis). Treatment is prolonged where the patient is co-infected with HIV. Table 2 describes the main doses and side effects of first- and second-line drugs.

The early institution of appropriate therapy is essential both to prevent the emergence of MDRTB and to treat it when it occurs (99). The WHO has adopted the DOTS strategy pioneered in studies performed in many parts of the world to treat drug-sensitive TB and prevent MDRTB developing and a DOTS Plus strategy to treat cases that do occur. Ensuring adherence and completion of therapy is the key aim and DOTS is one effective strategy for achieving it.

Table 2 Main doses and side effects of first-line anti-TB drugs (99–104)

Drug	Route[a]	Daily dose[b]	Intermittent (thrice weekly)	Major side effects[c]	Monitoring[d]
Isoniazid	PO IM IV	300 mg 5 mg/kg	15 mg/kg max: 900 mg	Peripheral neuropathy, hepatitis, CNS effects, increased phenytoin levels, interaction with drugs, hepatic enzyme elevation	LFT, levels of interacting drugs[e]
Rifampin	PO IV	600 mg 10 mg/kg	10 mg/kg max: 600 mg	GI upset, hepatitis, rash, bleeding problems, contact lens and body fluids coloured orange/pink, decreased serum levels of warfarin, methadone, contraceptive hormone, dapsone, ketoconazole, theophylline, flu-like symptoms	LFT, levels of interacting drugs
Pyrazinamide	PO	1.5–2.5 g 15/30 mg/kg	2–3 g 50–70 mg/kg	GI upset, increase in hepatic enzyme levels, rash, joint pain, hyperuricaemia (gout rarely), may complicate control of diabetes mellitus	LFT, uric acid (if needed)
Ethambutol	PO	2.5 g (max) 15–25 mg/kg	30 mg/kg	Red/green colour blindness, optic neuritis, decreased visual activity, rash	Colour vision, visual acuity
Streptomycin	IM IV	15 mg/kg	25 mg/kg	Nephrotoxicity, ototoxicity, hypokalaemia, hypomagnesaemia	Blood chemistry, renal function, audiometry

CNS central nervous system; GI gastrointestinal; IM intramuscular; IV intravenous; PO per os

[a] Possible routes of administration, in practice, all drugs are given orally if possible

[b] The daily dose is quoted for average adult weight; all doses are adjusted in accordance with a patient's weight

[c] Isoniazid causes increased elimination of pyridoxine, leading to peripheral neuropathy particularly in alcoholics, the malnourished, and in pregnancy. Daily doses of 10 mg of pyridoxine per day are sufficient to compensate for this loss

[d] Liver function tests (LFT); specific monitoring points are given. At appropriate intervals a patient should be monitored clinically, radiologically and bacteriologically. A full blood count (including platelets) should be performed if there is any bleeding tendency

[e] Streptomycin in patients over 60 years of age is more likely to lead to side effects; daily doses should be limited to 10 mg/kg with a maximum does of 750 mg. Closer observation of hearing loss and renal function may be necessary in this age group. Ethambutol is usually used in preference to streptomycin except in very young children where visual acuity cannot be determined readily

4.2 Drug Resistant Tuberculosis

The standardised treatment approach is greatly jeopardised by the presence of drug resistance. Single drug resistance to most first-line drugs can be successfully addressed by extension of therapy with first-line drugs or the addition of less commonly used first-line drugs (e.g. streptomycin) or the addition of some second-line drugs.

In the UK, management of drug resistance mainly follows the advice given by the British Thoracic Society, which was recently supported by the UK National Institute for Clinical Excellence (NICE) in the published guidelines of 2006.

The preferred treatment for isolated streptomycin, rifampin, ethambutol, and pyrazinamide resistance is as follows:

For isolated streptomycin resistance the standard treatment regimen still applies; for isolated ethambutol resistance (which is not common) the intensive phase remains 2 months of isoniazid, rifampin and ethambutol followed by 4 months of isoniazid and rifampin; for isolated pyrazinamide resistance (which is also uncommon when TB is caused by *M. tuberculosis* and is usually associated with *M. bovis* disease) the intensive phase remains 2 months of isoniazid, rifampin, and ethambutol followed by 7 months of isoniazid and rifampin.

The BTS guidelines (1998) recommend two approaches to isoniazid resistance depending on whether the resistance is identified before treatment is started or afterwards; if before, a regimen of rifampin, pyrazinamide, ethambutol, and streptomycin for 2 months followed by rifampin and ethambutol, for a further 7 months gives good results by directly observed therapy. If resistance is found after treatment has been started, isoniazid may be stopped and ethambutol, pyrazinamide, and rifampin should be given for 2 months followed by ethambutol and rifampin for a further 10 months.

Many practitioners have given a maximum of 9 months, therapy in all cases.

However, even a standard 6-month therapy may be sufficient as a study by Jindani et al. demonstrated (96). In this study the superiority of the 6-month rifampin-based regimen over the WHO-recommended 8-month regimen based on ethambutol and isoniazid for drug sensitive TB, was demonstrated in a subset of individuals with isoniazid mono-resistant TB which was only diagnosed after the completion of therapy where the cure rates were high nevertheless.

However resistance to rifampin and MDRTB create the greatest therapeutic difficulties: they are difficult to treat, remain infectious for long and pose a public health hazard. Resistance to rifampin alone is much less common than MDRTB, and patients are treated with 2 months of isoniazid, ethambutol and pyrazinamide followed by 16 months of isoniazid and ethambutol (104).

Ultimately patients are more likely to die although death from MDRTB disease is not inevitable (just as death from TB before the advent of chemotherapy was not a certainty). Survival is poor with standard first-line drug regimens (31, 105, 106). A key observation made over 20 years ago remains valid: "the largely forgotten fact that one-third of patients with advanced disease with positive sputum smears recover on their own, should be kept in mind when claims are made that an inappropriate drug regimen cured a patient with bacterial resistance" (107).

The standard approach in most industrialised countries today is to treat MDRTB with second-line, or reserve drugs. Main second-line drugs used in resistant cases are listed in Table 3.

With second-line drugs treatment success in MDRTB varies from 48% to more than 80% of patients cured (or probably cured) (110–112). For example Mitnick et al. (111) described the successful treatment of 75 MDRTB cases in Peru, despite resistance to a median of six drugs with identification of predictors of a poor outcome in a resource-poor setting. Of 66 patients who completed therapy 55 (83%) had a favourable outcome, while 5 (8%) died emphasising the importance of early initiation of an appropriate drug regimen and identifying predictors of poor outcome.

Death rates varied from 0 to 37% in studies of HIV-seronegative individuals, and up to 89% in HIV-seropositive populations (110, 112, 113). Even in high-income countries like the UK with access to individualised therapy, survival was relatively low (114) with a median survival time overall of 3.78 (3.66, 6.89) years. Median survival in patients treated with three drugs to which the bacterium was susceptible on in vitro testing ($n = 62$) was 5.66 years whereas in those not so treated ($n = 13$) survival was only 1.64 years. Several studies suggest that patients who are in poor clinical condition prior to treatment and who are infected with organisms resistant to a large number of drugs are associated with poor outcomes (110, 111, 114). In industrialised countries treatment in specialised centres with relatively unlimited resources will improve survival (115, 116). In a Turkish study, a cure rate of 77% was obtained in 158 consecutive patients infected with organisms that were resistant to a mean of 4.4 drugs, who were treated with at least three drugs to which the bacteria were susceptible and who had surgical resection performed in 36 patients. Thirty-eight percent of the patients with unsuccessful outcomes were infected with organisms that were resistant to more than five drugs; overall a successful outcome was independently associated with a younger age ($P = 0.013$) and the absence of previous treatment with ofloxacin ($P = 0.005$) (117). In all cases treatment should be directly observered for prolonged periods of at least 18–24 months.

Recent treatment strategies for MDRTB that include a quinolone may offer advantages over regimes that do not (93, 111, 118). In a 6-year retrospective study of the treatment of 229 MDRTB patients in Taiwan in which 51.2% were cured,

Table 3 Second-line drugs, dosages and side effects (55, 99, 104, 108, 109)

Drug	Route[a]	Daily dose	Major side effects	Notes
Ciprofloxacin	PO	500–1,000 mg (max: 1,500 mg) (2 doses)	GI upset, abdominal cramps, photosensitivity, headache, insomnia, interacts with warfarin and theophyllin, hypersensitivity	Antacids, iron supplements and sucralfate reduce gastrointestinal absorption
Ofloxacin	PO	600–800 mg	As above	As above
Moxifloxacin	PO	400 mg	GI upset, raised LFT, jaundice, CNS problems, photosensitivity	Monitor LFT and renal function
Amikacin[b]	IM IV	15 mg/kg (max: 1 g)	Ototoxicity, renal toxicity, occasional vestibular toxicity, hypokalaemiam hypomagnesaemia	Monitor auditory and renal function, blood chemistry
Prothionamide	PO	0.5–1 g (in 1–2 doses)	GI upset, raised hepatic enzymes, metallic taste, hypothyroidism (more likely if PAS given concurrently). Antacids/emetics may help but watch other drugs interactions	Monitor LFT. Start with 250 mg daily dose and increase as tolerated. Increase to bd quickly
Cycloserin	PO	0.5–1 g (in 1–2 doses)	Rash, psychosis, depression, seizures, headache, increases phenytoin levels. Avoid if underlying CNS problems or depression	Start with 250 mg daily and increase. Pyridoxine (50 mg) and each 250 mg may reduce CNS effects
Capreomycin	IM	15 mg/kg (max: 1 g)	Ototoxicity, renal toxicity, vestibular toxicity, hypokaliaemia, hypomagnesaemia, eosinophillia	Monitor auditory and renal function, blood chemistry
PAS	PO	8–12 g (divided doses)	GI upset, increased hepatic enzymes, decreased digoxin levels, increased phenytoin levels, haemolytic anaemia in glucose-6-phosphate dehydrogenase deficiency	Commence 1–2 g tds and increase as tolerated by patient. Tables create a high sodium load – monitor volume and electrolytes in cardiac and renal patients
Clarithromycin	PO IV	500 mg PO (2 doses)	GI upset, jaundice, hepatitis, interaction with many drugs including anticoagulants, antiepileptics, digoxin, rifabutin, usually by reducing liver enzyme activity	Only modest activity against TB, used principally to prevent emergence of drug resistance
Clofazamine	PO	100–300 mg	GI upset, causes skin darkening, abdominal pain, rare organ damage if drug crystal deposits occur	Avoid sunlight, dosing at mealtime may be helpful

CNS central nervous system; *GI* gastrointestinal; *IM* intramuscular; *IV* intravenous; *PAS para*-aminosalicyllic acid; *PO* per os

[a] Drugs are given daily, orally whenever possible. Treatment of drug resistant TB should be performed by those experienced in its management

[b] After bacteriological conversion, aminiglycosides can be given three times weekly

patients receiving ofloxacin were more likely to be cured, and were less likely to die, fail, and relapse (119). In a study of prognostic factors for the lung resection patients with MDRTB, those with a bacterial strain that was also ofloxacin resistant were more likely to experience treatment failure (120).

There has been limited data to support the use of one fluoroquinolone over another in terms of clinical outcome and unfortunately cross-resistance to one agent produces resistance to all in vitro and in murine models (121, 122). Follow-up duration and survival analyses in many of these studies are relatively short and many of the studies were conducted using a variety of methodologies and have outcomes (of cure, success, failure) that are defined in different ways making comparisons between studies difficult. No fluoroquinolone should be used without verifying that the bacterium is susceptible to it including the newer ones. One recent study in 106 patients with MDRTB demonstrated that levofloxacin was more effective overall than ofloxacin when incorporated into a multidrug regimen but the time to achieve sputum smear or culture conversion and rates of adverse effects were the same (118). These fluoroquinolones

might have an important place in the management of even drug sensitive TB. Moxifloxacin, for example, a relatively new fluoroquinolone has shown promise in vitro against drug sensitive TB using early bactericidal assays in vitro and in murine models (123–126); in the latter study the replacement of isoniazid with moxifloxacin offered the potential of reducing the duration of treatment by reducing the time needed to sterilise bacilli in murine models (126). Any combination that reduces duration of therapy is likely to improve adherence and likely to reduce the development of clinical resistance. Moxifloxacin has also shown promise against MDRTB in vitro, in murine models (127).

4.2.1 Low- and Middle-Income Countries

Whilst individualised treatment based on in vitro drug resistance analysis is probably the gold standard for MDRTB treatment the need for reliable but costly laboratory facilities for drug sensitivity means that the application of standardised second-line drug treatment has been advocated for middle-

and low-income countries. The latter strategy requires a detailed knowledge of likely drug resistance rates, particularly, MDRTB which demands recent surveys or surveillance of resistance. In all cases treatment should be directly observed for prolonged periods, for periods of at least 18–24 months.

In the last 2 years successful treatment of patients using second-line drugs in low-income countries, notably Peru, has been reported (111, 128).

Overall studies using standardised treatment approaches for MDRTB, have shown outcomes that are worse than for most studies using individualised treatment regimens in expert hands, but better results for individuals than either no treatment or treatment with first-line drugs alone (128).

4.2.2 Exrapulmonary Drug Resistant TB

Most attention has been given to understanding and treating pulmonary drug resistant and MDRTB cases as these are of greatest public health importance. For most extrapulmonary TB, treatment regimens are similar to those applied for pulmonary TB including drug resistant TB with the exception of TB meningitis. The high mortality associated with extra pulmonary MDRTB, particularly meningitis has been clearly demonstrated in the UK (114), the USA (129) and was strongly predictive of death in a series of 180 Vietnamese adults with MDRTB-associated meningitis (130).

4.3 Global Policy for MDRTB Therapy

At the global level, WHO has a global policy for managing MDRTB, and facilitates access to second-line anti-TB drugs through the Green Light Committee (GLC). The so called DOTS-Plus Projects approved by the GLC have access to quality-assured, second-line drugs at reduced prices and benefit from independent external monitoring. Between 2000 and 2005, the GLC approved treatment for almost 13,000 MDRTB patients. The Global Plan, the new Stop TB Strategy, the 2005 World Health Assembly resolution on sustainable financing for TB control and the new International Standards of TB Care document have all encouraged countries to expand their monitoring, diagnosis, and treatment programmes for drug-resistant TB reversing previous inadequate international support for addressing the MDRTB problem.

4.4 HIV and MDRTB

MDRTB carries a high mortality in the immunocompromised as described earlier. Three studies in the USA demonstrated an improved outcome with early treatment using at least three drugs to which the organism was susceptible on in vitro testing supporting the concept that early institution of appropriate treatment may extend survival even if individuals are HIV positive (112, 113, 131). Drug treatment strategies are similar to those employed for HIV-negative patients with anti-retroviral therapy considered at an early stage.

4.5 Therapeutic Alternatives: Immunotherapy

Immunotherapy or immunomodulation has remained largely experimental with a few notable exceptions. Strategies have usually combined a standard chemotherapeutic approach plus (1) adjunct recombinant immunomodulating cytokines (especially Th-1 and Th-1-like cytokines such as IFN-gamma, IL-2, IL-12, IL-18, and GM-CSF), (2) inhibitors of immunosuppressive cytokines (TGF-beta) and some proinflammatory tissue-damaging cytokines (TNF-alpha), and (3) immunomodulatory agents such as dexamethasone, imidazoquinoline, diethyldithiocarbamate, poloxamer, dibenzopyran, galactosylceramide, levamisole, and heat-killed *Mycobacterium vaccae* (132).

Adjunct steroid therapy has been part of general TB therapy, e.g. for TB meningitis, whereas other immunomodulators have been applied usually to refractory mycobacterial disease or MDRTB. Hopes for *Mycobacterium vaccae* (MV) have waned. Although some smaller trials of MV as an immunotherapeutic adjunct to chemotherapy in Argentina, Nigeria and Romania, for example, showed some benefit, larger trials notably in Southern Africa have largely been disappointing with little effect on treatment outcome and mortality. Some studies, erythrocytes sedimentation rates (ERS) however, have suggested an improvement in bacteriological conversion, reduction in erythrocytes sedimentation rates, recovery of body weight and radiographic appearance including lung cavity closure which might be of value as adjunct therapy for MDRTB patients (133). However, in an analysis of chest radiographs from 1,018 patients with pulmonary TB (478 HIV-positive; 540 HIV-negative) who had received a single injection of *M. vaccae* within the first 2 weeks of treatment as part of randomised placebo-controlled trials, there was no difference in radiographic improvement, deterioration or cavitary disease at the end of treatment or in follow-up when the *M. vaccae* and placebo groups were compared (134).

Nevertheless, the authors of a study, in Argentina, using multiple doses of heat-killed *Mycobacterium vaccae* (SRL 172) claimed that immunotherapy could reduce the overall period of chemotherapy. In this study a short-course, directly observed chemotherapy in 22 newly diagnosed HIV-negative pulmonary tuberculosis patients was supplemented with a triple dose of *M. vaccae*. Patients receiving immunotherapy showed a faster and more complete clinical improvement, accelerated disappearance of bacilli from sputum, better radiological clearance and a more rapid fall in ESR, than did those receiving placebo with a significantly faster return towards normal values in all the immunological parameters. The results were consistent with a regulatory activity on cellular immunity, reducing the influence of Th2 and enhancing Th1 to the benefit of the patients (135). If these results can be reproduced then there may be some benefit in shortening treatment, indirectly improving adherence and reducing the emergence of clinical resistance.

Cytokine therapy is possible but not always predictable in its outcome. Gamma-interferon (IFN) has been the most studied cytokine and its main properties are given in Table 4.

In a murine model, IFN potentiated macrophage killing of TB bacilli and in gamma-IFN gene-knockout mice normally sublethal bacterial doses killed the mice (136, 137). A murine study in which gamma-IFN was added prior to infection of mouse peritoneal macrophages with IgA-opsonised bacilli resulted in a synergistic increase of nitric oxide and TNF-alpha production and a 2- to 3-fold decrease in bacterial counts suggesting that combcined treatment with gamma-IFN and IgA could be developed as an adjunct to chemotherapy (141).

There is limited data on the clinical use of immunomodulating cytokines in drug sensitive or resistant TB unresponsive to standard chemotherapy. Following an early report (138) there has been one small open-label study in which five MDRTB smear- and culture-positive patients were given chemotherapy with aerosolised gamma-IFN and some symptomatic improvement was seen (142).

A later 6-month study used aerosolised gamma-IFN as adjuvant therapy in six patients with refractory MDRTB. The patients received 2 million international units of aerosolised gamma-IFN three times a week for 6 months while they continued on identical antituberculous chemotherapy. After gamma-IFN inhalation therapy, sputum smears remained persistently positive in all patients throughout the study period. Sputum cultures were transiently negative at the fourth month in two patients, but became positive again at the end of 6 months of gamma-IFN therapy. Five patients had radiological improvement including three patients who showed a decrease in the size of the cavitatory lesions. Resectional surgery could be performed in one patient in whom substantial clinical and radiological improvement was noted (143). An alternative approach has been to improve outcomes by trying to antagonise the effects of "over" production of beneficial cytokines such as tumour necrosis (TNF) factor alpha using thalidomide, with a modest clinical improvement (144). In a small study, thalidomide therapy was used on four children with paradoxical enlargement of intracranial tuberculomas and tuberculous brain abscesses despite being inadequate in antituberculosis treatment. Three of the four patients had relentless neurological deterioration, and all showed disease progression on neuroimaging. These lesions are frequently not responsive to standard treatment including steroids. Marked clinical and neuroradiologic improvement occurred after thalidomide was added (145).

Although immunomodulatory therapy is attractive, there remain serious problems including the high cost, occasionally with severe side effects, and, in many cases, only modest efficacy in potentiating host defence mechanisms, primarily because of the induction of macrophage-deactivating cytokines during the course of long-term administration of adjunctive agents.

4.6 Surgical Management

Although chemotherapy using multiple agents to which the bacterium is susceptible remains the gold standard for treatment, adjunct surgical resection is of value. In 205 patients treated at one expert centre in the USA (which had previously published a major series on treatment outcome of MDRTB patients recruited from 1973 to 1983 (110) and who were infected with bacterial strains resistant to a median of six drugs, an initial favourable response defined as at least three consecutive negative sputum cultures over a period of at least 3 months, was seen in 85% patients compared with 65% in the prior cohort (115). More importantly the latest cohort of patients had a greater long-term success rate of 75% versus 56%, and a lower tuberculosis death rate of 12% versus 22% previously. At the authors' centre, in the 1973–1983 period, only 7 of 171 (4%) patients had undergone resectional surgery; all 7 became consistently culture negative. In contrast, 130 of 205 (63%) of the patients in the 1984–1998 period underwent resectional surgery. Fluroquionolones were used in 80% of the patients, with greater use in the last 10 years

Table 4 Immunotherapy with cytokines

Cytokine[a]	Action
gamma-IFN	• Major immune activator
	• Induces expression MHC Class II molecules
Glycoproteins 40–70 kDa produced by CD4, CD8, NK cells	• Primes macrophage to release IL1
	• Activates macrophages for phagocytosis
	• Stimulates production reactive nitrogen species mainly via NO synthase
	• Augments antigen presentation
	• Increases responsiveness to IL2

Adapted from (136–140)

[a] Expensive but complex and potentially dangerous

compared with the first 5 years of the study period. Surgical resection, and to a smaller extent fluoroquinolone therapy, were associated with improved microbiological and clinical outcomes. The authors also advocated the use of therapeutic drug monitoring suggesting that it lessened or delayed toxicity and so favourably influenced treatment outcome.

Although resection appears to be of value in the management of MDRTB beyond the obvious restriction that there need to be sufficient post-resection residual lung capacity remaining for adequate respiratory function, the suitability of patients for surgery has only recently been evaluated. In a Korean study of 79 patients, low body mass index, resistance to ofloxacin, and cavitary lesions beyond the range of resection were identified as potentially poor prognostic factors for surgical lung resection in MDRTB patients (120).

4.7 Economic Value of Treating MDRTB

In wealthy industrialised countries, treatment for MDRT is individualised and based on the results of antimicrobial drug susceptibility testing. Recent studies have quantified the huge costs of diagnosing and treating MDRTB in the industrialised world. In the UK the minimum cost for treating MDRTB was estimated to be approximately 100,000 € (146) and higher values were reported in the USA in the 1990s.

As described above a standardised approach has been employed in areas with a high rate of MDRTB, a high absolute number of cases, and a lower income. There has been a long debate as to the economic appropriateness of treating MDRTB in low- and middle-income countries that led to a policy change at the WHO and the creation of the DOTS Plus pilot treatment projects.

The cost-effectiveness of these approaches has been analysed in different ways. Recently, a cost-effective analyses of a treatment programme in Peru of patients with MDRTB offered hope by suggesting that cases might be effectively treated under a standardised treatment approach for as little as approximately $2,400 per case, producing a cost per disability adjusted life year gained (DALY) of $211 – a figure not too dissimilar from what the World Bank has suggested should be viewed as an attractive investment in low-income countries (128). This important study also showed that such an approach might be feasible in some low-income settings and has been replicated in the middle-income country of Turkey (117).

A dynamic state-transition model of TB was developed using Peru as a model (i.e. a setting with a smear-positive TB incidence of 120 per 100,000 and 4.5% MDRTB among prevalent cases). Secondary analyses also considered other settings. Locally standardised second-line drugs for previously treated cases with confirmed MDRTB or comprehensive drug susceptibility testing and individualised treatment for previously treated cases, were cost-effective with a wide range of alternative assumptions about treatment costs, effectiveness, MDRTB prevalence, and transmission (147).

4.8 Infection Control Measures

The spread of MDRTB, particularly within institutions such as prisons, homeless shelters, and hospitals has been well documented internationally throughout the 1990s and is a particular concern when many highly vulnerable individuals, for example those infected with HIV, congregate (148, 149).

Prevention of nosocomial spread can be achieved through a combination of interventions and adequate training of all staff. Appropriate institutional infrastructure that ensures adequate and appropriate ventilation (e.g. negative pressure isolation rooms, air-filtration ultraviolet germicidal irradiation, biosafety cabinets in microbiology laboratories) and personal protection devices such as masks, and respirators are essential. Excellent guidelines to prevent nosocomial transmission between patients and staff, and in those working in laboratories ad pathology services are widely available in print and electronic form (150–153).

Studies using new gamma-INF assays here demonstrated high rates of TB infection in India (154) and in Russia (155). At the same time countries of the former Soviet Union also have very high rates of MDRTB in active disease, one can assume that when staff and patients are institutionally infected, infection is with a MDRTB strain. As care is primarily institutionalised in hospitals and prisons, interventions to prevent transmission must be a priority.

References

1. WHO. Global tuberculosis control: surveillance, planning, financing. Report, Geneva: World Health Organization, 2006 (WHO/HTM/TB/2006.362).
2. Drobniewski F, Balabanova Y, Ruddy M, et al. Rifampin- and multidrug-resistant tuberculosis in Russian civilians and prison inmates: dominance of the Beijing strain family. Emerg Infect Dis 2002;8(11):1320–6.
3. Dye C, Scheele S, Dolin P, Pathania V, Raviglione MC. Consensus statement. Global burden of tuberculosis: estimated incidence, prevalence, and mortality by country. WHO Global Surveillance and Monitoring Project. JAMA 1999;282(7):677–86.
4. WHO/IUALTD. Global project on anti-tuberculosis drug surveillance in the world. Report no. 3, Geneva: World Health Organization, 2004 (WHO/HTM/TB/2004.343).
5. Drobniewski F, Balabanova Y, Nikolayevsky V, et al. Drug-resistant tuberculosis, clinical virulence, and the dominance of the Beijing strain family in Russia. JAMA 2005;293(22):2726–31.
6. Toungoussova OS, Sandven P, Mariandyshev AO, Nizovtseva NI, Bjune G, Caugant DA. Spread of drug-resistant *Mycobacterium*

tuberculosis strains of the Beijing genotype in the Archangel Oblast, Russia. J Clin Microbiol 2002;40(6):1930–7.

7. Vareldzis BP, Grosset J, de Kantor I, et al. Drug-resistant tuberculosis: laboratory issues. World Health Organization recommendations. Tuber Lung Dis 1994;75:1–7.

8. Schwoebel V, Lambregts-van Weezenbeek CS, Moro ML, et al. Standardization of antituberculosis drug resistance surveillance in Europe. Recommendations of a World Health Organization (WHO) and International Union Against Tuberculosis and Lung Disease (IUATLD) Working Group. Eur Respir J 2000;16(2): 364–71.

9. WHO. Global project on anti-tuberculosis drug surveillance in the world. Report no. 2: prevalence and trends. Geneva: World Health Organisation, 2000.

10. WHO/IUALTD. Anti-tuberculosis drug resistance in the world. The WHO/IUALTD Global Project on anti-tuberculosis drug resistance surveillance. Geneva: World Health Organization, 1997.

11. Dye C, Espinal MA, Watt CJ, Mbiaga C, Williams BG. Worldwide incidence of multidrug-resistant tuberculosis. J Infect Dis 2002;185(8):1197–202.

12. Irish C, Herbert J, Bennett D, et al. Database study of antibiotic resistant tuberculosis in the United Kingdom, 1994–6. BMJ 1999;318(7182):497–8.

13. Rose AM, Watson JM, Graham C, et al. Tuberculosis at the end of the 20th century in England and Wales: results of a national survey in 1998. Thorax 2001;56(3):173–9.

14. Djuretic T, Herbert J, Drobniewski F, et al. Antibiotic resistant tuberculosis in the United Kingdom: 1993–1999. Thorax 2002;57(6):477–82.

15. Frieden TR, Fujiwara PI, Washko RM, Hamburg MA. Tuberculosis in New York City – turning the tide. N Engl J Med 1995;333:229–33.

16. Frieden TR, Sterling T, Pablos-Mendez A, Kilburn JO, Cauthen GM, Dooley SW. The emergence of drug-resistant tuberculosis in New York City. N Engl J Med 1993;328:521–6.

17. Munsiff SS, Li J, Cook SV, et al. Trends in drug-resistant *Mycobacterium tuberculosis* in New York City, 1991–2003. Clin Infect Dis 2006;42(12):1702–10.

18. Zignol M, Hosseini MS, Wright A, et al. Global incidence of multidrug-resistant tuberculosis. J Infect Dis 2006;194(4):479–85.

19. Kruuner A, Hoffner SE, Sillastu H, et al. Spread of drug-resistant pulmonary tuberculosis in Estonia. J Clin Microbiol 2001;39(9):3339–45.

20. Dewan P, Sosnovskaja A, Thomsen V, et al. High prevalence of drug-resistant tuberculosis, Republic of Lithuania, 2002. Int J Tuberc Lung Dis 2005;9(2):170–4.

21. Leimane V, Riekstina V, Holtz TH, et al. Clinical outcome of individualised treatment of multidrug-resistant tuberculosis in Latvia: a retrospective cohort study. Lancet 2005;365(9456): 318–26.

22. Skenders G, Fry AM, Prokopovica I, et al. Multidrug-resistant tuberculosis detection, Latvia. Emerg Infect Dis 2005;11(9): 1461–3.

23. EuroTB. Molecular surveillance of multi-drug resistant tuberculosis in Europe. Report no. 3. Euro Surveill, 2004, http://www.eurotb.org/mdr_tb_surveillance/pdf/MDR-TB_2005report.pdf.

24. Dewan PK, Arguin PM, Kiryanova H, et al. Risk factors for death during tuberculosis treatment in Orel, Russia. Int J Tuberc Lung Dis 2004;8(5):598–602.

25. Mokrousov I, Otten T, Vyazovaya A, et al. PCR-based methodology for detecting multidrug-resistant strains of *Mycobacterium tuberculosis* Beijing family circulating in Russia. Eur J Clin Microbiol Infect Dis 2003;22(6):342–8.

26. Ruddy M, Balabanova Y, Graham C, et al. Rates of drug resistance and risk factor analysis in civilian and prison patients with tuberculosis in Samara Region, Russia. Thorax 2005;60(2):130–5.

27. Kubica T, Agzamova R, Wright A, et al. The Beijing genotype is a major cause of drug-resistant tuberculosis in Kazakhstan. Int J Tuberc Lung Dis 2005;9(6):646–53.

28. Balabanova Y, Drobniewski F, Fedorin I, et al. The Directly Observed Therapy Short-Course (DOTS) strategy in Samara Oblast, Russian Federation. Respir Res 2006;7:44.

29. Coninx R, Pfyffer GE, Mathieu C, et al. Drug resistant tuberculosis in prisons in Azerbaijan: case study. BMJ 1998;316(7142):1423–5.

30. Toungoussova OS, Nizovtseva NI, Mariandyshev AO, Caugant DA, Sandven P, Bjune G. Impact of drug-resistant *Mycobacterium tuberculosis* on treatment outcome of culture-positive cases of tuberculosis in the Archangel oblast, Russia, in 1999. Eur J Clin Microbiol Infect Dis 2004;23(3):174–9.

31. Espinal MA, Kim SJ, Suarez PG, et al. Standard short-course chemotherapy for drug-resistant tuberculosis: treatment outcomes in 6 countries. JAMA 2000;283(19):2537–45.

32. CDC. Primary multidrug-resistant tuberculosis – Ivanovo Oblast, Russia, 1999. MMWR Morb Mortal Wkly Rep 1999;48(30):661–4.

33. Drobniewski FA, Balabanova YM. The diagnosis and management of multiple-drug-resistant-tuberculosis at the beginning of the new millenium. Int J Infect Dis 2002;6(Suppl 1):S21–31.

34. Kherosheva T, Thorpe LE, Kiryanova E, et al. Encouraging outcomes in the first year of a TB control demonstration program: Orel Oblast, Russia. Int J Tuberc Lung Dis 2003;7(11):1045–51.

35. Balabanova Y, Ruddy M, Hubb J, et al. Multidrug-resistant tuberculosis in Russia: clinical characteristics, analysis of second-line drug resistance and development of standardized therapy. Eur J Clin Microbiol Infect Dis 2005;24(2):136–9.

36. Canetti G, Fox W, Khomenko AG, et al. Advances in techniques of testing mycobacterial drug sensitivity, and the use of sensitivity tests in tuberculosis control programmes. Bull World Health Organ 1969;41:21–43.

37. Canetti G, Froman S, Grosset J, et al. Mycobacteria: laboratory methods for testing drug sensitivity and resistance. Bull World Health Organ 1963;29:565–78.

38. Drobniewski FA, Hoffner S, Rusch-Gerdes S, Skenders G, Thomsen V. Recommended standards for modern tuberculosis laboratory services in Europe. Eur Respir J 2006;28(5):903–9.

39. Gingeras TR, Ghandour G, Wang E, et al. Simultaneous genotyping and species identification using hybridization pattern recognition analysis of generic *Mycobacterium* DNA arrays. Genome Res 1998;8(5):435–48.

40. Saiki RK, Walsh PS, Levenson CH, Erlich HA. Genetic analysis of amplified DNA with immobilized sequence-specific oligonucleotide probes. Proc Natl Acad Sci U S A 1989;86(16):6230–4.

41. Watterson SA, Wilson SM, Yates MD, Drobniewski FA. Comparison of three molecular assays for rapid detection of rifampin resistance in *Mycobacterium tuberculosis*. J Clin Microbiol 1998;36(7):1969–73.

42. De Beenhouwer H, Lhiang Z, Jannes G, et al. Rapid detection of rifampicin resistance in sputum and biopsy specimens from tuberculosis patients by PCR and line probe assay. Tuber Lung Dis 1995;76(5):425–30.

43. Drobniewski FA, Watterson SA, Wilson SM, Harris GS. A clinical, microbiological and economic analysis of a national service for the rapid molecular diagnosis of tuberculosis and rifampicin resistance in *Mycobacterium tuberculosis*. J Med Microbiol 2000;49(3):271–8.

44. Mokrousov I, Filliol I, Legrand E, et al. Molecular characterization of multiple-drug-resistant *Mycobacterium tuberculosis* isolates from northwestern Russia and analysis of rifampin resistance using RNA/RNA mismatch analysis as compared to the line probe assay and sequencing of the rpoB gene. Res Microbiol 2002;153(4):213–9.

45. Nikolayevsky V, Brown T, Balabanova Y, Ruddy M, Fedorin I, Drobniewski F. Detection of mutations associated with isoniazid and rifampin resistance in *Mycobacterium tuberculosis* isolates

from Samara Region, Russian Federation. J Clin Microbiol 2004;42(10):4498–502.

46. Troesch A, Nguyen H, Miyada CG, et al. *Mycobacterium* species identification and rifampin resistance testing with high-density DNA probe arrays. J Clin Microbiol 1999;37(1):49–55.

47. Eltringham IJ, Drobniewski FA, Mangan JA, Butcher PD, Wilson SM. Evaluation of reverse transcription-PCR and a bacteriophage-based assay for rapid phenotypic detection of rifampin resistance in clinical isolates of *Mycobacterium tuberculosis*. J Clin Microbiol 1999;37(11):3524–7.

48. El-Hajj HH, Marras SA, Tyagi S, Kramer FR, Alland D. Detection of rifampin resistance in *Mycobacterium tuberculosis* in a single tube with molecular beacons. J Clin Microbiol 2001;39(11): 4131–7.

49. Piatek AS, Tyagi S, Pol AC, et al. Molecular beacon sequence analysis for detecting drug resistance in *Mycobacterium tuberculosis*. Nat Biotechnol 1998;16(4):359–63.

50. Riska PF, Jacobs WR, Jr. The use of luciferase-reporter phage for antibiotic-susceptibility testing of mycobacteria. Methods Mol Biol 1998;101:431–55.

51. Wilson SM, al-Suwaidi Z, McNerney R, Porter J, Drobniewski F. Evaluation of a new rapid bacteriophage-based method for the drug susceptibility testing of *Mycobacterium tuberculosis*. Nat Med 1997;3(4):465–8.

52. Albert H, Trollip AP, Mole RJ, Hatch SJ, Blumberg L. Rapid indication of multidrug-resistant tuberculosis from liquid cultures using FASTPlaqueTB-RIF, a manual phage-based test. Int J Tuberc Lung Dis 2002;6:523–8.

53. Sam IC, Drobniewski F, More P, Kemp M, Brown T. *Mycobacterium tuberculosis* and rifampin resistance, United Kingdom. Emerg Infect Dis 2006;12(5):752 9.

54. Caws M, Drobniewski FA. Molecular techniques in the diagnosis of *Mycobacterium tuberculosis* and the detection of drug resistance. Ann N Y Acad Sci 2001;953:138–45.

55. Drobniewski FA. Diagnosing multidrug resistant tuberculosis in Britain. Clinical suspicion should drive rapid diagnosis. BMJ 1998;317(7168):1263–4.

56. Walters SB, Hanna BA. Testing of susceptibility of *Mycobacterium tuberculosis* to isoniazid and rifampin by mycobacterium growth indicator tube method. J Clin Microbiol 1996;34(6):1565–7.

57. Pfyffer GE, Welscher HM, Kissling P, et al. Comparison of the Mycobacteria Growth Indicator Tube (MGIT) with radiometric and solid culture for recovery of acid-fast bacilli. J Clin Microbiol 1997;35(2):364–8.

58. Reisner BS, Gatson AM, Woods GL. Evaluation of mycobacteria growth indicator tubes for susceptibility testing of *Mycobacterium tuberculosis* to isoniazid and rifampicin. Diagn Microbiol Infect Dis 1995;22:325–9.

59. Scarparo C, Ricordi P, Ruggiero G, Piccoli P. Evaluation of the fully automated BACTEC MGIT 960 system for testing susceptibility of *Mycobacterium tuberculosis* to pyrazinamide, streptomycin, isoniazid, rifampin, and ethambutol and comparison with the radiometric BACTEC 460TB method. J Clin Microbiol 2004;42(3):1109–14.

60. Tortoli E, Benedetti M, Fontanelli A, Simonetti MT. Evaluation of automated BACTEC MGIT 960 system for testing susceptibility of *Mycobacterium tuberculosis* to four major antituberculous drugs: comparison with the radiometric BACTEC 460TB method and the agar plate method of proportion. J Clin Microbiol 2002;40(2):607–10.

61. Huang TS, Tu HZ, Lee SS, Huang WK, Liu YC. Antimicrobial susceptibility testing of *Mycobacterium tuberculosis* to first-line drugs: comparisons of the MGIT 960 and BACTEC 460 systems. Ann Clin Lab Sci 2002;32(2):142–7.

62. Adjers-Koskela K, Katila ML. Susceptibility testing with the manual mycobacteria growth indicator tube (MGIT) and the MGIT

960 system provides rapid and reliable verification of multidrug-resistant tuberculosis. J Clin Microbiol 2003;41(3):1235–9.

63. Ardito F, Posteraro B, Sanguinetti M, Zanetti S, Fadda G. Evaluation of BACTEC Mycobacteria Growth Indicator Tube (MGIT 960) automated system for drug susceptibility testing of *Mycobacterium tuberculosis*. J Clin Microbiol 2001;39(12):4440–4.

64. Bemer P, Palicova F, Rusch-Gerdes S, Drugeon HB, Pfyffer GE. Multicenter evaluation of fully automated BACTEC Mycobacteria Growth Indicator Tube 960 system for susceptibility testing of *Mycobacterium tuberculosis*. J Clin Microbiol 2002;40(1): 150 4.

65. Kruuner A, Yates M, Drobniewski F. Critical concentration setting and evaluation of MGIT 960 antimicrobial susceptibility testing to first- and second line antimicrobial drugs with clinical drug resistant strains of *Mycobacteirum tuberculosis*. J Clin Microbiol 2006;44(3):811–8.

66. Yagui M, Perales MT, Asencios L, et al. Timely diagnosis of MDR-TB under program conditions: is rapid drug susceptibility testing sufficient? Int J Tuberc Lung Dis 2006;10(8):838–43.

67. Banerjee A, Dubnau E, Quemard A, et al. inhA, a gene encoding a target for isoniazid and ethionamide in *Mycobacterium tuberculosis*. Science 1994;263:227–30.

68. Finken M, Kirschner P, Meier A, Wrede A, Bottger EC. Molecular basis of streptomycin resistance in *Mycobacterium tuberculosis*: alterations of the ribosomal protein S12 gene and point mutations within a functional 16S ribosomal RNA pseudoknot. Mol Microbiol 1993;9(6):1239–46.

69. Heym B, Honore N, Truffot-Perrot C, et al. Implications of multidrug resistance for the future of short course chemotherapy of tuberculosis: a molecular study. Lancet 1994;344:293–8.

70. Heym B, Alzari PM, Honore N, Cole ST. Missense mutations in the catalase-peroxidase gene, katG, are associated with isoniazid resistance in *Mycobacterium tuberculosis*. Mol Microbiol 1995;15(2):235–45.

71. Kapur V, Li LL, Hamrick MR, et al. Rapid *Mycobacterium* species assignment and unambiguous identification of mutations associated with antimicrobial resistance in *Mycobacterium tuberculosis* by automated DNA sequencing. Arch Pathol Lab Med 1995;119(2):131–8.

72. Zhang Y, Heym B, Allen B, Yung D, Cole S. The catalase-peroxidase gene and isoniazid resistance of *Mycobacterium tuberculosis*. Nature 1992;358:591–3.

73. Takiff HE, Salazar L, Guerrero C, et al. Cloning and nucleotide sequence of *Mycobacterium tuberculosis* gyrA and gyrB genes and detection of quinolone resistance mutations. Antimicrob Agents Chemother 1994;38(4):773–80.

74. Telenti A, Imboden P, Marchesi F, et al. Detection of rifampicin-resistance mutations in *Mycobacterium tuberculosis*. Lancet 1993;341(8846):647–50.

75. Williams DL, Waguespack C, Eisenach K, et al. Characterization of rifampin-resistance in pathogenic mycobacteria. Antimicrob Agents Chemother 1994;38(10):2380–6.

76. Baker L, Brown T, Maiden MC, Drobniewski F. Silent nucleotide polymorphisms and a phylogeny for *Mycobacterium tuberculosis*. Emerg Infect Dis 2004;10(9):1568–77.

77. Herrera L, Jimenez S, Valverde A, Garcia-Aranda MA, Saez-Nieto JA. Molecular analysis of rifampicin-resistant *Mycobacterium tuberculosis* isolated in Spain (1996–2001). Description of new mutations in the rpoB gene and review of the literature. Int J Antimicrob Agents 2003;21(5):403–8.

78. Heep M, Brandstatter B, Rieger U, et al. Frequency of rpoB mutations inside and outside the cluster I region in rifampin resistant clinical *Mycobacterium tuberculosis* isolates. J Clin Microbiol 2001;39(1):107–10.

79. Somoskovi A, Song Q, Mester J, et al. Use of molecular methods to identify the *Mycobacterium tuberculosis* complex (MTBC) and

other mycobacterial species and to detect rifampin resistance in MTBC isolates following growth detection with the BACTEC MGIT 960 system. J Clin Microbiol 2003;41(7):2822–6.

80. Parsons LM, Salfinger M, Clobridge A, et al. Phenotypic and molecular characterization of Mycobacterium tuberculosis isolates resistant to both isoniazid and ethambutol. Antimicrob Agents Chemother 2005;49(6):2218–25.

81. Baker LV, Brown TJ, Maxwell O, et al. Molecular analysis of isoniazid-resistant Mycobacterium tuberculosis isolates from England and Wales reveals the phylogenetic significance of the ahpC-46A polymorphism. Antimicrob Agents Chemother 2005;49(4):1455–64.

82. Brown TJ, Herrera-Leon L, Anthony RM, Drobniewski FA. The use of macroarrays for the identification of MDR Mycobacterium tuberculosis. J Microbiol Methods 2006;65(2):294–300.

83. Hellyer TJ, DesJardin LE, Hehman GL, Cave MD, Eisenach KD. Quantitative analysis of mRNA as a marker for viability of Mycobacterium tuberculosis. J Clin Microbiol 1999;37(2):290–5.

84. Jacobs WR, Jr., Barletta RG, Udani R, et al. Rapid assessment of drug susceptibilities of Mycobacterium tuberculosis by means of luciferase reporter phages. Science 1993;260(5109):819–22.

85. Hale YM, Pfyffer GE, Salfinger M. Laboratory diagnosis of myco-bacterial infections: new tools and lessons learned. Clin Infect Dis 2001;33(6):834–46.

86. Parsons LM, Somoskovi A, Urbanczik R, Salfinger M. Laboratory diagnostic aspects of drug resistant tuberculosis. Front Biosci 2004;9:2086–105.

87. WHO. Guidelines for drug susceptibility testing of second-line drugs for Mycobacterium tuberculosis. Geneva: World Health Organization, 2001.

88. Kim SJ, Espinal MA, Abe C, et al. Is second-line anti-tubercu-losis drug susceptibility testing reliable? Int J Tuberc Lung Dis 2004;8(9):1157–8.

89. Pfyffer GE, Bonato DA, Ebrahimzadeh A, et al. Multicenter laboratory validation of susceptibility testing of Mycobacterium tuberculosis against classical second-line and newer antimicro-bial drugs by using the radiometric BACTEC 460 technique and the proportion method with solid media. J Clin Microbiol 1999;37(10):3179–86.

90. Rusch-Gerdes S, Pfyffer GE, Casal M, Chadwick M, Siddiqi S. Multicenter laboratory validation of the BACTEC MGIT 960 tech-nique for testing susceptibilities of Mycobacterium tuberculosis to classical second-line drugs and newer antimicrobials. J Clin Microbiol 2006;44(3):688–92.

91. Sirgel FA, Fourie PB, Donald PR, et al. The early bactericidal activities of rifampin and rifapentine in pulmonary tuberculosis. Am J Respir Crit Care Med 2005;172(1):128–35.

92. Gosling RD, Heifets L, Gillespie SH. A multicentre compari-son of a novel surrogate marker for determining the specific potency of anti-tuberculosis drugs. J Antimicrob Chemother 2003;52(3):473–6.

93. Hu Y, Coates AR, Mitchison DA. Sterilizing activities of fluoroqui-nolones against rifampin-tolerant populations of Mycobacterium tuberculosis. Antimicrob Agents Chemother 2003;47(2):653–7.

94. Johansen IS, Larsen AR, Sandven P, et al. Drug susceptibility testing of Mycobacterium tuberculosis to fluoroquinolones: first experience with a quality control panel in the Nordic-Baltic col-laboration. Int J Tuberc Lung Dis 2003;7(9):899–902.

95. Combs DL, O'Brien RJ, Geiter LJ. USPHS tuberculosis short-course chemotherapy study trial 21: effectiveness, toxicity, and acceptability. The report of final results. Ann Intern Med 1990;112:397–406.

96. Jindani A, Nunn AJ, Enarson DA. Two 8-month regimens of chemotherapy for treatment of newly diagnosed pulmonary tuberculosis: international multicentre randomised trial. Lancet 2004;364(9441):1244–51.

97. East African/British Medical Research Councils. Controlled clinical trial of short-course (6-month) regimens of chemotherapy for treat-ment of pulmonary tuberculosis. Lancet 1972;1(7760):1079–85.

98. British Thoracic and Tuberculosis Association. Controlled trial of short-course chemotherapy in pulmonary tuberculosis. Lancet 1976;2(7995):1102–4.

99. Drobniewski F. Drug resistant tuberculosis in adults and its treat-ment. J R Coll Physicians Lond 1998;32(4):314–8.

100. British Thoracic Society JTC. Control and Prevention of Tuberculosis in the United Kingdom: Code of Practice 2000. Thorax 2000;55(11):887–901.

101. Frieden TR, Sterling TR, Munsiff SS, Watt CJ, Dye C. Tuberculosis. Lancet 2003;362(9387):887–99.

102. WHO. Global Tuberculosis Programme: treatment of tubercu-losis – guidelines for national programmes, 2nd edn. Geneva: World Health Organization, 1997.

103. NICE. Clinical Guideline N33. Tuberculosis: clinical diagnosis and management of tuberculosis, and measures for its prevention and control. National Institute for Health and Clinical Excellence, London, 2006, http://www.nice.org.uk/page.aspx?o=CG033.

104. British Thoracic Society, Ormerod P, Campbell I, et al. Chemotherapy and management of tuberculosis in the United Kingdom: recommendations 1998. Thorax 1998;53:536–48.

105. Coninx R, Mathieu C, Debacker M, et al. First-line tuberculosis therapy and drug-resistant Mycobacterium tuberculosis in pris-ons. Lancet 1999;353:969–73.

106. Migliori GB, Espinal M, Danilova ID, Punga VV, Grzemska M, Raviglione MC. Frequency of recurrence among MDR-tB cases 'successfully' treated with standardised short-course chemo-therapy. Int J Tuberc Lung Dis 2002;6(10):858–64.

107. Grzybowski S. Tuberculosis and its prevention. St Louis, MO: Warren H Green, Inc, 1983.

108. British Thoracic Society. Control and prevention of tubercu-losis in the United Kingdom: Code of Practice 1994. Joint Tuberculosis Committee of the British Thoracic Society. Thorax 1994;49(12):1193–200.

109. WHO. Treatment of tuberculosis: guidelines for national pro-grammes. Geneva: World Health Organization, 1997.

110. Goble M, Iseman MD, Madsen LA. Treatment of 171 patients with pulmonary tuberculosis resistant to isoniazid and rifampicin. N Engl J Med 1993;328:527–32.

111. Mitnick C, Bayona J, Palacios E, et al. Community-based therapy for multidrug-resistant tuberculosis in Lima, Peru. N Engl J Med 2003;348(2):119–28.

112. Park SK, Kim CT, Song SD. Outcome of chemotherapy in 107 patients with pulmonary tuberculosis resistant to isoniazid and rifampin. Int J Tuberc Lung Dis 1998;2:877–84.

113. Park MM, Davis AL, Schluger NW, Cohen H, Rom WN. Outcome of MDR-TB patients, 1983–1993. Prolonged survival with appropriate therapy. Am J Respir Crit Care Med 1996;153: 317–24.

114. Drobniewski F, Eltringham I, Graham C, Magee JG, Smith EG, Watt B. A national study of clinical and laboratory factors affecting the survival of patients with multiple drug resistant tuberculosis in the UK. Thorax 2002;57(9):810–6.

115. Chan ED, Laurel V, Strand MJ, et al. Treatment and outcome analysis of 205 patients with multidrug-resistant tuberculosis. Am J Respir Crit Care Med 2004;169:1103–09.

116. Hutchison DC, Drobniewski FA, Milburn HJ. Management of mul-tiple drug-resistant tuberculosis. Respir Med 2003;97(1):65–70.

117. Tahaoglu K, Torun T, Sevim T, et al. The treatment of multidrug-resistant tuberculosis in Turkey. N Engl J Med 2001;345:170–4.

118. Yew WW, Chan CK, Leung CC, et al. Comparative roles of levofloxacin and ofloxacin in the treatment of multidrug-resistant tuberculosis: preliminary results of a retrospective study from Hong Kong. Chest 2003;124(4):1476–81.

119. Chiang CY, Enarson DA, Yu MC, et al. Outcome of pulmonary multidrug-resistant tuberculosis: a six year follow-up study. Eur Respir J 2006;28:980–5.

120. Kim HJ, Kang CH, Kim YT, et al. Prognostic factors for surgical resection in patients with multidrug-resistant tuberculosis. Eur Respir J 2006;28:576–80.

121. Kam KM, Yip CW, Cheung TL, Tang HS, Leung OC, Chan MY. Stepwise decrease in moxifloxacin susceptibility amongst clinical isolates of multidrug-resistant *Mycobacterium tuberculosis*: correlation with ofloxacin susceptibility. Microb Drug Resist 2006;12(1):7–11.

122. Ginsburg AS, Sun R, Calamita H, Scott CP, Bishai WR, Grosset JH. Emergence of fluoroquinolone resistance in *Mycobacterium tuberculosis* during continuously dosed moxifloxacin monotherapy in a mouse model. Antimicrob Agents Chemother 2005;49(9):3977–9.

123. Miyazaki E, Miyazaki M, Chen JM, Chaisson RE, Bishai WR. Moxifloxacin (BAY12–8039), a new 8-methoxyquinolone, is active in a mouse model of tuberculosis. Antimicrob Agents Chemother 1999;43(1):85–9.

124. Gosling RD, Uiso LO, Sam NE, et al. The bactericidal activity of moxifloxacin in patients with pulmonary tuberculosis. Am J Respir Crit Care Med 2003;168(11):1342–5.

125. Johnson JL, Hadad DJ, Boom WH, et al. Early and extended early bactericidal activity of levofloxacin, gatifloxacin and moxifloxacin in pulmonary tuberculosis. Int J Tuberc Lung Dis 2006;10(6):605–12.

126. Nuermberger EL, Yoshimatsu T, Tyagi S, et al. Moxifloxacin-containing regimens of reduced duration produce a stable cure in murine tuberculosis. Am J Respir Crit Care Med 2004;170(10):1131–4.

127. Fattorini L, Tan D, Iona E, et al. Activities of moxifloxacin alone and in combination with other antimicrobial agents against multidrug-resistant *Mycobacterium tuberculosis* infection in BALB/c mice. Antimicrob Agents Chemother 2003;47(1):360–2.

128. Suarez PG, Floyd K, Portacarrero J, et al. Feasibility and cost-effectiveness of standardised second-line drug treatment for chronic tuberculosis patients: a national cohort study in Peru. Lancet 2002;359:1980–9.

129. Daikos GL, Cleary T, Rodriguez A, Fischl MA. Multidrug-resistant tuberculous meningitis in patients with AIDS. Int J Tuberc Lung Dis 2003;7(4):394–8.

130. Thwaites GE, Lan NT, Dung NH, et al. Effect of antituberculosis drug resistance on response to treatment and outcome in adults with tuberculous meningitis. J Infect Dis 2005;192(1):79–88.

131. Turett GS, Telzak EE, Torian LV, et al. Improved outcomes for patients with multidrug-resistant tuberculosis. Clin Infect Dis 1995;21:1238–44.

132. Tomioka H. Adjunctive immunotherapy of mycobacterial infections. Curr Pharm Des 2004;10(26):3297–312.

133. Stanford J, Stanford C, Grange J. Immunotherapy with *Mycobacterium vaccae* in the treatment of tuberculosis. Front Biosci 2004;9:1701–19.

134. Johnson JL, Nunn AJ, Fourie PB, et al. Effect of *Mycobacterium vaccae* (SRL172) immunotherapy on radiographic healing in tuberculosis. Int J Tuberc Lung Dis 2004;8(11):1348–54.

135. Dlugovitzky D, Fiorenza G, Farroni M, Bogue C, Stanford C, Stanford J. Immunological consequences of three doses of heat-killed *Mycobacterium vaccae* in the immunotherapy of tuberculosis. Respir Med 2006;100(6):1079–87.

136. Flynn JL, Chan J, Triebold KJ, Dalton DK, Stewart TA, Bloom BR. An essential role for interferon gamma in resistance to *Mycobacterium tuberculosis* infection. J Exp Med 1993;178(6):2249–54.

137. Flynn JL, Goldstein MM, Triebold KJ, Sypek J, Wolf S, Bloom BR. IL-12 increases resistance of BALB/c mice to *Mycobacterium tuberculosis* infection. J Immunol 1995;155(5):2515–24.

138. Holland SM, Eisenstein EM, Kuhns DB, et al. Treatment of refractory disseminated nontuberculous mycobacterial infection with interferon gamma. A preliminary report. N Engl J Med 1994;330(19):1348–55.

139. Cooper AM, Roberts AD, Rhoades ER, Callahan JE, Getzy DM, Orme IM. The role of interleukin-12 in acquired immunity to *Mycobacterium tuberculosis* infection. Immunology 1995;84(3):423–32.

140. Newport MJ, Huxley CM, Huston S, et al. A mutation in the interferon-gamma-receptor gene and susceptibility to mycobacterial infection. N Engl J Med 1996;335(26):1941–9.

141. Reljic R, Clark SO, Williams A, et al. Intranasal IFNgamma extends passive IgA antibody protection of mice against *Mycobacterium tuberculosis* lung infection. Clin Exp Immunol 2006;143(3):467–73.

142. Condos R, Rom WN, Schluger NW. Treatment of multidrug-resistant pulmonary tuberculosis with interferon-gamma via aerosol. Lancet 1997;349(9064):1513–5.

143. Koh WJ, Kwon OJ, Suh GY, et al. Six-month therapy with aerosolized interferon-gamma for refractory multidrug-resistant pulmonary tuberculosis. J Korean Med Sci 2004;19(2):167–71.

144. Tramontana JM, Utaipat U, Molloy A, et al. Thalidomide treatment reduces tumor necrosis factor alpha production and enhances weight gain in patients with pulmonary tuberculosis. Mol Med 1995;1(4):384–97.

145. Schoeman JF, Fieggen G, Seller N, Mendelson M, Hartzenberg B. Intractable intracranial tuberculous infection responsive to thalidomide: report of four cases. J Child Neurol 2006;21(4):301–8.

146. White VL, Moore-Gillon J. Resource implications of patients with multidrug resistant tuberculosis. Thorax 2000;55:962–3.

147. Resch SC, Salomon JA, Murray M, Weinstein MC. Cost-effectiveness of treating multidrug-resistant tuberculosis. PLoS Med 2006;3(7):e241.

148. Breathnach AS, de Ruiter A, Holdsworth GM, et al. An outbreak of multi-drug-resistant tuberculosis in a London teaching hospital. J Hosp Infect 1998;39(2):111–7.

149. Coronado VG, Beck-Sague CM, Hutton MD, et al. Transmission of multidrug-resistant *Mycobacterium tuberculosis* among persons with human immunodeficiency virus infection in an urban hospital: epidemiologic and restriction fragment length polymorphism analysis. J Infect Dis 1993;168:1052–5.

150. CDC. Guidelines for preventing the transmission of *Mycobacterium tuberculosis* in health-care settings. MMWR Morb Mortal Wkly Rep 2005;54:1–147

151. Advisory Committee on Dangerous Pathogens UHaSE. The management, design and operation of microbiological containment laboratories. London: ACDP, 2001.

152. Health and Safety Executive. Health Services Advisory Committee. Safe working and the prevention of infection in clinical laboratories and similar facilities. London: Health and Safety Executive, 2003.

153. CDC. National Institutes of Health. Biosafety in microbiological and biomedical laboratories. Washington: US Government Printing Office, 1999, HHS Publication No (CDC) 99-8395 (also available at http://www.cdc.gov/od/ohs/biosfty/bmbl4/bmbltoc.htm).

154. Pai M, Gokhale K, Joshi R, et al. *Mycobacterium tuberculosis* infection in health care workers in rural India: comparison of a whole-blood interferon gamma assay with tuberculin skin testing. JAMA 2005;293(22):2746–55.

155. Balabanova Y, Nikolayevskyy V, Fedorin I, et al. Occupational exposure and rates of latent tuberculosis infection among medical staff in Samara, Russia, Abstract from 27th Annual Congress of European Society of Mycobacteriology, London, 2007, Abstract: O12 2006.

Chapter 63
Drug Resistance by Non-Tuberculous Mycobacteria

Kathleen Horan and Gerard A. Cangelosi

1 Introduction

Non-tuberculous *Mycobacterium* species (NTM) cause disease in diverse animals as well as in susceptible humans. Antiretroviral therapy has decreased AIDS-associated NTM in many settings; however, the reported incidence of *M. avium* complex (MAC) infection of non-AIDS patients has increased in recent years, especially among women (1–4). Most NTMs are slowly growing mycobacteria like their close cousin, *M. tuberculosis*, with which they share many similarities in genomic composition, cellular physiology, and mechanisms of pathogenesis. Chemotherapeutic treatments, and mechanisms of resistance to these treatments, also bear many similarities to tuberculosis. However, there are critical distinctions, especially in the case of the most common NTM pathogen of humans, MAC. This chapter focuses on clinical aspects of NTM therapy and the biology of antimicrobial resistance by NTMs.

2 Clinical Presentations

NTM cause five major categories of human disease: skin, lymphadenitis, medical device and nosocomial infections, pulmonary disease, and disseminated disease. The type of infection has significant bearing on treatment decisions.

2.1 Skin and Soft Tissue Infections

M. marinum, isolated from fresh and salt water, is the prototypic NTM skin infection. The bacteria gain access to the skin through minor wounds from trauma and the first lesion is an erythematous papule which progresses into a violaceous plaque. Occasionally, the infection spreads along the lymphatic drainage of the initial inoculation site, resulting in a clinical presentation similar to sporotrichosis.

Rare skin lesions with *M. kansasii, M. scrofulaceum,* and *M. avium* complex have been reported (5). *M. ulcerans* causes the Buruli ulcer, a slowly developing, ulcerating subcutaneous nodule that is common in many tropical areas. Rarely cultured, Buruli ulcer is clinically diagnosed and treated with surgical excision (5). Rapidly growing mycobacteria such as *M. chelonae, M. fortuitum, and M. abscessus* are associated with myriad skin, soft tissue, and bone infections. Like *M. marinum*, the rapidly growing mycobacteria exploit minor trauma to cause disease ranging from cellulitis to subcutaneous abscesses (5).

2.2 Lymphadenitis

NTM lymphadenitis occurs in children of ages 1–5 years old without HIV. It presents with nontender, enlarging cervicofacial adenopathy which, left untreated, will form fistulas and drain via sinus tracts. The children often have weakly or strongly positive delayed hypersensitivity tuberculin skin tests (TST) without prior history of *M. tuberculosis* contacts (6). In North America, MAC is the agent most commonly implicated in NTM lymphadenitis, followed by *M. scrofulaceum*.

2.3 Medical Device and Nosocomial NTM Infections

NTM have been recognized since 1983 as etiologic agents in peritonitis and exit-site infections in patients receiving

G.A. Cangelosi (✉)
Department of Global Health, Seattle Biomedical Research Institute,
University of Washington, Seattle, WA, USA
jerry.cangelosi@sbri.org

D.L. Mayers (ed.), *Antimicrobial Drug Resistance*,
DOI 10.1007/978-1-60327-595-8_63, © Humana Press, a part of Springer Science+Business Media, LLC 2009

continuous ambulatory dialysis through peritoneal catheters (7). The most common agent in CAPD-related infections is *M. fortuitum* (8, 9), but other NTMs have also been documented (10–14). Since the first description of NTM peritonitis, it has been recommended to include NTM as a possible etiologic agent if peritoneal cultures are negative at 48 h with a clinical syndrome of CAPD-related peritonitis (7, 9). Mycobacteria have been shown to form biofilms on medical devices (15–17). Little is known about the drug susceptibility of biofilm mycobacteria, but device-related NTM infection usually requires removal of the offending device.

NTM have been implicated in other nosocomial and healthcare-related infections. Outbreaks of postinjection abscesses have been linked to injections in Netherlands, New England, Texas, and Colombia (18). Inadequate sterilization of the equipment and contamination of the injected material was implicated in these outbreaks. Surgical operations without implanted medical devices have been complicated by NTM infections. There are case reports of postoperative NTM infections after cardiac surgery, gastric cancer surgery, and Mohs micrographic dermatologic procedures (19, 20).

2.4 Pulmonary Disease

The American Thoracic Society (ATS) and Infectious Diseases Society of America (IDSA) released a joint statement reviewing the diagnosis and management of NTM disease in 2007 (21). Diagnosis of NTM pulmonary disease requires respiratory symptoms associated with radiographic evidence of cavities or nodular bronchiectasis, and culture of NTM from more than two sputa or a single bronchoalveolar lavage (21, 22).

In the U.S., the most common etiologic agent of NTM pulmonary infection is MAC, followed by *M. kansasii*. In the United Kingdom, *M. kansasii*, *M. malmoense*, MAC, and *M. xenopi* have geographic strongholds (22). NTM can present as fibrocavitary lung disease in patients with preexisting lung disease such as chronic obstructive pulmonary disease, and can complicate established bronchiectatic pulmonary disease as in *M. abscessus* disease in patients with cystic fibrosis (23). Slow-growing agents like MAC have also been isolated in middle and lingular lobe nodular bronchiectasis in older, nonsmoking generally female population without prior lung disease (24). In general, the fibrocavitary presentation has a faster rate of decline of respiratory function and a more predictable clinical course of decline. MAC disease presenting with nodular bronchiectasis has a less predictable course and requires clinical

judgment on the timing of the therapy, which is often poorly tolerated (25).

2.5 Disseminated Disease

In patients with HIV, disseminated infections with slow-growing agents like MAC and *M. kansasii* occur when CD4 counts drop below 100 cells/μL. Up to 40% of HIV patients with CD4 counts less than 50 cells/μL develop such infections. Disseminated MAC presents with fever, weight loss, diarrhea, adenopathy, and hepatosplenomegaly. Disseminated NTM infections are also seen in immunocompromised patients without HIV (26). Multiple host factors have been implicated in non-AIDS disseminated NTM infection including iatrogenic immunosuppression in solid organ and hematopoietic stem cell transplants (27), T-cell deficiencies (26), IFN-gamma receptor abnormalities (28), NRAMP1 polymorphisms (29), and IL-12 receptor defects (30, 31).

Crohn's disease. M. avium subspecies *paratuberculosis* (MAP) causes Johne's disease, a chronic and economically significant infection of ruminants. MAP also colonizes humans and has been implicated in Crohn's Disease, a debilitating inflammation of the bowel, but this link remains controversial (32–34).

3 Therapy

3.1 Drug Regimens

The ATS, ISDA, and British Thoracic Society (BTS) have outlined guidelines for NTM therapy and susceptibility testing (22, 25). Recommended drug regimens and treatment strategies outlined in Table 1 are adapted from several sources (4, 5, 25, 35, 36). Most recommendations are based on retrospective reviews and case studies; therefore, providers should remain vigilant for new therapies as well as multimodal approaches to therapy, such as intraperitoneal streptomycin for refractory CAPD catheters or surgical debridement in conjunction with anti-mycobacterial therapy (12).

3.2 Susceptibility Testing

Drug susceptibility testing remains controversial in NTM infection, in part because of paucity of data related to its efficacy. Evidence supports the use of drug susceptibilities in three specific settings: macrolide sensitivity in new MAC lung disease, rifamycin sensitivity in *M. kansasii*, and rapidly

Table 1   Treatment regimens for NTM disease

Disease state	Common etiology	Therapy	Alternative therapy	Duration	Outcome notes
Pulmonary Disease	*M. kansasii*	Isoniazid (300 mg) Rifampin (600 mg) EMB ((25 mg/kg) × 2mo, then 15 mg/kg)	Clarithromycin Moxifloxacin Surgical resection	18 months minimum with 12 months of culture negativity	Relapse rate: 0.8%
	M. avium complex	C 500–1,000 mg QD or AZ RIF 450–600 mg QD or RFB EMB (15 mg/kg) QD Streptomycin 2–3× week if tolerated	C1000 mg TIW or AZ 250mg-300 TIW* RIF 600 mg TIW* EMB 25 mg/kg TIW* Surgical resection	1 year after negative culture	Best outcome with therapy following ATS or BTS Guidelines
Disseminated Disease in HIV	*M. avium* complex	C 500–1,000 mg QD ± RFB 300 mg QD EMB 15 mg/kg QD HAART	AZ 500 mg QD + RFB + EMB (RCT with benefit to C over AZ) (44) Fluoroquinolones Amikacin	Lifelong if no HAART. 12 months if clinical response to HAART (46)	High mortality without concomitant HAART C + RFB + EMB improved survival (102)
	M. kansasii	Isoniazid 5 mg/kg (max 300 mg) RIF 10 mg/kg (max 600 mg) EMB 15 mg/kg HAART	Adjust RFB on PI or Clarithromycin Moxifloxacin	Lifelong if no HAART	High mortality without concomitant HAART
Disseminated Disease in Non-HIV	*M. avium* complex	C 500–1,000 mg QD ± rifamycin EMB 15 mg/kg QD	Azithromycin 250–500 mg QD	Consider adjunctive therapies and referral to specialty center	Not well characterized
Lymphadenitis	*M. avium complex* *M. scrofulaceum* *M. malmoense*	Surgical excision + C 500 mg PO BID if refractory or residual disease in parotid gland	Clarithromycin regimen alone (36)	2–6 months	Good outcome
Skin infections	*M. marinum*	C and EMB Add RIF for deep tissue involvement	Tetracyclines Trimethoprim/ sulfa Surgery for deep involvement Amikacin	12–24 weeks Continue 8 weeks after lesion resolves	No mortality; spontaneous resolution reported
	M. ulcerans	Surgical excision	May consider C + RIF postexcision	–	Antibiotics disappointing; excision can be deforming
	M. haemophilum	Combination therapy with C + Amikacin, Ciprofloxacin, and RIF or RFB	Consider surgical debridement	6–9 months	Not well characterized
	M. chelonae *M. fortuitum* *M. abscessus*	Macrolides, Amikacin, Cefoxitin (except *M. c*) Imipenam Quinolones (*M. f*), Linezolid	Consider surgical debridement	Minimum 4 months	Variable

C Clarithromycin; *AZ* azithromycin; *RIF* rifampin; *RFB* Rifabutin; *EMB* ethambutol; *HAART* highly active anti-retroviral therapy; *ATS* American Thoracic Society; *BTS* British Thoracic Society; *PI* protease inhibitor; *PO* by mouth; *BID* twice a day; *QD* every day; *TIW* thrice weekly

growing mycobacteria (RGM) (21). Macrolide susceptibility is an important determinant of treatment success and mortality; macrolide resistance without sputum conversion is associated with increased mortality (37). Macrolide resistance can develop on the recommended therapy including ethambutol and a rifamycin (4%), but it is less frequent in this situation than when macrolide monotherapy is given

(20%) (37). In vitro susceptibility predicted relapses in MAC disease when the MIC increased from ≤4.0 to ≥32 μg/mL (38). Gardner and colleagues found that 17% of HIV-associated MAC showed resistance to macrolides, and resistant isolates were more common in patients with prior macrolide exposure (39). Therefore, susceptibility testing for clarithromycin is recommended in newly diagnosed and relapsed cases of MAC disease (21). Similarly, resistance to rifamycins predicts treatment failure in *M. kansasii* disease. Resistance can develop on appropriate therapy including rifamycins; therefore, newly diagnosed and relapsed cases of *M. kansasii* should be assessed for sensitivity to rifamycins and resistant isolates should be tested more broadly to identify other agents for therapy (21). Drug susceptibility testing should be performed on all rapidly growing NTMs, as susceptibilities can vary intra- and interspecies (25).

3.3 Treatment Outcomes and Prognosis

Few specific NTM therapies have been evaluated in prospective, randomized controlled studies. Most treatment recommendations are derived from uncontrolled prospective studies or retrospective studies.

Prior to the use of rifampin, 4-month sputum conversion rates for *M. kansasii* therapy ranged from 52 to 81%, with relapse rates of 10% after completion of therapy (25). With the addition of rifampin to treatment regimens for *M. kansasii*, sputum conversion rates at 4 months approached 100% (25). In 180 patients treated with a regimen containing rifampin, only two patients developed resistance to rifampin while on therapy and had *M. kansasii* reappear in their sputa.

Prior to the era of highly active antiretroviral therapy (HAART), disseminated *M. kansasii* disease was usually progressive and fatal. A retrospective review comparing outcome of disseminated *M. kansasii* in HIV patients between 1991–1996 and 1997–2002 revealed a decrease in the total number of cases and 100% survival of patients treated with HAART and a rifamycin plus INH and ethambutol (40). Similar retrospective findings have been noted (35, 41) and new recommendations regarding length of therapy and prophylaxis have been published (42).

Macrolide therapy, which is ineffective against tuberculosis, has proven far more useful against MAC. In the pre-macrolide era, 4-month sputum conversion rates were dismally low in MAC lung disease, and relapse rates were frustratingly high. With the current recommended regimen of clarithromycin, ethambutol, and a rifamycin, sputum conversion rates of 90% have been seen (25). These reflect only the patients who are able to tolerate the regimen, and completion rates of NTM therapy are not well documented. In a retrospective review of 111 patients, Fujikane et al. (43) identified nutritional status and female gender as likely determinants of early sputum clearance on a clarithromycin-containing regimen. They found that long-term sputum negativity was associated with smaller radiographic lesions, a regimen that continued for 12 months after sputum clearance, and large lesions with early clearance.

To improve regimen tolerance in patients with a lower burden of disease, thrice weekly therapy with a macrolide, a

rifamycin, and ethambutol is recommended by the ATS/IDSA for MAC patients with nodular bronchiectatic, noncavitary disease. Thrice weekly therapy has been shown to have an acceptable sputum conversion rate in selected patients (21). Although macrolides have been shown to be crucial in MAC therapy, it is unclear in MAC pulmonary disease whether clarithromycin offers additional benefit over azithromycin. In HIV-related disseminated MAC disease, there is evidence of superiority of clarithromycin over azithromycin. In a randomized open-label study, Ward et al. (44) found that median time to sterilization of blood cultures in HIV patients with disseminated MAC was shorter in a clarithromycin/ethambutol-treated group compared to an azithromycin/ethambutol-treated group (4.38 weeks vs. >16 weeks). In MAC pulmonary disease with macrolide resistance, emerging data supports combination therapy with injectable aminoglycosides and surgical resection (37).

Surgical excision of affected lymph nodes has been the gold standard in treatment of pediatric NTM lymphadenitis, resulting in good outcome with low morbidity (36). Macrolide therapy may offer a nonsurgical option; a retrospective review by Luong et al. noted that 67% (30/45) of cases of NTM lymphadenitis in children resolved on antimycobacterials without surgical excision (36). The majority of these cases included clarithromycin as a single agent or in combination therapy. Macrolide therapy appeared to halt the stereotyped natural history of untreated NTM cervicofacial lymphadenitis and prevented fistulization. The advantages of a chemotherapeutic approach to NTM lymphadenitis must be weighed against the risk of adverse drug effects and, when monotherapy is used, the development of drug resistance.

Not surprisingly, the failure to follow the recommended guidelines (ATS or BTS) for therapy of NTM-related pulmonary disease led to a higher rate of treatment failure (76% vs. 26%, OR 7.7) in a retrospective study of NTM cases by Henry et al. (4). Two-year survival was lowest in patients with COPD and cystic fibrosis, although that was likely associated with the burden of the primary disease. Kim reported resolution of bronchiectasis in 30% of cases of NTM infection with treatment (45). Heterozygotes for the CF genotype are less likely to resolve bronchiectasis or cavitation associated with NTM infection (45).

3.4 Adjunctive Therapies

Host defense is an important variable in NTM infections. Human environments are teeming with NTM, and a normal human host can face a daily assault of NTM by showering, inhaling dirt, and eating contaminated foods. NTM are opportunistic pathogens that exploit known or unrecognized weaknesses in immunity. Therefore, diagnosis and therapy of a patient with NTM disease may require an examination of the host's immunity, and inclusion of adjunctive therapies for patients, especially those who are known to be immunodeficient.

Highly active anti-retroviral therapy (HAART) is a necessary adjunctive for patients with HIV coinfections. HAART has sharply decreased AIDS-associated disseminated MAC, which had previously been a leading cause of death in AIDS. Since the institution of HAART, revised guidelines call for the cessation of MAC therapy and prophylaxis in the HIV patient whose CD4 count rises above 100 cells/μL for 6 months or longer (42, 46, 47). In patients with refractory disease, despite maximal therapy including HAART (48), adjunctive therapy with immunomodulatory agents should be considered. HAART has been associated with immune reconstitution syndrome, in which the recovery of immune function is followed by an intense inflammatory reaction to previously subclinical MAC (49). The extent of this potential problem is not yet clear.

Cytokines like interferon-gamma are integral in the host defense against mycobacteria. Case studies have reported clinical success using adjunctive therapy with interferon-gamma in non-HIV patients with T-cell deficiencies and disseminated mycobacterial infections (26, 48, 50). Inhaled interferon-gamma has been used in refractory M. abscessus pulmonary disease, resulting in a clearance of the organism from the sputum (50). Other immunomodulatory agents, which have been considered for their role in antimycobacterial defense, include TNF-alpha, IL-12, and GM-CSF (47).

3.5 Emerging Antimicrobials

Multidrug-resistant tuberculosis has driven research in the area of antimycobacterials. Many of the agents discussed here have been used in tuberculous therapy, or were developed for antituberculosis therapy. Few have been tested clinically in the treatment of NTM diseases, but many of the agents show promising in vitro data for future therapeutic trials.

Linezolid, which has become an important tool against methicillin-resistant Staphylococcus aureus, has been reported to have in vitro activity (MIC ≤ 8 μg/mL) against rapidly growing mycobacteria and some slowly growing mycobacteria (51–54). In the study reported by Brown-Elliot et al. (52), the species most likely to be susceptible to linezolid included M. marinum, M. szulgai, M. gordonae, and M. kansasii. Unfortunately, most isolates of MAC, M. terrae complex, and M. simiae complex lacked susceptibility to linezolid with MIC ≥ 32 μg/mL. Linezolid has been reported as a salvage therapy in an immunosuppressed patient with cutaneous disease due to clarithromycin-resistant M. chelonae (55).

Moxifloxacin and other fluoroquinolones have swept into the antimycobacterial armamentarium, and they have activity against many NTMs including MAC and M. kansasii (Table 1). Levofloxacin has been shown to exhibit synergy in vitro when combined with ethambutol and clofazamine (56), but quinolone therapy combined with a macrolide is insufficient to prevent the development of macrolide resistance in MAC pulmonary disease (37).

3.6 Drug Toxicities and Intolerances

Killing NTMs with antimicrobials is only half the battle won. Many of the anti-NTM drugs have undesirable side effects and drug interactions. Mild side effects can be tolerated by patients for short courses, but it is difficult to ask a septuagenarian to tolerate daily nausea and vomiting for 12–18 months of treatment for a slowly progressive case of nodular bronchiectasis. Drug toxicities and intolerances are major contributing factors to the failure for the complete treatment. This, in turn, contributes to the development of drug resistance. Research aimed at overcoming these problems may be one way to reduce the problem of drug resistance NTM diseases. A brief summary of documented intolerances and side effects is given below.

Ethambutol is recognized to cause retrobulbar optic neuritis, which presents as loss of color discrimination and visual acuity. Griffith et al. noted that 6% of their study population, receiving daily ethambutol (25 mg/kg for the first 2 months, then 15 mg/kg), developed ocular toxicity, compared to none of their patients receiving every other day ethambutol therapy (25 mg/kg) (57). In the tuberculosis therapy literature, ethambutol ocular toxicity is dose related with an incidence of 5–6% at a dose of 25 mg/kg/day for 2 months and <1% at a dose of 15 mg/kg/day (57). The most recent guidelines have decreased the daily dosage of ethambutol in NTM disease, decreasing the likelihood of toxicity. Current recommendations call for periodic and symptomatic testing and ophthalmologic consultation for any visual complaints.

Clarithromycin and the other macrolides can cause nausea, vomiting, and diarrhea. In 1,178 HIV-positive patients enrolled in a study of MAC prophylaxis, 2.5% of patients taking clarithromycin alone could not eat for three days or experienced severe GI discomfort. When clarithromycin was combined with rifabutin, complaints of GI distress increased to 4.6% (58). Diarrhea occurred at similar frequencies. Clarithromycin inhibits hepatic metabolism of many drugs and may increase arrhythmias and toxicities in conjunction with Seldane™, digoxin, and other drugs (59).

The rifamycins cause orange staining of secretions and urine, which offers an excellent measure of compliance, but can be upsetting to patients. Other side effects include hepatitis, nausea, vomiting, and hypersensitivity reactions. The recent ATS/ISDA NTM statement recommends liver function testing (LFT) based on clinical symptoms, but does not endorse regular LFT monitoring while on therapy. The rifamycins can alter hepatic metabolism of many commonly prescribed drugs, including clarithromycin and the protease inhibitors that may be part of multidrug therapy for these patients. Rifabutin, often chosen in HIV patients receiving concomitant protease inhibitors, can cause leukopenia, uveitis, arthralgias, and myalgias.

The antimycobacterial aminoglycosides, including amikacin, streptomycin, and tobramycin, are all nephro- and ototoxic. Tetracyclines are not recommended in children under 8 years of age, as they are deposited in calicifying regions like the teeth and bones. They can lead to photosensitivity as well as nausea, vomiting, and diarrhea. Quinolones can also cause GI symptoms as well as the more unusual side effect of tendinopathies. Clofazamine should be considered carefully before use in HIV-infected patients, as increased mortality with clofazamine was seen prior to widespread HAART (60).

4 Prophylaxis and Prevention

Despite decreased mortality with the institution of HAART, NTM infections remain an important cause of HIV-related mortality and morbidity (61). Prophylactic macrolide therapy is recommended for patients with CD4 counts <50 cells/μL (42).

NTMs are environmental organisms that have evolved to survive many environmental threats including microbicides, elevations in temperature, and alterations in pH (62–65). Although elimination of NTM from water supplies can be difficult, viable counts of NTM in the treatment effluents are typically very low. Exposure may come about as a result of colonization of downstream sites, including end-user plumbing and taps. In some cases, NTM infections have been linked to the inadequate disinfection procedures. At a dialysis center in Louisiana, 25 of 140 patients developed *M. chelonae* infections before sampling of the water supply identified extensive contamination (66).

5 Mechanisms of Resistance

5.1 Primary and Acquired Resistance Associated with Genetic Alterations of Drug Targets

Resistance to commonly used antimycobacterial drugs may be primary (meaning that the patient was infected with a drug-resistant strain) or acquired (meaning that resistance developed during the course of the patient's treatment).

These mechanisms differ from those associated with intrinsic resistance, defined as the innate characteristics of some *Mycobacterium* species that exclude certain antibiotics from the antimycobacterial armamentarium.

In the case of *M. tuberculosis,* the genetic mechanisms of primary and acquired antimycobacterial drug resistance have been the subject of intensive study (67–70). *M. tuberculosis* strains are not known to carry exogenous (e.g., plasmid-borne) or trans-acting drug resistance genes. Instead, resistance results from mutations in genes coding for drug targets, or in genes required for the activation of prodrugs. For example, resistance to isoniazid can result from mutations in *katG*, which codes for the catalase activity required for INH activation, in *inhA*, a target enzyme in the mycolic acid biosynthetic pathway, or in other genes. Rifampin binds to the β-subunit of RNA polymerase, and resistance almost always results from point mutations in a short section of that protein's structural gene, *rpoB* (see Chaps. "Drug Resistance Assays for *Mycobacterium tuberculosis*" and "Drug Resistance by Non-tuberculous Mycobacteria" in this book). Multidrug resistance results from the accumulation of multiple individual resistance mutations, rather than from trans-acting mechanisms that affect multiple antibiotics.

Resistance of NTM isolates to individual drugs has been correlated with analogous altered-target phenomena. Rifampin resistance has been correlated with *rpoB* mutations in clinical isolates of *M. kansasii* (71), and to a much more limited extent, in *M. avium* (72). This mechanism was also reported in lab-generated rifampin-resistant clones of *M. ulcerans* (73). Similarly, missense mutations in the petidyltransferase region of the 23S rRNA gene have been correlated with macrolide resistance in *M. kansasii* (74), *M. chelonae* (75, 76), *M. abscessus* (76), and *M. avium* (77–79). Given the importance of macrolides for NTM treatment, it is unfortunate that most slowly growing bacteria have only one copy of the rRNA operon, a characteristic that may make them more susceptible than most bacteria to single-step mutations leading to macrolide resistance (76).

5. 2 Morphotypic Antibiotic Resistance of MAC

Among the most clinically significant treatment challenges associated with NTM infection is the multidrug resistance of MAC. Macrolides, fluoroquinolones, rifabutin, ethambutol, amikacin, and clofazamine are effective against primary isolates, but they lose effectiveness relatively quickly unless administered in combinations that often are poorly tolerated by patients.

There is a correlation between multidrug resistance and colony type of MAC. Virtually, all isolates form multiple colony morphotypes on laboratory media. Colony types vary with regard to infectivity and drug susceptibility. Reversible morphotypic switches are seen in virtually all the isolates of MAC, suggesting that they confer selective advantages. One such switch is opaque–transparent, in which transparent colony type variants are more resistant to multiple antibiotics than their opaque counterparts. Transparent variants also predominate in patient samples and grow better in animal and macrophage models of disease. Opaque variants grow better in laboratory media and predominate after passage in vitro. The molecular basis for the reversible opaque–transparent switch remains unknown (80–82).

An additional morphotypic switch, termed red–white, is visible among clinical isolates grown on media containing the lipoprotein stain Congo red (CR) (83, 84). The red–white switch operates independently of the opaque–transparent switch, such that red opaque (RO), red transparent (RT), white opaque (WO), and white transparent (WT) morphotypes can be distinguished by CR staining. White variants are more common than red variants in patient samples that have undergone minimal transfer and storage in vitro (84). White variants also grow better in animal and macrophage models of disease (83, 84). The white morphotype is expressed during infection and is likely to be relevant to disease and treatment outcomes. However, the red colony type can also be recovered from patient samples (84). White variants are more resistant than their red counterparts to multiple antibiotics in vitro (83). The list of affected drugs includes macrolides, rifamycins, penicillins, and quinolones.

The morphotypic multidrug resistance of MAC has been ascribed to the cell wall, although additional factors may contribute. Cell wall factors have been inferred from indirect observations. For example, the genetic markers of rifampin, macrolide, and streptomycin resistance seen in other mycobacteria are often missing in resistant MAC isolates (72, 78, 85, 86). Conditions that compromise cell wall integrity have been reported to increase the susceptibility of MAC to multiple drugs (87–89). More recently, mutational analysis identified gene products that are required for the multidrug resistance associated with the white and transparent morphotypes. Resistance to macrolides, quinolones, rifamycins, and penicillins was lost upon mutational knockout of a two-component regulatory system, *mtrAB*. Similar pan-susceptible phenotypes were seen in mutants defective in a protein that catalyzes the synthesis of mannosyl-β-1-phosphomycoketides (*pks12*), in a conserved hypothetical cell surface protein (Maa2520), and in other yet-to-be-characterized gene products (90, 91).

In order to study the genetics of morphotypic drug resistance in MAC, we have used uptake of the fluorescent nucleic acid stain SYTO16 as a surrogate marker of cell envelope permeability (92–94). Because the green fluorescence of SYTO16 is more than 40-fold enhanced upon binding to DNA, efficient staining requires permeation into the cytoplasm.

Cell populations of cultured MAC are morphotypically heterogeneous with regard to permeability, so we quantify staining as the percentage of cells that take up the stain (94). Briefly, growing bacteria are incubated with SYTO16 for 5 min at room temperature. After thorough washing to remove extracellular SYTO16, staining is assessed by using fluorescence microscopy and imaging software. A percentage is calculated based on the number of cells in each frame that fluoresce divided by the number of cells visible by light microscopy. Experiment-to-experiment variation is controlled by normalizing values to a WO control strain in each experiment.

Mutations leading to loss of morphotypic drug resistance, including those in *mtrAB*, *pks12*, and Maa2520, exhibited increased permeability to SYTO16 (reference (94) and unpublished results). The same correlation is seen in naturally occurring morphotypic variants of MAC strains, as illustrated in Fig. 1. Azithromycin and ciprofloxacin susceptibilities of WO, RO, RT, and WT variants of *M. avium* clinical isolate HMC02 were measured by E-test. MIC values are printed above the bar corresponding to the SYTO16 permeability of each clone in Fig. 1 (azithromycin above ciprofloxacin). The multidrug-resistant WT, WO, and RT forms excluded the stain, while the more drug-susceptible RO form was strongly stained. The red–white and opaque–transparent morphotypic switches are reversible and do not require drug selection, enabling these clones to toggle freely between multiresistant/impermeable and pan-sensitive/permeable forms. Relevant drug targets (23S rRNA and DNA gyrase) have not been sequenced in these clones to determine whether the resistant forms have mutations in the corresponding genes associated with resistance. Nonetheless, it is unlikely that such mutations can occur reversibly at high frequencies, especially in the absence of drug selection. Similar

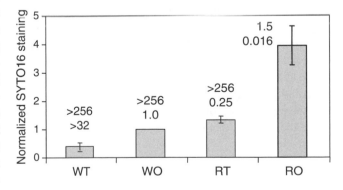

Fig. 1 Correlation between SYTO16 permeation and multidrug susceptibility. Naturally occurring WT, WO, RT, and RO morphotypic variants of *M. avium* clinical isolate HMC02 were assessed for SYTO16 uptake as described in the text and in (91). Data were normalized to the WO strain, and means and standard deviations of three measurements are shown. Numbers above each data bar are susceptibility in μg/mL to azithromycin (upper number) and ciprofloxacin (lower number) by E-test

morphotypic segregation into multiresistant/impermeable and pan-sensitive/permeable forms has been observed in eight other clinical isolates in addition to strain HMC02, indicating that this switching phenomenon is common among MAC strains (unpublished observations).

It is difficult to conceive a cell envelope permeability barrier that excludes structurally diverse antibiotics but not beneficial compounds. For MAC, the solution may be its morphotypic switches, which enable the organism to toggle between permeable and impermeable forms. Such a mechanism may help enable this environmental pathogen to survive and flourish in diverse environments.

A hypothetical permeability barrier is unlikely to be the only mechanism of drug resistance in MAC. Bacterial drug susceptibility can be impacted in cumulative fashion by multiple resistance mechanisms that function in a given cell. Thus, decreased permeability can function synergistically with increased expression of efflux pumps, resulting in reduced intracellular concentrations of a drug. This, in turn, can amplify the effects of missense mutations that reduce binding affinities of drug to the target (95). Any of these mechanisms might function in the multidrug resistance of individual MAC strains. However, a full understanding of the problem requires an understanding of how the bacterium regulates and maintains its morphotypic permeability barriers.

5.3 Intrinsic Drug Resistance

Mycobacterium species are innately resistant to many antibiotics that are commonly used to treat other bacterial infections. Penicillins and glycopeptides such as vancomycin are useless against most mycobacteria. NTMs may share environmental niches with related organisms, including the *Streptomyces* species that naturally produce many of the antibiotics that we use in the clinic. This could have led to the selection of the intrinsic antibiotic resistance seen in many environmental mycobacteria (95). The intrinsic resistance of *M. tuberculosis* to penicillins and macrolides, known from the earliest days of the clinical use of those drugs, may be a holdover from that pathogen's evolutionary roots in the environment.

Mechanisms of intrinsic resistance appear to vary among *Mycobacterium* species. For example, genomic comparisons *in silico* suggested that *M. tuberculosis* and MAC have different mechanisms of intrinsic resistance to macrolides and penicillins (90). A 23S rRNA methyltransferase gene, *erm*, is thought to function in the high-level resistance of *M. tuberculosis* to macrolides (96, 97). Expression of *erm* is controlled by WhiB7, a novel regulatory gene product, that controls the expression of multiple genes, including at least

some intrinsic drug resistance factors (98). WhiB7 is found in most or all *Mycobacterium* species, including soil saprophytes, consistent with an ancestral physiological function. Resistance of *M. tuberculosis* to penicillins is thought to be mediated by at least one major β-lactamase, *blaC*, and possibly by altered expression of several penicillin-binding proteins (99–102). The genome sequence of MAC strain 104 has homologs to penicillin-binding proteins and putative macrolide efflux pumps found in *M. tuberculosis,* but homologs to *ermMT* and *blaC* were not found in its genome (90). A laboratory-generated mutant of *M. tuberculosis* with a deletion of *pks12,* a gene required for morphotypic multidrug resistance in MAC, retained near-wild-type levels of intrinsic resistance to macrolides and penicillins (90).

6 Concluding Remarks

The incidence of NTM infection remains low in comparison to the major mycobacterial diseases of humans, tuberculosis and leprosy. However, the prevalence of NTM disease is elevated by the persistent nature of many such infections, and by the challenges associated with treatment in patient populations that often have impaired immune function. NTM infections, such as pulmonary MAC, are chronic, stubborn, and debilitating. As our population ages, the number of people susceptible to such infections may continue to rise. In order to meet this challenge, new drugs are needed and existing drugs must be preserved. It is imperative that we improve our understanding of intrinsic and acquired drug resistance in these pathogens. Given the diversity of drug resistance mechanisms seen among mycobacterial pathogens, such understanding cannot come solely from the intensive research efforts dedicated to fighting TB. It will come about only through direct genomic, molecular, and clinical investigation of the various NTM diseases themselves.

References

1. Chalermskulrat W, Gilbey JG, Donohue JF. Nontuberculous mycobacteria in women, young and old. Clin Chest Med 2002; (23):675–686
2. Falkinham JO, III. Epidemiology of infection by nontuberculous mycobacteria. Clin Microbiol Rev 1996; 9(2):177–215
3. Marras TK, Daley CL. Epidemiology of human pulmonary infection with nontuberculous mycobacteria. Clin Chest Med 2002; 23:553–567
4. Henry MT, Inamdar L, O'Riordain D, Schweiger M, Watson JP. Nontuberculous mycobacteria in non-HIV patients: epidemiology, treatment and response. Eur Respir J 2004; 23(5):741–746
5. Jogi R, Tyring SK. Therapy of nontuberculous mycobacterial infections. Dermatol Ther 2004; 17(6):491–498

6. Vu TT, Daniel SJ, Quach C. Nontuberculous mycobacteria in children: a changing pattern. J Otolaryngol 2005; 34 Suppl 1:40S–44S

7. Pulliam JP, Vernon DD, Alexander SR, Hartstein AI, Golper TA. Nontuberculous mycobacterial peritonitis associated with continuous ambulatory peritoneal dialysis. Am J Kidney Dis 1983; 2(6):610–614

8. White R, Abreo K, Flanagan R et al. Nontuberculous mycobacterial infections in continuous ambulatory peritoneal dialysis patients. Am J Kidney Dis 1993; 22(4):581–587

9. Youmbissi JT, Malik QT, Ajit SK, al Khursany IA, Rafi A, Karkar A. Non tuberculous mycobacterium peritonitis in continuous ambulatory peritoneal dialysis. J Nephrol 2001; 14(2):132–135

10. Giladi M, Lee BE, Berlin OG, Panosian CB. Peritonitis caused by *Mycobacterium kansasii* in a patient undergoing continuous ambulatory peritoneal dialysis. Am J Kidney Dis 1992; 19(6):597–599

11. Keenan N, Jeyaratnam D, Sheerin NS. *Mycobacterium simiae*: a previously undescribed pathogen in peritoneal dialysis peritonitis. Am J Kidney Dis 2005; 45(5):75-78

12. Sennesael JJ, Maes VA, Pierard D, Debeukelaer SH, Verbeelen DL. Streptomycin pharmacokinetics in relapsing *Mycobacterium xenopi* peritonitis. Am J Nephrol 1990; 10(5):422–425

13. Ellis EN, Schutze GE, Wheeler JG. Nontuberculous mycobacterial exit-site infection and abscess in a peritoneal dialysis patient. A case report and review of the literature. Pediatr Nephrol 2005; 20(7):1016–1018

14. Harro C, Braden GL, Morris AB, Lipkowitz GS, Madden RL. Failure to cure *Mycobacterium gordonae* peritonitis associated with continuous ambulatory peritoneal dialysis. Clin Infect Dis 1997; 24(5):955–957

15. Schulze-Röbbecke R, Fischeder R, Feldmann C, Janning B, Exner M, Wahl G. Dental units: an environmental study of sources of potentially pathogenic mycobacteria. Tuber Lung Dis 1995; 76:318–323

16. Schulze-Röbbecke R, Janning B, Fischeder R. Occurrence of mycobacteria in biofilm samples. Tuber Lung Dis 1992; 73:141–144

17. Hall-Stoodley L, Lappin-Scott H. Biofilm formation by the rapidly growing mycobacterial species *Mycobacterium fortuitum*. FEMS Microbiol Lett 1998; 168:77–84

18. Wallace RJ, Jr., Brown BA, Griffith DE. Nosocomial outbreaks/pseudo-outbreaks caused by nontuberculous mycobacteria. Annu Rev Microbiol 1998; 52:453–490

19. Fisher EJ, Gloster HM, Jr. Infection with mycobacterium abscessus after Mohs micrographic surgery in an immunocompetent patient. Dermatol Surg 2005; 31(7 Pt 1):790–794

20. Kasamatsu Y, Nakagawa N, Inoue K et al. Peritonitis due to *Mycobacterium fortuitum* infection following gastric cancer surgery. Intern Med 1999; 38(10):833–836

21. Griffith DE, Aksamit T, Brown-Elliott BA et al. An official ATS/IDSA statement: diagnosis, treatment, and prevention of nontuberculous mycobacterial diseases. Am J Respir Crit Care Med 2007; 175(4):367–416

22. Subcommittee of the Joint Tuberculosis Committee of the British Thoracic Society. Management of opportunist mycobacterial infections: Joint Tuberculosis Committee guidelines 1999. Thorax 2000; 55:210–218

23. Olivier KN, Weber DJ, Lee JH et al. Nontuberculous mycobacteria. II: nested-cohort study of impact on cystic fibrosis lung disease. Am J Respir Crit Care Med 2003; 167(6):835–840

24. Wickremasinghe M, Ozerovitch LJ, Davies G et al. Nontuberculous mycobacteria in patients with bronchiectasis. Thorax 2005; 60(12):1045–1051

25. American Lung Association and the American Thoracic Society. Diagnosis and treatment of disease caused by nontuberculous mycobacteria. Am J Respir Crit Care Med 1997; 156:S1-S25

26. Holland SM, Eisenstein EM, Kuhns DB et al. Treatment of refractory disseminated nontuberculous mycobacterial infection with interferon gamma. A preliminary report. N Engl J Med 1994; 330(19):1348–1355

27. Doucette K, Fishman JA. Nontuberculous mycobacterial infection in hematopoietic stem cell and solid organ transplant recipients. Clin Infect Dis 2004; 38(10):1428–1439

28. Jouanguy E, Lamhamedi-Cherradi S, Lammas D et al. A human IFNGR1 small deletion hotspot associated with dominant susceptibility to mycobacterial infection. Nat Genet 1999; 21(4):370–378

29. Koh WJ, Kwon OJ, Kim EJ, Lee KS, Ki CS, Kim JW. NRAMP1 gene polymorphism and susceptibility to nontuberculous mycobacterial lung diseases. Chest 2005; 128(1):94–101

30. Altare F, Durandy A, Lammas D et al. Impairment of mycobacterial immunity in human interleukin-12 receptor deficiency. Science 1998; 280(5368):1432–1435

31. de Jong R, Altare F, Haagen IA et al. Severe mycobacterial and Salmonella infections in interleukin-12 receptor-deficient patients. Science 1998; 280(5368):1435–1438

32. Hermon-Taylor J, Bull T. Crohn's disease caused by *Mycobacterium avium* subsp. *paratuberculosis*: a public health tragedy whose resolution is long overdue. J Med Microbiol 2002; 51:3–6

33. Shanahan F, O'Mahony J. The mycobacteria story in Crohn's disease. Am J Gastroenterol 2005; 100(7):1537–1538

34. Behr MA, Semret M, Poon A, Schurr E. Crohn's disease, mycobacteria, and NOD2. Lancet Infect Dis 2004; 4(3):136–137

35. Liao CH, Chen MY, Hsieh SM, Sheng WH, Hung CC, Chang SC. Discontinuation of secondary prophylaxis in AIDS patients with disseminated non-tuberculous mycobacteria infection. J Microbiol Immunol Infect 2004; 37(1):50–56

36. Luong A, McClay JE, Jafri HS, Brown O. Antibiotic therapy for nontuberculous mycobacterial cervicofacial lymphadenitis. Laryngoscope 2005; 115(10):1746–1751

37. Griffith DE, Brown-Elliott BA, Langsjoen B et al. Clinical and molecular analysis of macrolide resistance in *Mycobacterium avium* complex lung disease. Am J Respir Crit Care Med 2006; 174(8):928–934

38. Heifets L, Mor N, Vanderkolk J. *Mycobacterium avium* strains resistant to clarithromycin and azithromycin. Antimicrob Agents Chemother 1993; 37(11):2364–2370

39. Gardner EM, Burman WJ, DeGroote MA, Hildred G, Pace NR. Conventional and molecular epidemiology of macrolide resistance among new *Mycobacterium avium* complex isolates recovered from HIV-infected patients. Clin Infect Dis 2005; 41(7):1041–1044

40. Santin M, Alcaide F. *Mycobacterium kansasii* disease among patients infected with human immunodeficiency virus type 1: improved prognosis in the era of highly active antiretroviral therapy. Int J Tuberc Lung Dis 2003; 7(7):673–677

41. Marras TK, Morris A, Gonzalez LC, Daley CL. Mortality prediction in pulmonary *Mycobacterium kansasii* infection and human immunodeficiency virus. Am J Respir Crit Care Med 2004; 170(7):793–798

42. Karakousis PC, Moore RD, Chaisson RE. *Mycobacterium avium* complex in patients with HIV infection in the era of highly active antiretroviral therapy. Lancet Infect Dis 2004; 4(9):557–565

43. Fujikane T, Fujiuchi S, Yamazaki Y et al. Efficacy and outcomes of clarithromycin treatment for pulmonary MAC disease. Int J Tuberc Lung Dis 2005; 9(11):1281–1287

44. Ward TT, Rimland D, Kauffman C, Huycke M, Evans TG, Heifets L. Randomized, open-label trial of azithromycin plus ethambutol vs. clarithromycin plus ethambutol as therapy for *Mycobacterium avium* complex bacteremia in patients with human immunodeficiency virus infection. Veterans Affairs HIV Research Consortium. Clin Infect Dis 1998; 27(5):1278–1285

45. Kim JS, Tanaka N, Newell JD et al. Nontuberculous mycobacterial infection: CT scan findings, genotype, and treatment responsiveness. Chest 2005; 128(6):3863–3869

46. Kaplan JE, Masur H, Holmes KK. Guidelines for preventing opportunistic infections among HIV-infected persons – 2002. Recommendations of the U.S. Public Health Service and the Infectious Diseases Society of America. MMWR Recomm Rep 2002; 51(RR-8):1–52

47. Benson CA, Kaplan JE, Masur H, Pau A, Holmes KK. Treating opportunistic infections among HIV-exposed and infected children: recommendations from CDC, the National Institutes of Health, and the Infectious Diseases Society of America. MMWR Recomm Rep 2004; 53(RR-15):1–112

48. Sekiguchi Y, Yasui K, Yamazaki T, Agematsu K, Kobayashi N, Koike K. Effective combination therapy using interferon-gamma and interleukin-2 for disseminated *Mycobacterium avium* complex infection in a pediatric patient with AIDS. Clin Infect Dis 2005; 41(11):e104–106e

49. Race EM, Adelson-Mitty J, Kriegel GR et al. Focal mycobacterial lymphadenitis following initiation of protease-inhibitor therapy in patients with advanced HIV-1 disease. Lancet 1998; 351(9098):252–255

50. Hallstrand TS, Ochs HD, Zhu Q, Liles WC. Inhaled IFN-gamma for persistent nontuberculous mycobacterial pulmonary disease due to functional IFN-gamma deficiency. Eur Respir J 2004; 24(3):367–370

51. Alcaide F, Calatayud L, Santin M, Martin R. Comparative in vitro activities of linezolid, telithromycin, clarithromycin, levofloxacin, moxifloxacin, and four conventional antimycobacterial drugs against Mycobacterium kansasii. Antimicrob Agents Chemother 2004; 48(12):4562–4565

52. Brown-Elliott BA, Crist CJ, Mann LB, Wilson RW, Wallace RJ, Jr. In vitro activity of linezolid against slowly growing nontuberculous Mycobacteria. Antimicrob Agents Chemother 2003; 47(5):1736–1738

53. Guna R, Munoz C, Dominguez V et al. In vitro activity of linezolid, clarithromycin and moxifloxacin against clinical isolates of *Mycobacterium kansasii*. J Antimicrob Chemother 2005; 55(6):950–953

54. Wallace RJ, Jr, Brown-Elliott BA, Ward SC, Crist CJ, Mann LB, Wilson RW. Activities of linezolid against rapidly growing mycobacteria. Antimicrob Agents Chemother 2001; 45(3):764–767

55. Brown-Elliott BA, Wallace RJ, Jr, Blinkhorn R, Crist CJ, Mann LB. Successful treatment of disseminated *Mycobacterium chelonae* infection with linezolid. Clin Infect Dis 2001; 33(8):1433–1434

56. Rastogi N, Goh KS, Bryskier A, Devallois A. Spectrum of activity of levofloxacin against nontuberculous mycobacteria and its activity against the *Mycobacterium avium* complex in combination with ethambutol, rifampin, roxithromycin, amikacin, and clofazimine. Antimicrob Agents Chemother 1996; 40(11):2483–2487

57. Griffith DE, Brown-Elliott BA, Shepherd S, McLarty J, Griffith L, Wallace RJ, Jr. Ethambutol ocular toxicity in treatment regimens for *Mycobacterium avium* complex lung disease. Am J Respir Crit Care Med 2005; 172(2):250–253

58. Benson CA, Williams PL, Cohn DL et al. Clarithromycin or rifabutin alone or in combination for primary prophylaxis of *Mycobacterium avium* complex disease in patients with AIDS: a randomized, double-blind, placebo-controlled trial. The AIDS Clinical Trials Group 196/Terry Beirn Community Programs for Clinical Research on AIDS 009 Protocol Team. J Infect Dis 2000; 181(4):1289–1297

59. Midoneck SR, Etingin OR. Clarithromycin-related toxic effects of digoxin. N Engl J Med 1995; 333(22):1505

60. Chaisson RE, Keiser P, Pierce M et al. Clarithromycin and ethambutol with or without clofazimine for the treatment of bacteremic *Mycobacterium avium* complex disease in patients with HIV infection. AIDS 1997; 11(3):311–317

61. Miguez-Burbano MJ, Flores M, Ashkin D et al. Non-tuberculous mycobacteria disease as a cause of hospitalization in HIV-infected subjects. Int J Infect Dis 2006; 10(1):47–55

62. Falkinham JOI, Norton CD, LeChevallier MW. Factors influencing numbers of *Mycobacterium avium, Mycobacterium intracellulare,* and other mycobacteria in drinking water distribution systems. Appl Environ Microbiol 2001; 67:1225–1231

63. Falkinham JO III. Sources, transmission, and exposure of *M avium*. In: Bartram J, Rees G, editors. Pathogenic Mycobacteria in Water. Geneva: World Health Organization – U.S. Environmental Protection Agency; 2003

64. Falkinham JO, III. Factors influencing the chlorine susceptibility of *Mycobacterium avium, Mycobacterium intracellulare,* and *Mycobacterium scrofulaceum*. Appl Environ Microbiol 2003; 69(9):5685–5689

65. Taylor RH, Falkinham JOI, Norton CD, LeChevallier MW. Chlorine, chloramines, chlorine dioxide, and ozone susceptibility of *Mycobacterium avium*. Appl Environ Microbiol 2000; 66:1702–1705

66. Bolan G, Reingold AL, Carson LA et al. Infections with *Mycobacterium chelonei* in patients receiving dialysis and using processed hemodialyzers. J Infect Dis 1985; 152(5):1013–1019

67. Heifets L, Cangelosi GA. Antibiotic susceptibility testing of *Mycobacterium tuberculosis* – a neglected problem at the turn of the century. Int J Tuberc Lung Dis 2002; 3:564–581

68. Morris S, Gai BH, Suffys P, Portillo-Gomez L, Fairchok M, Rouse D. Molecular mechanisms of multiple drug resistance in clinical isolates of *Mycobacterium tuberculosis*. J Infect Dis 1995; 171:954–960

69. Somoskovi A, Parsons L, Salfinger M. The molecular basis of resistance to isoniazid, rifampin, and pyrazinamide in *Mycobacterium tuberculosis*. Respir Res 2001; 2(3):164–168

70. Garcia de Viedma D. Rapid detection of resistance in *Mycobacterium tuberculosis*: a review discussing molecular approaches. Clin Microbiol Infect 2003; 9(5):349–359

71. Klein JL, Brown TJ, French GL. Rifampin resistance in *Mycobacterium kansasii* is associated with rpoB mutations. Antimicrob Agents Chemother 2001; 45(11):3056–3058

72. Williams DL, Waguespack C, Eisenach K et al. Characterization of rifampin-resistance in pathogenic mycobacteria. Antimicrob Agents Chemother 1994; 38(10):2380–2386

73. Marsollier L, Honore N, Legras P et al. Isolation of three *Mycobacterium ulcerans* strains resistant to rifampin after experimental chemotherapy of mice. Antimicrob Agents Chemother 2003; 47(4):1228–1232

74. Burman WJ, Stone BL, Brown BA, Richard J, Bottger EC. AIDS-related *Mycobacterium kansasii* infection with initial resistance to clarithromycin. Diagn Microbiol Infect Dis 1998; 31(2):369–371

75. Vemulapalli RK, Cantey JR, Steed LL, Knapp TL, Thielman NM. Emergence of resistance to clarithromycin during treatment of disseminated cutaneous *Mycobacterium chelonae* infection: case report and literature review. J Infect 2001; 43(3):163–168

76. Wallace RJ, Jr, Meier A, Brown BA et al. Genetic basis for clarithromycin resistance among isolates of *Mycobacterium chelonae* and *Mycobacterium abscessus*. Antimicrob Agents Chemother 1996; 40(7):1676–1681

77. Nash KA, Inderlied CB. Rapid detection of mutations associated with macrolide resistance in *Mycobacterium avium* complex [published erratum appears in Antimicrob Agents Chemother 1996 Oct;40(10):2442]. Antimicrob Agents Chemother 1996; 40(7):1748–1750

78. Jamal MA, Maeda S, Nakata N, Kai M, Fukuchi K, Kashiwabara Y. Molecular basis of clarithromycin-resistance in *Mycobacterium avium-intracellulare* complex. Tuber Lung Dis 2000; 80(1):1–4

79. Meier A, Heifets L, Wallace RJ et al. Molecular mechanisms of clarithromycin resistance in *Mycobacterium avium*: observation of

multiple 23S rDNA mutations in a clonal population. J Infect Dis 1996; 174(2):354–360

80. Belisle JT, Brennan PJ. Molecular basis of colony morphology in *Mycobacterium avium*. Res Microbiol 1994; 145:237–242

81. Belisle JT, Klaczkiewicz K, Brennan PJ, Jacobs WR, Inamine JM. Rough morphological variants of *Mycobacterium avium*. J Biol Chem 1993; 268:10517–10523

82. Cangelosi GA, Clark-Curtiss JE, Behr M, Bull T, Stinear T. Biology of pathogenic mycobacteria in water. In: Bartram J, Rees G, Dufour A, Cotruvo JA, editors. Pathogenic Mycobacteria in Water. Geneva: World Health Organization – U.S. Environmental Protection Agency; 2004

83. Cangelosi GA, Palermo CO, Bermudez LE. Phenotypic consequences of red-white colony type variation in *Mycobacterium avium*. Microbiology 2001; 147:527–533

84. Mukherjee S, Petrofsky M, Yaraei K, Bermudez LE, Cangelosi GA. The white morphotype of *Mycobacterium avium-intracellulare* is common in infected humans and virulent in infection models. J Infect Dis 2001; 184:1480–1484

85. Obata S, Zwolska Z, Toyota E et al. Association of rpoB mutations with rifampicin resistance in *Mycobacterium avium*. Int J Antimicrob Agents 2006; 27(1):32–39

86. Portillo-Gomez L, Nair J, Rouse DA, Morris SL. The absence of genetic markers for streptomycin and rifampicin resistance in *Mycobacterium avium* complex strains. J Antimicrob Chemother 1995; 36:1049–1053

87. Rastogi N, Goh KS, Clavel-Seres S. Stazyme, a mycobacteriolytic preparation from a Staphylococcus strain, is able to break the permeability barrier in multiple drug resistant *Mycobacterium avium*. FEMS Immunol Med Microbiol 1997; 19(4):297–305

88. Jarlier V, Nikaido H. Mycobacterial cell wall: structure and role in natural resistance to antibiotics. FEMS Microbiol Lett 1994; 123:11–18

89. Nikaido H, Jarlier V. Permeability of the mycobacterial cell wall. Res Microbiol 1991; 142:437–443

90. Philalay JS, Palermo CO, Hauge KA, Rustad TR, Cangelosi GA. Genes required for intrinsic multidrug resistance in *Mycobacterium avium*. Antimicrob Agents Chemother 2004; 48(9):3412–3418

91. Cangelosi GA, Do JS, Freeman R, Bennett JG, Semret M, Behr MA. The two component regulatory system *mtrAB* is required for the morphotypic multi-drug resistance of *Mycobacterium avium*. Antimicrob Agents Chemother 2005; in press

92. Mailaender C, Reiling N, Engelhardt H, Bossmann S, Ehlers S, Niederweis M. The MspA porin promotes growth and increases antibiotic susceptibility of both *Mycobacterium bovis* BCG and *Mycobacterium tuberculosis*. Microbiology 2004; 150(4):853–864

93. Ibrahim P, Whiteley AS, Barer MR. SYTO16 labelling and flow cytometry of *Mycobacterium avium*. Lett Appl Microbiol 1997; 25:437–441

94. Cangelosi GA, Do JS, Freeman R, Bennett JG, Semret M, Behr MA. The two-component regulatory system mtrAB is required for morphotypic multidrug resistance in *Mycobacterium avium*. Antimicrob Agents Chemother 2006; 50(2):461–468

95. Nguyen L, Thompson CJ. Foundations of antibiotic resistance in bacterial physiology: the mycobacterial paradigm. Trends Micro 2006; 14(7):304–312

96. Buriankova K, Doucet-Populaire F, Dorson O et al. Molecular basis of intrinsic macrolide resistance in the *Mycobacterium tuberculosis* complex. Antimicrob Agents Chemother 2004; 48(1):143–150

97. Nash KA. Intrinsic macrolide resistance in *Mycobacterium smegmatis* is conferred by a novel erm gene, erm(38). Antimicrob Agents Chemother 2003; 47(10):3053–3060

98. Morris RP, Nguyen L, Gatfield J et al. Ancestral antibiotic resistance in *Mycobacterium tuberculosis*. Proc Natl Acad Sci 2005; 102(34):12200–12205

99. Voladri RK, Lakey DL, Hennigan SH, Menzies BE, Edwards KM, Kernodle DS. Recombinant expression and characterization of the major beta-lactamase of *Mycobacterium tuberculosis*. Antimicrob Agents Chemother 1998; 42(6):1375

100. Segura C, Salvado M, Collado I, Chaves J, Coira A. Contribution of beta-lactamases to beta-lactam susceptibilities of susceptible and multidrug-resistant *Mycobacterium tuberculosis* clinical isolates. Antimicrob Agents Chemother 1998; 42(6):1524–1526

101. Hackbarth CJ, Unsal I, Chambers HF. Cloning and sequence analysis of a class A beta-lactamase from *Mycobacterium tuberculosis* H37Ra. Antimicrob Agents Chemother 1997; 41(5):1182

102. Benson CA, Williams PL, Currier JS et al. A prospective, randomized trial examining the efficacy and safety of clarithromycin in combination with ethambutol, rifabutin, or both for the treatment of disseminated *Mycobacterium avium* complex disease in persons with acquired immunodeficiency syndrome. Clin Infect Dis 2003; 37(9):1234–1243

Section I
Fungal Drug Resistance – Clinical

Chapter 64
The Role of Resistance in *Candida* Infections: Epidemiology and Treatment

J.D. Sobel and R.A. Akins

1 Introduction

During the 1980s and 1990s there was a marked increase in the population of immunocompromised and severely ill individuals at risk of developing opportunistic fungal infections (1). In particular, the increased use of immunosuppressive agents particularly in organ transplant patients, chemotherapy and life-saving medical technology resulted in this increase of both superficial and serious invasive fungal infections (2–4).

The increase in fungal infections occurred at a time when there were few available, effective, systemic antifungal agents. The first fungal agent, griseofulvin, had been introduced in 1960 followed by the introduction of amphotericin B and these two agents represented the only two major systemic agents effective in antifungal therapy. Although topical azole antifungals were introduced in 1969, including miconazole and clotrimazole, parenteral and systemically active oral azoles only became available in the 1980s. Accompanying the introduction of these newer azoles, an explosion in the numbers of patients with AIDS at high risk of developing oropharyngeal and esophageal candidiasis was encountered.

It was during the 1990s that drug resistance became an important problem in virtually all populations of patients at risk, but predominantly in patients with AIDS (5–9). Reports of resistance to antifungal drugs are appearing with increased frequency. Confusion abounds as to how common *Candida* resistance is and whether patient isolates should be sent for susceptibility testing. Simultaneously, both clinical resistance and the increased incidence of fungal infections drove the development of new generations and classes of antifungal agents. Although extremely rare, prior to the 1990s, antifungal drug resistance has rapidly become a major problem in certain populations. The highest risk population has been the most vulnerable viz.; patients with HIV infection. Thus,

in the decade of the 1990s, up to a third of the AIDS patients, in an advanced stage, had drug resistant strains of *Candida albicans* isolated from the oral cavities. However, it is not only HIV-infected patients that have subsequently demonstrated major clinical problems with antifungal resistance (10). In particular, highly immunocompromised patients following both bone marrow and solid organ transplants have become a focus of rising antifungal resistance. The purpose of this chapter is to review the epidemiology, pathogenesis, risk factors for and treatment of resistant candidiasis. Understanding cellular and molecular mechanisms of antifungal drug resistance and associated risk factors is crucial to developing successful prophylactic and treatment strategies to prevent emergence of resistant fungi and is discussed in the accompanying chapter (29). Management of refractory fungal disease caused by resistant *Candida* species will be reviewed together with methods available to prevent further development of antifungal drug resistance in candidiasis.

2 Epidemiology of Candidiasis

Oropharyngeal candidiasis (OPC) is most prevalent in infants, the elderly and compromised hosts and is also associated with serious underlying conditions including diabetes, leukemia, neoplasia, steroid use, antimicrobial therapy, radiation therapy and chemotherapy. At least a quarter of cancer patients not receiving antifungal prophylaxis develop OPC (11), whereas other investigators have observed OPC in more than half of all immunocompromised patients. Prolonged neutropenia appears to be the single most important risk factor for both oropharyngeal colonization with a *Candida* species and subsequent symptomatic disease (12). Approximately 80–90% of patients with HIV infection will develop OPC at some stage of the disease (6) and 60% of untreated patients develop AIDS-related infection within 2 years of the appearance of OPC (13). *Candida albicans* remains the most common species responsible for OPC (14). A small unique population at high risk for developing azole antifungal

J.D. Sobel (✉)
Division of Infectious Diseases, Harper University Hospital, Detroit, MI, USA
jsobel@med.wayne.edu

D.L. Mayers (ed.), *Antimicrobial Drug Resistance*,
DOI 10.1007/978-1-60327-595-8_64, © Humana Press, a part of Springer Science+Business Media, LLC 2009

resistance are individuals with immune-deficiency related chronic mucocutaneous candidiasis (15, 16).

Vulvovaginal candidiasis is considered to be the second most common form of vaginitis worldwide, affecting millions of immunocompetent women. More than 90% of infections are caused by *Candida albicans* (17). The high prevalence of this infection in otherwise healthy females is responsible for significant morbidity and use of antifungal therapy.

During the 1980s, data from the National Center for Health Statistics (NCHS) reported that bloodstream infections was the 13th leading cause of death in the United States. *Candida* bloodstream infection has an attributable mortality of approximately 35% (1). Fungal infections, particularly due to *Candida* species, increased dramatically and accounted for 8–15% of all nosocomial bloodstream infections (18–20). The National Hospital Discharge Survey (NHDS) reported rates of oropharyngeal and disseminated candidiasis to have increased fourfold and 11-fold respectively between 1980 and 1989 (21). Bloodstream *Candida* infections previously predominantly seen in cancer patients became common in ICUs and pediatric wards (9, 22). In 1997, systemic mycoses ranked seventh as the underlying cause of death due to infections compared with being the tenth in the 1980 (23). The SCOPE study reported that for the 3-year period ending in 1998, *Candida* species remained the fourth most common cause of nosocomial bloodstream infection (1, 24). Risk factors for the increased incidence of candidemia have been reviewed (25, 26). Moreover, candidemia has the highest crude mortality (40–50%) of all nosocomial bloodstream infections (24, 27, 28). Autopsy studies have also confirmed the increase in the incidence of disseminated candidiasis (23). Candidemia is associated with prolongation of hospital stay of 70 versus the 40 days compared to matched nonfungemic patients (29) and as well as with considerable increase in costs of therapy (30).

At present, *C. albicans* accounts for ~40–60% of all nosocomial *Candida* infections, although a continued shift toward *Candida* species other than *C. albicans* has occurred, and is important because of the intrinsic or acquired antifungal resistance in several of these species (2, 27, 31–33).

3 Mechanism of Action of Antifungal Drugs (See Reviews) (34, 35)

3.1 Polyenes

The most important polyenes include amphotericin B and nystatin. Amphotericin B binds the primary fungal cell membrane to sterol-altering membrane permeability and ulti-

mately cell death. Amphotericin B also causes oxidative damage to fungal cells (see Chapter 25).

3.2 Fluoropyrimidines

Flucytosine, 5-fluorocytosine (5-FC) is a synthetic fluorinated pyrimidine. It is transported into susceptible fungal cells by the action of an enzyme cytosine permease and then converted by cytosine deaminase to fluorouracil. The latter molecule is incorporated into RNA in place of uracil. In addition, flucytosine blocks thymidylate synthetase, an essential enzyme for DNA synthesis (see Chapter 27).

3.3 Azoles

The azole antifungal agents in clinical use, contain either two or three nitrogens in the azole rank, are therefore classified as imidazoles (ketoconazole, miconazole, clotrimazole, econazole and butoconazole) or triazoles (itraconazole, fluconazole, terconazole). The newer azole agents include voriconazole posaconazole, ravuconazole and albaconazole. The azoles inhibit ergosterol synthesis in the fungal cell membrane through their action on the cytochrome P450-dependent enzyme lanosterol14 α-demethylase. Differences among various azoles relate primarily to their pharmacokinetics as well as their affinity for the target enzymes. There are also some differences in anti-fungal spectrum. The newest triazoles e.g., voriconazole, posaconazole have activity against many yeasts and filamentous fungi as well (see Chapter 26).

3.4 Echinocandins

This new class consists of parenteral caspofungin, micafungin, and anidulafungin. These agents inhibit the fungal cell wall synthesis of an enzyme 1, 3-β-D-glucan synthase, preventing the formation of 1, 3-β-D-glucan, an essential component of the fungal cell wall. These agents result in a weakened cell wall resulting in fungal cell lysis and are considered candidacidal (36) (see Chapter 28).

4 Definition of Resistance

4.1 Refractory Candidiasis

This, by no means uncommon, condition refers to treatment failure of symptomatic patients with antifungal agents. Only one of the many causes of therapeutic failure is due to the presence of in vitro confirmed resistant *Candida* spp. (Table 1) (Fig. 1). Treatment failure can also be the result of the failure of the antifungal agent to reach the target site of infection in sufficient concentrations due to inadequate dosing, impaired absorption (food, gastric pH), poor compliance, and drug interactions. Other causes of treatment failure include local factors that either interfere with drug action, e.g., purulent material in an undrained abscess, or prevent access to organisms seeking refuge in a biofilm e.g., prosthesis both intravascular or intraarticular (37, 38). A profoundly depressed immune system may also be responsible for failure. Both adequate numbers of functioning polymorphonuclear leukocytes and cell-mediated immunity are also essential in eradicating

Table 1 Causes of treatment failure resulting in refractory candidiasis

1. In vitro antifungal resistance
   Primary (intrinsic)
   Secondary
2. Failure of drug to reach site of infection in effective concentration
   Poor adherence
   Inadequate dosing
   Impaired oral absorption
   Drug interactions
3. Failure to drain abscess
4. Local protective mechanisms e.g., biofilm (catheter, prosthetic valve, device, foreign body)
5. Impaired host immune/defense mechanism
   PMNs
   CMI

Mechanisms 2–5 result in clinical resistance with failure associated with susceptible microorganisms

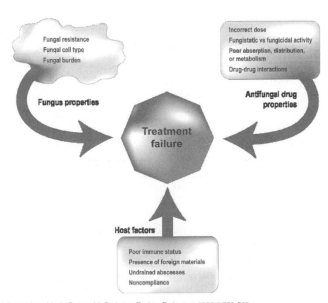

Adapted from Masia Canuto M, Gutierrez Rodero F. *Lancet.* 2002;2:550-563.

Fig. 1 Principal causes of failure of antifungal therapy

Candida infection. Clinical resistance refers to treatment failure despite microbial susceptibility in vitro.

4.2 Primary or Secondary Resistance

An organism that is resistant to a drug prior to exposure is defined as having intrinsic or primary resistance. Examples of primary resistance include *C. krusei* to fluconazole and *C. krusei* and *C. lusitaniae* to flucytosine. Acquired or secondary resistance develops during or after exposure to an antifungal agent e.g., HIV-infected patients with fluconazole-resistant OPC and esophageal candidiasis due to *C. albicans*. Cross-resistance refers to multidrug resistance either within the same class or may involve multiple classes. Heteroresistance refers to variable in vitro susceptibility of different colonies of the same isolate obtained from the same agar plate. All forms of in vitro resistance may be temporary, transient or irreversible.

5 Antifungal Susceptibility Tests

5.1 Methods

Acceptable testing methods and tentative breakpoints for antifungal agents have been suggested by Rex (37–40). These breakpoints are limited to yeast, particularly *Candida* and fluconazole and itraconazole (Table 2). Suggested breakpoints were based on the analysis of in vitro MIC (involving 883 isolates) and clinical data from 729 patients treated with these two antifungal agents. There appears to be general acceptance both of the method (M27-A) and of the breakpoints. Evidence of a correlation between antifungal susceptibility and clinical outcome has been established for fluconazole and itraconazole and oropharyngeal candidiasis due to *C. albicans* in HIV-infected individuals (37). The

Table 2 In vitro susceptibility of *Candida* spp. and interpretative breakpoints

Antifungal Agents	MIC (μg/mL)		
	Susceptible	Susceptible (dose-dependent)	Resistant
Fluconazole	≤8	16–32	≥64
Itraconazole	≤0.125	0.25–0.5	≥1
Flucytosine	≤4	8–16	≥32
Voriconazole	≤1	2	≥4
Posaconazole[a]	≤1	2	≥4
Ravuconazole[a]	≤1	2	≥4

[a]Unconfirmed

availability of standardized susceptibility testing has contributed enormously to predicting clinical outcome based upon in vitro testing (41). Susceptibility testing is increasingly used, although still not available or performed at all large hospitals.

Accordingly, in vitro measured resistance with MICs of fluconazole and itraconazole of ≥ 64 and ≥ 1 µg/mL, respectively, frequently correlates with failure in the treatment of clinical infections including OPC, esophageal candidiasis and systemic invasive candidiasis (37, 42).

The currently approved method of the National Committee for Clinical Laboratory Standards (NCCLS now CLSI) for yeast, antifungal susceptibility testing for yeasts M27-A was published in 1997, has resulted in a standardized reproducible method, which, as mentioned above, correlates with clinical response to antifungal therapy (43, 44). The M27-A methodology has limitations. Trailing growth seen utilizing azoles often makes consistent endpoint determination problematic (38). The susceptible-dose dependent designation, which was mainly intended to accommodate *C. glabrata*, implies that treatment with a dosage higher that usual, achieving higher serum or tissue concentration, might be effective against the specific strain. The aforementioned breakpoints and MICs correlated poorly with clinical and mycological response in vaginal candidiasis possibly due to unique in vivo growth conditions which enhanced azole activity (45, 46). Some studies of candidemia have found a good correlation between treatment failure and in vitro fluconazole resistance (42, 47). Breakpoints are now available for voriconazole.

NCCLS M27-A methodology has only a limited ability to measure MICs of *Candida* isolates to amphotericin B. Rex et al. recommended use of antibiotic medium 3 broth to measure resistance (48). In general, current methods are limited to identifying *Candida* isolates associated with clinical failure, although breakpoint MLCs (minimal lethal concentrations) and MICs of ≥ 1 µg/mL at 48 h has been recommended to predict mycologic *Candida* spp failure more accurately with amphotericin B (49). In a multicenter study

of candidemia in non-neutropenic patients, all blood isolates demonstrated amphotericin B MICs less than 1.0 µg/mL. As with fluconazole, clinical failures (10–15%) were all associated with in vitro susceptible isolates with low amphotericin B MICs (50).

The E-test is often used as an alternate to broth dilution methodology and certainly is useful in the setting of refractory clinical disease and no other testing method available. The E-test is considered suitable for testing *Candida* spp against amphotericin B or flucytosine, but less reliable for azole susceptibility (47, 51–55).

5.2 In vitro Susceptibility and Resistance of Candida Species (Table 3)

5.2.1 Azoles

The new triazoles, voriconazole, posaconazole and ravuconazole exhibit greater potency and spectrum than either fluconazole or itraconazole. The activity of these broad-spectrum triazoles extends to some fluconazole-resistant strains of *Candida*. The extensive use of fluconazole in the treatment and prophylaxis of candidiasis has led to concerns regarding the development of resistance, either the selection of intrinsically resistant species or the development of secondary resistance in normally susceptible species.

Primary and secondary azole resistance is species dependent and also shows marked geographic variation (56, 57). There is no clear evidence for a correlation between the agricultural use of azoles and an increase in antimycotic resistance in human pathogenic fungi. Primary resistance to azoles remains uncommon in candidiasis, with the exception of *Candida glabrata* and *Candida krusei*. Most acquired azole resistance emerged in AIDS patients with OPC and EC following prolonged azole therapy in the presence of advanced immunodeficiency. Azole resistance in other settings is uncommon (57, 58).

Table 3 Susceptibility of *Candida* spp. to antifungal agents

MIC$_{50}$	Amphotericin B	Fluconazole	Itraconazole	Voriconazole	Flucytosine	Caspofungin
C. albicans	0.5	0.5	0.12	0.03	≤0.25	0.12
C. tropicalis	0.25	1	0.06	0.06	≤0.25	0.25
C. glabrata	0.5	16	0.25	0.25	≤0.25	0.12
C. parapsilosis	0.25	1	0.12	0.03	≤0.25	1.0
C. krusei	0.25	64	0.5	0.5	16	0.5
C. lusitaniae	≥1	2	0.25	0.03	≤0.25	1.0

Shown are typical species-specific MIC$_{50}$s (µg/mL) adapted from reports describing collections of clinical isolates (50, 57, 59, 86, 208). MICs were obtained by the NCCLS M27 methodology (National Committee for Clinical Laboratory Standards 1995) for all drugs but amphotericin B. As this method fails to detect amphotericin B-resistant *Candida* (50), then-reported amphotericin B MICs were obtained by a more sensitive method based on use of Antibiotic Medium 3 in a agar-based testing format

1. *C. albicans*. Primary resistance to fluconazole, itraconazole, is extremely rare. Moreover outside the realm of AIDS, acquired or secondary resistance has likewise remained uncommon especially with regard to bloodstream isolates. Each year, thousands of randomly obtained BSI isolates from all over the world are tested in a single site (SENTRY) and over several years fluconazole resistant *C. albicans* remains <5% and shows no evidence of changing (58–60). In contrast, Antoniadou et al. reported that 9% of bloodstream isolates of *C. albicans* were resistant to fluconazole (MIC > 64 µg/mL) (61). Spontaneous fluconazole resistance in the absence of prior azole therapy has been reported in otherwise healthy adults (62). It has been reported, based upon molecular modeling studies, that certain mutations in *ERG* II result in significant levels of resistance to fluconazole and voriconazole but have less effect on the susceptibility of the organisms to itraconazole and posaconazole, possibly due to the more extensive binding of the latter agent to the target enzymes (63).

- *C. tropicalis*. Occasional strains of *C. tropicalis* demonstrate azole resistance, although MIC_{90} values indicate susceptibility. This species has a proclivity to produce trailing grown in vitro; often misinterpreted as resistance.
- *C. parapsilosis* strains are usually highly susceptible to all azoles (64).
- *C. krusei*. This species is intrinsically resistant to fluconazole and has higher MICs to itraconazole in the S-DD range. Voriconazole is, however, very active against *C. krusei* (59, 65). *C. krusei* incidence has remained stable over the last decade.
- *C. dubliniensis*. This species has been increasingly identified and implicated in OPC in HIV-infected agents and is usually identified as *C. albicans*. Most *C. dubliniensis* strains are susceptible to fluconazole although in vitro resistance can be induced. Acquired resistance appears much more rapidly than in *C. albicans*.
- *C. glabrata*. Among the pathogenic yeast species, *Candida glabrata*, which accounts for 5–40% of all yeast isolates depending on the studies, ranks second in all clinical forms of candidiasis today. This opportunistic pathogen is particularly relevant in immunocompromised patients including those receiving cytotoxic chemotherapy, undergoing transplantation or infected with HIV. This is the critical *Candida* species with regard to azole susceptibility and represents the Achilles' heel of the azole class (66, 67). *C. glabrata* isolates exhibit bimodal susceptibility to azoles with 10–15% of bloodstream isolates demonstrating fluconazole resistance (≥64 µg/mL) (59, 60). Patterns of fluconazole susceptibility vary by geographic area, patient population, risk factors and azole exposure (68). In particular, clini-

cal isolates obtained from patients with AIDS and OPC/EC and those with underlying malignancy show reduced susceptibility to fluconazole and itraconazole. Fluconazole resistance is lowest in Asia-Pacific and Latin-American regions (3–4%) and highest in North America (10–15%). Both the frequency of *C. glabrata* occurrence and azole susceptibility is profoundly affected by azole exposure, with 30–40% of isolates being S-DD. International surveillance reveals that recently submitted bloodstream isolates (2001–2005) of *C. parapsilosis* and *C. tropicalis* in contrast to *C. albicans* did reveal a slight increase in fluconazole resistance. A similar increase in resistance was observed for *C. glabrata* with sustained high rates of fluconazole resistance (14.3–18.3%) over this period (58). In general, whereas most *C. glabrata* isolates are still susceptible to voriconazole, most fluconazole-resistant *C. glabrata* isolates are resistant to itraconazole, and half are also resistant to voriconazole and posaconazole (59, 65, 69). Not surprisingly, several reports of voriconazole-resistant *C. glabrata* breakthrough fungemia in bone-marrow transplant recipients receiving long-term voriconazole prophylaxis have been reported (70).

5.2.2 Flucytosine

Intrinsic resistance among *C. albicans* has been described in 6.5–33% of isolates and is invariably associated with serotype B isolates (71). More recent studies have shown lower resistance frequency possibly due to infrequent use. Pfaller et al. studying 8,803 clinical isolates of *Candida* spp. reported susceptibility as follows: *C. albicans* (97%), *C. tropicalis* (92%), *C. guilliermondii* (100%), *C. dubliniensis* (100%), *C. parapsilosis* (99%), *C. glabrata* (99%) (60). The least susceptible species was *C. krusei* (5% susceptible, 67% intermediate, and 28% resistant). Barchiesi et al., in a smaller study reported that 82% of *C. glabrata* were susceptible to flucytosine (7). The pharmacokinetics and in vitro activity of flucytosine make the agent particularly useful for azole-resistant *Candida* infections in relatively inaccessible sites such as CSF and the genitourinary tract.

Secondary acquired resistance is common (30%) and is acquired rapidly to flucytosine when used as monotherapy. Accordingly, flucytosine is almost always used in combination with other antifungals.

5.2.3 Polyenes

Resistance to amphotericin B may be intrinsic or acquired (72). *C. albicans* resistance is extremely rare, although the NCCLS M27-A methodology may be underestimating its occurrence. For amphotericin B, NCCLS methodology generates a narrow MIC range limiting its ability to identify likely causes of therapeutic failure (49). Moreover, more important than resistance is the phenomenon of reduced susceptibility without frank resistance. Powderly et al. reported reduced amphotericin B sensitivity of blood isolates of *C. albicans* in neutropenic patients and correlated higher MICs with poor outcome (73). Fortunately, such strains are rare and secondary resistance is uncommon (74). Resistance in *C. parapsilosis* and *C. dubliniensis* but not *C. tropicalis* is rare (75). Although *C. glabrata* and *C. krusei* isolates are usually considered susceptible to amphotericin B, they tend to have higher MICs, justifying initial empiric use of amphotericin B at a higher dose of 1.0 mg/kg/day (76–78). Sterling reported the emergence of resistance to amphotericin B during therapy for *C. glabrata* infection in an immunocompetent host (79). Many but not all *C. lusitaniae* and some *C. guilliermondii* isolates demonstrate intrinsic resistance to amphotericin B (80, 81). Acquisition of secondary polyene-resistance in species, in addition to *C. albicans* include *C. lusitaniae* and *C. guilliermondii* during amphotericin B therapy especially in myelosuppressed patients (74, 82–84). Rare cases of fatal septicemia reported of amphotericin B-resistant *C. lusitaniae* (85). Resistance to amphotericin B desoxycholate implies that the organism will be resistant to the various lipid formulations of amphotericin B.

5.2.4 Echinocandins

Since caspofungin was the first licensed echinocandin in the US, most information describing *Candida* resistance to this new class of antifungals has been obtained with caspofungin although data on micafungin and anidulafungin are catching up. Reports of clinical and/or in vitro resistance to any of the echinocandin agents have been extremely rare to-date but have been reported. The in vitro activities of caspofungin against 3,959 isolates of *Candida* spp. from 95 different medical centers was determined and compared with fluconazole and itraconazole (86). No resistant strains of *C. albicans* were detected. Against all *Candida* species, 96% of MICs were ≤2 μg/mL. *C. albicans*, *C. dubliniensis*, *C. tropicalis* and *C. glabrata* were the most susceptible species and *C. guilliermondii* was the least susceptible, MIC$_{90}$ > 80 μg/mL. *C. parapsilosis* MIC$_{90}$ 2–4 μg/mL, versus *C. albicans* 0.25 μg/mL (86). Echinocandins remain very active against azole-resistant isolates of *C. albicans* and *C. glabrata* (99% of MICs were ≤1 μg/mL). There is no evidence of a significant impact of azole resistance mediated by CDR pumps on echinocandin resistance in clinical *Candida* isolates.

Similarly, large multinational *Candida* isolate collections have been used to evaluate in vitro resistance to micafungin and anidulafungin and almost identical and universal susceptibility has been reported and once more higher MICs of *C. parapsilo-*

sis emerged (58). Interestingly, caspofungin is not fungicidal for isolates of *C. parapsilosis* or *C. guilliermondii* (87).

Breakpoints for the echinocandin class of agents have only recently been established and in vitro and in vivo analysis has been hampered by a dearth of resistant isolates. Kartsonis et al. failed to establish any relationship between baseline caspofungin MICs and clinical outcome with isolates from both mucosal and invasive *Candida* infections (88). An echinocandin MIC of ≤ 2.0 μg/mL, a blood concentration easily achievable in vivo under normal dosing, would encompass 99.7% of all clinical isolates of *Candida* species (58).

While clinical failure due to echinocandin-resistant *Candida* isolates have been rare, acquired in vivo resistance following echinocandin exposure undoubtedly occurs and these resistant isolates fail appropriate therapy in animal models even if clinical failure was not reported (89). All the resistant isolates were shown to have homozygous mutations in the *FKS*1 gene. Nevertheless, clinical failures with all *Candida* species have also been reported (90, 91).

In 2004, Hernandez et al. reported a patient with azole-refractory OPC/EC which in spite of initial improvement eventually failed on caspofungin (92). Initial isolates exhibited low caspofungin MICs whereas a late isolate had higher MIC. The clinical response was reproduced in a murine model correlating MIC with the clinical response to caspofungin. Similarly, a case of progressive loss of echinocandin activity following prolonged use of treatment of *C. albicans* esophagitis was reported (93).

In 2005, Moudgal et al. described a patient with aortic valve endocarditis due to *C. parapsilosis* (94). After initially responding to combination therapy with caspofungin (MIC 2 μg/mL) and fluconazole, he cleared his fungemia and was discharged on fluconazole only. He returned 3 months later with recurrent *C. parapsilosis*, now resistant to both fluconazole and caspofungin (MIC > 16 μg/mL) and also to voriconazole and micafungin but not to anidulafungin. Similar, but infrequent case reports regarding acquired echinocandin resistance in *C. glabrata* are beginning to emerge (95). Additional surveillance is needed.

5.3 Correlation of in vitro Susceptibility Testing and Clinical Outcome of Treatment with Antifungal Agents

In vitro susceptibility is only one of the many factors that influence the outcome of therapy of fungal infections (38). A variety of pharmacokinetic, pharmacodynamic drug factors as well as a multitude of host factors (neutropenia, compliance, catheter presence, APACHE scores, abscess drainage) interact to impact upon clinical outcome(s). Even the definition of clinical outcome is controversial, ranging from clinical improvement, mycologic evaluation (short or long term) on patient survival (days or week). Nevertheless, in vitro susceptibility determination may serve as an objective, reproducible measure that can profoundly influence drug selection with physicians recognizing the limitations of in vitro susceptibility testing.

Establishing that an isolate is resistant to an antifungal agent in vitro is an immensely useful step in selecting therapy. Determining that the isolate is susceptible to antifungal agents in no way predicts survival or fungal eradication. Clinicians should recall the old 90–60 rule in which a clinical response of 90% or more can be expected when an in vitro sensitive strain is treated with an appropriate antibiotic in comparison to a 60% response when a resistant strain is treated with drugs showing reduced or no activity in vitro.

With regard to candidiasis, in vitro and clinical outcome correlations have mainly been applied to OPC/EC and candidemia, where the 90–60 rule appears to have been met, recognizing this is merely a minimal standard. The most important principle applied is that organisms deemed resistant in vitro are much less likely to respond in vivo. Yet within the candidemia RCTs involving hundreds of patients, almost all patients failing did so with highly susceptible strains. This emphasizes the principle that susceptibility in vitro does not guarantee successful therapy. Most studies evaluating the 90–60 rule have applied to azoles, specifically fluconazole and the best correlation was in OPC/EC in AIDS patients. The clinical predictability of amphotericin B susceptibility is less well established. Moreover, Sobel et al. found poor correlation between in vitro MICs and response to fluconazole therapy for VVC (45). Finally, any discussion of clinical correlation must distinguish resistance developing in a given strain of the same species from the problem of acquiring less susceptible strains from the same or different species.

5.4 Indications for Antifungal Susceptibility Testing in Candida Infections

Apart for reasons of: (1) periodic epidemiologic surveillance and resistance monitoring, routine susceptibility testing by any of the aforementioned methods is not indicated, (2) testing is justified for all *Candida* isolates associated with persistent breakthrough and recurrent candidemia and refractory mucosal candidiasis, (3) anticipated prolonged or critical therapy e.g., endocarditis, osteomyelitis especially with non-*albicans Candida* invasive infections, (4) selected non-*albicans Candida* species (*C. glabrata*) initially treated by non-azole regimens in whom a switch to oral therapy with either fluconazole or voriconazole is likely to complete therapy. Given the increase of parenteral echinocandins as

first-line therapy for candidemia only to have the remainder of the therapeutic course completed by oral triazoles, the Infectious Society of America now recommends that all first bloodstream isolates should be tested for antifungal susceptibility.

6 Pathogenesis of Resistant Candidiasis – Risk Factors

Does azole use select for antifungal drug resistance? In this context, clinical resistance is encountered with a) the presence of organisms with intrinsic, de novo resistance to antifungals usually seen with non-*albicans Candida* and rarely *C. albicans*, b) alternately, evolution of the initially sensitive strain to an identical strain that has undergone genetic and molecular changes, may occur or, c) there is replacement of the strain with a new resistant strain of the same species or finally replacement with a new strain of a different species.

Evidence links empirical, prophylactic and therapeutic use of azoles and selection for yeasts other than *C. albicans* that exhibit decreased susceptibility to azoles e.g., *C. glabrata* and *C. krusei* infections in patients receiving fluconazole prophylaxis (95–97). Most of the data, however, comes from AIDS patients. The emergence of antifungal-resistant *C. albicans* fungemia has been reported in bone marrow transplant recipients being administered on a long term with fluconazole prophylaxis (98). Similarly isolated reports of fluconazole resistant fungi in surgical ICUs are emerging (99).

While molecular changes in a single strain invariably reflect a single or more usually multiple genetic mutations, the dynamics of acquisition of a new strain or species is less well understood. New more resistant *Candida* strains or species may be acquired during hospitalization from medical staff carriers. This process has been well documented with *C. albicans* and *C. parapsilosis*, but *C. glabrata* is rarely identified on the hands of carriers or in hospital environment. It is hypothesized that patients may be colonized in the gastrointestinal tract simultaneously by multiple strains of *Candida*, including the possibility of multiple species. Routine culture only captures the dominant strain or species. After antifungal drug ingestion or pressure, more susceptible strains are eliminated or so reduced in number so as to allow growth and emergence and recognition of more resistant strains or species that have co-existed for a long time but were previously not recognized.

6.1 HIV/AIDS

AIDS patients have been the focal point of much of the scientific inquiry into fluconazole resistance. On the one hand, oral and esophageal candidiasis became extremely common as a clinical manifestation of AIDS in the 1980s. The availability of fluconazole as both treatment and subsequently prophylaxis in patients with recurrent disease was an enormous boon to care. Within a few short years, clinical and in vitro fluconazole resistance was widespread and caused major alarm among AIDS practitioners (6, 100). Several studies, mainly retrospective; identified risk factors for acquisition of fluconazole resistance (Table 4). In addition to the status of the immune system (CMI), i.e., CD4 lymphocyte count, most but not all studies concluded that patterns of fluconazole use were the dominant factors associated with resistance acquisition (101–104). In the majority of patients, mutation of a previously susceptible strain of *C. albicans* to a resistant strain is likely to have occurred, together with co-infection with *Candida* species resistant to fluconazole e.g., *C. glabrata* (105).

In a recent prospective, randomized, controlled trial conducted by the Mycoses Study Group, episodic treatment versus continuous prophylaxis with fluconazole was studied with particular reference to acquisition of resistance. The first conclusion was that overall acquisition of resistance was uncommon in this HAART-compliant study population. Secondly, the use of episodic compared to continuous fluconazole prophylaxis was not shown to be protective in preventing the emergence of resistance (106). In general, no pattern of fluconazole prescription or ingestion has been consistently identified as contributing to azole-resistance selection, although both dosing and duration have been widely implicated in the emergence of resistance. Most importantly, it has not been established whether lower doses used for longer periods of time lead to antifungal resistance and whether intermittent therapy, especially using higher doses for shorter periods prevents resistance (107, 108). In contrast to the above, resistant species were isolated in patients with HIV infection and with no prior exposure to fluconazole (109).

Table 4 Risk factors for azole resistance in candidiasis

HIV/AIDS
Advanced immunosuppression (low CD4 cells)
High viral load
Fluconazole administration
  Poor compliance
  Past fluconazole exposure
    Total dose
    Intermittent therapy
    Prophylaxis versus therapeutic
    Low dose
Hematologic malignancy/BM transplantation
  Azole exposure (prophylactic)
Prosthetic devices – foreign bodies
  Biofilm

6.2 Hematologic Malignancies and Transplant Patients

This growing population is the second focus of resistant candidiasis. Empiric systemic antifungals are widely used as empiric therapy for antibiotic-resistant fever in addition to azole prophylaxis both in neutropenic patients (usually fairly short-term) and non-neutropenic high-risk post-transplant patients (often long-term). Once more, azole exposure both oral and systemic is recognized as: a) infrequent cause of azole-resistant *C. albicans*, b) a more frequent and important cause of selection of non-*albicans Candida* species, both colonizing the gastrointestinal tract and as a cause of the ensuing infrequent invasive candidiasis (110, 111). Primary fluconazole resistance has been reported in patients with severe neutropenia (112, 113). Candidemia due to *C. krusei* has been associated with prior exposure to fluconazole (95, 114, 115).

6.3 Prosthetic Devices/in vivo Biofilm

Evidence has been presented based upon in vitro, animal models and clinical studies that *Candida* organisms found in biofilm may show significant reduced susceptibility to antifungal drugs (116). The implications are self-evident, since infections involving intravascular catheters, prosthetic valves and devices invariably fail intensive antifungal therapy and require surgical removal for cure. Clinical failure may also be due to failure of the antifungal drug to penetrate the biofilm and cell density of yeast cells found within the biofilm (117). The most important explanation for biofilm-related resistance appears to be the phenotypic and genotypic changes that are reported in biofilm containing yeast cells demonstrating in vitro antifungal resistance when compared to planktonic isotype cells. Nett et al. reported increased β-1,3 glucan content in *C. albicans* cell walls from biofilm compared to planktonic organisms thought to be responsible for polyene resistance and fluconazole resulting in limited intracellular penetration (118). It has been further suggested that biofilm-associated yeast cells are hence more susceptible to β-glucan inhibitors i.e., echinocandins (119).

6.4 Antifungal Drugs

While most of the information available on drug-induced resistance followed the use of fluconazole and ketoconazole, usually as oral agents, little is known about the potential for broader spectrum (itraconazole, voriconazole, posaconazole, caspofungin, micafungin, anidulafungin) or more active/potent in vitro drugs (voriconazole, posaconazole, echinocandins) or

Candida-cidal drugs (echinocandin) to select for less susceptible *C. albicans* or non-*albicans Candida* isolates.

Invasive infections due to amphotericin B-resistant *Candida* isolates have been increasingly reported in association with use of this agent (49, 73, 120, 121). Many *C. lusitaniae* and some *C. guilliermondii* isolates demonstrated primary resistance to amphotericin B but secondary resistance to amphotericin B appears to be uncommon. Acquired resistance associated with disseminated infections due to *C. glabrata, C. kruseii* and *C. albicans* that developed during therapy is reported (122). Resistance appears to be due to alteration or a decrease in the amount of ergosterol in the cell membrane. Yoon demonstrated in vitro, reversible switching of *C. lusitaniae* with acquired amphotericin B resistance (123). Nystatin-resistant *C. rugosa* was reported in a burn unit following extended use of prophylactic topical nystatin (124).

Data indicate that in individual patients, frequent exposure to azole may influence the emergence of non-albicans *Candida* species especially *C. glabrata* and may also select for acquired resistance in *C. albicans* strains particularly following prolonged exposure to subinhibitory azole concentrations (98, 110, 115). However, the overall effect of azoles on *Candida* species distribution and resistance development is incompletely understood (125, 126). Recently, Blott et al. reported that over an 11-year period in a single institution, the volume of fluconazole consumption did not correlate with *Candida* spp. distribution (125).

6.5 *Candida vaginitis*

In spite of widespread use and abuse of over-the-counter (OTC) imidazole antifungals, little evidence has emerged of azole resistance in *C. albicans* or selection of non-*albicans Candida* spp (127, 128). Similarly, prolonged use of long-term, low-dose (150 mg/week) fluconazole maintenance prophylaxis, in women with recurrent vulvovaginal candidiasis (RVVC) was not shown to select for non-*albicans Candida* spp. or to induce azole-resistant *C. albicans* in a large randomized controlled trials (RCT) (129). On the other hand, in a study of HIV-positive women with RVVC receiving fluconazole, some evidence did surface of emergence of *C. glabrata* as a more frequent pathogen (130, 131).

6.6 *Azole Cross-Resistance*

Given that the azole class of antifungal agents share a common mechanism of action in most cases of resistance, concerns for development of cross-resistance are justified.

When selecting antifungal treatment, it is essential to establish whether the patient has received previous antifungal therapy because patients may harbor *Candida* species resistant to multiple azole agents (132–134). Both in vitro and clinical studies have clearly demonstrated high frequency of azole-cross-resistance (135). Most of the early studies indicated cross-resistance to itraconazole, ketoconazole, and other imidazoles in isolates resistant to fluconazole (136). Most of the strains concerned were fluconazole-resistant isolates of *C. albicans* obtained from patients with advanced AIDS and refractory OPC (137, 138), i.e., mucosal candidiasis but others have reported cross-resistance in virtually all species of *Candida* exposed to non-fluconazole azoles e.g., itraconazole, ketoconazole (132, 133, 139, 140). Moreover, resistance found to first- and second-generation azoles may extend, even in the absence of exposure, to newer triazoles; voriconazole and posaconazole either as absolute resistance or more frequently as higher MIC values (136, 141–144). In general, fluconazole-resistant strains had higher MICs to voriconazole and posaconazole. Nevertheless, cross-resistance varies considerably among species hence most but not all *C. parapsilosis* and *C. albicans* isolates maintain susceptibility to itraconazole, posaconazole and voriconazole despite fluconazole resistance. Cross-resistance is often more predictable for *C. tropicalis* isolates and lack of cross-resistance is seen with *C. krusei*. The development of resistance to azoles invariably requires more than one mutation, hence isolates with resistance to both fluconazole and itraconazole exhibit multiple mechanisms or types of resistance and therefore are more likely to demonstrate resistance or reduced susceptibility to newer azole agents. Cross-resistance is a very common feature in azole-resistant *C. glabrata* isolates, especially in those that are capable of expressing multiple mechanisms of resistance (145).

Susceptibility testing of 6,970 *Candida* isolates from 200 centers worldwide by Pfaller et al. revealed that *C. albicans* and *C. glabrata* strains resistant to both fluconazole and itraconazole were less susceptible to posaconazole, ravuconazole and voriconazole (59). Slightly less than 50% of *Candida* species, isolates resistant to fluconazole maintained susceptibility to newer triazole agents (146). In a recent study of azole cross-resistance, fluconazole MICs of ≤32 µg/mL predicted susceptibility, and MICs of ≥64 µg/mL predicted resistance of *Candida* spp. to voriconazole and posaconazole (146). Voriconazole was active *C. krusei* regardless of azole susceptibility. While much has been written of fluconazole prophylaxis leading to widespread azole resistance, similarly itraconazole prophylaxis was shown to be associated with cross-resistance to fluconazole (133, 147). While much of the literature on azole-cross resistance has focused on mucosal candidiasis, similarly, large surveillance surveys of *Candida* spp. causing invasive infection including candidemia, have shown evidence of cross-resistance.

6.7 Drug Pharmacokinetics, Pharmacodynamics and Resistance in Candidiasis

Andes et al. reported the impact of fluconazole dosing regimens and pharmacodynamics on resistance development in *C. albicans* (148, 149). Fluconazole regimens that produced prolonged sub-MIC concentrations were associated with resistance development. The emergence of the resistant phenotype was associated with increased expression of *CDR1*- and *CDR2*-encoded efflux pumps but not *MDR1*-encoded pumps or *ERG-II* (148, 149). In a murine systemic candidiasis model the more frequently administered dosing regimens prevented the emergence of a resistant cell phenotype.

A correlation between in vitro susceptibility and response to therapy of non-mucosal candidiasis has been demonstrated in some studies (150, 151) but not others. Clancy et al. in 2003 evaluated 32 bloodstream *Candida* isolates and concluded that the geometric mean of MIC and the fluconazole dose/MIC ratio predicted clinical failure (152). Inadequate dosing of fluconazole (≤ 200 mg/d) and ratio <50 correlated with therapeutic failure, but not necessarily with resistance development.

7 Refractory Candidiasis: Clinical Resistance Syndromes and Their Management

7.1 Oropharyngeal and Esophageal Candidiasis

Refractory OPC and EC represent the most common manifestation of clinical azole resistance and failure that is supported by concomitant in vitro azole resistance. Most patients present with highly symptomatic episodes with oropharyngeal pain and debilitating dysphagia and odynophagia requiring hospitalization. The majority of patients with refractory upper gastrointestinal candidiasis have AIDS and advanced immunodeficiency. In the 1990s, the annual incidence of clinical failure of fluconazole in OPC was approximately 5% (102–104). Accordingly refractory superficial candidiasis peaked and became a major clinical problem during the decades of the 1990s prior to the availability of highly active antiretroviral therapy (HAART) (109, 153, 154). The majority of these patients have refractory disease caused by *C. albicans* (155). Only a minority have non-*albicans Candida* spp. usually *C. glabrata,* strains of which are usually resistant in vitro to fluconazole. Resistant strains of *C. albicans* and *C. glabrata* are frequently, but not invariably, cross-resistant

to itraconazole and ketoconazole (156). Refractory mucosal candidiasis has also been reportedly associated with *C. tropicalis* and *C. krusei* (5). In the absence of co-infection with non-*albicans Candida* species, refractory candidiasis is seen with both in vitro resistant and sensitive *C. albicans*. The reason for treatment failure caused by azole-sensitive *C. albicans* is usually the result of non-compliance with therapy drug underdosing or drug interactions. Another major factor is simply advanced immunodeficiency. With refractory esophagitis, it is important to exclude concomitant pathology such as CMV or HSV esophagitis. Other explanations for the in vitro-in vivo discrepancy in compliant patients relates to heteroresistance in individual colonies of *Candida*, with chance selection of a "susceptible" colony. Most patients with refractory OPC and EC almost always have the usual *Candida* spp. isolates with in vitro resistance.

Finally, some experts have questioned the virulence capacity of non-*albicans Candida* species to induce OPC and EC, let alone refractory disease (5, 157). It is true that refractory candidiasis in patients with AIDS from whom NAC strains are isolated, usually represent mixed infections with co-existent *C. albicans*, however resistant disease due to *C. glabrata* in the absence of *C. albicans* is now widely accepted.

The availability of HAART was rapidly followed by a marked decline in the frequency of refractory OPC and EC (158). It was assumed that enhanced mucosal immune function was responsible for this phenomenon. However this issue is more complex in that refractory disease resolved within days and weeks of the initiation of HAART, preceding demonstrable improvement or change in CD4 lymphocyte cell-count or any other marker of CMI, suggesting that some other beneficial effects might be responsible (159). Another observation, included the disappearance of azole-resistant strains of *C. albicans* and *C. glabrata* with the reappearance of azole-sensitive strains. How was improved mucosal CMI selecting susceptible strains of *Candida*? Another more recent hypothesis relates to a direct effect of HIV structural components in directly influencing genes carried by *Candida* responsible for virulence expression including development of azole resistance. Accordingly, HIV-gp 160 and gp 41 may influence *Candida* in vitro, selecting for azole resistance (160). According to this hypothesis, mucosal viral load (HIV RNA) would enhance *Candida* virulence in situ, and finally induce or select for azole resistance. Introduction of HAART and rapid decrease in viral load, before immune recovery, would explain early resolution of refractory mucosal candidiasis and re-emergence of azole-susceptible strains. Therapeutic protease inhibitors may further reduce *Candida* virulence by inhibiting fungal secretory aspartyl proteinases (161).

It follows that in the post-HAART era, the frequency of refractory disease as well as in vitro azole resistance declined substantially. The majority of patients with chronic and refractory disease are usually non-compliant AIDS patients infected with susceptible *C. albicans*. In a study of in-vitro susceptibility of oral isolates in the HAART era, Tacconelli showed a reduction in azole resistance from 37 to 7% (162). The explanation for the reduced or diminished at-risk population is thought to relate to reduced fluconazole exposure i.e., fewer low-dose regimens and less continuous long-term therapy, however, this hypothesis is unproven. Barchiesi et al. reported that most patients on HAART are colonized by strains of *C. albicans* susceptible to fluconazole (93% sensitive) (163). Most cases of OPC in the HAART era are caused by fluconazole-sensitive *C. albicans*.

A high prevalence of non-*albicans Candida* yeast (*C. albicans* 49%, *C. glabrata* 24%) with frequent resistance to fluconazole and itraconazole has also been reported in patients with advanced cancer, especially head and neck malignancy (164, 165). Another small but critically important patient population includes patients with the genetic variety of chronic mucocutaneous candidiasis such as autoimmune-polyendocrinopathy-candidiasis-ectodermal dystrophy (APECED) patients (166). Frequent decreased susceptibility of *C. albicans* to fluconazole is a common complication of prolonged fluconazole use in this population.

7.1.1 Treatment

Refractory Oropharyngeal Candidiasis

Clinical management requires evaluation and determination of etiological mechanisms responsible for clinical resistance, including CD4 count, compliance with HAART therapy, previous OPC and exposure to azoles, usually fluconazole (167). Finally, clinical resistance implies failure to respond despite adequate delivery of a tolerable therapeutic concentration of drugs. Once in vitro resistance is suspected, cultures are obtained and susceptibility of the responsible organisms is determined. Most commonly, *C. albicans* is present, sometimes together with a second species usually *C. glabrata*. While awaiting microbiology and susceptibility results, treatment is initiated. Therapeutic strategies are listed in Table 5. Initial options include progressively increasing doses of oral fluconazole from 100 to 400 mg/day, including fluconazole suspension (168) and Swish-and-swallow amphotericin B suspension (100 mg/mL, taken as 1 mL qid) (102–104, 169–171). Although cross-resistance with other triazoles is common, in the event of retained itraconazole sensitivity, itraconazole suspension (10 mg/mL, taken as 10 mL bid) is often effective, although usually on a temporary basis only (135, 172, 173). In the final analysis, in the absence of dramatically reversing the patient's immune status with effective HAART therapy, one

Table 5 Therapy of fluconazole-refractory oropharyngeal and esophageal candidiasis

High doses of fluconazole tablets
Fluconazole suspension
Itraconazole capsules/suspension
Amphotericin B oral suspension
IV amphotericin B/lipid formulation
Voriconazole oral/IV
Posaconazole oral
IV caspofungin
Immunomodulation
G-CSF
GM-CSF
α-interferon

may run out of topical options. Most of the fluconazole-resistant strains of *C. albicans* are highly susceptible to oral voriconazole (174). Oral voriconazole may be the last topical or oral option, although little data is published except for refractory esophageal candidiasis.

Parenteral antifungal now becomes the last resort employing intravenous amphotericin B, caspofungin or voriconazole (175). All these options may successfully control and eradicate acute symptomatic infection. However, unless immune reconstitution follows, relapse is inevitable. Potentially the aforementioned parenteral antifungals could be given on an intermittent maintenance basis.

While HAART therapy offers a definite solution in AIDS patients, the same cannot be said of CMC patients with progressive azole resistance starting with fluconazole, and extending sequentially to itraconazole and then to voriconazole with either *C. albicans* or *C. glabrata*. Intermittent parenteral echinocandins or lipid formulation of amphotericin B will be necessary.

Refractory Esophageal Candidiasis

As for refractory OPC, clinically resistant EC is mainly seen in untreated AIDS patients with advanced immunodeficiency, with a history of sporadic previous treatment with fluconazole. Refractory, especially chronic EC is associated with a profound impact on general health leading to weight loss, malnutrition and overall reduced general health status. Oral cultures usually reveal the *Candida* species responsible for esophageal disease; recognizing that more than one resistant species may coexist. Most cases of fluconazole-resistant EC are similarly resistant to itraconazole (176). Therapeutic options now include three classes of agents. Amphotericin B deoxycholate or lipid formulations can be used parenterally in hospitalized patients and while widely recognized as efficacious, there are little published data documenting efficacy. Cost with the use of lipid formulations and toxicity associated with conventional AmB remain issues. Regardless of which formulation is chosen, low dose regimens frequently fail in patients with azole-resistant *C. albicans* and/or *C. glabrata*. Response to IV therapy is frequently slow and >0.8 mg/kg AmB or 5 mg/kg of lipid AmB should be used.

Fortunately, additional less toxic options now exist in the form of oral/IV voriconazole 4 mg/kg bid or IV caspofungin 50 mg/day (177). Studies confirming similar efficacy with IV anidulafungin and micafungin daily are in press. Accordingly, caspofungin was found to have ~70% efficacy rate in treating patients with fluconazole-refractory EC (8, 175, 178, 179). No cross-resistance exists between azoles and echinocandins. Similar efficacy for refractory EC has been observed with voriconazole, also achieving ~70% response rates (180). An additional advantage over the echinocandins and polyenes exists with regard to converting parenteral voriconazole to oral therapy given the high bio-availability and absorption of this azole. The role of voriconazole in treating fluconazole-resistant *C. albicans* is still in its infancy, although in vitro studies have been completed. Numerous investigators have reported that more than 95% of fluconazole-resistant species, including *C. albicans*, *C. glabrata* and *C. krusei* are susceptible to voriconazole although the MIC_{90} values for fluconazole-resistant *Candida* isolates are considerably higher (58, 144). Table 2 shows the impact of fluconazole-resistant *C. albicans* on susceptibility to voriconazole, hence higher doses of voriconazole may well be indicated.

Regardless of the parenteral regimen selected, the dominant issue remains maintenance antifungal prophylaxis in these severely immunocompromised individuals. It cannot be emphasized sufficiently that the key to preventing further recurrences or inevitable relapses of refractory EC, lie with successful initiation of the HAART therapy. Recent studies indicated that relapse rates of EC are higher following initially successful echinocandin treatment (181). Until the HAART therapy reverses susceptibility, maintenance prophylaxis is best afforded with oral voriconazole.

7.2 Refractory Candida vaginitis (VVC)

Two forms of refractory VVC exist. In the first place, an individual episode of symptomatic vaginitis may not respond to conventional topical or oral antifungal therapy. The other form of refractory disease is found in a larger population of women with frequently recurring episodes of relapsing symptomatic vaginitis although each individual episode responds to conventional therapy (RVVC).

Failure to achieve clinical improvement and symptom resolution, i.e., azole-resistant vaginal *C. albicans* is extremely uncommon and has only occasionally been reported in either HIV-positive or -negative women (182). It is actually remarkable that resistance is not more frequent given the widespread use of low-dosage fluconazole as a single-dose therapy or once-weekly maintenance prophylaxis for RVVC. Nevertheless any patient with acute *Candida vaginitis*, failing to improve with a standard regimen of oral or topical azoles, with persistent symptoms, positive microscopy and cultures should be treated with topical boric acid 600 mg daily for 14 days. At the same time, the *C. albicans* isolate should be sent for azole susceptibility testing. As mentioned above, unresponsive *C. albicans* vaginitis is extremely rare. The same cannot be said for acute *C. glabrata* vaginitis which responds to azole agents with a 50% rate only (183). Acute *C. glabrata* vaginitis should be treated with topical boric acid 600 mg suppositories daily for 11–21 days with an anticipated clinical and mycological response rate of ~70% (183). Higher cure rates (>90%) can be obtained with topical 17% flucytosine intravaginal cream, 5 g nightly for 14 days, although the cream must be compounded and is not widely available, hence is expensive (183, 184). High cure rates also follow daily intravaginal amphotericin B 50 mg suppository for 14 days or in combination with topical flucytosine (185).

Acute vaginitis due to *C. krusei* although rare, will not surprisingly fail to respond to oral fluconazole, due to innate or primary resistance (186). Occasionally patients may respond to oral itraconazole or topical miconazole or clotrimazole prescribed for 14 days. *C. krusei* is also resistant to flucytosine and hence vaginitis due to this species is often extremely difficult to control.

It should be emphasized that refractory acute vaginitis is extremely rare, although busy practitioners might not agree. This is because of incorrect diagnosis on the part of practitioners who treat vaginitis on an empirical basis, invariably failing to measure pH, perform microscopy and obtain a vaginal culture. Several studies have confirmed the poor diagnostic acumen of practitioners. Self-diagnosis by women is no better. All other species of *Candida* can cause vaginitis, but tend to respond rapidly to azole therapy.

Much more common and affecting millions of women, in their child-bearing decades worldwide, is recurrent *Candida vaginitis* (RVVC), thought to affect 6–8 million women in the US Under these circumstances recurring episodes of vaginitis respond appropriately to antifungal therapy regardless of route, only for symptoms and signs to recur within a month or two but rarely monthly (187). RVVC is mostly caused by azole-sensitive *C. albicans* (>90%) and less commonly by *C. glabrata* (5%). RVVC is not a manifestation of drug resistance but of host factors that predispose to genital tract yeast colonization and a host immune response hyperreactivity to *Candida* antigens (187). RVVC is best controlled by fluconazole maintenance prophylaxis administered once weekly for 6 or more months (129), although other forms of suppressive azole therapy are effective but less convenient (188, 189). Boric acid has also been used effectively (190).

7.3 Refractory Candidemia and Disseminated Candidiasis

The incidence of bloodstream infections (BSI) due to *Candida* spp. has increased worldwide, with accompanying significant mortality. Fortunately, in parallel with this increase has been an increase in the therapeutic armamentarium for candidemia (Table 6). The purpose of this chapter is not to review management of candidemia, see reviews (77, 114, 191). Drug resistance is monitored by a variety of study organizations in multiple countries. Perhaps the most comprehensive antifungal susceptibility monitoring organization is the SENTRY system receiving more than 2,000 bloodstream *Candida* isolates annually from all over the world (58). Compiled data are shown in Table 7. Nevertheless, given the proportional and occasionally found absolute increase in cases of invasive candidiasis and candidemia due

Table 6 First-line antifungal drug therapy of candidemia (parenteral)

Amphotericin B (conventional-desoxycholate)
Lipid formulation AmB
Fluconazole (400 mg/d)
Fluconazole (800 mg/d)
Itraconazole
Voriconazole
Caspofungin
Micafungin
Anidulafungin
Amphotericin B + flucytosine
Amphotericin B + fluconazole

to non-albicans *Candida* species especially *C. glabrata*; together with the availability of safe and predictable effective echinocandins, guidelines from national and international Infectious Diseases societies have recently been issued which acknowledge the reduced azole susceptibility of non-albicans *Candida* species. Hence until information of the identity of the *Candida* species responsible for the bloodstream infection is available, echinocandins are considered drugs of first choice to be prescribed.

7.3.1 C. albicans

Despite the widespread use of fluconazole over the last 15 years, fluconazole resistance in *C. albicans* isolates remains below 5%, with no evidence of a progressive increased resistance with time or association with a specific geographic area (59). Hence candidemia due to drug-resistant *C. albicans* is rare, but has been rarely reported in patients with hematologic malignancy (98). *C. albicans* is no longer the most prevalent *Candida* species responsible for BSI but rarely is drug resistance a management issue. Should an azole-resistant *C. albicans* isolate be responsible for the candidemia the clinical manifestations include persistent candidemia on fluconazole therapy, relapsing candidemia or possibly increased mortality and finally breakthrough candidemia. In the last decade, results of at lease five randomized prospective controlled studies have been published involving fluconazole and other antifungal drugs (48, 192–196).

Table 7 Species Distribution of Candida from Cases of Invasive Candidiasis

Species	% of total no. of cases[a,b]					
	1997–1998	1999	2000	2001	2002	2003
C. albicans	73.3	69.8	68.1	65.4	61.4	62.3
C. glabrata	11.0	9.7	9.5	11.1	10.7	12.0
C. tropicalis	4.6	5.3	7.2	7.5	7.4	7.5
C. parapsilosis	4.2	4.9	5.6	6.9	6.6	7.3
C. krusei	1.7	2.2	3.2	2.5	2.6	2.7
C. guilliermondii	0.5	0.8	0.8	0.7	1.0	0.8
C. lusitaniae	0.5	0.5	0.5	0.6	0.5	0.6
C. kefyr	0.2	0.4	0.5	0.4	0.4	0.5
C. rugosa	0.03	0.03	0.2	0.7	0.6	0.4
C. famata	0.08	0.2	0.5	0.2	0.4	0.3
C. inconspicua			0.08	0.1	0.2	0.3
C. norvegensis			0.08	0.1	0.07	0.1
C. dubliniensis			0.01	0.08	0.1	0.05
C. lipolytica			0.06	0.06	0.06	0.08
C. zeylanoides			0.03	0.08	0.02	0.04
C. pelliculosa				0.06	0.05	0.04
Candida spp.[c]	3.9	6.0	3.7	3.3	7.9	4.9
Total no. of cases	22,533	20,998	11,698	21,804	24,680	33,002

[a] Data compiled from the ARTEMIS DISK Surveillance Program, 1997 to 2003 (221).
[b] Includes all specimen types and all hospitals from a total of 127 different institutions in 39 countries.
[c] *Candida* species not otherwise identified.

Attempts have been made to correlate clinical outcome with in vitro MICs. In none of the studies, has *C. albicans* antifungal resistance, specifically fluconazole emerged as a cause of drug failure (48, 192). The lack of fluconazole resistance in *C. albicans* BSI isolates after all these years remains reassuring, but the altered epidemiology is less so. In contrast in other studies, correlation between in vitro susceptibility and response to fluconazole therapy has been demonstrated, but rarely is persistent fungemia due to azole-resistant *C. albicans* but rather due to non-albicans *Candida* species (197).

7.3.2 *C. glabrata*

As evident in Table 3, candidemia due to *C. glabrata* has increased especially in North America and Europe. Fluconazole resistance in bloodstream isolates is evident in 7–10% of strains, with an addition of 27–30% of isolates considered S-DD implying reduced fluconazole susceptibility of *C. glabrata* isolates. Accordingly only 60–70% of *C. glabrata* bloodstream isolates are highly susceptible to fluconazole. Several studies involving *C. glabrata* have shown a similar susceptibility pattern (58, 60). In spite of the in vitro numbers, documented failure or suboptimal response to fluconazole and other antifungals have not been forthcoming in some studies but are impressively present in others (197). The explanation for this phenomenon is not apparent, but may simply reflect small numbers of patients with *C. glabrata* fungemia i.e., published studies have lacked the power to show any differences in outcome by *Candida* species.

Supporting the in vitro data are both anecdotal case reports of fluconazole failure to eradicate *C. glabrata* fungemia but it was responsive to parenteral polyene or echinocandin therapy as well as retrospective analysis of patients with persistent candidemia (150, 197). Accordingly, most experts would recommend avoiding any azoles, including voriconazole, initially in patients with candidemia caused by *C. glabrata* and initiate therapy with an echinocandin. In candidemia patients doing well on azoles, continued therapy with the azole would be perfectly reasonable.

8 Adjuvant Therapy for Resistant Candidiasis

The use of immune and non-immune adjuvants to treat refractory candidiasis is almost exclusively seen in patients with AIDS or chronic mucocutaneous candidiasis (CMC). Even with the latest generation of azoles (voriconazole, posaconazole) polyene and caspofungin use, refractory disease is still reported due to resistant *C. albicans, C. glabrata* and rarely other *Candida* species. There have been anecdotal successes reported with immunostimulators, mainly recombinant human granulocyte or macrophage colony-stimulating factor G-CSF or (rhu GM-CSF) (198, 199). Also, interferon gamma has occasionally been given (200). Unfortunately, investigators tend to publish only successful therapeutic endeavors and failures are more frequent (200, 201). Even so, long term use and success of these growth factors, especially associated with CMC, has not been forthcoming. The use of these agents, given these expenses, requires the performance of randomized controlled studies which are unlikely given the current infrequency of these refractory cases. The value of GM-CSF in invasive candidiasis has not been demonstrated but may have a role in persistently neutropenic patients. Monoclonal antibodies were shown to prevent disseminated candidiasis in a mouse model and has been the bases for vaccine development. Likewise, the administration of anti-*Candida* heat-shock antibodies may have an adjuvant role together with antifungals for resistant or refractory candidemia.

9 Prevention of Antifungal Resistance in *Candida* Species

In general standard principles of infection control that apply to all microorganisms and particularly nosocomial infections should be applied to prevent antifungal resistance.

Avoidance of prophylactic or suppressive therapy and a preference for repeated short course of azoles for OPC in the late stages of AIDS is an attractive but unproved measure for delaying the appearance of azole resistance. In a recent study conducted in patients with recurrent OPC and AIDS, episodic fluconazole therapy was compared to continuous fluconazole therapy aimed at evaluating likelihood of inducing fluconazole resistance and refractory oropharyngeal candidiasis (99). The study failed to show a difference in the two arms with regard to selection or induction of azole resistance. This somewhat disappointing result may reflect the fact that the study was conducted during the HAART era with relatively few individuals presenting with refractory mucosal disease, with advanced immunodeficiency and unavailability of HAART therapy. The outcome of the study is in sharp contrast to the clinical experience obtained in the pre-HAART era.

It goes without saying, that all unnecessary use of azoles should be avoided, whether as prophylaxis or therapy. Many clinicians prescribe a lower than recommended prophylactic dose of oral fluconazole in neutropenic patients i.e., 100 mg vs. 400 mg daily. To date, no evidence has emerged of increased fluconazole resistance as a specific consequence of this reduced daily dose. Nevertheless, many experts advise against use of azole prophylaxis in neutropenia of short duration. Paterson suggested that combining oral amphotericin B with azoles may prevent the emergence of resistant *Candida* species in neutropenic patients; however oral amphotericin B is poorly tolerated and non-compliance is common (202).

Studies have indicated that most *Candida* species are carried and readily transferred manually by nursing physicians and other medical personnel (203). Accordingly, adherence to strict hand washing principles applies equally to *Candida* and specifically the transfer of resistant strains of *C. albicans* and other *Candida* species (204, 205). In particular, *C. parapsilosis* is frequently isolated from hands in contrast to *C. glabrata* which appears to be endogenously acquired from GIT carriage only. Isolation of patients with resistant strains of *Candida* is not indicated in this era of universal precautions. Perhaps most controversial is the use of antifungal prophylaxis in selected high-risk patients in intensive care units. Several studies are currently under way to determine efficacy (206, 207).

10 Conclusion and Perspective

During the last two decades, enormous strides have been made in understanding the subcellular, molecular and genetic basis of antifungal resistance. All in all, clinically refractory candidiasis is uncommon. The explosion in clinically resistant cases of OPC and EC early in the AIDS epidemic has not stood the test of time with the arrival of antiretroviral therapy. Of course, resistant cases still occur and remain a therapeutic challenge but the majority of cases of mucosal disease are caused by azole-sensitive *Candida albicans*. There has been an increase in non-*albicans Candida* species causing invasive candidiasis. Much, but not all evidence points to widespread use of prophylactic, empirical and therapeutic use of fluconazole. Nevertheless, blood isolates of *C. albicans* remain remarkably and predictably susceptible to fluconazole and other azoles and this is a worldwide experience. There is no doubt that certain *Candida* species are less susceptible and/or resistant to fluconazole and show cross-resistance to all azoles. This species-specific (*C. krusei*, *C. glabrata*) azole resistance has a major influence in antifungal drug selection. These two species not only expose vulnerability of the azole class but require higher doses of polyenes. As such, fungal susceptibility tests are anything but routine and are infrequently and selectively used. The newer generations of azoles are often active against non-*albicans Candida* species (*C. glabrata* and *C. krusei*) and as such offer early confident broad spectrum therapy. Moreover, they are frequently active against fluconazole resistant *C. albicans*. The echinocandins have further eased the concern of azole resistance in candidiasis but time has yet to determine the potential for echinocandin-acquired resistance in candidiasis.

References

1. Edmond MB, Wallace SE, McClish DK, Pfaller MA, Jones RN, Wenzel RP. Nosocomial bloodstream infections in United States hospitals: a three-year analysis. Clin Infect Dis. 1999;29(2):239–244
2. Trick WE, Fridkin SK, Edwards JR, Hajjeh RA, Gaynes RP. Secular trend of hospital-acquired candidemia among intensive care unit patients in the United States during 1989–1999. Clin Infect Dis. 2002;35(5):627–630
3. Jarvis WR. Epidemiology of nosocomial fungal infections, with emphasis on *Candida* species. Clin Infect Dis. 1995;20(6):1526–1530
4. Kao AS, Brandt ME, Pruitt WR, Conn LA, Perkins BA, Stephens DS, et al. The epidemiology of candidemia in two United States cities: results of a population-based active surveillance. Clin Infect Dis. 1999;29(5):1164–1170
5. Baily GG, Perry FM, Denning DW, Mandal BK. Fluconazole-resistant candidosis in an HIV cohort. AIDS. 1994;8(6):787–792
6. Feigal DW, Katz MH, Greenspan D, Westenhouse J, Winkelstein W, Jr, Lang W, et al. The prevalence of oral lesions in HIV-infected homosexual and bisexual men: three San Francisco epidemiological cohorts. AIDS. 1991;5(5):519–525
7. Barchiesi F, Morbiducci V, Ancarani F, Scalise G. Emergence of oropharyngeal candidiasis caused by non-albicans species of *Candida* in HIV-infected patients. Eur J Epidemiol. 1993;9(4):455–456
8. Kontoyiannis DP, Lewis RE. Antifungal drug resistance of pathogenic fungi. Lancet. 2002;359(9312):1135–1144
9. Rowen JL, Tate JM, Nordoff N, Passarell L, McGinnis MR. Candida isolates from neonates: frequency of misidentification and reduced fluconazole susceptibility. J Clin Microbiol. 1999;37(11):3735–3737
10. Perea S, Patterson TF. Antifungal resistance in pathogenic fungi. Clin Infect Dis. 2002;35(9):1073–1080
11. Samonis G, Anaissie EJ, Rosenbaum B, Bodey GP. A model of sustained gastrointestinal colonization by *Candida albicans* in healthy adult mice. Infect Immun. 1990;58(6):1514–1517
12. Yeo E, Alvarado T, Fainstein V, Bodey GP. Prophylaxis of oropharyngeal candidiasis with clotrimazole. J Clin Oncol. 1985;3(12):1668–1671
13. Klein RS, Harris CA, Small CB, Moll B, Lesser M, Friedland GH. Oral candidiasis in high-risk patients as the initial manifestation of the acquired immunodeficiency syndrome. N Engl J Med. 1984;311(6):354–358
14. Coleman DC, Bennett DE, Sullivan DJ, Gallagher PJ, Henman MC, Shanley DB, et al. Oral *Candida* in HIV infection and AIDS: new perspectives/new approaches. Crit Rev Microbiol. 1993;19(2):61–82
15. Hay RJ, Clayton YM. Fluconazole in the management of patients with chronic mucocutaneous candidosis. Br J Dermatol. 1988;119(5):683–684
16. Horsburgh CR, Jr, Kirkpatrick CH. Long-term therapy of chronic mucocutaneous candidiasis with ketoconazole: experience with twenty-one patients. Am J Med. 1983;74(1B):23–29
17. Sobel JD, Faro S, Force RW, Foxman B, Ledger WJ, Nyirjesy PR, et al. Vulvovaginal candidiasis: epidemiologic, diagnostic, and therapeutic considerations. Am J Obstet Gynecol. 1998;178(2):203–211
18. Beck-Sague C, Jarvis WR. Secular trends in the epidemiology of nosocomial fungal infections in the United States, 1980–1990 National Nosocomial Infections. Surveillance System. J Infect Dis. 1993;167(5):1247–1251
19. Fridkin SK, Jarvis WR. Epidemiology of nosocomial fungal infections. Clin Microbiol Rev. 1996;9(4):499–511

20. Fraser VJ, Jones M, Dunkel J, Storfer S, Medoff G, Dunagan WC. Candidemia in a tertiary care hospital: epidemiology, risk factors, and predictors of mortality. Clin Infect Dis. 1992;15(3): 414–421

21. Fisher-Hoch SP, Hutwagner L. Opportunistic candidiasis: an epidemic of the 1980s. Clin Infect Dis. 1995;21(4):897–904

22. Rangel-Frausto MS, Wiblin T, Blumberg HM, Saiman L, Patterson J, Rinaldi M, et al. National epidemiology of mycoses survey (NEMIS): variations in rates of bloodstream infections due to *Candida* species in seven surgical intensive care units and six neonatal intensive care units. Clin Infect Dis. 1999;29(2):253–258

23. McNeil MM, Nash SL, Hajjeh RA, Phelan MA, Conn LA, Plikaytis BD, et al. Trends in mortality due to invasive mycotic diseases in the United States, 1980–1997. Clin Infect Dis. 2001;33(5):641–647

24. Wenzel RP, Edmond MB. Severe sepsis-national estimates. Crit Care Med. 2001;29(7):1472–1474

25. Blumberg HM, Jarvis WR, Soucie JM, Edwards JE, Patterson JE, Pfaller MA, et al. Risk factors for candidal bloodstream infections in surgical intensive care unit patients: the NEMIS prospective multicenter study. The National Epidemiology of Mycosis Survey. Clin Infect Dis. 2001;33(2):177–186

26. Bross J, Talbot GH, Maislin G, Hurwitz S, Strom BL. Risk factors for nosocomial candidemia: a case-control study in adults without leukemia. Am J Med. 1989;87(6):614–620

27. Pappas PG, Rex JH, Lee J, Hamill RJ, Larsen RA, Powderly W, et al. A prospective observational study of candidemia: epidemiology, therapy, and influences on mortality in hospitalized adult and pediatric patients. Clin Infect Dis. 2003;37(5):634–643

28. Gudlaugsson O, Gillespie S, Lee K, Vande Berg J, Hu J, Messer S, et al. Attributable mortality of nosocomial candidemia, revisited. Clin Infect Dis. 2003;37(9):1172–1177

29. Wey SB, Mori M, Pfaller MA, Woolson RF, Wenzel RP. Hospital-acquired candidemia. The attributable mortality and excess length of stay. Arch Intern Med. 1988;148(12):2642–2645

30. Rentz AM, Halpern MT, Bowden R. The impact of candidemia on length of hospital stay, outcome, and overall cost of illness. Clin Infect Dis. 1998;27(4):781–788

31. Girmenia C, Martino P, De Bernardis F, Gentile G, Boccanera M, Monaco M, et al. Rising incidence of *Candida parapsilosis* fungemia in patients with hematologic malignancies: clinical aspects, predisposing factors, and differential pathogenicity of the causative strains. Clin Infect Dis. 1996;23(3):506–514

32. Gumbo T, Isada CM, Hall G, Karafa MT, Gordon SM. *Candida glabrata* Fungemia. Clinical features of 139 patients. Medicine (Baltimore). 1999;78(4):220–227

33. Merz WG, Karp JE, Schron D, Saral R. Increased incidence of fungemia caused by *Candida krusei*. J Clin Microbiol. 1986;24(4):581–584

34. Ghannoum MA, Rice LB. Antifungal agents: mode of action, mechanisms of resistance, and correlation of these mechanisms with bacterial resistance. Clin Microbiol Rev. 1999;12(4):501–517

35. Masia Canuto M, Gutierrez Rodero F. Antifungal drug resistance to azoles and polyenes. Lancet Infect Dis. 2002;2(9):550–563

36. Bartizal K, Gill CJ, Abruzzo GK, Flattery AM, Kong L, Scott PM, et al. In vitro preclinical evaluation studies with the echinocandin antifungal MK-0991 (L-743,872). Antimicrob Agents Chemother. 1997;41(11):2326–2332

37. Rex JH, Pfaller MA, Galgiani JN, Bartlett MS, Espinel-Ingroff A, Ghannoum MA, et al. Development of interpretive breakpoints for antifungal susceptibility testing: conceptual framework and analysis of in vitro-in vivo correlation data for fluconazole, itraconazole, and candida infections. Subcommittee on Antifungal Susceptibility Testing of the National Committee for Clinical Laboratory Standards. Clin Infect Dis. 1997;24(2):235–247

38. Rex JH, Pfaller MA, Walsh TJ, Chaturvedi V, Espinel-Ingroff A, Ghannoum MA, et al. Antifungal susceptibility testing: practical aspects and current challenges. Clin Microbiol Rev. 2001;14(4):643–658

39. Rex JH, Pfaller MA, Rinaldi MG, Polak A, Galgiani JN. Antifungal susceptibility testing. Clin Microbiol Rev. 1993;6(4):367–381

40. Rex JH, Nelson PW, Paetznick VL, Lozano-Chiu M, Espinel-Ingroff A, Anaissie EJ. Optimizing the correlation between results of testing in vitro and therapeutic outcome in vivo for fluconazole by testing critical isolates in a murine model of invasive candidiasis. Antimicrob Agents Chemother. 1998;42(1):129–134

41. Espinel-Ingroff A, Warnock DW, Vazquez JA, Arthington-Skaggs BA. In vitro antifungal susceptibility methods and clinical implications of antifungal resistance. Med Mycol. 2000;38 Suppl 1:293–304

42. Clancy CJ, Kauffman CA, Morris A, et al. Correlation of fluconazole MIC and response to therapy for patients with candidemia due to *C. albicans* and non-*C. albicans* spp: results of a multicenter prospective study of candidemia. Proceedings of the 36th Annual Meeting of the Infectious Diseases Soceity of America. Denver, CO; 1998

43. National Committee for Clinical Laboratory Standards. Reference method for broth dilution antifungal susceptibility testing of yeasts: Approved Standards. National Committee for Clinical Laboratory Standards, Wayne, PA; 1997

44. Odds FC, Motyl M, Andrade R, Bille J, Canton E, Cuenca-Estrella M, et al. Interlaboratory comparison of results of susceptibility testing with caspofungin against *Candida* and *Aspergillus* species. J Clin Microbiol. 2004;42(8):3475–3482

45. Sobel JD, Zervos M, Reed BD, Hooton T, Soper D, Nyirjesy P, et al. Fluconazole susceptibility of vaginal isolates obtained from women with complicated *Candida vaginitis*: clinical implications. Antimicrob Agents Chemother. 2003;47(1):34–38

46. Moosa MY, Sobel JD, Elhalis H, Du W, Akins RA. Fungicidal activity of fluconazole against *Candida albicans* in a synthetic vagina-simulative medium. Antimicrob Agents Chemother. 2004;48(1):161–167

47. Clancy CJ, Nguyen MH. Correlation between in vitro susceptibility determined by E test and response to therapy with amphotericin B: results from a multicenter prospective study of candidemia. Antimicrob Agents Chemother. 1999;43(5):1289–1290

48. Rex JH, Pappas PG, Karchmer AW, Sobel J, Edwards JE, Hadley S, et al. A randomized and blinded multicenter trial of high-dose fluconazole plus placebo versus fluconazole plus amphotericin B as therapy for candidemia and its consequences in nonneutropenic subjects. Clin Infect Dis. 2003;36(10):1221–1228

49. Nguyen MH, Clancy CJ, Yu VL, Yu YC, Morris AJ, Snydman DR, et al. Do in vitro susceptibility data predict the microbiologic response to amphotericin B? Results of a prospective study of patients with *Candida fungemia*. J Infect Dis. 1998;177(2): 425–430

50. Rex JH, Cooper CR, Jr, Merz WG, Galgiani JN, Anaissie EJ. Detection of amphotericin B-resistant *Candida* isolates in a broth-based system. Antimicrob Agents Chemother. 1995;39(4): 906–909

51. Warnock DW, Johnson EM, Rogers TR. Multi-centre evaluation of the Etest method for antifungal drug susceptibility testing of *Candida* spp. and *Cryptococcus neoformans*. BSAC Working Party on Antifungal Chemotherapy. J Antimicrob Chemother. 1998;42(3):321–331

52. Pfaller MA, Messer SA, Bolmstrom A. Evaluation of E test for determining in vitro susceptibility of yeast isolates to amphotericin B. Diagn Microbiol Infect Dis. 1998;32(3):223–227

53. Arendrup M, Lundgren B, Jensen IM, Hansen BS, Frimodt-Moller N. Comparison of Etest and a tablet diffusion test with the NCCLS broth microdilution method for fluconazole and amphotericin B susceptibility testing of *Candida* isolates. J Antimicrob Chemother. 2001;47(5):521–526

54. Espinel-Ingroff A, Pfaller M, Erwin ME, Jones RN. Interlaboratory evaluation of E test method for testing antifungal susceptibilities of pathogenic yeasts to five antifungal agents by using Casitone agar and solidified RPMI 1640 medium with 2% glucose. J Clin Microbiol. 1996;34(4):848–852

55. Peyron F, Favel A, Michel-Nguyen A, Gilly M, Regli P, Bolmstrom A. Improved detection of amphotericin B-resistant isolates of *Candida lusitaniae* by E test. J Clin Microbiol. 2001;39(1):339–342

56. Johnson EM, Warnock DW. Azole drug resistance in yeasts. J Antimicrob Chemother. 1995;36(5):751–755

57. Ostrosky-Zeichner L, Rex JH, Pappas PG, Hamill RJ, Larsen RA, Horowitz HW, et al. Antifungal susceptibility survey of 2,000 bloodstream *Candida* isolates in the United States. Antimicrob Agents Chemother. 2003;47(10):3149–3154

58. Pfaller MA, Diekema DJ. Epidemiology of invasive candidiasis: a persistent public health problem. Clin Microbiol Rev. 2007;20(1):133–163

59. Pfaller MA, Diekema DJ. Twelve years of fluconazole in clinical practice: global trends in species distribution and fluconazole susceptibility of bloodstream isolates of *Candida*. Clin Microbiol Infect. 2004;10 Suppl 1:11–23

60. Pfaller MA, Diekema DJ, Jones RN, Messer SA, Hollis RJ. Trends in antifungal susceptibility of *Candida* spp. isolated from pediatric and adult patients with bloodstream infections: SENTRY Antimicrobial Surveillance Program, 1997 to 2000. J Clin Microbiol. 2002;40(3):852–856

61. Antoniadou A, Torres HA, Lewis RE, Thornby J, Bodey GP, Tarrand JP, et al. Candidemia in a tertiary care cancer center: in vitro susceptibility and its association with outcome of initial antifungal therapy. Medicine (Baltimore). 2003;82(5):309–321

62. Xu J, Ramos AR, Vilgalys R, Mitchell TG. Clonal and spontaneous origins of fluconazole resistance in *Candida albicans*. J Clin Microbiol. 2000;38(3):1214–1220

63. Xiao L, Madison V, Chau AS, Loebenberg D, Palermo RE, McNicholas PM. Three-dimensional models of wild-type and mutated forms of cytochrome P450 14alpha-sterol demethylases from *Aspergillus fumigatus* and *Candida albicans* provide insights into posaconazole binding. Antimicrob Agents Chemother. 2004;48(2):568–574

64. Hoban DJ, Zhanel GG, Karlowsky JA. In vitro susceptibilities of *Candida* and *Cryptococcus neoformans* isolates from blood cultures of neutropenic patients. Antimicrob Agents Chemother. 1999;43(6):1463–1464

65. Hazen KC, Baron EJ, Colombo AL, Girmenia C, Sanchez-Sousa A, del Palacio A, et al. Comparison of the susceptibilities of *Candida* spp. to fluconazole and voriconazole in a 4-year global evaluation using disk diffusion. J Clin Microbiol. 2003;41(12):5623–5632

66. Bodey GP, Mardani M, Hanna HA, Boktour M, Abbas J, Girgawy E, et al. The epidemiology of *Candida glabrata* and *Candida albicans* fungemia in immunocompromised patients with cancer. Am J Med. 2002;112(5):380–385

67. Fidel PL, Jr, Vazquez JA, Sobel JD. *Candida glabrata*: review of epidemiology, pathogenesis, and clinical disease with comparison to *C. albicans*. Clin Microbiol Rev. 1999;12(1):80–96

68. Safdar A, Chaturvedi V, Koll BS, Larone DH, Perlin DS, Armstrong D. Prospective, multicenter surveillance study of *Candida glabrata*: fluconazole and itraconazole susceptibility profiles in bloodstream, invasive, and colonizing strains and differences between isolates from three urban teaching hospitals in New York City (Candida Susceptibility Trends Study, 1998 to 1999). Antimicrob Agents Chemother. 2002;46(10):3268–3272

69. Ghannoum MA, Okogbule-Wonodi I, Bhat N, Sanati H. Antifungal activity of voriconazole (UK-109,496), fluconazole and amphotericin B against hematogenous *Candida krusei* infection in neutropenic guinea pig model. J Chemother. 1999;11(1):34–39

70. Imhof A, Balajee SA, Fredricks DN, Englund JA, Marr KA. Breakthrough fungal infections in stem cell transplant recipients receiving voriconazole. Clin Infect Dis. 2004;39(5):743–746

71. Stiller RL, Bennett JE, Scholer HJ, Wall M, Polak A, Stevens DA. Susceptibility to 5-fluorocytosine and prevalence of serotype in 402 *Candida albicans* isolates from the United States. Antimicrob Agents Chemother. 1982;22(3):482–487

72. Ellis D. Amphotericin B: spectrum and resistance. J Antimicrob Chemother. 2002;49 Suppl 1:7–10

73. Powderly WG, Kobayashi GS, Herzig GP, Medoff G. Amphotericin B-resistant yeast infection in severely immunocompromised patients. Am J Med. 1988;84(5):826–832

74. Nolte FS, Parkinson T, Falconer DJ, Dix S, Williams J, Gilmore C, et al. Isolation and characterization of fluconazole- and amphotericin B-resistant *Candida albicans* from blood of two patients with leukemia. Antimicrob Agents Chemother. 1997;41(1):196–199

75. Merz WG, Sandford GR. Isolation and characterization of a polyene-resistant variant of *Candida tropicalis*. J Clin Microbiol. 1979;9(6):677–680

76. Rex JH, Pfaller MA. Has antifungal susceptibility testing come of age? Clin Infect Dis. 2002;35(8):982–989

77. Pappas PG, Rex JH, Sobel JD, Filler SG, Dismukes WE, Walsh TJ, et al. Guidelines for treatment of candidiasis. Clin Infect Dis. 2004;38(2):161–189

78. Bhargava P. Amphotericin B-resistant *Candida krusei*? A comparison of standardized testing and time kill studies. 40th Interscience Confrence on Antimicrobial Agents and Chemotherapy; 2000; American Society for Microbiology, Toronto, ON, Canada; 2000

79. Sterling TR, Gasser RA, Jr, Ziegler A. Emergence of resistance to amphotericin B during therapy for *Candida glabrata* infection in an immunocompetent host. Clin Infect Dis. 1996;23(1):187–188

80. Minari A, Hachem R, Raad I. *Candida lusitaniae*: a cause of breakthrough fungemia in cancer patients. Clin Infect Dis. 2001;32(2):186–190

81. Hawkins JL, Baddour LM. *Candida lusitaniae* infections in the era of fluconazole availability. Clin Infect Dis. 2003;36(2):e14–8

82. Krcmery V, Jr, Oravcova E, Spanik S, Mrazova-Studena M, Trupl J, Kunova A, et al. Nosocomial breakthrough fungaemia during antifungal prophylaxis or empirical antifungal therapy in 41 cancer patients receiving antineoplastic chemotherapy: analysis of aetiology risk factors and outcome. J Antimicrob Chemother. 1998;41(3):373–380

83. Conly J, Rennie R, Johnson J, Farah S, Hellman L. Disseminated candidiasis due to amphotericin B-resistant *Candida albicans*. J Infect Dis. 1992;165(4):761–764

84. Pappagianis D, Collins MS, Hector R, Remington J. Development of resistance to amphotericin B in *Candida lusitaniae* infecting a human. Antimicrob Agents Chemother. 1979;16(2):123–126

85. Guinet R, Chanas J, Goullier A, Bonnefoy G, Ambroise-Thomas P. Fatal septicemia due to amphotericin B-resistant *Candida lusitaniae*. J Clin Microbiol. 1983;18(2):443–444

86. Pfaller MA, Diekema DJ, Messer SA, Hollis RJ, Jones RN. In vitro activities of caspofungin compared with those of fluconazole and itraconazole against 3,959 clinical isolates of *Candida* spp., including 157 fluconazole-resistant isolates. Antimicrob Agents Chemother. 2003;47(3):1068–1071

87. Barchiesi F, Spreghini E, Tomassetti S, Della Vittoria A, Arzeni D, Manso E, et al. Effects of caspofungin against *Candida guilliermondii* and *Candida parapsilosis*. Antimicrob Agents Chemother. 2006;50(8):2719–2727

88. Kartsonis N, Killar J, Mixson L, Hoe CM, Sable C, Bartizal K, et al. Caspofungin susceptibility testing of isolates from patients with esophageal candidiasis or invasive candidiasis: relationship of MIC to treatment outcome. Antimicrob Agents Chemother. 2005;49(9):3616–3623

89. Park S, Kelly R, Kahn JN, Robles J, Hsu MJ, Register E, et al. Specific substitutions in the echinocandin target Fks1p account for reduced susceptibility of rare laboratory and clinical *Candida* sp. isolates. Antimicrob Agents Chemother. 2005;49(8):3264–3273

90. Hakki M, Staab JF, Marr KA. Emergence of a *Candida krusei* isolate with reduced susceptibility to caspofungin during therapy. Antimicrob Agents Chemother. 2006;50(7):2522–2524

91. Cheung C, Guo Y, Gialanella P, Feldmesser M. Development of candidemia on caspofungin therapy: a case report. Infection. 2006;34(6):345–348

92. Hernandez S, Lopez-Ribot JL, Najvar LK, McCarthy DI, Bocanegra R, Graybill JR. Caspofungin resistance in *Candida albicans*: correlating clinical outcome with laboratory susceptibility testing of three isogenic isolates serially obtained from a patient with progressive *Candida esophagitis*. Antimicrob Agents Chemother. 2004;48(4):1382–1383

93. Laverdiere M, Lalonde RG, Baril JG, Sheppard DC, Park S, Perlin DS. Progressive loss of echinocandin activity following prolonged use for treatment of *Candida albicans* oesophagitis. J Antimicrob Chemother. 2006;57(4):705–708

94. Moudgal V, Little T, Boikov D, Vazquez JA. Multiechinocandin- and multiazole-resistant *Candida parapsilosis* isolates serially obtained during therapy for prosthetic valve endocarditis. Antimicrob Agents Chemother. 2005;49(2):767–769

95. Wingard JR, Merz WG, Rinaldi MG, Johnson TR, Karp JE, Saral R. Increase in *Candida krusei* infection among patients with bone marrow transplantation and neutropenia treated prophylactically with fluconazole. N Engl J Med. 1991;325(18):1274–1277

96. Wingard JR, Merz WG, Rinaldi MG, Miller CB, Karp JE, Saral R. Association of *Torulopsis glabrata* infections with fluconazole prophylaxis in neutropenic bone marrow transplant patients. Antimicrob Agents Chemother. 1993;37(9):1847–1849

97. Price MF, LaRocco MT, Gentry LO. Fluconazole susceptibilities of *Candida* species and distribution of species recovered from blood cultures over a 5-year period. Antimicrob Agents Chemother. 1994;38(6):1422–1424

98. Marr KA, White TC, van Burik JA, Bowden RA. Development of fluconazole resistance in *Candida albicans* causing disseminated infection in a patient undergoing marrow transplantation. Clin Infect Dis. 1997;25(4):908–910

99. Gleason TG, May AK, Caparelli D, Farr BM, Sawyer RG. Emerging evidence of selection of fluconazole-tolerant fungi in surgical intensive care units. Arch Surg. 1997;132(11):1197–1201; discussion 202

100. Law D, Moore CB, Denning DW. Amphotericin B resistance testing of *Candida* spp.: a comparison of methods. J Antimicrob Chemother. 1997;40(1):109–112

101. Maenza JR, Keruly JC, Moore RD, Chaisson RE, Merz WG, Gallant JE. Risk factors for fluconazole-resistant candidiasis in human immunodeficiency virus-infected patients. J Infect Dis. 1996;173(1):219–225

102. Fichtenbaum CJ, Powderly WG. Refractory mucosal candidiasis in patients with human immunodeficiency virus infection. Clin Infect Dis. 1998;26(3):556–565

103. Fichtenbaum CJ, Koletar S, Yiannoutsos C, Holland F, Pottage J, Cohn SE, et al. Refractory mucosal candidiasis in advanced human immunodeficiency virus infection. Clin Infect Dis. 2000;30(5):749–756

104. Fichtenbaum CJ, Zackin R, Rajicic N, Powderly WG, Wheat LJ, Zingman BS. Amphotericin B oral suspension for fluconazole-refractory oral candidiasis in persons with HIV infection. Adult AIDS Clinical Trials Group Study Team 295. AIDS. 2000;14(7):845–852

105. Cartledge JD, Midgley J, Gazzard BG. Non-albicans oral candidosis in HIV-positive patients. J Antimicrob Chemother. 1999;43(3):419–422

106. Goldman M. Randomized study of long-term chronic suppressive fluconazole vs. episodic fluconazole for patients with advanced HIV infection and history of oropharyngeal candidiasis. 42nd Interscience Conference on Antimicrobial Agents and Chemotherapy. American Society for Microbiology, San Diego, CA; 2002

107. Denning DW. Can we prevent azole resistance in fungi? Lancet. 1995;346(8973):454–455

108. Sobel JD, Ohmit SE, Schuman P, Klein RS, Mayer K, Duerr A, et al. The evolution of *Candida* species and fluconazole susceptibility among oral and vaginal isolates recovered from human immunodeficiency virus (HIV)-seropositive and at-risk HIV-seronegative women. J Infect Dis. 2001;183(2):286–293

109. Revankar SG, Dib OP, Kirkpatrick WR, McAtee RK, Fothergill AW, Rinaldi MG, et al. Clinical evaluation and microbiology of oropharyngeal infection due to fluconazole-resistant *Candida* in human immunodeficiency virus-infected patients. Clin Infect Dis. 1998;26(4):960–963

110. Hope W, Morton A, Eisen DP. Increase in prevalence of nosocomial non-*Candida albicans* candidaemia and the association of *Candida krusei* with fluconazole use. J Hosp Infect. 2002;50(1):56–65

111. Mahayni R, Vazquez JA, Zervos MJ. Nosocomial candidiasis: epidemiology and drug resistance. Infect Agents Dis. 1995;4(4):248–253

112. Goff DA, Koletar SL, Buesching WJ, Barnishan J, Fass RJ. Isolation of fluconazole-resistant *Candida albicans* from human immunodeficiency virus-negative patients never treated with azoles. Clin Infect Dis. 1995;20(1):77–83

113. Iwen PC, Kelly DM, Reed EC, Hinrichs SH. Invasive infection due to *Candida krusei* in immunocompromised patients not treated with fluconazole. Clin Infect Dis. 1995;20(2):342–347

114. Nguyen MH, Peacock JE, Jr, Morris AJ, Tanner DC, Nguyen ML, Snydman DR, et al. The changing face of candidemia: emergence of non-*Candida albicans* species and antifungal resistance. Am J Med. 1996;100(6):617–623

115. Abi-Said D, Anaissie E, Uzun O, Raad I, Pinzcowski H, Vartivarian S. The epidemiology of hematogenous candidiasis caused by different *Candida* species. Clin Infect Dis. 1997;24(6):1122–1128

116. Chandra J, Kuhn DM, Mukherjee PK, Hoyer LL, McCormick T, Ghannoum MA. Biofilm formation by the fungal pathogen *Candida albicans*: development, architecture, and drug resistance. J Bacteriol. 2001;183(18):5385–5394

117. Perumal P, Mekala S, Chaffin WL. Role for cell density in antifungal drug resistance in *Candida albicans* biofilms. Antimicrob Agents Chemother. 2007;51(7):2454–2463

118. Nett J, Lincoln L, Marchillo K, Massey R, Holoyda K, Hoff B, et al. Putative role of beta-1,3 glucans in *Candida albicans* biofilm resistance. Antimicrob Agents Chemother. 2007;51(2):510–520

119. Shuford JA, Rouse MS, Piper KE, Steckelberg JM, Patel R. Evaluation of caspofungin and amphotericin B deoxycholate against *Candida albicans* biofilms in an experimental intravascular catheter infection model. J Infect Dis. 2006;194(5):710–713

120. Dick JD, Merz WG, Saral R. Incidence of polyene-resistant yeasts recovered from clinical specimens. Antimicrob Agents Chemother. 1980;18(1):158–163

121. Fan-Havard P, Capano D, Smith SM, Mangia A, Eng RH. Development of resistance in *Candida* isolates from patients receiving prolonged antifungal therapy. Antimicrob Agents Chemother. 1991;35(11):2302–2305

122. White TC, Marr KA, Bowden RA. Clinical, cellular, and molecular factors that contribute to antifungal drug resistance. Clin Microbiol Rev. 1998;11(2):382–402

123. Yoon SA, Vazquez JA, Steffan PE, Sobel JD, Akins RA. High-frequency, in vitro reversible switching of *Candida lusitaniae*

clinical isolates from amphotericin B susceptibility to resistance. Antimicrob Agents Chemother. 1999;43(4):836–845

124. Dube MP, Heseltine PN, Rinaldi MG, Evans S, Zawacki B. Fungemia and colonization with nystatin-resistant *Candida rugosa* in a burn unit. Clin Infect Dis. 1994;18(1):77–82

125. Blot S, Janssens R, Claeys G, Hoste E, Buyle F, De Waele JJ, et al. Effect of fluconazole consumption on long-term trends in candidal ecology. J Antimicrob Chemother. 2006;58(2):474–477

126. Marchetti O, Bille J, Fluckiger U, Eggimann P, Ruef C, Garbino J, et al. Epidemiology of candidemia in Swiss tertiary care hospitals: secular trends, 1991 2000. Clin Infect Dis. 2004;38(3):311–320

127. Mathema B, Cross E, Dun E, Park S, Bedell J, Slade B, et al. Prevalence of vaginal colonization by drug-resistant *Candida* species in college-age women with previous exposure to over-the-counter azole antifungals. Clin Infect Dis. 2001;33(5):E23–27

128. Dorrell L, Edwards A. Vulvovaginitis due to fluconazole resistant *Candida albicans* following self treatment with non-prescribed triazoles. Sex Transm Infect. 2002;78(4):308–309

129. Sobel JD, Wiesenfeld HC, Martens M, Danna P, Hooton TM, Rompalo A, et al. Maintenance fluconazole therapy for recurrent vulvovaginal candidiasis. N Engl J Med. 2004;351(9):876–883

130. Schuman P, Sobel JD, Ohmit SE, Mayer KH, Carpenter CC, Rompalo A, et al. Mucosal candidal colonization and candidiasis in women with or at risk for human immunodeficiency virus infection. HIV Epidemiology Research Study (HERS) Group. Clin Infect Dis. 1998;27(5):1161–1167

131. Vazquez JA, Sobel JD, Peng G, Steele-Moore L, Schuman P, Holloway W, et al. Evolution of vaginal *Candida* species recovered from human immunodeficiency virus infected women receiving fluconazole prophylaxis: the emergence of *Candida glabrata*? Terry Beirn Community Programs for Clinical Research in AIDS (CPCRA). Clin Infect Dis. 1999;28(5):1025–1031

132. Myoken Y, Kyo T, Fujihara M, Sugata T, Mikami Y. Clinical significance of breakthrough fungemia caused by azole-resistant *Candida tropicalis* in patients with hematologic malignancies. Haematologica. 2004;89(3):378–380

133. Goldman M, Cloud GA, Smedema M, LeMonte A, Connolly P, McKinsey DS, et al. Does long-term itraconazole prophylaxis result in in vitro azole resistance in mucosal *Candida albicans* isolates from persons with advanced human immunodeficiency virus infection? The National Institute of Allergy and Infectious Diseases Mycoses study group. Antimicrob Agents Chemother. 2000;44(6):1585–1587

134. Muller FM, Weig M, Peter J, Walsh TJ. Azole cross-resistance to ketoconazole, fluconazole, itraconazole and voriconazole in clinical *Candida albicans* isolates from HIV-infected children with oropharyngeal candidosis. J Antimicrob Chemother. 2000;46(2):338–340

135. Cartledge JD, Midgley J, Gazzard BG. Clinically significant azole cross-resistance in *Candida* isolates from HIV-positive patients with oral candidosis. AIDS. 1997;11(15):1839–1844

136. Cuenca-Estrella M, Lee-Yang W, Ciblak MA, Arthington-Skaggs BA, Mellado E, Warnock DW, et al. Comparative evaluation of NCCLS M27-A and EUCAST broth microdilution procedures for antifungal susceptibility testing of *Candida* species. Antimicrob Agents Chemother. 2002;46(11):3644–3647

137. Vazquez JA, Lundstrom T, Dembry L, Chandrasekar P, Boikov D, Parri MB, et al. Invasive *Candida guilliermondii* infection: in vitro susceptibility studies and molecular analysis. Bone Marrow Transplant. 1995;16(6):849–853

138. Makarova NU, Pokrowsky VV, Kravchenko AV, Serebrovskaya LV, James MJ, McNeil MM, et al. Persistence of oropharyngeal *Candida albicans* strains with reduced susceptibilities to fluconazole among human immunodeficiency virus-seropositive children and adults in a long-term care facility. J Clin Microbiol. 2003;41(5):1833–1837

139. Davies A, Brailsford S, Broadley K, Beighton D. Resistance amongst yeasts isolated from the oral cavities of patients with advanced cancer. Palliat Med. 2002;16(6):527–531

140. Stevens DA, Stevens JA. Cross-resistance phenotypes of fluconazole-resistant *Candida* species: results with 655 clinical isolates with different methods. Diagn Microbiol Infect Dis. 1996;26(3–4):145–148

141. Cuenca-Estrella M, Diaz-Guerra TM, Mellado E, Monzon A, Rodriguez-Tudela JL. Comparative in vitro activity of voriconazole and itraconazole against fluconazole-susceptible and fluconazole-resistant clinical isolates of *Candida* species from Spain. Eur J Clin Microbiol Infect Dis. 1999;18(6): 432–435

142. Cuenca-Estrella M, Mellado E, Diaz-Guerra TM, Monzon A, Rodriguez-Tudela JL. Susceptibility of fluconazole-resistant clinical isolates of *Candida* spp. to echinocandin LY303366, itraconazole and amphotericin B. J Antimicrob Chemother. 2000;46(3):475–477

143. Bachmann SP, Patterson TF, Lopez-Ribot JL. In vitro activity of caspofungin (MK-0991) against *Candida albicans* clinical isolates displaying different mechanisms of azole resistance. J Clin Microbiol. 2002;40(6):2228–2230

144. Pelletier R, Loranger L, Marcotte H, De Carolis E. Voriconazole and fluconazole susceptibility of *Candida* isolates. J Med Microbiol. 2002;51(6):479–483

145. Sanguinetti M, Posteraro B, Fiori B, Ranno S, Torelli R, Fadda G. Mechanisms of azole resistance in clinical isolates of *Candida glabrata* collected during a hospital survey of antifungal resistance. Antimicrob Agents Chemother. 2005;49(2):668–679

146. Pfaller MA, Diekema DJ. Azole antifungal drug cross-resistance: mechanisms, epidemiology, and clinical significance. J Invasive Fungal Infect. 2007;1(3):74–92

147. McKinsey DS, Wheat LJ, Cloud GA, Pierce M, Black JR, Bamberger DM, et al. Itraconazole prophylaxis for fungal infections in patients with advanced human immunodeficiency virus infection: randomized, placebo-controlled, double-blind study. National Institute of Allergy and Infectious Diseases Mycoses Study Group. Clin Infect Dis. 1999;28(5):1049–1056

148. Andes D, Lepak A, Nett J, Lincoln L, Marchillo K. In vivo fluconazole pharmacodynamics and resistance development in a previously susceptible *Candida albicans* population examined by microbiologic and transcriptional profiling. Antimicrob Agents Chemother. 2006;50(7):2384–2394

149. Andes D, Forrest A, Lepak A, Nett J, Marchillo K, Lincoln L. Impact of antimicrobial dosing regimen on evolution of drug resistance in vivo: fluconazole and *Candida albicans*. Antimicrob Agents Chemother. 2006;50(7):2374–2383

150. Kovacicova G, Krupova Y, Lovaszova M, Roidova A, Trupl J, Liskova A, et al. Antifungal susceptibility of 262 bloodstream yeast isolates from a mixed cancer and non-cancer patient population: is there a correlation between in-vitro resistance to fluconazole and the outcome of fungemia? J Infect Chemother. 2000;6(4):216–221

151. Lee SC, Fung CP, Huang JS, Tsai CJ, Chen KS, Chen HY, et al. Clinical correlates of antifungal macrodilution susceptibility test results for non-AIDS patients with severe *Candida* infections treated with fluconazole. Antimicrob Agents Chemother. 2000;44(10):2715–2718

152. Clancy CJ, Yu VL, Morris AJ, Snydman DR, Nguyen MH. Fluconazole MIC and the fluconazole dose/MIC ratio correlate with therapeutic response among patients with candidemia. Antimicrob Agents Chemother. 2005;49(8):3171–3177

153. Maenza JR, Merz WG, Romagnoli MJ, Keruly JC, Moore RD, Gallant JE. Infection due to fluconazole-resistant *Candida* in patients with AIDS: prevalence and microbiology. Clin Infect Dis. 1997;24(1):28–34

154. Laguna F, Rodriguez-Tudela JL, Martinez-Suarez JV, Polo R, Valencia E, Diaz-Guerra TM, et al. Patterns of fluconazole susceptibility in isolates from human immunodeficiency virus-infected patients with oropharyngeal candidiasis due to *Candida albicans*. Clin Infect Dis. 1997;24(2):124–130

155. Quereda C, Polanco AM, Giner C, Sanchez-Sousa A, Pereira E, Navas E, et al. Correlation between in vitro resistance to fluconazole and clinical outcome of oropharyngeal candidiasis in HIV-infected patients. Eur J Clin Microbiol Infect Dis. 1996;15(1):30–37

156. Vazquez JA. Therapeutic options for the management of oropharyngeal and esophageal candidiasis in HIV/AIDS patients. HIV Clin Trials. 2000;1(1):47–59

157. Sangeorzan JA, Bradley SF, He X, Zarins LT, Ridenour GL, Tiballi RN, et al. Epidemiology of oral candidiasis in HIV-infected patients: colonization, infection, treatment, and emergence of fluconazole resistance. Am J Med. 1994;97(4):339–346

158. Martins MD, Lozano-Chiu M, Rex JH. Declining rates of oropharyngeal candidiasis and carriage of *Candida albicans* associated with trends toward reduced rates of carriage of fluconazole-resistant *C. albicans* in human immunodeficiency virus-infected patients. Clin Infect Dis. 1998;27(5):1291–1294

159. Zingman BS. Resolution of refractory AIDS-related mucosal candidiasis after initiation of didanosine plus saquinavir. N Engl J Med. 1996;334(25):1674–1675

160. Gruber A, Lukasser-Vogl E, Borg-von Zepelin M, Dierich MP, Wurzner R. Human immunodeficiency virus type 1 gp160 and gp41 binding to *Candida albicans* selectively enhances candidal virulence in vitro. J Infect Dis. 1998;177(4):1057–1063

161. Cassone A, De Bernardis F, Torosantucci A, Tacconelli E, Tumbarello M, Cauda R. In vitro and in vivo anticandidal activity of human immunodeficiency virus protease inhibitors. J Infect Dis. 1999;180(2):448–453

162. Tacconelli E, Bertagnolio S, Posteraro B, Tumbarello M, Boccia S, Fadda G, et al. Azole susceptibility patterns and genetic relationship among oral *Candida* strains isolated in the era of highly active antiretroviral therapy. J Acquir Immune Defic Syndr. 2002;31(1):38–44

163. Barchiesi F, Maracci M, Radi B, Arzeni D, Baldassarri I, Giacometti A, et al. Point prevalence, microbiology and fluconazole susceptibility patterns of yeast isolates colonizing the oral cavities of HIV-infected patients in the era of highly active antiretroviral therapy. J Antimicrob Chemother. 2002;50(6):999–1002

164. Bagg J, Sweeney MP, Lewis MA, Jackson MS, Coleman D, Al MA, et al. High prevalence of non-albicans yeasts and detection of anti-fungal resistance in the oral flora of patients with advanced cancer. Palliat Med. 2003;17(6):477–481

165. Silverman S, Jr, Luangjarmekorn L, Greenspan D. Occurrence of oral *Candida* in irradiated head and neck cancer patients. J Oral Med. 1984;39(4):194–196

166. Rautemaa R, Richardson M, Pfaller M, Koukila-Kahkola P, Perheentupa J, Saxen H. Decreased susceptibility of *Candida albicans* to azole antifungals: a complication of long-term treatment in autoimmune polyendocrinopathy-candidiasis-ectodermal dystrophy (APECED) patients. J Antimicrob Chemother. 2007;60(4):889–892

167. Darouiche RO. Oropharyngeal and esophageal candidiasis in immunocompromised patients: treatment issues. Clin Infect Dis. 1998;26(2):259–272; quiz 73–74

168. Martins MD, Rex JH. Fluconazole suspension for oropharyngeal candidiasis unresponsive to tablets. Ann Intern Med. 1997;126(4):332–333

169. Dewsnup DH, Stevens DA. Efficacy of oral amphotericin B in AIDS patients with thrush clinically resistant to fluconazole. J Med Vet Mycol. 1994;32(5):389–393

170. Grim SA, Smith KM, Romanelli F, Ofotokun I. Treatment of azole-resistant oropharyngeal candidiasis with topical amphotericin B. Ann Pharmacother. 2002;36(9):1383–1386

171. Nguyen MT, Weiss PJ, LaBarre RC, Miller LK, Oldfield EC, Wallace MR. Orally administered amphotericin B in the treatment of oral candidiasis in HIV-infected patients caused by azole-resistant *Candida albicans*. AIDS. 1996;10(14):1745–1747

172. Cartledge JD, Midgley J, Youle M, Gazzard BG. Itraconazole cyclodextrin solution – effective treatment for HIV-related candidosis unresponsive to other azole therapy. J Antimicrob Chemother. 1994;33(5):1071–1073

173. Eichel M, Just-Nubling G, Helm EB, Stille W. Itraconazole suspension in the treatment of HIV-infected patients with fluconazole-resistant oropharyngeal candidiasis and esophagitis. Mycoses. 1996;39 Suppl 1:102–106

174. Ruhnke M, Schmidt-Westhausen A, Trautmann M. In vitro activities of voriconazole (UK-109,496) against fluconazole-susceptible and -resistant *Candida albicans* isolates from oral cavities of patients with human immunodeficiency virus infection. Antimicrob Agents Chemother. 1997;41(3):575–577

175. Arathoon EG, Gotuzzo E, Noriega LM, Berman RS, DiNubile MJ, Sable CA. Randomized, double-blind, multicenter study of caspofungin versus amphotericin B for treatment of oropharyngeal and esophageal candidiases. Antimicrob Agents Chemother. 2002;46(2):451–457

176. Barbaro G, Barbarini G, Calderon W, Grisorio B, Alcini P, Di Lorenzo G. Fluconazole versus itraconazole for *Candida esophagitis* in acquired immunodeficiency syndrome. *Candida esophagitis*. Gastroenterology. 1996;111(5):1169–1177

177. Hegener P, Troke PF, Fatkenheuer G, Diehl V, Ruhnke M. Treatment of fluconazole-resistant candidiasis with voriconazole in patients with AIDS. AIDS. 1998;12(16):2227–2228

178. Villanueva A, Arathoon EG, Gotuzzo E, Berman RS, DiNubile MJ, Sable CA. A randomized double-blind study of caspofungin versus amphotericin for the treatment of candidal esophagitis. Clin Infect Dis. 2001;33(9):1529–1535

179. Villanueva A, Gotuzzo E, Arathoon EG, Noriega LM, Kartsonis NA, Lupinacci RJ, et al. A randomized double-blind study of caspofungin versus fluconazole for the treatment of esophageal candidiasis. Am J Med. 2002;113(4):294–299

180. Ally R, Schurmann D, Kreisel W, Carosi G, Aguirrebengoa K, Dupont B, et al. A randomized, double-blind, double-dummy, multicenter trial of voriconazole and fluconazole in the treatment of esophageal candidiasis in immunocompromised patients. Clin Infect Dis. 2001;33(9):1447–1454

181. Krause DS, Simjee AE, van Rensburg C, Viljoen J, Walsh TJ, Goldstein BP, et al. A randomized, double-blind trial of anidulafungin versus fluconazole for the treatment of esophageal candidiasis. Clin Infect Dis. 2004;39(6):770–775

182. Sobel JD, Vazquez JA. Symptomatic vulvovaginitis due to fluconazole-resistant *Candida albicans* in a female who was not infected with human immunodeficiency virus. Clin Infect Dis. 1996;22(4):726–727

183. Sobel JD, Chaim W, Nagappan V, Leaman D. Treatment of vaginitis caused by *Candida glabrata*: use of topical boric acid and flucytosine. Am J Obstet Gynecol. 2003;189(5):1297–1300

184. Horowitz BJ. Topical flucytosine therapy for chronic recurrent *Candida tropicalis* infections. J Reprod Med. 1986;31(9):821–824

185. White DJ, Habib AR, Vanthuyne A, Langford S, Symonds M. Combined topical flucytosine and amphotericin B for refractory vaginal *Candida glabrata* infections. Sex Transm Infect. 2001;77(3):212–213

186. Singh S, Sobel JD, Bhargava P, Boikov D, Vazquez JA. Vaginitis due to *Candida krusei*: epidemiology, clinical aspects, and therapy. Clin Infect Dis. 2002;35(9):1066–1070

187. Sobel JD. Pathogenesis and treatment of recurrent vulvovaginal candidiasis. Clin Infect Dis. 1992;14 Suppl 1:S148–S153

188. Spinillo A, Colonna L, Piazzi G, Baltaro F, Monaco A, Ferrari A. Managing recurrent vulvovaginal candidiasis. Intermittent prevention with itraconazole. J Reprod Med. 1997;42(2):83–87

189. Fong IW. The value of chronic suppressive therapy with itraconazole versus clotrimazole in women with recurrent vaginal candidiasis. Genitourin Med. 1992;68(6):374–377

190. Guaschino S, De Seta F, Sartore A, Ricci G, De Santo D, Piccoli M, et al. Efficacy of maintenance therapy with topical boric acid in comparison with oral itraconazole in the treatment of recurrent vulvovaginal candidiasis. Am J Obstet Gynecol. 2001;184(4):598–602

191. Eggimann P, Garbino J, Pittet D. Management of *Candida* species infections in critically ill patients. Lancet Infect Dis. 2003;3(12):772–785

192. Rex JH, Bennett JE, Sugar AM, Pappas PG, van der Horst CM, Edwards JE, et al. A randomized trial comparing fluconazole with amphotericin B for the treatment of candidemia in patients without neutropenia. Candidemia Study Group and the National Institute. N Engl J Med. 1994;331(20):1325–1330

193. Phillips P, Shafran S, Garber G, Rotstein C, Smaill F, Fong I, et al. Multicenter randomized trial of fluconazole versus amphotericin B for treatment of candidemia in non-neutropenic patients. Canadian Candidemia Study Group. Eur J Clin Microbiol Infect Dis. 1997;16(5):337–345

194. Mora-Duarte J, Betts R, Rotstein C, Colombo AL, Thompson-Moya L, Smietana J, et al. Comparison of caspofungin and amphotericin B for invasive candidiasis. N Engl J Med. 2002;347(25):2020–2029

195. Kulberg BJ, Sobel JD, Ruhke N, Pappas PG. A randomized, prospective, multicenter study of voriconazole versus a regimen of amphotericin B followed by fluconazole in the treatment of candidemia in non-neutropenic patients. Submitted

196. Anaissie EJ, Vartivarian SE, Abi-Said D, Uzun O, Pinczowski H, Kontoyiannis DP, et al. Fluconazole versus amphotericin B in the treatment of hematogenous candidiasis: a matched cohort study. Am J Med. 1996;101(2):170–176

197. Clancy CJ, Staley B, Nguyen MH. In vitro susceptibility of break through *Candida* bloodstream isolates correlates with daily and cumulative doses of fluconazole. Antimicrob Agents Chemother. 2006;50(10):3496–3498

198. Vazquez JA, Gupta S, Villanueva A. Potential utility of recombinant human GM-CSF as adjunctive treatment of refractory oropharyngeal candidiasis in AIDS patients. Eur J Clin Microbiol Infect Dis. 1998;17(11):781–783

199. Swindells S. Pilot study of adjunctive GM-CSF (yeast derived) for fluconazole-resistant oral candidiasis in HIV-infection. Infect Dis Clin Pract. 1997;6:278–279

200. Poynton CH, Barnes RA, Rees J. Interferon gamma and granulocyte-macrophage colony-stimulating factor for the treatment of hepatosplenic candidosis in patients with acute leukemia. Clin Infect Dis. 1998;26(1):239–240

201. Rokusz L, Liptay L, Kadar K. Successful treatment of chronic disseminated candidiasis with fluconazole and a granulocyte-macrophage colony-stimulating factor combination. Scand J Infect Dis. 2001;33(10):784–786

202. Paterson PJ, McWhinney PH, Potter M, Kibbler CC, Prentice HG. The combination of oral amphotericin B with azoles prevents the emergence of resistant *Candida* species in neutropenic patients. Br J Haematol. 2001;112(1):175–180

203. Fowler SL, Rhoton B, Springer SC, Messer SA, Hollis RJ, Pfaller MA. Evidence for person-to-person transmission of *Candida lusitaniae* in a neonatal intensive-care unit. Infect Control Hosp Epidemiol. 1998;19(5):343–345

204. Burnie JP, Lee W, Williams JD, Matthews RC, Odds FC. Control of an outbreak of systemic *Candida albicans*. Br Med J (Clin Res Ed). 1985;291(6502):1092–1093

205. Lupetti A, Tavanti A, Davini P, Ghelardi E, Corsini V, Merusi I, et al. Horizontal transmission of *Candida parapsilosis* candidemia in a neonatal intensive care unit. J Clin Microbiol. 2002;40(7):2363–2369

206. Ables A, Blumer NA, Valainis GT. Fluconazole prophylaxis of severe *Candida* infection in trauma and postsurgical patients: a porspective, double blind, randomized, placebo-controlled trial. Infect Dis Clin Pract. 2000;9:169–173

207. Garbino T. Fluconazole prevents severe *Candida* spp. infections in high risk critically ill patients. American Society of Microbiology, Washington DC; 1997

208. Pfaller MA, Diekema DJ. Role of sentinel surveillance of candidemia: trends in species distribution and antifungal susceptibility. J Clin Microbiol. 2002;40(10):3551–3557

Chapter 65
Antifungal Resistance: *Aspergillus*

P.H. Chandrasekar and Elias K. Manavathu

1 Introduction

Despite the availability of potent antifungal agents, systemic fungal infections continue to cause significant morbidity and mortality. While candida-related deaths have declined since the late 1980s, those due to aspergillosis remain high. Fifty to ninety percent of patients with invasive aspergillosis (IA) die despite treatment (1–3). Susceptible hosts, particularly cancer patients and transplant recipients, are profoundly immunocompromised with neutropenia and/or impaired monocyte/macrophage dysfunction; there is universal agreement that the outcome of IA is largely dictated by the host immune status (4–6). Regardless of the antifungal drug(s) employed, the poor outcome or failure of antifungal therapy is generally attributed to compromised host defenses and in most cases, not considered to be due to drug resistant fungi. Also, failure of antifungal drugs may be due to inappropriate dose, fungistatic activity, high protein binding, poor absorption/distribution and metabolism or drug interactions. Until recently, drug resistance in aspergillus was not adequately examined.

Cornerstone for the successful management of IA includes decrease in immunosuppression, immune restoration, surgical debridement and optimal antifungal drug therapy. The antifungal drugs available for therapy of IA are listed in Table 1. Data on aspergillus exhibiting resistance to drugs listed are limited. This limitation has largely been due to lack of interest in the past as the incidence of infection was low, amphotericin B was the only effective drug, the pathogen not readily recovered from most infected patients, lack of information on resistance to newer drugs, and more importantly, non-availability of a reliable susceptibility test method to correlate in vitro findings to clinical outcome.

P.H. Chandrasekar (✉)
Division of Infectious Diseases, Department of Internal Medicine, Wayne State University School of Medicine, Harper University Hospital, Detroit, MI, USA
pchandrasekar@med.wayne.edu

Rising incidence of aspergillosis, the recent availability of a standardized in vitro method to test susceptibility of filamentous fungi and the entry of new drugs have kindled the interest, and made it feasible to study the phenomenon of drug resistance in aspergillus (7).

2 In Vitro Resistance

2.1 Known Mechanisms of Resistance

Resistance can be described as primary (innate) when a fungal pathogen is intrinsically resistant to the antifungal drug, or secondary (acquired) when an organism develops resistance during drug exposure either due to spontaneous mutation or the acquisition of the resistance trait from an external source by genetic transfer. The known cellular and molecular mechanisms responsible for reduced in vitro and in vivo susceptibility to antifungal drugs fall into two broad categories, namely, reduced intracellular accumulation of the antifungal drug compared to that in the susceptible cells, and quantitative or structural alteration of the fungal drug target.

The reduced intracellular drug accumulation occurs either due to efflux of the drug from the cell mediated by efflux proteins, or due to reduced penetration of the drug into the cell because of selective drug-permeability barrier(s). The efflux proteins belong to two groups, *ATP Binding Cassette* (ABC) transporters and major facilitators. The efflux proteins pump out the drug accumulated in the cell at the expense of energy and maintain the concentration of the drug inside the cell below the level required for the inhibition of growth. Thus, even in the presence of high concentration of the drug outside the cell, the organism is able to grow and function physiologically more or less normally. The energy required for the expulsion of the drug is generally derived from hydrolysis of ATP. When an organism develops resistance to a certain drug due to efflux, the pump proteins are overproduced compared to the amount present in drug susceptible cells. In general, the efflux proteins are

Table 1 Drugs for invasive aspergillosis

A. Polyenes
  Amphotericin B deoxycholate (AmBD)
  Amphotericin B lipid complex (ABLC), Abelcet®
  Liposomal amphotericin B (LamB), Ambisome®
  Amphotericin B colloidal dispersion (ABCD), Amphocil®
B. Azoles
  Voriconazole, V-fend®
  Itraconazole, Sporanox®
  Posaconazole, Noxafil®
C. Echinocandins
  Caspofungin, Cancidas®
  Micafungin, Mycamine®
  Anidulafungin, Eraxis®

native to the cell carrying out essential nutrient transport but fortuitously adapted to perform transport of substances toxic to the cell, including antibiotics.

A second, less well-known mechanism for the reduced accumulation of antifungal drugs inside the fungal cell is diminished penetration of the drug because of selective permeability barrier(s). This type of mechanism is known to be responsible for low-level resistance to antibacterial drugs in Gram-negative bacteria such as the *Pseudomonas* species where the outer cell membrane or biofilm acts as a selective permeability barrier (8). In the case of fungi, the reduced penetration is often associated with other factors such as the chemical changes in the cell wall and production of hydrophobic compound such as pigment. Excessive production and incorporation of pigment(s) in the cell wall often act as a barrier for the penetration of toxic substances, including antifungal agents (9). Since the presence of cell wall pigment provides an added advantage to drug-resistant cells for survival in the presence of antifungal drugs compared to the susceptible ones, the synthesis of cell wall pigment(s) is often considered as a virulence factor (10).

Modification of the fungal drug target (with which the drug molecules interact to bring about their antifungal activity) is a well-known mechanism responsible for the emergence of antifungal drug resistance in medically important fungi. The modification of the drug target is achieved at two levels: quantitative and structural (qualitative). Quantitative drug target modification is obtained by the enhanced production of the drug target by upregulation of its synthesis or by the increased dosage of the gene(s) responsible for the synthesis of the drug target. In either case, the increased amount of the fungal drug target requires higher concentration of the drug to elicit an inhibitory effect. Thus, fungal cells with increased amount of the drug target will survive in the presence of increased amount of the drug compared to a susceptible cell that possesses the base level of the drug target. The structural modification of drug target occurs by the mutational acquisition of genetic variation affecting its synthesis or primary structure (protein). Variation of the primary structure of protein often leads to secondary and tertiary

structural changes that affect the binding and processing of drug molecules that mimic the natural substrate (in the case of enzyme target) or ligand (in the case of receptor molecules). Usually, drug target modification dependent mechanism alone or in combination with other resistance mechanism, leads to high-level cellular resistance to the antifungal drugs.

2.2 Resistance to Polyenes

Amphotericin B is a typical polyene antifungal drug approved for primary therapy against a wide variety of fungal infections since 1953 (11), and has remained as the unchallenged gold standard until recently. It is an amphoteric molecule composed of a hydrophilic polyhydroxyl chain along one side and a lipophilic polyene hydrocarbon chain on the other. It interacts with the fungal membrane-associated ergosterol forming channels or pores spanning across the plasma membrane disrupting the osmotic integrity and the selective permeability of the fungal plasma membrane. The loss of osmotic integrity and the selective permeability of the membrane result in leakage of essential intracellular cations such as calcium, potassium and magnesium as well as various metabolites (12). This indiscriminate massive loss of essential nutrients and ions is believed to be primarily responsible for the death of fungal cells when treated with amphotericin B, although other biochemical reaction such as oxidation of plasma membrane associated phospholipids and their derivatives affecting the proper functioning of the fungal plasma membrane may also play a major role for the fungicidal activity of amphotericin B (13).

In spite of the extensive use of amphotericin B as the primary antifungal drug against fungal infections over a period of nearly four decades, the emergence of high-level resistance to this compound in clinical isolates of fungi, including *Aspergillus* species, is very rare. The reason(s) for the lack of emergence of resistance to amphotericin B among clinical isolates of fungi is not understood. However, the occurrence of drug-target-modification-dependent acquired resistance to amphotericin B requires the synthesis of a modified ergosterol that is biologically functional, but unaffected by the inhibitory action of amphotericin B. The possibility of spontaneous emergence of such a sterol synthetic pathway capable of synthesizing an altered amphotericin B-resistant biologically functional ergosterol in fungi, including *Aspergillus* species, by genetic variation is remote. Hence it is not surprising that high-level amphotericin B resistance in fungi, including *Aspergillus* species, due to drug target modification is comparatively rare, although other mechanisms of antifungal resistance may occasionally confer reduced susceptibility to this antifungal drug. The clinical and laboratory isolates of *Aspergillus* species showing reduced in vitro or in vivo susceptibility to amphotericin B reported in the literature may belong to this group.

Few reports of low-level amphotericin B resistance among clinical isolates of *Aspergillus* species are available in the literature (Table 2) (14–18). When attempts were made to evaluate the in vitro resistance (defined as elevated MICs compared to that obtained for the susceptible isolates) to in vivo resistance using animal models, the correlation was poor (15, 16). On the other hand, when clinical outcome of amphotericin B treatment was retrospectively compared with the in vitro resis-

tance, there was good correlation between amphotericin B failure and elevated MIC of the drug. Because of the paucity of clinical isolates of *Aspergillus* species resistant to amphotericin B, Manavathu et al. (14) have selected *Aspergillus fumigatus* isolates showing low-to-medium level in vitro resistance to amphotericin B in the laboratory by UV irradiation followed by selection on Sabouraud dextrose agar containing amphotericin B. Using a murine pulmonary aspergillosis model, these investigators have demonstrated correlation between in vitro and in vivo resistance to amphotericin B (19).

Table 2 MIC of amphotericin B for *Aspergillus* isolates showing reduced in vitro susceptibility

Aspergillus isolate tested	MIC (μg/ml) range	Source of isolate	Possible resistance mechanism	Reference
Aspergillus fumigatus	4–16[a]	Selected in the laboratory following UV irradiation	Not studied	(14)
AB16.1				
AB16.2				
AB16.3				
AB16.4				
AF210	2[b]	Clinical isolate, susceptible to amphotericin B therapy	Not studied	(15)
AF65	1[b]	Clinical isolate, refractory to amphotericin B therapy	Not studied	(15)
AF10	2[b]	Clinical isolate	Not studied	(16)
Aspergillus flavus	≥100[c]	Laboratory isolate	Modification of cell wall	(17)
Aspergilllus udagawae	2–4	Clinical isolates	Not studied	(21)
Aspergillus terreus	2–4	Clinical isolates	Innately resistant	(18)
2624				
95–644				
96–1290				

[a]Determined in peptone yeast extract glucose broth. The MIC for the susceptible parent W73355 was 1 μg/ml
[b]Geometric mean MIC for susceptible isolates was ≤0.5 μg/ml
[c]Determined by a modified agar dilution technique. The MIC for the parent was ≤1 μg/ml

Table 3 MICs of various triazoles for selected *Aspergillus fumigatus* isolates showing in vitro resistance

Aspergillus fumigatus isolate	MIC (μg/ml)				Source of isolate	Possible resistance mechanism	Reference
	ITZ	PCZ	VCZ	RCZ			
AF72	≥16	ND	0.25	ND	Clinical isolate	CYP51Ap: G54E	(32)
RIT13	≥100	ND	ND	ND	Laboratory isolate	CYP51Ap: G54E and upregulation of *Afu*MDR3 and *Afu*MDR4	(33)
R7-1	≥32	≥16	0.25	ND	Laboratory isolate	CYP51Ap: G54W	(42)
ND202	≥32	≥16	0.25	ND	Clinical isolate	CYP51Ap: G54W	(42)
VCZ-F33	2	1	16	8	Laboratory isolate	CYP51Ap: G448S	(31)
VCZ-W42	2	1	8	4	Laboratory isolate	CYP51Ap: G448S	(31)
VCU-350	2	1	16	8	Clinical isolate	CYP51Ap: G448S	(41)
PCZ-W5	16	16	0.06	0.12	Laboratory isolate	CYP51Ap: G54R	(31)
PCZ-W8	16	8	0.062	0.062	Laboratory isolate	CYP51Ap: G54R	(31)
CM-1245	≥16	0.5–1	1	2–4	Clinical isolate	CYP51Ap: M220V	(34)
CM-2159	≥16	2	1–2	1–2	Clinical isolate	CYP51Ap: M220K	(34)
CM-2164	≥16	0.25–0.5	0.5–1	1–2	Clinical isolate	CYP51Ap: M220T	(34)
CM2627	8	4–8	4–8	0.5	Clinical isolate	CYP51Ap: L98H *plus* 32-bp repeat	(40)
CM3275	8	4–8	4–8	0.5	Clinical isolate	CYP51Ap: L98H *plus* 32-bp repeat	(40)

NB: The MICs of various triazoles for the susceptible *A. fumigatus* isolate range from 0.062 to 0.5 μg/ml. The amino acid change indicated is for P450 14α-sterol demethylase A of *A. fumigatus*

Although high-level amphotericin B resistance among clinical isolates of *Aspergillus fumigatus* is rare, *Aspergillus terreus* is inherently less susceptible to amphotericin B, perhaps due to innate resistance to this drug. Exact reason for its reduced susceptibility to amphotericin B is not known. Recently, Walsh et al. (18) have investigated the in vitro susceptibility of several clinical isolates of *A. terreus* by the CLSI broth microdilution method M-38A. The MIC of amphotericin B for these isolates ranged from 2 to 4 μg/ml, considerably higher than that of other susceptible *Aspergillus* species such as *A. fumigatus*. Moreover, when tested in an animal model (18), a representative of this group of organisms showed reduced susceptibility to amphotericin B therapy. Therefore, amphotericin B is not the preferred drug for the treatment of aspergillus infection caused by *A. terreus*.

In addition, Seo et al. (17) have selected an *A. flavus* isolate highly resistant to amphotericin B (MIC 100 μg/ml) in the laboratory by sequential transfer of a susceptible strain (MIC ≤ 1 μg/ml) to agar plates containing increasing concentrations of amphotericin B. Further investigation by these authors revealed that the resistant isolate had significant chemical modification to its cell wall which presumably results in poor penetration of the drug to the cell. Recently, Balajee et al. (20, 21) have shown that *A. lentulus* and *A. udagawae* previously erroneously identified as *A. fumigatus* are resistant to multiple antifungal drugs, including amphotericin B.

2.3 Resistance to Triazoles (Table 3)

The triazoles are second-generation members of the azole family of antifungal drugs characterized by the presence of a heterocyclic head region carrying three nitrogen atoms instead of the two found in imidazole molecules. The addition of an extra nitrogen atom to the imidazole ring moiety not only improved the spectrum of activity but also the potency of the molecule (22–24). This is not surprising since the heterocyclic ring moiety carrying the nitrogen atoms is the active functional group of the molecule while the hydrophobic aliphatic chain contributes significantly to the specificity and the pharmacologic properties of the molecule (25). Itraconazole and newer triazoles such as voriconazole (Pfizer Pharmaceuticals), posaconazole (Schering-Plough Pharmaceuticals), and ravuconazole (Bristol-Myers Squibb Pharmaceuticals) possess excellent in vitro and in vivo (clinical and/or animal models) activity against various *Aspergillus* species.

All triazoles are believed to have the same mode of action at clinically relevant concentrations. The primary molecular target of this group of compounds is the cytochrome P450-dependent 14α-sterol demethylase (P450$_{14DM}$), an enzyme responsible for the removal of the methyl group on carbon 14 of lanosterol. Although P450$_{14DM}$ is the primary molecular

target of triazoles, at high concentrations these drugs may have rather non-specific effect by directly interfering with the membrane function for which the mechanism is not understood. For instance, it is possible that these molecules, having the capacity to mimic certain sterols, could be inserted randomly into the membranes and as a result affect the function of the plasma membrane. Recently, it was noted that voriconazole has a second target in the sterol synthetic pathway, namely, 24-methylene dihydrolanosterol demethylation (26).

The *cyp*51 gene coding for P450$_{14DM}$ has been characterized from a wide variety of saprophytic and pathogenic fungi, including human pathogens (27–29). A comparison of the primary structure of P450$_{14DM}$ from various fungal species representing major groups of pathogenic fungi showed five highly conserved regions (Fig. 1) known to make an important contribution to either the enzyme activity or susceptibility of P450$_{14DM}$ to azole antifungal drugs. The role of two such highly conserved regions to triazole resistance in *A. fumigatus* has been examined recently. Proximal to the N terminus of the protein lies a region starting from amino acid P45 to F74 (amino acid residue numbering based on *A. fumigatus* P450$_{14DM}$) commonly known as the membrane-anchoring region (MAR) mainly consisting of hydrophobic amino acid residues. It is generally believed that this region of the polypeptide is responsible for anchoring the enzyme to the plasma membrane of the cell. The hydrophobic amino acid residues dominating this region facilitate the insertion of the polypeptide into the lipid bilayer of the membrane. The membrane anchoring places the enzyme molecule in the most favorable position to interact with the incoming substrate for binding to the active site for subsequent processing. Thus, plasma membrane-anchored P450$_{14DM}$ will be more efficient for rapid catalysis of the demethylation of lanosterol.

The most highly conserved region of the P450$_{14DM}$ is the heme-binding region located towards the carboxyl terminal portion (S441-Y461) of the protein. Since heme is an essential prosthetic group of all cytochrome P450 dependent enzymes, this region of the polypeptide is highly conserved in all P450$_{14DMS}$. Alignment of 25 P450$_{14DMS}$ from various sources ranging from *Homo sapiens* to the fungus *Cunninghemella elegans* showed that F447, G448, G450, R451, H452 and C454 are perfectly conserved at the core region of the HBR of P450$_{14DMS}$ (Fig. 2). Genetic and biochemical studies have shown that C470 in *S. cerevisiae* (C454 in *A. fumigatus*) is involved in substrate binding possibly by providing a sixth co-ordinate and presumed to be involved in the correct alignment of the incoming substrate molecule for maximum catalytic efficiency (23, 24). Mutant enzymes carrying variants of this residue lacks enzyme activity. Conservation of the critical amino acid residues at the heme-binding region is not only essential for the enzyme function, but also necessary for the maintenance of azole susceptibility of the protein. The exact role of each of the highly conserved amino acid

```
                                        MAR
A. fumigatus   31   LWNRTEPPMVFHWVPFLGSTISYGIDPYKFFFACREKYGDIFTFILLGQKTTVYL   85
P. italicum    37   -YNRKEPPVVFHWIPFIGSTIAYGMDPYQFFFASRAKYGDIFTFILLGKKTTVYL   90
U. maydis      55   T-PKNHPPVVFHFVPVTGSATYYGIDPYKFFFECREKYCDVFTFVLLGRKITVAL  108
C. albicans    43   L-RKDRAPLVFYWIPWFGSAASYGQQPYEFFESCRQKYGDVFSFMLLGKIMTVYL   96
C. elegans     41   K-NPNEPPNVFSLIPVLGNAVQFGMNPVAFLQECQKKYGDVFTFTMVGKRVTVCL   94
                     :  :* **   :*  :*::   :* :*   *: ::: ****:*:*  ::*:  ** *
```

```
                                        ASR I
A. fumigatus   86   GVQGNEFILNGKLKDVNAEEVYSPLTTPVFGSDVVYDCPNSKLMEQKKFIKYGLT  140
P. italicum    91   GVEGNEFILNGKLKDVNAEEVYGKLTTPVFGSDVVYDCPNSKLMEQKKFIKYGLS  145
U. maydis     109   GPKGSNLVFNAKHQQVTAEDAYTHLTTPVFGKEVVYDVPNAVFMEQKKFVKVGLS  163
C. albicans    97   GPKGHEFVFNAKLSDVSAEDAYKHLTTPVFGKGVIYDCPNSRLMEQKKFAKFALT  151
C. elegans     95   GADGNQFVFNSKQNLSSAAEAYNHMTKYVFGPDVVVYDAPHAVFMEQKKFIKAGLN  149
                     * :* :::::*:*    :*:::*  :*: *** :*:** *::  :****** * :*:
```

```
                                        ASR II
A. fumigatus  192   GQEVRSKLTAEFADLYHDLDKGFTPINFMLPWAPLPHNKK--RDAAHAR-MRSIY  243
P. italicum   197   GEEVRSKLTSEFADLFHDLDLGFSPINFMLPWAPLPHNASAIKHTTYARDLSGNY  251
U. maydis     219   GKEVRQGLDKSFAQLYHDLDSGFTPINFVIPNLPLPSN---FKRDRAQKKMSQFY  270
C. albicans   206   GDEMRRIFDRSFAQLYSDLDKGFTPINFVFPNLPLPHY---WRRDAAQKKISATY  257
C. elegans    198   GKEIRASLDGNVAKLYYDLDQGFKPINFIFPNLPLPSYR---RRDVACKKMADLY  249
                     *:*:*  ::  :: *:*: *** **:****::*  ***     ::   : :  *
```

```
                                        ASR III
A. fumigatus  293   AGQHSSSSISAWIMLRLASQPKVLEELYQEQLANLGPAGPDGSLPPLQYKDLDK-  346
P. italicum   304   AGQHSSSAISCWILLRLASQPEMAEKLHAEQIKNLGAD-----LPPLQYKDMDK-  352
U. maydis     325   AGQHTSSATSSWAFLRLASRPEIIEELYEEQLNVYSDGH--GGLRELDYETQKTS  377
C. albicans   307   GGQHSASTSAWFLLHLGKPHLQDVIYQEVVELLKEKG--GDLNDLTYEDLQK-  358
C. elegans    297   GGQHTSATTSAWTILELANRPDIIKALREEQIEKLGSLKAD-----LTFDNL-KD  345
                     :***:*::* *  :* :*  *:::*::  :  :*:      *  ::: :
```

```
                                        HBR
A. fumigatus  440   TSSPYLPFGAGRHRCIGEKFAYVNLGVILATIVRHLRLFNVDGKKGVPETDYSSL  494
P. italicum   445   TRSPYLPFGACRHRCIGEKFAYLNLEVIVATLVREFRFFNPEGMEGVPDTDYSSL  499
U. maydis     487   ANSPYLPFGAGRHRCIGEQFAYLQIGVILATFVRIFK-WHLDS-K-FPDPDYQSM  538
C. albicans   456   VSSPYLPFGGGRHRCIGEQFAYVQLGTILTTFVYNLR-WTIDGYK-VPDPDYSSM  508
C. elegans    444   SKSPFLPFCACRHRCIGEQFGYLQLKTVISTFIRTFDF-DLDG-KSVPKSDYTSM  496
                     :**:****:*********:*:*::  ::::*::  :    :: :  *::** *:
```

Fig. 1 Amino acid alignment of P450 14α-sterol demethylases (P450$_{14DMS}$) of representative organisms belonging to five major classes of fungi. The alignment was done by the DNA and Protein Sequence Analysis Program Omiga. The deduced amino acid sequences of various P450$_{14DMS}$ were obtained from the National Center for Biotechnology and Informatics (NCBI) protein data bank. *MAR* membrane-anchoring region; *HBR* heme-binding region; *ASR* azole susceptible region, i.e. enzyme with native sequence will be susceptible to the inhibitory action of azoles whereas variation of one or more amino acid in these regions would make the enzyme less susceptible to the azole antifungal drugs. The *numbers on the right* and *left* indicate the amino acid residue numbers of the polypeptide segments of various P450$_{14DMS}$ compared

```
Homo sapiens               YVPFGAGRHRCIGENFAYVQIKT   461
Sus scrofa                 YVPFGAGRHRCIGENFAYVQIKT   461
Rattus norvigicus          YVPFGAGRHRCIGENFAYVQIKT   461
Mus musculus               YVPFGAGRHRCVGENFAYVQIKT   461
Saccharomyces cerevisiae   YLPFGGGRHRCIGEHFAYCQLGV   482
Candida glabrata           YLPFGGGRHRCIGELFAYCQLGV   484
Candida albicans           YLPFGGGRHRCIGEQFAYVQLGT   482
Candida tropicalis         YLPFGGGRHRCIGEQFAYVQLGT   482
Issatchenkia orientalis    YLPFGGGRHRCT----------   414
Schizosaccharomyces pombe  YLPFGAGRHRCIGEQFAYMHLST   454
Aspergillus fumigatus      YLPFGAGRHRCIGEKFAYVNLGV   466
Aspergillus nidulans       YLPFGGGRHRCIGEKFAYVNLGV   463
Penicillium italicum       YLPFGAGRHRCIGEKFAYLNLEV   471
Penicillium digitatum      YLPFGAGRHRCIGEKFAYLNLGV   472
Uncinula necator           YLPFGAGRHRCIGEQFATLQLVT   481
Blumeria graminis          YLPFGAGRHRCIGEQFATVQLVT   479
Mollisia yallundae         YLPFGAGRHRCIGEQFANVQLIT   478
Mollisia acuformis         YLPFGAGRHRCIGEQFANVQLIT   478
Botryotinia fuckeliana     YLPFGAGRHRCIGEQFATVQLVT   468
Mycosphaerella graminicola YLPFGAGRHRCIGEQFAYVQLQT   490
Filabasidiella neoformans  YQPFGAGRHRCVGEQFAYTQLST   502
Ustilago maydis            YLPFGAGRHRCIGEQFAYLQIGV   513
Cunninghaemella elegans    FLPFGAGRHRCIGEQFGYLQLKT   470
Triticum aestivum          YISFGGGRHGCLGEPFAYLQIKA   407
Sorghum bicolor            YISFGGGRHGCLGEPFAYLQIKA   446
                           ** *** *
```

Fig. 2 Amino acid alignment of the heme-binding region of 25 P450$_{14DMS}$ from *Homo sapiens* to *C. elegans*. The highly conserved amino acid residues are marked by *asterisks*. The *numbers on the right* indicate the amino acid residue number. The alignment was done by DNA and Protein Sequence Analysis Program Omiga. The amino acid sequences were obtained from the NCBI protein data bank

residues for the binding and the processing of the substrate is not known at present due to the paucity of X-ray crystallographic data.

In contrast to pathogenic yeasts such as the *Candida* species in which there is a single gene coding for $P450_{14DM}$, in *A. fumigatus* there are two highly homologous genes *cyp*51A and *cyp*51B coding for P450 14α-sterol demethylases A (CYP51Ap) and B (CYP51Bp). Several reports of clinical and laboratory isolates of the *Aspergillus* species, primarily *A. fumigatus*, showing reduced susceptibility to triazoles have been published recently (21, 30–42). In several cases, resistance to one member of the triazole group failed to show cross-resistance to other triazole(s) (31, 37, 39, 41). Amino acid alteration of CYP51Ap appears to be the most commonly found mechanism of resistance to triazoles in *A. fumigatus*. Alteration of G54 of CYP51Ap to K, E or R confers resistance to itraconazole and posaconazole (31–33, 36, 41, 42) but not to voriconazole and ravuconazole (31, 41). In contrast, alteration of G448S primarily confers resistance to voriconazole and ravuconazole but only a modest reduction of susceptibility to posaconazole and itraconazole (31, 41). Modeling experiments (43–45) suggest that the heme-binding region is part of the active site of $P450_{14DM}$, and any amino acid change at the active site make the organism resistant to all triazoles to a lesser or greater degree. In contrast, amino acid variation at the putative membrane-anchoring region confers resistance to triazoles with a long aliphatic tail region. These results thus suggest that cross-resistance to triazoles in *A. fumigatus* is at least partly dependent on region-specific amino acid variation of $P450_{14DM}$. On the other hand, alteration of G138 to either C (38) or R (31) confers resistance to multiple triazoles. Initially Mellado et al. (34) and subsequently other investigators (35, 36) have noted that alteration of M220 in CYP51Ap to V, K, T (34) or I (35, 36) makes the organism harboring the mutant enzyme resistant to itraconazole. Interestingly, both G138 and M220 are located in the highly conserved ASRI and ASRII regions (Fig. 1) of CYP51Ap, respectively.

Recently, a novel mechanism for conferring resistance to multiple triazoles in an *A. fumigatus* isolate has been reported (40). The clinical isolate of *A. fumigatus* showing decreased susceptibility to multiple azoles had L98H mutation on CYP51Ap together with a 32-bp tandem repeat of nucleotide sequence at the promoter region. Neither the L98H mutation nor the 32-bp repeat alone had any effect on the susceptibility of this organism to triazoles. The concomitant presence of the amino acid alteration and the 32-bp repeat was needed for resistance to various triazoles.

Although the efflux mediated drug resistance is well documented in pathogenic yeasts (46–51), its contribution to drug resistance in pathogenic filamentous fungi, including *Aspergillus* species, is only at the early stages of investigation. In *A. fumigatus*, itraconazole is able to induce the expression of an ABC-transporter gene called *atr*F (35, 52),

but the role of this gene conferring resistance in clinical isolates to itraconazole is not established. Multiple drug resistance (MDR) membrane proteins called *afu*MDR1 and *afu*MDR2 were previously identified and characterized from *A. fumigatus* (53). But their actual function or contribution to antifungal drug resistance was not investigated. Recently, Nacimento et al. (33) have showed that AfuMDR1 and AfuMDR2 may not be involved in efflux mediated triazole resistance in this organism. On the other hand, AfuMDR3 and AfuMDR4 were over expressed in *A. fumigatus* resistant to itraconazole, but not AfuMDR1 and AfuMDR2 suggesting that AfuMDR3 and AfuMDR4 may play a role in efflux-mediated triazole resistance in *A. fumigatus*. However, these researchers were unable to document the accumulation of itraconazole in the resistant and susceptible isolates of *A. fumigatus*. By itraconazole uptake study in mycelia, Manavathu et al. (54) have previously demonstrated that the intracellular accumulation of radioactive itraconazole was significantly lower in laboratory-selected *A. fumigatus* isolates showing reduced in vitro susceptibility to itraconazole compared to that in the susceptible parent. The efflux of drug in combination with drug target modification have made laboratory-selected *A. fumigatus* isolates highly resistant (MIC ≥ 100 µg/ml) to itraconazole suggesting that multiple mechanisms of drug resistance may co-exist in the same cells to make them highly resistant to the drug (33). By expressing of *cyp*51A in an autonomously replicating multicopy plasmid, Osherov et al. (29) have transformed an itraconazole susceptible *A. fumigatus* to a drug resistant strain.

2.4 Resistance to Echinocandins

The echinocandins such as caspofungin, micafungin, and anidulafungin are semisynthetic cyclic lipohexapeptide antifungal drugs designed to render specific interaction with fungal cells with minimum level of toxicity to host cells at therapeutic doses. The molecular target of echinocandins is believed to be 1,3-β-D-glucan synthase (GS; E. C. 2.4.1.34; UDP Glucose: 1,3-β-D-glucan 3-β-D-glucosyltransferase), a multimeric membrane-bound enzyme that catalyzes the synthesis of β(1→3) glucan, even though there is no direct molecular evidence to support this view (55). However, it is safe to say that these compounds inhibit cell wall synthesis in a wide variety of fungi, and cell wall synthesis is the target of the echinocandin compounds. What distinguishes the members of the echinocandin family of antifungal drugs from the polyenes and the azoles is their specificity against fungi with relatively little mechanism-based toxicity against the host.

Recently, a pair of reports of echinocandin resistance in *Aspergillus* has been published. Gardiner et al. (56) have isolated two classes of *A. fumigatus* mutants in the laboratory showing reduced susceptibility to caspofungin. Site-directed mutation of the target gene coding for glucan synthase Fks1p, including the catalytic subunit, produced mutants showing low-level in vitro resistance (≈16-fold increase of MIC) to caspofungin. Subsequent characterization of one such mutant showed S678P alteration of Fks1p (57).

These investigators also isolated a number of spontaneous mutants of *A. fumigatus* in the laboratory showing a biphasic susceptibility pattern. At low concentrations of the drug (<0.5 µg/ml) these isolates were highly susceptible to the growth inhibitory effect of caspofungin. However, at drug concentrations >0.5 µg/ml but <16 µg/ml these spontaneous mutant isolates showed near normal growth pattern whereas at drug concentrations >16 µg/ml they showed partial susceptibility to growth inhibition. No target gene mutation or upregulation of Fks1p expression was noted in these isolates. These authors speculate that the biphasic pattern of susceptibility to caspofungin is caused by a novel mechanism of echinocandin resistance in *A. fumigatus* perhaps due to the remodeling of the cell wall components (56). In addition to the reports of the acquired resistance to caspofungin in *A. fumigatus* laboratory isolates, Balajee et al. (21) have shown that *A. lentulus* is intrinsically resistant to caspofungin.

2.5 Resistance to Allylamines

Terbinafine (Novartis Pharmaceuticals) is an allylamine antifungal drug that possesses excellent in vitro activity against *Aspergillus* species, including, *A. fumigatus*. The MICs of this compound against *Aspergillus* species is in the sub-microgram range, usually 2- to 4-fold lower than that of amphotericin B. Preliminary experiments indicate that terbinafine is a fungicidal agent against *Aspergillus* species (58–62). Only limited amount of in vivo data (animal models and case reports) is available at present and the indication is that it is less impressive in vivo than it is in vitro, perhaps because of poor availability of the drug due to the excessive protein binding.

The molecular target of terbinafine is squalene epoxidase (also known as squalene monooxygenase), an enzyme involved in the oxidation of squalene to 2,3-oxidosqualene (also called squalene 2,3-epoxide). The squalene epoxidase, in the presence of NADPH and oxygen, catalyzes the addition of an oxygen atom from molecular oxygen to the end of the squalene chain, forming an epoxide. The co-factor NADPH reduces the other oxygen atom to molecular oxygen and water. The inhibition of 2,3-oxidosqualene synthesis leads to the inhibition of ergosterol synthesis that eventually results in plasma membrane malfunction and fungal cell death.

The investigation of the effect of terbinafine on *Aspergillus* species is at its infancy, and an understanding of the spectrum of terbinafine resistance in *Aspergillus* species will be a few years away. To date, there are only three reports of terbinafine resistance in the *Aspergillus* species. In all three cases the resistant isolates were either genetically engineered or induced by UV-irradiation followed by selection in the presence of terbinafine. Liu et al. (62) have expressed multiple copies of the gene coding for squalene epoxidase in *A. fumigatus* using a multicopy plasmid. Transformants harboring multiple copies of squalene epoxidase gene showed decreased in vitro susceptibility to terbinafine.

Graminha et al. (63) have investigated terbinafine resistance in a laboratory isolate of *A. nidulans*. These investigators generated a number of terbinafine resistant mutant isolates of *A. nidulans* by UV-irradiation followed by selection in the presence of the drug. One such terbinafine resistant isolate was characterized by molecular genetic techniques. The resistant isolate had multiple copies of *salA*, a gene coding for salicylate 1-monooxygenase, an enzyme known to be responsible for the degradation of naphthalene ring structures in other microorganisms. So it is quite possible that the expression of multiple copies of *salA* may be responsible for the reduced susceptibility of *A. nidulans* to terbinafine.

In contrast to the gene dosage dependent terbinafine resistance in *A. nidulans* and *A. fumigatus*, Rocha et al. (64) have recently reported terbinafine resistance in a genetically engineered laboratory isolate of *A. fumigatus* harboring an altered squalene epoxidase gene. These investigators genetically engineered replacement of phenylalanine 389 of squalene epoxidase with leucine (F389L). This single amino acid change was sufficient to confer resistance to terbinafine in an isolate carrying the mutant enzyme. Since the terbinafine target is squalene epoxidase, an enzyme involved in the initial stage of ergosterol synthesis, spontaneous mutants resistant to terbinafine will ultimately emerge in nature with the increased use of this drug against aspergillus infection.

3 Animal Models

Animal models have been used extensively to study pathogenesis, host responses, disease transmission and therapy of aspergillus infection (65). Animal (mouse, rat, guinea pig and rabbit) models have been used to evaluate the in vivo efficacy of antimycotic drugs against pulmonary and disseminated aspergillosis caused by drug-susceptible and drug-resistant *Aspergillus* species (66–69). The selection of a particular animal model suitable for drug therapy study is dependent on the pharmacodynamics of the drug, ideally one that mimics the parameters in humans. Most data are from rodent, particularly, mouse models of aspergillosis. These models have been critical to the advancement of therapy. Using one or more of these animal models several investigators examined the efficacy of polyenes, triazoles, echinocandins and allylamines against *Aspergillus* isolates showing elevated MICs of the drug in vitro.

Using transiently immunocompromised murine (15, 16, 19) and guinea pig (16) models for disseminated (15, 16) and pulmonary (19) aspergillosis, the in vivo efficacy of amphotericin B against *Aspergillus fumigatus* isolates with either elevated amphotericin B MIC or isolate obtained from patients who failed amphotericin B therapy was examined. No consensus for the correlation of in vitro resistance to in vivo failure was obtained in these studies. For instance, Odds et al. (16) obtained no interpretable relationship either in mouse or guinea pig model when the MIC of amphotericin B was $\geq 2\,\mu g/ml$. In other words, no correlation of in vitro resistance to in vivo resistance was found. On the other hand, Verweij et al. (15) have investigated the efficacy of amphotericin B and caspofungin against two *A. fumigatus* clinical isolates (AF210 and AF65) with more or less similar amphotericin B MICs, although AF65 was obtained from a patient failing amphotericin B therapy. Amphotericin B treatment at doses 0.5, 2 and 5 mg/kg per day failed to improve the survival and reduction of fungal burden in the animals infected with *A. fumigatus* AF65, but not with AF210. Anidulafungin (LY303366) treatment at doses of 10 and 25 mg/kg per day was highly effective against AF210 and AF65 infections. These data suggest that even in the absence of elevated MIC, drug failure in the clinical situation is correlated with reduced therapeutic efficacy in the animal model. In contrast, Manavathu et al. (19) have investigated the in vivo efficacy of amphotericin B against a laboratory-selected *A. fumigatus* isolate with elevated amphotericin B MIC in a pulmonary aspergillosis model. Animals infected with the mutant isolate showing in vitro resistance also showed poor survival and increased fungal burden compared to those infected with the drug-susceptible parent. These conflicting limited data suggest the need for additional experiments to establish in vitro–in vivo correlation for amphotericin B resistance in *A. fumigatus* using animal models.

Recently, Walsh et al. (18) have examined the effect of conventional and liposomal amphotericin B on *Aspergillus terreus* infection utilizing an experimental invasive pulmonary aspergillosis model in transiently neutropenic rabbit. As mentioned previously, greater than 90% of the *A. terreus* isolates showed high-level in vitro resistance to amphotericin B (70). Treatment of rabbits infected with *A. terreus* with conventional and liposomal amphotericin B failed to improve survival and reduce fungal burden compared to those obtained for untreated animal controls, whereas treatment with posaconazole, and itraconazole improved survival with significant reduction of fungal burden. Thus, for *A. terreus* isolates, their innate in vitro resistance to amphotericin B is well correlated with lack of amphotericin B treatment efficacy in the rabbit model.

Among various triazoles that are effective against *Aspergillus* species, only itraconazole has been examined to assess the correlation of either in vitro or clinical resistance

by an animal model. Denning et al. (30) have investigated the susceptibility of a clinical isolate of *A. fumigatus* obtained from an immunocompromised patient with IA who failed itraconazole therapy. The clinical failure of this isolate was associated with elevated MIC for itraconazole with a modest rise of MICs for other triazoles. Itraconazole treatment of neutropenic mice infected with this isolate failed to improve survival and reduce fungal burden whereas the echinocandin anidulafungin was highly effective in prolonging the survival of the animal and significantly decreased the fungal burden. Likewise, micafungin was effective in neutropenic mice infected with an itraconazole-resistant strain of *A. fumigatus* and a strain of *A. terreus* demonstrating in vivo resistance to amphotericin B (71). In contrast, Odds et al. (16) have obtained no clearly interpretable results showing correlation between in vitro resistance and failure of drug treatment when the itraconazole MIC of the isolate was greater than $1\,\mu g/ml$. Once again, the paucity of sufficient data make it difficult to make any conclusion regarding the in vitro–in vivo correlation of triazole resistance in the animal model.

4 Clinical Data: Resistance

Primary resistance to antifungal drugs among the isolates of *A. fumigatus*, *A. flavus*, and *A. niger* is infrequent. Among the uncommon species, *A. ustus* is poorly susceptible to all antifungals and there are many case reports of *A. ustus* causing invasive aspergillosis with poor outcome, mostly in allogeneic stem cell recipients (71). Recently, *A. ustus* infection and zygomycosis have emerged as breakthrough infections in stem cell recipients receiving voriconazole and caspofungin (72, 73). *A. ustus* isolates were found resistant to amphotericin B, triazoles, and echinocandins.

4.1 Resistance to Polyenes

A. terreus appears innately resistant to amphotericin B, both in vitro and in animal models (18, 70). Available clinical data support such observations; in a 12-year retrospective analysis of IA caused by *A. terreus*, infection progressed rapidly resulting in a 91% mortality despite amphotericin B therapy (74). Steinbach and colleagues reported a mortality rate of 73% in patients with *A. terreus* infection, and treated mostly with a polyene (amphotericin B or amphotericin B lipid formulation) (75). The same investigators reported a significantly better survival (56%) in similar patients treated with voriconazole. Based on in vitro, animal, and limited clinical observations, it appears polyenes are best avoided and azoles are preferred agents in the therapy of *A. terreus* infection. Extremely limited clinical data exist for polyene resistance in non-terreus aspergillus species. In a retrospective study of

29 immunocompromised patients with IA and treated with amphotericin B, in vitro susceptibility to the drug predicted clinical outcome (76). Remarkably, 22 of 23 patients infected with aspergillus resistant to amphotericin B (MIC >2 µg/ml) (both *A. terreus* and non-terreus aspergillus) died, while none of the remaining 6 infected with susceptible aspergillus died. This study however used "older," non-standardized methods of susceptibility testing; furthermore, no details of clinical features were provided. Clinical failure with liposomal amphotericin B was noted during the treatment of severe cutaneous aspergillosis in two premature infants with extremely low birth weight; both infants were successfully treated with voriconazole (77).

Verweij et al. (15) described the recovery of amphotericin B-resistant *A. fumigatus* isolates from the lung of a patient with refractory infection treated with the same drug. Introducing the resistant isolate in the animal model, the investigators observed similar poor outcomes in those treated with amphotericin B and untreated controls. Also, a higher inoculum was required to produce disease in the animal model. Of interest, Lionakis et al. (78) found that pre-exposure of cancer patients to amphotericin B or triazoles was associated with increased frequency of recovery of non-fumigatus aspergillus species. Moreover, such post-exposure isolates was amphotericin B-resistant but not azole-resistant. Since clinical failures are common, emergence of aspergillus resistant to polyenes during therapy of invasive aspergillosis is of interest. Whether resistance to amphotericin B emerges is not clear since most clinical failures have been attributed to poor host factors and perhaps, infarcted tissue with poor drug penetration. Unlike with bacterial infections, difficulty in obtaining sequential isolates of the fungus during an episode of infection makes it hard to evaluate emergence of resistance. Available limited data suggest that the emergence of resistance to polyenes during therapy is uncommon (79–81).

4.2 Resistance to Azoles

Itraconazole, the first triazole effective against aspergillus, became available for clinical use in the mid-1990s. Data on resistance to itraconazole in the clinical context are limited, as shown in Table 4 (30, 37, 38, 82–89). Sporadic isolates of aspergillus resistant to itraconazole have been reported (90). It appears that both primary and secondary resistance to itraconazole does occur, and recent observations suggest an increase in azole-resistant *A. fumigatus* isolates. In a nationwide survey of 21 Dutch hospitals, no patients with multiple triazole resistant *A. fumigatus* were found (0 of 114 patients) during 1945–1998 as compared with 10 of 81 patients with such isolates since 2002 (*P* < 0.001) (88). Data on clinical significance of azole-resistant aspergillus isolates are steadily emerging. Noteworthy is a case report – a patient with chronic

granulomatous disease, who while receiving long-term prophylaxis with itraconazole, developed itraconazole-resistant invasive aspergillosis and required high-dose voriconazole for successful outcome (87). The *A. fumigatus* isolate had reduced susceptibility to other azoles (voriconazole, ravuconazole, and posaconazole) as well. Factors to explain the rise in azole-resistance among *A. fumigatus* isolates remain unclear. Such an emergence coinciding with the approval and increased use of voriconazole is noteworthy. However, azole-resistant infection has also occurred in patients who had not been previously treated with azoles suggesting that extensive azole use in agricultural environments may play a role (88).

In theory, "clinical resistance" may be anticipated during therapy with a polyene following exposure to azole, because the azole may have depleted the common target (i.e. ergosterol). No clinical study, however, has implicated prior azole exposure (as prophylaxis or therapy) as a cause for subsequent failure with polyene therapy, but such patients may need close observation. This situation may occur with increasing frequency with the standard use of voriconazole as primary therapy or prophylaxis against aspergillosis. Initial treatment with a polyene followed by an azole (as step-down or salvage) has been the common practice in the past. Voriconazole has been used with satisfactory results (~50% response) as salvage therapy in most patients initially treated with amphotericin B (91).

Given the suboptimal response with single drug use for invasive aspergillosis, particularly in profoundly compromised hosts (e.g. with persistent neutropenia), the strategy of drug combinations is increasingly employed. From previous in vitro observations, clinicians have been concerned about antagonism with the use of drug combinations, leading to clinical failure. However, recent data from in vitro studies and animal models suggest no antagonistic interactions when azoles are combined with polyenes or echinocandins (92–97). Retrospective data suggest synergistic efficacy with combination of azole (voriconazole) plus caspofungin (98, 99). Since no controlled clinical data are available from prospective studies of combination therapy, no firm recommendations can be made regarding simultaneous use of two or more drugs in the management of invasive aspergillosis. Whether emergence of resistance can be delayed or prevented with the strategy of combination therapy remains to be explored. Under desperate circumstances, clinicians employ multi-drug therapy in severe aspergillosis. Drug combinations are not always beneficial, may have antagonistic interactions and adverse effects of drugs, drug interactions, and drug costs are serious considerations.

4.3 Resistance to Echinocandins

No clinical data on aspergillus resistance to echinocandins are reported. Emergence of resistance is to be anticipated due

Table 4 Azole resistance in *Aspergillus*: human data

Reference/first author	Clinical data	Comments
(82)/Chryssanthou	*Three of 80 patients*: initially ITZ-susceptible, then ITZ-resistant *A. fumigatus* (ITZ use: 5 months–3 years)	No genotyping done (?Different strains)
(30)/Denning	*Patient 1*: Hodgkin's Disease – ITZ-susceptible *A. fumigatus* pleuropericarditis. Oral ITZ × 9 months, then Sputum: *A. fumigatus* (ITZ MIC > 16 µg/ml)	*A. fumigatus* strains with in vitro ITZ – resistance: good correlation in animal model
(84)/Oakley	*Patient 2*: AIDS-invasive aspergillosis due to *A. fumigatus*; AmB for 3 months; Relapsed infection (*A. fumigatus*[1] – recovered from sputum); improved with ITZ. Sputum culture – *A. fumigatus*[2]. Both *A. fumigatus*[1] and *A. fumigatus*[2] had ITZ MIC > 16 µg/ml *Animal model*: no decreased mortality in animals receiving ITZ for infection with ITZ-resistant aspergillus	Mechanism of resistance: primary or secondary
(85)/Dannaoui	*Patient*: bronchiectasis; sputum: ITZ-susceptible *A. fumigatus* Rx: ITZ × 5 months Relapse of infection; subsequent *A. fumigatus* ITZ MIC > 16 µg/ml *Animal model*: poor efficacy of ITZ in animals infected with ITZ-resistant aspergillus	Pre- and post-therapy isolates had similar RAPD patterns (i.e. same strain)
(86)/Verweij	*1945–1998*: collection of clinical isolates of aspergillus in the Netherlands from 114 patients (170 isolates)	Three ITZ-resistant *A. fumigatus* isolates recovered from a lung transplant recipient receiving ITZ
(87)/Balajee	1991–2000 (Seattle, USA) 10 of 128 *A. fumigatus* isolates: ITZ-resistant (MIC ≥ 1 µg/ml) Also, cross resistant with VCZ/caspofungin/amphotericin B	10 patients with ITZ-resistant *A. fumigatus* (No previous exposure to ITZ) Exact mechanisms of cross resistance unknown
88/Warris	*Patient*: chronic granulomatous disease *A. nidulans* infection → Successful therapy with VCZ; maintenance (6 years) on ITZ; subsequent aspergillosis with *A. fumigatus* (ITZ-resistant) Successful therapy with high-dose VCZ	*A. fumigatus* resistant to ITZ/RCZ, and reduced susceptibility to VCZ/PCZ
(37)/Howard	*Patient*: sarcoidosis with chronic cavitary aspergilloma (*A. fumigatus*); therapy with ITZ, then VCZ; some response to IV Caspofungin	*A. fumigatus* resistant to ITZ/VCZ/PCZ and RCZ Mutation (G138C) in the target gene (CYP51A) encoding 14α-sterol demethylase
(38)/Dannaoui	*Patient*: sarcoidosis complicated by aspergilloma; ITZ for 3 years; recovery of ITZ-resistant *A. fumigatus*, treated with VCZ (MIC 1 µg/ml) and obtained good response	Mutation (M220L) in CYP51A plus increased expression of multidrug transporters
(89)/Verweij	*Nine patients (13 isolates)*: 4 with primary IA and 5 with breakthrough IA (prior therapy with ITZ or VCZ); two died *A. fumigatus* resistant to ITZ/VCZ/PCZ/RCZ	Mutation (L98H) in CYP51A with a tandem repeat in the same promoter region (no clonal spread)
(90)/van Leer-Buter	*Patient*: Oropharyngeal carcinoma with pulmonary cavities *Bronchoalveolar lavage*: *A. fumigatus* and *A. niger*. Therapy with VCZ for about 10 days	Autopsy: *A. fumigatus* and *A. niger* *A. fumigatus*: azole-susceptible and azole-resistant (L98H in CYP51A and a tandem repeat in the promoter region) phenotypes

VCZ voriconazole; *ITZ* itraconazole; *PCZ* posaconazole; *RCZ* ravuconazole; *AmB* amphotericin B; *MIC* minimum inhibitory concentration

to the lack of cidal activity of echinocandins against aspergillus and the potential for point mutation resulting in altered glucan synthase. With the increased use of echinocandins for prophylaxis, empiric or definitive therapy, resistance to these drugs in aspergillus isolates needs to be closely monitored.

5 Conclusion

Unlike the situation with candida, data on drug resistance in aspergillus are limited. Recent standardization of susceptibility testing for filamentous fungi has made it possible to study the phenomenon of resistance. Of the four drug classes, aspergillus resistance in azoles is most commonly described; resistance to polyene class has remained remarkably low. Mechanisms of azole resistance in aspergillus are better understood. With the increasing incidence of aspergillosis and the widespread use of orally administered anti-aspergillus drugs for prolonged periods in different settings (prophylaxis or therapy), particularly in compromised hosts or in those with a heavy burden of the organism, the emergence of drug resistance in aspergillus is likely to escalate.

References

1. McNeil MM, Nash SL, Hajjeyh RA, Phelan MA, Conn LA, Pkikaytis BD, et al. Trends in mortality due to invasive mycotic diseases in the United States. 1980–1997. *Clin Infect Dis* 2001; 33:641–647.

2. Baddley JW, Stroud TP, Salzman D, Pappas PG. Invasive mold infections in allogeneic bone marrow transplant recipients. *Clin Infect Dis* 2001; 232:1319–1324.

3. Marr KA, Carter RA, Crippa F, Wald A, Corey L. Epidemiology and outcome of mould infections in hematopeictic stem cell transplant recipients. *Clin Infect Dis* 2002; 34:909–917.

4. Denning DW, Invasive aspergillosis in immunocompromised patients. *Curr Opin Infect Dis* 1994; 7:456–462.

5. Schaffner A, Douglas H, Braude A. Selective protection against conidia by mononuclear and against mycelia by polymorphonuclear phagocytes in resistance to *Aspergillus*. Observations on these two lines of defense in vivo and in vitro with human and mouse phagocytes. *J Clin Invest* 1982; 69:617–631.

6. Schneemann M, Schaffner A. Host defense mechanism in *Aspergillus fumigatus* infections. *Contrib Microbiol* 1999; 2:57–68.

7. National Committee for Clinical Laboratory Standards. Reference method for broth dilution antifungal susceptibility testing of filamentous fungi: approved standard (NCCLS document M38-A). Wayne, PA: National Committee for Clinical Laboratory Standards, 2002.

8. Stewart PS. Mechanisms of antibiotic resistance in bacterial biofilms. *Int J Med Microbiol* 2002; 292:107–113

9. Youngchim S, Morris-Jones R, Hay RJ, Hamilton AJ. Production of melanin by *Aspergillus fumigatus*. *J Med Microbiol* 2004; 53:175–181.

10. Langfelder K, Streibel M, Jahn B, Haase G, Brakhage AA. Biosynthesis of fungal melanins and their importance for human pathogenic fungi. *Fungal Genet Biol* 2003; 38:143–158.

11. Sugar AM. The polyene macrolide antifungal drugs. In P.K. Peterson and J. Verhoef (eds.), *Antimicrobial Agents*, vol. 1, pp 229–244. Elsevier, Amsterdam, the Netherlands, 1986.

12. Kerridge D. The plasma membrane of *Candida albicans* and its role in the action of antifungal drugs. In G. W. Gooday, D. Lloyd, and A.P.J. Trinci (eds.), *The Eukaryotic Microbial Cell*, p 103. Cambridge University Press, Cambridge, England, 1980.

13. Brajtburg J, Powderly WG, Kobayashi GS, Medoff G. Amphotericin B: current understanding of mechanisms of action. *Antimicrob Agents Chemother* 1990; 34:183–188.

14. Manavathu EK, Alangaden GJ, Chandrasekar PH. In-vitro isolation and antifungal susceptibility of amphotericin B-resistant mutants of *Aspergillus fumigatus*. *J Antimicrob Chemother* 1998; 41:615–619.

15. Verweij PE, Oakley KL, Morrissey J, Morrissey G, Denning DW. Efficacy of LY303366 against amphotericin B-susceptible and

16. Odds FC, Gerven FV, Espinel-Ingroff A, Bartlett MS, et al. Evaluation of possible correlations between antifungal susceptibilities of filamentous fungi in vitro and antifungal treatment outcomes in animal infection models. *Antimicrob Agents Chemother* 1998; 42:282–288.

17. Seo K, Akiyoshi H, Ohnishi Y. Alteration of cell wall composition leads to amphotericin B resistance in *Aspergillus flavus*. *Microbiol Immunol* 1999; 43:1017–1025.

18. Walsh TJ, Petraitis V, Petraitiene R, Field-Ridley A, et al. Experimental pulmonary aspergillosis due to *Aspergillus terreus*: pathogenesis and treatment of an emerging fungal pathogen resistant to amphotericin B. *J Infect Dis* 2003; 188:305–319.

19. Manavathu EK, Cutright JL, Chandrasekar PH. In vivo resistance of a laboratory-selected *Aspergillus fumigatus* isolate to amphotericin B. *Antimicrob Agents Chemother* 2005; 49:428–430.

20. Balajee SA, Gribskov JL, Hanley E, Nickle D, Marr KA. *Aspergillus lentulus* sp. nov. a new sibling species of *A. fumigatus*. *Eukaryot Cell* 2005; 4:625–632.

21. Balajee SA, Nickle D, Varga J, Marr KA. Molecular studies reveal frequent misidentification of *Aspergillus fumigatus* by morphotyping. *Eukaryot Cell* 2006; 5:1705–1712.

22. Vanden Bossche H, Lauwers W, Willemsens G, Marichal P, et al. Molecular basis for the antimycotic and antibacterial activity of N-substituted immidazoles and triazoles: the inhibition of isoprenoid biosynthesis. *Pest Sci* 1984; 15:188–198

23. Yoshida Y, Ayoma Y. Interaction of azole antifungal agents with cytochrome $P450_{14DM}$ purified from *Saccharomyces cerevisiae* microsomes. *Biochem Pharmacol* 1987; 36:229–235.

24. Tuck SF, Aoyama Y, Yoshida Y, Ortiz de Montellano PR. Active site topology of *Saccharomyces cerevisiae* lanosterol 14α-demethylase (CYP51) and its G301Δ mutant (cytochrome $P450_{3G1}$). *J Biol Chem* 1992; 267:13175–13179.

25. Vanden Bossche H. Biochemical targets for antifungal azole derivatives: hypothesis on the mode of action. In M. R McGinnis (ed.), *Current Topics in Medical Mycology*, pp 313–351, Springer, New York, 1985.

26. Sabo JA, Abdel-Rahman SM. Voriconazole: a new triazole antifungal. *Ann Pharmacother* 2000; 34:1032–1043.

27. Manavathu EK, Baskaran I, Alangaden GJ, Chandrasekar PH. Molecular characterization of the P450-dependent lanosterol demethylase gene from clinical isolates of *Aspergillus fumigatus*. In Abstracts of the 101st General Meeting of the American Society for Microbiology, May 20–24, 2001, Orlando, FL. Abstract F-20.

28. Mellado E, Diaz-Guerra TM, Cuenca-Estrella M, Rodriguez-Tudela JL. Identification of two different 14α-sterol demethylase-related genes (*cyp*51A and *cyp*51B) in *Aspergillus fumigatus* and other *Aspergillus* species. *J Clin Microbiol* 2001; 39:2431–2438.

29. Osherov N, Kontoyiannis DP, Romans A, May GS. Resistance to itraconazole in *Aspergillus nidulans* and *Aspergillus fumigatus* is conferred by extra copies of the *A. nidulans* P-450 14α-demethylase gene, pdmA. *J Antimicrob Chemother* 2001; 48:75–81.

30. Denning DW, Venkateswarlu K, Oakley KL, Anderson MJ, et al. Itraconazole resistance in *Aspergillus fumigatus*, *Antimicrob Agents Chemother* 1997; 41:1364–1368.

31. Manavathu EK, Abraham OC, Chandrasekar PH. Isolation and in vitro susceptibility of voriconazole-resistant laboratory isolates of *Aspergillus fumigatus*. *Clin Microbiol Infect* 2001; 7:130–137.

32. Diaz-Guerra TM, Mellado E, Cuenca-Estrella M, Rodriguez-Tudela JL. A point mutation in the 14α-sterol demethylase gene cyp51A contributes to itraconazole resistance in *Aspergillus fumigatus*. *Antimicrob Agents Chemother* 2003; 47:1120–1124.

33. Nascimento AM, Goldman GH, Park S, Marras SAE, et al. Multiple resistance mechanisms among *Aspergillus fumigatus* mutants with

high-level resistance to itraconazole. *Antimicrob Agents Chemother* 2003; 47:1719–1726.

34. Mellado E, Garcia-Effron G, Alcazar-Fuoli L, Cuenca-Estrella M, Rodriguez-Tudela JL. Substitutions at methionine 220 in the 14α-sterol demethylase (Cyp51A) of *Aspergillus fumigatus* are responsible for resistance in vitro to azole antifungal drugs. *Antimicrob Agents Chemother* 2004; 48:2747–2750.

35. da Silva Ferreira ME, Capellaro JL, dos Reis Marques E, Malavazi I, Perlin D, Park S, Anderson JB, Colombo AL, Arthington-Skaggs BA, Goldman MH, Goldman GH. In vitro evolution of itraconazole resistance in *Aspergillus fumigatus* involves multiple mechanisms of resistance. *Antimicrob Agents Chemother* 2004; 48:4405–4413.

36. Chen J, Li H, Li R, Bu D, Wan Z. Mutations in the cyp51A gene and susceptibility to itraconazole in *Aspergillus fumigatus* serially isolated from a patient with lung aspergilloma. *J Antimicrob Chemother* 2005; 55:31–37.

37. Dannaoui ED, Garcia-Hemoso D, Naccache JM, Meneau I, Sanglard D, Bouges-Michel C, Valeyre D, Lortholary O. Use of voriconazole in a patient with aspergilloma caused by an itraconazole-resistant strain of *Aspergillus fumigatus*. *J Med Microbiol* 2006; 55:1457–1459.

38. Howard SJ, Webster I, Moore CB, Gardiner RE, Park S, Perlin DS, Denning DW. Multiazole resistance in *Aspergillus fumigatus*. *Int J Antimicrob Agents* 2006; 28:450–453.

39. Kaya AD, Kiraza N. In vitro susceptibilities of *Aspergillus* spp. Causing otomycosis to amphotericin B, voriconazole, and itraconazole. *Mycoses* 2007; 50:447–450.

40. Mellado E, Garcia-Effron G, Alcázar-Fuoli L, Melchers WJG, Verweij PE, Cuenca-Estrella M, Rodríguez-Tudela JL. A new *Aspergillus fumigatus* resistance mechanism conferring in vitro cross-resistance to azole antifungals involves a combination of *cyp51A* alterations. *Antimicrob Agents Chemother* 2007; 51:1897–1904.

41. Manavathu EK, Espinel-Ingroff A, Alangaden GJ, Chandrasekar PH. Molecular studies on voriconazole-resistance in a clinical isolate of *Aspergillus fumigatus*. 43rd ICAAC 2003, Abstract M-392.

42. Mann PA, Parmegiani RM, Wei SO, Mendrick CA, et al. Mutations in *Aspergillus fumigatus* resulting in reduced susceptibility to posaconazole appear to be restricted to a single amino acid in the cytochrome P450 14α-demethylase. *Antimicrob Agents Chemother* 2003; 47:577–581.

43. Xiao L, Madison V, Chau AS, Loebenberg D, et al. Three-dimensional models of wild-type and mutated forms of cytochrome P450 14α-sterol demethylases from *Aspergillus fumigatus* and *Candida albicans* provide insights into posaconazole binding. *Antimicrob Agents Chemother* 2004; 48:568–574.

44. Boscott PE, Grant GH. Modeling of cytochrome P450 14α-demethylase (*Candida albicans*) from P450cam. *J Mol Graph* 1994; 12:185–193.

45. Podust LM, Stojan J, Poulos TL, Watermann MR. Substrate recognition sites in 14α-sterol demethylase from comparative analysis of amino acid sequences and X-ray structure of *Mycobacterium tuberculosis* CYP51. *J Inorg Biochem* 2001; 87:227–235.

46. White TC. Increased mRNA levels of ERG16, CDR, and MDR1 correlate with increases in azole resistance in *Candida albicans* isolates from a patient infected with human immunodeficiency virus. *Antimicrob Agents Chemother* 1997; 41:1482–1487.

47. Sanglard D, Kuchler K, Ischer F, Pagani JL, et al. Mechanisms of resistance to azole antifungal agents in *Candida albicans* isolates from AIDS patients involve specific multidrug transporters. *Antimicrob Agents Chemother* 1995; 39;2378–2386.

48. Prasad R, Wergifosse P, Goffeau A, Balzi E. Molecular cloning and characterization of *Candida albicans*, CDR1, conferring multiple resistance to drugs and antifungals. *Curr Genet* 1995; 27:320–329.

49. Parkinson T, Falconer DJ, Hitchcock CA. Fluconazole resistance due to energy-dependent drug efflux in *Candida glabrata*. *Antimicrob Agents Chemother* 1995; 39;1696–1699.

50. Venkateswarlu K, Denning DW, Manning NJ, Kelly SL. Resistance to fluconazole in *Candida albicans* from AIDS patients correlated with reduced intracellular accumulation of drug. *FEMS Microbiol Lett* 1995; 131:337–341.

51. Albertson GD, Niimi M, Cannon RD, Jenkinson HF. Multiple efflux mechanisms are involved in *Candida albicans* fluconazole resistance. *Antimicrob Agents Chemother* 1996; 40:2835–2841.

52. Slaven JW, Anderson MJ, Sanglard D, Dixson GK, et al. Increased expression of a novel *Aspergillus fumigatus* ABC transporter gene, atrF, in the presence of itraconazole in itraconazole resistant clinical isolate. *Fungal Genet Biol* 2002; 36:199–206.

53. Latge JP. *Aspergillus fumigatus* and aspergillosis. *Clin Microbiol Rev* 1999; 12:310–350.

54. Manavathu EK, Vasquez JA, Chandrasekar PH. Reduced susceptibility in laboratory-selected mutants of *Aspergillus fumigatus* to itraconazole due to decreased intracellular accumulation of the antifungal agent. *Int J Antimicrob Agents* 1999; 12:213–219.

55. Douglas CM, D'Ippolito JA, Shei GJ, Meinz M, et al. Identification of the FKS1 gene of *Candida albicans* as the essential target of 1,3-β-D-glucan synthase inhibitors. *Antimicrob Agents Chemother* 1997; 41:2471–2479.

56. Gardiner RE, Souteropoulos P, Park S, Perlin DS. Characterization of *Aspergillus fumigatus* mutants with reduced susceptibility to caspofungin. *Med Mycol* 2005; 43 Suppl 1:S299–S305.

57. Rocha EMF, Garcia-Effron G, Park S, Perlin DS. A Ser678Pro substitution in Fks1p confers resistance to echinocandin drugs in *Aspergillus fumigatus*. *Antimicrob Agents Chemother* 2007; 51:4174–4176.

58. Petranyi G, Petraitiene R, Sarafandi AA, Kelaher AM, et al. Antifungal activity of the allylamine derivative terbinafine in vitro. *Antimicrob Agents Chemother* 1987; 31:1365–1368.

59. Ryder NS, Leiner I. Synergistic interaction of terbinafine with triazoles or amphotericin B against *Aspergillus* species. *Med Mycol* 2001; 39:91–95.

60. Ryder NS, Favre B. Antifungal activity and mechanism of action of terbinafine. *Rev Contemp Pharmacother* 1997; 8:275–287.

61. Mosquera J, Moore CB, Warn PA, Denning DW. In vitro interaction of terbinafine with itraconazole, fluconazole, amphotericin B and 5-flucytosine against *Aspergillus* species. *J Antimicrob Chemother* 2002; 50:189–194.

62. Liu W, May GS, Lionakis MS, Lewis RE, et al. Extra copies of the *Aspergillus fumigatus* squalene epoxidase gene confer resistance to terbinafine: genetic approach to studying gene dose-dependent resistance to antifungals in *A. fumigatus*. *Antimicrob Agents Chemother* 2004; 48:2490–2496.

63. Graminha MAS, Rocha EMF, Prade RA, Martinez-Rossi NM. Terbinafine resistance mediated by salicylate 1-monooxygenase in *Aspergillus nidulans*. *Antimicrob Agents Chemother* 2004; 48:3530–3535.

64. Rocha EMF, Gardiner RE, Park S, Martinez-Rossi NM, Perlin DS. A Phe389Leu substitution in ErgA confers terbinafine resistance in *Aspergillus fumigatus*. *Antimicrob Agents Chemother* 2006; 50:2533–2536.

65. Clemons KV, Stevens DA. The contribution of animal models of aspergillosis to understanding pathogenesis, therapy and virulence. *Med Mycol* 2005; 43: (Suppl 1):S101–S110.

66. Van Etten EW, Stearne-Cullen LE, ten Kate M, Bakker-Woudenberg IA. Efficacy of liposomal amphotericin B with prolonged circulation in blood in treatment of severe pulmonary aspergillosis in leukopenic rats. *Antimicrob Agents Chemother* 2000; 44:540–545.

67. Murphy M, Bernard EM, Ishimaru T, Armstrong D. Activity of voriconazole (UK-109,496) against clinical isolates of *Aspergillus* species and its effectiveness in an experimental model of invasive pulmonary aspergillosis. *Antimicrob Agents Chemother* 1997; 41:696–698.

68. Van Cutsem J, Janssen PJ. In vitro and in vivo models to study the activity of antifungals against *Aspergillus*. In H. Vanden Bossche,

D.W.R. MacKenzie, and G. Cauwenbergh (eds.), *Aspergillus and Aspergillosis*, pp 215–227. Plenum, New York, NY.

69. Chakrabarti A, Jatana M, Sharma SC. Rabbit as an animal model of paranasal sinus mycoses. *J Med Vet Mycol* 1997; 35:295–297.

70. Sutton DA, Sanche SE, Revankar SG, Fothergill AQ, Rinaldi MG. *In vitro* amphotericin B resistance in clinical isolates of *Aspergillus terreus*, a head-to-head comparison of voriconazole. *Clin Infect Dis* 2004; 39:743–746.

71. Warn PA, Morrissey G, Morrissey J, Denning DW. Activity of micafungin (FK463) against an itraconazole-resistant strain of *Aspergillus fumigatus* and a strain of *Aspergillus terreus* demonstrating in vivo resistance to amphotericin B. *J Antimicrob Chemother* 2003; 51:913–919.

72. Iwen PC, Rupp ME, Bishop MR, Rinaldi MG, Sutton DA, Tarantolo S, Hinrichs SH. Disseminated aspergillosis caused by *Aspergillus ustus* in a patient following allogcneic peripheral stem cell transplantation. *J Clin Microbiol* 1998; 36:3713–3717.

73. Pavie J, Lacroix C, Hermoso DG, Robin M, Ferry C, Bergeron A, Feuilhade M, Dromer F, Gluckman E, Molina J-M, Ribaud P. Breakthrough disseminated *Aspergillus ustus* infection in allogeneic hematopoietic stem cell transplant recipients receiving voriconazole or caspofungin prophylaxis. *J Clin Microbiol* 2005; 43:4902–4904.

74. Imhof A, Balajee SA, Fredricks DN, Englund JA, Marr KA. Breakthrough fungal infections in stem cell transplant recipients receiving voriconazole. *Clin Infect Dis* 2004; 39:743–746.

75. Iwen PC, Rupp ME, Langnas AN, Reed EC, Hinrichs SH. Invasive pulmonary aspergillosis due to *Aspergillus terreus*: 12-year experience and review of the literature. *Clin Infect Dis* 1998; 26:1092–1097.

76. Steinbach WJ, Benjamin DK Jr., Kontoyiannis DP, Perfect FR, Lutsar I, Marr KA, et al. Infections due to *Aspergillus terreus*: a multicenter retrospective analysis of 83 cases. *Clin Infect Dis* 2004; 39:192–198.

77. Lass-Florl C, Kofler G, Kropshofcr G, et al. *In vitro* testing of susceptibility of amphotericin B is reliable predictor of clinical outcome in invasive aspergillosis. *J Antimicrob Chemother* 1998; 42:497–502.

78. Frankenbusch K, Eifinger F, Kribs A, Rengelshauseu J, Roth B. Severe primary cutaneous aspergillosis refractory to amphotericin B and the successful treatment with systemic voriconazole in two premature infants with extremely low birth weight. *J Perinatol* 2006; 26:511–514.

79. Lionakis MS, Lewis RE, Torres HA, Albert ND, Raad II, Kontoyiannis DP. Increased frequency of non-*fumigatus Aspergillus* species in amphotericin B- or triazole-pre-exposed cancer patients with positive cultures for aspergilli. *Diagn Microbiol Infect Dis* 2005; 52:15–20.

80. Moosa MY, Alangaden GJ, Manavathu EK, Chandrasekar PH. Resistance to amphotericin B does not emerge during treatment for invasive aspergillosis. *J Antimicrob Chemother* 2002; 49:209–213.

81. Dannaoui E. Meletiadis J, Tortorano AM, et al. Susceptibility testing of sequential isolates of *Aspergillus fumigatus* recovered from treated patients. *J Med Microbiol* 2004; 53:129–134.

82. Paterson PJ, Seaton S, Prentice HG, Kibbler CC. Treatment failure in invasive aspergillosis: susceptibility of deep tissue isolates following treatment with amphotericin B. *J Antimicrob Chemother* 2003; 52:873–876.

83. Chrysssanthou E. In vitro susceptibility of respiratory isolates of *Aspergillus* species to itraconazole and amphotericin B acquired resistance to itraconazole. *Scand J Infect Dis* 1997; 29:509–512.

84. Oakley KL, Morrissey G, Denning DW. Efficacy of SCH-56592 in a temporarily neutropenic murine model of invasive aspergillosis with an itraconazole-susceptible and an itraconazole-resistant isolate of *Aspergillus fumigatus*. *Antimicrob Agents Chemother* 1997; 41:1504–1507.

85. Dannaoui E, Borel E, Monier MR, Piens MA, et al. Acquired itraconazole resistance in *Aspergillus fumigatus*. *J Antimicrob Chem* 2001; 47:333–340.

86. Verweij PE, TE Dorsthorst DTA, Rijs AJMM, et al. Nationwide survey of in vitro activities of itraconazole and voriconazole against clinical *Aspergillus fumigatus* isolates cultured between 1945 and 1998. *J Clin Microb* 2002; 47:2648–2650.

87. Balajee SA, Weaver M, Imhof A, et al. *Aspergillus fumigatus* variant with decreased susceptibility to multiple antifungals. *Antimicrob Agents Chemother* 2004; 48:1197–1203.

88. Warris A, Weemaes CM, Verweij PE. Multidrug resistance in *Aspergillus fumigatus*. *N Engl J Med* 2002; 347:2173–2174.

89. Verweij PE, Mellado E, Melchers WJ. Multiple-triazole-resistant aspergillosis. *N Engl J Med* 2007; 356:1481–1483.

90. van Leer-Buter C, Takes RP, Hebeda KM, Melchers WJG, Verweij PE. Aspergillosis-and a misleading sensitivity result. *Lancet* 2007; 370:102.

91. Dannaoui E, Persat F, Monier MR, Borel E, Piens MA, Picot S. In vitro susceptibility of *Aspergillus* spp. Isolates to amphotericin B and itraconazole. *J Antimicrob Chemother* 1999; 44:553–555.

92. Denning DW, Ribaud P, Milpied N, Caillot D, Herbrecht R, Thiel E, et al. Efficacy and safety of voriconazole in the treatment of acute invasive aspergillosis. *Clin Infect Dis* 2002; 34:563–571.

93. Denning DW, Hanson LH, Perlman AM, Stevens DA. In vitro susceptibility and synergy studies of *Aspergillus* species to conventional and new agents. *Diagn Microbiol Infect Dis* 1992; 15:21–34.

94. Maesaki S, Kohno S, Kaku M, Koga H, Hara K. Effects of antifungal agent combinations administered simultaneously and sequentially against *Aspergillus fumigatus*. *Antimicrob Agents Chemother* 1994; 38:2843–2845.

95. Arikan S, Lozano-Chiu M, Paetznick V, Rex JH. In vitro synergy of caspofungin and amphotericin B against *Aspergillus* and *Fusarium* spp. *Antimicrob Agents Chemother* 2002; 46:245–247.

96. Perea S, Gonzalez G, Fothergill AW, Kirkpatrick WR, Rinaldi MG, Patterson TF. In vitro interaction of caspofungin acetate with voriconazole against clinical isolates of *Aspergillus* spp. *Antimicrob Agents Chemother* 2002; 46:3039–3041.

97. Kirkpatrick WR, Perea S, Coco BJ, Patterson TF. Efficacy of caspofungin alone and in combination with voriconazole in a Guinea pig model of invasive aspergillosis. *Antimicrob Agents Chemother* 2002; 46:2564–2568.

98. Petraitis V, Petraitiene R, Sarafandi AA, Kelaher AM, Lyman CA, Casler HE, et al. Combination therapy in treatment of experimental pulmonary aspergillosis: synergistic interactions between an antifungal triazole and an echinocandin. *J Infect Dis* 2003; 187:1834–1843.

99. Marr KA, Boeckh M, Carter RA, Kim HW, Corey L. Combination antifungal therapy for invasive aspergillosis. *Clin Infect Dis* 2004; 39:797–802.

Chapter 66
Drug Resistance in *Cryptococcus neoformans*

Kimberly E. Hanson, Barbara D. Alexander, and John Perfect

1 Introduction

Cryptococcus neoformans is an encapsulated yeast known to cause disease in both immunosuppressed as well as seemingly immunocompetent hosts. The infection begins after inhalation of the yeast into the lung which may be followed by hematogenous spread to extrapulmonary tissue (1). The five most common anatomic sites of cryptococcal involvement are the lungs, central nervous system (CNS), skin, prostate, and eye. Importantly, *C. neoformans* has a unique predilection for neural tissue and causes severe and often fatal meningoencephalitis. Most patients present themselves with subacute signs and symptoms of the central nervous system disease such as fever, headache, mental status changes, lethargy, or coma (1).

There are two species of pathogenic cryptococcus with five major serotypes based on various capsular epitopes. Nearly all infections in patients with AIDS involve the *C. neoformans* variety *grubii* (serotype A) except in Europe where *Cryptococcus neoformans* var. *neoformans* (serotype D) and some A/D hybrid strains also cause clinical diseases. *C. gattii* (serotypes B and C) is confined to the tropics and subtropics and primarily causes infection in immunocompetent individuals. Despite serological evidence for widespread infection in select human populations, cryptococcosis is an uncommon disease in individuals with a healthy immune system. Life-threatening infections caused by this pathogen have been increasingly recognized worldwide, largely due to the AIDS epidemic and the expanded use of immunosuppressive drugs and chemotherapeutic agents. Progress in the fields of organ transplantation and management strategies in hematology–oncology have led to decreased patient mortality and to an increased number of immunosuppressed survivors at risk for invasive fungal infections. Although precise estimates of the incidence of cryptococcal disease are not available, the disease was thought to affect between 6 and 10% of AIDS patients in the United States, Australia, and western Europe prior to the advent of highly active antiretroviral therapy (HAART). Currently, between 15 and 30% of AIDS patients in sub-Saharan Africa are affected (1, 2). The incidence of cryptococcosis is particularly high in the southeastern US and equatorial Africa (1, 2).

Cryptococcal disease in both HIV-positive and HIV-negative hosts continues to be associated with significant morbidity and mortality. Successful treatment has historically relied on the use of amphotericin B, flucytosine, and fluconazole. Despite the availability of new antifungal agents and HAART, treatment failures continue to occur for a variety of reasons including direct antifungal drug resistance. AIDS patients with cryptococcal meningitis who survive beyond initial induction therapy may require prolonged maintenance therapy to prevent disease relapse. This treatment setting in conjunction with the prolonged use of antifungal agents for other fungal infections has generated concern that the less susceptible cryptococcal strains may emerge.

The potentially devastating clinical ramifications of antifungal drug resistance have led to intensified efforts to better define the scope of the resistance problem. To this end, a significant amount of work has gone toward improving and standardizing systems capable of identifying fungal resistance when it occurs, delineating the molecular mechanisms responsible for the development of drug resistance, and designing new and improved strategies to treat patients with resistant cryptococcosis. The aim of this review is to summarize the current understanding of clinical resistance in *Cryptococcus neoformans* and to discuss future directions for the prevention and management of clinical resistance when it occurs.

2 Definitions

Drug resistance is an important clinical problem in a variety of infectious diseases. Classically, the term resistance is used to describe an in vitro phenomenon in which a microorganism

J. Perfect (✉)
Acting Chief, Division Infections Diseases,
Duke University Medical Center, Durham, NC, USA
perfe001@mc.duke.edu

D.L. Mayers (ed.), *Antimicrobial Drug Resistance*,
DOI 10.1007/978-1-60327-595-8_66, © Humana Press, a part of Springer Science+Business Media, LLC 2009

displays relative insensitivity to a specified antimicrobial agent as compared with other isolates of the same species. Resistance can either be primary or secondary. Primary resistance occurs in microorganisms never exposed to the drug of interest. Primary resistance in *C. neoformans* is relatively uncommon but has been reported to occur with flucytosine (3) and possibly fluconazole (4). Secondary resistance, also known as acquired resistance, results from previous drug exposure. This form of drug resistance has been increasingly observed in *C. neoformans* with the azole class of antifungals (5–10). Secondary resistance to flucytosine was primarily a concern in the 1970s when this agent was used as monotherapy for the treatment of cryptococcal meningitis, but with the use of the combination of flucytosine and amphotericin B, this development to flucytosine resistance is unusual (11). Intrinsic resistance has been defined as an inherent resistance of all isolates of one species to a certain drug. This type of resistance in *C. neoformans* has been described for the echinocandin class of drugs which target the 1,3 beta-glucan synthetase (12). The relatively low efficacy of caspofungin, the first commercially available echinocandin, may be a result of limited drug activity against the *C. neoformans* glucan synthetase (2). Clinical resistance has also been termed clinical failure. Clinical resistance describes an in vivo phenomenon in which a microorganism continues to cause/show evidence of the disease despite therapeutic concentrations of an appropriate antibiotic at the site of infection.

2.1 Clinical Resistance

The reasons for clinical treatment failure are many and include: (1) host factors such as immune status; (2) site of infection; (3) drug characteristics including bioavailability and toxicity profile; (4) fungal factors such as the virulence of the infecting strain as well as the minimum inhibitory concentration (MIC). Arguably, the most important long-term prognostic factor for the successful treatment of cryptococcosis is the ability to treat the patient's underlying disease process (3).

2.1.1 Clinical Resistance Patterns in Patients Without HIV Infection

Treatment failure as a result of impaired host defenses has been clearly described in the setting of neoplastic disease. In the classic prognostic analysis conducted by Diamond and Bennett in 1974, patients who died on amphotericin B therapy were more likely to have an underlying lymphoreticular malignancy and/or to have received corticosteroid therapy (13). Furthermore, patients with cryptococcal meningitis who relapsed after antifungal therapy were more

likely to have received 20 mg or more of prednisone a day. Improved clinical outcomes were noted if the corticosteroids were reduced to below 20 mg of prednisone daily.

Outcomes related to invasive cryptococcal disease in HIV-negative patients have been reevaluated in the era of effective azole therapy. Overall mortality was 30%, and mortality attributable to cryptococcal meningitis was 12% in a study of 306 HIV-negative patients conducted at 15 United States medical centers from 1990 through 1996 (14). Cause-specific mortality was highest for patients with organ failure syndromes (34%), and second highest for patients with hematologic malignancies (21%) (14). Although solid organ transplant (SOT) recipients are at risk for developing cryptococcal disease, SOT recipients in this study were not shown to have poorer outcomes as compared with other groups. Other investigators, however, have reported higher mortality rates for SOT recipients who develop cryptococcosis. In a MEDLINE review through 1998, Husain et al. (15) identified a total of 178 cases of *C. neoformans* infection in SOT recipients and reported an overall mortality rate of 42% (72/172). Another observational study of 31 SOT recipients with *C. neoformans* infection quoted a mortality rate of 50% (16). More studies are needed in solid organ transplant recipients to know whether this group may be at a higher risk for death from cryptococcal disease.

2.1.2 Clinical Resistance Patterns in Patients With HIV Infection

Currently recommended antifungal treatment regimens in conjunction with HAART have improved the prognosis for patients with HIV-associated cryptococcosis, however, the acute mortality remains unacceptably high (17). Robinson and colleagues (18) reported that 37% of 204 evaluable AIDS patients with cryptococcal meningitis enrolled between 1986 and 1993 failed to have a negative CSF culture after 10 weeks of the combination therapy with amphotericin B (AmB) and flucytosine. Twenty-nine deaths were reported within the first 2 weeks of the study and a total of 62 deaths occurred prior to the 10-week assessment. Multivariate analysis identified the CD4 cell count as one of the characteristics associated with the treatment outcome at 10 weeks.

2.1.3 Clinical Resistance and Pharmacologic Limitations

The location of cryptococcal infection in combination with the pharmacologic properties of currently available antifungal drugs also plays a role in clinical outcome. A vivid example of this was the observation that fluconazole incompletely eradicated cryptococcus from the genitourinary tract of patients with prostatic involvement and HIV infection (19).

Similarly, ketoconazole with its inconsistent oral absorption and limited penetration into the central nervous system has been shown to be ineffective for treating cryptococcal meningitis in spite of in vitro activity (20). Drug side-effect profiles and patient adherence are also important considerations in treatment failure. Nephrotoxicity and infusion-related side effects, for example, can limit the clinical effectiveness of AmB, and the development of bone marrow and gastrointestinal side effects have been a problem with flucytosine therapy.

2.1.4   Cryptococcal Virulence Factors and Clinical Resistance

Cryptococcal pathogenicity also influences clinical resistance patterns. Intrinsic virulence differences among *C. neoformans* strains have been shown to exist under controlled conditions in animal models (21) and cryptococcal infection in humans may be linked to the infecting strain's inherent virulence characteristics. Mitchell and colleagues (22) performed a retrospective review of patients with cerebral cryptococcosis in Australia between 1985 and 1992. Infection with *C. neoformans var gattii* was associated with a poorer prognosis despite prolonged AmB administration and careful management of increased intracranial pressure. In addition to the cryptococcal variety, the yeast's ability to produce a melanin-like pigment in vitro has also been linked to pathogenesis (23). Melanin may protect the yeast from UV damage, extremes in temperature, oxidative stresses, and host macrophages (24). Van Duin et al. (25) demonstrated that melanization reduced the susceptibility of *C. neoformans* to AmB and caspofungin using in vitro killing assays. The work of Odom and colleagues (26) has shown that calcineurin is required for *C. neoformans* virulence in warm temperatures that mimic the host environment. The cryptococcal capsule has also been shown to play a key role in virulence. Acapsular mutants are typically avirulent, whereas encapsulated organisms display varying degrees of pathogenicity. Buchanan and Murphy (23) have provided an extensive review of cryptococcal disease pathogenesis.

We have highlighted several of the host characteristics, pharmacologic limitations, and fungal virulence factors thought to be an integral part of cryptococcal clinical resistance. In addition to these variables, the in vitro antimicrobial susceptibility of *C. neoformans* has been shown in both animal models and clinical practice to be an important predictor of clinical outcome in cryptococcal infection (22, 25, 27–29). Primary and secondary antifungal drug resistance have both become clinically important issues as the number of immunocompromised patients requiring long-term antifungal therapy has grown. The remainder of this review will focus on the identification of resistant cryptococcal isolates in the microbiology laboratory in addition to a review of the epidemiology and molecular mechanisms of antifungal drug resistance in *C. neoformans*.

3 Susceptibility Testing

Antifungal susceptibility testing has accrued substantial interest in recent years as the incidence of invasive fungal infections and the number of available antifungal agents have increased. A great deal of effort has gone into the development of a reproducible and clinically relevant reference method for the susceptibility testing of yeast. This collaborative work has promoted standardization across laboratories and, although imperfect, it has given clinicians an in vitro benchmark to assist in the selection of antifungal therapy. The National Committee for Clinical Laboratory Standards (NCCLS) has published laboratory standards (M27-A2 and M44-A) for the susceptibility testing of yeast.

The M27 document has been revised multiple times beginning with a proposed version (M27-P) in 1992, followed by a tentative document (M27-T) in 1995, and the approved guidelines (M27-A) published in 1997 with a second edition (M27-A2) accepted in August of 2002. The M27-A2 broth dilution method specifies inoculum preparation, culture medium, incubation parameters, and MIC endpoints for flucytosine and the azoles. NCCLS endorses both broth macrodilution methodology in addition to a microdilution adaptation, as a substantial body of work has shown excellent correlation between the two techniques (30, 31). The microdilution method, which is less labor intensive, has become the broth dilution technique of choice in most microbiology laboratories.

The M44-A document, which replaced M44-P in 2004, provides methodology for disk diffusion testing of *Candida* spp. with interpretive breakpoints for fluconazole. One significant advantage of this method is that qualitative results can usually be determined after 20–24h incubation as opposed to 72h with M27. M44 methods and breakpoints have been extended to *Cryptococcus*. Pfaller et al. compared fluconazole disk diffusion zone diameters to MICs determined by M27-A2 (32). A total of 276 clinical *C. neoformans* isolates were tested and method comparisons yielded an overall categorical agreement of 86%, with 0% very major errors, 2% major errors, and 12% minor errors.

3.1 Modifications to the M27-A2 Document

One concern has been that some *C. neoformans* isolates grow slowly or suboptimally in the NCCLS M27 recommended RPMI-1640 medium. Additionally, the recommended incubation time of 72h is felt by some to be too long for practical purposes. Amendments to the M27-A2 methods are provided by the NCCLS that may enhance the performance of drug susceptibility testing for *C. neoformans*. The use of Yeast Nitrogen Base (YNB) in place of the standard RPMI-1640 medium may facilitate the growth of *C. neoformans* and improve the clinical relevance of the MIC. This alteration was first suggested by Ghannoum et al. (33). A subsequent study showed strong inter-laboratory agreement between the NCCLS M27-P microdilution method and the YNB-based method proposed by Ghannoum when tested at three separate sites (2).

3.2 The E-Test for Antifungal Susceptibility Testing

Several investigators have compared the E-test and NCCLS microdilution methods for determining susceptibility of *C. neoformans* isolates. The results of these investigations have been somewhat mixed. Using RPMI 1640 medium with 2% glucose (RPG agar) for the E-test, Aller et al. (34) reported that fluconazole and flucytosine MICs measured by the E-test showed good agreement with broth microdilution methods (81.1 and 89.2% ± 2 dilutions agreement, respectively). Only fluconazole, however, showed a statistically significant agreement between methods. Itraconazole and AmB MICs showed poor correlation (54% and 13.5% ± 2 dilutions agreement, respectively). No itraconazole or AmB-resistant isolates were included for analysis. Using the same medium, Maxwell and colleagues (35) showed good agreement between the E-test and microdilution methods for voriconazole (94%) and AmB (99%).

Lozano-Chiu et al. (31) reported that antibiotic 3 medium was superior to both the YNB and the RPMI-1640 media for consistently identifying AmB-resistant cryptococcal isolates in broth by the M27-A2 methods. When these investigators used an E-test agar diffusion method, both the RPMI-1640 and the antibiotic 3 medium allowed ready detection of the amphotericin B-resistant isolates. In addition, the investigators reported a high level of agreement between the broth and E-test methods.

The etiology of discrepancy in AmB results between these studies is unclear. Based on available data, the E-test is likely to be a useful alternative to the M27 microdilution technique for determining the susceptibility of *C. neoformans* to flucytosine, fluconazole, voriconazole, and possibly AmB. The E-test may be especially helpful for detecting AmB-resistant isolates.

3.3 Interpretive Breakpoints

Interpretative breakpoints have only been established for *Candida* species, and correlate most strongly with the treatment of esophageal candidiasis in HIV-infected patients. Even though recent refinements in susceptibility testing have

provided clearer MIC cut-off data, continued technical variability and lack of a standardized test medium have prevented the establishment of interpretive breakpoints for *C. neoformans* by the NCCLS broth dilution. At this time, there is no exact MIC or zone size endpoint to identify resistant *C. neoformans* phenotypes. Additional prospective studies are required to identify accurate clinical endpoint determinations for antifungal drug resistance. The interpretive breakpoints for resistance used by our laboratory for *C. neoformans*, based on clinical experience and knowledge of the clinical pharmacology of available antifungal agents, are: a MIC ≥ 16 µg/mL for fluconazole, ≥1 µg/mL for itraconazole, ≥32 µg/mL for flucytosine, and ≥1 µg/mL for AmB. Others have used zone diameters of ≤14 mm as a threshold for resistance. These breakpoints are merely guidelines, and must be interpreted cautiously in the context of the clinical scenario.

3.4 Clinical Relevance of In Vitro Fungal Susceptibility

Several studies have found a correlation between susceptibility testing results, and clinical responses in cryptococcal disease (25, 27–29). The majority of these studies have focused on the clinical predictive value of fluconazole minimal inhibitory concentrations (MICs). Aller et al. (27) reviewed 25 episodes of predominantly AIDS-related cryptococcal infection in 25 patients from 1994 to 1996 from the U.S. and Seville, Spain. Therapeutic failure was observed in 5 of 24 patients with AIDS. There was a statistically significant association between high MICs to fluconazole (≥16 µg/mL) and mortality rate as well as treatment failure. Susceptibility testing in this study was performed following the microdilution guidelines described in document M27-A. Menichetti et al. (28) conducted a study of high-dose fluconazole therapy in 14 consecutive AIDS patients with cryptococcal meningitis. The reported median time to the first negative CSF culture was 56 days for patients who had an isolate with a fluconazole MIC of 4 µg/mL and 16 days for patients with an isolate MIC of <4 µg/mL. Although the difference in median time to CSF sterilization did not reach statistical significance, 40 days, difference may have clinical relevance. An analysis correlating clinical outcome with fluconazole MIC was not conducted in this study.

Witt and colleagues (29), using both the microdilution technique of Ghannoum (36) as well as the M27-P macrodilution method (37), attempted to determine whether or not in vitro cryptococcal susceptibility to fluconazole in conjunction with clinical variables might predict treatment outcome for patients with acute AIDS-associated cryptococcal meningitis. The study population consisted of patients who had enrolled in one of two clinical trials evaluating varying doses of fluconazole with or without flucytosine. The treatment was considered successful if the patient was alive with a sterile CSF culture at the end of 10 weeks of therapy. The mean log MIC for fluconazole was significantly higher for the isolates from patients who failed therapy as compared to those that had treatment success. This was only true, however, when the MIC was measured by the modified microdilution method. There was no statistically significant difference in the mean log MIC distribution when the MIC was measured by the standard M27 macrodilution technique. The authors suggested this discrepancy may be due in part to enhanced growth in the YNB medium as compared to the RPMI used for the macrodilution technique.

There are relatively few published reports of AmB resistance in *C. neoformans* (38–41). Similarly, there is a paucity of data correlating AmB MIC with clinical outcome. Powderly et al. (42) evaluated four serial isolates from a single patient with AIDS-associated cryptococcal meningitis. They described a rise in AmB MICs from 0.4 to 1.6 μg/mL that correlated with clinical relapse. Alternatively, others have described susceptibilities of serial *Cryptococcus neoformans* isolates from patients with relapsed meningitis whose isolates showed no increase in amphotericin resistance relative to the initial isolate (43). Reasons for the lack of data on AmB resistance in *Cryptococcus* may be several-fold. Difficulties with the current reference methods for AmB broth susceptibility testing may be a factor limiting the identification and reporting of resistance in cryptococcal isolates. Regardless of the susceptibility testing method employed, AmB resistance appears to be relatively uncommon in clinical practice.

Finally, it must be emphasized that the MIC is not an ultimate predictor of clinical response. The MIC should always be evaluated in the context of the clinical setting. In any case of treatment failure, one must carefully consider specific host factors such as level of immune competence, site of infection, therapeutic regimen (i.e., drug doses, available serum drug concentrations, potential drug–drug interactions), and medication adherence in addition to in-vitro susceptibility data.

4 Epidemiology of Cryptococcal Antifungal Drug Resistance

A few extensive studies have examined the prevalence of resistant cryptococcal strains in clinical practice (44–47). Brandt and colleagues (44) reported on the largest, population-based, active surveillance program to date. This study was conducted by the Centers for Disease Control and Prevention (CDC) in four metropolitan areas of the United States between 1992–1994 and 1996–1998. A total of 732 isolates from 522 patients were evaluated as part of this surveillance. In vitro susceptibilities for AmB were measured using the E-test and MICs for flucytosine, fluconazole, and itraconazole were measured by the NCCLS broth microdilution method. A broad range of MICs were observed over the study period. Interestingly, the MIC_{50} and MIC_{90} for the four drugs did not change by more than a 1 log dilution between the first 3 years of surveillance as compared to the follow-up 3-year period. No geographical differences were noted. The AmB MIC was ≥2 μg/mL for only two isolates in the entire study. Both isolates were identified in the 1996–1998 surveillance period. Individual histories of AmB exposure were not described for these isolates. Six isolates (0.6%) collected between the years of 1992 and 1994, and four isolates (1.6%) collected between 1996 and 1998, had flucytosine MICs ≥32 μg/mL. The incident isolate MIC for fluconazole was ≥64 μg/mL for 6 of 253 patients (2.4%) between 1992 and 1994, and ≥64 μg/mL for 2 of 269 patients (0.7%) between 1996 and 1998. The investigators also compared fluconazole susceptibilities for 172 serial isolates of *C. neoformans* collected at least 1 month apart from 71 patients. Thirteen of the 71 (18%) patients with follow-up isolates had a fourfold or greater increase in fluconazole MIC as compared with the initial isolate. The remaining 58 patients (82% of serial isolates) showed either no change in MIC (33 patients) or up to a 1 log dilution change (25 patients). Clinically, this is an interesting observation given that the group of patients with serial isolates available for comparison had presumably been receiving fluconazole maintenance therapy.

Yildiran et al. (46) investigated the in vitro susceptibilities of 213 cerebrospinal fluid isolates from 192 patients against fluconazole, voriconazole, and posaconazole using the M27-A macrodilution method. This *C. neoformans* collection was comprised of isolates previously submitted to the University of Texas Health Science Center in San Antonio between 1990 and 1999. The MIC_{50} and MIC_{90} for each of the triazoles studied remained essentially unchanged over the 10-year observation period. Overall, posaconazole was the most active triazole (MIC_{90}, 0.06 μg/mL) followed by voriconazole (MIC_{90}, ≤ 0.125 μg/mL) and then fluconazole (MIC_{90}, 8 μg/mL). Twenty patients with relapsing meningitis who had serial isolates submitted at least 1 month apart were reviewed. Nine patients (45%) had the same fluconazole MICs (± 1 dilution) for the initial as compared to the final isolates; six patients (30%) had a 4- to 16-fold rise in the fluconazole MIC; and the remaining five patients (25%) had a 4- to 16-fold decrease in MICs. The voriconazole MICs remained unchanged over time (± 1 dilution). Sixteen patients (80%) had equivalent (± 1 dilution) posaconazole MICs for the original and final isolate; 2 (10%) patients had a fourfold rise in MICs; and the final 2 (10%) had a 4- to 16-fold decrease. The observed changes in fluconazole MICs over time did not necessarily predict the directional changes observed in the posaconazole MIC. Proposed explanations for the decrease in posaconazole MICs seen over time in some isolates include speculation that a different cryptococcal strain could be causing relapse. Previous studies, however, have shown that relapses are most often caused by the initial infecting strain. Yildiran suggests that another possible explanation can be derived from the work of Mondon et al. (48) who described transient changes in the expression of azole susceptibility under different growth conditions.

In vitro susceptibility of *Cryptococcus neoformans* has also been studied in the UK. Davey et al. (45) reviewed 263 isolates and also found a broad range of MICs to both fluconazole and itraconazole. Their review consisted of 143 clinical isolates submitted to a reference laboratory in Bristol between 1994 and 1996, 77 isolates collected between 1971 and 1989 from the UK National Collection of Pathogenic Fungi, and 43 isolates collected from Ugandan AIDS patients in 1996 who had not received azole treatment. Eight of 143 (5.6%) isolates collected from 1994 to 1996 had fluconazole MICs $\geq 64\,\mu g/L$ compared with 2 of 41 (4.9%) isolates collected between 1986 and 1989. The MICs for UK isolates were similar to the MICs for the Ugandan isolates. Six AIDS patients were identified in whom an 8- to 32-fold rise in fluconazole MIC occurred with serial blood or CSF isolates.

Results from a global surveillance study of yeast susceptibilities to fluconazole and voriconazole were also recently reported (47). Using standardized disk diffusion testing, 2,230 *C. neoformans* isolates collected from 134 study sites in 40 countries were tested over an 8.5-year period. Interpretive breakpoints (zone diameters) for fluconazole were: susceptible $\geq 19\,mm$ and resistant $\leq 14\,mm$. For voriconazole, $\geq 17\,mm$ was considered susceptible and $\leq 13\,mm$ resistant. Overall, 10.4% of isolates were resistant to fluconazole while only 1.7% were resistant to voriconazle. A significant proportion of fluconazole-resistant isolates (13.6%) showed cross-resistance to voriconazole.

Taken together, these relatively large studies provide us with some insight into the prevalence of cryptococcal drug resistance over diverse geographic regions. Although the majority of isolates in the studies outlined above appear to be susceptible to a variety of antifungal agents in vitro, acquired azole resistance has clearly been demonstrated and continues to be reported (5–8, 10, 19). In many parts of the developing world, the fungicidal combination of AmB and flucytosine for cryptococcal meningitis (CM) is precluded by cost, availability, and difficulties with drug administration and monitoring. In South Africa, like many resource-limited settings, fluconazole monotherapy has primarily been the standard initial treatment for CM. Bicanic et al. recently described 32 episodes of relapsed CM in 27 HIV-positive subjects after initial treatment with fluconazole (400 mg daily) (49). Seventy-six percent of culture-positive relapses ($n = 21$)

were associated with isolates that had reduced susceptibility to fluconazole and these cases carried a high associated mortality regardless of whether or not the patient was on HAART. Interestingly, 44% of patients infected with fluconazole-resistant isolates had been receiving rifampicin without adjustment of fluconazole dose. Rifampicin is known to induce fluconazole metabolism.

In summary, continued surveillance with documentation of clinical outcomes in relation to MIC is warranted. This is especially important in instances of relapsed cryptococcosis.

5 Antifungal Drugs and Molecular Mechanisms of Resistance

There are a limited number of antifungal agents available for the treatment of cryptococcosis. The major classes of drugs in use today are the polyenes, azoles, and fluoropyrimidines. Recent studies have also evaluated the activity of echinocandin analogs alone and in combination with other antifungal agents against *C. neoformans*. The mode of action of the antifungal agents used to treat cryptococcosis can be divided into three broad categories which include: (1) fungal plasma membrane disruption (polyenes and azoles), (2) DNA and RNA synthesis inhibition (fluoropyrimidines), 3) 1,3 β-D-glucan synthase inhibitors (echinocandins). The development of drug resistance can occur at several sites along the fungal metabolic pathway. Research on the mechanisms of antifungal drug resistance has focused on several areas such as alterations of the drug target, impairment of drug entry into the cell, drug efflux out of the cell, and inactivation of drug within the target cell (50–53).

5.1 Polyenes

Amphotericin B deoxycholate was first discovered in 1956 by Gold and coworkers while working with the aerobic actinomycete *Streptomyces nodosus* (50). AmB was licensed for use in 1959 and is active against a variety of fungi including *Cryptococcus neoformans*. The polyene antifungals, including AmB and the newer less toxic lipid formulations, are fungicidal agents. These drugs work by targeting ergosterol, the principal sterol in most fungal plasma membranes. Ergosterol is important for maintaining structural integrity (53). It has been hypothesized that 8–10 molecules of drug bind to form a pore within the fungal lipid bilayer, thus promoting spillage of potassium ions and disruption of the cellular proton gradient (33, 51). In addition to the cell membrane effects, polyenes are also thought to induce oxidative damage in fungal cells (33).

Several investigators have described potential mecha-nisms for AmB resistance (38–41). Kelly et al. (41) described two *C. neoformans* isolates collected from a patient with AIDS-associated cryptococcal meningitis who had failed therapy with AmB and fluconazole. When the pre- and post-treatment isolates were compared, the investigators found the post-treatment isolate to have depleted cell membrane ergosterol concentrations as a result of a newly acquired defect in sterol delta$^{8 \rightarrow 7}$ isomerase. This target defect conferred AmB resistance but did not affect the post-treatment isolates' susceptibility to fluconazole.

Ghannoum et al. (54) also described characteristics of cryptococcal sterol composition in relation to amphotericin B and fluconazole susceptibilities. They evaluated 13 iso-lates from five patients with recurrent cryptococcal meningi-tis. Strain typing with DNA probes showed that the initial and relapse isolates were identical. All five patients had received fluconazole, and three of the five had also received AmB in the interval between initial diagnosis and relapse of infection. Relapse isolates differed from the initial isolates in sterol composition. None of the relapse isolates had a change in AmB susceptibility, but several relapse isolates did differ in their susceptibility to fluconazole (43, 54). The investiga-tors concluded that the sterol changes could have been a result of the selective pressure of the antifungal regimen or potentially a result of unidentified in vivo host selection pressures.

The use of azole antifungals, which also inhibit fungal ergosterol synthesis, may theoretically result in a lack of a binding site for AmB. Joseph-Horne and colleagues (39) identified *C. neoformans* mutants that were cross-resistant to azoles and AmB but found that this cross-resistance was not related to sterol biosynthesis. The frequency with which the cross-resistant phenotype was detected in their study was 10^{-8}. The authors suggest that a single mutation may be responsible for the cross-resistance, and hypothesize that reduced cellular content of drug could account for the observed multi-drug resistance. Unfortunately, no direct measure of AmB drug accumulation could be performed in this investigation. In another study, the same investigators (40) were able to isolate, in vitro, a series of *C. neoformans* mutants resistant to AmB that retained the ability to accumu-late ergosterol. They postulated that there are at least three categories of AmB-resistant mutants found among *C. neo-formans* isolates. These categories include: (1) sterol mutants; (2) AmB and azole cross-resistant mutants; and (3) AmB-resistant mutants exhibiting no azole cross-resistance.

An animal study conducted by Currie et al. (38) suggests that host factors may also play a role in the development of antifungal drug resistance. In this study, serial passage of five environmental *C. neoformans* isolates in a mouse resulted in statistically significant increases in AmB MIC$_{50s}$ for all isolates, but no significant differences in the flucon-azole MICs were noted. Mouse passage was associated with changes in cell membrane sterol content and composition for all five of the passed cryptococcal isolates. Paradoxically, ergosterol content increased in four of the five isolates, all of which were more resistant to AmB after serial passage. This finding highlights the complexity of AmB resistance mecha-nisms and suggests, at least in the murine model, that drug-resistant variants may arise in vivo without prior drug exposure. As of yet, there has not been a report of primary amphotericin B resistance in a *C. neoformans* strain isolated from a human.

5.2 Fluoropyrimidines

Flucytosine (5-FC) is a fluorinated pyrimidine that was dis-covered in 1957 as part of a search for novel chemotherapeu-tics. 5-FC is structurally similar to both fluorouracil (5-FU) and floxuridine (50). 5-FC is an oral antifungal agent with minimal protein binding and excellent penetration into body fluids (51). Flucytosine was first introduced in 1968 with subsequent FDA approval in 1971 for the treatment of inva-sive mycoses.

5-FC is taken up into fungal cells by a cytosine permease. The drug is then deaminated to 5-FU by cytosine deaminase, an enzyme not present in human tissues. Intracellularly, the deam-inated compound is converted to a nucleoside triphosphate termed fluorouridine triphosphate (FUTP). FUTP is incorporated into fungal RNA where it causes miscoding and ultimately abnormal protein synthesis (33, 50). 5-FU may also be converted to a deoxynucleoside capable of disrupting DNA synthesis (33, 50).

Inherent resistance to 5-FC has been demonstrated in *C. neoformans* (55) and is thought to result from one of sev-eral mechanisms (53). First, a loss of cytosine permease or deaminase activity may lead to decreased uptake or deami-nation of the drug (11). These enzymatic defects confer intrinsic resistance to 5-FC (53). The next mechanisms of resistance are defects in the activity of uracil phosphoribo-syltransferase or uridine-5-monophosphate pyrophosphory-lase, enzymes integral to the pyrimidine salvage pathway (11, 53). Block et al. (11) found that cryptococcal isolates resistant to 5-FC also acquired significant resistance to 5-FU. This cross-resistance suggested an abnormality in the protein or genes associated with uracil phosphoribosyltransferase or uridine-5-monophosphate pyrophosphorylase.

Whelan (56) first demonstrated that 5-FC resistance may arise de novo in *C. neoformans* as a result of mutations in either of two non-linked genes. The genes named FCY1 and FCY2 act as simple Mendelian determinants which recom-bine freely, but have not yet been specifically isolated or sequenced. Studies have examined the frequency of the appearance of 5-FC resistant mutants within susceptible clinical isolates (57). In an in vitro experiment, resistant mutants appeared in <0.001% of randomly selected colonies. The average mutation rate was 70 ± 17.9 mutants per 10^7 cryptococcal cells, suggesting that 5-FC resistance is possibly a single mutational event. These data also suggest that the mutation rate is such that 5-FC resistance could easily be selected for at infection sites such as the CSF, where the burden of yeast can reach 10^7 CFU/mL or greater (57, 58).

Hespenthal and Bennett (59) published their early experience with 5-FC as monotherapy for cryptococcal meningitis. Their data, collected before the first AmB/5-FC trials, showed that secondary resistance occurred in six of 13 patients who did not respond to therapy or relapsed. In the isolates that developed secondary resistance, 5-FC MICs rose from ≤ 2.5 to $>320 \mu g/mL$ and remained at this level for all subsequent testing. The overall treatment failure rate for flucytosine monotherapy in this study was 57% (13 out of 23 patients).

The combination of AmB and 5-FC for the treatment of cryptococcal meningitis diminished the frequency of 5-FC resistance in relapse strains (60). Clinical experience has shown that 5-FC should always be used in combination with other antifungal drugs such as AmB or fluconazole for the treatment of life-threatening cryptococcosis because of the high rate of secondary drug resistance (61).

5.3 Azoles

Discovery of the azole derivatives in the late 1960s marked a major therapeutic advance for the treatment of invasive mycoses. This class of antifungal agents is totally synthetic, and consists of two groups, the imidazoles and the triazoles. The triazoles have three nitrogen molecules within the azole ring while the imidazoles have two nitrogen atoms. The azoles are fungistatic drugs. The newer azole compounds (voriconazole and posaconazole) have a broadened spectrum of antifungal activity including activity against most yeast as well as some filamentous fungi (33). Itraconazole, fluconazole, ketoconazole, voriconazole, and posaconazole have all been shown to have in vitro activity against environmental isolates of C. neoformans (62).

5.3.1 Sterol Biosynthesis

Like the polyenes, the azole class of antifungal drugs act by interrupting sterol biosynthesis, a multi-step process involved in the conversion of lanosterol to ergosterol. Specifically, azoles inhibit lanosterol 14α-demethylase ($P450_{14dm}$), a cytochrome P450-dependent enzyme containing a heme moiety in its active site. Azole compounds function by binding to the iron atom within the $P450_{14dm}$ heme group through an unhindered nitrogen in the azole ring. The azole–heme complex prevents the demethylation of lanosterol required for ergosterol formation. Resultant ergosterol depletion in conjunction with the accumulation of lanosterol and other methylated sterol precursors, interferes with fungal membrane structure and function (33, 51, 53, 55).

Several investigators have attempted to better delineate the mechanisms responsible for azole drug resistance in C. neoformans. There appear to be multiple processes that play a role in azole resistance which include changes in the affinity of the target enzyme (sterol 14α-demethylase), inhibition of 3-ketosteroid reductase, drug uptake defects, over-expression of the target enzyme, and genetic mutations encoding for multidrug efflux pumps. Each will be reviewed here.

Venkateswarlu and colleagues (63) evaluated 11 Cryptococcus neoformans isolates in an attempt to determine the biochemical basis of tolerance to fluconazole. The investigators focused on a variability in sterol composition, inhibition of $P450_{14dm}$ by fluconazole, and the cellular concentration of fluconazole. Sterol analysis was conducted in the presence and absence of fluconazole. Exposure to fluconazole produced a decrease in ergosterol levels to below 20% of normal in all isolates. All treated isolates accumulated obtusifolione and eburicol, indicative of the inhibition of 3-ketosteroid reductase (a NADPH-dependent enzyme catalyzing C-4 demethylation required for ergosterol biosynthesis) and $P450_{14dm}$, respectively. Eburicol and obtusifolione can not support cell growth because they are methylated at the C-4 position, and it has been postulated that optimal membrane function requires C-4 demethylation. The investigators suggest that the inhibition of 3-ketosteroid reductase and $P450_{14dm}$ may result from direct azole effects or possibly from the retention of a C-14α-methyl group in the substrate. Inhibition of $P450_{14dm}$ was tested by measuring the incorporation of $[2-^{14}C]$ mevalonate into C-14 demethylated sterols in cell extracts. It was noted that only the isolates with low-level fluconazole resistance displayed decreased $P450_{14dm}$ sensitivity to fluconazole. Finally, cellular concentrations of fluconazole were measured using radiolabeled drug. The most resistant strains were observed to have a 10- to 20-fold reduction in drug accumulation. The authors hypothesize this could have resulted from the presence of multidrug resistance transporters similar to those found in azole-resistant strains of C. albicans. In summary, these data suggest low-level fluconazole resistance may be related to changes in the affinity of the $P450_{14dm}$ target enzyme for fluconazole while high-level fluconazole resistance may result from decreases in the cellular concentration of fluconazole.

Lamb et al. (64) also studied the P450 system of C. neoformans in relation to azole tolerance. In their analysis, sterol composition did not change in the azole-tolerant clinical isolates. All strains accumulated approximately 70%

ergosterol, similar to previous sterol analyses of wild type *C. neoformans*. The investigators also evaluated P450 using microsomal fractions. The specific P450 content was observed to be higher in the azole-tolerant isolates, with approximately twice the P450 content of the susceptible strains. They also noticed that the intracellular concentration of fluconazole was reduced in all of the tolerant isolates, but the drug concentration remained in excess of the microsomal P450 content per cell, suggesting ample drug was available to exert antifungal effect. Lamb's group concluded that alterations in drug target cytochrome P450 may be responsible for azole tolerance, and that this alteration could result in diminished affinity for drug at the enzyme's active site.

5.3.2 14α-Demethylase (ERG11)

Complimentary to the body of work contributing to an improved understanding of the biochemical basis for azole drug resistance in *C. neoformans*, recent attention has also turned to the potential genetic mechanisms of azole drug resistance in *C. neoformans*. The gene encoding 14α-demethylase (ERG11) has been evaluated to determine whether molecular modifications such as mutation or overexpression may lead to antifungal drug resistance in yeast. The majority of this work has been done with *C. albicans*. Mellado and colleagues (65) studied the role of ERG11 alteration in the development of fluconazole resistance in *C. neoformans* by examining five isolates from one AIDS patient with recurrent cryptococcal meningitis exposed to fluconazole over a 14-month period. DNA fingerprinting showed that all five isolates were the same strain. Isolates 1 through/to 4 were considered susceptible to fluconazole (MIC 1–2 μg/mL) while the fifth isolate showed an MIC of 16 μg/mL and was considered resistant. PCR amplification and gene sequencing of ERG11 for the first four isolates did not show any base changes. The fifth strain displayed a point mutation (g1855t) in a highly conserved region of the ERG11 protein. An equivalent substitution has been described at the G464S position in *C. albicans* and has been linked previously to fluconazole resistance in this organism. This analysis is one of the first studies to link a point mutation to drug resistance in *C. neoformans*.

5.3.3 Multi-Drug Efflux Pumps

Posteraro et al. (66) designed a cDNA subtraction library technique to compare gene expression between a fluconazole-resistant mutant and its original azole-susceptible clinical isolate. The azole-resistant mutant was generated by in vitro exposure to fluconazole. The resistant phenotype, with a fluconazole MIC of 64 μg/mL, was stable after 20 consecutive sub-cultures on a drug-free medium. DNA fingerprinting was performed on the two strains, yielding identical RFLP patterns. The investigators then identified cDNA expressed in the resistant mutant but not the fluconazole-susceptible parental strain. Sequence analysis revealed that a portion of cDNA expressed only in the resistant mutant was homologous to known members of the ATP binding cassette (ABC) transporter super-family. ABC transporters are a group of genes known to code for multi-drug efflux pumps. The unique mutant cDNA was then used as a probe to isolate the entire gene from the *C. neoformans* genomic library. Subsequent sequencing identified an ABC transporter gene that encodes a protein with a significant degree of similarity to other ABC transporters. The researchers named the gene *C. neoformans* Antifungal Resistance 1 (*CnAFR1*, GenBank accession number AJ428201). The *CnAFR1* locus in the resistant isolate was disrupted by homologous recombination to determine whether *CnAFR1* is involved in fluconazole resistance. Disruption of the gene resulted in improved susceptibility to fluconazole in the null mutant. Furthermore, reintroduction of *CnAFR1* led to restoration of the resistance phenotype.

Thornewell et al. (67) also identified a *C. neoformans* gene encoding a protein related to the ABC transporter multidrug resistance proteins. However, the cellular function of this CneMDR1 protein has not been clearly established and the investigators concluded further experiments are required to determine whether CneMDR1 is actively involved in antifungal drug resistance.

5.3.4 Heteroresistance

Strains of *C. neoformans* expressing variable susceptibility to azoles in vitro have recently been described. Xu and colleagues (68) examined patterns of fluconazole resistance in 21 strains of *C. neoformans* selected for their inability to grow on plates impregnated with 8 μg/mL of fluconazole. They found significant heterogeneity in mutation rates and fluconazole susceptibilities among strains as well as among progeny of the same strain. These results support the idea that subpopulations with varying fluconazole MICs exist among offspring derived from a single colony. This in vitro phenomenon has been termed heteroresistance. Interestingly, in Xu's study there was no correlation between mutation rate and the original MIC and the resistant phenotype of the putative mutants was stable upon subculture to fluconazole-free medium. Mondon et al. (48) also described heterogeneity in fluconazole MICs among the clonal subpopulations of a single isolate derived from a HIV-negative man, who had never been treated with antifungal drugs. In addition, these investigators outlined steadily increasing fluconazole MICs among six sequential isolates from an AIDS patient with recurrent meningitis. When single colonies obtained from the isolates of both patients were grown on medium containing 64 µg/mL of fluconazole, a homogeneous population of resistant cells was observed. Upon return to a drug-free medium the majority of these sub-clones lost their resistance and reverted to the initial heteroresistant phenotype.

Yamazumi et al. (69) investigated the prevalence of heteroresistance in clinical cryptococcal isolates obtained over a broad geographic distribution. In their report, 4.7% (5 of 107 isolates) exhibited heteroresistance to fluconazole. Similar to previous work, fluconazole resistance was selected for by exposure to fluconazole. This resistance was sensitive to incubation temperatures and reversible after serial subcultures back to a drug-free medium.

The results of these studies are interesting and suggest that mutation rates and selection pressures leading to fluconazole resistance in vitro are likely to be heterogeneous processes. The stability of fluconazole resistance described by Xu is contrasted by findings of back reversion to susceptible phenotype on subculture by Mondon and Yamazumi. This may suggest differing underlying mechanisms of resistance between studies. Further work is warranted to help establish the molecular mechanisms responsible for heteroresistance in vitro, as well as to determine the clinical significance of fluconazole heteroresistance and the role it might play in treatment failure.

5.4 Glucan Synthesis Inhibitors

The fungal cell wall has also been an attractive focus of antifungal drug research and development. Although the composition of the cell wall varies among fungal species, there are common pathways not found in mammalian cells which have been evaluated as potential antifungal drug targets. The general components of these synthesis pathways include chitin, mannoproteins, and 1,3-β-glucan (70). The echinocandins are cyclic hexapeptides which inhibit the biosynthesis of 1,3-β-glucan. Specifically, these compounds function as non-competitive inhibitors of 1,3-β-D-glucan synthase, an enzyme involved in the production of glucan polymers in the fungal cell wall (12, 71). The current generation of echinocandin includes caspofungin, anidulafungin, and micafungin. These agents have potent activity against a variety of fungi including *Candida* species, *Aspergillus* species, and *Pneumocystis carinii,* but limited activity against *C. neoformans* (12). It has been hypothesized that the lack of anti-cryptococccal activity displayed by the echinocandins may result from few 1,3-β-D-glucan linkages in the cryptococcal cell wall, absent or low levels of the target enzyme, or limited binding of the synthase inhibitors to the target enzyme.

Feldmesser et al. (72) undertook an ultra-structural analysis of the cryptococcal cell wall in an attempt to better define glucan linkages, and thereby investigate one of the proposed

mechanisms of echinocandin drug resistance in *C. neoformans. C. neoformans* cells were grown with and without caspofungin in cell culture. Affinity purified rabbit antiserum against 1,3-β- and 1,6-β-D-glucan were used to determine whether these epitopes were present in the cell wall of *C. neoformans* cells. Using immunoelectron microscopy and gold particle quantitation, the investigators were able to show that both 1,3-β- and 1,6-β-D-glucan linkages were present in *C. neoformans* cells grown in vitro as well as in infected murine pulmonary tissue. The researchers detected fewer glucan epitopes when the *C. neoformans* cells were grown in caspofungin concentrations typically fungicidal for other fungal species. The group concluded that the absence of 1,3-β-D-glucan linkages does not explain the relative lack of efficacy of caspofungin. They also found that caspofungin partially inhibited the formation of 1,3-β-D-glucan linkages as measured by epitope detection. The authors suggest that *C. neoformans* 1,3-β-D-glucan synthase may be relatively resistant to inhibition by caspofungin and offer this as an explanation for the drug's lack of efficacy against *C. neoformans.*

Previous studies of *C. albicans* and *S. cerevisiae* mutants have identified the transmembrane subunit of the 1,3-β-D-glucan synthase as the target for the echinocandins. The enzyme is a heteromeric complex consisting of two subunits, a large 215-kDa catalytic subunit in the plasma membrane, and a small GTP-binding subunit which activates the catalytic portion of the enzyme (71). Fks1p is the proposed catalytic subunit, and is encoded by two homologous genes FKS1 and FKS2. Single disruptions of either gene in *S. cerevisiae* have not been shown to affect fungal viability, however, a double disruption is lethal (73). Similar FKS genes have been identified in *C. albicans* and *Aspergillus* species (74).

Thompson et al. (75) cloned and sequenced the FKS1 homolog from a *C. neoformans* strain by cross hybridization to *S. cerevisiae.* Sequence analysis of the cryptococcal Fks1p protein was 58% identical to both *C. albicans* and *S. cerevisiae* FKS1, and 62% homologous to *A. fumigatus* FKS1. Only one copy of FKS was found in the *C. neoformans* isolates. Amino acid sequences known to be essential for echinocandin susceptibility in *S. cerevisiae* were conserved in the cryptococcal analysis. Thompson's group then disrupted the FKS1 gene in order to evaluate its role in cryptococcal viability. Homologous integrative transformation with a plasmid equally capable of integrating into one of the two unique positions within the FKS1 gene was employed to statistically show the essentiality of the gene products for viability. Only one of the two possible integration orientations was capable of disrupting gene function. The demonstration of essentiality derives from exclusive recovery of integrations in the non-disrupting orientation. The investigators observed 23 homologous recombination events in the non-disrupting orientations and no integrations in the disrupting orientation. The probability of this result, assuming an equal chance of recombination in either orientation, is 1.19×10^{-7}. The authors felt this was a strong statistical argument for the essentiality of the FKS1 gene in *C. neoformans*. They also concluded that the gene encoding 1,3-β-D-glucan synthase is present in *C. neoformans* and that glucan synthesis is required for fungal viability. Further evaluation of the biochemical differences among fungal glucan synthases may provide additional information regarding the relative lack of anti-cryptococcal activity displayed by the echinocandins.

As for the notion that limited drug access may play a role in echinocandin resistance, Thompson et al. (75) also demonstrated that acapsular *C. neoformans* strains have caspofungin MICs similar to the capsular isolates described in previous studies. The cryptococcal polysaccharide capsule does not appear to play a significant role in the relative lack of efficacy of caspofungin against *C. neoformans*.

6 Strategies to Overcome Drug Resistance in *Cryptococcus neoformans*

Effective strategies to prevent antifungal drug resistance are needed. Plans for the management of existing drug resistance, especially fluconazole resistance, are paramount. This section focuses on six strategies that should be considered in the clinical approach to the prevention and/or management of antifungal drug resistance in *C. neoformans*.

6.1 Primary Prophylaxis

The simplest and most cost-effective strategy to manage cryptococcal drug resistance is to prevent infection entirely. *Cryptococcus* var. *gattii* has been found in association with several species of eucalyptus and other trees while varieties *neoformans* and *grubii* have been isolated from fruit, trees, and bird excreta. Patients at high risk for cryptococcal infection should avoid these environments entirely. Complete elimination of all yeast exposure, however, is highly unlikely. Prevention of the development of cryptococcosis could also involve either chemoprophylaxis or immunization, targeting individuals at the highest risk for the disease. Unfortunately, adoption of a prophylactic strategy in high-risk patients has the potential to increase the incidence of drug resistance as a result of prolonged exposure to antifungal drugs while cryptococcal vaccines await the results of clinical trials in humans.

Several studies have assessed the efficacy of azole prophylactic therapy for the prevention of cryptococcal disease in high risk AIDS patients. Both fluconazole and itraconazole are effective for preventing cryptococcosis (76, 77). None of the prevention trials, however, have shown a survival benefit. In addition, the expense, potential for selection of resistant fungi (both *Candida* and *Cryptococcus* species), and possible drug–drug interactions make most physicians reluctant to use azoles for primary prophylaxis (78). Also, current use of HAART and its associated immune reconstitution have significantly reduced the risk for cryptococcosis in patients with HIV infection. Currently, the recommendations from the Infectious Disease Society of America (IDSA) and U.S. Public Health Service (USPHS) do not endorse primary prophylaxis for fungal disease in patients with AIDS (79).

A polysaccharide-protein conjugate vaccine composed of cryptococcal capsular glucuronoxylomannan covalently coupled to tetanus toxoid has been developed and was first described by Devi et al. in 1991 (80). Subsequently, the vaccine has been shown to produce a protective antibody response in mice with high levels of capsular antibodies identified after active and passive immunization (81). The finding that the antibodies to the capsular polysaccharide glucuronoxylomannan could mediate protection against infection has led to substantial excitement in the cryptococcal vaccination field. A phase I clinical trial evaluating the safety and immunogenicity of a protective antibody in healthy and HIV-infected volunteers has been completed at the National Institutes of Health. The results, as of yet, have not been published. Currently, there are no fungal vaccines or serotherapeutics available for routine clinical use (82).

6.2 Host Immune Function Modulation

A significant proportion of the drug resistance problems associated with *C. neoformans* are related to clinical resistance. Enhancing the overall immune function of the host with HAART or the reduction of immunosuppressive agents, if possible, for transplant and autoimmune disease patients, is likely the most effective means of preventing cryptococcosis. Effective augmentation of the host immune response along with appropriate fungicidal therapy capable of promoting rapid tissue sterilization is an ideal strategy for preventing antifungal drug resistance.

6.2.1 Cytokine Therapy

A significant amount of work in the last decade has gone toward defining the host cell signaling through cytokines in addition to the potential of antibody-based therapies (50). Commercially available cytokines include granulocyte, granulocyte–macrophage, and macrophage colony stimulating factors (G-CSF, GM-CSF, and M-CSF) (83–85), as well as γ-inferferon (86), interleukin 12 (IL-12) (87, 88), IL-18 (88), and IL-2 (89). These agents have produced remarkable results in vitro, particularly when used in combination with antifungal agents. The best-studied of the cytokines has been γ-inferferon. A clinical study comparing two different doses of γ-inferferon three times per week versus no cytokine treatment as adjunctive therapy in patients receiving standard drugs for cryptococcal meningitis was recently conducted (90). More needs to be done using cytokines in the treatment of human cryptococcosis before the clinical utility of these agents can be fully realized.

6.2.2 Antibody Therapy

Casadevall (91) has written a cogent review of antibody-based therapies for emerging infectious diseases. Theoretical benefits of antibody-based therapy include pathogen-specific targeting of therapy, toxin neutralization, the enhancement of host effector cell function, and exploitation of favorable pharmacokinetic profiles as has been seen with human IgG (i.e., long half-life, good tissue penetration, and positive safety and tolerability record) (91). Potential problems with antibody-derived therapy include the emergence of antibody-resistant variants, triggering neutralizing antibody production and/or allergic response, limited CNS penetration, and cost (91). Several experimental studies have shown that monoclonal antibodies to *C. neoformans* capsular glucuron-oxylomannan can enhance the therapeutic efficacy of 5-FC (92), AmB (93), and fluconazole (94) in mouse models. Passive immunization with melanin-binding monoclonal antibodies have also been shown to improve survival and reduce fungal burden in *C. neoformans* infected mice (95). Although studies evaluating the safety of adjunctive sero-therapy with monoclonal antibodies for treatment of human cryptococcosis have been performed, human efficacy data are lacking at present (52).

6.3 Pharmacotherapeutic Strategies

Optimal pharmacologic therapy should be individualized, and several variables need to be considered when attempting to curtail the emergence of antifungal drug resistance. These variables include drug selection and dose, drug administration schedule, duration of therapy, site of infection, and host immune status (53, 55). Although none of these factors have been evaluated specifically for their contribution to antifungal drug resistance in cryptococcosis, we can make some inferences based on our experience with pharmacotherapeutic efficacy and antimicrobial drug resistance in other disease states.

6.3.1 Drug Dosing

One might hypothesize that the use of less toxic antifungal drugs at high doses for as brief a time as possible would optimally reduce the emergence of resistance. Amphotericin B has transformed cryptococcal meningitis from a uniformly fatal infection to one that is potentially curable. Recent studies have suggested that treatment regimens containing a higher daily dose of AmB (0.7 mg/kg/d) are associated with more rapid CSF sterilization (17, 96) and may decrease short-term mortality in AIDS patients with meningitis as compared with regimens employing lower doses of the polyene (96).

6.3.2 Drug Selection

One limitation to the high-dose AmB has been the increased incidence of toxic side effects. Lipid preparations can be given at higher doses with fewer adverse side effects. Currently, the most clinical experience exists with liposomal amphotericin B (Ambisome) at doses of 4 mg/kg/d for the treatment of AIDS-associated cryptococcal meningitis. Ambisome appears at least clinically equivalent to conventional AmB (97, 98).

The favorable therapeutic index of the azoles makes dose escalation an attractive option to promote cure and prevent the emergence of antifungal drug resistance. Although optimal dosing for the acute treatment of cryptococcosis is not precise, doses of 800 mg/d for meningitis and 400 mg/d for pulmonary disease are likely to give maximal results (13, 52). A review by Duswald et al. (99) illustrates that higher daily doses of fluconazole than are currently approved may be well-tolerated and improve clinical outcomes in selected patient populations for a variety of indications. Furthermore, as we better understand the relationship between MIC and clinical outcomes, the use of newer azole preparations may become important additions to the armamentarium of anti-cryptococcal agents.

In vitro studies comparing the newer triazoles to fluconazole and itraconazole against clinical isolates of *C. neoformans* have been very encouraging. Independent studies have found that the new triazoles appear to be highly active in vitro against *C. neoformans*. Pfaller et al. (100) evaluated 566 clinical isolates from the US and Africa and found voriconazole to be more active against *Cryptococcus* isolates than either fluconazole or itraconazole. As the fluconazole MICs increased in this study, so did the MICs of itraconazole and voriconazole. Despite this finding, 65% of the isolates with fluconazole MICs in the range of 16–32 µg/mL remained highly susceptible to voriconazole (MIC ≤ 0.12 µg/mL) and 99% of isolates with fluconazole MICs ≥ 16 µg/mL were inhibited by ≤ 1 µg of voriconazole per mL. These results suggest there is not automatic cross-resistance among the azoles for *C. neoformans*. Unfortunately, recent studies with voriconazole in patients with refractory cryptococcosis have a reported success rate of only 39% (101). This represents a very select group of patients meeting strict criteria for treatment failure and it is possible that certain patients are refractory to all azole therapy. Further clinical studies need to be done to confirm the promising in vitro results described with voriconazole (100, 102), ravuconazole (103), and posaconazole (104) for cryptococcosis. We need to better define which patients may benefit most from treatment with the new triazoles. Future clinical research efforts should not only evaluate specific drugs and dosing regimens, but also explore the role of the host immune status in the development of antifungal resistance.

6.4 Combination Therapy

Therapeutic regimens utilizing antifungal drug combinations offer multiple potential advantages: (1) a more rapid fungicidal response; (2) reduced resistance development; (3) enhanced spectrum of activity prior to identification of drug susceptibilities; and (4) reduced relapse rates (52). Several antifungal combinations have been critically evaluated for the treatment of cryptococcal disease, and the IDSA has published comprehensive practice guidelines which include the currently recommended drug combinations (61).

6.4.1 Amphotericin B Plus Flucytosine

Amphotericin B combined with 5-FC for 2 weeks, followed by 8 weeks of treatment with either itraconazole or fluconazole for the initial treatment of AIDS-associated cryptococcal meningitis has been evaluated in a randomized double-blind multicenter trial (96). The addition of 5-FC to induction therapy with AmB followed by fluconazole consolidation was independently associated with CSF sterilization and reduced relapse rates. Another study using quantitative yeast counts in the CSF showed that AmB plus 5-FC more rapidly sterilized the CSF of patients compared with patients receiving AmB alone, AmB plus fluconazole, or all three drugs together (105).

6.4.2 Fluconazole Plus Flucytosine

Flucytosine plus fluconazole has also been evaluated in human studies. A prospective randomized open-label trial of 58 Ugandan patients with AIDS showed that the combination of fluconazole, 200 mg once a day for 2 months in combination with 5-FC at a dose of 150 mg/kg/d for the first

2 weeks, improved survival at 180 days as compared to fluconazole monotherapy (106). In a non-comparative prospective open-label pilot study of 32 subjects with AIDS, the clinical success rate of fluconazole combined with 5-FC at 10 weeks was reported to be greater than previous reports of either of the drugs alone (107).

6.4.3 Other Combinations

Amphotericin B and fluconazole given in combination are not a part of the formal recommendations set forth in the IDSA treatment guidelines; rather, it is recommended that these agents be given sequentially (61). Our personal experience with polyenes and azoles administered concomitantly for the treatment of cryptococcosis has not shown antagonism, nor have we noticed an increase in the incidence of antifungal drug resistance (52). Rex and colleagues have shown in a well-designed, randomized, and blinded multicenter trial that the combination of AmB and fluconazole was not antagonistic for the treatment of candidemia in non-neutropenic adult patients as compared to fluconazole alone (108).

Several other interesting drug combinations have been evaluated in vitro. Fugita et al. (109) have shown the combination of AmB and rifampin to be synergistic in vitro. The echinocandins have not proven to be effective against *C. neoformans* when used alone, but Franzot and Casadevall (110) showed the combination of caspofungin and AmB in vitro can be strongly synergistic. When fluconazole was combined with caspofungin in this analysis, the effects were less impressive. Barchiesi et al. (111) used checkerboard methodology to evaluate the in vitro interactions of 5-FC and posaconazole in addition to a murine model for in vivo efficacy. In this study, combination therapy with posaconazole and 5-FC was more active in vitro than either of the agent alone. Although a survival benefit was not demonstrated in vivo, tissue burden experiments showed a reduction in number of cryptococcal cells for those mice receiving combination therapy. The reader is referred to a recent comprehensive publication by Neely and Ghannoum for an additional review of combination antifungal therapy (112).

6.5 Surgical Intervention

Another strategy that may be useful, in the appropriate clinical setting, to treat drug-resistant infections is surgical excision or debulking. Surgical intervention has been described for the management of large intracerebral mass lesions >3 cm (113) and large pulmonary cryptococcomas (114), particularly with variety *gattii,* unresponsive to conventional pharmocotherapy.

Continued systemic antifungal therapy is required since surgery alone is unlikely to completely eradicate infection.

6.6 New Drug Targets and Drug Development

The development of new antifungal drugs is likely the most important long-term strategy to manage the problem of antifungal drug resistance. In addition to the agents already mentioned, there are other classes of compounds with demonstrated anti-cryptococcal activity in vitro. These novel agents diversify the range of drug targets and thus broaden therapeutic options. Several of these investigational agents will be discussed here.

6.6.1 Benzimidazole Compounds

In vitro studies have shown *C. neoformans* to be quite susceptible to selected antihelmintic benzimidazole compounds. Benzimidazoles work by binding free β-tubulin, thereby inhibiting polymerization required for the microtubule-dependent uptake of glucose. Cruz and Edlin (115) characterized β-tubulin genes and their expression in *C. neoformans*. They also identified a likely benzimidazole target in this fungal pathogen. Del Poeta et al. (116) have described two bis-benzimidazole compounds with potent in vitro activity against yeast.

6.6.2 Immunophilins and the Inhibition of Signal Transduction Pathways

The immunosuppressants cyclosporin A (CsA), FK506 (tacrolimus), and rapamycin (sirolimus) are natural products that have revolutionized the field of transplantation. These compounds are known to have antimicrobial properties and have been shown to possess activity against *C. neoformans* (26, 117–120). Husain et al. (121) have shown that SOT recipients who developed cryptococcosis while receiving tacrolimus were statistically less likely to have CNS involvement as compared to all other transplant recipients not receiving this drug.

The immunosuppressive properties of these agents result from inhibition of cellular signal transduction pathways required for T cell activation (122). All three agents diffuse into cells and bind to intracellular immunophilins present in human lymphocytes as well as yeast. CsA binds to cyclophilin A while FK506 and rapamycin bind to FKBP12. The drug–immunophilin complex targets various proteins required for signal transduction and cell proliferation. In

humans as well as *C. neoformans,* the cyclophilin A-CsA and FKBP12–FK506 complexes target calcineurin, a calcium-regulated protein phosphatase (26). Calcineurin has been shown to be essential for the virulence of *C. neoformans* and is required for its growth at 37° (26). FKBP12-rapamycin does not affect calcineurin. Instead, the FKBP12–rapamycin complex inhibits TOR kinases integral in cell-cycle regulation (117).

Recent work has focused on identifying non-immunosuppressive analogs of these drugs and testing them in vitro against *C. neoformans* (118–120). The results of these studies have been promising. Novel non-immunosuppressive analogs have been found and appear to retain some anti-cryptococcal activity in vitro. Further examination of CsA, FK506, and rapamycin analogs are needed. These compounds may have promise for development as antifungal drugs for use either alone or in combination with other agents.

6.6.3 ATPase Activity and H⁺ Transport

The bafilomycins are a group of macrolide antibiotics that inhibit vacuolar-type proton translocating ATPases (V-ATPases) with high affinity (123). Bafilomycin A_1 has also been shown to inhibit plasma membrane ATPase (P-ATPase) as well as the ATP-binding cassette (ABC) transporters (124). ATPase inhibition reduces cellular ability to withstand cation stress and has been identified as a potential new antifungal target. Manavathu and colleagues (125) examined the in vitro susceptibility of *C. neoformans* to NC1175, a novel conjugated styryl ketone with ATPase inhibitory properties in *Candida* and *Aspergillus* species. The MIC values for NC1175 were three- to four-fold higher than those of AmB and various azoles (NC1175 MIC_{90} = 1 mg/L). The authors state that this compound displays fungicidal activity against *C. neoformans* in vitro, although these data were not shown, and suggest the mechanism of action is at least partly due to inhibition of P-ATPase-mediated extrusion of intracellular protons.

Studies with *Saccharomyces cerevisiae* have shown that mutants with impaired structure or function of V-ATPase were nonviable if the yeast also had cellular defects in calcineurin (126). Del Poeta et al. (127) have taken this observation a step further and explored the in vitro effects of combining the calcineurin inhibitor FK506 or its non-immunosuppressive analogue with bafilomycin A_1 against *C. neoformans*. They found that FK506 in combination with bafilomycin displayed dramatic synergistic antifungal activity. In combination, the dose of both agents could be reduced and still retain an inhibitory endpoint. This is potentially important given the immunosuppressive effects of FK506 which are integral to host outcomes. The nonimmunosuppressive analog combined with bafilomycin was not synergistic against the wild-type

C. neoformans strains tested. Interestingly, the combination of FK506 plus caspofungin was synergistic in vitro. Again, additional studies in animal models are needed to better define the clinical potential for these novel drugs and drug combinations.

6.6.4 Sordarins

The sordarins are another new class of antifungal drugs which selectively inhibit protein synthesis in a variety of yeast. Sordarin derivatives have been reported to show antifungal activity against *C. neoformans* (128). The mechanism of action is thought to be inhibition of fungal elongation factor 2, an essential step in protein synthesis.

6.6.5 Novel Drug Combinations

Recent interest has also focused on the potential role of drug efflux pump inhibitors used in combination with antifungal agents. There is emerging evidence that some drug resistance observed in *C. neoformans* may be related to the presence of efflux pumps capable of extruding antifungal drugs from the cell (63, 66). Analogous to the combination of β-lactam antibiotics with a β-lactamase inhibitor, compounds capable of inhibiting efflux machinery in fungi could potentially be combined with antifungal drugs to increase efficacy. A compound with anti-efflux properties has been identified (MC-510,027) and has been shown to decrease the MIC of three azoles against several *Candida* species (129). We are not aware of any published studies looking at the utility of this compound, or others like it, in combination with standard antifungal agents against *Cryptococcus*.

In addition to efflux inhibitors, several other drugs have been evaluated as possible adjunctive agents in the treatment of cryptococcosis. Chloroquine at low concentrations has been shown to enhance the activity of human mononuclear phagocytes against *C. neoformans* (122). The antifungal activity of chloroquine is enhanced at higher concentrations likely to be found within the acidic environment of cryptococcal phagosomes (130). A related compound, quinacrine, was found to be between 10- and 100-fold more active against *Cryptococcus* than cholorquine on a molar basis (130). These findings have potential clinical applicability as both drugs have proven to be safe and tolerable when administered orally and they are available in the developing world. Furthermore, the benefits of chloroquine in murine models of cryptococcosis have been demonstrated (131). Experiments examining whether chloroquine and quinacrine have additive or synergistic activity when combined with other agents will bolster our understanding of the utility

of these, and possibly other related compounds, for the treatment of cryptococcosis.

7 Conclusions

The last 10 years have seen an explosion in laboratory and clinical work focused on the medically important fungi, as these organisms have recently emerged as a significant group of opportunistic pathogens. With more widespread use of antifungal therapy for maintenance and/or prophylactic purposes in immunosuppressed patient populations, the problem of antifungal drug resistance is likely to continue to be an important issue. The future of cryptococcal therapy will almost certainly include novel and existing drugs used in combination to maximize fungal killing and minimize the ramifications of antifungal drug resistance. As our understanding of the molecular mechanisms of drug resistance improves, new drug targets will be identified and therapeutic strategies individualized. Conventional antifungal drugs may also eventually be combined with immunoactive cytokines or antibodies to help enhance the host's immune response to cryptococcal disease. Finally, continued clinical laboratory experience, improved microbiologic techniques, and laboratory standardization will enhance our ability to predict clinical outcome based on data such as MICs. The foundations for a productive future in cryptococcal research and clinical care have been firmly established, and we expect the field to continue to flourish in the next few decades.

References

1. Mitchell TG, Perfect JR. Cryptococcosis in the era of AIDS – 100 years after the discovery of *Cryptococcus neoformans*. Clin Microbiol Rev 1995; 8(4):515–548
2. Sanati H, Messer SA, Pfaller M et al. Multicenter evaluation of broth microdilution method for susceptibility testing of *Cryptococcus neoformans* against fluconazole. J Clin Microbiol 1996; 34(5):1280–1282
3. Cuenca-Estrella M, Diaz-Guerra TM, Mellado E, Rodriguez-Tudela JL. Flucytosine primary resistance in *Candida* species and *Cryptococcus neoformans*. Eur J Clin Microbiol Infect Dis 2001; 20(4):276–279
4. Orni-Wasserlauf R, Izkhakov E, Siegman-Igra Y, Bash E, Polacheck I, Giladi M. Fluconazole-resistant *Cryptococcus neoformans* isolated from an immunocompetent patient without prior exposure to fluconazole. Clin Infect Dis 1999; 29(6):1592–1593
5. Armengou A, Porcar C, Mascaro J, Garcia-Bragado F. Possible development of resistance to fluconazole during suppressive therapy for AIDS-associated cryptococcal meningitis. Clin Infect Dis 1996; 23(6):1337–1338
6. Berg J, Clancy CJ, Nguyen MH. The hidden danger of primary fluconazole prophylaxis for patients with AIDS. Clin Infect Dis 1998; 26(1):186–187

7. Birley HDL, Johnson EM, Mcdonald P, Parry C, Carey PB, Warnock DW. Azole drug-resistance as a cause of clinical relapse in AIDS patients with cryptococcal meningitis. Int J STD AIDS 1995; 6(5):353–355

8. Currie BP, Ghannoum M, Bessen L, Casadevall A. Decreased fluconazole susceptibility of a relapse *Cryptococcus neoformans* isolate after fluconazole treatment. Inf Dis Clin Pract 1995; 4(4):318–319

9. Friese G, Discher T, Fussle R, Schmalreck A, Lohmeyer J. Development of azole resistance during fluconazole maintenance therapy for AIDS-associated cryptococcal disease. AIDS 2001; 15(17):2344–2345

10. Viard JP, Hennequin C, Fortineau N, Pertuiset N, Rothschild C, Zylberberg H. Fulminant cryptococcal infections in HIV-infected patients on oral fluconazole. Lancet 1995; 346(8967):118

11. Block ER, Jennings AE, Bennett JE. 5-fluorocytosine resistance in *Cryptococcus neoformans*. Antimicrob Agents Chemotherapy 1973; 3(6):649–656

12. Walsh TJ. Echinocandins – an advance in the primary treatment of invasive candidiasis. N Engl J Med 2002; 347(25):2070–2072

13. Perfect JR, Casadevall A. Cryptococcosis. Infect Dis Clin North Am 2002; 16(4):837

14. Pappas PG, Perfect JR, Cloud GA et al. Cryptococcosis in human immunodeficiency virus-negative patients in the era of effective azole therapy. Clin Infect Dis 2001; 33(5):690–699

15. Husain S, Wagener MM, Singh N. *Cryptococcus neoformans* infection in organ transplant recipients: Variables influencing clinical characteristics and outcome. Emerg Infect Dis 2001; 7(3):375–381

16. Singh N, Alexander BD, Gupta KL. Characteristics and outcome of *Cryptococcus neoformans* infection of the central nervous system in organ transplant recipients: a prospective, multicenter study. 42nd ICAAC, 392, San Diego, CA, 2002

17. Robinson PA, Bauer M, Leal ME et al. Early mycological treatment failure in AIDS-associated cryptococcal meningitis. Clin Infect Dis 1999; 28(1):82–92

18. Diamond RD, Bennett JE. Prognostic factors in cryptococcal meningitis. A study in 111 cases. Ann Intern Med 1974; 80(2):176–181

19. Larsen RA, Bozzette S, Mccutchan JA, Chiu J, Leal MA, Richman DD. Persistent *Cryptococcus neoformans* infection of the prostate after successful treatment of meningitis. Ann Intern Med 1989; 111(2):125–128

20. Perfect JR, Durack DT, Hamilton JD, Gallis HA. Failure of ketoconazole in *cryptococcal meningitis*. JAMA 1982; 247(24): 3349–3351

21. Mitchell DH, Sorrell TC, Allworth AM et al. Cryptococcal disease of the CNS in immunocompetent hosts – influence of cryptococcal variety on clinical manifestations and outcome. Clin Infect Dis 1995; 20(3):611–616

22. Velez JD, Allendoerfer R, Luther M, Rinaldi MG, Graybill JR. Correlation of in vitro azole susceptibility with in-vivo response in a murine model of cryptococcal meningitis. J Infect Dis 1993; 168(2):508–510

23. Buchanan KL, Murphy JW. What makes *Cryptococcus neoformans* a pathogen? Emerg Infect Dis 1998; 4(1):71–83

24. Casadevall A, Rosas AL, Nosanchuk JD. Melanin and virulence in *Cryptococcus neoformans*. Curr Opin Microbiol 2000; 3(4):354–358

25. van Duin D, Casadevall A, Nosanchuk JD. Melanization of *Cryptococcus neoformans* and *Histoplasma capsulatum* reduces their susceptibilities to amphotericin B and caspofungin. Antimicrob Agents Chemother 2002; 46(11):3394–3400

26. Odom A, Muir S, Lim E, Toffaletti DL, Perfect J, Heitman J. Calcineurin is required for virulence of *Cryptococcus neoformans*. EMBO J 1997; 16(10):2576–2589

27. Aller AI, Martin-Mazuelos E, Lozano F et al. Correlation of fluconazole MICs with clinical outcome in cryptococcal infection. Antimicrob Agents Chemother 2000; 44(6):1544–1548

28. Menichetti F, Fiorio M, Tosti A et al. High-dose fluconazole therapy for cryptococcal meningitis in patients with AIDS. Clin Infect Dis 1996; 22(5):838–840

29. Witt MD, Lewis RJ, Larsen RA et al. Identification of patients with acute AIDS-associated cryptococcal meningitis who can be effectively treated with fluconazole: the role of antifungal susceptibility testing. Clin Infect Dis 1996; 22(2):322–328

30. Barchiesi F, Colombo AL, Mcgough DA, Rinaldi MG. Comparative-study of broth macrodilution and microdilution techniques for in-vitro antifungal susceptibility testing of yeasts by using the National-Committee-For-Clinical-Laboratory-Standards Proposed Standard. J Clin Microbiol 1994; 32(10):2494–2500

31. Lozano-Chiu M, Paetznick VL, Ghannoum MA, Rex JH. Detection of resistance to amphotericin B among *Cryptococcus neoformans* clinical isolates: performances of three different media assessed by using E-test and National Committee for Clinical Laboratory Standards M27-A methodologies. J Clin Microbiol 1998; 36(10):2817–2822

32. Pfaller MA, Messer SA, Boyken L et al. Evaluation of the NCCLS M44-P disk diffusion method for determining susceptibilities of 276 clinical isolates of *Cryptococcus neoformans* to fluconazole. J Clin Microbiol 2004; 42(1):380–383

33. Georgopapadakou NH, Walsh TJ. Antifungal agents: chemotherapeutic targets and immunologic strategies. [Review] [300 refs]. Antimicrob Agents Chemother 1996; 40(2):279–291

34. Aller AI, Martin-Mazuelos E, Gutierrez MJ, Bernal S, Chavez M, Recio FJ. Comparison of the Etest and microdilution method for antifungal susceptibility testing of *Cryptococcus neoformans* to four antifungal agents. J Antimicrob Chemother 2000; 46(6):997–1000

35. Maxwell MJ, Messer SA, Hollis RJ, Diekema DJ, Pfaller MA. Evaluation of Etest method for determining voriconazole and amphotericin B MICs for 162 clinical isolates of *Cryptococcus neoformans*. Journal of Clinical Microbiology 2003; 41(1):97–99

36. Ghannoum MA, Ibrahim AS, Fu Y, Shafiq MC, Edwards JE, Criddle RS. Susceptibility testing of *Cryptococcus neoformans* – a microdilution technique. J Clin Microbiol 1992; 30(11):2881–2886

37. EspinelIngroff A, Kish CW, Kerkering TM et al. Collaborative comparison of broth macrodilution and microdilution antifungal susceptibility tests. J Clin Microbiol 1992; 30(12):3138–3145

38. Currie B, Sanati H, Ibrahim AS, Edwards JE, Jr, Casadevall A, Ghannoum MA. Sterol compositions and susceptibilities to amphotericin B of environmental *Cryptococcus neoformans* isolates are changed by murine passage. Antimicrob Agents Chemother 1995; 39(9):1934–1937

39. Joseph-Horne T, Hollomon D, Loeffler RS, Kelly SL. Cross-resistance to polyene and azole drugs in *Cryptococcus neoformans*. Antimicrob Agents Chemother 1995; 39(7):1526–1529

40. Joseph-Horne T, Loeffler RS, Hollomon DW, Kelly SL. Amphotericin B resistant isolates of *Cryptococcus neoformans* without alteration in sterol biosynthesis. J Med Vet Mycol 1996; 34(3):223–225

41. Kelly SL, Lamb DC, Kelly DE et al. Resistance to fluconazole and cross-resistance to amphotericin B in *Candida albicans* from AIDS patients caused by defective sterol delta5,6-desaturation. FEBS Lett 1997; 400(1):80–82

42. Powderly WG, Keath WJ, Sokol-Anderson M, et al. Amphotericin B-resistant *Cryptococcus neoformans* in a patient with AIDS. Infect Dis Clin Pract 1992; 1:314–316

43. Casadevall A, Spitzer ED, Webb D, Rinaldi MG. Susceptibilities of serial *Cryptococcus neoformans* isolates from patients with recurrent cryptococcal meningitis to amphotericin B and fluconazole. Antimicrob Agents Chemother 1993; 37(6):1383–1386

44. Brandt ME, Pfaller MA, Hajjeh RA et al. Trends in antifungal drug susceptibility of *Cryptococcus neoformans* Isolates in the United States: 1992 to 1994 and 1996 to 1998. Antimicrob Agents Chemother 2001; 45(11):3065–3069

45. Davey KG, Johnson EM, Holmes AD, Szekely A, Warnock DW. In-vitro susceptibility of *Cryptococcus neoformans* isolates to fluconazole and itraconazole. J Antimicrob Chemother 1998; 42(2):217–220

46. Yildiran ST, Fothergill AW, Sutton DA, Rinaldi MG. In vitro susceptibilities of cerebrospinal fluid isolates of *Cryptococcus neoformans* collected during a ten-year period against fluconazole, voriconazole and posaconazole (SCH56592). Mycoses 2002; 45(9–10):378–383

47. Pfaller MA, Diekema DJ, Gibbs DL et al. Results from the ARTEMIS DISK Global Antifungal Surveillance study, 1997 to 2005: an 8.5-year analysis of susceptibilities of *Candida* species and other yeast species to fluconazole and voriconazole determined by CLSI standardized disk diffusion testing. J Clin Microbiol 2007; 45(6):1735–1745

48. Mondon P, Petter R, Amalfitano G et al. Heteroresistance to fluconazole and voriconazole in *Cryptococcus neoformans*. Antimicrob Agents Chemother 1999; 43(8):1856–1861

49. Bicanic T, Harrison T, Niepieklo A, Dyakopu N, Meintjes G. Symptomatic relapse of HIV-associated cryptococcal meningitis after initial fluconazole monotherapy: the role of fluconazole resistance and immune reconstitution. Clin Infect Dis 2006; 43(8):1069–1073

50. Alexander BD, Perfect JR. Antifungal resistance trends towards the year 2000 – implications for therapy and new approaches. Drugs 1997; 54(5):657–678

51. Loeffler J, Stevens DA. Antifungal drug resistance. Clin Infect Dis 2003; 36:S31–S41

52. Perfect JR, Cox GM. Drug resistance in *Cryptococcus neoformans*. Drug Resist Updat 1999; 2(4):259–269

53. White TC, Marr KA, Bowden RA. Clinical, cellular, and molecular factors that contribute to antifungal drug resistance. Clin Microbiol Rev 1998; 11(2):382–402

54. Ghannoum MA, Spellberg BJ, Ibrahim AS et al. Sterol composition of *Cryptococcus neoformans* in the presence and absence of fluconazole. Antimicrob Agents Chemother 1994; 38(9):2029–2033

55. Balkis MM, Leidich SD, Mukherjee PK, Ghannoum MA. Mechanisms of fungal resistance: an overview. Drugs 2002; 62(7):1025–1040

56. Whelan WL. The genetic basis of resistance to 5-fluorocytosine in *Candida* species and *Cryptococcus neoformans*. Crit Rev Microbiol 1987; 15(1):45–56

57. Perfect JR, Durack DT, Gallis HA. Cryptococcemia. Medicine 1983; 62(2):98–109

58. Perfect JR, Cox GM. Drug resistance in *Cryptococcus neoformans*. Drug Resist Updat 1999; 2(4):259–269

59. Hospenthal DR, Bennett JE. Flucytosine monotherapy for cryptococcosis. Clin Infect Dis 1998; 27(2):260–264

60. Bennett JE, Dismukes WE, Duma RJ et al. Comparison of amphotericin-B alone and combined with flucytosine in the treatment of cryptococcal meningitis. N Engl J Med 1979; 301(3):126–131

61. Saag MS, Graybill RJ, Larsen RA et al. Practice guidelines for the management of cryptococcal disease. Infectious Diseases Society of America. Clin Infect Dis 2000; 30(4):710–718

62. Yildiran ST, Saracli MA, Fothergill AW, Rinaldi MG. In vitro susceptibility of environmental *Cryptococcus neoformans* variety neoformans isolates from Turkey to six antifungal agents, including SCH56592 and voriconazole. Eur J Clin Microbiol Infect Dis 2000; 19(4):317–319

63. Venkateswarlu K, Taylor M, Manning NJ, Rinaldi MG, Kelly SL. Fluconazole tolerance in clinical isolates of *Cryptococcus neoformans*. Antimicrob Agents Chemother 1997; 41(4):748–751

64. Lamb DC, Corran A, Baldwin BC, Kwon-Chung J, Kelly SL. Resistant P45051A1 activity in azole antifungal tolerant *Cryptococcus neoformans* from AIDS patients. FEBS Lett 1995; 368(2):326–330

65. Mellado E, Rodero L, Rodriquez C, et al. G484S amino acid substitution of 14-alpha lanosterol demethylase (ERG11) related to fluconazole resistance in recurrent *Cryptococcus neoformans* clinical isolate. 43rd ICAAC, 443, Chicago, IL, 2003

66. Posteraro B, Sanguinetti M, Sanglard D et al. Identification and characterization of a *Cryptococcus neoformans* ATP binding cassette (ABC) transporter-encoding gene, CnAFR1, involved in the resistance to fluconazole. Mol Microbiol 2003; 47(2): 357–371

67. Thornewell SJ, Peery RB, Skatrud PL. Cloning and characterization of CneMDR1: a *Cryptococcus neoformans* gene encoding a protein related to multidrug resistance proteins. Gene 1997; 201(1–2):21–29

68. Xu J, Onyewu C, Yoell HJ, Ali RY, Vilgalys RJ, Mitchell TG. Dynamic and heterogeneous mutations to fluconazole resistance in *Cryptococcus neoformans*. Antimicrob Agents Chemother 2001; 45(2):420–427

69. Yamazumi T, Pfaller MA, Messer SA et al. Characterization of heteroresistance to fluconazole among clinical isolates of *Cryptococcus neoformans*. J Clin Microbiol 2003; 41(1):267–272

70. Anaissie. EJ, McGinnis MR, Pfaller MA. *Clinical Mycology*. Philadelphia: 2003

71. Denning DW. Echinocandins: a new class of antifungal. [Review] [17 refs]. J Antimicrob Chemother 2002; 49(6).889–891

72. Feldmesser M, Kress Y, Mednick A, Casadevall A. The effect of the echinocandin analogue caspofungin on cell wall glucan synthesis by *Cryptococcus neoformans*. J Infect Dis 2000; 182(6):1791–1795

73. Mazur P, Morin N, Baginsky W et al. Differential expression and function of two homologous subunits of yeast 1,3-beta-D-glucan synthase. Mol Cell Biol 1995; 15(10):5671–5681

74. Mio T, Adachi Shimizu M, Tachibana Y et al. Cloning of the *Candida albicans* homolog of *Saccharomyces cerevisiae* GSC1/FKS1 and its involvement in beta-1,3-glucan synthesis. J Bacteriol 1997; 179(13):4096–4105

75. Thompson JR, Douglas CM, Li W et al. A glucan synthase FKS1 homolog in *Cryptococcus neoformans* is single copy and encodes an essential function. J Bacteriol 1999; 181(2):444–453

76. Havlir DV, Dube MP, Mccutchan JA et al. Prophylaxis with weekly versus daily fluconazole for fungal infections in patients with AIDS. [see comment]. Clin Infect Dis 1998; 27(6):1369–1375

77. McKinsey DS, Wheat LJ, Cloud GA et al. Itraconazole prophylaxis for fungal infections in patients with advanced human immunodeficiency virus infection: randomized, placebo-controlled, double-blind study. National Institute of Allergy and Infectious Diseases Mycoses Study Group. Clin Infect Dis 1999; 28(5):1049–1056

78. Kovacs JA, Masur H. Prophylaxis against opportunistic infections in patients with human immunodeficiency virus infection. N Engl J Med 2000; 342(19):1416–1429

79. Kaplan JE, Masur H, Holmes KK et al. An overview of the 1999 US Public Health Service/Infectious Diseases Society of America guidelines for preventing opportunistic infections in human immunodeficiency virus-infected persons. Clin Infect Dis 2000; 30(Suppl 1):S15–S28

80. Devi SJ, Schneerson R, Egan W et al. *Cryptococcus neoformans* serotype A glucuronoxylomannan-protein conjugate vaccines: synthesis, characterization, and immunogenicity. Infect Immun 1991; 59(10):3700–3707

81. Devi SJ. Preclinical efficacy of a glucuronoxylomannan-tetanus toxoid conjugate vaccine of *Cryptococcus neoformans* in a murine model. [erratum appears in Vaccine 1996 Sep;14(13):1298]. [Review] [29 refs]. Vaccine 1996; 14(9):841–844

82. Deepe GS, Jr Prospects for the development of fungal vaccines. [Review] [114 refs]. Clin Microbiol Rev 1997; 10(4):585–596

83. Brummer E, Nassar F, Stevens DA. Effect of macrophage colony-stimulating factor on anticryptococcal activity of bronchoalveolar macrophages: synergy with fluconazole for killing. Antimicrob Agents Chemother 1994; 38(9):2158–2161

84. Chiller T, Farrokhshad K, Brummer E, Stevens DA. Effect of granulocyte colony-stimulating factor and granulocyte-macrophage colony-stimulating factor on polymorphonuclear neutrophils, monocytes or monocyte-derived macrophages combined with voriconazole against Cryptococcus neoformans. Med Mycol 2002; 40(1):21–26

85. Tascini C, Vecchiarelli A, Preziosi R, Francisci D, Bistoni F, Baldelli F. Granulocyte-macrophage colony-stimulating factor and fluconazole enhance anti-cryptococcal activity of monocytes from AIDS patients. AIDS 1999; 13(1):49–55

86. Herrmann JL, Dubois N, Fourgeaud M, Basset D, Lagrange PH. Synergic inhibitory activity of amphotericin-B and gamma interferon against intracellular Cryptococcus neoformans in murine macrophages. J Antimicrob Chemother 1994; 34(6):1051–1058

87. Pietrella D, Kozel TR, Monari C, Bistoni F, Vecchiarelli A. Interleukin-12 counterbalances the deleterious effect of human immunodeficiency virus type 1 envelope glycoprotein gp120 on the immune response to Cryptococcus neoformans. J Infect Dis 2001; 183(1):51–58

88. Zhang T, Kawakami K, Qureshi MH, Okamura H, Kurimoto M, Saito A. Interleukin-12 (IL-12) and IL-18 synergistically induce the fungicidal activity of murine peritoneal exudate cells against Cryptococcus neoformans through production of gamma interferon by natural killer cells. Infect Immun 1997; 65(9):3594–3599

89. Levitz SM. Activation of human peripheral blood mononuclear cells by interleukin-2 and granulocyte-macrophage colony-stimulating factor to inhibit Cryptococcus neoformans. Infect Immun 1991; 59(10):3393–3397

90. Pappas PG, Bustamante B, Ticona E, et al. Adjuvant interferon gamma for the treatment of Cryptococcal meningitis: a randomized double blind pilot trial. 41st ICAAC. 2001

91. Casadevall A. Antibody-based therapies for emerging infectious diseases. [Review] [68 refs]. Emerg Infect Dis 1996; 2(3):200–208

92. Feldmesser M, Mukherjee J, Casadevall A. Combination of 5-flucytosine and capsule-binding monoclonal antibody in the treatment of murine Cryptococcus neoformans infections and in vitro. J Antimicrob Chemother 1996; 37(3):617–622

93. Mukherjee J, Zuckier LS, Scharff MD, Casadevall A. Therapeutic efficacy of monoclonal antibodies to Cryptococcus neoformans glucuronoxylomannan alone and in combination with amphotericin B. Antimicrob Agents Chemother 1994; 38(3):580–587

94. Mukherjee J, Feldmesser M, Scharff MD, Casadevall A. Monoclonal antibodies to Cryptococcus neoformans glucuronoxylomannan enhance fluconazole efficacy. Antimicrob Agents Chemother 1995; 39(7):1398–1405

95. Rosas AL, Nosanchuk JD, Casadevall A. Passive immunization with melanin-binding monoclonal antibodies prolongs survival of mice with lethal Cryptococcus neoformans infection. Infect Immun 2001; 69(5):3410–3412

96. van der Horst CM, Saag MS, Cloud GA et al. Treatment of cryptococcal meningitis associated with the acquired immunodeficiency syndrome. National Institute of Allergy and Infectious Diseases Mycoses Study Group and AIDS Clinical Trials Group [see comment]. N Engl J Med 1997; 337(1):15–21

97. Coker RJ, Viviani M, Gazzard BG et al. Treatment of cryptococcosis with liposomal amphotericin B (AmBisome) in 23 patients with AIDS. AIDS 1993; 7(6):829–835

98. Leenders AC, Reiss P, Portegies P et al. Liposomal amphotericin B (AmBisome) compared with amphotericin B both followed by oral fluconazole in the treatment of AIDS-associated cryptococcal meningitis. AIDS 1997; 11(12):1463–1471

99. Duswald KH, Penk A, Pittrow L. High-dose therapy with fluconazole > or = 800 mg day-1. Mycoses 1997; 40(7–8):267–277

100. Pfaller MA, Zhang J, Messer SA et al. In vitro activities of voriconazole, fluconazole, and itraconazole against 566 clinical isolates of Cryptococcus neoformans from the United States and Africa. Antimicrob Agents Chemother 1999; 43(1):169–171

101. Perfect JR, Marr KA, Walsh TJ et al. Voriconazole treatment for less-common, emerging, or refractory fungal infections. Clin Infect Dis 2003; 36(9):1122–1131

102. Nguyen MH, Yu CY. In vitro comparative efficacy of voriconazole and itraconazole against fluconazole-susceptible and -resistant Cryptococcus neoformans isolates. Antimicrob Agents Chemother 1998; 42(2):471–472

103. Yamazumi T, Pfaller MA, Messer SA, Houston A, Hollis RJ, Jones RN. In vitro activities of ravuconazole (BMS-207147) against 541 clinical isolates of Cryptococcus neoformans. Antimicrob Agents Chemother 2000; 44(10):2883–2886

104. Pfaller MA, Messer SA, Hollis RJ, Jones RN. In vitro activities of posaconazole (Sch 56592) compared with those of itraconazole and fluconazole against 3,685 clinical isolates of Candida spp. and Cryptococcus neoformans. Antimicrob Agents Chemother 2001; 45(10):2862–2864

105. Brouwer AE, Rajanuwong A, Chierakul W. Combination antifungal therapies for HIV-associated cryptococcal meningitis: feasibility and powers of quantitative CSF cultures to determine fungicidal activity. Lancet (in press)

106. Mayanja-Kizza H, Oishi K, Mitarai S et al. Combination therapy with fluconazole and flucytosine for cryptococcal meningitis in Ugandan patients with AIDS. [see comment]. Clin Infect Dis 1998; 26(6):1362–1366

107. Larsen RA, Bozzette SA, Jones BE et al. Fluconazole combined with flucytosine for treatment of cryptococcal meningitis in patients with AIDS. Clin Infect Dis 1994; 19(4):741–745

108. Rex JH, Pappas PG, Karchmer AW et al. A randomized and blinded multicenter trial of high-dose fluconazole plus placebo versus fluconazole plus amphotericin B as therapy for candidemia and its consequences in nonneutropenic subjects.[see comment]. Clin Infect Dis 2003; 36(10):1221–1228

109. Fujita NK, Edwards JE, Jr. Combined in vitro effect of amphotericin B and rifampin on Cryptococcus neoformans. Antimicrob Agents Chemother 1981; 19(1):196–198

110. Franzot SP, Casadevall A. Pneumocandin L-743,872 enhances the activities of amphotericin B and fluconazole against Cryptococcus neoformans in vitro. Antimicrob Agents Chemother 1997; 41(2):331–336

111. Barchiesi F, Schimizzi AM, Najvar LK et al. Interactions of posaconazole and flucytosine against Cryptococcus neoformans. Antimicrob Agents Chemother 2001; 45(5):1355–1359

112. Neely MN, Ghannoum MA. The exciting future of antifungal therapy. [Review] [208 refs]. Eur J Clin Microbiol Infect Dis 2000; 19(12):897–914

113. Fujita NK, Reynard M, Sapico FL, Guze LB, Edwards JE, Jr. Cryptococcal intracerebral mass lesions: the role of computed tomography and nonsurgical management. Ann Intern Med 1981; 94(3):382–388

114. Hammerman KJ, Powell KE, Christianson CS et al. Pulmonary cryptococcosis: clinical forms and treatment. A Center for Disease Control cooperative mycoses study. Am Rev Respir Dis 1973; 108(5):1116–1123

115. Cruz MC, Edlind T. beta-Tubulin genes and the basis for benzimidazole sensitivity of the opportunistic fungus Cryptococcus neoformans. Microbiology 1997; 143(Pt 6):2003–2008

116. Del Poeta M, Bixel AS, Barchiesi F et al. In-vitro activity of dicationic aromatic compounds and fluconazole against Cryptococcus neoformans and Candida spp. J Antimicrob Chemother 1999; 44(2):223–228

117. Cruz MC, Cavallo LM, Gorlach JM et al. Rapamycin antifungal action is mediated via conserved complexes with FKBP12 and TOR kinase homologs in *Cryptococcus neoformans*. Mol Cell Biol 1999; 19(6):4101–4112

118. Cruz MC, Del Poeta M, Wang P et al. Immunosuppressive and nonimmunosuppressive cyclosporine analogs are toxic to the opportunistic fungal pathogen *Cryptococcus neoformans* via cyclophilin-dependent inhibition of calcineurin. Antimicrob Agents Chemother 2000; 44(1):143–149

119. Cruz MC, Goldstein AL, Blankenship J et al. Rapamycin and less immunosuppressive analogs are toxic to Candida albicans and *Cryptococcus neoformans* via FKBP12-dependent inhibition of TOR. Antimicrob Agents Chemother 2001; 45(11): 3162–3170

120. Odom A, Del Poeta M, Perfect J, Heitman J. The immunosuppressant FK506 and its nonimmunosuppressive analog L-685,818 are toxic to *Cryptococcus neoformans* by inhibition of a common target protein. Antimicrob Agents Chemother 1997; 41(1):156–161

121. Husain S, John G, Singh N. Changing spectrum of *C. neoformans* infection in organ transplant recipients in the era/area of calcineurin-inhibitor based immunosuppression (tacrolimus and cyclosporine, CsA). 42nd ICAAC, 392, 2002

122. Cardenas ME, Sanfridson A, Cutler NS, Heitman J. Signal-transduction cascades as targets for therapeutic intervention by natural products. [Review] [71 refs]. Trends Biotechnol 1998; 16(10):427–433

123. Drose S, Altendorf K. Bafilomycins and concanamycins as inhibitors of V-ATPases and P-ATPases. [Review] [69 refs]. J Exp Biol 1997; 200(Pt 1):1–8

124. Hunke S, Dose S, Schneider E. Vanadate and bafilomycin A1 are potent inhibitors of the ATPase activity of the reconstituted bacterial ATP-binding cassette transporter for maltose (MalFGK2). Biochem Biophys Res Commun 1995; 216(2):589–594

125. Manavathu EK, Dimmock JR, Vashishtha SC, Chandrasekar PH. Inhibition of H(+)-ATPase-mediated proton pumping in *Cryptococcus neoformans* by a novel conjugated styryl ketone. J Antimicrob Chemother 2001; 47(4):491–494

126. Garrett-Engele P, Moilanen B, Cyert MS. Calcineurin, the Ca2+/calmodulin-dependent protein phosphatase, is essential in yeast mutants with cell integrity defects and in mutants that lack a functional vacuolar H(+)-ATPase. Mol Cell Biol 1995; 15(8):4103–4114

127. Del Poeta M, Cruz MC, Cardenas ME, Perfect JR, Heitman J. Synergistic antifungal activities of bafilomycin A(1), fluconazole, and the pneumocandin MK-0991/caspofungin acetate (L-743,873) with calcineurin inhibitors FK506 and L-685,818 against *Cryptococcus neoformans*. Antimicrob Agents Chemother 2000; 44(3):739–746

128. Dominguez JM, Kelly VA, Kinsman OS, Marriott MS, Gomez de las HF, Martin JJ. Sordarins: A new class of antifungals with selective inhibition of the protein synthesis elongation cycle in yeasts. Antimicrob Agents Chemother 1998; 42(9):2274–2278

129. Chamberlin S, Blais J, Cotter DP, et al. Impact of MC-510,027, a fungal efflux pump inhibitor, on the susceptibility of clinical isolates of Candida spp. to antifungal agents. 39th ICAAC, 1999

130. Harrison TS, Griffin GE, Levitz SM. Conditional lethality of the diprotic weak bases chloroquine and quinacrine against *Cryptococcus neoformans*. J Infect Dis 2000; 182(1):283–289

131. Mazzolla R, Barluzzi R, Brozzetti A et al. Enhanced resistance to *Cryptococcus neoformans* infection induced by chloroquine in a murine model of meningoencephalitis. Antimicrob Agents Chemother 1997; 41(4):802–807

Chapter 67
Antifungal Drug Resistance in Histoplasmosis

L. Joseph Wheat, Patricia Connolly, Melinda Smedema, and P. David Rogers

1 Introduction

Histoplasma capsulatum var. *capsulatum* is an ascomycete from the Arthrodermataceae family, and the causative agent of histoplasmosis. It is found in soil, particularly in microfoci of bat or starling guano, growing as a mold (1). The mold consists of hyphae bearing both macroconidia and the infectious microconidia. *H. capsulatum* grows as a yeast at temperatures exceeding 35°C. It is the yeast form that is primarily found in the infected host. The organism is endemic to certain parts of North America, primarily the Ohio and Mississippi River valleys.

Infection with *H. capsulatum* is initiated upon inhalation of microconidia, which germinate into yeasts upon engulfment by macrophages and activate the host innate immune response (2). The organism survives within macrophages, which are believed to play a role in dissemination. T-cell immunity is critical to mounting an effective immune response to *H. capsulatum*. Individuals with underlying immune defects, such as acquired immunodeficiency syndrome (AIDS), are at greater risk of developing more severe forms of histoplasmosis. In areas of the US where *H. capsulatum* is endemic, disseminated histoplasmosis occurs in approximately 5% of AIDS patients.

In the absence of underlying immune disorders, most symptomatic cases of infection are acute and self-limited as is the case for acute pulmonary histoplasmosis (3). In some cases, presumably following high inoculum exposure, acute pulmonary histoplasmosis may be diffuse, causing respiratory difficulty (4). Chronic pulmonary histoplasmosis represents a progressive pulmonary form of disease, as seen in tuberculosis, and causes loss of lung function. This manifestation is more often observed in patients with underlying obstructive lung disease. Progressive disseminated histoplasmosis (PDH) represents a progressive clinical illness with extrapulmonary spread of infection. Risk factors for PDH include underlying immunosupressive disorders, treatment with corticosteroids or other immunosuppressive medications, and the extremes of age (3). Recently, treatment of inflammatory disorders with tumor necrosis factor (TNF) inhibitors has been recognized to predispose to severe forms of histoplasmosis (5).

2 Treatment

Amphotericin B was the drug of choice for the management of histoplasmosis for many years, dating back to early reports of Furcolow (6) and Putnam (7). The advent of the azole antifungals expanded the options for treatment significantly. The availability of these agents in an oral formulation has allowed for the management of this disease on an outpatient basis. Likewise, the introduction of the lipid-based amphotericin B formulations and intravenous formulations of the newer triazoles has expanded the options for management of this disease in the inpatient setting.

2.1 Amphotericin B

In the early retrospective studies of patients with PDH, mortality was 83% in untreated patients contrasted to 23% in those receiving amphotericin B (6). In a more recent review, mortality approached 50% in patients treated with amphotericin B with AIDS and severe PDH manifested by respiratory failure or shock (8). In most cases, renal impairment that was present at baseline or that developed after initiation of treatment resulted in dosage reduction or skipped doses of amphotericin B (8). This high failure rate was the reason for performing a double-blind trial comparing liposomal vs. deoxycholate amphotericin B (9). This formulation was chosen because it achieves highest concentrations in the blood and brain, and is

L.J. Wheat (✉)
MiraVista Diagnostics/MiraBella Technologies,
Indianapolis, IN, USA,
jwheat@miravistalabs.com

D.L. Mayers (ed.), *Antimicrobial Drug Resistance*,
DOI 10.1007/978-1-60327-595-8_67, © Humana Press, a part of Springer Science+Business Media, LLC 2009

the least nephrotoxic of the amphotericin B preparations. In a study in patients with AIDS who had PDH, resolution of fever and improvement of symptoms occurred in a higher proportion of patients treated with the liposomal formulation at a dosage of 3 mg/kg/d than with the standard deoxycholate preparation at a dose of 0.7 mg/kg/d (9). Survival also was better with the liposomal preparation. Thus, liposomal amphotericin B may be preferred in patients with severe or moderately severe PDH, Table 1. Interestingly, however, clearance of fungemia was similar with both preparations.

Liposomal amphotericin B appears to act more rapidly than itraconazole in patients with PDH. By comparison of the data from the study evaluating liposomal amphotericin B (10) and the earlier study evaluating itraconazole (11), fungemia cleared more rapidly with amphotericin B (12), supporting a hypothesis that induction therapy with an amphotericin B product might be more effective than with itraconazole. Treatment can usually be changed to itraconazole within 1–2 weeks, after the patient defervesces and exhibits improvement in other signs or symptoms.

2.2 Itraconazole

Itraconazole is the preferred oral agent in patients with milder manifestations who are not felt to require hospitalization, for completion of therapy following response to amphotericin B, and for those who are unable to tolerate any amphotericin B preparation. In noncomparative trials, itraconazole was successful in 85–100% of the cases (11, 13) compared to 56–70% for ketoconazole (14, 15). If itraconazole is used as initial therapy for patients with moderately severe or severe manifestations of histoplasmosis, the intravenous formulation should be used to accelerate achievement of therapeutic concentrations, and potentially improve the response to therapy. Causes for the failure of itraconazole therapy include inability to absorb itraconazole, drug interactions accelerating its metabolism, and administration to patients with severe infection.

Table 1 Selection of antifungal agents and duration of therapy

Severity	Antifungal agent
Severe disease	Amphotericin B 0.7–1 mg/kg/d, or Liposomal amphotericin B 3 mg/kg/d
Mild disease	Itraconazole 200 mg once or twice daily
Condition	**Duration**
Progressive disseminated	12 months
Severe immunodeficiency	Life-long
Chronic pulmonary	12–24 months
Acute pulmonary	1.5–3 months

2.3 Fluconazole

Fluconazole is less effective than itraconazole in histoplasmosis, on the basis of data from an experimental model of histoplasmosis (16) and experience in humans (10). It was effective in 12 out of 14 (86%) non-AIDS patients with disseminated histoplasmosis, but two relapsed (17). In another study, although 74% of patients with AIDS who had mild or moderately severe manifestations of histoplasmosis responded to 800 mg daily of fluconazole, one-third relapsed over the next 6 months while receiving 400 mg daily for chronic maintenance therapy (18). Fourfold or greater increases in the minimum inhibitory concentration (MIC) to fluconazole occurred in the isolates from over half of failing patients (18), but cross-resistance to itraconazole was not observed (19). Also, the clearance of fungemia was more rapid during induction therapy with itraconazole than with fluconazole (10). Fluconazole is not recommended except in persons who cannot take itraconazole.

2.4 New Agents

H. capsulatum is very susceptible to posaconazole (20, 21), which was also highly effective in experimental infection (21, 22). Others have shown voriconazole to be active against *H. capsulatum* (20, 23), but animal studies have not been conducted. Furthermore, activity of voriconazole against fluconazole-resistant strains remains to be studied. In vitro susceptibility to the echinocandins and in vivo effectiveness in the experimental infection remains unclear. While caspofungin (24) and anidulofungin (Wheat, unpublished observation, 2004) were not effective in our studies, others reported greater in vitro susceptibility (20, 25) and a more favorable outcome of experimental infection using caspofungin (25). Variable susceptibility was observed with nikkomycin Z, and its effectiveness in the mouse model correlated with MIC in our laboratory (26), but greater in vitro activity and in vivo efficacy was observed by others (27, 28).

2.5 Combination Therapy

While there are no data with human, we have studied combination therapy in a murine model. In two studies, antagonism was noted using the combination of amphotericin B and fluconazole (16, 29). While itraconazole was not antagonistic to amphotericin B, the outcome was no better than with amphotericin B alone. Nikkomycin Z and fluconazole, used at relatively low doses, exhibited additive activity in an experimental model of histoplasmosis (27).

3 Resistance

3.1 Susceptibility Testing

We have shown that the susceptibility to fluconazole correlated with the treatment outcome in humans (30) and susceptibility to nikkomycin Z in our murine model (26). These findings suggest that susceptibility testing could be used to identify drugs for further evaluation in histoplasmosis, and for evaluating the cause for treatment failure in patient management. We have used the yeast in our studies because it is the form found in the tissues, but conversion of the mold, the form commonly isolated in the clinical laboratory, to the yeast for susceptibility testing may be difficult and time-consuming.

We have adapted the NCCLS method for yeast for susceptibility testing of *H. capsulatum* (31). First, the *Histoplasma* inoculum was standardized by comparison to McFarland standard of 5 at 530 nm, then diluted 1:100, while the *Candida parapsilosis* ATCC 90018 control was prepared according to the NCCLS method, by comparison to a 0.5 McFarland standard, then diluted 1:2,000. This modification was required because of the slower growth rate of *H. capsulatum*. The second modification of the NCCLS protocol was prolongation of the incubation time for *Histoplasma* to 96–120 h of incubation at 37°C, again based upon the slower growth rate of *H. capsulatum*. Growth of *H. capsulatum* was scored by comparison to controls grown without the presence of drug. Inhibition of at least 80%, as compared to that with no drug control, was defined as the MIC for the azoles only.

We find that *H. capsulatum* yeast is susceptible to amphotericin B and most triazoles (16, 21, 30). Small amount of strains were susceptible to nikkomycin Z; however (26), and none were susceptible to the echinocandins caspofungin (24) or anidulofungin (Wheat, unpublished, 2004). We also have noted resistance to 5-fluorocytosine with MICs > 64 μg/mL in all the 20 strains tested (Wheat, unpublished observation, 2004).

However, using mold others have noted greater susceptibility to the echinocandins (20, 25) and nikkomycin Z (27). Studies are needed to investigate the differences in susceptibility and response to therapy between the mold and yeast to define the optimal form for susceptibility testing and experimental infection.

3.2 Resistance as a Cause for Failure

Resistance as a cause for treatment failure only has been reported for fluconazole (19, 30). Most failures with amphotericin B and itraconazole are caused by the inadequate drug exposure or delayed therapy, and not by the resistance. In fact, there are no reports of resistance to itraconazole or amphotericin B, and we have also not observed the same in our laboratory.

We have reported resistance to fluconazole. In the initial case (19), the fluconazole MIC increased from 0.62 μg/mL in the pretreatment isolate to 20 μg/mL in an isolate obtained at relapse 16 weeks later. In a subsequent analysis, susceptibility of pretreatment isolates was compared for 37 patients who responded to treatment and 28 who failed to treatment (30). Fluconazole MICs were significantly lower for patients who responded to therapy as compared to those who did not (Fig. 1). Likewise, in 17 sets of pretreatment and posttreatment isolates from patients failing therapy, ten exhibited at least a fourfold increase in fluconazole MIC (Fig. 2). Cross-resistance to itraconazole was not observed, and the activity of the newer triazoles against these strains is under investigation.

The activity of the echinocandins against *H. capsulatum* has been inconsistent. In vitro susceptibility testing using the yeast revealed MICs of 16 μg/mL or greater in over 90% of

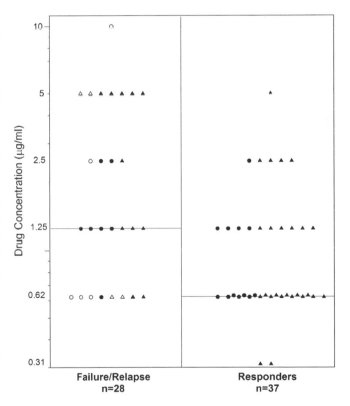

Fig. 1 Comparison of MICs to fluconazole for pretreatment isolates between patients who fail induction or relapse during maintenance therapy (N = 28) to those from responders (N = 37). Each point represents the isolate from one patient, and the horizontal line represents the median for the group. The circles represent version 1 patients and the triangles version 2 patients. On the left panel, induction failures are depicted by an open symbol and maintenance failures (relapses) by a closed symbol (obtained with permission of Clinical Infectious Diseases)

isolates, and the therapy in an experimental infection model was ineffective in our laboratory (24). Others reported higher activity (20, 25), and greater effectiveness in the experimental model (25). In one report, the geometric mean MIC for five mold isolates was 1.3 µg/mL for caspofungin and 3.6 µg/mL for anidulofungin (20). The MIC of the mold isolate used in the experimental model reporting the effectiveness of caspofungin was 0.25 µg/mL (25). Whether the differences in susceptibility and outcomes of experimental infection are related to differences in pathogenicity of the yeast versus mold or some strain-specific property remain to be determined.

Nikkomycin Z was active against some strains of *H. capsulatum* and effective against one susceptible strain in our experimental model (26). In this study, the MIC was 4 µg/mL in 6 out of 20 isolates, but ranged from 8 to 64 µg/mL or greater in 14, with an MIC_{90} of ≥ 64 µg/mL. While nikkomycin Z 20 mg/kd twice daily did not prolong survival or reduce fungal burden in mice infected with an isolate with an MIC of ≥ 64 µg/mL, that dose was as effective as amphotericin B against a strain with an MIC of 4 µg/mL. Nikkomycin Z 100 mg/kg twice daily was somewhat effective against the

isolate with the MIC of ≥ 64 µg/mL. In another study using a mold with an MIC of 0.5 µg/mL, nikkomycin Z 2.5 to 25 mg/kg twice daily improved survival and reduced fungal burden in the spleen (27).

3.3 Mechanisms of Antifungal Resistance

The biochemical basis of acquired resistance to fluconazole has been examined in a single series of *H. capsulatum* isolates obtained from an AIDS patient who failed fluconazole therapy (19). Fluconazole and itraconazole MICs for these isolates are shown in Table 2. Molecular genetic studies revealed the similarity of these isolates using RAPD PCR fingerprinting. The effects of both fluconazole and itraconazole on growth and ergosterol content in these isolates were then examined. The IC_{50} for fluconazole was threefold greater for the relapse isolate as compared to that of the parent isolate. Likewise, with regard to ergosterol content, the IC_{50} for fluconazole was fivefold greater for the relapse isolate as compared to that of the parent isolate. Unexpectedly, itraconazole was more potent against the relapse than the parent isolate with respect to both growth inhibition and ergosterol content. When sterol biosynthesis was more closely examined using [^{14}C] acetate (Fig. 3), similar differences in the potency of both the azoles were observed between the parent and relapse isolate, consistent with the differences observed in growth inhibition and ergosterol content.

Ergosterol and ergosta-5, 22-diene-3-β-ol remained the predominant sterols formed in both the parent and relapse isolates in the absence of drug. Inhibition of ergosterol biosynthesis by both the azoles resulted in accumulation of eburicol and obtusifolione in the parent isolate; however, in the relapse isolate less of these sterols accumulated in response to fluconazole whereas more of these sterols accumulated in response to itraconazole. This suggests that the cytochrome P-450-dependent enzymes 14α demethylase and 3-ketosteroid reductase became less sensitive to fluconazole and more sensitive to itraconazole in the relapse isolate. Further examination is needed to determine the molecular basis for the change in sensitivity of these enzymes to fluconazole and itraconazole.

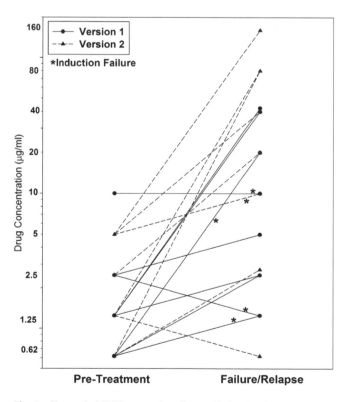

Fig. 2 Change in MIC between baseline and induction failure or maintenance relapse isolates. *Solid lines* represent version 1 cases (induction dose 600 mg followed by maintenance dose 200 mg daily) and the *broken lines* represent version 2 cases (induction dose 800 mg followed by maintenance dose 400 mg daily). The *asterisks* mark induction failures, all others are maintenance relapses (obtained with permission of Clinical Infectious Diseases)

Table 2 MICs of fluconazole and itraconazole for a matched series of *H. Capsulatum* isolates representing the acquisition of resistance to fluconazole

Time during therapy at which the isolate was obtained	MICs (µg/mL)	
	Fluconazole	Itraconazole
Pretreatment	0.62	0.004
Week 8	1.25	0.004
Week 12	2.5	0.004
Week 16 (replace)	20.0	0.004

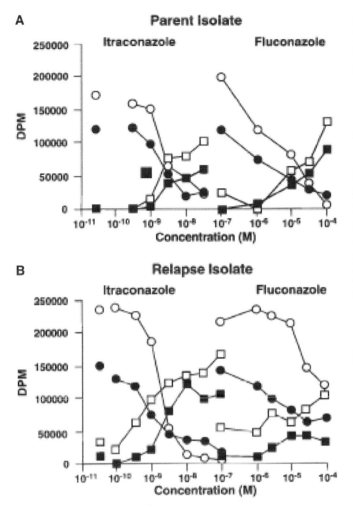

A Parent Isolate

B Relapse Isolate

Fig. 3 Effects of itraconazole (ITZ) and fluconazole (FCZ) on ergosterol synthesis from [14C] acetate by the parent and relapse isolates. Time of incubation was 48 h in GY medium. Drug and [14C] acetate were added immediately before inoculation. Sterols formed are: ergosterol (*open circle*), ergosta-5, 22-diene-3-ol (*closed circle*), obtusifolione (*open square*), and eburicol (24-methylene dihydrolanosterol) (*closed square*). Results for controls (ergosterol synthesis in the presence of solvent DMSO) are depicted inside the left-hand margin by the datum points that are not connected by lines. Results are mean values from four experiments (presented with the permission of Antimicrobial Agents and Chemotherapy)

Recently, the effects of melanin synthesis on antifungal susceptibility in *H. capsulatum* have been investigated (32). *H. capsulatum* has been shown to produce melanin both in vitro and in vivo (33). The susceptibilities of melanized and nonmelenaized isolates of *H. capsulatum* to amphotericin B, caspofungin, fluconazole, itraconazole, and 5-fluorocytosine were examined using the NCCLS macrodilution protocol for yeasts. Using this method, no differences in antifungal susceptibility were observed. However, when these antifungal agents were examined using a killing assay, melanization was found to reduce the susceptibilities of *H. capsulatum* to both amphotericin B and caspofungin. These effects may be due to the binding of amphotericin B and caspofungin to

melanin. The clinical relevance of these findings are unclear. Further examination of the effects of melanin on susceptibility to these antifungal agents, particularly amphotericin B, is warranted.

4 Conclusion

In conclusion, the liposomal formulation of amphotericin B and itraconazole appear to be the drugs of choice for the treatment of histoplasmosis. Of the newer agents, posaconazole is the most promising. Antifungal resistance limits the effectiveness of fluconazole in histoplasmosis. Susceptibility testing appears to be helpful in preclinical evaluation of antifungal agents and perhaps the investigation of treatment failure despite adequate drug exposure.

References

1. Cano M, Hajjeh RA. The epidemiology of histoplasmosis: a review. Semin Resp Infect 2001; 16:109 118
2. Newman SL. Cell-mediated immunity to *Histoplasma capsulatum*. Semin Resp Infect 2001; 16:102–108
3. Wheat LJ, Kauffman CA. Histoplasmosis. Infect Dis Clin North Am 2003; 17:1–19, vii
4. Wheat LJ, Conces D, Allen SD, Blue-Hindy D, Loydlen J. Pulmonary histoplasmosis syndromes: recognition, diagnosis, and management. Semin Respir Crit Care Med 2004; 25:129–144
5. Wood KL, Hage CA, Knox KS et al. Histoplasmosis after treatment with anti-TNF-{alpha} therapy. Am J Respir Crit Care Med 2003; 167:1279–1282
6. Furcolow ML. Comparison of treated and untreated severe histoplasmosis. JAMA 1963; 183:121–127
7. Putnam LR, Sutliff WD, Larkin JC et al. Histoplasmosis cooperative study: chronic pulmonary histoplasmosis treated with amphotericin B alone and with amphotericin B and triple sulfonamide. Am Rev Respir Dis 1968; 97:96–102
8. Wheat L. Histoplasmosis in the acquired immunodeficiency syndrome. Curr Top Med Mycol 1996; 7:7–18
9. Johnson PC, Wheat LJ, Cloud GA et al. Safety and efficacy of liposomal amphotericin B compared with conventional amphotericin B for induction therapy of histoplasmosis in patients with AIDS. Ann Intern Med 2002; 137:105–109
10. Wheat LJ, Connolly P, Haddad N, Le Monte A, Brizendine E, Hafner R. Antigen clearance during treatment of disseminated histoplasmosis with itraconazole versus fluconazole in patients with AIDS. Antimicrob Agents Chemother 2002; 46:248–250
11. Wheat J, Hafner R, Korzun AH et al. Itraconazole treatment of disseminated histoplasmosis in patients with the acquired immunodeficiency syndrome. Am J Med 1995; 98:336–342
12. Wheat LJ, Cloud G, Johnson PC et al. Clearance of fungal burden during treatment of disseminated histoplasmosis with liposomal amphotericin B versus itraconazole. Antimicrob Agents Chemother 2001; 45:2354–2357
13. Dismukes WE, Bradsher RW, Jr, Cloud GC et al. Itraconazole therapy for blastomycosis and histoplasmosis. Am J Med 1992; 93:489–497

14. Slama TG. Treatment of disseminated and progressive cavitary histoplasmosis with ketoconazole. Am J Med 1983;70–73

15. Dismukes WE, Cloud G, Bowles C et al. Treatment of blastomycosis and histoplasmosis with ketoconazole: Results of a prospective randomized clinical trial. Ann Intern Med 1985; 103:861–872

16. LeMonte A, Washum K, Smedema M, Schnizlein-Bick C, Kohler R, Wheat LJ. Amphotericin B combined with itraconazole or fluconazole for treatment of histoplasmosis. J Infect Dis 2000;545–550

17. McKinsey DS, Kauffman CA, Pappas PG et al. Fluconazole therapy for histoplasmosis. Clin Infect Dis 1996; 23:996–1001

18. Wheat J, MaWhinney S, Hafner R et al. Treatment of histoplasmosis with fluconazole in patients with acquired immunodeficiency syndrome. Am J Med 1997; 103:223–232

19. Wheat J, Marichal P, Vanden Bossche H, Le Monte A, Connolly P. Hypothesis on the mechanism of resistance to fluconazole in *Histoplasma capsulatum*. Antimicrob Agents Chemother 1997; 41:410–414

20. Espinel-Ingroff A. Comparison of in vitro activities of the new triazole SCH56592 and the echinocandins MK-0991 (L-743,872) and LY303366 against opportunistic filamentous and dimorphic fungi and yeasts. J Clin Microbiol 1998; 36:2950–2956

21. Connolly P, Wheat J, Schnizlein-Bick C et al. Comparison of a new triazole antifungal agent, Schering 56592, with itraconazole and amphotericin B for treatment of histoplasmosis in immunocompetent mice. Antimicrob Agents Chemother 1999; 43:322–328

22. Connolly P, Wheat LJ, Schnizlein-Bick C et al. Comparison of a new triazole, posaconazole, with itraconazole and amphotericin B for treatment of histoplasmosis following pulmonary challenge in immunocompromised mice. Antimicrob Agents Chemother 2000; 44:2604–2608

23. Li RK, Ciblak MA, Nordoff N, Pasarell L, Warnock DW, McGinnis MR. In vitro activities of voriconazole, itraconazole, and amphotericin B against *Blastomyces dermatitidis*, *Coccidioides immitis*, and *Histoplasma capsulatum*. Antimicrob Agents Chemother 2000; 44:1734–1736

24. Kohler S, Wheat LJ, Connolly P et al. Comparison of the echinocandin caspofungin with amphotericin B for treatment of histoplasmosis following pulmonary challenge in a murine model. Antimicrob Agents Chemother 2000; 44:1850–1854

25. Graybill JR, Najvar LK, Montalbo EM, Barchiesi FJ, Luther MF, Rinaldi MG. Treatment of histoplasmosis with MK-991 (L-743,872). Antimicrob Agents Chemother 1998; 42:151–153

26. Goldberg J, Connolly P, Schnizlein-Bick C et al. Comparison of nikkomycin Z with amphotericin B and itraconazole for treatment of histoplasmosis in a murine model. Antimicrob Agents Chemother 2000; 44:1624–1629

27. Graybill JR, Najvar LK, Bocanegra R, Hector RF, Luther MF. Efficacy of nikkomycin Z in the treatment of murine histoplasmosis. Antimicrob Agents Chemother 1998; 42:2371–2374

28. Hector RF, Zimmer BL, Pappagianis D. Evaluation of nikkomycins X and Z in murine models of coccidioidomycosis, histoplasmosis, and blastomycosis. Antimicrob Agents Chemother 1990; 34:587–593

29. Haynes RR, Connolly PA, Durkin MM et al. Antifungal therapy for central nervous system histoplasmosis, using a newly developed intracranial model of infection. J Infect Dis 2002; 185:1830–1832

30. Wheat LJ, Connolly P, Smedema M et al. Emergence of resistance to fluconazole as a cause of failure during treatment of histoplasmosis in patients with acquired immunodeficiency disease syndrome. Clin Infect Dis 2001; 33:1910–1913

31. Waitz, J. A., Bartlett, M. S., Ghannoum, M. A., Espinel-Ingroff, A., Lancaster, M. V., Odds, F. C., Pfaller, M. A., Rex, J. H., Rinaldi, M. G., Walsh, T. J., Galgiani, J. N. *Reference Method of Broth Dilution Antifungal Susceptibility Testing of Yeasts*; Approved Standard. M27-A (ISBN 1–56238–328–0), 1–29. 1997. Wayne, PA, National Committee on Clinical Laboratory Standards

32. Van Duin D, Casadevall A, Nosanchuk JD. Melanization of *Cryptococcus neoformans* and *Histoplasma capsulatum* reduces their susceptibilities to amphotericin B and caspofungin. Antimicrob Agents Chemother 2002; 46:3394–3400

33. Nosanchuk JD, Gomez BL, Youngchim S et al. *Histoplasma capsulatum* synthesizes melanin-like pigments in vitro and during mammalian infection. Infect Immun 2002; 70:5124–5131

Chapter 68
Drug Resistance in *Pneumocystis jirovecii*

Jannik Helweg-Larsen, Thomas Benfield, Joseph Kovacs, and Henry Masur

1 Introduction

Pneumocystis jirovecii (previously known as *Pneumocystis carinii*) is an opportunistic fungus that causes pneumonia, Pneumocystis pneumonia (PCP), in immunocompromised individuals. Before 1982, PCP was relatively rare and primarily diagnosed among patients with congenital immunodeficiencies, and patients receiving potent immunosuppressive therapy as part of an antineoplastic regimen. However, with the AIDS pandemic PCP emerged as the most common AIDS-defining diagnosis in industrialized countries. The peak incidence of PCP was observed in the late 1980s and early 1990s. Subsequently, there has been a decline in the incidence of PCP because of the widespread introduction of PCP chemoprophylaxis and the introduction of increasingly potent HIV-1 antiretroviral regimens. However, PCP remains a serious opportunistic infection among heavily immunosuppressed patients who are not receiving appropriate chemoprophylaxis.

2 The Organism

Pneumocystis were identified early in the last century in guinea pigs by Chagas and in rat lungs by Carini (1, 2). These investigators mistakenly considered the organisms as a new form of *Trypanozoma cruzi*. In 1912, Pneumocystis was recognized as a new species and named in honor of Carini (3). Pneumocystis was first described in humans in 1942 by two Dutch investigators, van der Meer and Brug, who described it in three cases: a 3-month-old infant with congenital heart disease and in 2 of 104 autopsy cases – a 4-month-old infant and a 21-year-old adult (4). However, *Pneumocystis* was first established as a human pathogen when Jirovec in 1952 identified the organism as the cause of interstitial plasma cell pneumonia among premature or malnourished infants in orphanages (5).

For most of the twentieth century, *Pneumocystis* was considered as a protozoon and single species based on its morphologic features, its resistance to classical antifungal agents and the effectiveness of certain drugs used to treat protozoan infections. However, in 1988, based on the work by Edman and colleagues (6), phylogenetic analysis of ribosomal RNA (rRNA) sequences and observations of genome size placed *P. carinii* in the fungal kingdom. Functional and phylogenetic comparisons of several other genes have since confirmed its position (7–9). Phylogenetic data suggest that *Pneumocystis* is an ancient organism without any close relatives. It has been suggested that the *Pneumocystis* species represent an early divergent line in the fungal kingdom, which may have branched coincident with the bifurcation of the basidiomycete and ascomycete lineages. The organism has recently been placed in a group of fungi entitled the Archiascomycetes (10). In contrast to most other fungi, *Pneumocystis* possesses only one copy of the nuclear ribosomal RNA locus, has a fragile cell wall and contains little or no ergosterol (11).

Pneumocystis organisms have been identified in most mammalian species in which it has been searched for. Genetic and antigenic analyses have shown that *Pneumocystis* includes a broad family of organisms, with species specificity among its mammalian hosts (11–13). Remarkably, the level of genetic divergence between *Pneumocystis* organisms infecting different mammals is greater than the degree of divergence observed between certain fungi classified as distinct species (14, 15). Phylogenetic comparisons of DNA sequences in organisms from 18 different nonhuman primate species have demonstrated that sequence divergence correlates with the phylogenetic difference between the host species, which suggests that *Pneumocystis* species have evolved together with their hosts (16).

In 1994, an interim trinomial name change was adopted with the name *P. carinii* f.sp. *hominis* for *Pneumocystis* infecting humans and *P. carinii* f.sp. *carinii* for one of the two species infecting rats (17). Subsequently, in 2002,

J. Helweg-Larsen (✉)
Department of Infectious Diseases, Rigshospitalet,
Copenhagen University Hospital, Copenhagen, Denmark
jhelweg@dadlnet.dk

D.L. Mayers (ed.), *Antimicrobial Drug Resistance*,
DOI 10.1007/978-1-60327-595-8_68, © Humana Press, a part of Springer Science+Business Media, LLC 2009

993

because of the recognition of its genetic and functional distinctness, the organism infecting humans was renamed *Pneumocystis jirovecii,* in honor of Otto Jirovec, who was among the first to describe the microbe in humans (18–20).

3 Transmission and Infection

Since *P. jirovecii* organism cannot be cultured in vitro, knowledge about its biology has been difficult to obtain. However, the development of molecular and immunological techniques has permitted considerable insight into this organism and on how it interacts with its various animal hosts. Antibody and PCR findings indicate that primary infection with *P. jirovecii* happens in early childhood with a uniform high incidence in all geographic areas, and suggest that *P. jirovecii* organisms are ubiquitous. Its environmental source is, however, unknown. Organisms may be coming from inanimate environmental sources, or may be spread by healthy humans. Studies have not conclusively demonstrated the environmental niche.

It was previously though that the infection was carried life-long and that clinical infection was a result of reactivation in immunocompromised hosts. PCR findings have questioned this view and support a more complex picture of transmission and infection.

When the organism is obtained initially as a primary infection, it is not clear whether an immunocompetent host develops a transient disease. Various investigators have proposed that primary infection might correlate with the development of upper or lower respiratory manifestations, or with the development of sudden infant death syndrome (21–23). Following primary infection, the presumption, based on murine models, has been that the organism becomes latent, later manifesting clinically if the patient becomes profoundly immunosuppressed.

More recent data, however, suggests that human hosts can be infected with more than one strain of *Pneumocystis jirovecii,* raising the possibility that infection can be acquired on multiple occasions, leading to latency with a variety of distinct organisms (24). The clinical disease PCP may, therefore, occur as a reactivation of a prior latent organism, or as a result of recent acquisition of an airborne pathogen.

As noted above, the environmental source of *Pneumocystis* has not been identified. Since most infants acquire antibody against *Pneumocystis* during the first year of life, the organism must be ubiquitous. Whether the organism is being shed into the environment regularly by healthy hosts, or whether the organism is introduced into the environment from an inanimate environmental source such as trees or grass is unknown. However, nonhuman animals are not the source, because, as mentioned above, each animal species is infected with a different strain of *Pneumocystis,* and there is no cross-species infection that has been identified.

Pneumocystis has specific tropism for the lung, where it exists in the alveoli. In rare cases organism have been detected in other organs, but it seldom causes disease at extrapulmonary sites. After inhalation, the organism attaches tightly to the surface of type I alveolar cells (25). Adherence is primarily mediated by the major surface glycoprotein (MSG) (26, 27). This protein is the most abundant antigen on the surface of *Pneumocystis* and is encoded by a multicopy gene family. MSG represents a family of proteins that are highly polymorphic, repeated and distributed among all the chromosomes of *Pneumocystis*. MSG shows high level of antigenic variation by switching the expression of multiple MSG genes, with a system that resembles the antigenic system used for antigenic variation in *Trypanozoma cruzi* (28, 29). It is likely that this antigenic variation in MSG serves for avoiding the host immune response. There is no detailed knowledge of the life cycle and the mode of replication has not been definitely established, but both asexual and sexual life cycles have been proposed (30, 31). Recently, several genes, which in other fungi are involved in mating, pheromone responsiveness, and responses to environmental changes, have been demonstrated in *Pneumocystis*, suggesting that the organism has a sexual replication cycle that responds to environmental changes in the lung (32, 33).

4 Drug Treatment

The major drug classes used for treatment and prophylaxis of PCP include antifolate drugs, diamines, atovaquone, and macrolides (Tables 1 and 2). Most traditional antifungal agents have no activity against *Pneumocystis*. As *Pneumocystis* was originally believed to be a protozoon, initial drug testing focused on drugs with activity against protozoan infections.

In 1958, pentamidine isethionate was the first drug used to successfully treat PCP (34). In the 1960s, the combination of sulfadoxine and pyrimethamine was used for the prevention of epidemic infantile pneumocystosis in Iran (35). In 1966, Rifkind treated two patients with sulfadiazine and pyrimethamine; both patients died, but two patients were successfully treated 4 years later (36). Between 1974 and 1977, studies led by Hughes et al. established that the combination of trimethoprim–sulfamethoxazole (TMP–SMX) is effective for both treatment and prophylaxis of murine and then human PCP (37–39). TMP–SMX is as effective as intravenous pentamidine for therapy, and is still the treatment of choice. Additionally, TMP–SMX is the most effective chemoprophylaxis for PCP, and therefore the standard for prevention.

Table 1 Regimens for prophylaxis against Pneumocystis pneumonia

Drug	Oral or aerosol dose
First choice	
Trimethoprim–sulfamethoxazole	1 DS or SS daily
Alternatives	
Trimethoprim–sulfamethoxazole	1 DS three times per week
Dapsone	50 mg twice daily or 100 mg twice weekly
Dapsone with	50 mg daily
Pyrimethamine plus	50 mg weekly
Leucovorin	25 mg weekly
Dapsone with	200 mg weekly
pyrimethamine plus	75 mg weekly
Leucovorin	25 mg weekly
Pentamidine aerosolized	300 mg monthly via nebulizer system
Atovaquone	1,500 mg daily
[a]Pyrimethamine plus	25–75 mg qd
Sulfadiazine	0.5–2.0 g q6h

DS: double strength = 800 mg sulfamethoxazole, 160 mg trimethoprim; SS: single strength = 400 mg sulfamethoxazole, 80 mg trimethoprim.
[a]This regimen only for use in case of concurrent toxoplasmosis

Other drugs have proven activity for therapy, including sulfadiazine plus pyrimethamine, atovaquone, clindamycin plus pyrimethamine, trimetrexate, dapsone and aerosolized pentamidine. Not all drugs that are effective for therapy are also effective for chemoprophylaxis. Dapsone, dapsone–trimethoprim, atovaquone and aerosolized pentamidine are also effective for prophylaxis. Intravenous pentamidine and clindamycin–primaquine have not been shown to be effective for chemoprophylaxis. There are other drugs that have in vitro activity or anecdotal anti-PCP activity in humans and could have a role in managing human disease if all other alternatives were not feasible. These include azithromycin, doxycycline, and caspofungin.

5 Prophylaxis

Among HIV-infected patients, the occurrence of PCP is closely related to the CD4 count: With lower CD4 counts, the risk of PCP increases. While a count of 200 cells/mm³ is often used as an indicator or susceptibility, HIV-infected patients do in fact develop PCP at counts higher than 200 cells/mm³, although at a frequency lower than that at 200, 100, or 50 cells/mm³.

Patients with congenital immunodeficiencies, particularly X-linked immunodeficiency with hyper-immunoglobulin M and SCID, patients receiving long-term and high-dose corticosteroid therapy, and patients receiving certain chemotherapeutic regimens for cancer therapy or transplantation are at the risk of developing PCP. Interestingly, some chemotherapeutic agents such as fludarabine or antithymocyte globulin

produce a much higher risk of PCP than other regimens (40–43). In patients without HIV, CD4 counts are not a reliable marker of susceptibility. Several studies have shown that the occurrence of PCP is not as predictable with these markers in diseases unrelated to HIV (42).

Systemic chemoprophylaxis against PCP was introduced by Dutz in Iran in the early 1950s. He showed that outbreaks of PCP could be aborted with the use of sulfadoxine plus pyrimethamine (44). Hughes et al. followed this observation with a classic study of children with acute lymphocytic leukemia (ALL); they showed that PCP could be virtually eliminated by TMP–SMX prophylaxis (39) Subsequently this prophylaxis was used for other populations of cancer and transplant recipients with a very high success rate. With the advent of the AIDS epidemic, PCP prophylaxis was used sporadically in the 1980s. After the publication of a convincing study by Fischl et al., PCP prophylaxis became a standard of care for HIV-infected patients with CD4 counts less than 200 cells/mm³ in 1989 (45). The identification of additional risk factors for the development of PCP has led to expanded recommendations for the use of PCP chemoprophylaxis details are provided in Table 3. HIV-1 infected patients with oral candidiasis or a CD4 count less than 200 cells/μL, should be offered primary prophylaxis. Secondary prophylaxis should be offered to all patients following an episode of PCP. In HIV patients receiving prophylaxis; prophylaxis can safely be interrupted if immune function is improved above a CD4 count of 200 cells/μL for at least 3 months following antiretroviral therapy. If the patient subsequently fails antiretroviral therapy and the CD4 declines to below 200 cells/μL, prophylaxis should be restarted.

In non-HIV infected individuals, conditions such as organ transplantation, high-dose steroid treatment and/or high-dose chemotherapy may confer a high risk of PCP. Prophylaxis should be offered as shown in Table 3. Several prophylactic regimens are available. The most efficient, cheap and widely used regimen is daily TMP–SMX. TMP–SMX prophylaxis is relatively well tolerated by most non-HIV patients; in contrast, HIV patients have a high frequency of adverse effects, in particular rash and myelosuppression. Before the advent of antiretroviral therapy, 50% of patients experienced an adverse effect after 12 months of prophylaxis with double-strength TMP–SMX (160/800 mg), and half would have switched to other types of prophylaxis after 3 years (46). Fortunately, 80/400 mg TMP–SMX daily appears to be equally effective and is associated with fewer side effects than 160/800 mg daily (47). Because of its efficacy, ease of administration and cost, every effort should be tried to maintain patients at risk of PCP on TMP–SMX. For patients, who have reacted to TMP SMX, it has been shown to be safe to reintroduce TMP–SMX by dose escalation (48, 49). A variety of dosing regimens can be used with similar efficacy. Tolerability may improve with the lower dose or the intermittent regimens.

Table 2 Drug regimens for the treatment of PCP

Drug	Route	Dose	Toxicity	Advantages	Disadvantages
First choice					
Trimethoprim–sulfamethoxazole	By mouth	2 DS every 8 h	Rash and fever Anemia and neutropenia Hyperkalemia	Superior efficacy Inexpensive Oral and iv	Rash common
	Intravenous	Trimethoprim 5 mg/kg with sulfamethoxazole 20 mg/kg every 8 h	Hepatitis Nephritis Anaphylactoid reaction	Bacterial and anti-toxoplasmosis activity	
Alternatives					
Dapsone plus trimethoprim	By mouth	100 mg daily	Rash, nausea and vomiting and fever Methemoglobinemia, leukopenia and haemolytic anemia	Inexpensive	No iv formulation
	By mouth	320 mg every 8 h	Liver function abnormalities; headache Dapsone may cause hemolysis in patients with G-6PD		
Clindamycin plus primaquine	By mouth, intravenous	300–450 mg every 6 h 30 mg daily	*Clostridium difficile* diarrhea, nausea and vomiting. Primaquine may cause hemolysis in patients with G-6PD deficiency		No iv formulation for primaquine
Pentamidine	Intravenous	4 mg/kg day	High incidence of adverse effects, particularly hypoglycemia and nephrotoxicity Pancreatitis and IDDM. Hypotension with short infusion time Pancytopenia Q-T prolongation	Highly effective	Toxicity common. Only iv formulation
Atovaquone	By mouth	750 mg twice daily	Rash, nausea, diarrhea and headache (20%) Fever, increased transaminases and neutropenia	Well tolerated	Expensive Useful for mild disease
Adjunctive therapy Prednisone in patients with room air pAO$_2$ < 70 mmhg (9.3 kPa)	By mouth, intravenous	40 mg twice daily for 5 days 40 mg daily, days 6 through 11 20 mg daily, days 12 through 21 while on anti-PCP therapy	Standard of care for moderate or severe disease	Metabolic problems, especially glucose and electrolyte changes	

6 Treatment of PCP

Untreated PCP is invariably fatal. In the beginning of the HIV epidemic, the mortality rate of PCP was reported to be 30–40% (50, 51), increasing to 70–90% among patients who progressed to respiratory failure (52). Over the past decade, mortality rates have dropped to 5–15% (53–58). This appears to be a consequence of earlier recognition of the infection, the introduction of adjuvant corticosteroids to patients with moderate-to-severe PCP as defined by a PaO$_2$ of less than

Table 3 Recommendations for PCP prophylaxis and risk identification in selected diseases

Disease	Risk identification	Duration of prophylaxis	Comment
HIV-1 infection	Prior PCP	Lifelong unless CD4 count >200 × >3 months due to ART	Prophylaxis improves survival
CD4 cell count<200			Restart prophylaxis if CD4 count falls to < 200 despite ART
Oropharyngeal candidiasis			
CD4 cell count <14%			
Prior AIDS-defining illness			
Organ transplantation			
Kidney	Depends on intensity of immunosuppression and occurrence of graft versus host disease or rejection	General: minimum 6 month after transplantation:	Need for PCP prophylaxis determined by clinical experience. CD4 count is not a reliable predictor
Lung		At least 6 months	
Heart/Liver		Indefinitely	
Autologous BMT		6-12 month	
Allogenic BMT		6–12 month	
Rejection		Minimum 1 year	
Graft versus Host disease		Reinstate	
		Reinstate	
Malignancy			
Acute lymphoblastic leukemia (ALL)	During and subsequent to combination chemotherapy	During severe immunosuppression	Need for PCP prophylaxis determined by clinical experience with each chemotherapeutic regimen. CD4 count is not a reliable predictor
		Continue during maintenance therapy for childhood ALL	
Chronic lymphatic leukemia (CLL)	Treatment with Fludarabine or Alemtuzumab (Campath, anti-CD52)	Minimum 2 months after discontinuation or until CD4>200	
		3–6 month post chemotherapy	
Lymphoma	Certain chemotherapeutic regimens e.g. PROMACE-CYTABOM		

BMT bone marrow transplantation; ART antiretroviral therapy

70 mmHg, better diagnostic and therapeutic abilities related to concomitant processes, and improved ICU supportive measures.

The importance of educating patients to seek medical attention early, when symptoms are still mild, must be an emphasis of patient management programs. Both patients and health care professionals must recognize that mild symptoms such as dyspnea, cough, or low-grade fever can be the initial manifestation of PCP, especially in patients with CD4+ T lymphocyte counts below 200 cells/mm³. Thus, clinicians should not wait for all the features of PCP to be present, or for the chest radiograph to be abnormal, before initiating a workup for PCP. Moreover, once there is a high suspicion therapy should be instituted promptly if the diagnostic procedures will be delayed.

The choice of specific chemotherapy is also important. The most potent drugs for PCP treatment are antifolate drugs, which act by blocking de novo synthesis of folates through inhibition of dihydroperoate synthase (DHPS) or dihydrofolate reductase (DHFR) (Fig. 1).

DHPS catalyzes the condensation of *p*-aminobenzoic acid (PABA) and hydroxymethyl dihydropterin–pryophospate to produce dihydropteroate, which is later converted to dihy-drofolate by dihydrofolate synthase. Subsequently, dihydrofolate is reduced by dihydrofolate reductase (DHFR) into tetrahydrofolate. Sulfa drugs are structural analogs of PABA and inhibit DHPS.

The earliest clinical trials to treat PCP were performed with sulfadiazine plus pyrimethamine on the assumption that these drugs would have synergistic action against pneumocystis, as against plasmodia. When the commercial combination of sulfamethoxazole plus trimethoprim was developed to treat bacterial infections, this preparation was assessed for PCP therapy and prophylaxis since commercial sponsorship of studies could be obtained. At that time, there was no knowledge about the relative potency of various sulfonamide preparations against pneumocystis, nor was there information about the relative potency of various DHFR inhibitors. Subsequently, it was found that sulfamethoxazole is probably as potent as any of the other commercially available sulfonamide preparations as discussed below. However, trimethoprim is not as potent as other available DHFR inhibitors, as also described below.

In Table 2, drug treatment options for PCP are listed together with the most important advantages and toxicities of each drug regimen. During the 1980s several trials investigated

Fig. 1 Emergence of DHPS since 1989, worldwide

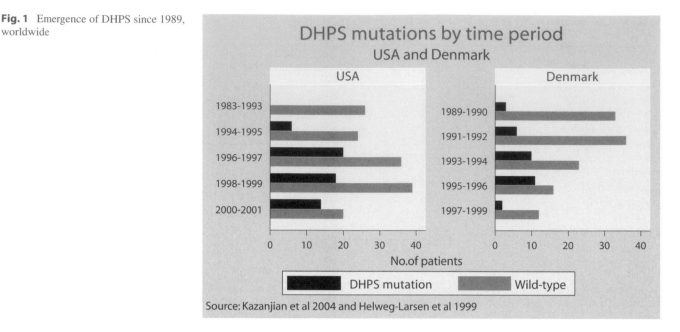

the efficacy of TMP–SMX compared to pentamidine (59–62). In the only noncrossover trial ($n = 70$) (61), TMP–SMX was associated with a better survival than pentamidine. However, when all the trials are considered, TMP–SMX and pentamidine appear to have roughly comparable efficacy (59). Drug toxicity occurs in 24–57% of HIV-infected patients treated with TMP–SMX (63).

Adverse effects generally occur after 7 days of therapy and most commonly include rash, fever and leukopenia. Hepatotoxicity characterized by elevated transaminases also occurs. There are cases of sulfamethoxazole-induced interstitial nephritis, renal calculus formation, anaphylactoid reactions and pancreatitis reported. Trimethroprim can be associated with hyperkalemia. These toxicities are usually not life threatening, although fatal cases of Stevens–Johnson syndrome have occurred.

Pentamidine is associated with a high frequency of toxicities, some of which are treatment-limiting. Early experiences with rapid infusions of pentamidine were associated with hypotension and death, so this route of administration was abandoned. Intramusuclar injections were better tolerated in terms of blood pressure, but they caused a high frequency of sterile abscesses. Therapy was then administered by slow intravenous infusion, which is the best tolerated route. Inhaled pentamidine has been used for therapy, and is well tolerated, but efficacy is poor. Pentamidine is nephrotoxic and causes predictable glomerular and tubular damage to the kidney. Pentamidine is toxic to the pancreas; its initial effects cause a surge of insulin release that often manifests as hypoglycemia. Hypoglycemia can occur days or weeks after starting therapy, and may occur many days after stopping therapy. Leukopenia can also occur. Pentamidine prolongs the QT interval, and cases of torsades de pointe have been reported.

Treatment-limiting toxicities with pentamidine treatment occur in 13–80% of patients.

Alternatives for the therapy to TMP–SMX and pentamidine include dapsone–pyrimethamine, clindamycin–primaquine, and atovaquone (Table 2). Trimetrexate has activity, but is no longer commercially available. Dapsone has not been studied as a single drug and thus should not be used alone for treatment. Dapsone–trimethoprim is effective, however, and probably has potency that is comparable to TMP–SMX. However, since this combination does not come as a fixed-dose combination, is only available orally, and cross-reacts with sulfa in 50% of allergic patients, this regimen does not offer many advantages over TMP–SMX.

Clindamycin–primaquine appears to work on a metabolic pathway different from that of TMP–SMX. Two comparative trials of clindamycin/primaquine with TMP–SMX in moderate-to-severe PCP demonstrated apparent equivalence for clindamycin–primaquine, but both trials were underpowered (64, 65). Clindamycin causes a relatively high incidence of hepatitis, rash and diarrhea in HIV-infected patients. Primaquine can only be given orally.

Atovaquone is well tolerated and acts on a metabolic pathway different from that of TMP–SMX. However, this drug is also only available orally, and does not appear to be as potent as TMP–SMX (66). This is a good alternative to TMP–SMX for patients with mild disease who cannot tolerate TMP–SMX.

Efficacy of dapsone–pyrimethamine has only been demonstrated for mild-to-moderate PCP and for atovaquone only for mild PCP (64, 66–68). Both must be administered orally.

The optimal duration of therapy for PCP has never been properly tested. Usual recommendations are that

HIV-negative patients should receive 2 weeks and HIV-positive patients three weeks of drug treatment.

Many patients experience progressive oxygen desaturation during the first 4–5 days of therapy. This deterioration appears to be caused by the drug-induced death of *Pneumocystis* organisms with exacerbation of alveolar inflammation. This inflammation can be reduced by corticosteroids. Four randomized, controlled trials demonstrated that corticosteroids could reduce mortality in patients with moderate or severe disease (69–72). On the basis of these results, adjunctive steroids are now recommended for all patients with severe disease (PaO$_s$ < 70 mmgh).

7 Sulfonamide Resistance

The widespread use of TMP–SMX and dapsone for therapy and prophylaxis of PCP among HIV patients has led to the concern that sulfa (sulfonamide or sulfone) resistance could develop in *P. jirovecii*.

In many pathogenic bacteria and parasites, resistance to sulfonamides has increased as a consequence of selective pressure, and has limited the efficacy of sulfonamides (73). Widespread use of sulfa drugs for malaria and bacterial infection in Africa has produced high rates of resistance in *P. falciparum* and many bacterial species (74). In San Francisco, the increasing use of PCP prophylaxis among HIV patients led to a marked increase in trimethoprim–sulfamethoxazole resistance among isolates of *Staphylococcus aureus* and seven genera of Enterobacteriaceae (75). In a retrospective study, trimethoprim–sulfamethoxazole resistance was more than twice as likely in blood culture isolates from HIV patients receiving trimethoprim–sulfamethoxazole compared to patients not receiving this prophylaxis (76).

In pathogens such as *Escherichia coli, Neisseria meningitidis, Mycobacterium leprae* and *Plasmodium falciparum*, sulfonamide resistance is caused by mutations in the primary sequence of the DHPS gene (77–79). The mutations that confer resistance are localized within a highly conserved active site of the DHPS protein. In *Pneumocystis*, the DHPS protein is part of a trifunctional protein along with dihydroneopterin aldolase and hydroxymethyldihydropterin pyrophosphokinase, that together are encoded by the multidomain *FAS* gene (80).

In 1997, Lane and co-workers were the first to identify non-synonymous (resulting in changes in the encoded amino acid) DHPS mutations in *Pneumocystis jirovecii* (81). The most frequent DHPS mutations occur at nucleotide positions 165 and 171, which lead to an amino acid change at positions 55 (Thr to Ala) and 57 (Pro to Ser). The homologous Thr and Pro are highly conserved across species, including *Pneumocystis* infecting other hosts. Thus, these variants appear to represent true mutations rather than allelic polymorphisms. Either

mutation can occur alone. The Th55 is homologous to Thr62 of *E. coli* DHPS, which based on its crystal structure, binds the pterin substrate. It is hypothesized that the Thr55Ala and Pro57Ser affect the position of Arg56 (whose homologue in *E. coli* is involved in binding pterin as well as sulfa drugs), decreasing its ability to bind sulfa drugs and resulting in a consequent reduction in sulfa drug sensitivity (82, 83).

However, frequently both mutations are seen in the same isolate. While the association with sulfa exposure is consistent with the concept that these mutations represent resistance that developed under drug pressure, documenting resistance is very difficult partly because *Pneumocystis* cannot be cultured, and partly because functional enzymes (recombinant or native) are unavailable.

Recently, *Saccharomyces cerevisiae* has been used as a model to study *P. jirovecii* DHPS resistance. The DHPS enzyme of *S. cerevisiae* has high functional and genetic similarity to the DHPS of *P. jirovecii*. This enzyme from Saccharomyces is also trifunctional. By site-directed mutagenesis, the in vitro effects of mutations identical to the DHPS mutations in *P. jirovecii* can be investigated. Using this model, two recent studies reported that the double DHPS mutations Thr55Ala and Pro57Ser result in an absolute requirement for PABA, consistent with resistance being associated with altered substrate binding (84, 85). Interestingly, the single mutation Pro57Ser conferred resistance to sulfadoxine, which is supported by clinical observations suggesting a specific association of this mutation with sulfadoxine resistance in PCP (84). However, one study showed an increase in sensitivity of the double mutations to sulfamethoxazole, suggesting that this approach may not accurately reflect the effect of these mutations in *P. jirovecii*.

Several clinical studies have investigated the frequency and significance of DHPS mutations in *P. jirovecii*. Table 4 provides a summary of the studies reporting frequencies of mutations in sulfa-exposed and sulfa-unexposed patients. Although the studies vary considerably in size (13–158 patients) and in definitions of sulfa exposure, a clear association between previous exposure to sulfa drugs (primarily for prophylaxis rather than therapy) and DHPS mutations has been shown in all studies. Large geographical variation in the prevalence of DHPS mutations has been reported, ranging from 7 to 69% of isolates. In the US, the incidence of mutations was lower in Indianapolis and Denver compared to San Francisco, where one study reported that more than 80% of patients were infected with mutant strains (86). Wide variations have also been observed in studies from Europe with a particularly low incidence in Italy; in one study, an 8% frequency of mutations was found among 107 HIV patients between 1994 and 2001 (87). Mutations have rarely been found in clinical isolates obtained prior to the early 1990s, but seem to have increased in frequency recently, presumably as a consequence of increasing selective pressure caused by the

Table 4 Prevalence of DHPS mutations and association with sulfa exposure

Study	Country (year)	Number of DHPS mutations/no. of PCP episodes	DHPS mutations/ sulfa exposed	DHPS mutations/ no sulfa exposure	Risk ratio (95%CI)
Santos (112)	France (1993–1998)	11/20 (55%)	5/5 (100%)	3/12 (25%)	4. 0 (1.5–10.7)
Helweg-Larsen et al. (90)	Denmark (1989–1999)	31/152 (20%)	18/29 (62%)	13/123 (11%)	5.87 (3.26–10.57)
Ma et al. (99)	USA (1985–1998)	16/37 (43%)	11/16 (69%)	3/15 (20%)	3.44 (1.19–9.97)
Huang et al. (113)[a]	USA (1996–1999)	76/111 (69%)	57/71 (80%)	19/40 (48%)	1.69 (1.20–2.39)
Ma et al. (87)	Italy (1994–2001)	9/107 (8%)	6/31	3/76	4.90 (1.31–18.38)
Beard et al. (114)[a]	USA (1995–1998)	152/220 (69%)	np	np	Na
Takahashi et al. (115)	Japan (1994–1999)	6/24 (25%)	2/3 (33%)	4/24 (19%)	4.00 (1.20–13.28)
Costa et al. (116)	Portugal (1994–2001)	24/89 (27%)	5/16 (31%)	19/73	1.20 (0.53–2.73)
Visconti et al. (117)	Italy (1992–1997)	7/20 (35%)	3/4	3/14	3.50 (1.11–11.07)
Zingale et al. (118)	Italy (1996–2002)	25/64 (39%)	21/29	4/35	6.34 (2.45–16.37)
Nahimana et al. (94)	France (1993–1996)	57/158 (36%)	25/29	32/129	3.48 (2.49–4.85)
Kazanjian et al. (89)	USA (1983–2001)	58/145 (40%)	38/56	20/89	3.02 (1.97–4.62)
Kazanjian et al. (89)	China (1998–2001)	0/15	0/0	1/15	Na
Totet et al. (119)	France (1996–2001)	0/13	0/0	2/13	Na
Crothers et al. (120)	USA (1997–2002)	175215	65/72	110/143	2.12 (1.05–4.27)
Valerio et al. (121)	Italy (1994–2004)	14/154 (9%)	4/38	10/116	1.22 (0.41–3.67)

Treatment according to current or previous exposure to sulfone drugs (trimethoprim–sulfamethoxazole, dapsone or sulfadiazine) at diagnosis of PCP. *F* France; *DK* Denmark; *I* Italy; *P* Portugal; *Np* not provided; *Na* not applicable
[a]Overlap of patients in these studies

widespread use of sulfa drugs for prophylaxis (they were widely used for treatment in the 1980s) of PCP (88–90), Fig. 1. Importantly, DHPS mutations have also been increasingly found in patients without any previous exposure to sulfa drugs, suggesting person-to-person spread of mutant strains.

On the basis of a genetic analysis of multiple loci, it appears that the mutations arose independently in multiple strains of *Pneumocystis* (91). In a genotype study of 13 European HIV patients with recurrent episodes of PCP, a switch from wild-type to mutant DHPS occurred in five of seven patients who had a recurrence of the otherwise same molecular type of *P. jirovecii* (92). All patients had received treatment or secondary prophylaxis with trimethoprim–sulfamethoxazole or dapsone. These findings suggest that DHPS mutants may be selected in vivo (within a given patient) under the pressure of trimethoprim–sulfamethoxazole or dapsone. The emergence of DHPS mutations appears to be specific for *P. jirovecii* because only wild-type *Pneumocystis* DHPS has been found in other primate species (93).

The clinical significance of DHPS mutations, specifically with regard to response to prophylaxis and therapy using a sulfa-based regimen (primarily trimethoprim–sulfamethoxazole or dapsone), has been controversial. Several studies have reported a significant association of DHPS mutations with failure of low-dose sulfa prophylaxis (Table 4). However, the extent to which this association reflects actual drug resistance or failure to comply with prescribed prophylaxis is unknown. Hence, in spite of the emergence of mutant DHPS strains, current clinical experience supports the efficacy of trimethoprim–sulfamethoxazole prophylaxis when taken regularly. However,

there is evidence to suggest a contributory role for DHPS mutations in breakthrough PCP in patients using alternative sulfa prophylaxis. Hauser et al. found a significant association with the failure of pyrimethamine–sulfadoxine prophylaxis and the Pro57Ser mutation: all the 14 patients failing this type of prophylaxis harboured this mutation (94). Further, a relatively high number of prophylaxis failures associated with DHPS mutations have been described in patients receiving dapsone prophylaxis. Thus, available data currently suggest that DHPS mutations contribute to low-level sulfa resistance, and may be the most important in failure of second-line sulfa prophylaxis. However, the major reason for PCP breakthrough continues to be the poor adherence to chemoprophylaxis (95).

Studies assessing the impact of DHPS mutations on response to therapeutic, high-dose trimethoprim–sulfamethoxazole have been conflicting, as shown in Fig. 2. While initial case reports suggested that patients with mutant DHPS strains had increased risk of failing sulfa therapy or prophylaxis (96), subsequent studies have not supported such a conclusion. A Danish study of 152 patients with AIDS-related PCP found that the presence of DHPS mutations was an independent predictor of decreased 3-month survival, when compared to patients harboring wild-type DHPS (90). However, two more recent studies have found either no effect or a trend for lower death rate when comparing patients with DHPS mutation to wild-type (86, 94). There are several possible reasons for the discrepancy between the studies, including methodological differences in the definitions of survival endpoints or prophylaxis and treatment failures, or other confounding factors related to the difficulties in assessing

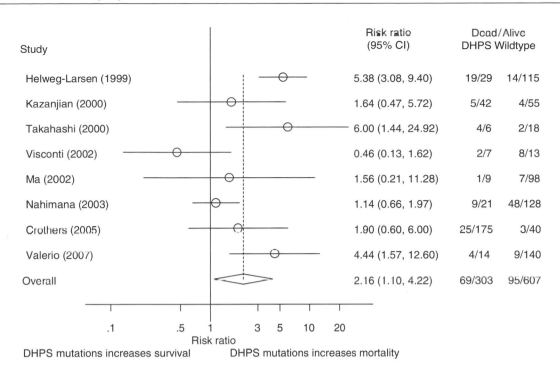

Fig. 2 Risk of deaths with DHPS mutation compared to wild-type in published observation studies. Forest plot of DHPS mutations and survival in HIV-positive patients. DerSimonian random effects analysis

clinical resistance (see **Box 1**). Moreover, even in studies reporting an association of DHPS mutations with failure of sulfa therapy, the majority of patients with mutant DHPS strains have been successfully treated with trimethoprim–sulfamethoxazole or dapsone–trimethoprim. These observations suggest that the currently identified DHPS mutations may confer only low-level sulfa resistance, allowing PCP to occur in the setting of prophylactic doses of sulfa drugs, that is overcome by the higher doses used for therapy. Given that *Pneumocystis* has already demonstrated an ability to mutate under antibiotic pressure, a major concern is that additional mutations may develop that produce high-level resistance.

8 DHFR Resistance

The diaminopyrimidines, trimethoprim and pyrimethamine, are competitive inhibitors of dihydrofolate reductase (DHFR), which catalyzes the reduction of the biologically inactive 7,8-dihyfrofolate to the active 5,6,7,8-tetrahydrofolate in the presence of NADPH and is essential for the biosynthesis of purine/pyrimidine nucleotides, thymidylate and certain amino acids. They are used in combination with sulfonamides.

Interestingly, in animal models trimethoprim does not add any potency to sulfonamides, and thus may not be contributing at all to the anti-PCP efficacy of TMP–SMX (97). The

amino acid sequence of DHFR from *P. jirovecii* differs from rat-derived *P. carinii* by 38%. Recently, Ma and Kovacs evaluated the activity of DHFR inhibitors by using a yeast assay expressing *P. jirovecii* DHFR and observed that the human *Pneumocystis*-derived DHFR had ~10-fold increase in sensitivity to trimetrexate and trimethoprim compared to rat *Pneumocystis*-derived DHFR. For the human *Pneumocystis*-derived DHFR yeast strain, trimethoprim and pyrimethamine were both weak inhibitors, with IC_{50}s in the micromolar range; trimetrexate was about 10- and 40-fold more potent than trimethoprim and pyrimethamine, respectively (Table 5). Given that trimetrexate is much more potent against PCP than trimethoprim in vitro, the combination of trimetrexate and sulfamethoxazole may be a more potent combination than trimethoprim plus sulfamethoxazole. However, there are currently no clinical data to support this.

In several bacterial and parasitic species, resistance to DHFR inhibitors has emerged as a consequence of selective pressure by DHFR inhibitors. In this way, resistance of *P. falciparum* and *P. vivax* to pyrimethamine has emerged and is now widespread (98). However, despite the widespread use of trimethoprim in combination with sulfamethoxazole for the prevention and treatment of PCP, only relatively few DHFR mutations have been identified in *Pneumocystis* DHFR (99–102). Ma et al. detected only a single synonymous DHFR mutation in specimens obtained from 32 patients, of whom 22 had previous exposure to TMP–SMX therapy or prophylaxis (99). Takahashi et al. found four mutations in *P. jirovecii*

Box 1 Limitations to the study of drug resistance in *Pneumocystis*

Compared to other pathogenic fungi, the study of drug resistance in *P. jirovecii* has been and continues to be difficult. In spite of many attempts there exists no in vitro culture system for propagation of *Pneumocystis*. The absence of a culture system precludes standard susceptibility testing and has greatly limited the understanding of many fundamental aspects of the organism and impeded investigations into the mechanisms of drug resistance. Since the knowledge of the metabolic pathways is limited, most drug development has been empiric and the currently available treatment options for PCP have been unchanged during the last 15 years. Experimental systems have mainly relied on immuno-suppressed animal, in particular the rat model of *Pneumocystis*.

Another problem is that no consistent definition of clinical failure exists. In other fungal infections, clinical resistance is classically defined as the persistence or progression despite the administration of appropriate antimicrobial treatment. However, this definition is problematic when applied to PCP. First, persistence of *Pneumocystis* organisms may happen in spite of a successful treatment response. Studies using repeat bronchoscopy during and immediately after successful treatment of PCP have shown that clearance of organisms is slow, with approximately half of patients still harboring *Pneumocystis* at the end of three weeks of treatment in spite of a successful treatment response (122–125). Although infection is eventually cleared and the viability of organisms detected at the end of treatment is uncertain, it is clear that the detection of organisms during or at the end of treatment cannot be interpreted as a proxy for resistance. Second, host inflammatory response, rather than resistance to antimicrobial drug treatment, may cause an apparent absence of response to treatment. PCP is characterized by marked pulmonary inflammation that in severe cases results in alveolar damage and respiratory failure. Although an efficient immune response is required to control the infection, it has also been demonstrated that an excessive inflammatory response, rather than direct effects of *Pneumocystis* organisms, is crucial for the pulmonary injury (126, 127). Therefore, a severe inflammatory response with respiratory distress, rather than drug resistance, may cause treatment failure. Third, treatment of PCP is associated with a high incidence of adverse effects including fever. In clinical practice, it may be difficult to know whether a slow treatment response with continuing fever is caused by the infection or by the treatment. Given the difficulties in defining clinical failure, reported failure rates for primary trimethoprim–sulfamethoxazole treatment in AIDS patients have varied considerably, ranging from 10 to 40% of cases (38, 53, 55).

In addition, the contribution of nonadherence in presumed failure of prophylaxis may be difficult to assess. The most important reason for prophylaxis failure continues to be nonadherence to prescribed prophylaxis (95, 128, 129). Clinical resistance has been investigated by genotyping of *P. jirovecii* isolates from patients who develop PCP in spite of prescribed chemoprophylaxis. However, in most studies assessment of adherence to prophylaxis has been based on chart reviews, which may fail to disclose nonadherence to a drug regimen. The likelihood of developing *P. jirovecii* resistance within a patient is likely to be higher with inadequate or interrupted dosing. Hence, in theory resistance mutations could be markers of poor adherence, rather than the direct cause of treatment failure.

Table 5 Inhibitory concentrations (50%, IC$_{50}$) of DHFR inhibitors from a yeast complementation assay

DHFR inhibitor	IC$_{50}$ (nM) Human-derived *P. jiroveci* DHFR	Rat-derived *P. carinii* DHFR
Trimethoprim	5,700	81,000
Pyrimethamine	20,500	33,200
Trimetrexate	490	4,200
Adapted (94)		

DHFR from 27 patients, of whom only three had previous exposure to TMP–SMX (100). Two of these mutations were nonsynonymous and were not associated with prior exposure to TMP–SMX. In both studies, patients were successfully treated with TMP–SMZ. Nahimana et al. documented non-synonymous substitutions in 9 of 15 patients receiving a DHFR inhibitor as part of their prophylactic regimen compared to 2 of 18 not receiving a DHFR inhibitor (101). Interestingly, 5 of 7 patients receiving pyrimethamine had nonsynonymous substitutions, suggesting a greater selective pressure of this drug. A South African study found nonsynonymous DHFR mutations in samples obtained between 2001 and 2003 in 3 of 27 patients. None had long-term exposure to TMP–SMX before developing PCP (102). Finally, Matos and coworkers from Portugal recently reported a 27% rate of DHFR mutations in 128 PCP episodes, without association to failure of PCP prophylaxis (103).

In conclusion, although several studies have reported DHFR mutations, there is so far no evidence that the widespread use of trimethoprim or pyrimethamine have caused emergence of clinical significant resistance to DHFR inhibitors.

8.1 Atovaquone

Atovaquone (2-[*trans*-4-(4′-chlorphenyl)cyclohexyl]-3-hydroxy-1,4-hydroxynaphthoquinone) is used to prevent and treat disease caused by *P. jirovecii*, *Plasmodium* spp., *Toxoplasma gondii* and *Bebesia* spp. (104). Atovaquone is structurally similar to the mitochondrial protein ubiquinone (coenzyme Q), and competitively binds to the cytochrome bc_1 complex. The bc_1 complex catalyzes electron transfer from ubiquinone to cytochrome c and thereby proton translocation across the mitochondrial membrane resulting in the generation of ATP. Binding of atovaquone to the ubiquinol oxidation pocket of the bc_1 complex and the Rieske iron–sulphur protein disrupts electron transport and leads to collapse of the mitochondrial membrane potential (105). Eventually, this presumably results in the depletion of ATP within *Pneumocystis* and leads to killing of the organism (106). Mutations of the cytochrome b gene have been identified in *Plasmodium* spp., *Toxoplasma gondii* and *Pneumocystis*. In vitro studies of Plasmodium and Toxoplasma show that these mutations confer resistance to atovaquone. Since *Pneumocystis* cannot be propagated in vitro, similar susceptibility testing cannot be done. In vitro studies of the *Saccharomyces cerevisiae* cytochrome bc_1 complex and atovaquone have demonstrated binding to the ubiquitol pocket. Introduction of mutations near the binding pocket led to decreased activity of atovaquone (105). Introduction of seven mutations observed in isolates of *Pneumocystis* from atovaquone-experienced patients into *S. cervisiae* cytochrome b increased the inhibitory concentration from 25 to >500 nM (107, 108).

Results from two clinical studies have been published. In the first, sequencing of the cytochrome b gene of *Pneumocystis* from ten patients showed sequence variations in four patients (109). Three of four patients receiving atovaquone as prophylaxis demonstrated such variations. Notably, two of them had nonsynonymous changes leading to amino acid substitutions within the ubiquitol pocket. Similar mutations in other microorganisms are associated with resistance to atovaquone. One patient, who had not received atovaquone prophylaxis, had a synonymous change that did not confer any change in amino acid sequence. In the second study, a nested case-control study, significantly more patients who previously had been exposed to atovaquone (5 of 15 patients) had mutations compared to unexposed patients (3 of 45) (110). Five different mutations near the ubiquitol pocket were described bringing the total number to seven. The high number of mutations is unusual but may be explained by a higher mutational rate and impaired proofreading of mitochondrial genes. Survival from PCP did not differ between patients with or without mutations. Overall, these findings are consistent with the development of atovaquone resistance after selective pressure is exerted.

9 Pentamidine and Clindamycine–Primaquine

Pentamidine and clindamycine–primaquine are used for prevention and treatment of PCP, but possible resistance mechanisms have yet to be discovered and reported.

10 Conclusion

In spite of the inability to culture the organisms, it is now clear that mutations involved in sulfa and atovaquone drug resistance have emerged in *P. jirovecii* as a result of selective pressure by the widespread use of PCP prophylaxis. Currently, the clinical effect of the described mutations seems modest. DHPS mutations at codon 55 and 57 are implicated in the failure of low-dose sulfaprophylaxis, but there is no firm evidence that DHPS mutations result in significant resistance to high-dose sulfa therapy. However, it is possible that if additional mutations arise, then high-level sulfa resistance could emerge and lead to diminished efficacy of TMP–SMX. This would lead to the loss of the most efficient and inexpensive therapy for PCP.

The increasing HIV epidemic and use of TMP–SMX in the third world may significantly increase the risk for the development of high-level resistance. Therefore, investigations into the mechanisms of drug resistance and identification of new molecular targets are continuing. A promising advance will be the completion of the *Pneumocystis* Genome Project, which was initiated in 1997. Complete physical maps and gene sequences are being determined for the genomes of *P. carinii* (111). These data will be crucial for further understanding of the infection and will enable identification of new polymorphic regions and drug targets and may eventually also lead to the development of a culture system.

Acknowledgements We thank Philippe Hauser for providing additional data (94).

References

1. Carini A. Formas de eschizogonia de *Trypanosoma lewisii*. Arch Soc Med Ci Sao Paulo 1910;204
2. Chagas C. Nova trypanomiazaea humanan. Über eine neue Trypanomiasis der Menchen. Mem Inst Osvaldo Cruz 1909;1:159–218
3. Delanoe P, Delanoe M. Sur les supports des kystes *Pneumocystis carinii* du poumon des rats avec *Tryponosoma lewisi*. C R Acad Sci (Paris) 1912;155:658–660
4. van der Meer MG, Brug SL. Infection à Pneumocystis chez l'homme et chez les animaux. Am Soc Belge Méd Trop 1942;22:301–309

5. Vanek J, Jirovec O. Parasitäre Pneumonie "Interstitielle" plasma-zellenpneumonie der Frühgeburten, verursacht durch *Pneumocystis carinii*. Zbl Bakt I Abt Orig 1952;158:120–127

6. Edman JC, Kovacs JA, Masur H, Santi DV, Elwood HJ, Sogin ML. Ribosomal RNA sequence shows *Pneumocystis carinii* to be a member of the fungi. Nature 1988;334(6182):519–522

7. Edman U, Edman JC, Lundgren B, Santi DV. Isolation and expression of the *Pneumocystis carinii* thymidylate synthase gene. Proc Natl Acad Sci U S A 1989;86:6503–6507

8. Stringer JR, Walzer PD. Molecular biology and epidemiology of *Pneumocystis carinii* infection in AIDS. AIDS 1996;10(6):561–571

9. Cushion MT. Pneumocystis: unraveling the cloak of obscurity. Trends Microbiol 2004;12(5):243–249

10. Haase G. *Pneumocystis carinii* Delanoe and Delanoe (1912) has been placed in the Archiascomycetales, a class of the Ascomycota. Infect Immun 1997;65(10):4365–4366

11. Stringer JR. *Pneumocystis carinii*: what is it, exactly? Clin Microbiol Rev 1996;9(4):489–498

12. Gigliotti F, Harmsen AG, Haidaris CG, Haidaris PJ. *Pneumocystis carinii* is not universally transmissible between mammalian species. Infect Immun 1993;61(7):2886–2890

13. Bauer NL, Paulsrud JR, Bartlett MS, Smith JW, Wilde CE. *Pneumocystis carinii* organisms obtained from rats, ferrets, and mice are antigenically different. Infect Immun 1993;61(4): 1315–1319

14. Cushion MT, Kaselis M, Stringer SL, Stringer JR. Genetic stability and diversity of *Pneumocystis carinii* infecting rat colonies. Infect Immun 1993;61(11):4801–4813

15. Lundgren B, Cotton R, Lundgren JD, Edman JC, Kovacs JA. Identification of *Pneumocystis carinii* chromosomes and mapping of five genes. Infect Immun 1990;58(6):1705–1710

16. Demanche C, Berthelemy M, Petit T, Polack B, Wakefield AE, Dei-Cas E et al. Phylogeny of *Pneumocystis carinii* from 18 primate species confirms host specificity and suggests coevolution. J Clin Microbiol 2001;39(6):2126–2133

17. Revised nomenclature for *Pneumocystis carinii*. The pneumocystis workshop. J Eukaryot Microbiol 1994;41(5):121S–122S

18. Frenkel JK. *Pneumocystis pneumonia*, an immunodeficiency-dependent disease (IDD): a critical historical overview. J Eukaryot Microbiol 1999;46(5):89S–92S

19. Stringer JR, Beard CB, Miller RF, Wakefield AE. A new name (*Pneumocystis jiroveci*) for pneumocystis from humans. Emerg Infect Dis 2002;8(9):891–896

20. Vanek J, Jirovec O. Parasitäre pneumonie "Interstitielle" plasma-zellenpneumonie der Frühgeburten, verursacht durch *Pneumocystis carinii*. Zbl Bakt I Abt Orig 1952;158:120–127

21. Vargas SL, Ponce CA, Hughes WT, Wakefield AE, Weitz JC, Donoso S et al. Association of primary *Pneumocystis carinii* infection and sudden infant death syndrome. Clin Infect Dis 1999;29(6):1489–1493

22. Vargas SL, Hughes WT, Santolaya ME, Ulloa AV, Ponce CA, Cabrera CE et al. Search for primary infection by *Pneumocystis carinii* in a cohort of normal, healthy infants. Clin Infect Dis 2001 15;32(6):855–861

23. Larsen HH, von Linstow ML, Lundgren B, Hogh B, Westh H, Lundgren JD. Primary pneumocystis infection in infants hospitalized with acute respiratory tract infection. Emerg Infect Dis 2007;13(1):66–72

24. Helweg-Larsen J, Lundgren B, Lundgren JD. Heterogeneity and compartmentalization of *Pneumocystis carinii* f. sp. hominis genotypes in autopsy lungs. J Clin Microbiol 2001;39(10): 3789–3792

25. Benfield TL, Prento P, Junge J, Vestbo J, Lundgren JD. Alveolar damage in AIDS-related *Pneumocystis carinii* pneumonia. Chest 1997;111(5):1193–1199

26. Lundgren B, Lipschik GY, Kovacs JA. Purification and characterization of a major human *Pneumocystis carinii* surface antigen. J Clin Invest 1991;87:163–170

27. Mei Q, Turner RE, Sorial V, Klivington D, Angus CW, Kovacs JA. Characterization of major surface glycoprotein genes of human *Pneumocystis carinii* and high-level expression of a conserved region. Infect Immun 1998;66(9):4268–4273

28. Angus CW, Tu A, Vogel P, Qin M, Kovacs JA. Expression of variants of the major surface glycoprotein of *Pneumocystis carinii*. J Exp Med 1996;183(3):1229–1234

29. Stringer JR, Keely SP. Genetics of surface antigen expression in *Pneumocystis carinii*. Infect Immun 2001;69(2):627–639

30. Matsumoto Y, Yoshida Y. Sporogony in *Pneumocystis carinii*: synaptonemal complexes and meiotic nuclear divisions observed in precysts. J Protozool 1984;31(3):420–428

31. Cushion MT, Ruffolo JJ, Walzer PD. Analysis of the developmental stages of *Pneumocystis carinii*, in vitro. Lab Invest 1988;58(3):324–331

32. Smulian AG, Sesterhenn T, Tanaka R, Cushion MT. The ste3 pheromone receptor gene of *Pneumocystis carinii* is surrounded by a cluster of signal transduction genes. Genetics 2001;157(3):991–1002

33. Kottom TJ, Limper AH. *Pneumocystis carinii* cell wall biosynthesis kinase gene CBK1 is an environmentally responsive gene that complements cell wall defects of cbk-deficient yeast. Infect Immun 2004;72(8):4628–4636

34. Ivady G, Paldy L. A new method of treating interstitial plasma cell pneumonia in premature infant with 5-valent antimony & aromatic diamidines. Monatsschr Kinderheilkd 1958;106(1):10–14

35. Post C, Fakouhi T, Dutz W, Bandarizadeh B, Kohout EE. Prophylaxis of epidemic infantile pneumocystosis with a 20:1 sulfadoxine+pyrimethamine combination. Curr Ther Res Clin Exp 1971;13(5):273–279

36. Kirby HB, Kenamore B, Guckian JC. *Pneumocystis carinii* pneumonia treated with pyrimethamine and sulfadiazine. Ann Intern Med 1971;75(4):505–509

37. Hughes WT, McNabb PC, Makres TD, Feldman S. Efficacy of trimethoprim and sulfamethoxazole in the prevention and treatment of *Pneumocystis carinii* pneumonitis. Antimicrob Agents Chemother 1974;5(3):289–293

38. Hughes WT, Feldman S, Sanyal SK. Treatment of *Pneumocystis carinii* pneumonitis with trimethoprim–sulfamethoxazole. Can Med Assoc J 1975 14;112(13 Spec No):47–50

39. Hughes WT, Kuhn S, Chaudhary S, Feldman S, Verzosa M, Aur RJ et al. Successful chemoprophylaxis for *Pneumocystis carinii* pneumonitis. N Engl J Med 1977;297(26):1419–1426

40. Selik RM, Starcher ET, Curran JW. Opportunistic diseases reported in AIDS patients: frequencies, associations, and trends. AIDS 1987;1(3):175–182

41. Yale SH, Limper AH. *Pneumocystis carinii* pneumonia in patients without acquired immunodeficiency syndrome: associated illness and prior corticosteroid therapy. Mayo Clin Proc 1996;71(1):5–13

42. Mansharamani NG, Balachandran D, Vernovsky I, Garland R, Koziel H. Peripheral blood CD4 + T-lymphocyte counts during *Pneumocystis carinii* pneumonia in immunocompromised patients without HIV infection. Chest 2000;118(3):712–720

43. Byrd JC, Hargis JB, Kester KE, Hospenthal DR, Knutson SW, Diehl LF. Opportunistic pulmonary infections with fludarabine in previously treated patients with low-grade lymphoid malignancies: a role for *Pneumocystis carinii* pneumonia prophylaxis. Am J Hematol 1995;49:135–142

44. Dutz W, Post C, Jennings-Khodadad E, Fakouhi T, Kohout E, Bandarizadeh B. Therapy and prophylaxis of *Pneumocystis carinii* pneumonia. Natl Cancer Inst Monogr 1976;43:179–185

45. Fischl MA, Dickinson GM, La Voie L. Safety and efficacy of sulfamethoxazole and trimethoprim chemoprophylaxis for *Pneumocystis carinii* pneumonia in AIDS. JAMA 1988;259:1185–1189

46. Bozzette SA, Finkelstein DM, Spector SA, Frame P, Powderly WG, He W et al. A randomised trial of three antipneumocystis agents in patients with advanced human immunodeficiency virus infection. N Engl J Med 1995;332:693–699

47. Schneider MM, Nielsen TL, Nelsing S, Hoepelman AI, Eeftinck S, van der Graaf Y et al. Efficacy and toxicity of two doses of trimethoprim–sulfamethoxazole as primary prophylaxis against *Pneumocystis carinii* pneumonia in patients with human immunodeficiency virus. Dutch AIDS Treatment Group. J Infect Dis 1995;171(6):1632–1636

48. Leoung GS, Stanford JF, Giordano MF, Stein A, Torres RA, Giffen CA et al. Trimethoprim–sulfamethoxazole (TMP–SMZ) dose escalation versus direct rechallenge for *Pneumocystis Carinii* pneumonia prophylaxis in human immunodeficiency virus-infected patients with previous adverse reaction to TMP–SMZ. J Infect Dis 2001;184(8):992–997

49. Para MF, Finkelstein D, Becker S, Dohn M, Walawander A, Black JR. Reduced toxicity with gradual initiation of trimethoprim–sulfamethoxazole as primary prophylaxis for *Pneumocystis carinii* pneumonia: AIDS Clinical Trials Group 268. J Acquir Immune Defic Syndr 2000;24(4):337–343

50. Brenner M, Ognibene FP, Lack EE, Simmons JT, Suffredini AF, Lane HC et al. Prognostic factors and life expectancy of patients with acquired immunodeficiency syndrome and *Pneumocystis carinii* pneumonia. Am Rev Respir Dis 1987;136(5):1199–1206

51. Kales CP, Murren JR, Torres RA, Crocco JA. Early predictors of in-hospital mortality for *Pneumocystis carinii* pneumonia in the acquired immunodeficiency syndrome. Arch Intern Med 1987;147(8):1413–1417

52. Murray JF, Felton CP, Garay SM, Gottlieb MS, Hopewell PC, Stover DE et al. Pulmonary complications of the acquired immunodeficiency syndrome. Report of a National Heart, Lung, and Blood Institute workshop. N Engl J Med 1984;310(25):1682–1688

53. Bauer T, Ewig S, Hasper E, Rockstroh JK, Luderitz B. Predicting in-hospital outcome in HIV-associated *Pneumocystis carinii* pneumonia. Infection 1995;23(5):272–277

54. Ewig S, Bauer T, Schneider C, Pickenhain A, Pizzulli L, Loos U et al. Clinical characteristics and outcome of *Pneumocystis carinii* pneumonia in HIV-infected and otherwise immunosuppressed patients. Eur Respir J 1995;8(9):1548–1553

55. Bennett CL, Horner RD, Weinstein RA, Kessler HA, Dickson GM, Pitrak DL et al. Empirically treated *Pneumocystis carinii* pneumonia in Los Angeles, Chicago, and Miami: 1987–1990. J Infect Dis 1995;172:312–315

56. Lundgren JD, Barton SE, Katlama C, Ledergerber B, Gonzalez-Lahoz J, Pinching AJ et al. Changes in survival over time after a first episode of *Pneumocystis carinii* pneumonia for European patients with acquired immunodeficiency syndrome. Multicentre Study Group on AIDS in Europe. Arch Intern Med 1995;155(8):822–828

57. Cohn SE, Klein JD, Weinstein RA, Shapiro MF, Dehovitz JD, Kessler HA et al. Geographic variation in the management and outcome of patients with AIDS-related *Pneumocystis carinii* pneumonia. J Acquir Immune Defic Syndr Hum Retrovirol 1996;13:408–415

58. Bang D, Emborg J, Elkjaer J, Lundgren JD, Benfield TL. Independent risk of mechanical ventilation for AIDS-related *Pneumocystis carinii* pneumonia associated with bronchoalveolar lavage neutrophilia. Respir Med 2001;95(8):661–665

59. Siegel SE, Wolff LJ, Baehner RL, Hammond D. Treatment of *Pneumocystis carinii* pneumonitis. A comparative trial of sulfamethoxazole–trimethoprim v pentamidine in pediatric patients with cancer: report from the Children's Cancer Study Group. Am J Dis Child 1984;138(11):1051–1054

60. Wharton JM, Coleman DL, Wofsy CB, Luce JM, Blumenfeld W, Hadley WK et al. Trimethoprim–sulfamethoxazole or pentamidine for *Pneumocystis carinii* pneumonia in the acquired immunodeficiency syndrome. A prospective randomized trial. Ann Intern Med 1986;105(1):37–44

61. Sattler FR, Cowan R, Nielsen DM, Ruskin J. Trimethoprim–sulfamethoxazole compared with pentamidine for treatment of *Pneumocystis carinii* pneumonia in the acquired immunodeficiency syndrome: a prospective, noncrossover study. Ann Intern Med 1988;109:280–287

62. Klein NC, Duncanson FP, Lenox TH, Forszpaniak C, Sherer CB, Quentzel H et al. Trimethoprim–sulfamethoxazole versus pentamidine for *Pneumocystis carinii* pneumonia in AIDS patients: results of a large prospective randomized treatment trial. AIDS 1992;6(3):301–305

63. Hughes WT, Lafon SW, Scott JD, Masur H. Adverse events associated with trimethoprim–sulfamethoxazole and atovaquone during the treatment of AIDS-related *Pneumocystis carinii* pneumonia. J Infect Dis 1995;171:1295–1301

64. Safrin S, Finkelstein DM, Feinberg J, Frame P, Simpson G, Wu A et al. Comparison of three regimens for treatment of mild to moderate *Pneumocystis carinii* pneumonia in patients with AIDS: a double-blind, randomized trial of oral trimethoprim–sulfamethoxazole, dapsone-trimethoprim, and clindamycin–primaquine. Ann Intern Med 1996;124:792–802

65. Toma E, Thorne A, Singer J, Raboud J, Lemieux C, Trottier S et al. Clindamycin with primaquine vs. trimethoprim–sulfamethoxazole therapy for mild and moderately severe *Pneumocystis carinii* pneumonia in patients with AIDS: a multicenter, double-blind, randomized trial (CTN 004). CTN-PCP Study Group. Clin Infect Dis 1998;27(3):524–530

66. Hughes W, Leoung G, Kramer F, Bozzette SA, Safrin S, Frame P et al. Comparison of atovaquone (566C80) with trimethoprim–sulfamethoxazole to treat *Pneumocystis carinii* pneumonia in patients with AIDS. N Engl J Med 1993 27;328(21):1521–1527

67. Medina I, Mills J, Leoung G, Hopewell PC, Lee B, Modin G et al. Oral therapy for *Pneumocystis carinii* pneumonia in the acquired immunodeficiency syndrome. A controlled trial of trimethoprim–sulfamethoxazole versus trimethoprim–dapsone. N Engl J Med 1990;323(12):776–782

68. Rosenberg DM, McCarthy W, Slavinsky J, Chan CK, Montaner J, Braun J et al. Atovaquone suspension for treatment of *Pneumocystis carinii* pneumonia in HIV-infected patients. AIDS 2001;15(2):211–214

69. Montaner JS, Lawson LM, Levitt N, Belzberg A, Schechter MT, Ruedy J. Corticosteroids prevent early deterioration in patients with moderately severe *Pneumocystis carinii* pneumonia and the acquired immunodeficiency syndrome (AIDS) [see comments]. Ann Intern Med 1990;113(1):14–20

70. Bozzette SA, Sattler FR, Chiu J, Wu AW, Gluckstein D, Kemper C et al. A controlled trial of early adjunctive treatment with corticosteroids for *Pneumocystis carinii* pneumonia in the acquired immunodeficiency syndrome. N Engl J Med 1990;323:1451–1457

71. Gagnon S, Boota AM, Fischl MA, Baier H, Kirksey OW, La VL. Corticosteroids as adjunctive therapy for severe *Pneumocystis carinii* pneumonia in the acquired immunodeficiency syndrome. A double-blind, placebo-controlled trial. N Engl J Med 1990;323(21):1444–1450

72. Nielsen TL, Eeftinck Schattenkerk JKM, Jensen BN, Lundgren JD, Gerstoft J, Van Steenwijk RP et al. Adjunctive corticosteroid therapy for *Pneumocystis carinii* pneumonia in AIDS: A randomized European multicenter open label study. J Acquir Immune Defic Syndr 1992;5:726–731

73. Skold O. Sulfonamide resistance: mechanisms and trends. Drug Resist Updat 2000;3(3):155–160

74. Feikin DR, Dowell SF, Nwanyanwu OC, Klugman KP, Kazembe PN, Barat LM et al. Increased carriage of trimethoprim/sulfamethoxazole-resistant *Streptococcus pneumoniae* in Malawian children after treatment for malaria with sulfadoxine/pyrimethamine. J Infect Dis 2000;181(4):1501–1505

75. Martin JN, Rose DA, Hadley WK, Perdreau-Remington F, Lam PK, Gerberding JL. Emergence of trimethoprim–sulfamethoxazole resistance in the AIDS era. J Infect Dis 1999;180(6): 1809–1818

76. Wininger DA, Fass RJ. Impact of trimethoprim–sulfamethoxazole prophylaxis on etiology and susceptibilities of pathogens causing human immunodeficiency virus-associated bacteremia. Antimicrob Agents Chemother 2002;46(2):594–597

77. Swedberg G, Fermer C, Skold O. Point mutations in the dihydropteroate synthase gene causing sulfonamide resistance. Adv Exp Med Biol 1993;338:555–558

78. Fermer C, Kristiansen BE, Skold O, Swedberg G. Sulfonamide resistance in *Neisseria meningitidis* as defined by site-directed mutagenesis could have its origin in other species. J Bacteriol 1995;177(16):4669–4675

79. Williams DL, Spring L, Harris E, Roche P, Gillis TP. Dihydropteroate synthase of *Mycobacterium leprae* and dapsone resistance. Antimicrob Agents Chemother 2000;44(6):1530–1537

80. Volpe F, Ballantine SP, Delves CJ. The multifunctional folic acid synthesis fas gene of *Pneumocystis carinii* encodes dihydroneopterin aldolase, hydroxymethyldihydropterin pyrophosphokinase and dihydropteroate synthase. Eur J Biochem 1993;216(2):449–458

81. Lane BR, Ast JC, Hossler PA, Mindell DP, Bartlett MS, Smith JW et al. Dihydropteroate synthase polymorphisms in *Pneumocystis carinii*. J Infect Dis 1997;175:482–485

82. Achari A, Somers DO, Champness JN, Bryant PK, Rosemond J, Stammers DK. Crystal structure of the anti-bacterial sulfonamide drug target dihydropteroate synthase. Nat Struct Biol 1997;4(6):490–497

83. Armstrong W, Meshnick S, Kazanjian P. *Pneumocystis carinii* mutations associated with sulfa and sulfone prophylaxis failures in immunocompromised patients. Microbes Infect 2000;2(1):61–67

84. Meneau I, Sanglard D, Bille J, Hauser PM. Pneumocystis jiroveci dihydropteroate synthase polymorphisms confer resistance to sulfadoxine and sulfanilamide in *Saccharomyces cerevisiae*. Antimicrob Agents Chemother 2004;48(7):2610–2616

85. Iliades P, Meshnick SR, Macreadie IG. Dihydropteroate synthase mutations in *Pneumocystis jiroveci* can affect sulfamethoxazole resistance in a *Saccharomyces cerevisiae* model. Antimicrob Agents Chemother 2004;48(7):2617–2623

86. Navin TR, Beard CB, Huang L, del Rio C, Lee S, Pieniazek NJ et al. Effect of mutations in *Pneumocystis carinii* dihydropteroate synthase gene on outcome of *P. carinii* pneumonia in patients with HIV-1: a prospective study. Lancet 2001;358(9281):545–549

87. Ma L, Kovacs JA, Cargnel A, Valerio A, Fantoni G, Atzori C. Mutations in the dihydropteroate synthase gene of human-derived *Pneumocystis carinii* isolates from Italy are infrequent but correlate with prior sulfa prophylaxis. J Infect Dis 2002;185(10):1530–1532

88. Kazanjian P, Locke AB, Hossler PA, Lane BR, Bartlett MS, Smith JW et al. *Pneumocystis carinii* mutations associated with sulfa and sulfone prophylaxis failures in AIDS patients. AIDS 1998;12(8):873–878

89. Kazanjian PH, Fisk D, Armstrong W, Shulin Q, Liwei H, Ke Z et al. Increase in prevalence of *Pneumocystis carinii* mutations in patients with AIDS and *P. carinii* pneumonia, in the United States and China. J Infect Dis 2004;189(9):1684–1687

90. Helweg-Larsen J, Benfield TL, Eugen-Olsen J, Lundgren JD, Lundgren B. Effects of mutations in *Pneumocystis carinii* dihydropteroate synthase gene on outcome of AIDS-associated *P. carinii* pneumonia. Lancet 1999;354(9187):1347–1351

91. Ma L, Kovacs JA. Genetic analysis of multiple loci suggests that mutations in the *Pneumocystis carinii* f. sp. hominis dihydropteroate synthase gene arose independently in multiple strains. Antimicrob Agents Chemother 2001;45(11):3213–3215

92. Nahimana A, Rabodonirina M, Helweg-Larsen J, Meneau I, Francioli P, Bille J et al. Sulfa resistance and dihydropteroate synthase mutants in recurrent *Pneumocystis carinii* pneumonia. Emerg Infect Dis 2003;9(7):864–867

93. Demanche C, Guillot J, Berthelemy M, Petitt T, Roux P, Wakefield AE. Absence of mutations associated with sulfa resistance in *Pneumocystis carinii* dihydropteroate synthase gene from non-human primates. Med Mycol 2002;40(3):315–318

94. Nahimana A, Rabodonirina M, Zanetti G, Meneau I, Francioli P, Bille J et al. Association between a specific *Pneumocystis jiroveci* dihydropteroate synthase mutation and failure of pyrimethamine/sulfadoxine prophylaxis in human immunodeficiency virus-positive and -negative patients. J Infect Dis 2003;188(7): 1017–1023

95. Lundberg BE, Davidson AJ, Burman WJ. Epidemiology of *Pneumocystis carinii* pneumonia in an era of effective prophylaxis: the relative contribution of non-adherence and drug failure. AIDS 2000;14(16):2559–2566

96. Mei Q, Gurunathan S, Masur H, Kovacs JA. Failure of co-trimoxazole in *Pneumocystis carinii* infection and mutations in dihydropteroate synthase gene. Lancet 1998;351(9116):1631–1632

97. Walzer PD, Kim CK, Foy JM, Linke MJ, Cushion MT. Inhibitors of folic acid synthesis in the treatment of experimental *Pneumocystis carinii* pneumonia. Antimicrob Agents Chemother 1988;32(1):96–103

98. Roper C, Pearce R, Nair S, Sharp B, Nosten F, Anderson T. Intercontinental spread of pyrimethamine-resistant malaria. Science 2004 20;305(5687):1124

99. Ma L, Borio L, Masur H, Kovacs JA. *Pneumocystis carinii* dihydropteroate synthase but not dihydrofolate reductase gene mutations correlate with prior trimethoprim–sulfamethoxazole or dapsone use. J Infect Dis 1999;180(6):1969–1978

100. Takahashi T, Endo T, Nakamura T, Sakashitat H, Kimurat K, Ohnishit K et al. Dihydrofolate reductase gene polymorphisms in *Pneumocystis carinii* f. sp. hominis in Japan. J Med Microbiol 2002;51(6):510–515

101. Nahimana A, Rabodonirina M, Francioli P, Bille J, Hauser PM. *Pneumocystis jirovecii* dihydrofolate reductase polymorphisms associated with failure of prophylaxis. J Eukaryot Microbiol 2003;50 Suppl:656–657

102. Robberts FJ, Chalkley LJ, Weyer K, Goussard P, Liebowitz LD. Dihydropteroate synthase and novel dihydrofolate reductase gene mutations in strains of *Pneumocystis jirovecii* from South Africa. J Clin Microbiol 2005;43(3):1443–1444

103. Costa MC, Esteves F, Antunes F, Matos O. Genetic characterization of the dihydrofolate reductase gene of *Pneumocystis jirovecii* isolates from Portugal. J Antimicrob Chemother 2006;58(6):1246–1249

104. Baggish AL, Hill DR. Antiparasitic agent atovaquone. Antimicrob Agents Chemother 2002;46(5):1163–1173

105. Kessl JJ, Lange BB, Merbitz-Zahradnik T, Zwicker K, Hill P, Meunier B et al. Molecular basis for atovaquone binding to the cytochrome bc1 complex. J Biol Chem 2003;278(33):31312–31318

106. Cushion MT, Collins M, Hazra B, Kaneshiro ES. Effects of atovaquone and diospyrin-based drugs on the cellular ATP of *Pneumocystis carinii* f. sp. carinii. Antimicrob Agents Chemother 2000;44(3):713–719

107. Hill P, Kessl J, Fisher N, Meshnick S, Trumpower BL, Meunier B. Recapitulation in *Saccharomyces cerevisiae* of cytochrome b mutations conferring resistance to atovaquone in *Pneumocystis jiroveci*. Antimicrob Agents Chemother 2003;47(9):2725–2731

108. Kessl JJ, Hill P, Lange BB, Meshnick SR, Meunier B, Trumpower BL. Molecular basis for atovaquone resistance in *Pneumocystis jirovecii* modeled in the cytochrome bc(1) complex of *Saccharomyces cerevisiae*. J Biol Chem 2004;279(4): 2817–2824

109. Walker DJ, Wakefield AE, Dohn MN, Miller RF, Baughman RP, Hossler PA et al. Sequence polymorphisms in the *Pneumocystis carinii* cytochrome b gene and their association with atovaquone prophylaxis failure. J Infect Dis 1998;178(6):1767–1775

110. Kazanjian P, Armstrong W, Hossler PA, Huang L, Beard CB, Carter J et al. *Pneumocystis carinii* cytochrome b mutations are associated with atovaquone exposure in patients with AIDS. J Infect Dis 2001;183(5):819–822

111. Pneumocystis Genome Project. http://pneumocystis uc edu/html/genome_pro html 2003; Available from: URL: http://pgp.cchmc.org/

112. Santos LD, Lacube P, Latouche S, Kac G, Mayaud C, Marteau M et al. Contribution of dihydropteroate synthase gene typing for *Pneumocystis carinii* f. sp. hominis epidemiology. J Eukaryot Microbiol 1999;46(5):133S–4S

113. Huang L, Beard CB, Creasman J, Levy D, Duchin JS, Lee S et al. Sulfa or sulfone prophylaxis and geographic region predict mutations in the *Pneumocystis carinii* dihydropteroate synthase gene. J Infect Dis 2000;182(4):1192–1198

114. Beard CB, Carter JL, Keely SP, Huang L, Pieniazek NJ, Moura IN et al. Genetic variation in *Pneumocystis carinii* isolates from different geographic regions: implications for transmission. Emerg Infect Dis 2000;6(3):265–272

115. Takahashi T, Hosoya N, Endo T, Nakamura T, Sakashita H, Kimura K et al. Relationship between mutations in dihydropteroate synthase of *Pneumocystis carinii* f. sp. Hominis isolates in Japan and resistance to sulfonamide therapy. J Clin Microbiol 2000;38(9):3161–3164

116. Costa MC, Helweg-Larsen J, Lundgren B, Antunes F, Matos O. Mutations in the dihydropteroate synthase gene of *Pneumocystis jiroveci* isolates from Portuguese patients with Pneumocystis pneumonia. Int J Antimicrob Agents 2003;22(5):516–520

117. Visconti E, Ortona E, Mencarini P, Margutti P, Marinaci S, Zolfo M et al. Mutations in dihydropteroate synthase gene of *Pneumocystis carinii* in HIV patients with *Pneumocystis carinii* pneumonia. Int J Antimicrob Agents 2001;18(6):547–551

118. Zingale A, Carrera P, Lazzarin A, Scarpellini P. Detection of *Pneumocystis carinii* and characterization of mutations associated with sulfa resistance in bronchoalveolar lavage samples from human immunodeficiency virus-infected subjects. J Clin Microbiol 2003;41(6):2709–2712

119. Totet A, Duwat H, Magois E, Jounieaux V, Roux P, Raccurt C et al. Similar genotypes of *Pneumocystis jirovecii* in different forms of *Pneumocystis* infection. Microbiology 2004;150(Pt 5):1173–1178

120. Crothers K, Beard CB, Turner J, Groner G, Fox M, Morris A et al. Severity and outcome of HIV-associated Pneumocystis pneumonia containing *Pneumocystis jirovecii* dihydropteroate synthase gene mutations. AIDS 2005;19(8):801–805

121. Valerio A, Tronconi E, Mazza F, Fantoni G, Atzori C, Tartarone F et al. Genotyping of Pneumocystis jiroveci pneumonia in Italian AIDS patients. Clinical outcome is influenced by dihydropteroate synthase and not by internal transcribed spacer genotype. J Acquir Immune Defic Syndr 2007;45(5):521–528

122. Shelhamer JH, Ognibene FP, Macher AM, Tuazon C, Steiss R, Longo D et al. Persistence of *Pneumocystis carinii* in lung tissue of acquired immunodeficiency syndrome patients treated for Pneumocystis pneumonia. Am Rev Respir Dis 1984;130(6):1161–1165

123. O'Donnell WJ, Pieciak W, Chertow GM, Sanabria J, Lahive KC. Clearance of *Pneumocystis carinii* cysts in acute *P. carinii* pneumonia: assessment by serial sputum induction. Chest 1998;114(5):1264–1268

124. Roger PM, Vandenbos F, Pugliese P, DeSalvador F, Durant J, LeFichoux Y et al. Persistence of *Pneumocystis carinii* after effective treatment of *P. carinii* pneumonia is not related to relapse or survival among patients infected with human immunodeficiency virus. Clin Infect Dis 1998;26(2):509–510

125. Epstein LJ, Meyer RD, Antonson S, Strigle SM, Mohsenifar Z. Persistence of *Pneumocystis carinii* in patients with AIDS receiving chemoprophylaxis. Am J Respir Crit Care Med 1994;150:1456–1459

126. Benfield TL. Clinical and experimental studies on inflammatory mediators during AIDS associated *Pneumocystis carinii* pneumonia. Dan Med Bull 2003;50(2):161–176

127. Thomas CF, Jr, Limper AH. Current insights into the biology and pathogenesis of Pneumocystis pneumonia. Nat Rev Microbiol 2007;5(4):298–308

128. Schneider MME, Hoepelman AIM, Schattenkerk JKME, Nielsen TL, Graaf Y, Frissen JPHJ et al. A controlled trial of aerosolized pentamidine or trimethoprim–sulfamethoxazole as primary prophylaxis against *Pneumocystis carinii* pneumonia in patients with human immunodeficiency virus infection. N Engl J Med 1992;327:1836–1841

129. Klein MB, Lalonde RG. The continued occurrence of primary *Pneumocystis carinii* pneumonia despite the availability of prophylaxis. Clin Infect Dis 1997;24(3):522–523

Chapter 69
Antiviral Resistance in Influenza Viruses: Clinical and Epidemiological Aspects

Frederick G. Hayden[1]

1 Introduction

Two classes of anti-viral agents, the M2 ion channel inhibitors (amantadine, rimantadine) and neuraminidase (NA) inhibitors (oseltamivir, zanamivir) are available for treatment and prevention of influenza in most countries of the world. The principle concerns about emergence of antiviral resistance in influenza viruses are loss of drug efficacy, transmission of resistant variants, and possible increased virulence or transmissibility of resistant variants (1). Because seasonal influenza is usually an acute, self-limited illness in which viral clearance occurs rapidly due to innate and adaptive host immune responses, the emergence of drug-resistant variants would be anticipated to have modest effects on clinical recovery, except perhaps in immunocompromised or immunologically naïve hosts, such as young infants or during the appearance of a novel strain. In contrast to the limited impact of resistance emergence in the treated immunocompetent individual, the epidemiologic impact of resistance emergence and transmission could be considerable, including loss of both prophylactic and therapeutic activity for a particular drug, at the household, community, or perhaps global level. Influenza epidemiology in temperate climates is expected to provide some protection against widespread circulation of resistant variants, as viruses do not persist between epidemics but rather are re-introduced each season and new variants appear often (2, 3).

However, the emergence and circulation of M2 ion channel inhibitor-resistant variants has been an important concern given their transmission fitness, detection in some animal

influenza viruses and many human isolates of avian A(H5N1) virus, their frequent emergence during therapy in humans, and the increasing use of amantadine in regions of the globe like China that may be the sites for emergence of new drift variants or possibly pandemic strains. Indeed, the recent observations of global spread of M2 inhibitor-resistant A(H3N2) viruses, initially recognized in Asia (4, 5), illustrates the public health consequences of antiviral resistance in influenza viruses and has led to changes in policies for use of this antiviral class of drugs in many countries. The more recent and unexpectedly rapid dissemination of oseltamivir-resistant A(H1N1) viruses highlights the unpredictability of antiviral resistance emergence and spread (6, 6a). Antiviral resistance and its consequences are key factors that need to be considered by health authorities and governments when making decisions regarding the stockpiling of antivirals for response to pandemics or other influenza threats (7), although concerns about antiviral resistance, particularly to NA inhibitors, should not dissuade countries from developing adequate antiviral inventories for pandemic response (1, 8).

Factors that influence the clinical and epidemiologic importance of drug-resistant influenza viruses include the magnitude of phenotypic resistance, its frequency and rapidity of emergence, its stability and ability of resistant variants to compete with wild-type viruses in the absence of selective drug pressure, and the effects of resistance mutations on viral replication competence, pathogenicity, and transmissibility *in vivo*. In general, data to date indicate that mutations conferring either NA or M2 inhibitor resistance are not associated with worsened viral virulence, atypical influenza, or enhanced transmissibility in humans. In contrast to M2 inhibitor resistance, most but not all NA mutations conferring resistance in clinical isolates have been associated with reduced infectivity, replication, and pathogenicity in animal models of influenza. However, changes in other influenza genes segments, such as antigenic change in the hemagglutinin (HA), or perhaps compensatory mutations in the target genes may enhance viral fitness and be associated with widespread transmission

F.G. Hayden (✉)
Department of Medicine, University of Virginia School of Medicine, Charlottesville, VA, USA,
fgh@virginia.edu

[1]The author was a staff member of the World Health Organization during the writing of this chapter. The author alone is responsible for the views expressed in this publication and they do not necessarily represent the decisions or the stated policy of the World Health Organization.

D.L. Mayers (ed.), *Antimicrobial Drug Resistance*,
DOI 10.1007/978-1-60327-595-8_69, © Humana Press, a part of Springer Science+Business Media, LLC 2009

and illness. The following sections/chapters review clinical and epidemiological data on antiviral resistance for the two classes of available anti-influenza agents. Information from experimental animal models of influenza is incorporated to supplement the limited data derived from clinical studies.

2 M2 Ion Channel Inhibitors (Amantadine, Rimantadine)

Amantadine was initially approved in the United States in 1966 for influenza A(H2N2) infections and then for all influenza A viruses in 1976; rimantadine was used in the former Soviet Union for decades and later approved for use in the United States in 1993. Rapid selection of drug-resistant variants was demonstrated over 30 years ago in early laboratory studies employing in vitro and in vivo passage in the presence of amantadine (9, 10), and the study of resistance was used to determine the mechanism of antiviral action of M2 inhibitors (reviewed in (11)). For human influenza viruses, resistance was shown to be due to point mutations in the M gene and corresponding single amino acid substitutions in the transmembrane region of the M2 protein (positions 26, 27, 30, 31, 34) that resulted in marked loss of phenotypic susceptibility in vitro. The clinical implications of resistance became apparent in studies during the 1980s of treated children (12), in whom a high frequency of resistance emergence was documented, and subsequently of households and nursing homes, where transmission of drug-resistant variants was implicated in failures of drug prophylaxis (13–15). Phenotypic resistance to M2 inhibitors is high-level and generally leads to loss of antiviral activity in vivo.

2.1 Detection of Resistance

Detection of M2 inhibitor resistance has usually relied on virus isolation from respiratory samples and susceptibility testing of virus in cell culture. Several assays have been described including plaque reduction, yield reduction, and ELISA (16). Following phenotypic analysis, genotypic M2 inhibitor resistance has been confirmed by nucleotide sequence analysis of the M2 gene and detection of the characteristic mutations. Genotypic detection can be accomplished quickly by the use of PCR-restriction length polymorphism (RFLP) analysis of the RNA extracted from respiratory samples using commercially available endonucleases for discrimination of point mutations in the M2 gene (17). Greater sensitivity in detecting resistant clones has been described with reverse transcription-polymerase chain reaction amplification of the RNA followed by sequencing of multiple clones (18). Recently the rapid pyro-

sequencing technique has been shown to be a reliable, high-throughput method for detecting genotypic resistance in large numbers of community isolates (4, 5). Following treatment, approximately 70–90% of amino acid substitutions in resistant viruses occur at position 31 and about 10% each are found at positions 27 and 30 (17). The distribution of resistance mutations depends on influenza A subtype, such that Ser31Asn predominates in A(H3N2) subtype whereas Val27Ala occurs with increased frequency in A(H1N1) subtype viruses (19). M2 proteins show considerable evolution in human and swine viruses, and the H3 and H1 subtype viruses have phylogenetically different M2 proteins (20). This may influence the mutations that are more advantageous for conferring M2 inhibitor resistance. Of note, the Ser31Asn mutation has been responsible for the resistant A(H3N2) and A(H1N1) variants that have recently circulated globally (4, 5).

2.2 Susceptibility of Field Isolates

Pandemic strains, including reassortants bearing the M gene of the 1918 virus (21), and earlier prototype epidemic viruses (13) have been susceptible to amantadine and rimantadine. Until recently, studies of community isolates of A(H3N2) viruses generally revealed low levels of primary resistance, approximately 1–3% (Table 1). A survey of 2,017 isolates from 43 countries during 1991–1995 detected resistance in only 0.8%; of the 16 persons with resistant isolates, two were receiving drug and four others were in potential contact with drug recipients (22). Of note, 4.5% of 198 isolates from Australia, collected between 1989 and 1995, showed resistance for unexplained reasons. Another survey of 1,813 field isolates collected 1968–1999 in the United Kingdom found resistance in 1.5% (23). Amantadine was approved of for use in Japan in 1998, and a Japanese study found resistant isolates in 3.4% of 179 children before starting antiviral treatment in the 1999–2000 season, although not in the preceding or succeeding seasons (24). A survey of 1,096 community isolates collected over four seasons in Canada from 1998 to 2002 found that 0.7% showed resistance mutations (Li, unpublished observations). During the same period, 20% of 138 viruses isolated during nursing home outbreaks, in which amantadine was often used for control, were resistant. Resistant isolates have also been reported without known drug exposure in nursing home residents (25).

However, the incidence of resistance in field isolates of A(H3N2) viruses increased dramatically in 2003 in isolates from China, perhaps related to increased use of over-the-counter amantadine after the emergence of severe acute respiratory syndrome (SARS) (4, 8). During the 2004–2005 influenza season, approximately 70% of the A(H3N2) isolates from China and Hong Kong and nearly 15% of those from

Table 1 Representative studies of M2 inhibitor susceptibility of influenza A field isolates from adults and children

	Site	Period	Method	Number tested by subtype	No. (%) resistant
Belshe et al. (13)	US	1978–1988	EIA, S	65 H1N1	0
				181 H3N2	5 (2.0%)[a]
Valette et al. (162)	France	1988–1990	EIA	28 H1N1	0
				77 H3N2	0
Ziegler et al. (22)	43 countries	1991–1995	EIA, S, PCR-RFLP	2,017	16 (0.8%)[b]
Dawson (23)	UK	1968–1999	EIA, Plaque	1,813	28 (1.5%)
Suzuki et al. (24)	Japan	1993–1998	Not stated	55	0
		1999–2000	Not stated	179	6 (3.4%)
Li 2003 (personal communication)	Canada	1998–2002	PCR-RFLP	1,096	8 (0.7%)
Shih et al. (163)	Taiwan	1996–1998	Plaque, S	84	1(1.2%)
Bright et al. (4)	Global	1994–2005	S	6,525 H3N2	392 (6.0%)
		1994–2002			0.3–1.8%
		2003–2005			12.3–13.3%[c]
		1998–2004		589 H1N1	2 (0.3%)
Bright et al. (5)	US	2005–2006	S	205 H3N2	193 (92.3%)
				8 H1N1	2 (25%)
Saito et al. (164)	Japan	2005–2006	S	354 H3N2	231 (65.3%)
Saito et al. (165)				61 H1N1	0
		2006–2007	S	632 H3N2	566 (89.6%)
				120 H1N1	77 (64.2%)
Barr et al. (27)	Australia, New Zealand, Asia, South Africa	2005	S	102 H3N2	43 (42%)
				37 H1N1	0
Deyde (28, 29)	Asia	2006–2007	S	235 H3N2	156 (66.4%)
				118 H1N1	87 (73.7%)
	Europe			71 H3N2	25 (35.2%)
				45 H1N1	27 (60.0%)
	North America			481 H3N2	327 (68.0%)
				519 H1N1	15 (2.9%)
	South America			77 H3N2	73 (94.8%)
				29 H1N1	0 (0)

Abbreviations: S = M2 gene sequence analysis; PCR–RFLP = polymerase chain reaction–restriction length polymorphism; *EIA* enzyme immunoassay

[a] All resistant viruses from family members receiving rimantadine

[b] Over 80% of tested isolates were H3N2 subtype and all resistant ones were of this subtype. Separate analysis found that 9 (4.5%) of 198 strains from Australia, 1989–1995, were resistant

[c] In 2004–2005 the frequencies of resistance in H3N2 viruses were 73.8% in China, 69.6% in Hong Kong, 22.7% in Taiwan, 15.1% in South Korea, 4.3% in Japan, 30.0% in Canada, 19.2% in Mexico, 14.5% in USA, and 4.7% in Europe

the United States and Europe showed resistance due to a Ser31Asn mutation, and this frequency increased to over 90% in the United States during the 2005–2006 season (5). Resistant A(H3N2) viruses have spread widely in countries without substantial M2 inhibitor use (Table 1). This unprecedented global spread of A(H3N2) viruses with a specific mutation (Ser31Asn) has occurred despite the absence of a sustained selective drug pressure, possibly because the resistant M gene was incorporated into efficiently spreading HA antigenic variants, so-called "hitch-hiking" of a resistance marker (26). Initial phylogenetic analyses of the M2 and other viral genes, particularly HA, suggested a common lineage of these viruses (26, 27), but testing of greater numbers of resistant strains over several seasons has found no signature amino acid changes in the HA (28, 29). This experience clearly indicates that this

resistance mutation does not reduce transmissibility. Recently an increased frequency of resistant A(H1N1) viruses harboring this mutation, particularly in Asia, has also been recognized (Table 1). The public health consequence has been to make this class of antiviral drugs unreliable for prophylaxis or treatment currently. It remains to be seen to what extent the emergence of new antigenic variants will lead to the returned circulation of susceptible viruses, but almost all A(H3N2) viruses isolated in late 2008 continued to show adamantane resistance.

2.2.1 Swine and Avian Viruses

In addition, a characteristic feature of A(H1N1), A(H1N2), and A(H3N2) swine viruses circulating in Europe since 1987 has been the presence of a Ser31Asn mutation, as well as Val27Ala in some isolates, that confers resistance to M2 inhibitors (30, 31); such isolates have caused occasional human infections and are now present in Asia (32). Some swine isolates from the 1930s were found to harbor the same resistance mutation (Bean, unpublished observations). The introduction of human and avian genes and genetic reassortment among co-circulating subtypes has been found in swine influenza isolates in different parts of the world (31, 31a). The postulated role of the swine as intermediate hosts in the emergence of some novel human viruses highlight the potential risk of a new human epidemic or pandemic strains harboring primary M2 inhibitor resistance.

In addition, direct inter-species transmission of virus from birds or a reassortment event leading to acquisition of an M gene encoding resistance in a human strain provides another route for acquisition of the M2 inhibitor resistance in a human virus. One survey of avian isolates found that M2 inhibitor-resistant variants were not detected among 1979–1983 isolates, whereas 31% of H5 and 11% of H9 strains from Southeast Asia isolated in 2000–2004 carried M2 resistance mutations (33). In North America, resistant variants occurred among 16% of H7 viruses only, whereas H6 viruses were amantadine-sensitive. Resistance due to the Ser31Asn mutation was also confirmed in poultry A(H5N1) isolates collected between 2002 and 2005 in Northern China, which perhaps related to use of amantadine in chicken food or water (34). One highly pathogenic avian A(H7N7) isolate from a fatal human case in Holland in 2003 was resistant to amantadine in cell culture and in experimentally infected mice; resistance was linked to the HA protein and not to mutations in M2 (34a).

2.2.2 A(H5N1) Viruses

Although the initial human isolates of avian A(H5N1) viruses in Hong Kong in 1997 were M2 inhibitor susceptible (34b), more recent human isolates of clade 1 viruses have been resistant to M2 inhibitors (35, 36). One sequence analysis of 638 M2 genes of avian and human isolates of A(H5N1) viruses from 1996 to 2005 found resistance due to dual Ser31Asn and Leu26Ile mutations in almost all clade 1 isolates from Vietnam, Thailand, and Cambodia since 2003, observations that were consistent with a single introduction (37). M2 inhibitor-resistance due to the Ser31Asn mutation, or less often mutations at positions 27 or 30, was seen in a minority of isolates from China and Hong Kong SAR starting in 2003 and in only 2 of 32 Indonesian viruses. In 2005 the frequency of resistance detection was 83% in Vietnam but only 7% in China. Another survey of 55 avian A(H5N1) isolates from Southeast Asian countries found that all of the A(H5N1) viruses from Vietnam, Malaysia

and Cambodia contained dual-resistance mutations (L26I and S31N), while 4 of 6 strains from Indonesia were sensitive (38). However, subsequent studies indicate that an increasing proportion of Clade 2.1 isolates from Indonesia have been resistant (over 80% in 2006–2007), whereas over 90% clade 2.2 and 2.3 isolates from Eurasia, Africa, and China have been susceptible (A. Klimov, personal communication). These observations highlight the need for continued surveillance of drug susceptibility in new human and animal influenza viruses.

2.3 Resistance in Posttreatment Isolates

The rapid emergence of resistant variants in M2 inhibitor-treated patients has been found also in studies of experimentally infected animals. In a study using a chicken A(H5N2) virus, resistant viruses are detectable by 2–3 days after starting drug administration and persisted thereafter (39). A study in ferrets inoculated with a human influenza A(H3N2) virus detected M2 inhibitor resistance mutations in four of the nine amantadine-treated animals by day 6 after inoculation; in each instance two or more M2 gene mutations were identified (40). In contrast, intranasal zanamivir did not select for known neuraminidase resistance mutations under similar conditions.

2.3.1 Immunocompetent Patients

Resistant variants arise commonly and rapidly in M2 inhibitor-treated children and adults with acute influenza (Table 2). One study of adults found that resistant virus could be detected in 50% of six rimantadine recipients by day three of treatment, although the nasal lavage titers were lower than in placebo recipients shedding susceptible virus (41). Another study found that 33% of 24 adult and pediatric household members receiving rimantadine shed resistant virus on day 5 of treatment; none were positive when tested five days later (41). A larger pediatric trial found emergence of resistant virus in 27% of 37 rimantadine recipients, including 45% of those still virus positive on day 7, compared to 6% of 32 acetaminophen recipients (12). Resistant virus was detected as early as day 3 but was usually present on days 5–7. A study of Japanese children treated with amantadine found that 30% of 81 in the 1999–2000 season and 23% of 30 during the following season had resistant virus detected on day 3–5 after a 3-day course (19). Resistant variants were detected more frequently in A(H3N2)-infected children (33%) than in A(H1N1)-infected ones (20%). Another study employing sensitive molecular cloning detection methods found mutations conferring resistance in 80% of 15 hospitalized children

Table 2 Recovery of resistant influenza A during M2 inhibitor treatment

Study	Seasons	Patient group	Treatment	Number treated	No. (%) shedding resistant viruses
Hall et al. (12)	1983	Children	Rimantadine	37	10 (27%) H3N2
Hayden et al. (41)	1987–1989	Children	Rimantadine	21	6 (29%) H3N2
Hayden et al. (41)	1988–1989	Adults	Rimantadine	13	5 (38%) H3N2
Betts, personal communication		Elderly	Rimantadine	26	3 (11%)
Englund et al. (42)	1993–1994	Immunocompromised	Amantadine, Rimantadine	15	5 (33%) H3N2
Saito et al. (19)	1999–2001	Children	Amantadine	111	22 (33%) H3N2 9 (20%) H1N1
Shirashi et al. (18)	1999–2001	Children (hospitalized)	Amantadine	15	8 (100%) H3N2 4 (57%) H1N1

during or immediately after amantadine treatment (18). Nine (75%) of 12 children had 2–4 different resistance mutations detected in clones from a single sample, sometimes mixed with a wild-type virus. Viruses with the Ser31Asn mutation were more prevalent in A(H3N2)-infected children and those with Val27Ala in A(H1N1)-infected ones compared to other mutations, suggesting that they had greater replication competence in these subtypes (18).

2.3.2 Immunocompromised Hosts

Resistant influenza A viruses may be shed for prolonged periods in immunocompromised hosts, who can serve as a reservoir for nosocomial transmission. One study of adult bone marrow transplant and acute leukemia patients recovered resistant virus in 5 (33%) of 15 M2 inhibitor-treated patients and in five (83%) of six patients with illness who shed virus for ≥3 days (42). The median time between first and last virus isolation was 7 days with range up to 44 days. Death associated with influenza occurred in two of the five (40%) patients with resistant virus, compared to 5 of the 24 (21%) without, and prolonged illness was noted in several with protracted shedding. Other reports have documented prolonged shedding of resistant variants in immunocompromised hosts with or without continued drug exposure, including one transplanted SCID child who shed resistant virus for 5 weeks and one adult leukemia patient who shed resistant virus for ≥1 week off therapy (43). Another case report documented recovery of resistant virus >1 month after cessation of a course of amantadine, as well as shedding of mixtures of wild-type virus and variants with different resistance genotypes (44). Heterogeneous populations of resistant variants with sequential or dual mutations have been found in several immunocompromised hosts (42, 43). One stem cell transplant recipient shed the dually M2 inhibitor and oseltamivir-resistant virus for at least 5 months and probably over a period of 1 year (45). The prolonged shedding of resistant variants in immunocompromised hosts is consistent with the genetic stability of such variants observed in experimental

animal models (39). However, early amantadine or rimantadine treatment in acute leukemia or hematopoietic stem cell transplant patients with drug-susceptible influenza A can be clinically beneficial and was associated with a significant reduction (35% versus 76%) in the risk of progression to pneumonia in one report (46).

2.4 Transmissibility of Resistant Variants

The transmissibility of M2 inhibitor-resistant viruses has been demonstrated in animal models and in several clinical settings. Competition-transmission studies with an avian A/chicken/Pennsylvania/1370/83(H5N2) virus compared the transmissibility of wild-type virus with resistant variants possessing M2 substitutions at positions 27, 30, or 31 (39). Contact birds shedding resistant virus due to earlier incorporation of amantadine in the drinking water of donors (four days only) were caged with birds shedding susceptible virus, and the virus was allowed to transmit through three more sets of contact birds in the absence of selective drug pressure. Resistant virus was detected from the final set of contact birds in three of four experiments over four cumulative transmission cycles.

2.4.1 Households

Both amantadine and rimantadine are effective for postexposure prophylaxis of illness due to susceptible strains in household contacts, when ill index cases are not given concurrent treatment (Table 3). In contrast, two studies have found no significant reduction in secondary influenza illness in household contacts receiving either amantadine or rimantadine for postexposure prophylaxis, when the ill index cases received treatment with the same drug. One of these documented failures of prophylaxis due to infection by drug-resistant variants, most likely transmitted from the treated index cases (14). These findings indicate that the strategy of using M2

Table 3 Influenza prevention in households with postexposure prophylaxis (PEP)

Study	Drug (age of contacts)	Season (predominant virus)	Index case treated	Influenza A illness in contacts No./total evaluable (%)		PEP efficacy (%)
				Active	Control	
Galbraith et al. (166)	Amantadine (≥2 years)	1967–1968 (A/H2N2)	No	0/91 (0%)	12/90 (13%)	100
Bricaire (167)	Rimantadine (≥1 year)	1988–1989 (A/not stated)	No	8/151[a] (5%)	26/150[a] (17%)	70
Monto et al. (168)	Zanamivir (≥5 years)	2000–2001 (A/H3N2, B)	No	12/661 (2%)	55/630 (9%)	82
Welliver et al. (169)	Oseltamivir (≥13 years)	1998–1999 (A/H3N2, B)	No	4/493 (1%)	34/462 (7%)	89
Galbraith et al. (170)	Amantadine (≥2 years)	1968–1969 (A/H3N2)	Yes	5/43 (12%)	6/42 (14%)	6
Hayden et al. (14)	Rimantadine (≥1 year)	1987–1989 (A/H3N2, A/H1N1)	Yes	11/61 (18%)	10/54 (19%)	3
Hayden et al. (171)	Zanamivir (≥5 years)	1998–1999 (A/H3N2, B)	Yes	7/414 (2%)	40/423 (9%)	82
Hayden et al. (172)	Oseltamivir (≥1 year)	2000–2001 (A/H3N2, B)	Yes	11/400 (3%)	40//392 (10%)	73

[a]Clinical influenza

inhibitors for both index case treatment and postexposure prophylaxis in households should be avoided.

2.4.2 Chronic Care Facilities

Transmission of M2 inhibitor-resistant viruses is well documented in nursing home outbreaks of influenza A and may be manifested by a persistent or an increasing number of virus-positive patients despite amantadine prophylaxis. The recovery of the same genotype of resistant virus from multiple patients on prophylaxis or from patients or staff not receiving drug indicate ongoing transmission in this setting (15, 47). This is particularly true with multiple isolations of a less commonly observed resistant variant, as was found with nine isolates of a Leu26Phe variant in one nursing home outbreak (47). The frequency of instances in which amantadine or rimantadine have failed to control outbreaks because of resistance emergence is not well defined. In Canada amantadine was used for outbreak control in 29 influenza A outbreaks in chronic care facilities over 11 influenza seasons studied between 1989 and 2000 (48). In 22 (76%) instances, transmission was stopped within 2–3 days, whereas the outbreak was not controlled in seven (24%) instances. Susceptibility testing found emergence of M2 inhibitor resistance in three of six outbreaks with ongoing transmission; amantadine failure was associated with simultaneous prophylactic and therapeutic use of the drug and with treatment of a higher proportion of ill persons in the facility. Continuing outbreaks due to resistant virus were associated with a higher proportion of cases in shared rooms compared to those due to susceptible virus. During the 1999–2000 season another study found that only 59% of 200 influenza A outbreaks were controlled by amantadine (49); four of five amantadine outbreak failures were associated with circulation of susceptible virus, perhaps because of use of reduced amantadine doses in an effort to avoid side effects (50). Such findings emphasize the importance of proper isolation of treated persons and of

using NAI for treatment of ill/sick persons. However, failures of rimantadine prophylaxis due to resistant virus have been observed in nursing home residents despite use of oseltamivir treatment of ill/sick residents (51). Uncontrolled clinical experiences indicate that prophylaxis with inhaled zanamivir (47, 52) or oral oseltamivir (48, 50) are both effective in terminating such outbreaks. One controlled comparative study found that inhaled zanamivir prophylaxis was superior to oral rimantadine in protecting nursing home residents, largely because of the high frequency of M2 inhibition resistance in the nursing homes (53).

Resistant viruses have been recovered occasionally from patients receiving long-term amantadine for Parkinsonism (54). One study during the 1998–1999 season in Japanese nursing homes detected resistant viruses by PCR–RLFP analysis in elderly residents with influenza-like illness in 24% of 141 PCR positive nasopharyngeal samples, over 90% of which were due to Ser31Asn substitutions (17). Only 18% of the 34 patients with resistance detected were receiving amantadine at the time of sampling. The average frequency of resistance detection was nonsignificantly higher in the four homes using amantadine for therapy of ILI (28%) than in the four homes where it was used for Parkinsonism (16%). Such findings indicate that patients receiving amantadine for noninfluenza indications may serve as a source of drug-resistant virus under certain circumstances.

2.5 Pathogenicity

M2 inhibitor-resistant influenza A viruses appear to cause typical influenza illness without obviously enhanced or attenuated symptoms (14, 16, 41). Illness occurs in both the presence or absence of the drug, a finding that indicates the loss of antiviral effectiveness in vivo. In temporal relationship to increasing frequencies of M2 inhibitor resistance in Japan during the 2003–2006 seasons, amantadine treatment was found to have decreasing clinical effectiveness, whereas that of oseltamivir did not change (55). In nursing home outbreaks residents developing influenza due to resistant strains have experienced serious illness, including fatal outcomes in some instances (56). Patients with infections caused by M2 inhibitor-resistant variants have no obvious reductions in the risks of pneumonia, hospitalization, or death compared to those with wild-type illness. One study of higher-risk patients during the 2004–2005 season found no differences in the number of symptoms, duration of illness, or frequency of hospitalization in comparing outcomes among 80 patients with A(H3N2) illness due to M2 inhibitor-susceptible virus to 72 patients infected with resistant viruses (57). While the M gene mutations do not appear to attenuate or potentiate the virulence of human influenza viruses, more subtle effects on biologic fitness cannot be excluded by studies to date. Occasionally wild-type virus replaces resistant variants after cessation of amantadine (18). As noted for some avian H7 viruses, this reversion in the absence of selective drug pressure suggests diminished replication competence of some resistant genotypes. However, the most common resistant variants with Ser31Asn have no apparent loss of replication competence or transmissibility.

Animal model studies have found that mutations in the M2 protein do not appear to attenuate or potentiate the virulence of influenza viruses compared to wild-type virus in the absence of drug administration. Resistant variants of an avian influenza A/chicken/Pennsylvania/1370/83(H5N2) with position 27, 30, or 31 substitutions were comparable to drug-susceptible virus in causing mortality in experimentally infected birds, although virulence in both susceptible and resistant viruses varied (39). As expected, amantadine administration protected against death in birds inoculated with wild-type virus but not a resistant variant. Studies with three pairs of epidemiologically linked human A(H3N2) subtype isolates, representing resistant variants with M2 substitutions at Val27Ala, Ala30Val, or Ser31Asn, found no differences in febrile responses, peak nasal viral titers, and nasal inflammatory cell counts in experimentally infected ferrets between the resistant variants and corresponding wild-type viruses (58). The variants retained their resistance phenotype during the short-term passage in ferrets. In an A/Udorn/307/72(H3N2) virus background, the Ser31Asn and Val27Thr mutations were associated with replication in cell culture and mice comparable to wild-type virus (59). Studies of a laboratory virus A/WSN(H1N1) that was genetically engineered to harbor different M2 resistance mutations found that none were associated with reduced replication in cell culture or diminished virulence in mice, and several mutations, including Ser31Asn and particularly the combination of Ser31Asn with Val27Ala were associated with increased weight loss and mortality in mice compared to susceptible virus (60). In general, it appears that M2 inhibitor resistant human influenza A viruses that emerge in vivo do not differ substantially in replication ability or pathogenicity from drug-susceptible wild-type viruses.

In treated patients the emergence of resistant virus may be associated with persistence of viral shedding and in some studies delays in resolution of illness in immunocompetent persons. Retrospective analysis of rimantadine-treated adult and pediatric family members infected with influenza A(H3N2) virus found that the third who had emergence of the resistant virus on therapy, experienced somewhat longer times to resolution of symptoms, fever, and possibly functional impairment compared to the two-thirds that did not shed resistant virus (41). However, both groups had more rapid illness recovery than placebo-treated persons. Another study of influenza A(H3N2) illness found that rimantadine-treated children had lower frequencies and titers of detectable virus on the second day of treatment but higher values on days 6 and 7 after treatment and a mean 1-day longer period of viral shedding, principally related to the emergence of resistant variants (12). Among rimantadine recipients, illness measures were initially improved compared to placebo, but 41% became worse on later days compared to 18% in the placebo. Rimantadine recipients with resistant virus tended to have increased illness scores on days 5 and 6 compared to those without. Although such studies do not prove that resistance emergence caused the delay in recovery, the persistence of symptoms combined with emergence of resistance could contribute to transmission of resistant virus from such persons, especially young children.

2.6 Treatment Alternatives

Amantadine and rimantadine share susceptibility and resistance, so that resistance to one M2 inhibitor confers high-level cross-resistance to the other one and to date the entire class of compounds targeting M2 protein. Because of their different mechanism of antiviral action, NA inhibitors (discussed below) retain full activity against M2 inhibitor-resistant viruses and are appropriate choices for both prophylaxis and treatment of suspected M2 inhibitor-resistant infections. Both oseltamivir and zanamivir have been used with apparent success in terminating ongoing institutional outbreaks in which amantadine-resistance was implicated (47, 48, 50, 52). One unanswered clinical question is whether combined treatment with an M2 and NA inhibitor reduces the likelihood of resistance emergence to either class of drugs. In vitro studies indicate that the combination reduces this risk (61). One small study comparing oral rimantadine monotherapy to rimantadine combined with aerosolized zanamivir in hospitalized adults found that the only M2 inhibitor-resistant variants were detected in the rimantadine monotherapy group (62), and further studies of combination therapy are warranted in serious infections including those due to A(H5N1), when the infecting virus is known or likely to be M2 inhibitor susceptible (63, 63a).

The synthetic nucleoside ribavirin is also inhibitory for M2-inhibitor resistant influenza A and B viruses and is a therapeutic consideration. Aerosolized ribavirin has been studied in uncomplicated influenza and used in treating individuals with influenza pneumonia (reviewed in (64)). High (8.4 g in 2 days) but not low (1 g/day) dose oral ribavirin appears to reduce clinical illness in uncomplicated influenza (65, 66), and intravenous ribavirin has been used in severe infections with uncertain benefit (67). Other potential inhibitors have been reviewed (68, 69, 69a) and are briefly discussed below.

3 Neuraminidase Inhibitors (Zanamivir, Oseltamivir)

Antiviral resistance studies with the neuraminidase (NA) inhibitors were initiated shortly after their discovery. Initial efforts utilizing sequential passage in cell culture to select resistant variants found that changes in either viral HA or NA could confer resistance in vitro (reviewed in (70, 71)). The frequency and possible importance of resistance emergence during drug administration have been studied largely in the context of controlled clinical trials conducted in the late 1990s that served as the basis for approval of zanamivir and oseltamivir. Due to differences in drug binding interactions and structural differences in the enzyme active site, NA inhibitors show varying susceptibility patterns that depend on virus type and subtype (reviewed in (72, 73)). For example, several studies found that zanamivir is on average 3- to 10-fold more potent against influenza B NAs than oseltamivir but somewhat less active against influenza A N2s (74, 75). While the possible clinical importance of such differences is uncertain, the lower oseltamivir carboxylate susceptibility of influenza B relative to A NAs may have clinical consequences. Several Japanese studies have reported that oseltamivir therapy is somewhat less effective for treatment of influenza B compared to influenza A, particularly in younger children, as measured by time to defervescence and by reductions in viral titers in the upper respiratory tract (76, 77). In contrast, inhaled zanamivir appears comparably effective in influenza A and B infections (78). Zanamivir and oseltamivir have been available in many countries since 1999, but their actual extent of clinical use has been quite limited, except recently in Japan (79, 80). Consequently, the possible epidemiologic importance of resistance emergence and transmission has received limited direct study to date.

3.1 Detection of Resistance

Several phenotypic and genotypic assays are used to detect NA inhibitor resistance (6a). As noted above, changes in either NA or HA can result in antiviral resistance to NA inhibitors under laboratory conditions (reviewed in (70, 72)). This relates to the functional balance between the receptor binding activity of HA and the receptor-destroying activity of NA, such that HA mutations causing decreased dependence on NA action for viral elution from cells can lead to in vitro resistance to NA inhibitors. Furthermore, both the target enzyme and inhibitors exert extra-cellular effects. Unlike the situation for M2 inhibitors, cell-culture-based assays have not been validated for detecting phenotypic resistance in clinical isolates, in part because of the differences in cellular receptor specificity between human respiratory epithelium and most available cell culture types (reviewed in (71)). Recent, low passage clinical isolates often appear resistant to NA inhibitors in laboratory cell lines. Madin Darby canine kidney (MDCK) cell line that are stably transfected with human 2,6-sialyltransferase (SIAT1) to enhance expression of alpha 2,6-linked sialic acid and reduce that of alpha 2,3-linked ones overcome this limitation but has not been widely utilized to date (81, 82). Based on plaque size determinations, oseltamivir susceptibility in SIAT1-MDCK cells increases and appears to correlate well with the results in enzyme inhibition assays for clinical isolates (82). However, the levels of resistance observed in yield reduction assays with such cells may be much less than observed in enzyme inhibition assays for viruses with several clinically relevant oseltamivir resistance mutations, and some resistant variants (e.g., Arg292Lys) may not replicate sufficiently for assay (83).

HA binding efficiency and associated susceptibility to NA inhibitors are affected by amino acids in the receptor binding pocket, location and presence of oligosaccharide chains, and the structure of cellular receptors (84). Changes in HA that alter binding to the α2,3-linked sialic acid residues on typical MDCK cells may reduce susceptibility to NA inhibitors in vitro but not change binding to human cells expressing α2,6-linked residues. Consequently, HA mutations have been looked for in clinical isolates usually by comparing the sequence of pre- and posttherapy isolates and in some instances by examining changes in receptor affinity. HA variants that have reduced receptor affinity show cross-resistance in vitro to all NA inhibitors but in general retain susceptibility to NA inhibitors in animal models (71, 85). Of note, altering the HA receptor binding site of a clade 1 A(H5N1) virus by reverse genetics, including switch from α2,3 to α2,6 specificity, did not affect NA inhibitor susceptibility of the engineered viruses in differentiated human bronchial epithelial cells, although many receptor variants were less susceptible in MDCK and SIAT1-MDCK cells (85a).

In order to detect changes in NA susceptibility, most studies have utilized enzyme inhibition assays for phenotyping and sequence analysis of the NA gene to detect relevant mutations (6a). Real-time RT PCR using labeled probes and more recently pyro-sequencing methods have been used to rapidly detect specific NA mutations (86, 86a). Both fluorometric and chemiluminescent NA inhibition assays are available, but all assays have limitations and may not reliably detect resistant subpopulations (87). No clinically validated thresholds for resistance (absolute concentrations or fold-changes compared to wild-type) have been determined for the different NA inhibitors using NA inhibition assays. Depending on the drug, virus strain, and assay inhibitory concentrations for clinically and laboratory selected NA variants have shown at least 10-fold to over 1,000-fold reductions in susceptibility (87).

The NA mutation conferring resistance depends on the drug and virus type and subtype. For oseltamivir, His274Tyr confers resistance in N1 but not N2-containing viruses (88), whereas Arg292Lys and Glu119Val are the most common resistance mutations in N2-containing viruses. Because of the differences in interaction among drugs with the active enzyme site, varying patterns of cross-resistance are found for particular NA mutations. Importantly, zanamivir retains full inhibitory activity against variants with either the His274Tyr or Glu119Val mutation and partial activity against the Arg292Lys variant (87, 89).

3.2 Susceptibility of Field Isolates

Studies utilizing both phenotypic susceptibility testing and NA sequence analysis have rarely documented primary (de novo) resistance to the NA inhibitors in community isolates of human influenza viruses until the 2007–2008 season (below). Natural variation occurs in susceptibility patterns, and the range of inhibitory concentrations may vary by tenfold or more within an NA type or subtype. The possible clinical importance of such differences is unknown. Both zanamivir and oseltamivir have also been shown to be active in vitro and in vivo against virus containing the neuraminidase of the 1918 pandemic strain (21) and against A(H5N1) and other avian viruses (90–92). Both drugs are active against the nine NA subtypes recognized in nature (92).

3.2.1 Surveillance Studies to 2006

Assays of large numbers of pretreatment isolates and those from placebo recipients during controlled clinical trials in both adults and children (reviewed in (93)) did not detect naturally occurring resistant variants to either zanamivir or oseltamivir. One large survey of 1,054 influenza isolates collected between 1996 and 1999 through the World Health Organization's Global Influenza Surveillance Network (GISN) found no instances of neuraminidase

resistance to zanamivir or oseltamivir in enzyme inhibition assays (Table 4) (94). Sequence analysis of isolates with inhibition values above the 95% confidence limits and other isolates found variation in some previously conserved resides but no recognized resistance mutations. Similarly, no resistance was observed in over 3,000 pretreatment isolates collected in clinical trials of oseltamivir (95).

Since introduction of the drugs into clinical practice, continued surveillance detected phenotypic resistance to oseltamivir in 8 of 2,287 community isolates (0.35%) collected during the influenza seasons from 1999 to 2002 (Table 4), four of which showed reduced susceptibility to zanamivir (80). Three isolates had a recognized resistance mutation (His274Tyr in H1N1; Asp198Glu and Ile222Thr in B) but other several new NA mutations were detected that might have contributed to reduced susceptibility. As these viruses were not obtained from persons taking a NA inhibitor, the results would indicate that either transmission of resistant variants was occurring from treated persons or that low level of de novo resistance occurs. Similarly, an Australian study of 532 strains collected between 1998 to 2002 (Table 4) found only one instance of apparent resistance (75), an influenza B/Perth/211/2001 isolate that contained a mixed population with resistant variants harboring a Asp198Glu mutation (reported above) (96, 97). A survey of 1,550 isolates collected worldwide in 2000–2002 reported very few outlier results and no confirmed isolates with resistance (98). A study in France did not find changes in A(H3N2) susceptibility to either agent nor recognized resistant variants over 3 years from 2002 to 2005, although four variants with deficient NA and resistance to both drugs in cell culture were described (99). Surveys of community isolates in Japan, which has had the highest per capita use of oseltamivir in the world, have found low frequencies of oseltamivir-resistance in influenza A (79) and B (100, 101) viruses. During the 2003–2004 season 0.3% of 1,180 H3N2 isolates harbored oseltamivir resistance mutations (79), whereas no resistance was found in influenza B viruses that season or in A(H3N2) and A(H1N1) isolates during the subsequent season (Table 4). However, 3.0% of 132 H1N1 isolates during the 2005–2006 season had the His274Tyr mutation that confers oseltamivir resistance (102). During the 2004–2005 season 1.7% of 422 influenza B isolates from untreated persons showed reduced susceptibility to neuraminidase inhibitors; four of these persons were likely infected in the community and three through household contact (100). These findings likely indicate low-level transmission of resistant variants in the community during periods of substantial oseltamivir use.

In addition to examining the frequencies of resistant variants in community isolates, most studies have not found evidence for secular trends indicating reduced NAI suscepti-

Table 4 Representative studies of oseltamivir and zanamivir susceptibility of field isolates of influenza A and B viruses to 2006-7

Study	Location	Seasons	Assay	No. tested	No. (%) resistant	Mutations detected
McKimm-Breschkin et al. (94)	Worldwide	1999–2002	NAI-FA, NAI-CL, S	139 A/N1	0	
				767 A/N2	0	
				148 B	0	
Hurt et al. (75)	Australia, South East Asia, Oceania	1998–2002	NAI-FA	235 A/N1	0	
				169 A/N2	0	
				128 B	1[a]	Asp197Glu
Hurt et al. (173)		2001–2006	NAI-FA	288 A/N1	1	His274Tyr
				540 A/N2	0	
				270 B	1[a]	Asp197Glu
Bovin and Goyette (74)	Canada	1999–2000	NAI-CL	38 H3N2	0	
				40 H2N1	0	
				23 B	0	
Mungall et al. (98)	Worldwide	2000–2002	NAI-CL	567 A/N2	0	
				271 A/N1	0	
				712 B	0	
Monto et al. (80)	Worldwide	1999–2002	NAI-CL, S	922 A/N2	3 (0.3%)	Gln41Gly, Gln226His
				622 A/N1	3 (0.5%)	His274Tyr, Tyr155His, Gly248Arg
				743 B	2 (0.3%)	Asp198Glu, Ile222Thr
Ferraris et al. (99)	France	2002–2005	NAI-FA, S	788 H3N2	0[b]	
Escuret et al. (99a)	France	2005–2006		151 H1N1	3 (2.0%)	1 His274Tyr, 2[c]
				225 B	1	1Asp198Tyr
NISN (79)	Japan	2003–2004	NAI-CL, S	1,180 H3N2	3 (0.3%)	2 Glu119Val, 1 Arg292Lys
				171 B	0	
Hatakeyama et al. (100)	Japan	2004–2005	NAI-FA, S	422 B	7 (1.7%)	3 Asp198Asn, 3 Ile222Thr, 1 Ser250Gly[d]
NISN (102)	Japan	2004–2005	NAI-CL, S	558 H3N2	0	
				60 H1N1	0	
		2005–2006	S	250 H3N2	0	
				132 H1N1	4 (3.0%)	4 His274Tyr
				61B	0	
		2006–2007	S	54 H1N1	0	
				134 H3N2	0	
				119 B	0	

NAI neuraminidase inhibition; *CL* chemiluminescence; *FA* fluorescence; *S* sequence analysis of neuraminidase gene; *NISN* Neuraminidase Inhibitor Susceptibility Network. Amino acid numbering based on N2 neuraminidase.

[a] One B/Perth/211/2001 isolate had 7- to 9-fold reduced susceptibility to zanamivir and 14- to18-fold to oseltamivir compared to the mean inhibitory concentrations of influenza B strains and contained a mixed population including resistant variants with a Asp197Glu mutation (96)

[b] Four isolates (0.5%) with NA deficiency were found to be resistant to NA inhibitors in cell culture-based assays

[c] Two A(H1N1) isolates had 9- and 30-fold reduced susceptibility to zanamivir but no loss of oseltamivir susceptibility nor apparent NA mutation (99a).

[d] Asp198Asn confers resistance to both oseltamivir and zanamivir, Ile222Thr to oseltamivir, and Ser250Gly to zanamivir (100).

bility of influenza NAs since the drugs have been introduced into practice. However, one survey in the United Kingdom found that the susceptibility of influenza B, but not influenza A, NAs to both oseltamivir and zanamivir had decreased by over 50% since 1997 (101). Such changes may be related to natural genetic evolution in viral NA unrelated to drug use but emphasize the importance of continued surveillance.

3.2.2 A(H1N1) Viruses

In January 2008, WHO was notified about a high prevalence (75%) of oseltamivir resistance due to the His274Tyr muta-

tion in seasonal influenza A(H1N1) viruses in Norway (6, 6a). Depending on the assay methods, this mutation is associated with 350-fold to >1,500-fold reductions in N1 susceptibility in enzyme inhibition assays (87, 89, 103, 104) and lack of response in vivo (104a, 119, 120). Subsequent surveillance through WHO's GISN and the European Influenza Surveillance Scheme (EISS) found an overall 16% frequency of resistance in community A(H1N1) isolates during the 2007–8 northern hemisphere season (105, 105a). However, many countries were unaffected and wide variations in resistance prevalence existed within Europe and in different regions of the world. In comparison, no viruses with the His274Tyr mutation were detected among 139 A(H1N1) isolates collected globally through GISN from 1996 to 1999 (94) and this mutation was rarely detected in community isolates subsequently, except for the 2005-6 season in Japan (Table 4) (80, 102). The unexpected high prevalence of oseltamivir resistance in A(H1N1) viruses in many parts of the world within a single season indicated efficient person-person transmission. Available evidence indicated that selective drug pressure was not driving this phenomenon, and Japan had a notably low rate of resistant A(H1N1) viruses. Although several oseltamivir-resistant A(H1N1) variants belonging to clade 2B were detected globally, a predominate antigenic drift variant A/Brisbane/59/2007(H1N1) lineage, that is resistant to oseltamivir but susceptible to zanamivir and M2 inhibitors (105, 105a) emerged and continued to circulate in the southern hemisphere and subsequently northern hemispheres in 2008–2009. These viruses replicated efficiently and caused typical influenza illness including severe and sometimes fatal infections (104a). The circulation of H1N1 viruses naturally resistant to oseltamivir emphasizes that genetic variations may result in variations in sensitivity to oseltamivir in the absence of apparent selective drug pressure.

Sporadic zanamivir resistance occurs at low frequency in community A(H1N1) isolates (80, 99a). Variants that show about 100-fold less susceptibility to zanamivir but sensitivity to oseltamivir, related to a Q136K mutation in NA, have been reported from the Philippines and Australia (106).

3.2.3 A(H5N1) Viruses

Almost all avian A(H5N1) viruses isolated from birds and humans have been susceptible to NA inhibitors. However, one survey of avian A(H5N1) isolates collected between 2004 and 2006 in Southeast Asia found that two of 55 viruses showed approximately 4- to 16-fold reduced susceptibility to oseltamivir and one of these had 63 fold decreased susceptibility to zanamivir (107). Novel NA mutations of potential significance (Ile117Val, Val116Ala) were detected in these isolates. In addition, rare avian isolates harboring the His274Tyr mutation have been detected (108, 109), and one study reported that recent avian A(H5N1) positive samples have preexisting resistant subpopulations possessing this mutation (109). One clade 1 A/Vietnam/JP36-2/05 virus was transmissible in ferrets and showed apparent emergence of the H274Y mutation in an infected recipient animal (109a). Avian A(H5N1) viruses possessing an Asn294Ser NA mutation that confers 12- to 15-fold or greater reductions in oseltamivir susceptibility have been detected in two fatal cases before initiation of oseltamivir therapy and also in some isolates from birds (110).

Most clade 1 A(H5N1) viruses from 2004 to 2005 appear to have increased susceptibility to oseltamivir carboxylate compared to 1997 isolates from Hong Kong or human

A(H1N1) viruses in enzyme inhibition and cell culture assays (111, 112, 114, 114a, 114b). The increased oseltamivir susceptibility has been postulated to be related to amino acid changes at residues 248 and 252 surrounding the active site (111). The susceptibility of A(H5N1) viruses to oseltamivir, but not to zanamivir, varies up to 30-fold in enzyme inhibition assays with clade 2 viruses being less susceptible than early clade 1 viruses (113, 113a). While the clinical importance of such susceptibility variations is uncertain, these differences in in vitro susceptibility correspond to some extent with the dose levels of oseltamivir needed to reduce replication in murine and ferret treatment models (114). Despite increased susceptibility of some clade 1 viruses, their virulence and rapid replication kinetics require higher oseltamivir doses to inhibit replication in animal models (112, 114, 114a, 114b). Resistance emergence has been documented very uncommonly in murine and ferret treatment models to date (63a, 112, 114a, 114b).

3.2.4 HA Mutations

Clinical isolates possessing HA mutations that induce cross-resistance to NA inhibitors in cell culture, but no NA changes, have been described. One such HA variant (Arg229Ile) showed reduced binding to MDCK cell receptors and over 100-fold reduced susceptibility in MDCK cells but full susceptibility in ferrets (85). Similarly, apparent reductions in the zanamivir susceptibility of circulating A(H3N2) viruses in MDCK cell culture are linked to specific changes in HA (Leu226Ile/Val) that alter receptor binding without associated NA mutations (115), but zanamivir has been shown to be effective against H3N2 viruses in controlled clinical trials.

3.3 Resistance in Posttreatment Isolates

Oseltamivir-resistant viruses with NA mutations have been detected in clinical trials when the drug has been used for influenza treatment (reviewed in (95)) (Table 5). No zanamivir-resistant viruses have been recovered in zanamivir-treated immunocompetent hosts, although the number of paired isolates studied has been low and limited by the need for pharyngeal or lower respiratory isolates (71, 116). For both zanamivir and oseltamivir, no resistant variants have been detected in immunocompetent persons receiving drug for chemoprophylaxis of seasonal influenza to date (117).

3.3.1 Immunocompetent Hosts

In natural infections, oseltamivir-resistant variants have been detected much more commonly in treated children than adults

Table 5 Frequency of resistance emergence to oseltamivir or zanamivir during treatment of influenza A and B virus infections

Drug/Study	Population	Assay	Virus type	Number of isolates tested	No. (%) resistant	Mutations detected
Oseltamivir						
Gubareva et al. (119)	Adults	NAI, S	A/H1N1	54	2 (4%)	2 His274 Tyr
Roberts et al. (118)	Adults	NAI, S	A/H3N2	418	5 (1%)	4 Arg292Lys, 1 Glu119Val
Whitley et al. (123)[a]	Children – outpatient	NAI, S	A & B	150 A 66 B	10 (6.7 %) 0	8 Arg292Lys, 1 Glu119Val, 1 His274Tyr
Kiso et al. (124)[a]	Children – outpatient + hospitalized	Cloning + S	A/H3N2	50	9 (18%)	6 Arg292Lys, 2 Glu119Val, 1 Asn294Ser
Ward et al. (122)[a]	Children – outpatient + hospitalized	NAI, S	A/H1N1	43	7 (16%)	7 His274Tyr
Hatakeyama et al. (100)	Children – outpatient	NAI, S	B	74	1 (1.4%)	Gly402Ser
Democratis et al. (125)	Children – outpatient	S	A/H1N1	11	3 (27%)	3 His274Tyr
			A/H3N2	34	1 (3%)	Arg292Lys
			B	19	0	
Zanamivir						
Barnett et al. (116)	Adults	NAI, S	A + B	41	0	

[a] These pediatric studies used a 2 mg/kg dose of oseltamivir that has been shown to give reduced drug exposure because of more rapid clearance in children under the age of 5 years. Insufficient drug exposure may have contributed to resistance emergence in these studies

[b] This influenza B isolate showed 7-fold and 4-fold reduced susceptibility to zanamivir and oseltamivir, respectively and high IC50 values to oseltamivir (100).

(Table 5). Analysis of samples from over 2,500 influenza patients treated with oseltamivir as outpatients indicates that the frequency of resistance detection has been about 10-fold lower in adults than children (118) (Table 4). Resistance may emerge more readily in influenza A infections but has been reported in influenza B (100). In contrast to in vitro observations, no HA resistance mutations have been detected in those with NA mutations conferring oseltamivir resistance (118).

Among 54 volunteers experimentally infected with an A(H1N1) virus, oseltamivir-resistant variants with His274Tyr mutation were detected in two subjects in association with apparent rebounds in viral replication (119). In addition, this study found that oseltamivir-treated subjects were less likely than placebo to have late viral isolates showing reversion of the egg-adapted inoculum virus to a human receptor HA genotype. The His274Tyr finding suggests that HA mutations with reduced affinity for human receptors might have a replication advantage over viruses with human receptor preference during oseltamivir use in humans. This mutation has also been detected in infected children (Table 5), immunocompromised hosts (below) and in several patients infected with A(H5N1) virus (120, 121). One study of A(H1N1)-infected children from Japan reported a frequency of 16% resistance emergence with this mutation (122). In two A(H5N1) patients, including the one who was treated within 2 days of the onset of illness onset and had resistant virus detected on day four of the treatment, and the emergence of the His274Tyr resistance mutation in the upper respiratory tract was associated temporally with persistent viral replication and fatal outcome (121). Another A(H5N1)-infected patient had emergence of resistant

clones with this mutation during oseltamivir administration at prophylactic doses but survived and had a cleared virus after the dose was increased (120).

One treatment study of outpatient children, most of whom had influenza A(H3N2) illness, detected resistant variants in 5.5% of 182 patients who were culture positive and for whom adequate data were obtained (Table 5) (123). The resistant variants were all influenza A, typically detected on day 6, and were not recovered on day 10. The clinical course of oseltamivir-treated patients who shed resistant variants has not differed appreciably from those who did not shed such variants (117, 123). Another Japanese study of mostly hospitalized children that utilized molecular techniques for detection of resistant clones found that 18% of 50 influenza A(H3N2)-infected children harbored viruses with NA mutations conferring resistance (124). The viruses with NA mutations fully replaced the wild-type in three cases and co-existed with wild-type in six others; they emerged as early as on day 4 of the treatment, persisted to day 7, and appeared to be associated with more prolonged shedding. The use of weight-based dosing for children in Japan, as contrasted with unit dosing in most countries, is associated with lower drug exposure in young children and has been postulated to be a major factor in the higher frequency of resistance detected in these studies. However, a recent study found the His274Tyr mutation emerge in 3(27%) of 11 A(H1N1)-infected children receiving weight-adjusted doses (125), although the frequencies of influenza A/H3N2 and B virus resistance detection were low in this trial (Table 4). The higher frequency of resistance emergence in young children, likely experiencing their first or second influenza infection, may be relevant to the expected frequency of resistance during NA inhibitor use in a pandemic or outbreak due to a novel virus (124).

3.3.2 Immunocompromised Hosts

Several case reports have documented the emergence of NA resistance in highly immunocompromised hosts with influenza but the risk has not been well defined. During several weeks of therapy with inhaled zanamivir, one 18-month-old bone marrow transplant recipient had prolonged shedding of an influenza B virus, first with an HA mutation (Thr198Ile) that reduced affinity for human cell receptors and altered antigenicity and later with a dual variant that also possessed an NA catalytic site mutation (Arg152Lys) conferring 1,000-fold reduction in neuraminidase susceptibility by enzyme inhibition assay (126). Of note, the later isolate showed a tenfold increase in susceptibility to zanamivir in several cell cultures, a finding that demonstrates the unreliability of cell culture-based phenotypic assays. A 23-year-old male who underwent bone marrow transplantation for acute lymphocytic leukemia documented persistent influenza A infection of the upper respiratory tract for 18 months despite sequential courses of amantadine, oseltamivir, rimantadine, and ultimately zanamivir (45). An influenza A(H1N1) isolate with dual resistance to M2 inhibitors and oseltamivir, but not zanamivir, and possessing an His274Tyr substitution in NA was documented for the last six months of his life. Several immunocompromised patients have experienced emergence of influenza A(H3N2) viruses harboring both Glu119Val in NA and M2 inhibitor resistance mutations, perhaps fostered by sequential antiviral therapy (127, 128). One of these patients died with continued replication of dually resistant virus, whereas two others survived, including one who had persistent excretion of resistant virus for eight months after cessation of oseltamivir (128). In addition, one instance of apparent failure of oseltamivir prophylaxis for influenza B with subsequent emergence of a resistant variant with an Asp198Asn has been reported (127). Quasi-species of resistant and susceptible subpopulations may be present. However, the frequency of resistance emergence is undefined in such patients, and oseltamivir appears to be a useful therapy in most immunocompromised patients (129, 129a). One prospective study of 38 bone marrow transplant patients with acute influenza treated with oseltamivir, including 12 before engraftment, reported only two episodes of pneumonia and no influenza-related deaths (129). Antigen positivity was detected for 7 days or more in 8% of those treated but no resistance studies were performed. Oseltamivir is also active in an immunocompromised SCID mouse model, although resistant variants arise in some treated animals (129b). In a study of seven bone marrow transplant patients given

inhaled zanamivir, treatment was continued until excretion of virus ceased (median 15 days, range 5–44 days) (130); despite four presenting with evidence for lower respiratory involvement, symptoms resolved promptly and no influenza mortality occurred. Careful virologic monitoring of immunocompromised hosts treated with anti-influenza agents is warranted to document clearance of infection.

3.4 Transmissibility of Resistant Variants

Human to-human transmission of NA inhibitor resistant variants appeared to be rare until the 2007–2008 season, although the number of studies examining this question was small and the surveys of community isolates discussed above show the potential. One study during an influenza B epidemic in Japan provided strong epidemiologic and virologic evidence for transmission of oseltamivir-resistant variants among siblings in three households (100). However, in contrast to M2 inhibitors, oral oseltamivir and inhaled zanamivir are both effective for postexposure prophylaxis of influenza in household settings, whether the ill index cases are treated or not with the same drug (Table 3). However, the oseltamivir-resistant A(H1N1) viruses with His274Tyr mutation spread efficiently during the 2007–2009 seasons and caused household transmission and several nosocomial outbreaks (6).

The reduced fitness and replication competence of certain NA mutations appears to correlate with reduced transmissibility in animal models. One study inoculated ferrets intranasally with comparable infectious doses of a clinical isolate of wild-type influenza A/Sydney/5/97(H3N2) virus or its oseltamivir-resistant variant containing the Arg292Lys substitution and found that the mutant virus was associated with lower infectivity (50% versus 100%), 10- to 100-fold lower nasal viral titers, and lack of transmission to susceptible contact animals, in contrast to 100% transmission with wild-type virus (131). One donor ferret inoculated with the Arg292Lys-containing resistant virus transmitted wild-type virus to several contacts, but it is unclear whether this resulted from reversion of the resistant variant, emergence of a wild-type subpopulation, or cross-contamination during the experiment. In contrast, similar studies with an influenza A(H3N2) virus possessing the Glu119Val resistance substitution found that the variant was as transmissible as the parental, wild-type virus and resulted in comparable nasal viral titers in both donor and recipient animals (132). In guinea pigs recombinant human influenza A/H3N2 viruses with the Glu119Val or dual Glu119Val and Iso222Val mutations had similar infectivity as wild-type and were transmitted efficiently by direct contact; however, in contrast to wild-type virus, the oseltamivir-resistant viruses transmitted poorly or not at all by aerosol (132a). An influenza A(H1N1)

Table 6 Effects of NA mutations that confer oseltamivir resistance on viral fitness measures in representative influenza A and B viruses

Virus (subtype) (reference)	Mutation	Enzyme activity or stability (% of parental virus)	Infectivity in mice/ ferret	Replication in ferret	Transmissibility in ferret
A/Wuhan/359/95(H3N2) Yen et al. (83) A/Wuhan-like/98(H3N2) Herlocher et al. (132)	Glu119Val	↓	↓/–[a]	–	–
A/Wuhan/359/95(H3N2) Yen et al. (83) A/Sydney/5/97(H3N2) Herlocher et al. (131); Carr et al. (133)	Arg292Lys	↓↓ (2%)	↓ (>100-fold) / ↓ (>100-fold)	↓↓ Reversion to wild-type observed	0 or ↓↓
A/Texas/36/91(H1N1) Ives et al. (135) A/New Caledonia-like/01(H1N1) Herlocher et al. (132)	His 274 Tyr	–	↓ (>1,000-fold) / ↓ (>100-fold)	– or ↓[b]	– (1–2 day delay)
A/WSN/33(H1N1) Abed et al. (104)	His 274 Tyr	NR	–/NR	NR	NR
	Asn294Ser	NR	↓/NR	NR	NR
A/Puerto Rico/8/34(H1N1) Yen et al. (136)	His274Tyr	↓[c]	–/NR	NR	NR
	Asn294Ser	↓[c]	–/NR	NR	NR
A/Hanoi/30408/05(H5N1) Le et al. (120) A/Vietnam/1203/04(H5N1) Yen et al. (136)	His274Tyr	↓	–/–	↓	NR
	Asn294Ser	↓	–/–	NR	NR
B/Rochester/02/2001 Mishin et al. (89)	Asp198Asn	NR	NR	–	NR
B/Memphis/20/96 Gubareva et al. (126) B/Beijing/1/87 Jackson et al. (139)	Arg152Lys	↓↓ (3–5%)	NR / ↓	↓	NR

– no change compared to wild-type; ↓ decreased; *O* absent; *NR* not reported

[a] One ferret study reported that infectivity was decreased at least 100- to 1,000-fold, and the resistant variant reverted to wild-type (175) but another study indicate full retention of replication and transmissibility in ferrets (132)

[b] Differing results from two studies with different A(H1N1) viruses

[c] Despite reductions, the A(H5N1) neuraminidase retained high levels of enzymatic activity that greatly exceeded that of A/PR8(H1N1) virus (136)

harboring the His274Tyr mutation required a 100-fold higher inoculum to infect donor ferrets, but once infected, they transmitted infection to contact animals with a delay of 1–3 days compared to wild-type virus. These studies indicate that the degree of compromise in transmissibility varies with the particular NA mutation and ranges from the severely to the minimally compromised. The oseltamivir-resistant A(H1N1) viruses that have extensively transmitted during the 2007–2008 season remain to be studied in such models.

3.5 Pathogenicity

The highly conserved nature of the NA enzyme active site and the lack of circulating influenza strains in which NA is absent are postulated reasons that NA mutations would likely reduce the biologic fitness of the virus (95, 117). Detailed studies of the infectivity and virulence of clinical isolates possessing different NA mutations have been con-ducted in experimentally infected animals. Most, but not all, of these NA variants show markedly reduced enzyme activity or stability and reduced fitness in animals compared to their drug-susceptible parents (Table 6). An influenza B virus with an Arg152Lys mutation showed only 3–5% of the enzymatic activity of its parent and was less infectious and associated with lower nasal viral titers in infected animals (126). Even when inoculated into ferrets at an infectious dose ratio of 60:1 (mutant:parent), the susceptible parent outgrew the mutant in the absence, but not in the presence, of zanamivir treatment. An A/Sydney/5/97(H3N2) virus containing a Arg292Lys substitution, replicated as well as a wild-type in MDCK cell culture but showed approximately 100-fold reduced infectivity and 10- to 1,000-fold lower lung viral titers in experimentally infected mice (133). In ferrets the resistant variant was approximately 100-fold less infectious than the wild-type and was associated with significantly lower nasal viral titers, nasal inflammatory cell counts, and for lower viral inocula, febrile responses. Similarly, an A/Victoria/3/75(H3N2) variant possessing both the Arg292Lys mutation and hemagglutinin substitutions was about 10,000-fold less infectious in mice (134). In comparison, an influenza A(H3N2) with the Glu119Val mutation appears to replicate to comparable levels and cause similar febrile responses compared to its respective parental viruses (132) (Table 6).

Oseltamivir-resistant A(H1N1) viruses that circulated in the 2007–2008 season replicated in vitro as well as susceptible strains (134a) and caused typical influenza illness including complications, hospitalizations, fatalities in previously healthy and high-risk hosts (6, 104a). Findings with clinical isolates of influenza A(H1N1) virus possessing the His274Tyr mutation have varied in animal model studies (Table 6). One found that an A/Texas/36/91(H1N1) variant replicated less well in MDCK cell culture and that its infectivity and/or replication were severely compromised in mice and ferrets (135) (Table 6). In addition, inocula that resulted in comparable levels of replication in the upper respiratory tract were associated with reduced nasal inflammatory cell and febrile responses in ferrets compared to the wild-type virus. In contrast, a study of an A/New Caledonia(H1N1) variant found that, although less infectious for ferrets, infected animals had similar nasal viral titers and febrile responses as those infected with the wild-type virus (132). A laboratory virus A/WSN(H1N1) genetically engineered to posses the His274Tyr mutation was as virulent and replication competent in mice as the parental virus (104). However, a clone from a clinical H5N1 isolate with this mutation grew less well in ferrets (>10-fold reduction in lung titers) and was less pathogenic compared to an oseltamivir susceptible clone (120). Of note, while oseltamivir inhibited replication of the susceptible virus in the ferret model, it had no effect on replication of resistant virus. As predicted by in vitro susceptibility testing, zanamivir was inhibitory for both viruses. However, studies of another clade 1 A(H5N1) virus harboring the His274Tyr mutation found no differences in viral replication levels or lethality compared to susceptible, wild-type virus in mice (136).

The Asn294Ser mutation has been recognized in both N2 and N1-containing viruses; it is associated with much greater loss of in vitro susceptibility in N2 than N1 viruses but retains susceptibility to zanamivir (104, 120). For one laboratory adapted A(H1N1) virus, this mutation has been associated with reduced replication in cell culture and in mice, as well as reduced lethality in mice (104). Lower infectivity, replication, and pathogenicity for ferrets has been reported following infection by an A(H3N2) virus with this mutation (presented by J Oxford, 9th ISRVI, Hong Kong, March 2007). Studies of an A(H5N1) virus with this mutation indicated no reduction in pulmonary viral replication or lethality in mice (136).

3.6 Treatment Alternatives

The patterns of NA inhibitor cross-resistance vary by virus type and subtype, such that zanamivir retains inhibitory generally activity for the most common resistant variants that emerge during therapeutic use of oseltamivir. Zanamivir is fully inhibitory for oseltamivir-resistant variants possessing the Glu119Val substitution in N2 or His274Tyr or Asn294Ser in N1 (87, 104). Depending on the virus and assay, zanamivir is partially inhibitory for resistant variants with Arg292Lys substitution in N2, in that the loss of susceptibility is about 5- to 25-fold compared to the wild type (83, 87, 89, 104, 138). Inhaled zanamivir has been used in treating immunocompromised hosts (130), including a few who had virologic failure on oseltamivir (104a, 138), but it has not been systematically studied in oseltamivir-resistant infections. Patients with pneumonia may not respond (138a). Oseltamivir is not inhibitory for the Arg152Lys mutation in influenza B NA that confers reduced susceptibility to zanamivir (139).

Parenterally administered NA inhibitors are under clinical investigation at present. Of note, zanamivir is highly active after intravenous administration (140), which provides peak plasma concentrations that are approximately 100-fold higher than those achieved after oral oseltamivir administration. Peramivir retains at least partial inhibitory activity against many variants with oseltamivir resistance mutations (103) and has been shown to be active after intravenous or intramuscular injection in animal models of influenza (137, 141), including infections due to A(H5N1) viruses (142). Phase 2 human trials of parenteral peramivir are in progress (69a). Other NA inhibitors inhibitory for most oseltamivir-resistant variants and zanamivir dimers that have prolonged duration of antiviral effect after topical application are currently under development (143). These may provide NA inhibitor prevention and perhaps treatment alternatives in the future.

Because of their differing mechanism of antiviral action, M2 inhibitors generally retain activity against influenza A viruses resistant to NA inhibitors and would be appropriate agents for prophylaxis or treatment of suspected NA inhibitor-resistant infections, if the circulating strain was known to be susceptible. Ribavirin would also be expected to be inhibitory for influenza A and B viruses resistant to the NA inhibitors, but there are no reports of its use in human influenza infections due to such variants. Ribavirin combined with a neuraminidase inhibitor exerts additive to synergistic antiviral activity in vitro (144, 145). In mice experimentally infected with influenza A, the combination of orally administered ribavirin and peramivir was associated with improved survival relative to ribavirin alone but not to peramivir alone (144). A combination of ribavirin and oseltamivir was no more effective than ribavirin alone against a lethal influenza A(H1N1) infection but superior to single agents against influenza B (146), whereas this combination showed additive effects against two highly pathogenic H5N1 influenza viruses in mice (114a). Further studies of such ribavirin-NA inhibitor combinations are warranted to determine whether this strategy offers the possibility of treating severe influenza, particularly that due to M2 inhibitor-resistant viruses.

4 Modeling Studies

Various mathematical models have been developed to estimate the emergence and transmission of drug-resistant influenza viruses and the associated implications for antiviral effectiveness (147–150). At the population level, the transmission fitness of resistant variants is the key determinant of their impact, in addition to the frequency of resistance emergence (148, 149). In addition to out-competing the wild-type virus in the presence of selective drug pressure, substantial transmission of resistant variants would require that their absolute transmissibility be sufficient to enable sustained spread. During seasonal influenza, even high rates of oseltamivir use are predicted to not cause substantial resistance transmission in the community as long as viral fitness is compromised (151). When this model assumed a 10% relative transmissibility of oseltamivir-resistant variants compared to the wild-type virus, even extensive use of oseltamivir for treatment (40% coverage of ill persons) resulted in low levels of resistant variants circulating in the community after several seasons of use (151). A closed population outbreak model predicted that the combination of antiviral treatment and prophylaxis would reduce the total number of infected persons but increase the fraction of resistant infections compared to treatment only of ill persons (149). Some of these models have attempted to determine the importance of drug resistance emergence by making linkages between viral replication dynamics at the individual level and transmission of resistant virus in particular populations (152, 153). Resistance emergence at the individual level depends strongly on specific within-host dynamics of influenza infections, including viral mutation rate, the fitness costs of resistance mutations, and the effects of host immune responses and antiviral administration on replication.

In a pandemic scenario, the ability of antiviral interventions to lower attack rates depends heavily on the magnitude of antiviral effectiveness, the timing of their application, the fitness costs, if any, of resistance and development of compensatory mutations (153a). Very early antiviral treatment, particularly prophylaxis, would be predicted to reduce the risk of resistance emergence in some models (152, 153). However, even very low rates of resistance emergence in persons receiving antiviral treatment or prophylaxis would strongly promote the spread of resistant

variants in a pandemic (150). Prophylaxis, by eliminating competition from drug-susceptible virus, might increase substantially the number of resistant cases, if resistant variants have sufficient transmission fitness (149, 150). The extent of antiviral use is predicted to affect the extent of resistance transmission, in part because inhibiting the spread of drug-susceptible strains with antiviral interventions in the absence of an effective vaccine would keep a pool of susceptibles to resistant strains. Modeling predicts that when two drugs are available, allocating different drugs to cases and contacts is likely to be most effective at constraining resistance emergence (147). Resistance concerns indicate the importance of stockpile diversification.

However, many assumptions used in these models have been based primarily on observations from experimental influenza infections of immunocompetent young adults and sometimes animals, so that they require validation by studies in seasonal influenza, whenever possible. Furthermore, their predictive values in pandemic influenza are uncertain. For example, in a pandemic the emergence of resistant variants that are transmissible is more likely with a higher intrinsic reproduction number (R_0) of the wild-type virus (152). In addition, it is possible that an initially less fit resistant variant will acquire further compensatory mutations that would allow it to replicate as well as be a susceptible, wild-type virus in the absence of selective drug pressure. The recent experiences with widespread circulation of M2 inhibitor-resistant A(H3N2) and A(H1N1) viruses and of oseltamivir-resistant A(H1N1) viruses underline this potential.

5 Implications and Future Research Directions

The available evidence indicates that future pandemic and epidemic influenza A viruses may show de novo resistance to M2 inhibitors, whereas it is much less likely that such a strain would show primary resistance to NA inhibitors (1). Of concern, M2 inhibitor resistance has been documented in high frequencies of recent A(H3N2) and A(H1N1) clinical isolates, selected swine isolates resulting in human infection, and in many recent human isolates of avian influenza A(H5N1) viruses. Furthermore, the frequency of resistance emergence during therapy is substantially higher with M2 inhibitors than NA inhibitors and, for both classes, is higher in children than adults. Higher frequencies of antiviral resistance emergence would be expected in treatment of pandemic compared to interpandemic influenza. However, the recent circulation of oseltamivir-resistant A(H1N1) viruses in the absence of selective drug pressure highlights the uncertainty with regard to future neuraminidase inhibitor susceptibility patterns. Thus, the clinical and epidemiologic implications of antiviral resistance in a future pandemic influenza virus cannot be predicted with confidence, and mechanisms to rapidly monitor the susceptibility patterns of circulating strains are needed to guide recommendations for antiviral use in both seasonal and pandemic influenza.

5.1 Current Clinical Use of Antivirals

Because of high antiviral resistance frequencies in epidemic influenza A strains, M2 inhibitors are not reliable for prophylaxis or treatment at present. They remain valuable agents for prophylaxis of influenza A illness, providing that the circulating strain is likely to be susceptible, and are an option for treatment of oseltamivir-resistant A(H1N1) illnesses when zanamivir cannot be used, as with recently circulating oseltamivir-resistant A(H1N1) viruses. They are also an option for combined treatment with NA inhibitors in serious infections when the locally circulating strains are susceptible. This strategy also applies for A(H5N1) virus infections (63, 63a, 154).

M2 and NA inhibitors retain activity against variants resistant to the other class, although dual resistance has emerged in highly immunocompromised hosts. Consequently, NA inhibitors can be used for treatment and prevention of M2 inhibitor-resistant virus infections and, when circulating strains are M2 inhibitor susceptible, vice versa. While M2 inhibitor resistance confers resistance to all drugs in this class, NA inhibitor resistance patterns vary with drug and virus type/subtype, such that zanamivir retains activity for many, including His274Tyr and Asn294Ser in N1, Glu119Val in N2, and Iso222Thr in B, but not all oseltamivir-resistant variants. Several influenza B (e.g., Asp198Asn, Asp198Asn, Arg152Lys) and A/N1 (Tyr155His) mutations result in cross-resistance, and the Arg292Lys mutation in N2 causes substantially reduced zanamivir susceptibility. Zanamivir is an important alternative for prophylaxis and treatment in uncomplicated illness, especially when resistance to other available agents is suspected. However, the effectiveness of inhaled zanamivir in serious lower respiratory illness including A(H5N1) disease is uncertain, and resistance to zanamivir has also been reported rarely in community isolates of A(H1N1). These uncertainties reinforce the importance of continued monitoring of community isolates to assess whether increasing frequencies of resistance might affect drug effectiveness.

5.2 Future Research Directions

A substantial number of unanswered questions remain regarding antiviral drug resistance in influenza viruses. New NA mutations in N1, N2, and B neuraminidases continue to

be recognized and their associated phenotypic susceptibility and fitness consequences require study (6a, 174). The role of compensatory mutations in the target proteins that enhance viral fitness are not well understood. Further data on the duration and levels of drug-resistant variants in the upper and lower respiratory tract of treated persons, in comparison to those observed in nontreated persons or in those treated with the other class of antivirals would be helpful in predicting the likelihood of transmission and whether there are differences between drug-susceptible and resistant viruses for either M2 or NA inhibitors. From a therapeutic perspective it remains to be established whether alternative dosing regimens or, especially in seriously ill persons, combinations of antivirals might be able to prevent or mitigate the frequency of resistance emergence and improve clinical outcomes. For management of individual patients, particularly seriously ill or immunocompromised hosts, the development of improved assays to rapidly detect resistant variants would enable selection of appropriate initial antivirals for treatment and therapeutic monitoring. Continued surveillance of antiviral susceptibility patterns in human and animal influenza viruses, especially community isolates in countries with higher antiviral use, and for resistance transmission in high-risk epidemiologic settings is needed.

The development of antiviral agents with activity against viruses resistant to currently available agents remains a priority. In addition to the parenteral neuraminidase inhibitors discussed above, other potential inhibitors with activity in animal models, including activity against A(H5N1) virus, include the polymerase inhibitor T-705 (155, 156), neutralizing antibodies (157–159), and the receptor-destroying sialidase DAS181 (160, 161). These approaches are entering into clinical study at present (69a).

References

1. Hayden FG, Monto AS, Webster R, Zambon M. NISN Statement on antiviral resistance in influenza viruses. Weekly Epidemiological Record 2004; 79(33):306–308
2. Russell CA, Jones TC, Barr IG et al. The global circulation of seasonal influenza A (H3N2) viruses. science 2008; 320(5874): 340–346
3. Rambaut A, Pybus OG, Nelson MI, Viboud C, Taubenberger JK, Holmes EC. The genomic and epidemiological dynamics of human influenza A virus. Nature 2008; 453:615–619
4. Bright RA, Medina Mj, Xu X et al. Incidence of adamantane resistance among influenza A (H3N2) viruses isolated worldwide from 1994 to 2005: a cause for concern. The Lancet 2005; 366:1175–1181
5. Bright RA, Shay DK, Shu B, Cox NJ, Klimov AI. Adamantane resistance among influenza A viruses isolated early during the 2005–2006 influenza season in the United States. JAMA: The Journal of American Medical Association-Express (online) (doi:10.1001/jama.295.8.joc60020), 295. 2–2–2006.
6. WHO/ECDC. WHO/ECDC Frequently Asked Questions for Oseltamivir Resistance. http://www.who.int/csr/disease/influenza/oseltamivir_faqs/en/index.html. 2008.

6a. Lackenby A, Thompson CI, Democratis J. The potential impact of neuraminidase inhibitor resistant influenza. Current Opinion in Infectious Diseases 2008, 21:626–638

7. WHO Departmentof Communicable Disease Surveillance and Response. WHO Guidelines on the Use of Vaccines and Antivirals during Influenza Pandemics. 2004. http://www.who.int/csr/resources/publications/influenza/WHO_CDS_CSR_RMD_2004_8

8. Hayden FG. Antiviral resistance in influenza viruses – implications for management and pandemic response. The New England Journal of Medicine 2006; 354(8):785–788

9. Cochran KW, Maassab HF, Tsunoda A, Berlin BS. Studies on the antiviral activity of amantadine hydrochloride. Annals of the New York Academy of Sciences 1965; 130:432–43910.

10. Oxford JS, Logan IS. In vivo selection of an influenza A2 strain resistant to amantadine. Nature 1970; 226:82–83

11. Hay AJ. Amantadine and rimantadine – mechanisms. In: Richman DD, editor. Antiviral Drug Resistance. Chichester, England: John Wiley & Sons Ltd, 1996: 43–58

12. Hall CB, Dolin R, Gala CL et al. Children with influenza A infection: treatment with rimantadine. Pediatrics 1987; 80(2):275–282

13. Belshe RB, Burk B, Newman F, Cerruti RL, Sim IS. Resistance of influenza A virus to amantadine and rimantadine: results of one decade of surveillance. Journal of Infectious Diseases 1989; 159(3):430–435

14. Hayden FG, Belshe RB, Clover RD, Hay AJ, Oakes MG, Soo W. Emergence and apparent transmission of rimantadine-resistant influenza A virus in families. New England Journal of Medicine 1989; 321(25):1696–1702

15. Mast EE, Harmon MW, Gravenstein S et al. Emergence and possible transmission of amantadine-resistant viruses during nursing home outbreaks of influenza A (H3N2). Am J Epidemiol 1991; 134(9):988–997

16. Hayden FG. Amantadine and rimantadine – clinical aspects. In: Richman DD, editor. Antiviral Drug Resistance. Chichester, England: John Wiley & Sons Ltd, 1996: 59–77

17. Saito R, Oshitani H, Masuda H, Suzuki H. Detection of amantadine-resistant influenza A virus strains in nursing homes by PCR-Restriction fragment length polymorphism analysis with nasopharyngeal swabs. Journal of Clinical Microbiology 2002; 40:84–88

18. Shiraishi K, Mitamura K, Sakai-Tagawa Y, Goto H, Sugaya N, Kawaoka Y. High frequency of resistant viruses harboring different mutations in amantadine-treated children with influenza. Journal of Infectious Diseases 2003; 188:57–61

19. Saito R, Sakai T, Sato I et al. Frequency of amantadine-resistant influenza A viruses during two seasons featuring cocirculation of H1N1 and H3N2. Journal of Clinical Microbiology 2003; 41(5):2164–2165

20. Ito T, Gorman OT, Kawaoka Y, Bean WJ, Webster RG. Evolutionary analysis of the influenza A virus M gene with comparison of the M1 and M2 proteins. Journal of Virology 1991; 65(10):5491–5498

21. Tumpey TM, Garcia-Sastre A, Mikulasova A et al. Existing antivirals are effective against influenza viruses with genes from the 1918 pandemic virus. Proceedings of the National Academy of Sciences of the United States of America 2002; 99(21): 13849–13854

22. Ziegler T, Hemphill ML, Ziegler ML et al. Low incidence of rimantadine resistance in field isolates of influenza A viruses. Journal of Infectious Diseases 1999; 180(4):935–939

23. Dawson J. Neuraminidase inhibitor and amantadine. Lancet 2000; 355:2254

24. Suzuki H, Saito R, Oshitani H. Excess amantadine use and resistant viruses. Lancet 2001; 358:1910

25. Houck P, Hemphill M, LaCroix S, Hirsh D, Cox N. Amantadine-resistant influenza A in nursing homes. Identification of a resistant virus prior to drug use. Archives of Internal Medicine 1995; 155(5):533–537

26. Simonsen L, Viboud C, Grenfell BT et al. The genesis and spread of reassortment human influenza A/H3N2 viruses conferring adamantane resistance. Molecular Biology and Evolution 2007; 24(8):1811–1820

27. Barr IG, Hurt AC, Iannello P, Tomasov C, Deed N, Komadina N. Increased adamantane resistance in influenza A(H3) viruses in Australia and neighbouring countries in 2005. Antiviral Research 2007; 73(2):112–117

28. Deyde VM, Xu X, Bright RA et al. Surveillance of Resistance to adamantanes among influenza A(H3N2) and A(H1N1) viruses isolated worldwide. The Journal of Infectious Diseases 2007; 196(2):249–257

29. Deyde V, Garten R, Sheu T, Gubareva L, Klimov A. Reply to Saito et al. The Journal of Infectious Diseases 2008; 197(4):632–633

30. Schmidtke M, Zell R, Bauer K et al. Amantadine resistance among porcine H1N1, H1N2, and H3N2 influenza A viruses isolated in Germany between 1981 and 2001. Intervirology 2006; 49(5):286–293

31. Marozin S, Gregory V, Cameron K et al. Antigenic and genetic diversity among swine influenza A H1N1 and H1N2 viruses in Europe. Journal of General Virology 2002; 83(Pt 4):735–745

31a. Olsen CW, Karasin AI, Carman S, Li YCW, et al. Triple reassortant H3N2 influenza A viruses, Canada, 2005. Emerging Infectious Diseases 2006; 12(7):1132–1135.

32. Gregory V, Lim W, Cameron K et al. Infection of a child in Hong Kong by an influenza A H3N2 virus closely related to viruses circulating in European pigs. Journal of General Virology 2001; 82:1397–1406

33. Ilyushina NA, Govorkova EA, Webster RG. Detection of amantadine-resistant variants among avian influenza viruses isolated in North America and Asia. Virology 2005; 341:102–106.

34. He G, Qiao J, Dong C, He C, Zhao L, Tian Y. Amantadine-resistance among H5N1 avian influenza viruses isolated in Northern China. Antiviral Research 2008; 77(1):72–76

34a. Ilyushina NA, Govorkova EA, Russell CJ, Hoffmann E, Webster RG. Contribution of H7 haemagglutinin to amantadine resistance and infectivity of influenza virus. Journal of General Virology 2007; 88:1266–1274.

34b. Writing Committee of the World Health Organization (WHO) Consultation on Human Influenza A/H5. Current Concepts: Avian influenza A (H5N1) infection in humans. N Engl J Med 2005;353:1374–1385.

35. Hien TT, Liem NT, Dung NT et al. Avian influenza A (H5N1) in 10 patients in Vietnam. New England Journal of Medicine 2004; 350(12):1179–1188

36. Peiris JS, Yu WC, Leung CW et al. Re-emergence of fatal human influenza A subtype H5N1 disease. Lancet 2004; 363:617–619

37. Cheung CL, Rayner JM, Smith GJD et al. Distribution of amantadine-resistant H5N1 avian influenza variants in Asia. The Journal of Infectious Diseases 2006; 193(12):1626–1629

38. Hurt AC, Selleck P, Komadina N, Shaw R, Brown L, Barr IG. Susceptibility of highly pathogenic A(H5N1) avian influenza viruses to the neuraminidase inhibitors and adamantanes. Antiviral Research 2007; 73(3):228–231

39. Bean WJ, Threlkeld SC, Webster RG. Biologic potential of amantadine-resistant influenza A virus in an avian model. Journal of Infectious Diseases 1989; 159(6):1050–1056

40. Herlocher ML, Truscon R, Fenton R et al. Assessment of development of resistance to antivirals in the ferret model of influenza virus infection. Journal of Infect Diseases 2003; 188: 1355–1361

41. Hayden FG, Sperber SJ, Belshe RB, Clover RD, Hay AJ, Pyke S. Recovery of drug-resistant influenza A virus during therapeutic use of rimantadine. Antimicrobial Agents & Chemotherapy 1991; 35(9):1741–1747

42. Englund JA, Champlin RE, Wyde PR et al. Common emergence of amantadine and rimantadine resistant influenza A viruses in symptomatic immunocompromised adults. Clinical Infectious Disease 1998; 26(6):1418–1424

43. Klimov AI, Rocha E, Hayden FG, Shult PA, Roumillat LF, Cox NJ. Prolonged shedding of amantadine-resistant influenzae A viruses by immunodeficient patients: detection by polymerase chain reaction-restriction analysis. Journal of Infectious Diseases 1995; 172(5):1352–1355

44. Boivin G, Goyette N, Bernatchez H. Prolonged excretion of amantadine-resistant influenza A virus quasi species after cessation of antiviral therapy in an immunocompromised patient. Clinical Infectious Disease 2002; 34:e23–e25

45. Weinstock DM, Gubareva LV, Zuccotti G. Prolonged shedding of multidrug-resistant influenza A virus in an immunocompromised patient. New England Journal of Medicine 2003; 348(9): 867–868

46. La Rosa AM, Malik S, Englund JA et al. Influenza A in hospitalized adults with leukemia and hematopoietic stem call transplant (HSCT) recipients; risk factors for progression to pneumonia. Abstracts of the 39th Annual Meeting of the Infectious Diseases Society of America, San Francisco, CA, October 25–28, 2001, 111, Abstract #418

47. Lee C, Loeb M, Phillips A et al. Zanamivir use during transmission of amantadine-resistant influenza A in a nursing home. Infection Control & Hospital Epidemiology 2000; 21(11):700–704

48. Tamblyn SE. Antiviral use during influenza outbreaks in long-term care facilities. In: Osterhaus A, Cox N, Hampson A, editors. Options for the Control of Influenza IV. New York: Excerpta Medica, 2001: 817–822

49. Pohani G, Henry B, Nsubuga J. Summary report of the 1999/00 Ontario influenza season. Public Health and Epidemiology Report Ontario 2000; 11(7):136–154

50. Bowles SK, Lee W, Simor AE et al. Use of oseltamivir during influenza outbreaks in Ontario nursing homes, 1999–2000. Journal of American Geriatrics Society 2002; 50:608–616

51. Drinka PJ, Haupt T. Emergence of rimantadine-resistant virus within 6 days of starting rimantadine prophylaxis with oseltamivir treatment of symptomatic cases. Journal of the American Geriatrics Society 2007; 55(6):923–926

52. Hirji Z, O'Grady S, Bonham J et al. Utility of zanamivir for chemoprophylaxis of concomitant influenza A and B in a complex continuing-care population. Canada Communicable Disease Report 2001; 27(3):21–24

53. Gravenstein SMMC, Drinka PM, Osterweil DM et al. Inhaled zanamivir versus rimantadine for the control of influenza in a highly vaccinated long-term care population. Journal of the American Medical Directors Association 2005; 6(6):359–366

54. Iwahashi J, Tsuji K, Ishibashi T et al. Isolation of amantadine-resistant influenza A viruses (H3N2) from patients following administration of amantadine in Japan. Journal of Clinical Microbiology 2001; 39(4):1652–1653

55. Kawai N, Ikematsu H, Iwaki N, Kawamura K, Kawashima T, Kashiwagi S. A change in the effectiveness of amantadine for the treatment of influenza over the 2003–2004, 2004–2005, and 2005–2006 influenza seasons in Japan. Journal of Infection and Chemotherapy 2007; 13(5):314–319

56. Degelau J, Somani SK, Cooper SL, Guay DR, Crossley KB. Amantadine-resistant influenza A in a nursing facility. Archives of Internal Medicine 1992; 152(2):390–392

57. Rahman M, Bright RA, Kieke BA et al. Adamantane-resistant influenza infection during the 2004–05 season. Emerging Infectious Diseases 14(1):173–6, 2008

58. Sweet C, Hayden FG, Jakeman KJ, Grambas S, Hay AJ. Virulence of rimantadine-resistant human influenza A (H3N2) viruses in ferrets. Journal of Infectious Diseases 1991; 164(5):969–972

59. Watanabe T, Watanabe S, Ito H, Kida H, Kawaoka Y. Influenza A virus can undergo multiple cycles of replication without M2 ion channel activity. Journal of Virology 75(12):5656–62, 2001

60. Abed Y, Goyette N, Boivin G. Generation and characterization of recombinant influenza A (H1N1) viruses harboring amantadine resistance mutations. Antimicrobial Agents & Chemotherapy 2005; 49(2):556–559

61. Ilyushina NA, Bovin NV, Webster RG, Govorkova EA. Combination chemotherapy, a potential strategy for reducing the emergence of drug-resistant influenza A variants. Antiviral Research 2006; 70(3):121–131

62. Ison MG, Gnann JW Jr, Nagy-Agren S et al. Safety and efficacy of nebulized zanamivir in hospitalized patients with serious influenza. Antiviral Therapy 2003; 8:183–190

63. Writing Committee of the Second World Health Organization Consultation on Clinical Aspects of Human Infection with Avian Influenza A (H5N1) Virus. Current Concepts: Update on Avian Influenza A (H5N1) Virus Infection in Humans. N Engl J Med 2008;358:261–73.

63a. Ilyushina NA, Hoffmann E, Salomon R, Webster RG, Govorkova EA. Amantadine-oseltamivir combination therapy for H5N1 influenza infection in mice. Antiviral Ther 2007; 12:263–370.

64. Knight V, Gilbert BE. Ribavirin aerosol treatment of influenza. [Review]. Infectious Disease Clinics of North America 1987; 1(2):441–457

65. Smith CB, Charette RP, Fox JP, Cooney MK, Hall CE. Lack of effect of oral ribavirin in naturally occurring influenza A virus (H1N1) infection. Journal of Infectious Diseases 1980; 141(5):548–554

66. Stein DS, Creticos CM, Jackson GG et al. Oral ribavirin treatment of influenza A and B. Antimicrobial Agents & Chemotherapy 1987; 31(8):1285–1287

67. Hayden FG, Sable CA, Connor JD, Lane. Intravenous ribavirin by constant infusion for serious influenza and parainfluenzavirus infection. Antiviral Therapy 1996; 1(1):51–56

68. De Clercq E. Antiviral agents active against influenza A viruses. Nature Reviews: Drug Discovery 2006; 5(12):1015–1025

69. Beigel J, Bray M. Current and future antiviral therapy of severe seasonal and avian influenza. Antiviral Research 2008; 78(1):91–102

69a. Hayden F. Developing new antiviral agents for influenza treatment: What does the future hold? Clin Infect Dis 2009; 48:S3–S13.

70. McKimm-Breschkin JL. Resistance of influenza viruses to neuraminidase inhibitors – a review. Antiviral Research 2000; 47:1–17

71. Tisdale M. Monitoring of viral susceptibility: new challenges with the development of influenza NA inhibitors. Reviews in Medical Virology 2000; 10:45–55

72. Zambon M, Hayden FG. Position statement: global neuraminidase inhibitor susceptibility network. Antiviral Research 2001; 49:147–156

73. McKimm-Breschkin JL. Neuraminidase inhibitors for the treatment and prevention of influenza. Expert Opinion on Pharmacotherapy 2002; 3(2):103–112

74. Boivin G, Goyette N. Susceptibility of recent Canadian influenza A and B virus isolates to different neuraminidase inhibitors. Antiviral Research 2002; 54(3):143–147

75. Hurt AC, Barr IG, Hartel G, Hampson AW. Susceptibility of human influenza viruses from Australasia and South East Asia to the neuraminidase inhibitors zanamivir and oseltamivir. Antiviral Research 2004; 62(1):37–45

76. Sugaya N, Mitamura K, Yamazaki M et al. Lower clinical effectiveness of oseltamivir against influenza B contrasted with influenza A infection in children. Clinical Infectious Disease 2007; 44(2):197–202

77. Kawai N, Ikematsu H, Iwaki N et al. Factors influencing the effectiveness of oseltamivir and amantadine for the treatment of influenza: a multicenter study from Japan of the 2002–2003 influenza season. Clinical Infectious Disease 2005; 40(9):1309–1316

78. Kawai N, Ikematsu H, Iwaki N et al. Zanamivir treatment is equally effective for both influenza A and influenza B. Clinical Infectious Disease 2007; 44(12):1666

79. NISN. Use of influenza antivirals during 2003–2004 and monitoring of neuraminidase inhibitor resistance. Weekly Epidemiological Record 2005; 80(17):156

80. Monto AS, Kimm-Breschkin JL, Macken C et al. Detection of influenza viruses resistant to neuraminidase inhibitors in global surveillance during the first 3 years of their use. Antimicrobial Agents & Chemotherapy 50(7):2395–402, 2006

81. Matrosovich M, Matrosovich T, Carr J, Roberts NA, Klenk HD. Overexpression of the alpha-2,6-sialyltransferase in MDCK cells increases influenza virus sensitivity to neuraminidase inhibitors. Journal of Virology 2003; 77(15):8418–8425

82. Hatakeyama S, Sakai-Tagawa Y, Kiso M et al. Enhanced expression of an {alpha}2,6-linked sialic acid on MDCK cells improves isolation of human influenza viruses and evaluation of their sensitivity to a neuraminidase inhibitor. Journal of Clinical Microbiology 2005; 43(8):4139–4146

83. Yen HL, Herlocher LM, Hoffmann E et al. Neuraminidase inhibitor-resistant influenza viruses may differ substantially in fitness and transmissibility. Antimicrobial Agents & Chemotherapy 2005; 49(10):4075–4084

84. Gubareva LV. Molecular mechanisms of influenza virus resistance to neuraminidase inhibitors. Virus Research 2004; 103(1–2):199–203

85. Abed Y, Bourgault AM, Fenton RJ et al. Characterization of 2 influenza A(H3N2) clinical isolates with reduced susceptibility to neuraminidase inhibitors due to mutations in the hemagglutinin gene. Journal of Infectious Diseases 2002; 186(8):1074–1080

85a. Ilyushina NA, Govorkova EA, Gray TE, Bovin NV, Webster RG. Human-like receptor specificity does not affect the neuraminidase inhibitor susceptibility of H5N1 influenza viruses. PLoS Pathogens 2008; 4(4):e1000043.

86. Chutinimitkul S, Suwannakarn K, Chieochansin T et al. H5N1 Oseltamivir-resistance detection by real-time PCR using two high sensitivity labeled TaqMan probes. Journal of Virological Methods 2007; 139(1):44–49

86a. Carr MJ, Sayre N, Duffy M, Connell J, Hall WW. Rapid molecular detection of the H275Y oseltamivir resistance gene mutation in circulating influenza A (H1N1) viruses. Journal of Virological Methods 2008;153:257–262.

87. Wetherall NT, Trivedi T, Zeller J et al. Evaluation of neuraminidase enzyme assays using different substrates to measure susceptibility of influenza virus clinical isolates to neuraminidase inhibitors: report of the neuraminidase inhibitor susceptibility network. Journal of Clinical Microbiology 2003; 41(2):742–750

88. Wang MZ, Tai CY, Mendel DB. Mechanism by which mutations at his274 alter sensitivity of influenza a virus N1 neuraminidase to oseltamivir carboxylate and zanamivir. Antimicrobial Agents & Chemotherapy 2002; 46(12):3809–3816

89. Mishin VP, Hayden FG, Gubareva LV. Susceptibilities of antiviral-resistant influenza viruses to novel neuraminidase inhibitors. Antimicrobial Agents & Chemotherapy 2005; 49(11):4515–4520

90. Gubareva LV, McCullers JA, Bethell RC, Webster RG. Characterization of influenza A/HongKong/156/97 (H5N1) virus in a mouse model and protective effect of zanamivir on H5N1 infection in mice. Journal of Infectious Diseases 1998; 178(6):1592–1596

91. Leneva IA, Goloubeva O, Fenton RJ, Tisdale M, Webster RG. Efficacy of zanamivir against avian influenza A viruses that possess genes encoding H5N1 internal proteins and are pathogenic in mammals. Antimicrobial Agents & Chemotherapy 2001; 45(4):1216–1224

92. Govorkova EA, Leneva IA, Goloubeva OG, Bush K, Webster RG. Comparison of efficacies of RWJ-270201, zanamivir, and oseltamivir against H5N1, H9N2, and other avian influenza viruses. Antimicrobial Agents & Chemotherapy 2001; 45(10):2723–2732

93. Cooper NJ, Sutton AJ, Abrams KR, Wailoo A, Turner D, Nicholson KG. Effectiveness of neuraminidase inhibitors in treatment and prevention of influenza A and B: systematic review and meta-analyses of randomised controlled trials. British Medical Journal 2003; 326(7401):1235–1239

94. McKimm-Breschkin J, Trivedi T, Hampson A et al. Neuraminidase sequence analysis and susceptibilities of influenza virus clinical isolates to zanamivir and oseltamivir. Antimicrobial Agents & Chemotherapy 2003; 47(7):2264–2272

95. Aoki FY, Boivin G, Roberts N. Influenza virus susceptibility and resistance to oseltamivir. Antiviral Therapy 2007; 12(4 Pt B): 603–616

96. Hurt AC, Iannello P, Jachno K et al. Neuraminidase inhibitor-resistant and -sensitive influenza B viruses isolated from an untreated human patient. Antimicrobial Agents & Chemotherapy 2006; 50(5):1872–1874

97. Hurt AC, McKimm-Breschkin JL, McDonald M, Barr IG, Komadina N, Hampson AW. Identification of a human influenza type B strain with reduced sensitivity to neuraminidase inhibitor drugs. Virus Research 2004; 103(1–2):205–211

98. Mungall BA, Xu X, Klimov A. Surveillance of influenza isolates for susceptibility to neuraminidase inhibitors during the 2000–2002 influenza seasons. Virus Research 2004; 103(1–2): 195–197

99. Ferraris O, Kessler N, Valette M, Lina B. Evolution of the susceptibility to antiviral drugs of A/H3N2 influenza viruses isolated in France from 2002 to 2005. Vaccine 2006; 24(44–46): 6656–6659

99a. Escuret V, Frobert E, Bouscambert-Duchamp M, Sabatier M, et al. Detection of human influenza A (H1N1) and B strains with reduced sensitivity to neuraminidase inhibitors. Journal of Clinical Virology 2008; 41:25–28.

100. Hatakeyama S, Sugaya N, Ito M et al. Emergence of influenza B viruses with reduced sensitivity to neuraminidase Inhibitors. JAMA: The Journal of the American Medical Association 2007; 297(13):1435–1442

101. Lackenby A, Baldevarona J, Democratis J et al. Decreasing sensitivity of influenza B viruses. Abstract Book – Options for the Control of Influenza VI, Toronto, ON, Canada, June 17–23, 2007, 238, Abstract #P930

102. Neuraminindase Inhibitor Susceptibility Network. Monitoring of neuraminidase inhibitor resistance among clinical influenza virus isolates in Japan during the 2003–2006 influenza seasons. Weekly Epidemiological Record 2007; 82(17):149–150

103. Gubareva LV, Webster RG, Hayden FG. Comparison of the activities of zanamivir, oseltamivir, and RWJ-270201 against clinical isolates of influenza virus and neuraminidase inhibitor-resistant variants. Antimicrobial Agents & Chemotherapy 2001; 45(12):3403–3408

104. Abed Y, Baz M, Boivin G. Impact of neuraminidase mutations conferring influenza resistance to neuraminidase inhibitors in the N1 and N2 genetic backgrounds. Antiviral Therapy 2006; 11(8):971–976

104a. van der Vries E, van den Berg B, Schutten M. Fatal oseltamivir-resistant influenza virus infection. N Engl J Med 2008; 359(10):1074–1076.

105. World Health Organization. Influenza A(H1N1) virus resistance to oseltamivir. http://www.who.int/csr/disease/influenza/h1n1_table/en/index.html. 2008. http://www.who.int/csr/disease/influenza/h1n1_table/en/print.html

105a. World Health Organization. Influenza A(H1N1) virus resistance to oseltamivir, last quarter 2007 to first quarter 2008, Preliminary summary and future plans. 2008. http://www.who.int/csr/disease/influenza/oseltamivir_summary/en/index.html

106. Hurt AC, Barr IG. Novel mutations in the '150-cavity' of N1 neuraminidase confer reduced sensitivity to the neuraminidase inhibitors. Abstract Book – Options for the Control of Influenza VI, Toronto, ON, Canada, June 17–23, 2007, 48 Abstract #067, 2008

107. Hurt AC, Selleck P, Komadina N, Shaw R, Brown L, Barr IG. Susceptibility of highly pathogenic A(H5N1) avian influenza viruses to the neuraminidase inhibitors and adamantanes. Antiviral Research 73(3):228–31, 2007

108. Yatsyshina S, Shestopalov A, Evseyenko V et al. Isolation and molecular characterization of the influenza A/H5N1 viruses isolated during the outbreaks of avian influenza among birds in the European part of Russia in 2005: a virus strain with ozeltamivir-resistance mutation was found. Molecular Genetics, Microbiology and Virology 2008; 23(1):31–41

109. Rayner JM, Cheung CL, Smith GJD et al. Naturally occurring antiviral drug resistance in avian H5N1 virus. Abstract Book – Options for the Control of Influenza VI, Toronto, ON, Canada, June 17–23, 2007, 48 Abstract #068

109a. Yen HL, Lipatov AS, Ilyushina NA, Govorkova EA, Franks J, Yilmaz N, et al. Inefficient transmission of H5N1 influenza viruses in a ferret contact model. J Virol 2007 81(13):6890–6398.

110. Saad MD, Boynton BR, Earhart KC et al. Detection of oseltamivir resistance mutation N294S in humans with influenza A H5N1. Abstract Book – Options for the Control of Influenza VI, Toronto, ON, Canada, June 17–23, 2007, 228 Abstract # P909

111. Rameix-Welti MA, Agou F, Buchy P et al. Natural variation can significantly alter the sensitivity of influenza A (H5N1) viruses to oseltamivir. Antimicrobial Agents & Chemotherapy 2006; 50(11):3809–3815

112. Yen HL, Monto AS, Webster RG, Govorkova EA. Virulence may determine the necessary duration and dosage of oseltamivir treatment for highly pathogenic A/Vietnam/1203/04 (H5N1) influenza virus in mice. Journal of Infectious Diseases 2005; 192(4):665–672

113. McKimm-Breschkin J, Selleck P, Usman TB, Johnson M. Reduced sensitivity of influenza A (H5N1) to oseltamivir. Emerging Infectious Diseases 2007; 13(9):1354–1357

113a. Le MTQ, Wertheim HFL, Nguyen HD, Taylor W, et al. Influenza A H5N1 clade 2.3.4 virus with a different antiviral susceptibility profile replaced clade 1 virus in humans in Northern Vietnam. PLoS ONE 2008; 3(10):e3339.

114. Govorkova EA, Ilyushina NA, Boltz DA, Douglas A, Yilmaz N, Webster RG. Efficacy of oseltamivir therapy in ferrets inoculated with different clades of H5N1 influenza virus. Antimicrobial Agents & Chemotherapy 2007; 51(4):1414–1424

114a. Ilyushina NA, Hay A, Yilmaz N, Boon ACM, Webster RG, Govorkova EA. Oseltamivir-ribavirin combination therapy for highly pathogenic H5N1 influenza virus Infection in mice. Antimicrobial Agents Chemother 2008; 52(11):3889–3897.

114b. Boltz DA, Rehg JE, McClaren J, Webster RG, Govorkova EA. Oseltamivir prophylactic regimens prevent H5N1 influenza morbidity and mortality in a ferret model. Journal of Infectious Diseases 2008; 197:1315–1323

115. Thompson CI, Barclay WS, Zambon MC. Changes in in vitro susceptibility of influenza A H3N2 viruses to a neuraminidase inhibitor drug during evolution in the human host. Journal of Antimicrobial Chemotherapy 2004; 53(5):759–765

116. Barnett J, Cadman A, Gor D et al. Zanamivir susceptibility monitoring and characterization of influenza virus clinical isolates obtained during phase II clinical efficacy studies. Antimicrobial Agents & Chemotherapy 2000; 44(1):78–87

117. Jackson HC, Roberts N, Wang Z, Belshe R. Management of influenza Use of new antivirals and resistance in perspective. Clinical Drug Investigation 2000; 20(6):447–454

118. Roberts N. Treatment of influenza with neuraminidase inhibitors: virological implications. Philosophical Transactions of the Royal Society 2001; 356(1416):1895–1897

119. Gubareva LV, Kaiser L, Matrosovich MN, Soo-Hoo Y, Hayden FG. Selection of influenza virus mutants in experimentally infected volunteers treated with oseltamivir. Journal of Infectious Diseases 2001; 183:523–531

120. Le QM, Kiso M, Someya K et al. Avian flu: isolation of drug-resistant H5N1 virus. Nature 2005; 437(7062):1108

121. Menno D. de Jong MD, Thanh TT, Khanh TH, Hien VM, et al. Oseltamivir resistance during treatment of influenza A (H5N1) infection. N Engl J Med 2005;353;2667–2672.

122. Ward P, Small I, Smith J, Suter P, Dutkowski R. Oseltamivir (Tamiflu(R)) and its potential for use in the event of an influenza pandemic. J Antimicrob Chemother 2005; 55(Suppl_1):i5–21

123. Whitley RJ, Hayden FG, Reisinger K et al. Oral oseltamivir treatment of influenza in children. Pediatric Infectious Disease Journal 2001; 20(2):127–133

124. Kiso M, Mitamura K, Sakai-Tagawa Y et al. Resistant influenza A viruses in children treated with oseltamivir: descriptive study. Lancet 2004; 364(9436):759–765

125. Democratis J, Lakenby A, McNally T et al. A prospective study to assess the emergence and transmissibility of resistance to oseltamivir following treatment of children with influenza. Abstract Book – Options for the Control of Influenza VI, Toronto, ON, Canada, June 17–23, 2007, 228, Abstract # P923

126. Gubareva LV, Matrosovich MN, Brenner MK, Bethell R, Webster RG. Evidence for zanamivir resistance in an immunocompromised child infected with influenza B virus. Journal of Infectious Diseases 1998; 178(5):1257–1262

127. Ison MG, Hayden FG, Mishin V, Braciale TJ, Gubareva L. Comparative activities of oseltamivir and A-322278 in immunocompetent and immunocompromised murine models of influenza virus infection. Journal of Infect Diseases 2006; 193:765–772

128. Baz M, Abed Y, McDonald J, Boivin G. Characterization of multidrug-resistant influenza A/H3N2 viruses shed during 1 year by an immunocompromised child. Clinical Infectious Disease 2006; 43(12):1555–1561

129. Machado CM, Boas L, Mendes A et al. Use of oseltamivir to control influenza complications after bone marrow transplantation. Bone Marrow Transplantation 2004; 34(2):111–114

129a. Chemaly RF, Torres HA, Aguilera EA, Mattiuzzi G, et al. Neuraminidase inhibitors improve outcome of patients with leukemia and influenza: an observational study. Clin Infect Dis 2007; 44:964–967.

129b. Ison MG, Mishin VP, Braciale TJ, Hayden FG, Gubareva LV. Comparative activities of oseltamivir and A-322278 in immunocompetent and immunocompromised murine models of influenza virus infection. Journal of Infectious Diseases 2006; 193:765–72

130. Johny AA, Clark A, Price N, Carrington D, Oakhill A, Marks DI. The use of zanamivir to treat influenza A and B infection after allogeneic stem cell transplantation. Bone Marrow Transplantation 2002; 29(2):113–115

131. Herlocher ML, Carr J, Ives J et al. Influenza virus carrying an R292K mutation in the neuraminidase gene is not transmitted in ferrets. Antiviral Research 2002; 54(2):99–111

132. Herlocher ML, Truscon R, Elias S et al. Influenza viruses resistant to the antiviral drug oseltamivir: transmission studies in ferrets. The Journal of Infectious Diseases 2004; 190(9):1627–1630

132a. Bouvier NM, Lowen AC, Palese P. Oseltamivir-resistant influenza A viruses are transmitted efficiently among guinea pigs by direct contact but not by aerosol. J Virol 2008; 82(20):10052–10058.

133. Carr J, Ives J, Kelly L et al. Influenza virus carrying neuraminidase with reduced sensitivity to oseltamivir carboxylate has altered properties in vitro and is compromised for infectivity and replicative ability in vivo. Antiviral Research 2002; 54(2):79–88

134. Tai CY, Escarpe PA, Sidwell RW et al. Characterization of human influenza virus variants selected in vitro in the presence of the neuraminidase inhibitor GS 4071. Antimicrobial Agents & Chemotherapy 1998; 42(12):3234–3241

134a. Rameix-Welti M-A, Enouf V, Cuvelier F, Jeannin P, van der Werf S. Enzymatic properties of the neuraminidase of seasonal H1N1 influenza viruses provide insights for the emergence of natural resistance to oseltamivir. PLoS Pathogens 2008; 4(7):e1000103

135. Ives JAL, Carr JA, Mendel DB et al. The H274Y mutation in the influenza A/H1N1 neuraminidase active site following oseltamivir phosphate treatment leave virus severely compromised both in vitro and in vivo. Antiviral Research 2002; 55:307–317

136. Yen HL, Ilyushina NA, Salomon R, Hoffmann E, Webster RG, Govorkova EA. Neuraminidase inhibitor-resistant recombinant A/Vietnam/1203/04 (H5N1) influenza viruses retain their replication efficiency and pathogenicity in vitro and in vivo. Journal of Virology 2007; 81(22):12418–12426

137. Mishin VP, Hayden FG, Signorelli KL, Gubareva LV. Evaluation of methyl inosine monophosphate (MIMP) and peramivir activities in a murine model of lethal influenza A virus infection. Antiviral Research 71(1):64–8, 2006

138. Gubareva LV. Characterization of influenza A and B viruses recovered from immunocompromised patients treated with antivirals. In: Kawaoka Y, editor. Options for the Control of Influenza V. Amsterdam: Elsevier BV, 2004: 126–129

138a. Medeiros R, Rameix-Welti AM, Lorin V, Ribaud P, et al. Failure of zanamivir therapy for pneumonia in a bone-marrow transplant recipient infected by a zanamivir-sensitive influenza A (H1N1) virus. Antiviral Ther 2007;12:571–576.

139. Jackson D, Barclay W, Zurcher T. Characterization of recombinant influenza B viruses with key neuraminidase inhibitor resistance mutations. The Journal of Antimicrobial Chemotherapy 2005; 55(2):162–169

140. Calfee DP, Peng AW, Cass L, Lobo M, Hayden FG. Safety and efficacy of intravenous zanamivir in preventing experimental human influenza A virus infection. Antimicrobial Agents & Chemotherapy 1999; 43(7):1616–1620

141. Bantia S, Arnold CS, Parker CD, Upshaw R, Chand P. Anti-influenza virus activity of peramivir in mice with single intramuscular injection. Antiviral Research 2006; 69(1):39–45

142. Yun NE, Linde NS, Zacks MA et al. Injectable peramivir mitigates disease and promotes survival in ferrets and mice infected with the highly virulent influenza virus, A/Vietnam/1203/04 (H5N1). Virology 2008; 374(1):198–209

143. Makoto Yamashita M, Tomozawa T, Kakuta M, Tokumitsu A, Nasu H, and Kubo S. CS-8958, a prodrug of the new neuraminidase inhibitor R-125489, shows long-acting anti-influenza virus activity. Antimicrob Agents Chemother 2009; 53(1):186–192

144. Smee DF, Bailey KW, Morrison A, Sidwell RW. Combination treatment of influenza A virus infections in cell culture and in mice with the cyclopentane neuraminidase inhibitor RWJ-270201 and ribavirin. Chemotherapy 2002; 48:88–93

145. Madren LK, Shipman C Jr, Hayden FG. In vitro inhibitory effects of combinations of anti-influenza agents. Antiviral Chemistry & Chemotherapy 1995; 6(2):109–113

146. Smee D, Wong MH, Bailey KW, Sidwell RW. Activities of oseltamivir and ribavirin used alone and in combination against infections in mice with recent isolates of influenza A(H1N1) and B viruses. Antiviral Chemistry & Chemotherapy 2006; 17(4): 185–192.

147. McCaw JM, Wood RG, McCaw CT, McVernon J. Impact of emerging antiviral drug resistance on influenza containment and spread: Influence of subclinical infection and strategic use of a stockpile containing one or two drugs. PLoS ONE 2008; 3(6): e2362

148. Stilianakis NI, Perelson AS, Hayden FG. Emergence of drug resistance during an influenza epidemic: Insights from a mathematical model. Journal of Infectious Diseases 1998; 177:863–873

149. Regoes RR, Bonhoeffer S. Emergence of drug-resistant influenza virus: population dynamical considerations. Science 2006; 312(5772):389–391

150. Lipsitch M, Cohen T, Murray M, Levin BR. Antiviral resistance and the control of pandemic influenza. PLoS Medicine/Public Library of Science 2007; 4(1):e15

151. Ferguson NM, Mallett S, Jackson H, Roberts N, Ward P. A population-dynamic model for evaluating the potential spread of drug-resistant influenza virus infections during community-based use of antivirals. Journal of Antimicrobial Chemotherapy 2003; 51:977–990

152. Alexander ME, Bowman CS, Feng Z et al. Emergence of drug resistance: implications for antiviral control of pandemic influenza. Proceedings of the Royal Society of London – Series B: Biological Sciences 274(1619):1675–84, 2007

153. Handel A, Longini IM, Jr., Antia R. Neuraminidase inhibitor resistance in influenza: assessing the danger of its generation and spread. PLoS Computational Biology 2007; 3(12):e240

153a. Moghadas SM, Bowman CS, Ro G, Wu J. Population-wide emergence of antiviral resistance during pandemic influenza. PLoS ONE 2008: 3(3): e1839

154. WHO. Clinical management of human infection with avian influenza A(H5N1) virus 2007. http://www.who.int/csr/disease/avian_influenza/guidelines/clinicalmanage07/en/index.html

155. Furuta Y, Takahashi K, Fukuda Y et al. In vitro and in vivo activities of anti-influenza virus compound T-705. Antimicrobial Agents & Chemotherapy 2002; 46(4):977–81

156. Sidwell RW, Barnard DL, Day CW et al. Efficacy of orally administered T-705 on lethal avian influenza A (H5N1) virus infections in mice. Antimicrobial Agents & Chemotherapy 2007; 51(3):845–851

157. Lu J, Guo Z, Pan X et al. Passive immunotherapy for influenza A H5N1 virus infection with equine hyperimmune globulin F(ab')2 in mice. Respiratory Research 2006; 7:43

158. Simmons CP, Bernasconi NL, Suguitan AL et al. Prophylactic and therapeutic efficacy of human monoclonal antibodies against H5N1 influenza. PLoS Medicine 2007; 4(5):e178

159. Hanson B, Boon A, Lim A, Webb A, Ooi E, Webby R. Passive immunoprophylaxis and therapy with humanized monoclonal antibody specific for influenza A H5 hemagglutinin in mice. Respiratory Research 2006; 7(1):126

160. Belser JA, Lu X, Szretter K et al. DAS181, A novel sialidase fusion protein, protects mice from lethal avian influenza H5N1 virus infection. Journal of Infect Diseases 2007; 196(10):1493–1499

161. Malakhov MP, Aschenbrenner LM, Smee DF et al. Sialidase fusion protein as a novel broad-spectrum inhibitor of influenza virus infection. Antimicrobial Agents & Chemotherapy 2006; 50(4):1470–1479

162. Valette M, Allard JP, Aymard M, Millet V. Susceptibilities to rimantadine of influenza A/H1N1 and A/H3N2 viruses isolated during the epidemics of 1988 to 1989 and 1989 to 1990. Antimicrobial Agents & Chemotherapy 1993; 37(10):2239–2240

163. Shih S, Lee C, Tsai H, Chen G, Tsao K. Amantadine-resistant influenza A virus in Taiwan. Journal of Formosa Medical Association 2001; 100(9):608–612

164. Saito R, Li D, Suzuki H. Amantadine-resistant influenza A (H3N2) virus in Japan, 2005–2006. The New England Journal of Medicine 2007; 356(3):312–313

165. Saito R, Suzuki Y, Li D et al. Increased incidence of adamantane-resistant influenza A(H1N1) and A(H3N2) viruses during the 2006–2007 influenza season in Japan. The Journal of Infectious Diseases 2008; 197(4):630–632

166. Galbraith AW, Oxford JS, Schild GC, Watson GI. Protective effect of 1-adamantanamine hydrochloride on influenza A2 infections in the family environment: a controlled double-blind study. Lancet 1969; 2(629):1026–1028

167. Bricaire F, Hannoun C, Boissel JP. Prevention of influenza A: Effectiveness and tolerance of rimantadine hydrochloride. La Presse Medicale 1990; 19(2):69–72.

168. Monto AS, Pichichero ME, Blanckenberg SJ et al. Zanamivir prophylaxis: an effective strategy for the prevention of influenza types A and B within households. Journal of Infectious Diseases 2002; 186:1582–1588

169. Welliver R, Monto AS, Carewicz O et al. Effectiveness of oseltamivir in preventing influenza in household contacts: a randomized controlled trial. JAMA: The Journal of American Medical Association 2001; 285(6):748–754

170. Galbraith AW, Oxford JS, Schild GC, Watson GI. Study of 1-adamantanamine hydrochloride used prophylactically during the Hong Kong influenza epidemic in the family environ-ment. Bulletin of the World Health Organization 1969; 41(3): 677–682

171. Hayden FG, Gubareva LV, Monto AS et al. Inhaled zanamivir for preventing influenza in families. New England Journal of Medicine 2000; 343(18):1282–1289

172. Hayden FG, Belshe R, Villanueva C et al. Management of influenza in households: a prospective, randomized com-parison of oseltamivir treatment with or without post-expo-sure prophylaxis. Journal of Infectious Diseases 2004; 189: 440–449

173. Hurt AC, Barr IG. Influenza viruses with reduced sensitivity to the NA inhibitor drugs in untreated young children. Community Drug Intelligence 2008; 32(1):57–62

174. Ferraris O, Lina B. Mutations of neuraminidase implicated in neuraminidase inhibitors resistance. Journal of Clinical Virology 2008; 41:13–19

175. Carr J, Ives J, Tai CY et al. An oseltamivir-treatment selected influenza A/Wuhan/359/95 virus with an E119V mutation in the neuraminidase gene has reduced infectivity in vivo. Abstracts of the II International Symposium on Influenza and other Respiratory Viruses, Grand Cayman, Cayman Islands, British West Indies, December 10–12, 1999

Chapter 70
Herpesvirus Resistance

G. Boivin and W.L. Drew

1 Antiviral Agents for Herpesvirus Infections

Three antiviral agents and a prodrug are currently available for the systemic treatment of human cytomegalovirus (HCMV) infections. Ganciclovir (GCV, Cytovene, Hoffmann LaRoche) is a deoxyguanosine analog and was the first drug to be approved in 1988. Since then, it has remained the first-line treatment for HCMV infections in immunocompromised patients. Upon entry in HCMV-infected cells, GCV is selectively phosphorylated by a viral protein kinase homolog (the product of the UL97 gene, pUL97). Subsequently, cellular kinases convert GCV-monophosphate into GCV triphosphate, which acts as a potent inhibitor of the HCMV DNA polymerase (pol) by competing with deoxyguanosine triphosphate on the enzyme binding site (Fig. 1). Ganciclovir is also incorporated into the viral DNA, where it slows down and eventually stops chain elongation (1–3). Ganciclovir formulations are available for intravenous (IV) or oral administration and as ocular implants for the local treatment of HCMV retinitis. Because of its poor bioavailability (~6%), efforts were made to develop prodrugs of GCV. Valganciclovir (VGCV, Valcyte, Hoffmann LaRoche) is a new valyl ester formulation of GCV exhibiting about 10 times the bioavailability of GCV following oral administration (4).

The other two compounds approved for systemic treatment of HCMV infections are also potent inhibitors of the viral DNA pol. However, owing to their toxicity profiles, they are usually reserved for patients failing or not tolerating GCV therapy. Cidofovir (CDV, Vistide, Gilead Sciences) is a nucleotide analog of cytidine (also called acyclic nucleoside phosphonate) that only requires activation (phosphorylation) by cellular enzymes to exert its antiviral activity (5). Once in its diphosphate form, CDV inhibits the HCMV DNA pol by a mechanism similar to that of GCV (Fig. 1). Foscarnet (FOS, Foscavir, AstraZeneca), a pyrophosphate analog, differs from the two previous antivirals both by its mechanism of action and by the fact that it does not require any activation step to exert its antiviral activity. Foscarnet binds to and blocks the pyrophosphate binding site on the viral polymerase, thereby preventing incorporation of incoming deoxyribonucleotide triphosphates (dNTPs) into viral DNA (Fig. 1) (6). Finally, formivirsen (Vitravene, Novartis) is a 21-nt-long antisense oligonucleotide with sequence complementary to the HCMV immediate-early-2 mRNA that interferes with HCMV replication at an early stage during the replication cycle (7). Its only current indication is for the local treatment of HCMV retinitis in AIDS patients.

In addition to the treatment of established HCMV disease, antivirals have also been used to prevent such symptomatic episodes, especially in transplant recipients. The first strategy, defined as prophylaxis, consists of administering an antiviral to patients during the first 3 months or so after transplantation. The second strategy, referred to as "preemptive therapy", consists of using short courses of antivirals only for high-risk patients on the basis of evidence of active viral replication (e.g., detection of early HCMV antigens such as the pp65 protein or sufficient amounts of viral DNA/mRNA) (8). These preventive strategies have shown efficacy in preventing HCMV disease in both solid organ transplant (SOT) and hematopoietic stem cell transplant (HSCT) patients (9–11). However, some studies suggest that "prevention" may only delay, rather than truly prevent, the onset of HCMV disease in predisposed patients (10, 12–15).

Antiviral agents currently licensed for the treatment of herpes simplex virus (HSV) and varicella-zoster (VZV) infections include acyclovir (ACV, Zovirax, GlaxoSmithKline) and its valyl-ester prodrug valacyclovir (VACV, Valtrex, GlaxoSmithKline); famciclovir (FCV, Famvir, Novartis), which is the valyl-ester prodrug of penciclovir (PCV); and FOS. Acyclovir and PCV are deoxyguanosine analogs that must be phosphorylated by the thymidine kinase (TK) of HSV (UL23) and VZV (ORF36) and then by cellular kinases to exert their antiviral activity (1, 16). The triphosphate forms are competitive inhibitors of the viral DNA pol. In addition,

G. Boivin (✉)
Centre de Recherche en Infectiologie of Université Laval, Québec City, QC, Canada
Guy.Boivin@crchul.ulaval.ca

D.L. Mayers (ed.), *Antimicrobial Drug Resistance*,
DOI 10.1007/978-1-60327-595-8_70, © Humana Press, a part of Springer Science+Business Media, LLC 2009

Fig. 1 Mechanisms of action of currently available antiviral agents with activity against human cytomegalovirus herpesviruses. From (37)

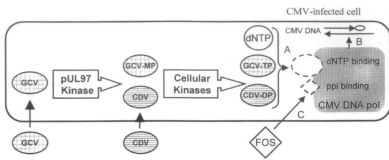

incorporation of ACV triphosphate into the replicating viral DNA chain stops synthesis (1). The pyrophosphate analog FOS is usually indicated for ACV- or PCV-resistant HSV or VZV infections (17, 18). Episodic (short term) or suppressive (continuous) therapy with the deoxyguanosine analogs can be used in the management of recurrent HSV infections (1).

2 Human Cytomegalovirus Resistance

2.1 *Phenotypic and Genotypic Assays to Evaluate HCMV Drug Susceptibility*

Two different albeit complementary approaches have been developed to assess HCMV drug resistance. In the phenotypic method, the virus is grown in the presence of various concentrations of an antiviral in order to determine the concentration of drug that will inhibit a percentage (more commonly 50%) of viral growth in cell culture. In this assay, a standardized viral inoculum is inoculated in different wells. The virus is then allowed to grow for a few days (typically 7–10 days) in the presence of serial drug dilutions before staining the cells. The number of viral plaques per concentration is first determined. Then, the percentage of viral growth, as compared to a control well without antiviral, is plotted against drug concentrations to determine the concentration that will inhibit the growth of 50% of viral plaques (50% inhibitory concentration or IC_{50}). Even though recent efforts have been made to standardize this assay (19), the inter-assay and inter-laboratory variability is still problematic. In addition to the relative subjectivity of this method, there are some differences in the cut-off values defining drug resistance depending on the laboratory. Similar assays, either based on detection of HCMV DNA by hybridization (20) or quantitative polymerase chain reaction (PCR) or the detection of specific HCMV antigens by enzyme-linked immunosorbent assay (ELISA) (21), flow cytometry (22, 23), immunofluorescence (24), or immunoperoxidase (25) have also been developed. Among those, a commercial DNA:DNA hybridization assay (Hybriwix probe system/cytomegalovirus susceptibility test kit) developed by

Diagnostic Hybrids (Athens, Ohio) has shown good correlation with the plaque reduction assay (26–28). Even though the readout method is more objective, cut-off values defining resistance are still a matter of debate. Altogether, phenotypic assays are time consuming, are subject to possible selection bias introduced during viral growth of mixed viral populations in cell culture (29, 30), and may lack sensitivity to detect low-level resistance or minor resistant subpopulations (29, 31).

In contrast to phenotypic assays, which directly measure drug susceptibility of viral isolates, genotypic assays detect the presence of viral mutations known to be associated with drug resistance. Those assays are based on restriction fragment length polymorphism (RFLP) of PCR-amplified DNA fragments or on DNA sequencing of viral genes (UL97 and UL54) that are the sites of HCMV resistance to antivirals. One of the advantages of these assays is that they can be performed directly on clinical specimens (32, 33), thereby reducing considerably the time required to obtain results. By omitting the need to grow the virus, such methods also minimize the risks of introducing a selection bias. The limited number of UL97 mutations responsible for GCV resistance has allowed the development of rapid RFLP assays to detect their presence in clinical samples (34, 35). Indeed, approximately 70% of GCV-resistant clinical isolates contain mutations in one of three UL97 codons (460, 594, and 595) (36). Typically, the presence of a given mutation will either obliterate an existing restriction site or create a new one. The difference in RFLP patterns can then be visualized following gel electrophoresis. The major advantages of this assay include its short turn-around time (2–4 days) and its ability to detect as little as 10–20% of a mutant virus in a background of wild-type viruses (34). However, because of reports of resistance mutations at other codons, DNA sequence of the entire UL97 region involved in GCV resistance should be determined for a comprehensive analysis. For genotypic analysis of UL54 DNA polymerase mutations, DNA sequencing is required because of the large number of mutations reported within all conserved regions of this gene (37). Genotypic approaches are fast but their interpretation is not always straightforward (i.e., discriminating between mutations associated with natural polymorphisms (38, 39) from those related to drug resistance). In order to prove that a new mutation is associated with drug resistance, recombinant viruses need to be generated using either overlapping cosmid/plasmid inserts (40) or by marker transfer experiments of the mutated gene in a wild-type (41–43) or genetically engineered (31, 44) virus prior to testing of this mutant virus in phenotypic assays.

2.2 Clinical Significance, Incidence, and Risk Factors for Drug-Resistant HCMV Infections

Drug resistant HCMV strains first emerged as a significant problem in patients with AIDS. Numerous studies have documented the emergence of drug-resistant HCMV strains (detected by phenotypic or genotypic methods) and their correlation with progressive or recurrent HCMV disease (mainly retinitis) during therapy (Fig. 2) (33, 41, 43, 45–49). The first study to evaluate the prevalence of GCV resistance in AIDS patients was conducted by evaluating the excretion of GCV-resistant strains in urine of 31 patients with AIDS treated with IV GCV for HCMV retinitis. In this study, no resistant isolates were recovered in patients treated for ≤3 months, whereas 38% of those excreting the virus in their urine after more than 3 months of GCV had a resistant isolate, representing 8% of the entire cohort of patients (50). Since then, larger studies have evaluated the temporal emergence of GCV-resistant strains using either phenotypic (26) or genotypic (36) assays. In all studies, GCV resistance (defined by an IC_{50} value ≥ 6 μM) at the initiation of treatment was a rare event (≤ 2.7% of tested strains). Phenotypic evaluation of blood or urine isolates from 95 patients treated with GCV (mostly IV) for HCMV retinitis revealed that 7, 12, 27, and 27% of patients excreted a GCV-resistant strain after a drug exposure of 3, 6, 9, and 12 months, respectively (26). On the other hand, a more recent study of 148 AIDS

patients treated for HCMV retinitis with oral VGCV has identified the presence of GCV resistance mutations in 2, 7, 9, and 13% of patients after 3, 6, 9, and 12 months of therapy, respectively (36). The lower incidence of GCV resistance in the latter study despite the use of sensitive genotypic methods might be explained by differences in the study population, notably improvement in HIV therapy. Owing to their less frequent use in clinic, fewer data have been reported on the temporal emergence of FOS- and CDV-resistant HCMV strains in HIV-infected individuals. One small study found an incidence of phenotypic resistance to FOS of 9, 26, 37, and 37% after 3, 6, 9, and 12 months of therapy using an IC_{50} cut-off value of 400 μM (27), whereas another one reported rates of 13, 24, and 37% after 6, 9, and 12 months using an IC_{50} cut-off value of 600 μM (28). The data on CDV resistance (IC_{50} value ≥ 2–4 μM) are even more limited but they seem to indicate a resistance rate similar to what has been observed with GCV and FOS (27). Proposed risk factors for the development of HCMV resistance in this patient population include inadequate tissue drug concentrations due to poor tissue penetration (e.g., the eyes) or poor bioavailability (e.g., oral GCV), a sustained and profound immunosuppression status (CD4 counts <50 cells/μL), frequent discontinuation of treatment due to toxicity, and a high pretherapy HCMV load (51, 52).

HCMV resistance to GCV appears to be an emerging problem in SOT recipients and has been associated with an increased number of asymptomatic and symptomatic viremic episodes, earlier onset of HCMV disease, graft loss, and an increased risk of death (53). Owing to the different HCMV preventive strategies and immunosuppressive regimens in use at different centers and considering the heterogeneity of the transplant populations, it has been difficult to precisely evaluate the temporal emergence of HCMV resistance in that setting. Lung transplant recipients appear to have the highest incidence of CMV resistance development with rates of 3.6–9% after median cumulative GCV exposures ranging from 79 to 100 days (54–56). In two of those studies, the incidence of resistance increased to 15.8–27% in D+/R− patients (55, 56) and occurred as a late complication, i.e., a median of 4.4 months after transplantation (55). As opposed to what has been reported in lung transplant recipients, the incidence of GCV resistance in other SOT populations has been much lower in D+/R− patients (12, 56) and very rare in R+ subjects (56). More specifically, Lurain and colleagues studied two cohorts of SOT patients including heart, liver, and kidney recipients at two US centers (56). Phenotypic evaluation for HCMV resistance prompted by either clinical suspicion or positive blood cultures indicated that the rates of resistance were generally low (e.g., <0.5%) at one center and varied from 2.2 to 5.6% at another center depending on the transplanted organ. Another retrospective study by Limaye and colleagues evaluated 240 SOT patients including 67 D+/R− patients but

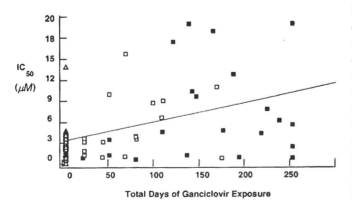

Fig. 2 Relationship between total days of ganciclovir exposure and in vitro antiviral sensitivity of cytomegalovirus (CMV) isolates to ganciclovir in patients with CMV retinitis and AIDS (data from 102 patients). From (45)

excluded lung transplant recipients (12). In their cohort, GCV-resistant HCMV disease developed only in D+/R– patients, with resistance rates of 7% in these patients. HCMV resistance was more frequently seen among recipients of kidney/pancreas or pancreas alone (21%) than among kidney (5%) or liver (0%) recipients. Of note, cases of GCV-resistant HCMV infections occurred at a median of 10 months after transplantation with a median total drug exposure of 194 days (129 days of oral GCV) including two to three treatment courses for HCMV disease per patient. Importantly, GCV-resistant HCMV infections accounted for 20% of HCMV diseases that occurred during the first year after transplantation (12).

The first prospective study evaluating the emergence of GCV resistance in SOT recipients was recently reported by Boivin et al. (57) In this study, molecular methods were used to assess the emergence of UL97 and UL54 mutations associated with GCV resistance in D+/R– patients (175 liver, 120 kidney, 56 heart, 11 kidney/pancreas, and 2 liver/kidney recipients) receiving HCMV prophylaxis with either oral GCV (1 g TID) or oral VGCV (900 mg OD). Among 301 evaluable patients, the incidence of GCV resistance at the end of the prophylactic period (day 100 post transplant) was very low in both arms (0 and 1.9% for the VGCV and oral GCV arms, respectively). During the first year following transplantation, GCV-resistance-associated mutations were found in none compared to 6.1% of patients at the time of suspected HCMV disease after receiving VGCV and oral GCV prophylaxis, respectively. Of note, however, no lung transplant and only a small number of kidney/pancreas recipients were included in the study, which might explain at least partly the low emergence of GCV resistance in this study as compared to previous ones. Interestingly, detection of known GCV resistance mutations was not necessarily associated with adverse clinical consequences in the latter study (57). Documented risk factors for the emergence of GCV resistance in SOT patients include the lack of HCMV-specific immunity (as encountered in the D+/R– group) (58, 59), lung or kidney/pancreas transplantation, longer drug exposure (prophylaxis > preemptive therapy), suboptimal plasma or tissue drug concentrations (as seen with oral GCV), potent immunosuppressive regimens, a high HCMV viral load, and frequent episodes of HCMV disease (12, 53, 55, 60).

Limited data from small-scale studies suggest that the incidence of GCV resistance in the bone marrow transplant (BMT)/HSCT population might not be as high as observed in SOT recipients and AIDS patients, perhaps because of the more limited immunosuppression exposure. In a study published by Gilbert et al., molecular methods were used to detect the presence of the most common UL97 mutations associated with GCV resistance in blood samples of HSCT patients selected on the basis of having a positive HCMV PCR despite ≥14 days of preemptive IV GCV or a second viremic episode within the first 98 days after transplantation.

No UL97 mutations associated with GCV resistance were detected in this cohort of 50 patients (ten of them fulfilling the above criteria for genotypic testing) (61). However, this was a small study and resistance would be unlikely after just a short period of preemptive treatment. In another study designed to evaluate risk factors and outcomes associated with rising HCMV antigenemia levels during the first 2–4 weeks of preemptive therapy, Nichols and colleagues (62) prospectively evaluated 119 HSCT patients receiving preemptive GCV or FOS therapy following a positive pp65 antigenemia test. Among these subjects, 47 (39%) exhibited a significant rise in antigenemia levels despite antiviral administration and 15 had at least one isolate available for susceptibility testing. Only one GCV-resistant isolate was identified in a patient who received 4 weeks of GCV therapy (62). In contrast, Erice et al. (63) reported genotypic or phenotypic evidences of infection with a GCV-resistant HCMV strain in two out of five selected patients who had received GCV for a median of 58 days. However, all five patients had also received ACV prophylaxis for a median of 47 days, which could have predisposed to the selection of a GCV-resistant HCMV strain (64). Of note, the impact of prior ACV in selecting for GCV resistance has not been confirmed by another group (65). Even though short courses of GCV therapy appear to be relatively safe in adult BMT patients, the situation might differ in pediatric patients receiving T-cell-depleted unrelated transplants as reported by Eckle and colleagues (66). In their study of 42 such patients, 3 showed genotypic evidences of GCV resistance, followed by the excretion of a resistant strain after 30–93 days of GCV exposure. Of note, in the same study, none of the 37 patients who underwent a similar procedure, but who received their transplant from a mismatched related donor, developed GCV resistance (66). Rapid emergence of GCV resistance was also documented in 4/5 children with congenital immunodeficiency disorders who underwent T-cell-depleted BMT (67). In those patients, genotypic evidence of GCV resistance was demonstrated after only 7–24 days (median 10 days) of cumulative GCV therapy. Finally, the emergence of GCV-resistant strains has been recently associated with previously uncommon central nervous system HCMV disease and retinitis occurring late after HSCT (30, 68).

2.3 Role of HCMV UL97 and UL54 Mutations in Drug-Resistant Clinical Strains

Cumulative results obtained in three recent studies that have documented the emergence of UL97 mutations in clinical isolates (56, 69) or in blood samples (36) from 61 AIDS and SOT patients are in general agreement with the proposed frequency of UL97 mutations based on characterization of

Table 1 Susceptibility to ganciclovir and UL97 sequence data for clinical CMV isolates

Specimen no	Ganciclovir IC$_{50}$ (pM)	Restriction diagnosis	Sequence diagnosis
179	0.9	Neg	Wt
190	1.7	Neg	Wt
198	1.8	Neg	Wt
177	2.3	Neg	Wt
176	3.0	Neg	Wt
173	3.3	Neg	Wt
195	3.5	Neg	Wt
188	6.0	Neg	Wt
197	6.6	Neg	Wt
180	6.7	Neg	Q520
184	7.2	Neg	Wt
194	7.4	Neg	G596
191	7.6	Δ460, Δ594	V460, V594
193	7.7	Neg	G592
186	7.8	Δ460, Δ594	I460, V594
196	7.8	S595	S595
199	7.8	Δ594	V594
192	8.5	Δ594, S595	V594, S595
189	9.4	Δ460, Δ594	V460, V594
200	9.8	Δ460	V460
201	9.8	Δ460	V460
187	10.1	Δ594	Deletion 591–599 S510
178	10.5	Δ460, Δ594 S595	I460, V594, S595
181	12.4	S595	S595
323	12.5	Δ460	I460
182	12.8	Neg	V591, W595
183	19.0	Δ460	V460
395	19.0	Δ460, S594	I460, S595
175	24.0	Δ594	V594
174	50.0	Δ594	V594

Neg no restriction site change detected; *Wt* wild-type sequence in regions analyzed
From (70)

76 independent UL97 mutants gathered in a single laboratory over years (31). Those data suggest that mutations A594V (30–34.5%), L595S (20–24%), M460V (11.5–14.5%), and H520Q (5–11.5%) represent the most frequent UL97 mutations present in GCV-resistant mutants (Table 1) (70). Other frequent UL97 mutations associated with resistance include C592G and C603W. On the basis of marker transfer experiments, mutations M460V (7×) (34), C603W (8×) (43), deletion of codons 595–603 (8.4×) (71), H520Q (10×) (35), L595S (4.9–11.5×) (31, 34), A594V (10.7×) (34), C607Y (12.5×) (72), and deletion of codon 595 (13.3×) (41) appear to be associated with the highest increase in GCV resistance over the parental strain, whereas mutations C592G, A594T, E596G and deletion of codon 600 seem to confer only modest decreases in susceptibility (31). Interestingly, analysis of the GCV-phosphorylating activity of mutated UL97

Table 2 CMV DNA polymerase (pol) mutations and cross-resistance

Resistance mutations in codons	Drug resistance due to pol mutations
395–540	GCV, CDV
696–845	Foscarnet
756–809	GCV, Foscarnet
978–988	GCV, CDV ± Foscarnet

Since pol mutations are usually accompanied by UL 97 mutations, strains harboring pol mutations are usually resistant to ganciclovir, even when the pol mutation itself does not convey ganciclovir resistance
From (70)

genes expressed in a recombinant vaccinia virus expression system would have predicted mutations H520Q and M460V to confer the greatest decrease in GCV susceptibility (73).

Among the most frequent DNA pol mutations associated with drug resistance, there are V715M, V781I, and L802M conferring FOS resistance and F412C, L501I/F, and P522S conferring GCV/CDV resistance (Table 2) (70). Mutation A809V conferring GCV/FOS resistance has also been reported with some frequency. Importantly, some mutations (E756K, V812L, and del981–982) have been associated with resistance to all three antivirals (44, 74). With regard to the levels of resistance, mutations L501I, K513N, and deletion of codons 981–982 have been associated with a 6- to 8-fold decrease in GCV susceptibility (40, 44, 74) and mutations F412C/V, K513N, and A987G with a 10- to 18-fold decrease in CDV susceptibility (40, 43, 74), whereas mutations D588N, V715M, E756K, L802M, and T821I seem to confer a 5.5- to 21-fold resistance to FOS (40, 42–44, 75). A few UL54 mutations have been studied in marker transfer experiments for their effect on viral fitness. Among those, mutations T700A and V715M (conserved region II) (42), K513N (δ region C) (74), and D301N (Exo I motif) (44) were shown to significantly reduce the yield of progeny virus in cell culture supernatants, whereas some others (D413E, T503I, L516R, and E756K/D) were associated with only a modest attenuation of viral replication (44). In the case of HCMV DNA pol mutants selected during GCV therapy, it should be noted that UL97 mutations have been generally shown to emerge first and to confer a low level of resistance (IC$_{50}$ <30 μM), whereas subsequent emergence of UL54 mutations usually leads to a high level of drug resistance (IC$_{50}$ >30 μM) (76–78).

2.4 When and How to Monitor for HCMV Resistance

HCMV resistance to antivirals should be suspected in patients failing treatment who have been exposed to an antiviral for substantial periods of time (typically >3–4 months of treatment in AIDS patients and after long-term prophylaxis in transplant recipients), especially if some risk factors are present (i.e., D+/R− SOT, lung or kidney/pancreas transplant, AIDS patients with CD4 counts <50 cells/μL). Resistance should be suspected in pediatric patients with shorter periods of drug exposure if they had T-cell depletion. Clinical resistance is more likely if active viral replication (high or increasing levels of DNAemia/antigenemia or viremia) persists or recurs despite maximum IV doses of the antivirals (52, 60). On the other hand, rising antigenemia levels during the first two weeks of antiviral therapy in HSCT recipients have not been associated with antiviral resistance, but rather with host and other transplant-related factors (62, 79). Whenever antiviral resistance is suspected, phenotypic and/or genotypic investigation for resistance should be undertaken. As discussed above, genotypic methods are fast and more convenient and provide useful information for selection of an alternative treatment. However, identification of mutations of unknown significance remains problematic and, for that reason, phenotypic assays may still be necessary. Furthermore, genotypic assays do not quantitate the degree of resistance while phenotypic assays do. The choice of the sample to analyze may also have some importance. Some studies have reported that there is a good correlation between genotypes detected in the eyes and the blood (93.5%) (80) or between blood and urine isolates (87.5%) (77) of AIDS patients with HCMV retinitis. However, there have been at least some reports of resistant HCMV strains restricted to specific body compartments (66, 81). This suggests that resistance assessment based solely on blood or urine samples may be suboptimal in some cases.

2.5 Management of Infections Caused by Resistant HCMV Strains

Resistance is more likely when stable or rising viral loads (especially DNAemia levels) or persistence of clinical symptoms are observed more than 2 weeks after initiating appropriate full-dose IV antiviral therapy. In this context, clinical decisions on disease management should be based on genotypic analysis of UL97 and UL54 genes (when available), the patient's immune status (e.g., high risk D+/R− recipients, lung transplant recipients) and disease severity (i.e., sight- or life-threatening conditions) (51, 60). Despite the limitation mentioned above, genotypic resistance testing is more practical and rapid (results in 72–96 h) than phenotypic assays. Thus, rescue therapy should be ideally based on results of the genotypic assays. In centers where genotypic testing is unavailable or performed infrequently, initial management should avoid the use of drugs with similar pathways of resistance. For instance, patients failing GCV should be given FOS in the absence of any sequencing data due to possible UL54 mutations that confer resistance to both GCV and CDV. On the other hand, if UL97 and UL54

sequencing data are available and indicate that only UL97 mutations are present, then CDV therapy can be attempted. Other empiric options for patients failing GCV therapy could consist of reinducing the patient with higher than normal doses of GCV (up to 10 mg/kg IV BID) or combination therapy with reduced doses of GCV and FOS (82, 83), although these strategies are associated with significant toxicity and can be clinically risky in patients with life- or sight-threatening diseases. Whenever possible, improvement of the patient's immune status (i.e., reduction of immunosuppressive regimen in transplant patients or aggressive antiretroviral therapy in AIDS patients) should also be considered. HCMV viral load should be carefully monitored (once weekly) to quantitate a response to the change in therapy.

3 Herpes Simplex Virus and Varicella-Zoster Virus Resistance

3.1 Phenotypic and Genotypic Assays to Evaluate HSV and VZV Drug Susceptibility

Phenotypically, HSV resistance to ACV is related to one of the following mechanisms: (a) a complete deficiency in viral TK activity (TK deficient), (b) a decreased production of viral TK (TK low producer), (c) a viral TK protein with altered substrate specificity (TK altered), i.e., the enzyme is able to phosphorylate thymidine, the natural substrate, but does not phosphorylate ACV, and finally (d) a viral DNA pol with altered substrate specificity (DNA pol altered). Alteration or absence of the TK protein is the most frequent mechanism seen in the clinic, probably because TK is not essential for viral replication in most tissues and cultured cells (84, 85). However, several reports have demonstrated that at least some TK activity is needed for HSV reactivation from latency in neural ganglia (86–88). The TK phenotype can be determined by the selective incorporation of iododeoxycytidine (IdC) and thymidine into infected cells using plaque autoradiography (89). However, it can be difficult to evaluate residual TK activity in HSV isolates of immunocompromised patients in whom heterogenous populations (TK-competent/TK-deficient) may coexist (85, 90). Recently, the HSV TK gene was expressed in the protozoan parasite *Leishmania*, normally devoid of TK activity, in order to evaluate the role of specific mutations in conferring resistance to nucleoside analogs (91). Although such expression systems do not allow the determination of the resistance levels conferred by a specific TK mutation, they may facilitate the discrimination between resistance-associated mutations and polymorphic alterations. Only approximately 10% of ACV-resistant HSV strains have polymerase mutations (92). Resistance to FOS and to CDV is conferred by specific mutations within the viral DNA pol, which is the ultimate target of all current antiviral drugs. Depending upon the locus of the pol mutation, there may or may not be cross-resistance between ACV, FOS, and CDV (93). At the present time, no simple enzymatic assay has been described to rapidly assess the DNA polymerase activity of alphaherpesviruses.

Levels of drug resistance (IC50 values) are best measured by cell-based (phenotypic) assays. Such assays are more practical in the case of HSV (and to some extent VZV) than for HCMV considering the more rapid replication kinetics of the former viruses. However, HSV resistance cut-offs to ACV have varied in the literature, from 4.4 to 13.2 μM, according to the method selected, i.e., plaque reduction or dye uptake assays, and various other factors (94–98). For this reason, a susceptibility index is said to be a better measure of viral resistance. The ratio of the IC_{50} of the patient's isolate should be 10× or greater than the IC_{50} of a known, sensitive HSV control (99). An alternative to phenotypic assays is genotyping by sequence analysis. For a comprehensive genotypic analysis, the whole TK gene as well as the conserved regions of the HSV DNA pol gene should be determined because of the large number of TK mutations (substitutions, deletions, and additions) as well as DNA pol mutations associated with drug resistance (100). Different systems can be used to generate HSV recombinant viruses and evaluate specific HSV mutations such as transfection of a set of overlapping viral cosmids and plasmids allowing rapid site-directed mutagenesis (93) and the cloning of the viral genome into bacterial artificial chromosomes.

Acyclovir-resistant VZV infections are defined from a clinical point of view by the persistence of lesions after 7–10 days of ACV therapy. Susceptibility of VZV to acyclovir can be tested in plaque reduction assays using fibroblastic cell lines such as MRC-5 (101). The end point for detecting resistance is a susceptibility index of greater than or equal to 4, i.e., the test strain has an IC_{50} greater than 4 times that of a control, known sensitive strain, e.g., the OKA strain. As regards absolute values, three resistant strains from a single series had mean ACV IC_{50} values of 85 μM vs. 3.3 μM for the OKA strain (102). Recently, Shali et al. have developed a rapid phenotypic assay for assessing ACV-resistant VZV strains following expression of the viral TK gene in a TK-deficient bacterium (*tdk* mutant) (103). VZV TK activity can thus be indirectly evaluated by reduction of colony formation in the presence of the nucleoside analog 5-fluorodeoxyuridine (FudR).

3.2 Clinical Significance, Incidence, and Risk Factors for Drug-Resistant HSV and VZV Infections

Antiviral drugs against herpesviruses provide some of the best examples of effective and selective antiviral therapy.

However, drug-resistant viruses have been rapidly selected in the laboratory and also identified in the clinic. Contrasting with HCMV resistance data, no extensive survey has been performed to evaluate the rate of emergence of drug-resistant HSV isolates according to the duration of antiviral therapy. Such study would be a difficult task considering that oral and topical ACV formulations are widely used. Moreover, no uniform agreement has been reached on a standardized method to measure HSV susceptibility to antiviral agents. Thus, it is difficult to compare data from different laboratories and define the true incidence of HSV resistance in specific patient populations.

In immunocompetent hosts, HSV resistance to ACV is not a clinically important problem. Studies have shown that 0.1 to 0.6% of HSV isolates recovered from untreated, prophylaxed, or treated immunocompetent subjects harbor a resistant phenotype to ACV ($IC_{50} \geq 8.8 \mu$M) as assessed by a plaque reduction assay, and this seems to reflect the natural occurrence of TK-deficient mutants in a viral population (104–109). Except for two notable cases (110, 111), the occasional recovery of ACV-resistant HSV-2 from immunocompetent hosts has not been associated with clinical failure and proved to be transient (104). However, ACV-resistant HSV strains are more often isolated in immunocompromised hosts and such isolates have been associated with persistent and/or disseminated diseases (95, 96, 105, 112–117). In the few clinical surveys reported, the rate of ACV-resistant HSV isolates has varied from 4.3 to 14% among all immunocompromised groups (96, 105, 109, 118–120). More specifically, Christopher et al. reported that 6.5% of HSV isolates obtained from patients with cancer were resistant to ACV compared to 10% from heart or lung transplant recipients and 6% from AIDS patients (105). Similarly, Englund et al. showed that 7% of HSV isolates recovered from AIDS patients were resistant to ACV compared to 5–14% from diverse SOT and BMT recipients (96). In another study, 8% of allogeneic cell transplant recipients demonstrated persistent HSV excretion despite ACV therapy, whereas 5% of HSV isolates showed significant level of ACV resistance in vitro (121). Morfin et al. reported that patients receiving either autologous or allogenic bone marrow have a similar incidence, i.e., 9%, of HSV infection but resistance occurred only in allogenic transplants, reaching a prevalence of 30% (100). The severity of immunosuppression and the prolonged use of ACV are considered two important factors for the development of drug resistance. The importance of the severity of immunosuppression is underscored by Langston et al., who studied adult patients undergoing lymphocyte-depleted hematopoietic progenitor cell transplant from HLA-matched family donors (122). All seven evaluable, HSV-1 or -2 seropositive patients reactivated at a median of 40 days post transplant, and the five strains tested were all resistant to ACV. Furthermore, FOS resistance developed rapidly in the three patients treated with this drug (122). Importantly, the prevalence of ACV-resistant HSV isolates has remained stable in immunocompromised patients over the past two decades (105, 109) and there has been no unequivocal evidence of transmission of a resistant HSV strain from person to person.

Sparse data are available regarding the incidence of ACV-resistant VZV isolates in the clinic but some studies have shown that such resistant viruses have been mainly found in AIDS patients with low CD4 cell counts who presented with atypical, disseminated, or relapsing zoster lesions (102, 123, 124).

Only a few FOS-resistant HSV ($IC_{50} \geq 330 \mu M$, or a threefold increase in IC_{50} value compared to the parental susceptible strain) and VZV isolates have been reported in the clinic (125–130). Nine FOS-resistant HSV clinical isolates from HIV-infected subjects in whom ACV and FOS therapy sequentially failed have been described (129). These isolates contained single-base substitutions in conserved regions (II, III, or VI) and in nonconserved regions (between I and VII) of the DNA pol gene. Interestingly, most of these isolates retained susceptibility or, at the most, borderline levels of susceptibility to ACV and CDV (129, 131).

3.3 Management of Infections Caused by Resistant HSV and VZV Strains

With the increased incidence of ACV-resistant HSV infections observed in patients with AIDS and other immunocompromised hosts, several studies have examined the utility of alternative antiviral agents and treatment regimens. Standard doses of IV or oral ACV have no clinical benefit if the HSV isolate is resistant to ACV in vitro. Most ACV-resistant strains isolated from immunocompromised patients are TK deficient and are therefore also resistant to VACV and FCV. In the presence of suspected or confirmed resistance to ACV (or its prodrug VACV), the options are either to switch to high-dose oral drug (e.g., VACV) or intravenous ACV, or to use second-line agents such as FOS or CDV. If lesions do not begin to respond to high-dose oral VACV or intravenous ACV within 5–7 days, one of the other options should be chosen.

Acyclovir-resistant HSV strains remain susceptible in vitro to vidarabine, which is phosphorylated without TK, and to FOS, which does not require phosphorylation for activity. Studies have confirmed that FOS is superior to vidarabine in the treatment of these TK-deficient, drug-resistant HSV infections (18, 132, 133). The dosage of FOS used for the treatment of ACV-resistant HSV infections is 40 mg/kg every 8 h (with reduction in dose for renal dysfunction). Continuous-infusion ACV therapy has been effective in a few patients with severe ACV-resistant HSV infection. Acyclovir has been administered at a dosage of 1.5–2.0 mg/kg/h for 6 weeks, and complete resolution of ACV-resistant HSV proctitis has been reported (134).

Cidofovir, in a 1–3% ointment, is effective in about 50% of patients, when applied daily for 5 days (135). Intravenous CDV 5 mg/kg once weekly has also been effective (136, 137). A final option for topical therapy is trifluorothymidine (TFT) as ophthalmic solution, which may be applied to the affected area three to four times a day until the lesion is completely healed (138, 139).

As with many opportunistic infections in AIDS patients, there is a high incidence of recurrent HSV disease after successful treatment of drug-resistant HSV. Some (but not all) relapses in this setting have been due to drug-resistant strains, suggesting that these mutant viruses are capable of causing latency in the immunocompromised host. Chronic prophylaxis with daily ACV, VACV, FCV, or FOS can be considered in patients who have been treated successfully for drug-resistant HSV, although there are no data to confirm efficacy in this setting. Foscarnet-resistant strains of HSV have been reported, raising concerns over the possible selection for multidrug-resistant HSV with suppressive therapy (129, 140).

Drug-resistant VZV strains have been identified in patients with AIDS. These patients may present with atypical-appearing cutaneous lesions that shed VZV intermittently despite ongoing high-dose antiviral therapy. Such strains have been isolated from patients previously treated with ACV for recurrent VZV or HSV infection, and these strains may be resistant to ACV, VACV, and FCV by the deficiency of the TK enzyme (123, 124, 141). Foscarnet has been shown to be effective in small studies, but as with HSV, cross-resistance between ACV and FOS may occur owing to viral DNA polymerase mutations (130). The intravenous dosage used has been 40 mg/kg three times daily.

4 Conclusions

With the increasing number of immunocompromised subjects and the prolonged administration of antiviral agents, the problem of drug-resistance among herpesviruses is not expected to fade. Clearly, some drug-resistant mutants of HCMV and HSV are pathogenic and can result in significant morbidity and mortality among severely immunocompromised patients. Considerable advances have been made during recent years in our understanding of the mechanisms of herpesvirus resistance, although significant work needs to be done to evaluate the impact of specific mutations on the virus-replicating capacities (fitness) both in vitro and in vivo. It is anticipated that a better knowledge of the molecular mechanisms of drug resistance as well as rapid laboratory methods for detecting viral mutant sequences directly in clinical samples will result in more rational therapeutic strategies. On the other hand, since all currently available anti-herpetic agents target the viral DNA pol, there is an urgent need to develop and evaluate new antivirals with different mechanisms of action. In that regard, a few alternative compounds with broad or selective anti-herpetic activity have been recently described, although none is in a late stage of development (142–144).

In addition to efforts that are being made to develop oral formulation of CDV (145), new compounds with anti-HCMV activity are currently being developed. These drugs belong to different classes that include benzimidazoles derivatives, 4-sulfonamides-substituted naphthalene derivatives, benzathidazine-modified acyclonucleosides, tricyclic inhibitors, indolocarbazoles, and an experimental immunosuppressive agent (146, 147). Among promising candidates, maribavir (1263W94) is an L-ribofuranosyl derivative of BDCRB (benzimidazole derivative) that has been shown to have good bioavailability and toxicity profile in humans (148, 149) associated with a potent inhibitory effect on HCMV replication in vitro (148, 150) and in vivo (151). Maribavir is thought to prevent the exit of nucleocapsids from the nucleus (nuclear egress) and DNA replication by direct inhibition of pUL97 (150, 152), and mutations conferring resistance to this drug have been mapped to this gene (150) as well as the gene UL27 (153, 154). Other promising compounds include another derivative of the prototype BDCRB, the D-ribopyranosyl derivative GW275175X, as well as the nonnucleosidic 4-sulfonamides-substituted naphthalene derivative, tomeglovir (BAY-384766). Both compounds showed good inhibitory activity against HCMV replication (144, 155, 156) and seem to interfere with cleavage of concatameric DNA molecules and encapsidation which involve pUL89 and pUL56, respectively (156).

References

1. Balfour HH, Jr. Antiviral drugs. N Engl J Med 1999;340:1255–1268
2. Biron KK, Stanat SC, Sorrell JB, et al. Metabolic activation of the nucleoside analog 9-[(2-hydroxy-1- (hydroxymethyl)ethoxy] methyl)guanine in human diploid fibroblasts infected with human cytomegalovirus. Proc Natl Acad Sci U S A 1985;82:2473–2477
3. Sullivan V, Talarico CL, Stanat SC, Davis M, Coen DM, Biron KK. A protein kinase homologue controls phosphorylation of ganciclovir in human cytomegalovirus-infected cells. Nature 1992;358:162–164
4. Pescovitz MD, Rabkin J, Merion RM, et al. Valganciclovir results in improved oral absorption of ganciclovir in liver transplant recipients. Antimicrob Agents Chemother 2000;44:2811–2815
5. Cihlar T, Chen MS. Identification of enzymes catalyzing two-step phosphorylation of cidofovir and the effect of cytomegalovirus infection on their activities in host cells. Mol Pharmacol 1996;50:1502–1510
6. Chrisp P, Clissold SP. Foscarnet. A review of its antiviral activity, pharmacokinetic properties and therapeutic use in immunocompromised patients with cytomegalovirus retinitis. Drugs 1991;41:104–129
7. Mulamba GB, Hu A, Azad RF, Anderson KP, Coen DM. Human cytomegalovirus mutant with sequence-dependent resistance to

the phosphorothioate oligonucleotide fomivirsen (ISIS 2922). Antimicrob Agents Chemother 1998;42:971–973
8. Boeckh M, Boivin G. Quantitation of cytomegalovirus: methodologic aspects and clinical applications. Clin Microbiol Rev 1998;11:533–5541
9. Boeckh M, Leisenring W, Riddell SR, et al. Late cytomegalovirus disease and mortality in recipients of allogeneic hematopoietic stem cell transplants: importance of viral load and T-cell immunity. Blood 2003;101:407–414
10. Lowance D, Neumayer HH, Legendre CM, et al. Valacyclovir for the prevention of cytomegalovirus disease after renal transplantation. N Engl J Med 1999;340:1462–1470
11. Paya CV, Wilson JA, Espy MJ, et al. Preemptive use of oral ganciclovir to prevent cytomegalovirus infection in liver transplant patients: a randomized, placebo-controlled trial. J Infect Dis 2002;185:854–860
12. Limaye AP, Corey L, Koelle DM, Davis CL, Boeckh M. Emergence of ganciclovir-resistant cytomegalovirus disease among recipients of solid-organ transplants. Lancet 2000;356:645–649
13. Nguyen Q, Champlin R, Giralt S, et al. Late cytomegalovirus pneumonia in adult allogeneic blood and marrow transplant recipients. Clin Infect Dis 1999;28:618–623
14. Razonable RR, Rivero A, Rodriguez A, et al. Allograft rejection predicts the occurrence of late-onset cytomegalovirus (CMV) disease among CMV-mismatched solid organ transplant patients receiving prophylaxis with oral ganciclovir. J Infect Dis 2001;184:1461–1464
15. Zaia JA, GallezHawkins GM, Tegtmeier BR, et al. Late cytomegalovirus disease in marrow transplantation is predicted by virus load in plasma. J Infect Dis 1997;176:782–785
16. Fyfe JA, Keller PM, Furman PA, Miller RL, Elion GB. Thymidine kinase from herpes simplex virus phosphorylates the new antiviral compound, 9-(2-hydroxyethoxymethyl)guanine. J Biol Chem 1978;253:8721–8727
17. Safrin S, Ashley R, Houlihan C, Cusick PS, Mills J. Clinical and serologic features of herpes simplex virus infection in patients with AIDS. AIDS 1991;5:1107–1110
18. Safrin S, Crumpacker C, Chatis P, et al. A controlled trial comparing foscarnet with vidarabine for acyclovir-resistant mucocutaneous herpes simplex in the acquired immunodeficiency syndrome. N Engl J Med 1991;325:551–555
19. Landry ML, Stanat S, Biron K, et al. A standardized plaque reduction assay for determination of drug susceptibilities of cytomegalovirus clinical isolates. Antimicrob Agents Chemother 2000;44:688–692
20. Dankner WM, Scholl D, Stanat SC, Martin M, Sonke RL, Spector SA. Rapid antiviral DNA–DNA hybridization assay for human cytomegalovirus. J Virol Methods 1990;28:293–298
21. Tatarowicz WA, Lurain NS, Thompson KD. In situ ELISA for the evaluation of antiviral compounds effective against human cytomegalovirus. J Virol Methods 1991;35:207–215
22. Kesson A, Zeng F, Cunningham A, Rawlinson W. The use of flow cytometry to detect antiviral resistance in human cytomegalovirus. J Virol Methods 1998;71:177–186
23. McSharry JM, Lurain NS, Drusano GL, et al. Flow cytometric determination of ganciclovir susceptibilities of human cytomegalovirus clinical isolates. J Clin Microbiol 1998;36:958–964
24. Telenti A, Smith TF. Screening with a shell vial assay for antiviral activity against cytomegalovirus. Diagn Microbiol Infect Dis 1989;12:5–8
25. Gerna G, Baldanti F, Zavattoni M, Sarasini A, Percivalle E, Revello MG. Monitoring of ganciclovir sensitivity of multiple human cytomegalovirus strains coinfecting blood of an AIDS patient by an immediate-early antigen plaque assay. Antivir Res 1992;19:333–345

26. Jabs DA, Enger C, Dunn JP, Forman M. Cytomegalovirus retinitis and viral resistance: ganciclovir resistance. J Infect Dis 1998;177:770–773

27. Jabs DA, Enger C, Forman M, Dunn JP. Incidence of foscarnet resistance and cidofovir resistance in patients treated for cytomegalovirus retinitis. The Cytomegalovirus Retinitis and Viral Resistance Study Group. Antimicrob Agents Chemother 1998;42:2240–2244

28. Weinberg A, Jabs DA, Chou S, et al. Mutations conferring foscarnet resistance in a cohort of patients with acquired immunodeficiency syndrome and cytomegalovirus retinitis. J Infect Dis 2003;187:777–784

29. Gilbert C, Boivin G. Discordant phenotypes and genotypes of cytomegalovirus (CMV) in patients with AIDS and relapsing CMV retinitis. AIDS 2003;17:337–341

30. Hamprecht K, Eckle T, Prix L, Faul C, Einsele H, Jahn G. Ganciclovir-resistant cytomegalovirus disease after allogeneic stem cell transplantation: pitfalls of phenotypic diagnosis by in vitro selection of an UL97 mutant strain. J Infect Dis 2003;187:139–143

31. Chou S, Waldemer RH, Senters AE, et al. Cytomegalovirus UL97 phosphotransferase mutations that affect susceptibility to ganciclovir. J Infect Dis 2002;185:162–169

32. Boivin G, Chou S, Quirk MR, Erice A, Jordan MC. Detection of ganciclovir resistance mutations and quantitation of cytomegalovirus (CMV) DNA in leukocytes of patients with fatal disseminated CMV disease. J Infect Dis 1996;173:523–528

33. Wolf DG, Smith IL, Lee DJ, Freeman WR, Flores Aguilar M, Spector SA. Mutations in human cytomegalovirus UL97 gene confer clinical resistance to ganciclovir and can be detected directly in patient plasma. J Clin Invest 1995;95:257–263

34. Chou S, Erice A, Jordan MC, et al. Analysis of the UL97 phosphotransferase coding sequence in clinical cytomegalovirus isolates and identification of mutations conferring ganciclovir resistance. J Infect Dis 1995;171:576–583

35. Hanson MN, Preheim LC, Chou S, Talarico CL, Biron KK, Erice A. Novel mutation in the UL97 gene of a clinical cytomegalovirus strain conferring resistance to ganciclovir. Antimicrob Agents Chemother 1995;39:1204–1205

36. Boivin G, Gilbert C, Gaudreau A, Greenfield I, Sudlow R, Roberts NA. Rate of emergence of cytomegalovirus (CMV) mutations in leukocytes of patients with acquired immunodeficiency syndrome who are receiving valganciclovir as induction and maintenance therapy for CMV retinitis. J Infect Dis 2001;184:1598–1602

37. Gilbert C, Bestman-Smith J, Boivin G. Resistance of herpesviruses to antiviral drugs: clinical impacts and molecular mechanisms. Drug Resist Updat 2002;5:88–114

38. Chou S, Lurain NS, Weinberg A, Cai GY, Sharma PL, Crumpacker CS. Interstrain variation in the human cytomegalovirus DNA polymerase sequence and its effect on genotypic diagnosis of antiviral drug resistance. Antimicrob Agents Chemother 1999;43:1500–1502

39. Lurain NS, Weinberg A, Crumpacker CS, Chou S. Sequencing of cytomegalovirus UL97 gene for genotypic antiviral resistance testing. Antimicrob Agents Chemother 2001;45:2775–2780

40. Cihlar T, Fuller M, Cherrington J. Characterization of drug resistance-associated mutations in the human cytomegalovirus DNA polymerase gene by using recombinant mutant viruses generated from overlapping DNA fragments. J Virol 1998;72:5927–5936

41. Baldanti F, Silini E, Sarasini A, et al. A three-nucleotide deletion in the UL97 open reading frame is responsible for the ganciclovir resistance of a human cytomegalovirus clinical isolate. J Virol 1995;69:796–800

42. Baldanti F, Underwood MR, Stanat SC, et al. Single amino acid changes in the DNA polymerase confer foscarnet resistance and slow-growth phenotype, while mutations in the UL97-encoded phosphotransferase confer ganciclovir resistance in three double-resistant human cytomegalovirus strains recovered from patients with AIDS. J Virol 1996; 70:1390–1395

43. Chou S, Marousek G, Guentzel S, et al. Evolution of mutations conferring multidrug resistance during prophylaxis and therapy for cytomegalovirus disease. J Infect Dis 1997;176:786–789

44. Chou S, Lurain NS, Thompson KD, Miner RC, Drew WL. Viral DNA polymerase mutations associated with drug resistance in human cytomegalovirus. J Infect Dis 2003;188:32–39

45. Drew WL, Stempien MJ, Andrews J, et al. Cytomegalovirus (CMV) resistance in patients with CMV retinitis and AIDS treated with oral or intravenous ganciclovir. J Infect Dis 1999;179:1352–1355

46. Chou S, Marousek G, Parenti DM, et al. Mutation in region III of the DNA polymerase gene conferring foscarnet resistance in cytomegalovirus isolates from 3 subjects receiving prolonged antiviral therapy. J Infect Dis 1998;178:526–530

47. Smith IL, Shinkai M, Freeman WR, Spector SA. Polyradiculopathy associated with ganciclovir-resistant cytomegalovirus in an AIDS patient: phenotypic and genotypic characterization of sequential virus isolates. J Infect Dis 1996;173:1481–1484

48. Smith IL, Taskintuna I, Rahhal FM, et al. Clinical failure of CMV retinitis with intravitreal cidofovir is associated with antiviral resistance. Arch Ophthalmol 1998;116:178–185

49. Wolf DG, Lee DJ, Spector SA. Detection of human cytomegalovirus mutations associated with ganciclovir resistance in cerebrospinal fluid of AIDS patients with central nervous system disease. Antimicrob Agents Chemother 1995;39:2552–2554

50. Drew WL, Miner RC, Busch DF, et al. Prevalence of resistance in patients receiving ganciclovir for serious cytomegalovirus infection. J Infect Dis 1991;163:716–719

51. Drew W. Cytomegalovirus Disease in the Highly Active Antiretroviral Therapy Era. Curr Infect Dis Rep 2003;5:257–265

52. Nichols W, Boeckh M. Cytomegalovirus Infections. Curr Treat Opt Infect Dis 2001;3:78–91

53. Bhorade SM, Lurain NS, Jordan A, et al. Emergence of ganciclovir-resistant cytomegalovirus in lung transplant recipients. J Heart Lung Transplant 2002;21:1274–1282

54. Kruger RM, Shannon WD, Arens MQ, Lynch JP, Storch GA, Trulock EP. The impact of ganciclovir-resistant cytomegalovirus infection after lung transplantation. Transplant 1999;68:1272–1279

55. Limaye AP, Raghu G, Koelle DM, Ferrenberg J, Huang ML, Boeckh M. High incidence of ganciclovir-resistant cytomegalovirus infection among lung transplant recipients receiving preemptive therapy. J Infect Dis 2002;185:20–27

56. Lurain NS, Bhorade SM, Pursell KJ, et al. Analysis and characterization of antiviral drug-resistant cytomegalovirus isolates from solid organ transplant recipients. J Infect Dis 2002;186:760–768

57. Boivin G, Goyette N, Gilbert C, et al. Absence of cytomegalovirus-resistance mutations after valganciclovir prophylaxis, in a prospective multicenter study of solid-organ transplant recipients. J Infect Dis 2004;189:1615–1618

58. Baldanti F, Lilleri D, Campanini G, et al. Human cytomegalovirus double resistance in a donor-positive/recipient-negative lung transplant patient with an impaired CD4-mediated specific immune response. J Antimicrob Chemother 2004;53:536–539

59. Benz C, Holz G, Michel D, et al. Viral escape and T-cell immunity during ganciclovir treatment of cytomegalovirus infection: case report of a pancreatico-renal transplant recipient. Transplant 2003;75:724–727

60. Limaye AP. Ganciclovir-resistant cytomegalovirus in organ transplant recipients. Clin Infect Dis 2002;35:866–872

61. Gilbert C, Roy J, Bélanger R, et al. Lack of emergence of cytomegalovirus UL97 mutations conferring ganciclovir (GCV) resistance following preemptive GCV therapy in allogeneic stem cell transplant recipients. Antimicrob Agents Chemother 2001;45:3669–3671

62. Nichols WG, Corey L, Gooley T, et al. Rising pp65 antigenemia during preemptive anticytomegalovirus therapy after allogeneic

hematopoietic stem cell transplantation: risk factors, correlation with DNA load, and outcomes. Blood 2001;97:867–874

63. Erice A, Borrell N, Li W, Miller WJ, Balfour HH, Jr. Ganciclovir susceptibilities and analysis of UL97 region in cytomegalovirus (CMV) isolates from bone marrow recipients with CMV disease after antiviral prophylaxis. J Infect Dis 1998;178:531–534

64. Michel D, Hohn S, Haller T, Jun D, Mertens T. Aciclovir selects for ganciclovir-cross-resistance of human cytomegalovirus in vitro that is only in part explained by known mutations in the UL97 protein. J Med Virol 2001;65:70–76

65. Drew WL, Anderson R, Lang W, Miner RC, Davis G, Lalezari J. Failure of high-dose oral acyclovir to suppress CMV viruria or induce ganciclovir-resistant CMV in HIV antibody positive patients. J Acquir Immune Defic Syndr Hum Retrovirol 1995;8:289–291

66. Eckle T, Prix L, Jahn G, et al. Drug-resistant human cytomegalovirus infection in children after allogeneic stem cell transplantation may have different clinical outcomes. Blood 2000;96:3286–3289

67. Wolf DG, Yaniv I, Honigman A, Kassis I, Schonfeld T, Ashkenazi S. Early emergence of ganciclovir-resistant human cytomegalovirus strains in children with primary combined immunodeficiency. J Infect Dis 1998;178:535–538

68. Wolf DG, Lurain NS, Zuckerman T, et al. Emergence of late cytomegalovirus central nervous system disease in hematopoietic stem cell transplant recipients. Blood 2003;101:463–465

69. Jabs DA, Martin BK, Forman MS, et al. Longitudinal observations on mutations conferring ganciclovir resistance in patients with acquired immunodeficiency syndrome and cytomegalovirus retinitis: The Cytomegalovirus and Viral Resistance Study Group Report Number 8. Am J Ophthalmol 2001;132:700–710

70. Drew WL, Paya CV, Emery V. Cytomegalovirus (CMV) resistance to antivirals. Am J Transplant 2001;1:307–312

71. Chou S, Meichsner CL. A nine-codon deletion mutation in the cytomegalovirus UL97 phosphotransferase gene confers resistance to ganciclovir. Antimicrob Agents Chemother 2000;44:183–185

72. Baldanti F, Underwood MR, Talarico CL, et al. The Cys607→Tyr change in the UL97 phosphotransferase confers ganciclovir resistance to two human cytomegalovirus strains recovered from two immunocompromised patients. Antimicrob Agents Chemother 1998;42:444–446

73. Baldanti F, Michel D, Simoncini L, et al. Mutations in the UL97 ORF of ganciclovir-resistant clinical cytomegalovirus isolates differentially affect GCV phosphorylation as determined in a recombinant vaccinia virus system. Antiviral Res 2002;54:59–67

74. Cihlar T, Fuller MD, Mulato AS, Cherrington JM. A point mutation in the human cytomegalovirus DNA polymerase gene selected in vitro by cidofovir confers a slow replication phenotype in cell culture. Virology 1998;248:382–393

75. Mousavi-Jazi M, Schloss L, Drew WL, et al. Variations in the cytomegalovirus DNA polymerase and phosphotransferase genes in relation to foscarnet and ganciclovir sensitivity. J Clin Virol 2001;23:1–15

76. Erice A, Gil-Roda C, Perez JL, et al. Antiviral susceptibilities and analysis of UL97 and DNA polymerase sequences of clinical cytomegalovirus isolates from immunocompromised patients. J Infect Dis 1997;175:1087–1092

77. Jabs DA, Martin BK, Forman MS, et al. Mutations conferring ganciclovir resistance in a cohort of patients with acquired immunodeficiency syndrome and cytomegalovirus retinitis. J Infect Dis 2001;183:333–337

78. Smith IL, Cherrington JM, Jiles RE, Fuller MD, Freeman WR, Spector SA. High-level resistance of cytomegalovirus to ganciclovir is associated with alterations in both the UL97 and DNA polymerase genes. J Infect Dis 1997;176:69–77

79. Gerna G, Sarasini A, Lilleri D, et al. In vitro model for the study of the dissociation of increasing antigenemia and decreasing DNAemia and viremia during treatment of human cytomegalovirus infection with ganciclovir in transplant recipients. J Infect Dis 2003;188:1639–1647

80. Hu H, Jabs DA, Forman MS, et al. Comparison of cytomegalovirus (CMV) UL97 gene sequences in the blood and vitreous of patients with acquired immunodeficiency syndrome and CMV retinitis. J Infect Dis 2002;185:861–867

81. Liu W, Kuppermann BD, Martin DF, Wolitz RA, Margolis TP. Mutations in the cytomegalovirus UL97 gene associated with ganciclovir-resistant retinitis. J Infect Dis 1998;177:1176–1181

82. Mylonakis E, Kallas WM, Fishman JA. Combination antiviral therapy for ganciclovir-resistant cytomegalovirus infection in solid-organ transplant recipients. Clin Infect Dis 2002;34:1337–1341

83. Studies, AIDS. Combination foscarnet and ganciclovir therapy vs monotherapy for the treatment of relapsed cytomegalovirus retinitis in patients with AIDS. The Cytomegalovirus Retreatment Trial. Arch Ophthalmol 1996;114:23–33

84. Morfin F, Souillet G, Bilger K, Ooka T, Aymard M, Thouvenot D. Genetic characterization of thymidine kinase from acyclovir-resistant and -susceptible herpes simplex virus type 1 isolated from bone marrow transplant recipients. J Infect Dis 2000;182:290–293

85. Gaudreau A, Hill E, Balfour HH, Erice A, Boivin G. Phenotypic and genotypic characterization of acyclovir-resistant herpes simplex viruses from immunocompromised patients. J Infect Dis 1998;178:297–303

86. Coen DM, Kosz-Vnenchak M, Jacobson JG, et al. Thymidine kinase-negative herpes simplex virus mutants establish latency in mouse trigeminal ganglia but do not reactivate. Proc Natl Acad Sci U S A 1989;86:4736–4740

87. Tenser RB, Hay KA, Edris WA. Latency-associated transcript but not reactivatable virus is present in sensory ganglion neurons after inoculation of thymidine kinase-negative mutants of herpes simplex virus type 1. J Virol 1989;63:2861–2865

88. Wilcox CL, Crnic LS, Pizer LI. Replication, latent infection, and reactivation in neuronal culture with a herpes simplex virus thymidine kinase-negative mutant. Virology 1992;187:348–352

89. Martin JL, Ellis MN, Keller PM, et al. Plaque autoradiography assay for the detection and quantitation of thymidine kinase-deficient and thymidine kinase-altered mutants of herpes simplex virus in clinical isolates. Antimicrobial Agents and Chemotherapy 1985;28:181–187

90. Sasadeusz JJ, Sacks SL. Spontaneous reactivation of thymidine kinase-deficient, acyclovir-resistant type-2 herpes simplex virus: masked heterogeneity or reversion? J Infect Dis 1996;174:476–482

91. Bestman-Smith J, Schmit I, Papadopoulou B, Boivin G. Highly reliable heterologous system for evaluating resistance of clinical herpes simplex virus isolates to nucleoside analogues. J Virol 2001;75:3105–3110

92. Chibo D, Druce J, Sasadeusz J, Birch C. Molecular analysis of clinical isolates of acyclovir resistant herpes simplex virus. Antiviral Res 2004;61:83–91

93. Bestman-Smith J, Boivin G. Drug resistance patterns of recombinant herpes simplex virus DNA polymerase mutants generated with a set of overlapping cosmids and plasmids. J Virol 2003;77:7820–7829

94. Collins P, Ellis MN. Sensitivity monitoring of clinical isolates of herpes simplex virus to acyclovir. J Med Virol 1993;Suppl:58–66

95. Erlich KS, Mills J, Chatis P, et al. Acyclovir-resistant herpes simplex virus infections in patients with the acquired immunodeficiency syndrome. N Engl J Med 1989;320:293–296

96. Englund JA, Zimmerman ME, Swierkosz EM, Goodman JL, Scholl DR, Balfour HH, Jr. Herpes simplex virus resistant to acyclovir. A study in a tertiary care center. Ann Intern Med 1990;112:416–422

97. Safrin S, Kemmerly S, Plotkin B, et al. Foscarnet-resistant herpes simplex virus infection in patients with AIDS. J Infect Dis 1994;169:193–196

98. Chatis PA, Crumpacker CS. Analysis of the thymidine kinase gene from clinically isolated acyclovir-resistant herpes simplex viruses. Virology 1991;180:793–797

99. Sarisky RT, Crosson P, Cano R, et al. Comparison of methods for identifying resistant herpes simplex virus and measuring antiviral susceptibility. J Clin Virol 2002;23:191–200

100. Morfin F, Thouvenot D. Herpes simplex virus resistance to antiviral drugs. J Clin Virol 2003;26:29–37

101. Fillet AM, Dumont B, Caumes E, et al. Acyclovir-resistant varicella-zoster virus: phenotypic and genetic characterization. J Med Vir 1998;55:250–254

102. Saint-Leger E, Caumes E, Breton G, et al. Clinical and virologic characterization of acyclovir-resistant varicella-zoster viruses isolated from 11 patients with acquired immunodeficiency syndrome. Clin Infect Dis 2001;33:2061–2067

103. Sahli R, Andrei G, Estrade C, Snoeck R, Meylan PR. A rapid phenotypic assay for detection of acyclovir-resistant varicella-zoster virus with mutations in the thymidine kinase open reading frame. Antimicrob Agents Chemother 2000;44:873–878

104. Whitley RJ, Gnann JW, Jr. Acyclovir: a decade later. N Engl J Med 1992;327:782–789

105. Christophers J, Clayton J, Craske J, et al. Survey of resistance of herpes simplex virus to acyclovir in northwest England. Antimicrob Agents Chemother 1998;42:868–872

106. Fife KH, Crumpacker CS, Mertz GJ, Hill EL, Boone GS. Recurrence and resistance patterns of herpes simplex virus following cessation of ≥6 years of chronic suppression with acyclovir. J Infect Dis 1994;169:1338–1341

107. Mertz GJ, Jones CC, Mills J, et al. Long-term acyclovir suppression of frequently recurring genital herpes simplex virus infection. A multicenter double-blind trial. JAMA 1988;260:201–206

108. Boon RJ, Bacon TH, Robey HL, et al. Antiviral susceptibilities of herpes simplex virus from immunocompetent subjects with recurrent herpes labialis: a UK-based survey. J Antimicrob Chemother 2000;46:1051

109. Danve-Szatanek C, Aymard M, Thouvenot D, et al. Surveillance network for herpes simplex virus resistance to antiviral drugs: 3-year follow-up. J Clin Microbiol 2004;42:242–249

110. Kost RG, Hill EL, Tigges M, Straus SE. Brief report: recurrent acyclovir-resistant genital herpes in an immunocompetent patient. N Engl J Med 1993;329:1777–1782

111. Swetter SM, Hill EL, Kern ER, et al. Chronic vulvar ulceration in an immunocompetent woman due to acyclovir-resistant, thymidine kinase-deficient herpes simplex virus. J Infect Dis 1998;177:543–550

112. Hill EL, Hunter GA, Ellis MN. In vitro and in vivo characterization of herpes simplex virus clinical isolates recovered from patients infected with human immunodeficiency virus. Antimicrob Agents Chemother 1991;35:2322–2328

113. Safrin S, Assaykeen T, Follansbee S, Mills J. Foscarnet therapy for acyclovir-resistant mucocutaneous herpes simplex virus infection in 26 AIDS patients: preliminary data. J Infect Dis 1990;161:1078–1084

114. Morfin F, Thouvenot D, Aymard M, Souillet G. Reactivation of acyclovir-resistant thymidine kinase-deficient herpes simplex virus harbouring single base insertion within a 7 Gs homopolymer repeat of the thymidine kinase gene. J Med Virol 2000;62:247–250

115. Wade JC, Newton B, McLaren C, Flournoy N, Keeney RE, Meyers JD. Intravenous acyclovir to treat mucocutaneous herpes simplex virus infection after marrow transplantation: a double-blind trial. Ann Intern Med 1982;96:265–269

116. Boivin G, Erice A, Crane DD, Dunn DL, Balfour HH. Acyclovir susceptibilities of herpes simplex virus strains isolated from solid organ transplant recipients after acyclovir or ganciclovir prophylaxis. Antimicrob Agents Chemother 1993;37:357–359

117. Chen Y, Scieux C, Garrait V, et al. Resistant herpes simplex virus type 1 infection: an emerging concern after allogeneic stem cell transplantation. Clin Infect Dis 2000;31:927–935

118. Levin MJ, Bacon TH, Leary JJ. Resistance of herpes simplex virus infections to nucleoside analogues in HIV-infected patients. Clin Infect Dis 2004;39 Suppl 5:S248–S257

119. Reyes M, Shaik NS, Graber JM, et al. Acyclovir-resistant genital herpes among persons attending sexually transmitted disease and human immunodeficiency virus clinics. Arch Intern Med 2003;163:76–80

120. DeJesus E, Wald A, Warren T, et al. Valacyclovir for the suppression of recurrent genital herpes in human immunodeficiency virus-infected subjects. J Infect Dis 2003;188:1009–1016

121. Chakrabarti S, Pillay D, Ratcliffe D, Cane PA, Collingham KE, Milligan DW. Resistance to antiviral drugs in herpes simplex virus infections among allogeneic stem cell transplant recipients: risk factors and prognostic significance. J Infect Dis 2000;181:2055–2058

122. Langston AA, Redei I, Caliendo AM, et al. Development of drug-resistant herpes simplex virus infection after haploidentical hematopoietic progenitor cell transplantation. Blood 2002;99:1085–1088

123. Morfin F, Thouvenot D, De Turenne-Tessier M, Lina B, Aymard M, Ooka T. Phenotypic and genetic characterization of thymidine kinase from clinical strains of varicella-zoster virus resistant to acyclovir. Antimicrob Agents Chemother 1999;43:2412–2416

124. Boivin G, Edelman CK, Pedneault L, Talarico CL, Biron KK, Balfour HH, Jr. Phenotypic and genotypic characterization of acyclovir-resistant varicella-zoster viruses isolated from persons with AIDS. J Infect Dis 1994;170:68–75

125. Collins P, Larder BA, Oliver NM, Kemp S, Smith IW, Darby G. Characterization of a DNA polymerase mutant of herpes simplex virus from a severely immunocompromised patient receiving acyclovir. J Gen Virol 1989;70:375–382

126. Bendel AE, Gross TG, Woods WG, Edelman CK, Balfour HH, Jr. Failure of foscarnet in disseminated herpes zoster. Lancet 1993;341:1342

127. Fillet AM, Visse B, Caumes E, Dumont B, Gentilini M, Huraux JM. Foscarnet-resistant multidermatomal zoster in a patient with AIDS. Clin Infect Dis 1995;21:1348–1349

128. Hwang CB, Ruffner KL, Coen DM. A point mutation within a distinct conserved region of the herpes simplex virus DNA polymerase gene confers drug resistance. J Virol 1992;66:1774–1776

129. Schmit I, Boivin G. Characterization of the DNA polymerase and thymidine kinase genes of herpes simplex virus isolates from AIDS patients in whom acyclovir and foscarnet therapy sequentially failed. J Infect Dis 1999;180:487–490

130. Safrin S, Berger TG, Gilson I, et al. Foscarnet therapy in five patients with AIDS and acyclovir-resistant varicella-zoster virus infection. Ann Intern Med 1991;115:19–21

131. Bestman-Smith J, Boivin G. Herpes simplex virus isolates with reduced adefovir susceptibility selected in vivo by foscarnet therapy. J Med Virol 2002;67:88–91

132. Chatis PA, Miller CH, Schrager LE, Crumpacker CS. Successful treatment with foscarnet of an acyclovir-resistant mucocutaneous infection with herpes simplex virus in a patient with acquired immunodeficiency syndrome. N Engl J Med 1989;320:297–300

133. Erlich KS, Jacobson MA, Koehler JE, et al. Foscarnet therapy for severe acyclovir-resistant herpes simplex virus type-2 infections in patients with the acquired immunodeficiency syndrome (AIDS). An uncontrolled trial. Ann Intern Med 1989; 110:710–713

134. Engel JP, Englund JA, Fletcher CV, Hill EL. Treatment of resistant herpes simplex virus with continuous-infusion acyclovir. JAMA 1990;263:1662–1664

135. Lalezari J, Schacker T, Feinberg J, et al. A randomized, double-blind, placebo-controlled trial of cidofovir gel for the treatment of acyclovir-unresponsive mucocutaneous herpes simplex virus infection in patients with AIDS. J Infect Dis 1997;176:892–898

136. Lalezari JP, Drew WL, Glutzer E, et al. Treatment with intravenous (S)-1-[3-hydroxy-2-(phosphonylmethoxy)propyl]-cytosine of acyclovir-resistant mucocutaneous infection with herpes simplex virus in a patient with AIDS. J Infect Dis 1994;170:570–572

137. Kopp T, Geusau A, Rieger A, Stingl G. Successful treatment of an aciclovir-resistant herpes simplex type 2 infection with cidofovir in an AIDS patient. Br J Dermatol 2002;147:134–138

138. Chilukuri S, Rosen T. Management of acyclovir-resistant herpes simplex virus. Dermatol Clin 2003;21:311–320

139. Kessler HA, Hurwitz S, Farthing C, et al. Pilot study of topical trifluridine for the treatment of acyclovir-resistant mucocutaneous herpes simplex disease in patients with AIDS (ACTG 172). AIDS Clinical Trials Group. J Acquir Immune Defic Syndr Hum Retrovirol 1996;12:147–152

140. Snoeck R, Andrei G, Gerard M, et al. Successful treatment of progressive mucocutaneous infection due to acyclovir- and foscarnet-resistant herpes simplex virus with (S)-1-(3-hydroxy-2-phosphonylmethoxypropyl)cytosine (HPMPC) Clin Infect Dis 1994;18:570–578

141. Jacobson MA, Berger TG, Fikrig S, et al. Acyclovir-resistant varicella zoster virus infection after chronic oral acyclovir therapy in patients with the acquired immunodeficiency syndrome (AIDS). Ann Intern Med 1990;112:187–191

142. Duan J, Liuzzi M, Paris W, et al. Antiviral activity of a selective ribonucleotide reductase inhibitor against acyclovir-resistant herpes simplex virus type 1 in vivo. Antimicrob Agents Chemother 1998;42:1629–1635

143. Liuzzi M, Deziel R, Moss N, et al. A potent peptidomimetic inhibitor of HSV ribonucleotide reductase with antiviral activity in vivo. Nature 1994;372:695–698

144. McSharry JJ, McDonough A, Olson B, et al. Susceptibilities of human cytomegalovirus clinical isolates to BAY38–4766, BAY43–9695, and ganciclovir. Antimicrob Agents Chemother 2001;45:2925–2927

145. Bidanset DJ, Beadle JR, Wan WB, Hostetler KY, Kern ER. Oral activity of ether lipid ester prodrugs of cidofovir against experimental human cytomegalovirus infection. J Infect Dis 2004;190:499–503

146. Emery VC, Hassan-Walker AF. Focus on new drugs in development against human cytomegalovirus. Drugs 2002;62:1853–1858

147. Michel D, Mertens T. The UL97 protein kinase of human cytomegalovirus and homologues in other herpesviruses: impact on virus and host. Biochim Biophys Acta 2004;1697:169–180

148. Koszalka GW, Johnson NW, Good SS, et al. Preclinical and toxicology studies of 1263W94, a potent and selective inhibitor of human cytomegalovirus replication. Antimicrob Agents Chemother 2002;46:2373–2380

149. Wang LH, Peck RW, Yin Y, Allanson J, Wiggs R, Wire MB. Phase I safety and pharmacokinetic trials of 1263W94, a novel oral anti-human cytomegalovirus agent, in healthy and human immunodeficiency virus-infected subjects. Antimicrob Agents Chemother 2003;47:1334–1342

150. Biron KK, Harvey RJ, Chamberlain SC, et al. Potent and selective inhibition of human cytomegalovirus replication by 1263W94, a benzimidazole L-riboside with a unique mode of action. Antimicrob Agents Chemother 2002;46:2365–2372

151. Lalezari JP, Aberg JA, Wang LH, et al. Phase I dose escalation trial evaluating the pharmacokinetics, anti-human cytomegalovirus (HCMV) activity, and safety of 1263W94 in human immunodeficiency virus infected men with asymptomatic HCMV shedding. Antimicrob Agents Chemother 2002;46:2969–2976

152. Krosky PM, Baek MC, Coen DM. The human cytomegalovirus UL97 protein kinase, an antiviral drug target, is required at the stage of nuclear egress. J Virol 2003;77:905–914

153. Chou S, Marousek GI, Senters AE, Davis MG, Biron KK. Mutations in the human cytomegalovirus UL27 gene that confer resistance to maribavir. J Virol 2004;78:7124–7130

154. Komazin G, Ptak RG, Emmer BT, Townsend LB, Drach JC. Resistance of human cytomegalovirus to the benzimidazole L-ribonucleoside maribavir maps to UL27. J Virol 2003;77:11499–11506

155. Reefschlaeger J, Bender W, Hallenberger S, et al. Novel non-nucleoside inhibitors of cytomegaloviruses (BAY 38–4766): in vitro and in vivo antiviral activity and mechanism of action. J Antimicrob Chemother 2001;48:757–767

156. Underwood MR, Ferris RG, Selleseth DW, et al. Mechanism of action of the ribopyranoside benzimidazole GW275175X against human cytomegalovirus. Antimicrob Agents Chemother 2004;48:1647–1651

Chapter 71
Clinical Implications of HIV-1 Drug Resistance

Douglas L. Mayers

1 Overview

The human immunodeficiency virus type 1 (HIV-1) is a retrovirus that has developed a replication strategy that allows it to effectively escape from immune selection pressure and establish lifelong infection in infected persons. This replication strategy involves production of 10^7–10^9 virions per day, each with a half-life of only 1–2 days (1–3). HIV-1 utilizes an error-prone reverse transcriptase enzyme that lacks proofreading activity and generates 3×10^{-5} errors per base pair per replication cycle (1). Each patient is infected with a swarm of closely related viruses called a quasispecies. Since there are roughly 9,000 base pairs per virion, every possible single and double mutant virus is created every day in an untreated patient. This strategy allows the virus to escape immune selection pressure and is very efficient at generating drug-resistant viruses in those patients whose drug regimens do not completely suppress viral replication or who are poorly compliant with a fully suppressive regimen.

Since single-base drug-resistant mutants pre-exist in every patient at low frequencies, they can emerge as the predominant circulating virus in as little as 14 days if monotherapy is utilized. This is seen with drugs such as lamivudine (with a M184V mutation) or non-nucleoside reverse transcriptase inhibitors (NNRTIs) such as efavirenz or nevirapine (with K103N or Y181C mutations) where single-point mutations cause high-level drug resistance. Alternatively, some drugs have a higher barrier to resistance because of the need for multiple mutations to cause high-level resistance, which can take months to develop. A small group of drugs develop low levels of resistance slowly, possibly because their primary resistance mutations have low replication capacities (Table 1).

Additionally, each virion contains two strands of genomic RNA, and the reverse transcriptase enzyme can jump from one RNA template strand to the other when replicating the viral genome (4–6). If two strains of HIV-1, each resistant to one agent, are circulating in a patient, the virus can use recombination to generate a new virus resistant to both drugs. The clinical relevance of recombination in generating drug-resistant HIV-1 has not been established, although it has been demonstrated in both *in vitro* experiments and in clinical viruses (7, 8).

2 Epidemiology

With the HIV-1 quasispecies replication strategy it is critical that patients be given a drug regimen that is expected to fully suppress all viral replication. This goal was not achievable for most patients in the early years of HIV-1 therapy, when regimens containing only nucleoside agents were available. Many patients developed viruses with progressively higher levels of nucleoside resistance and broad resistance to all agents in the nucleoside class. This nucleoside resistance often limited the durability of responses to subsequent combination regimens that combined nucleoside agents with protease inhibitors (PIs) or NNRTIs as they became available. Additionally, the early combination regimens were composed of agents with a high pill burden, multiple doses per day, and significant side effects, which reduced patients' ability to take the pills as prescribed. Thus, a large population of patients with resistance to multiple classes of HIV-1 agents was created in the late 1980s and 1990s. The more recent development of simple, once- or twice-a-day regimens of highly active antiretroviral therapy (HAART) with NNRTIs or boosted PIs appears to improve patient compliance and may result in more durable antiviral responses, with reduced numbers of patients harboring viruses with resistance to multiple classes of antiretroviral drugs in the future.

D.L. Mayers (✉)
Executive Vice President & Chief Medical Officer, Idenix
Pharmaceuticals, Cambridge, MA, USA
mayers.douglas@idenix.com

D.L. Mayers (ed.), *Antimicrobial Drug Resistance*,
DOI 10.1007/978-1-60327-595-8_71, © Humana Press, a part of Springer Science+Business Media, LLC 2009

Table 1 Patterns of HIV-1 drug resistance emergence

Level of resistance	High	High	Low
Time course	Weeks	Months to years	Months to years
Mechanism of resistance	Single-point mutation	Accumulation of mutations	Complex or unclear[a]
Drugs	Lamivudine (3TC)	Zidovudine (AZT)	Didanosine (ddI)
	Emtricitabine (FTC)	Abacavir (ABC)	Zalcitabine (ddC)
	Efavirenz (EFV)	Saquinavir (SQV)	Stavudine (d4T)
	Nevirapine (NVP)	Indinavir (IDV)	Tenofovir (TDF)
		Ritonavir (RTV)	
		Nelfinavir (NFV)	
		Amprenavir (APV)	
		Tipranavir (TPV)	
		Darunavir (DRV)	
		Etravirine (ETV)	

[a]Selected viral mutants may have low replication capacities

3 Prevalence

A series of studies of the prevalence of drug-resistant HIV-1 in treated patients were conducted in North America and Europe between 1996 and 2003 (Table 2) (9–12). Investigators in the United States evaluated a random representative sample of treated patients and estimated that 63% of treated patients had viremia of >500 copies/mL (9). Among viremic patients, the overall rate of any drug resistance was very consistent across the cohorts at 69–80% of treated patients. Rates of resistance to nucleoside reverse transcriptase inhibitors (NRTI) ranged from 64 to 78%, NNRTIs from 25 to 61%, and PIs from 31 to 62%. Three classes of drug resistance (multidrug-resistant (MDR) viruses) were detected in 13–25% of viremic treated patients. The most common NRTI mutations detected were M184V associated with lamivudine use and T215Y/F associated with zidovudine use. The rates of NNRTI and PI resistance were driven by general use in the treated population, with NNRTI resistance increasing from 1996 to 2003 as NNRTI use became more widespread (9–12). The most common NNRTI mutation was K103N. PI mutations varied with differential use in the different countries.

Factors associated with the development of HIV drug resistance have included host factors such as advanced HIV disease and low CD4 count at the time of initiation of treatment, viral factors such as high baseline viral load and primary drug resistance, drug regimen factors related to adherence, and the potency and composition of the antiretroviral regimen given (9, 13, 14).

4 Transmission

HIV-1 is transmitted predominantly through sexual contact, blood exposure/transfusion, and from mother to child. Factors associated with the risk of HIV transmission include high viral load, concomitant sexually transmitted diseases, host genetic factors, and high-risk behaviors. Persons with drug-resistant HIV-1 can transmit the virus to their partners.

Interestingly, differential transmission of drug resistance mutations has been observed. Viruses containing the M184V mutation in reverse transcriptase or major protease mutations appear underrepresented in newly infected patients compared to the frequency in prevalently infected populations (12, 15). This could be due to reduced replication capacity combined with lower viral loads in the potentially transmitting patients with these viruses (12).

The sexual transmission of zidovudine-resistant virus was first reported in 1993 (16). Surveys of HIV-1 drug resistance have subsequently demonstrated different patterns of transmitted drug resistance over time with some evidence of geographic variability (17–28). Representative studies, in which prevalent and incident HIV-1 drug resistance can be compared, are presented in Table 2. In the period from 1995 to 1998 in North America and Europe, the predominant resistance in transmitted HIV-1 was to nucleoside antiretroviral agents (NRTIs), with rates ranging from 8.5 to 13.4% and low levels of transmission of viruses resistant to NNRTIs (1.7–2.6%) or PIs (0.9–2.8%). In more recent surveys in North America and Europe from 1999 to 2002, rates of NRTI resistance have ranged from 6.3 to 15.9%, NNRTIs from 6.6 to 13.2%, and PIs from 3.2 to 9.1%. The incidence of newly infected patients with drug-resistant virus ranges from approximately 10–27%, with MDR viruses estimated to be present in 0–4% (18–20, 22, 29). As was seen with prevalent HIV drug resistance, transmitted NNRTI resistance has progressively increased from 1996–1997 to 2000–2001 (18–20, 22). A Centers for Disease Control (CDC) survey of 1,082 treatment-naïve, newly diagnosed patients who did not have AIDS showed that 8.6% of these patients had genotypic evidence of drug-resistant HIV-1 and 1.3% had MDR virus (30). Transmitted drug-resistant viruses can persist for long

Table 2 Prevalence and incidence of HIV-1 drug resistance

Prevalence of drug resistance in treated patients with viremia

Location	Years	N	Any-R	NRTI-R	NNRTI-R	PI-R	3 class-R	References
USA	1996–1998	1,797	76.0	71.0	25.0	41.0	13.0	Richman et al. (9)
Canada	1997–2003	552	69.0	>70	61.0	62.0	NA	Turner et al. (12)
France	1997–2002	2,248	80.0	78.0	29.0	47.	25.0	Tamalet et al. (11)
UK	1998–2000	275	80.0	64.0	36.0	31.0	14.0	Scott et al. (10)
Switzerland	1999–2001	373	72.0	67.0	28.0	37.0	16.0	Yerly et al. (21)

Incidence of drug resistance in newly HIV-infected persons

Location	Years	# Samples	Any-R	NRTI-R	NNRTI-R	PI-R	3 class-R	References
North America	1995–1998	264	8.0	8.5	1.7	0.9	NA	Little et al. (18)
North America	1999–2000	113	22.7	15.9	7.3	9.1	NA	Little et al. (18)
New York	1995–1998	154	13.2	11.8	2.6	1.3	2.6	Simon et al. (19)
New York	1999–2001	78	19.7	14.5	6.6	5.	4.0	Simon et al. (19)
San Francisco	1996–1997	40	25.0	10.0	0.0	2.5	0.0	Grant et al. (20)
San Francisco	1998–1999	94	18.1	4.2	6.	5.3	0.0	Grant et al. (20)
San Francisco	2000–2001	91	27.4	12.1	13.2	7.7	1.2	Grant et al. (20)
Europe (SPREAD)	1996–1998	217	13.50	13.4	2.3	2.8	NA	Wensing et al. (22)
Europe (SPREAD)	1999–2000	448		9.8	3.1	4.4	NA	Wensing et al. (22)
Europe (SPREAD)	2001–2002	95		6.3	9.2	3.2	NA	Wensing et al. (22)
Switzerland	1999–2001	220	10.5	8.6	0.9	2.3	0.0	Yerly et al. (21)

periods of time in the absence of treatment in comparison to the reversion to wild-type (drug-sensitive) viruses that occurs in patients who develop drug-resistant virus on treatment and then stop therapy (31–35). It is not clear whether these viruses have altered pathogenicity from the available data (33, 36–38). The median time to virologic suppression is longer in patients with primary drug-resistant viruses who receive combination therapy than in patients who are infected with drug-sensitive virus (20).

The high prevalence of drug resistance in newly infected patients has led to guideline recommendations that all patients should have drug-resistance testing prior to initiating antiretroviral therapy, if testing is available (39–42).

5 Prevention of Mother-to-Child Transmission

Mother-to-child transmission of HIV-1 remains a major problem in the developing world. Initial studies showed that zidovudine given antepartum, and intrapartum to the mother and to the newborn for six weeks, could reduce the rate of mother-to-child transmission by 67% (43). Subsequently, the HIVNET 012 study in Uganda showed that a single-dose nevirapine given perinatally to mother and child could reduce mother-to-child transmission of HIV-1 to 15.7% compared to 25.8% at 18 months of follow-up in a breast-feeding population (44). The simple, effective, single-dose nevirapine regimen has become widely used throughout the developing world. Subsequently, it was shown that single-dose nevirapine would induce NNRTI-resistant virus in 20–25% of mothers and 46% of exposed HIV-infected infants using population sequencing (45, 46). If more sensitive measurements of NNRTI resistance mutations are used, higher levels of NNRTI resistance can be detected. If these mothers require treatment with a nevirapine-containing regimen within 6 months after exposure to single-dose nevirapine, treatment responses to nevirapine-containing regimens are significantly reduced (47, 48). Longitudinal studies have shown that the prevalence of NNRTI-resistant virus in the mothers exposed to single-dose nevirapine declines over time (46, 49), and mothers who require treatment more than 6 months after prior exposure to single-dose nevirapine have treatment response rates similar to women who have not been previously exposed to nevirapine (48). The development of drug-resistant virus with regimens to prevent mother-to-child transmission of HIV-1 has driven the use of short-term combination treatment in the developed world. As combination antiretroviral therapy becomes more widely available, the ultimate solution will be to provide chronic, fully suppressive combination therapy to all HIV-1-infected mothers.

6 Clinical Significance

The emergence of drug-resistant HIV-1 during treatment has been associated with rising plasma HIV RNA levels, declining CD4 cell counts, and reduced responses to subsequent courses of antiretroviral therapy (50, 51). Development of MDR HIV-1 is associated with disease progression and death (52).

Some patients who develop drug-resistant HIV-1 while on a protease inhibitor-containing regimen can maintain low levels of plasma HIV RNA and stable CD4 cell counts for several years (53). This may be due to reduced levels of replication capacity (viral fitness) in the viruses that emerge on these regimens. Ultimately, many of these patients will experience CD4 decline and HIV-1 disease progression with MDR virus.

7 Resistance to HIV Nucleotide Reverse Transcriptase Inhibitors

HIV Nucleoside Reverse Transcriptase Inhibitors (NRTIs) block HIV replication by chain termination of the growing DNA strand (54). Resistance to these agents occurs via mutations that selectively block incorporation of the incoming NRTI, such as L74 V for didanosine, V75T for d4T, and M184V for 3TC resistance, or alternatively via thymidine analog mutations (TAMs) associated with zidovudine use at positions M41L, D67N, K70R, L210W, T215Y/F, and K219Q/E that allow the reverse transcriptase to selectively excise the incorporated NRTI by increased phosphorolysis (55, 56). Generally, increasing numbers of NRTI mutations in the reverse transcriptase enzyme are associated with higher levels of drug resistance and broadened resistance to agents in the NRTI class (57). Multi-NRTI resistance is most commonly produced by sequential accumulation of TAMs with M184V and additional NRTI-resistance-associated mutations (58). Less commonly, virus can develop the Q151M mutation (often combined with A62V, V75I, F77L, and F116Y) or by amino acid insertion(s) at position 69S combined with multiple TAMs to produce broad resistance to agents of the NRTI class (59–62). HIV-1 NRTI resistance is reviewed extensively in Chap. 33.

8 Resistance to HIV-1 Non-nucleoside Reverse Transcriptase Inhibitors

HIV-1 Non-nucleoside Reverse Transcriptase Inhibitors (NNRTIs) all bind to a common pocket and block the action of HIV RT in a noncompetitive way (63, 64). HIV-2 viruses and HIV-1 clade O viruses found in West Africa are naturally resistant to all available NNRTIs (65). In all other HIV-1 clades, resistance to the first-generation HIV-1 NNRTIs, nevirapine and efavirenz, is generally produced by a single-point mutation at position K103N or Y181C/I resulting in high-level resistance and/or a transient response with rapid viral rebound to members of the NNRTI class (66, 67). If these agents are continued after viral rebound occurs, additional mutations at positions L100I, V106A/M, V108I, Y188C/L/H, G190S/A, and P225H can be selected (66, 67).

Recently, a new second-generation NNRTI, etravirine, has been introduced into clinical practice to treat patients with NNRTI-resistant virus. This agent is active against viruses with the common K103N mutation. Resistance to etravirine is associated with mutation at positions V90I, A98G, L100I, K101E/P, V106I, V179D/F, Y181C/I/V and G190S/A usually in combination with Y181C (68). Additionally, responses are reduced when multiple NNRTI-associated resistance mutations are present in the circulating virus. This strongly suggests that patients should not be maintained on a nevirapine- or efavirenz-containing regimen after virologic rebound to prevent development of resistance to the newer second-generation NNRTIs. HIV-1 NNRTI resistance is reviewed extensively in Chap. 33.

9 Resistance to HIV-1 Protease Inhibitors

HIV Protease Inhibitors (PIs) act by preventing the HIV protease enzyme from cleaving the Gag protein, an essential step of the viral maturation process (69). Resistance to HIV PIs is a multistep process involving the development of primary mutations in the active site of the protease enzyme responsible for drug resistance and the appearance of compensatory mutations away from the active site which increase the protease enzymatic efficiency (70–72). The accumulation of multiple primary protease resistance mutations (D30N, G48V, I50V, V82A/F/T/S, I84 V, or L90M) alters the protease-enzyme-binding pocket, leading to increasing and broadened PI resistance (73). Recently, second-generation PIs active against viruses resistant to the first-generation PIs have been developed. These include the agents tipranavir and darunavir.

Many viruses adapt to the altered drug-resistant protease enzyme by mutating their Gag cleavage sites to fit altered enzyme-binding pocket (74, 75). When this occurs, the virus becomes "locked" into the altered enzyme configuration since reversion of resistance would require simultaneous reversion of the protease resistance mutations and the gag cleavage site mutations.

HIV-1 PI resistance is reviewed extensively in Chap. 34.

10 Resistance to HIV-1 Entry Inhibitors

HIV-1 entry inhibitors prevent the HIV envelope proteins gp120 and gp41 from interacting with their cellular receptors and fusing with the host cell membrane.

Enfuvirtide (T-20) blocks the fusion of the viral and host cell membranes mediated by gp41 (76). The mutations that produce enfuvirtide resistance usually occur at codons 36–45 in the first heptad repeat region (HR1) of gp41 and are not detected with conventional genotypic or phenotypic HIV resistance assays (77). Patients are generally assumed to have virus sensitive to enfuvirtide if the drug has not been administered previously, and are assumed to have virus with enfuvirtide resistance if they have received enfuvirtide previously and experienced viral rebound on the agent.

Maraviroc, a CCR5 inhibitor, blocks the interaction of the HIV-1 gp 120 envelop protein with the CCR5 molecule on the surface of host cells (78). The virus gp120 envelope initially binds to CD4 followed by secondary binding to either CCR5 or CXCR4 on the host cell surface. Viruses that are R5-tropic (bind CCR5 to enter host cells) are inhibited by maraviroc, while viruses that are X4-tropic (bind CXCR4 to enter host cells) or have a mixed R5/X4 tropism are not inhibited. R5-tropism predominates at the time of infection and during the early stages of HIV disease when patients are asymptomatic. As HIV disease progresses and CD4 cells decline, viruses with a mixed R5/X4-tropism or X4-tropism become more common. Since maraviroc is currently indicated for treatment-experienced patients, a tropism assay should be obtained to confirm the presence of R5-tropic virus before the drug is given. Patients whose virus rebounds in the presence of maraviroc therapy are generally assumed to be resistant but a susceptibility/tropism assay can be conducted to confirm decreased susceptibility.

HIV-1 entry inhibitor resistance is reviewed extensively in Chap. 35.

11 Resistance to HIV Integrase Inhibitors

Raltegravir, an HIV-1 integrase inhibitor, blocks the strand transfer reaction that the HIV integrase uses to insert the HIV genome into host cell DNA (79). Resistance to raltegravir is mediated by two pathways of resistance in the HIV-1 integrase gene: Q148H/K/R combined with either L74M + E138A, E138K, or G140S; or N155H combined with either L74M, E92Q, T97A, E92Q + T97A, Y143H, G163K/R, V151I, or D232N (80). Since the integrase gene is not contained in the standard HIV drug resistance assays, patients who are naïve to raltegravir are generally assumed to have sensitive virus and those who have taken raltegravir with viral rebound are assumed to have the drug-resistant virus. HIV-1 integrase inhibitor resistance is reviewed extensively in Chap. 36.

12 Mutational Interactions

Some drug resistance mutations in the HIV genome can interact to result in resensitization of the virus to an antiviral drug to which it was previously resistant. For instance, if a virus is resistant to zidovudine with multiple TAMs and a T215Y/F mutation and develops a L74V mutation due to exposure to didanosine (81) or a Y181C mutation due to nevirapine exposure (82), the virus can show zidovudine sensitivity on a phenotypic sensitivity assay. Viruses with multiple TAMs from nucleoside exposure can demonstrate hypersusceptibility to NNRTI agents and this has been shown to result in better responses to efavirenz-containing regimens when the next round of therapy is given (provided adequate background therapy is available to combine with the NNRTI) (83–86). Knowledge of mutational interactions can sometimes be used to obtain an enhanced response from a component of a combination regimen in treatment-experienced patients. It should be kept in mind that most of these mutational interactions can be overcome by the virus moving to an alternative resistance pathway so that they are only of clinical benefit if a fully suppressive next regimen can be designed.

13 Viral Fitness (Replication Capacity)

Viral fitness or the ability to replicate in host cells can be reduced owing to the presence of drug resistance mutations which decrease a viral enzyme's functional activity as the cost of developing resistance. In the patient, the predominant circulating virus is the one that grows best in the presence of the current drug selection pressure but this virus can often be rapidly overgrown by wild-type virus if the drugs are stopped. Diminished fitness is seen clinically when a patient's virus rebounds in the presence of a drug regimen but the viral load remains well below baseline levels and the CD4 cell count stays up despite the emergence of drug-resistant virus (53). Some patients can remain clinically stable for extended periods of time until the virus develops additional mutations which either increase drug resistance or compensate for the drug resistance mutations and allow the virus to replicate more efficiently. When this occurs, CD4 cells will decline and disease progression can occur.

Some drug resistance mutations such as those associated with lamivudine resistance (M184V in reverse transcriptase) or primary protease inhibitor resistance (D30N) have been associated with decreased viral fitness as manifested by lower viral loads in treated patients who experience viral rebound on therapy and reduced transmission to newly infected patients (12).

Viral fitness or replication capacity is determined by dividing the amount of viral growth of the clinical HIV-1 isolate in the no-drug well of an *in vitro* drug resistance assay by the amount of growth of the wild-type (drug-sensitive) control virus in the no-drug wells from the same assay. There have been several recent reviews of the implications of HIV viral fitness on drug resistance, disease progression, transmission, and global epidemic evolution (87, 88).

14 Clades

Most of current knowledge of HIV-1 drug resistance has been developed from patients infected with clade B virus, which is the predominant strain of virus circulating in North America and Europe (89). However, most of the patients infected with HIV-1 in the developing world have non-clade B viruses (such as clade A/E viruses in Asia and clade C viruses in Sub-Saharan Africa) (89, 90). The resistance pathways for antiviral drugs are generally similar in non-clade B to those seen in patients with clade B viruses but different primary pathways and profiles can occur (90). For example, patients receiving nelfinavir with clade B virus often develop a D30N mutation in their virus, whereas those with clade C virus develop a L90M mutation more often than the D30N (91). Similarly, patients who receive nevirapine with clade B virus often develop a secondary V106A mutation, whereas those with clade C virus with a 106 mutation usually develop a V106M mutation (92, 93).

The effect of different genetic backgrounds on drug resistance pathways in different regions of the world is currently under investigation. As more information becomes available, resistance algorithms developed in the developed world will need to be expanded to improve interpretation for the non-clade B viruses which predominate in the developing world and now account for up to 24–30% of new infections in Europe (22, 94–96).

15 Laboratory Diagnosis of HIV-1 Drug Resistance

Zidovudine (AZT) resistant virus was detected using an MT-2 syncytial assay in 1989 (97). Soon thereafter, it was shown that phenotypic resistance to zidovudine was associated with mutations in reverse transcriptase at positions M41L, D67N, K70R, T215Y/F, and K219Q/E (98). As each new antiretroviral drug was developed, viruses with phenotypic drug resistance were detected soon afterwards and the viral genetic mutations associated with drug resistance and/or viral breakthrough were then determined.

Clinical investigators developed a standardized HIV-1 phenotypic drug resistance assay using peripheral blood mononuclear cells which could be applied to the majority of clinical HIV-1 isolates to determine the clinical significance of HIV phenotypic drug resistance (99). This assay was slow and labor intensive requiring cultivation of HIV-1 *in vitro*, quantitation of the viral stock to produce a standardized inoculum, and then viral replication in the presence of multiple drug levels to obtain an EC_{50} value (the concentration of drug required to reduce viral replication by 50% compared to a no-drug control well). The whole process took 4 to 6 weeks and could be conducted only in a research laboratory. Subsequently, commercial laboratories developed HIV phenotypic resistance assays utilizing recombinant viruses containing polymerase chain reaction (PCR) amplified segments of clinical HIV-1 isolates that could be automated and produce highly reproducible results with a 2-week turnaround. Use of HIV-1 phenotypic assays is described in detail in Chap. 83 (Table 3).

The development of high-throughput genotypic sequencing allowed the commercial development of sequencing of a PCR-amplified segment containing the HIV-1 protease gene and a portion of the reverse transcriptase gene to detect mutations associated with phenotypic HIV-1 drug resistance and/or viral rebound in the clinic (Table 3). Databases of these mutations and listings of these mutations are updated regularly (100–102). Interpretative algorithms for resistance resulting from the combinations of drug resistance mutations produced by currently available antiretroviral drug regimens have become complex and are generally generated using computer algorithms. These are then translated into a user-friendly report in which susceptibility to each agent is generally interpreted as sensitive, partially resistant, or resistant. Use of HIV-1 genotypic assays is described in detail in Chap. 86 (Table 3).

Several groups have provided guidance on the use and interpretation of HIV drug resistance assays (40–42, 103). The patients for whom resistance testing is recommended are listed in Table 4. Numerous websites contain current information on HIV drug resistance (104). Some useful websites are listed in Table 5.

There are several important caveats to the interpretation of HIV-1 drug resistance assays. The assays all report the results for the predominant circulating virus at each time point and will not detect minority viral species that are present at levels below 20–25% although novel assays are being developed to detect minority populations of drug-resistant virus. Additionally, virus populations can turn over rapidly if antiretroviral drugs are discontinued or drug regimens are

Table 3 Comparison of genotypic and phenotypic drug resistance testing

	Genotypic drug resistance testing	Phenotypic drug resistance testing
Strengths	Rapid turnaround	Direct measure of drug susceptibility
	Less expensive	Can provide a measure of viral replication capacity
	Widely available	
	Clinically validated in multiple clinical trials	
Weaknesses	Interpretative algorithms are not standardized	Lack of availability of standardized clinical cutoffs
	Indirect measure of resistance	More expensive
	Difficulty interpreting complex mutation patterns	Slower turnaround
	Difficulty interpreting resistance to novel agents	Less widely available
	Cannot detect minority variants (<20% of all viruses)	Cannot detect minority variants

Table 4 Indications for obtaining an HIV drug resistance test

Primary/acute or recent HIV infection[a,b,c,d]
Initiation of antiretroviral therapy[a,b,c,d]
Poor response to initial antiretroviral therapy[a]
Viral rebound on antiretroviral treatment[a,b,c,d]
Pregnancy if detectable plasma virus[a,b,c]
Postexposure prophylaxis[c]
Pediatric patients initiating antiretroviral treatment[b,c]

[a]IAS-USA recommendations (40, 103)
[b]US DHHS Treatment Guidelines (42)
[c]European Guidelines (41)
[d]British HIV Association (39)

Table 5 HIV drug resistance websites

Stanford HIV Drug Resistance Database	http://hivdb.stanford.edu/
Los Alamos HIV Drug Resistance Database	http://resdb.lanl.gov/Resist_DB
Stephen Hughes, HIV Drug Resistance Program, National Cancer Institute (structural database)	http://www.retrovirus.info/rt/
European HIV Resistance Network	http://www.umcutrecht.nl/ subsite/spread-programme/
HIV Drug Resistance Initiative	http://www.hiv-dri.org/
HIV InSite – genotypic testing for HIV drug resistance	http://hivinsite.ucsf.edu/ InSite?page = kbr-03–02–07
Geno2pheno website	http://www.geno2pheno.org/
IAS-USA website	http://www.iasusa.org/ resistance_mutations/ index.html

changed. Thus, patients who are considering switching anti retroviral therapy should have a resistance test performed while on treatment and not after stopping drugs for a period of time. Importantly, when considering drugs to utilize in a new antiretroviral regimen for patients who have received prior antiretroviral therapy, the clinician needs to consider all prior drugs given and all prior antiretroviral resistance results since these earlier viruses will continue to be present as archived viral DNA in HIV-1 infected cells and can rapidly re-emerge under the appropriate antiviral selection pressure.

16 Treatment of Drug-Resistant HIV-1

16.1 Initial Treatment of HIV-1

Treatment is initiated for HIV-1 infection with different guidelines in different regions of the world (39, 42, 103, 105). All guidelines agree that treatment should be initiated for patients with symptomatic HIV-1 disease or CD4 counts less than 200 cells/μL. In North America and Europe, guidelines are moving to earlier treatment with CD4 cell counts <350 cells/μL, and some investigators are advocating near-universal treatment of all HIV-infected persons. Initial treatment is typically with two nucleoside drugs and an NNRTI, or two nucleosides with a protease inhibitor. Data showing that approximately 10–27% of newly HIV-1-infected persons have a virus with genotypic evidence of drug resistance and up to 4% of these patients may harbor an MDR virus has led to the recommendation that all HIV-infected persons should have a resistance test prior to initiating therapy. Patients who do not have a brisk antiviral response in plasma HIV RNA to combination antiretroviral treatment during the first 2 months of treatment should be evaluated for treatment adherence and be considered for genotypic resistance testing at that time.

The goal of combination therapy for treatment of HIV-1 disease is to obtain complete suppression of HIV replication, which is measured by a plasma HIV RNA level of less than 50 copies/mL. The challenge for the treating physician and patient is to maintain high levels of adherence to taking the drug regimen over decades of treatment since the most common cause of virological rebound is poor adherence or discontinuation of treatment. If the patient has evidence of a rising plasma HIV RNA value, the clinician should carefully review patient adherence to taking the medications, side effects of treatment that could reduce adherence, concomitant medications such as rifampin which can lower the levels of HIV NNRTI and protease inhibitors, and new onset gastrointestinal disorders such as nausea, vomiting, or diarrhea to determine if there is any modifiable issue that can be resolved in order to fully suppress the virus. If the plasma HIV RNA remains elevated after these measures are taken, a resistance test should be considered to guide the next round of treatment. Allowing patients to remain on a combination antiretroviral regimen despite active HIV-1 replication manifested by detectable HIV RNA levels will result in increasing levels of resistance to the drugs administered and broadened resistance to the remaining drugs from the classes of drugs used in the regimen (106).

16.2 Treatment of Drug-Resistant HIV-1

Patients who have experienced virologic breakthrough after initial or early rounds of antiretroviral treatment usually have active drugs available to develop an effective combination treatment regimen. It is critical for each new round of therapy to combine at least two and preferably three active antiretroviral drugs together to ensure that a fully suppressive regimen is used. Adding less than three active drugs often leads to rapid viral breakthrough with resistance to the new class of drugs. HIV drug resistance testing has shown short-term clinical benefit in helping to select active drugs for treatment-experienced patients and should be considered (107–110). Treatment decisions need to take into account prior drug exposure, drug toxicities on prior antiviral regimens, prior resistance test results and the resistance data while on the most recent antiretroviral drug regimen, and patient wishes (Table 6). Where available, advice from an expert with experience treating patients with MDR HIV-1 should be obtained (108, 110).

16.3 Salvage Therapy for Drug-Resistant HIV-1

The goals of HIV treatment can change for patients who have virus resistant to most or all currently available drugs. The benefits of drug resistance testing may be limited in this group of patients. These patients should be maintained on antiretroviral treatment since discontinuing all treatment results in disease progression. For patients who are asymptomatic with stable CD4 cell counts, the clinician may elect to continue the current regimen, if it is well tolerated, or switch to a simpler, more easily tolerated combination drug regimen if drug toxicities are present. The goal in these patients is no longer complete viral suppression but to maintain immune status

Table 6 Factors in choosing drug regimens for treatment-experienced patients

Number and duration of prior antiretroviral drugs
Toxicity while receiving prior antiretroviral drugs
Current and prior HIV drug resistance test results
Ability to develop a combination drug regimen with at least two and
    preferably three drugs active against the current circulating virus
Patient desires

(especially a CD4 count above 200 cells/μL) and patient functioning until active drugs become available to develop a fully active antiviral regimen (111).

Structured treatment interruptions (STIs) to allow sensitive virus to re-emerge and overgrow the MDR circulating virus are not recommended. Studies have shown that re-emergence of wild-type, drug-sensitive virus is associated with increasing viral loads and CD4 declines potentially resulting in disease progression events (112–114). Re-initiation of combination therapy after an STI results in a transient improvement of antiviral responses compared to continued treatment, but the decreased CD4 counts can remain depressed for more than a year compared to continued therapy (113). Discontinuation of antiviral treatment has been associated with increased risk of opportunistic disease or death from any cause including cardiovascular, renal, and hepatic disease (115, 116).

Some investigators have tried "mega-HAART" regimens to treat patients using five to eight antiretroviral drugs (117–119). While some short-term antiviral benefits have been observed, the toxicity of these regimens has limited their utility in general practice.

16.4 Novel Classes of Antiretroviral Drugs

Recently, the availability of second-generation HIV protease inhibitors (tipranavir and darunavir), a second-generation NNRTI (etravirine), enfuvirtide (T-20), and two new classes of HIV-1 inhibitors: maraviroc, a CCR5 inhibitor, and raltegravir, an HIV integrase inhibitor, have greatly expanded the potential treatment options for patients whose virus is resistant to multiple classes of antiretroviral drugs. Combinations of these drugs have made complete viral suppression possible for patients with the most resistant viruses and have led to a standard goal of therapy to achieve undetectable virus (plasma HIV RNA < 50 copies/mL) for all stages of HIV treatment. It is critical in these patients to combine two to three active antiretroviral drugs together to ensure that a fully suppressive regimen is used. These decisions in patients with limited options for use of NRTI, NNRTI, and PI classes of drugs may benefit from use of both genotypic and phenotypic HIV drug resistance tests (120). Advice from an expert with experience in treating patients with MDR HIV-1 should be obtained, if possible (120).

16.5 Prevention of HIV-1 Drug Resistance

The most effective method to prevent emergence of HIV-1 drug resistance and block further transmission of HIV-1 is to fully suppress HIV replication with combination therapy in all

HIV-infected persons (121). Once fully suppressive therapy is given, high patient adherence to the prescribed regimen determines the ultimate durability of each drug regimen. Recent advances utilizing daily fixed-dose combination regimens with well-tolerated agents have significantly increased the success rates and durability of initial antiretroviral treatment.

The development of second-generation NNRTIs and PIs for patients with MDR virus and the additional development of the entry inhibitors, enfuvirtide and maraviroc, as well as the integrase inhibitor, raltegravir, offer the potential for patients with HIV-1 resistant to multiple classes of antiretroviral drugs to fashion fully suppressive combination drug regimens and obtain durable treatment responses. This should reduce the potential for transmission of MDR viruses to the next generation of HIV-1 infected patients.

Preliminary data suggest that the availability of fully suppressive combination therapy for HIV-1 has the potential to lower the rates of HIV-1 transmission along with both prevalent and incident HIV-1 drug resistance rates (122). Additionally, prevention programs encouraging safe sex practices and needle exchange can prevent transmission of HIV and should be developed in conjunction with the local communities to reduce the number of new HIV infections.

References

1. Coffin JM. HIV population dynamics in vivo: implications for genetic variation, pathogenesis, and therapy. Science 1995; 267:483–489
2. Ho DD, Neumann AU, Perelson AS, Chen W, Leonard JM, Markowitz M. Rapid turnover of plasma virions and CD4 lymphocytes in HIV-1 infection. Nature 1995; 373:123–126
3. Perelson AS, Neumann AU, Markowitz M, Leonard JM, Ho DD. HIV-1 dynamics in vivo: virion clearance rate, infected cell lifespan, and viral generation time. Science 1996; 271:1582–1586
4. Hu W-S, Temin H. Genetic consequences of packaging two RNA genomes in one retroviral particle: pseudodiploidy and high rate of genetic recombination. Proc Natl Acad Sci U S A 1990; 87:1556–1560
5. Chen J, Powell D, Hu W-S. High frequency of genetic recombination is a common feature of primate lentivirus replication. J Virol 2006; 80:9651–9658
6. Robertson DL, Sharp PM, McCutchan FE, Hahn BH. Recombination of HIV-1. Nature 1995; 374:124–126
7. Gu Z, Gao Q, Faust EA, Wainberg MA. Possible involvement of cell fusion and viral recombination in generation of human immunodeficiency virus variants that display dual resistance to AZT and 3TC. J Gen Virol 1995; 76:2601–2605
8. Tamara N, Charpentier C, Tenaillon O, Hoede C, Clavel F, Hance AJ. Contribution of recombination to the evolution of human immunodeficiency viruses expressing resistance to antiretroviral treatment. J Virol 2007; 81:7620–7628
9. Richman DD, Morton SC, Wrin T, et al. The prevalence of antiretroviral drug resistance in the United States. AIDS 2004; 18:1393–1401
10. Scott P, Arnold E, Evans B, et al. Surveillance of HIV antiretroviral drug resistance in treated individuals in England: 1998–2000. J Antimicrob Chemother 2004; 53:469–473

11. Tamalet C, Fantini J, Tourres C, Yahi N. Resistance of HIV-1 to multiple antiretroviral drugs in France: a 6-year survey (1997–2002) based on an analysis of over 7000 genotypes. AIDS 2003; 17:2383–2388
12. Turner D, Brenner B, Routy JP, et al. Diminished representation of HIV-1 variants containing select drug resistance-conferring mutations in primary HIV-1 infection. J Acquir Immune Defic Syndr 2004; 37:1627–1631
13. Demeter LM, Hughes MD, Coombes RW, et al. Predictors of virologic and clinical outcomes in HIV-1 infected patients receiving concurrent treatment with indinavir, zidovudine, and lamivudine. Ann Intern Med 2001; 135:954–964
14. Harrigan PR, Hogg RS, Dong WW, et al. Predictors of HIV drug-resistance mutations in a large antiretroviral-naive cohort initiating triple antiretroviral therapy. J Infect Dis 2005; 191:339–347
15. de Mendoza C, Rodriguez C, Corral A, del Romero J, Gallego O, Soriano V. Evidence of differences in the sexual transmission efficiency of HIV strains with distinct drug resistance genotypes. Clin Infect Dis 2004; 39:1231–1238
16. Erice A, Mayers D, Strike D, et al. Brief report: primary infection with zidovudine resistant HIV-1. N Engl J Med 1993; 328:1163–1165
17. Little SJ, Daar ES, D'Aquila RT, et al. Reduced antiretroviral drug susceptibility among patients with primary HIV infection. JAMA 1999; 282:1142–1149
18. Little SJ, Holte S, Routy JP, et al. Antiretroviral-drug resistance among patients recently infected with HIV. N Engl J Med 2002; 347:385–394
19. Simon V, Vanderhoeven J, Hurley A, et al. Evolving patterns of HIV-1 resistance to antiretroviral agents in newly infected individuals. AIDS 2002; 16:1511–1519
20. Grant RM, Hecht FM, Warmerdam M, et al. Time trends in primary HIV-1 drug resistance among recently infected persons. JAMA 2002; 288:181–188
21. Yerly S, Jost S, Talenti A, et al. Study SHC. Infrequent transmission of HIV-1 drug resistant variants. AntivirTher 2004; 9:375–384
22. Wensing AM, van de Viver D, Angarano G, et al. Prevalence of drug resistant HIV-1 variants in untreated individuals in Europe: implications for clinical management. J Infect Dis 2005; 192:958–966
23. Soares MA, Brindeiro RM, Tanuri A. Primary HIV-1 drug resistance in Brazil. AIDS 2004; 18 (Suppl 3):S9–S13
24. Ammaranond P, Cunningham P, Oelrichs R, et al. No increase in protease resistance and a decrease in reverse transcriptase resistance mutations in primary HIV-1 infection: 1992–2001. AIDS 2003; 17:264–267
25. Chaix ML, Descamps D, Harzic M, et al. Stable prevalence of genotypic drug resistance mutations but increase in non-B virus among patients with primary HIV-1 infection in France. AIDS 2003; 17:2635–2643
26. Descamps D, Calvez V, Izopet J, et al. Prevalence of resistance mutations in antiretroviral-naive chronically HIV-infected patients in 1998: a French nationwide study. AIDS 2001; 15:1777–1782
27. Brindeiro RM, Diaz RS, Sabino EC, et al. Brazilian Network for HIV Drug Resistance Surveillance (HIV-BResNet): a survey of chronically infected individuals. AIDS 2003; 17:1063–1069
28. Ammaranond P, Cunningham P, Oelrichs R, et al. Rates of transmission of antiretroviral drug resistant strains of HIV-1. J Clin Virol 2003; 26:153–161
29. Grossman Z, Lorber M, Maayan S, et al. Drug-resistant HIV infection among drug-naive patients in Israel. Clin Infect Dis 2005; 40:294–302
30. Weinstock HS, Zaidi I, Heneine W, et al. The epidemiology of antiretroviral drug resistance among drug-naive HIV-1-infected persons in 10 US cities. J Infect Dis 2004; 189:2174–2180
31. Brenner BG, Routy JP, Petrella M, et al. Persistence and fitness of multidrug-resistant human immunodeficiency virus type 1 acquired in primary infection. J Virol 2002; 76:1753–1761

32. Smith DM, Wong JK, Shao H, et al. Long-term persistence of transmitted HIV drug resistance in male genital tract secretions: implications for secondary transmission. J Infect Dis 2007; 196:356–360

33. Chan KC, Galli RA, Montaner JS, Harrigan PR. Prolonged retention of drug resistance mutations and rapid disease progression in absence of therapy after primary HIV infection. AIDS 2003; 17:1256–1258

34. Barbour JD, Hecht FM, Wrin T, et al. Persistence of primary drug resistance among recently HIV-1 infected adults. AIDS 2004; 18:1683–1689

35. Delaugerre C, Morand-Joubert L, Chaix M-L, et al. Persistence of multidrug-resistant HIV-1 without antiretroviral treatment 2 years after sexual transmission. Antivir Ther 2004; 9:415–421

36. Markowitz M, Mohri H, Mehandru S, et al. Infection with multidrug resistant, dual-tropic HIV-1 and rapid progression to AIDS: a case report. Lancet 2005; 365:1031–1038

37. Hecht FM, Grant RM, Petropolis CJ, et al. Sexual transmission of an HIV-1 variant resistant to multiple reverse-transcriptase and protease inhibitors. N Engl J Med 1998; 339:307–311

38. CASCADE Virology Collaboration. The impact of transmitted drug resistance on the natural history of HIV infection and response to first-line therapy. AIDS 2006; 20:21–28

39. Gazzard B, Bernard AJ, Boffito M, et al. British HIV Association guidelines for treatment of HIV-infected adults with antiretroviral therapy. HIV Med 2006; 7:487–503

40. Hirsch MS, Brun-Vezinet F, Clotet B, et al. Antiretroviral resistance testing in adults infected with human immunodeficiency virus type 1: 2003 recommendations of an international IAS Society-USA panel. Clin Infect Dis 2003; 37:113–128

41. Vandamme AM, Sonnerborg A, it-Khaled M, et al. Updated European recommendations for the clinical use of HIV drug resistance testing. Antivir Ther 2004; 9:829–848

42. Panel on antiretroviral guidelines for adult and adolescents. Guidelines for the use of antiretroviral agents in HIV-infected adults and adolescents. Department of Health and Human Services. January 29, 2008; 1–134. Available at http://aidsinfo.nih.gov/contentfiles/AdultandAdolescentGL.pdf

43. Connor EM, Sperling RS, Gelber R, et al. Reduction of maternal-infant transmission of human immunodeficiency virus type 1 with zidovudine treatment. Pediatric AIDS Clinical Trials Group Protocol 076 Study Group. N Engl J Med 1994; 331:1173–1180

44. Jackson JB, Musoke P, Fleming T, et al. Intrapartum and neonatal single dose nevirapine compared with zidovudine from prevention of mother-to-child transmission of HIV-1 in Kampala, Uganda: 18 month follow-up of the HIVNET 012 randomised trial. Lancet 2003; 362:859–868

45. Jackson JB, Becker-Pergola G, Guay LA, et al. Identification of the K103N resistance mutation in Ugandan women receiving nevirapine to prevent HIV-1 vertical transmission. AIDS 2000; 14:F111-F115

46. Eshleman SH, Mracna M, Guay LA, et al. Selection and fading of resistance mutations in women and infants receiving nevirapine to prevent HIV-1 vertical transmission (HIVNET 012). AIDS 2001; 15:1951–1957

47. Jourdain G, Ngo-Giang-Houng N, Le Coeur S, et al. Group PHPT. Intrapartum exposure to nevirapine and subsequent maternal responses to nevirapine-based antiretroviral therapy. N Engl J Med 2004; 351:229–240

48. Lockman S, Shapiro RL, Smeaton LM, et al. Response to antiretroviral therapy after a single, peripartum dose of nevirapine. N Engl J Med 2007; 356:135–147

49. Flys T, Nissley DV, Claasen CW, et al. Sensitive drug-resistance assays reveal long-term persistence of HIV-1 variants with the K103N nevirapine (NVP) resistance mutation in some women and infants after the administration of single-dose NVP: HIVNET 012. J Infect Dis 2005; 192:24–29

50. D'Aquila RT, Johnson VA, Welles SL, et al. Zidovudine resistance and HIV-1 disease progression during antiretroviral therapy. AIDS Clinical Trials Group Protocol 116B/117 Team and the Virology Committee Resistance Working Group. Ann Intern Med 1995; 122:401–408

51. Japour AJ, Welles S, D'Aquila RT, et al. Prevalence and clinical significance of zidovudine resistance mutations in human immuno-deficiency virus isolated from patients after long-term zidovudine treatment. AIDS Clinical Trials Group 116B/117 Study Team and Virology Committee Resistance Working Group. J Infect Dis 1995; 171:1172–1179

52. The Plato Collaboration. Predictors of trend in CD4-positive T-cell count and mortality among HIV-1 infected individuals with virological failure to all three antiretroviral-drug classes. Lancet 2004; 364:51–62

53. Deeks SG, Barbour JD, Martin JN, Swanson MS, Grant RM. Sustained CD4 + T cell response after virologic failure of protease inhibitor-based regimens in patients with human immunodeficiency virus infection. J Infect Dis 2000; 181:946–953

54. De Clercq E. HIV inhibitors targeted at the reverse transcriptase. AIDS Res Hum Retroviruses 1992; 8:119–134

55. Gotte M, Wainberg MA. Biochemical mechanisms involved in overcoming HIV resistance to nucleoside inhibitors of reverse transcriptase. Drug Resist Updat 2000; 3:30–38

56. Sluis-Cremer N, Arion D, Parniac MA. Molecular mechanisms of HIV-1 resistance to nucleoside reverse transcriptase inhibitors (NRTIs). Cell Mol Life Sci 2000; 57:1408–1422

57. Mayers DL, Japour AJ, Arduino JM, Hammer SM, et al. Dideoxynucleoside resistance emerges with prolonged zidovudine montherapy. Antimicrob Agents Chemother 1994; 38:307–314

58. Winters MA, Baxter JD, Mayers DL, et al. Frequency of antiretroviral drug resistance mutations in HIV-1 strains from patients failing triple drug regimens. The Terry Beirn Community Programs for Clinical Research on AIDS. Antivir Ther 2000; 5:57–63

59. Iverson AK, Shafer RW, Wehrly K, et al. Multidrug-resistant human immunodeficiency virus type 1 strains resulting from combination therapy. J Virol 1996; 70:1086–1090

60. Winters MA, Merigan TC. Insertions in the Human Immunodeficiency Virus type 1 protease and reverse transcriptase genes: clinical impact and molecular mechanisms. Antimicrob Agents Chemother 2005; 49:2575–2582

61. Shirasaka T, Kavlick MF, Ueno T, et al. Emergence of human immunodeficiency virus type 1 variants with resistance to multiple dideoxynucleosides in patients receiving therapy with dideoxynucleosides. Proc Natl Acad Sci U S A 1995; 92:2398–2404

62. Larder BA, Bloor S, Kemp SD, et al. A family of insertion mutations between codons 67 and 70 of human immunodeficiency virus type 1 reverse transcriptase confer multinucleoside analog resistance. Antimicrob Agents Chemother 1999; 43:1961–1967

63. Esnouf R, Ren J, Ross C, Jones Y, Stammers D, Stuart D. Mechanism of inhibition of HIV-1 RT by non-nucleoside inhibitors. Struct Biol 1995; 2:303–308

64. Spence RA, Kati WM, Anderson KS, Johnson KA. Mechanism of inhibition of HIV-1 reverse transcriptase by non-nucleoside inhibitors. Science 1995; 267:988–993

65. Descamps D, Collin G, Loussert-Ajaka I, Saragosti S, Simon F, Brun-Vezinet F. HIV-1 group O sensitivity to antiretroviral drugs.. AIDS 1995; 9:977–978

66. Richman D, Havlir D, Corbeil J, et al. Nevirapine resistance mutations of human immunodeficiency virus type 1 selected during therapy. J Virol 1994; 68:1660–1666

67. Batchelor LT, Anton ED, Kudish P, Baker D, Bunville J, et al. HIV-1 mutations selected in patients failing EFV combination therapy. Antimicrob Agents Chemother 2000; 44:475–484

68. Vingerhoets J, Buelens A, Peeters M, et al. Impact of baseline NNRTI mutations on the virological response to TMC125 in the

phase III clinical trials DUET-1 and DUET-2. Antiviral Ther 2007; 12:S34

69. McQuade TJ, Tomasselli AG, Liu L, et al. A synthetic HIV-1 protease inhibitor with antiviral activity arrests HIV-like particle maturation. Science 1990; 247:454–456

70. Molla A, Korneyeva M, Gao Q, et al. Ordered accumulation of mutations in HIV protease confers resistance to ritonavir. Nat Med 1996; 2:760–766

71. Condra JH, Holder DJ, Schlief WA, Blahey OM, et al. Genetic correlates of in vivo resistance to indinavir, a human immunodeficiency virus type 1 protease inhibitor. J Virol 1996; 70:8270–8276

72. Turner D, Schapiro JM, Brenner BG, Wainberg MA. The influence of protease inhibitor resistance profiles on selection of HIV therapy in treatment-naive patients. Antivir Ther 2004; 9:301–314

73. Condra JH. Virological and clinical implications of resistance to HIV-1 protease inhibitors. Drug Resist Updat 1998; 1:292–299

74. Doyon L, Croteau G, Thibeault D, Poulin F, Pilote L, Lamarre D. Second locus involved in human immunodeficiency virus type 1 resistance to protease inhibitors. J Virol 1996; 70:3763–3769

75. Cote HC, Brumme ZL, Harrigan PR. Human immunodeficiency virus type 1 protease cleavage site mutations associated with protease inhibitor cross resistance selected by indinavir, ritonavir and saquinavir. J Virol 2001; 75:589–594

76. Wild CT, Greenwell T, Matthews T. A synthetic peptide from HIV-1 gp41 is a potent inhibitor of virus-mediated cell-cell fusion. AIDS Res Hum Retroviruses 1993; 9:1051–1053

77. Sista PR, Melby T, Davison D, et al. Characterization of determinants of genotypic and phenotypic resistance to enfuvirtide in baseline and on-treatment HIV-1 isolates. AIDS 2004; 18: 1787–1794

78. Dorr P, Wesby S, Dobbs S, et al. Maraviroc (UK-427,857), a potent, orally bioavailable and selective small-molecule inhibitor of chemokine receptor CCR5 with broad-spectrum anti-human immunodeficiency virus type 1 activity. Antimicrob Agents Chemother 2005; 49:4721–4732

79. Hazuda DJ, Felock P, Witmer M, Wolfe A, et al. Inhibitors of strand transfer that prevent integration and inhibit HIV-1 replication in cells. Science 2000; 287:646–650

80. Hazuda DJ, Miller MD, Nguyen BY, Zhao J. for the P005 Study Team. Resistance to the HIV-integrase inhibitor raltegravir: analysis of protocol 005, a phase II study in patients with triple-class resistant HIV-1 infection. Antiviral Ther 2007; 12:S10

81. St Clair MH, Martin JL, Tudor-Williams G, et al. Resistance to ddI and sensitivity to AZT induced by a mutation in HIV-1 reverse transcriptase. Science 1991; 253:1557–1559

82. Larder BA. 3″-azido-3″-deoxythymidine resistance suppressed by a mutation conferring human immunodeficiency virus type 1 resistance to nonnucleoside reverse transcriptase inhibitors. Antimicrob Agents Chemother 1992; 36:2664–2669

83. Whitcomb JM, Huang W, Limolo K, Paxinos E, et al. Hypersusceptibility to NNRTIs in HIV-1: clinical, phenotypic and genotypic correlates. AIDS 2002; 16:F41–F47

84. Shulman NS, Bosch RJ, Mellors JW, Albrecht MA, Katzenstein DA. Genetic correlates of efavirenz hypersusceptibility. AIDS 2004; 18:1781–1785

85. Haubrich RH, Kemper CA, Hellman NS, Keiser PH, et al. The clinical relevance of NNRTI hypersusceptibility: a prospective cohort analysis. AIDS 2002; 16:33–40

86. Shulman N, Zalopa AR, Passaro D, Shafer RW, et al. Phenotypic hypersusceptibility to NNRTIs in treatment-experienced HIV-infected patients: impact on virological response to efavirenz-based therapy. AIDS 2001; 15:25–32

87. Quinones-Mateu ME, Moore-Dudley DM, Jegede O, Weber J, Arts EJ. Viral resistance and fitness. Adv Pharmacol 2008; 56:257–296

88. Dykes C, Demeter LM. Clinical significance of human immunodeficiency virus type 1 replication fitness. Clin Microbiol Rev 2007; 20:550–578

89. Kantor R, Katzenstein D. Drug resistance in non-subtype B HIV-1. J Clin Virol 2004; 29:152–159

90. Spira S, Wainberg MA, Loemba H, Turner D, Brenner BG. Impact of clade diversity on HIV-1 virulence, antiretroviral drug sensitivity and drug resistance. J Antimicrob Chemother 2003; 51:229–240

91. Grossman Z, Paxinos EE, Averbach D, et al. Mutation D30N is not preferentially selected by human immunodeficiency virus type 1 subtype C in the development of resistance to nelfinavir. Antimicrob Agents Chemother 2004; 48:2159–2165

92. Brenner B, Turner D, Oliveira M, et al. A V106M mutation in HIV-1 clade C viruses exposed to efavirenz confers cross-resistance to non-nucleoside reverse transcriptase inhibitors. AIDS 2003; 17:F1–F5

93. Grossman Z, Istomin V, Averbuch D, et al. Genetic variation at NNRTI resistance-associated positions in patients infected with HIV-1 subtype C. AIDS 2004; 18:909–915

94. Rhee S-Y, Kantor R, Katzenstein D, et al. for the International Non Subtype B HIV-1 Working Group. HIV-1 pol mutation frequency by subtype and treatment experience: extension of the HIVseq program to seven non-B subtypes. AIDS 2006; 20:643–651

95. Kantor R, Katzenstein DA, Efron B, et al. Impact of HIV-1 subtype and antiretroviral therapy on protease and reverse transcriptase genotype: results of a global collaboration. PLoS Med 2005; 2:325–337

96. Descamps D, Chaix ML, Andre P, et al. French national sentinel survey of antiretroviral drug resistance in patients with HIV-1 primary infection and in antiretroviral-naive chronically infected patients in 2001–2002. J Acquir Immune Defic Syndr 2005; 38:545–552

97. Larder BA, Darby G, Richman DD. HIV with reduced sensitivity to zidovudine (AZT) isolated during prolonged therapy. Science 1989; 243:1731–1734

98. Larder BA, Kemp SD. Multiple mutations in HIV-1 reverse transcriptase confer high-level resistance to zidovudine (AZT). Science 1989; 246:1155–1158

99. Japour AJ, Mayers DL, Johnson VA, et al. A standardized peripheral blood mononuclear cell culture assay for the determination of drug susceptibilities of clinical human immunodeficiency virus-1 isolates. Antimicrob Agents Chemother 1993; 37:1095–1101

100. Johnson VA, Brun-Vezinet F, Clotet B, et al. Update of the drug resistance mutations in HIV-1: 2007. Top HIV Med 2007; 15:119–125

101. Rhee S-Y, Gonzales MJ, Kantor R, Betts BJ, Ravela J, Shafer RW. Human immunodeficiency virus reverse transcriptase and protease sequence database. Nucleic Acids Res 2003; 31:298–303

102. Shafer RW, Rhee S-Y, Pillay D, et al. HIV-1 protease and reverse transcriptase mutations for drug resistance surveillance. AIDS 2007; 21:215–223

103. Hammer SM, Saag MS, Schechter M, et al. Treatment for Adult HIV Infection. 2006 Recommendations of the International AIDS Society–USA Panel. JAMA 2006; 296:827–843

104. Liu TF, Shafer RW. Web resources for HIV type 1 genotypic resistance test interpretation. Clin Infect Dis 2006; 42:1608–1618

105. Antiretroviral therapy for HIV infection in adults and adolescents: recommendations for a public health approach. 2006 revision, Geneva, Switzerland: WHO Press, 2006; 1–128. Available at http://www.who.int/hiv/pub/guidelines/en/

106. Cozzi-Lepri A, Phillips AN, Ruiz L, et al. Evolution of drug resistance in HIV-infected patients remaining on a virologically

failing combination antiretroviral therapy regimen. AIDS 2007; 21:721–732

107. Durant J, Clevenbergh P, Halfon P, et al. Drug-resistance genotyping in HIV-1 therapy: the VIRADAPT randomized controlled trial. Lancet 1999; 353:2195–2199

108. Baxter JD, Mayers DL, Wentworth DN, et al. A randomized study of antiretroviral management based on plasma genotypic antiretroviral resistance testing in patients failing therapy: CPCRA 046 Study Team for the Terry Beirn Community Programs for Clinical Research on AIDS. AIDS 2000; 14:F83–F93

109. Cohen C, Hunt S, Sension M, et al. and the VIRA3001 Study Team. A randomized trial assessing the impact of phenotypic resistance testing on antiretroviral therapy. AIDS 2002; 16:579–588

110. Tural C, Ruiz L, Holtzer C, et al., Havana Study Group. Clinical utility of HIV-1 genotyping and expert advice: the Havana trial. AIDS 2002; 16:209–218

111. The PLATO Collaboration. Predictors of trend in CD4-positive T-cell count and mortality among HIV-1-infected individuals with virological failure to all three antiretroviral-drug classes. Lancet 2004; 364:51–62

112. Deeks SG, Wrin T, Hoh R, et al. Virologic and immunologic consequences of discontinuing combination antiretroviral drug therapy in HIV-infected patients with detectable viremia. N Engl J Med 2001; 344:472–480

113. Lawrence J, Mayers DL, Huppler Hullsiek K, et al. for the 064 Study Team of the Terry Beirn Community Programs for Clinical Research on AIDS Structured treatment interruption in patients with multidrug-resistant human immunodeficiency virus. N Engl J Med 2003; 349 837–846

114. Ghosn J, Wirden M, Ktorza N, et al. No benefit of a structured treatment interruption based on genotypic resistance in heavily pretreated HIV-infected patients. AIDS 2005; 19:1643–1647

115. The Strategies for Management of Antiretroviral Therapy (SMART) Study Group CD4 + count-guided interruption of antiretroviral therapy. N Engl J Med 355:2283–2296

116. Kousignian I, Abgrall S, Grabar S, et al., Clinical Epidemiology Group of the French Hospital Database on HIV. Maintaining antiretroviral therapy reduces the risk of AIDS-defining events in patients with uncontrolled viral replication and profound immunodeficiency. Clin Infect Dis 2008; 46:296–304

117. Miller V, Cozzi-Lepri A, Hertogs K, et al. HIV drug susceptibility and treatment response to mega-HAART regimen in patients from the Frankfurt HIV cohort. Antivir Ther 2000; 5:49–55

118. Montaner JS, Harrigan PR, Jahnke N, et al. Multiple drug rescue therapy for HIV-infected individuals with prior virologic failure on multiple regimens. AIDS 2001; 15:61–69

119. Youle M, Tyrer M, Fisher M, et al. Brief report: two year outcome of a multidrug regimen in patients who did not respond to a protease inhibitor regimen. J Acquir Immune Defic Syndr 2002; 29:58–61

120. Hirsch HH, Drechsler H, Holbro A, et al. Genotypic and phenotypic resistance testing of HIV-1 in routine clinical care. Eur J Clin Microbiol Infect Dis 2005; 24:733–738

121. Routy JP, Machouf N, Edwardes MD, et al. Factors associated with a decrease in the prevalence of drug resistance in newly HIV-1 infected individuals in Montreal. AIDS 2004; 18:2305–2312

122. de Mendoza C, Rodreiguez C, Eiros JM, et al. Antiretroviral recommendations may influence the rate of transmission of drug-resistant HIV type 1. Clin Infect Dis 2005; 41:227–232

Chapter 72
Clinical Implications of Resistance for Patients with Chronic Hepatitis B

Nathaniel A. Brown

1 Scientific Background, Natural History, and Treatment Goals in Chronic Hepatitis B: Similarities and Contrasts with HIV Infection

Chronic infections with human immunodeficiency virus (HIV), hepatitis B virus (HBV), and hepatitis C virus (HCV) are widely prevalent, affecting, in *toto,* some 600–700 million people worldwide, and continue to be associated with significant morbidity and mortality despite advances in antiviral therapy.

Progress in antiviral therapy for HIV infection began 20 years ago with zidovudine (Retrovir™, AZT), the first in a series of nucleoside-type inhibitors of the HIV reverse transcriptase (RT). In roughly the same time period, progress in the treatment of hepatitis B and hepatitis C began with alpha-interferon treatment. While providing important evidence that such severe chronic viral infections can be successfully treated in some patients, the overall durable response rates to these early antiviral treatment regimens were relatively low due to the emergence of drug-resistant viral strains within several months after initiating nucleoside monotherapies, in the case of HIV infection, and to a high rate of intrinsic resistance to interferon's beneficial effects in hepatitis B and C patients, a phenomenon which is still poorly understood.

During the past two decades, increasing scientific understanding of HIV infection has supported a series of important therapeutic advances, involving the development of potent HIV inhibitors from several different mechanistic classes, and the concurrent use of these antiviral agents in combination treatment regimens. Today, with the improved efficacy and reduced resistance offered by such combination antiviral regimens (often termed "Highly Active Antiretroviral Therapy," i.e., HAART regimens), over 70% of newly treated HIV patients can expect to have profound virologic responses to de novo combination treatment with such multi-drug antiviral regimens,

achieving and maintaining PCR-nondetectable serum HIV RNA for years, with associated survival benefits (1, 2).

As anti-HBV and anti-HCV therapeutics progress beyond interferon monotherapy into an era of increasing availability of direct-acting, orally administered anti-HBV and anti-HCV agents, it is appropriate to consider the key lessons from progress in HIV therapeutics – and their applicability to advancing treatment for hepatitis B and C. Before delving into clinical aspects of HBV resistance, the subject of this chapter, it is worthwhile to consider the virologic and pathogenetic similarities and differences between HIV and HBV infection, which result in differences in natural history and treatment goals, as well as the potential lessons from advances in HIV therapy that may be relevant to optimizing HBV therapy.

Several important scientific and clinical similarities and contrasts between HIV infection and HBV infection are summarized in Table 1.

2 Contrasts in Natural History and Treatment Goals for Patients with Chronic HBV Infection vs. HIV Infection

The distinct biologic features of HIV and HBV infection summarized in Table 1 result in substantial differences in the natural history of these two globally important chronic viral infections, with implications for differences in patient management with antiviral therapy. The natural history of chronic HIV infection is characterized by relentless progression, with a somewhat variable time course, to immunologic failure and endstage multi-organ complications. In contrast, after perinatal acquisition (the most common mode), the natural history of chronic HBV infection is characterized by three pathogenetic phases, which have a widely variable course in individual patients: the "immune tolerance" phase, the "immune clearance" phase, and the "inactive carrier" phase (3–5). The initial, immune tolerance phase is characterized by high HBV

N.A. Brown (✉)
Antiviral Development Consultants LLC, Weston, MA, USA
nat.brown@comcast.net

D.L. Mayers (ed.), *Antimicrobial Drug Resistance*,
DOI 10.1007/978-1-60327-595-8_72, © Humana Press, a part of Springer Science+Business Media, LLC 2009

Table 1 Scientific and clinical features of chronic HIV and HBV infections

Feature	HIV	HBV
Polymerase fidelity	Low: 100-fold higher error rate for HIV reverse transcriptase (RT) compared to most eukaryotic DNA polymerases	Intermediate: 10-fold higher error rate for HBV polymerase/reverse transcriptase (Pol/RT) compared to eukaryotic DNA polymerases
Persistent genomic forms	Integrated double-stranded DNA, reverse-transcribed from HIV RNA templates	Covalently closed circular DNA (cccDNA), maintained as episomal mini-chromosomes
Replication kinetics in untreated patients	Large daily virion turnover, ca. 10^9–10^{10} virions/day; virion half-life ca. 6 h	Large daily virion turnover, ca. 10^{11}–10^{12} virions/day; virion half-life ca. 12–24 h
Tissue tropism	Relatively wide: lymphocytes, R–E system, nerve cells, epithelial cells. Progressive irrevocable depletion of CD4 lymphocytes is key to immune failure	Relatively narrow: hepatocytes; ? lymphoid cells and/or R–E system? Hepatocytes regenerable, relatively short-lived (ca. 10- to 100-day half-life for HBV-infected hepatocytes)
Transmission	Predominantly sexual; IV drug use; perinatal transmission declining with antiviral treatment of mother and infant	Predominantly perinatal in endemic regions, such as Asia. Predominantly sexual and IV drug use in non-endemic settings
Natural history, untreated	Average 10–15 years to endstage clinical complications, which potentially occur in virtually all HIV carriers if untreated. Spontaneous resolution rare, if at all	10–50 years to endstage complications, which occur in 15–40% of chronic HBV carriers. Spontaneous resolution to inactive carrier state in 3–15% per year, primarily during "immune clearance phase" (typically second to fifth decades of life), after perinatal acquisition
Functional consequences of viral breakthrough with drug-resistant virus	Loss of CD4 cells, including memory CD4 cells and potentially other non-regenerable cells	Loss of hepatocytes; potentially regenerable if cirrhosis not advanced
Vaccine availability	No	Yes

replication, with detectable serum hepatitis B "e" antigen (HBeAg) and high serum HBV DNA levels (averaging 6–10 $\log_{10}$ genome copies/mL), but with normal serum ALT levels and negligible liver inflammation. As immunologic tolerance of HBV antigens is lost or partially lost with age, the subsequent immune clearance phase is characterized initially by continuing high HBV replication (HBeAg positive, with high-to-moderate HBV DNA levels) with onset of signs of immune-mediated liver injury, reflected by chronic necroinflammatory changes on liver biopsy and persistently or intermittently elevated serum aminotransferase (ALT, AST) levels reflecting hepatocyte necrosis. In some HBV carriers, the immune clearance phase eventually results in clearance of detectable serum HBeAg, usually with gain of detectable antibody to HBeAg (termed "HBeAg seroconversion") and transition to the third (inactive carrier) phase. For those who achieve it, the inactive carrier phase comprises a state of substantially lower HBV replication, with serum HBV DNA levels usually below 5 $\log_{10}$ copies/mL and sometimes nondetectable by sensitive PCR methods. Some of these HBeAg-seroconverted patients eventually lose detectable serum hepatitis B surface antigen (HBsAg) as well, at which time HBV DNA is typically nondetectable in the peripheral blood although usually still detectable in liver biopsy specimens (6).

In contrast to perinatally acquired HBV infection, adolescent and adult patients with horizontally acquired chronic HBV infection (via sexual transmission, IV drug use, or contaminated blood products or medical sharps), experience no immune tolerant phase and enter directly into the immune clearance phase, with or without eventual transition to the inactive carrier phase and clearance of clinically significant levels of HBV replication.

The course of chronic HBV infection in individual carriers is highly variable with regard to progression through the disease phases and the development of clinical consequences. Rarely, perinatally acquired or horizontally acquired chronic HBV infection can progress to cirrhosis and/or hepatocellular carcinoma rather quickly, e.g., during the first 10–20 years after infection. More commonly 20–50 years are required for progression to endstage disease (cirrhosis or hepatocellular carcinoma). In many HBV carriers, the immune clearance phase is short or clinically inapparent, with little or no lasting liver injury before progression to the inactive carrier phase, while in others the immune clearance phase persists without durable HBeAg seroconversion and with persistent high-level HBV replication and associated necroinflammatory liver damage progressing to endstage disease. In some patients there is a fourth disease phase, i.e., reactivation from the inactive carrier phase, sometimes after many years, with return to high levels of HBV replication and with recrudescence of HBV-associated necroinflammatory liver damage (3). HBV reactivation can occur spontaneously, or in conjunction with recognized risk factors such as cancer (or cancer chemotherapy) and various forms of immunodebilitation.

Finally, it should be noted that, in some patients with chronic hepatitis B, loss of detectable HBeAg reflects, not immune clearance, but rather the emergence, usually during the third to the sixth decades of life, of HBV strains with mutations in pre-core/core gene sequences that abrogate HBeAg expression but do not affect HBV virion production since the abrogated HBeAg peptide is not a virion component. In these patients with "HBeAg-negative" chronic hepatitis B, virion production can continue at clinically significant levels, reflected by serum HBV DNA levels typically in the range of 4–9 $\log_{10}$ copies/mL, about 1.5–2 $\log_{10}$ below the levels observed during wild-type (HBeAg-positive) HBV infection but still enough to cause progressive liver disease.

Because of the distinct phases and variable clinical course of chronic HBV infection, optimal clinical management of hepatitis B patients requires considerations of each patient's phase of disease and risk factors for progression to endstage complications. This natural history of HBV infection contrasts with HIV infection, where essentially all patients can be assumed to need continuous antiviral treatment due to a risk for CD4 lymphocyte depletion and clinical disease progression.

Patients in the immune tolerant phase of HBV infection, with persistently normal ALTs, have been found to have a generally favorable prognosis despite high levels of HBV replication. Since current anti-HBV therapy is usually not eradicative of HBV infection, and liver disease and treatment-induced HBeAg seroconversion are negligible in immune tolerant patients, antiviral therapy for chronic HBV infection is currently reserved primarily for patients in the immune clearance phase of HBV infection, with substantial HBV DNA levels coupled with evidence of an ongoing immune response producing necroinflammatory liver injury, with elevated serum ALT levels and histologic evidence of "interface hepatitis." The histologic hallmark of interface hepatitis is chronic inflammatory cells breaking out of the peri-portal areas and into the interportal and intralobular areas of hepatic architecture (5, 7, 8). The essential treatment goal for most patients with chronic HBV infection is therefore to suppress HBV replication and minimize liver injury during the immune clearance phase, with an adjunctive goal to induce HBeAg clearance if possible. In HBeAg-positive patients HBeAg clearance, denoted by HBeAg loss or seroconversion (HBeAg loss with gain of detectable HBeAb), can result in a durable transition to the inactive carrier state, during which patients need continual monitoring but usually do not need antiviral treatment.

A current treatment controversy concerns the quantitative degree of HBV suppression needed to minimize liver injury in patients with chronic hepatitis B during periods of active HBV replication. Large seroepidemiologic studies suggest that significant hepatic disease progression can occur in HBV carriers with persistent serum HBV DNA levels exceeding 3–4 $\log_{10}$ copies/mL (9–13). Such cross-sectional studies include HBV carriers with and without concurrent liver disease, however, and some experts have suggested that, in patients with established HBV-associated chronic liver disease, i.e., with chronic hepatitis B, HBV replication should be reduced as much as possible, preferably to PCR-nondetectable serum HBV DNA levels.

3 Implications for Viral Resistance (HBV vs. HIV)

The biologic similarities and differences between HBV and HIV infection noted in Table 1 also bear directly on the prospects for the evolution of drug-resistant viral variants during antiviral therapy and the clinical consequences of antiviral drug resistance. High daily virion production and error-prone viral polymerase activities result in a high likelihood of spontaneous emergence of drug-resistant viral mutants during both HIV and HBV infection. However, clinical experience with antiviral nucleosides in hepatitis B patients indicates slower/lower emergence of viral resistance compared to HIV patients treated with the same agent, as illustrated by the prototypical data for lamivudine in HIV and HBV patients. During the HIV trials of lamivudine monotherapy in the mid-1990s, HIV resistance was nearly universal within 3–6 months after starting lamivudine monotherapy, while viral resistance emerged more slowly with lamivudine monotherapy in trials with hepatitis B patients (14–32% of patients at 1 year, and 50% of patients at 3 years) (14–16). The clinical import of these HBV vs. HIV differences is that potent nucleoside/tide monotherapies can produce marked suppression of HBV replication in many patients with chronic hepatitis B, with responses typically lasting 2–3 years or longer, while this duration of virologic response to antiviral monotherapies was not observed historically for any anti-HIV agent.

Presumably the biologic features of HBV infection responsible for this slower/lower emergence of viral resistance include not only the tenfold lower error rate with the HBV Pol/RT but also the overall narrower tissue tropism, with HBV's primary tropism for a relatively short-lived cell type (hepatocytes), which results in a need for continual HBV polymerase activity and tissue re-infection to maintain the cccDNA templates that allow for HBV persistence, including the spontaneously mutated cccDNA templates encoding drug-resistant HBV strains. Additionally, for unclear reasons presumably related to the dynamics of the phosphorylated nucleoside/tide inhibitors in the active domain of the viral polymerase, and to overall virus/host dynamics (e.g., including immunologic features), hepatitis B patients treated with nucleosides/tides are likely to have large multi-log reductions in serum HBV DNA levels, while HIV patients treated with the same nucleoside/tide (e.g., with lamivudine and adefovir as prototypes) typically experience only a ca. 1-log$_{10}$ reduction in serum HIV RNA levels. This more rapid and more quantitative suppression of viral replication in hepatitis B patients reduces the chance for emergence of viral variants carrying drug resistance mutations, compared to the lesser degree of viral suppression achieved in HIV patients treated with the same nucleoside/tide. Indeed de novo combination regimens with multi-class anti-HIV agents became the standard-of-care for HIV therapy because of the inability to fully suppress HIV replication to PCR-nondetectable levels with nucleosides alone.

Although hepatitis B patients achieve quantitatively better antiviral efficacy with nucleosides/tide monotherapies compared to HIV patients, prolonged treatment with nucleoside/tide monotherapies in hepatitis B patients has, predictably, been associated with the eventual emergence of drug-resistant HBV strains in cumulatively increasing proportions of patients over prolonged periods of time (years), as will be further discussed below. To further improve HBV therapy with direct antivirals, should de novo combination regimens be used in hepatitis B patients, similar to HIV therapy? While drug-resistant viral variants can arise spontaneously for any antiviral agent, the probability of a single viral strain arising endogenously, with resistance mutations to multiple agents in a combination regimen, is small and requires a longer timeframe. Therefore, de novo combination treatment, with two or more potent agents having complementary (non-overlapping) viral resistance mutations, is always preferable in principle for all chronic viral infections, including HIV and HBV infections, toward the treatment goals of maximal viral suppression and minimal chance for emergence of drug-resistant viral strains. De novo combination therapy is certainly needed for HIV infection, when many patients presenting for treatment are young and essentially all patients are at risk for potentially fatal progression of the disease within 10–15 years and all monotherapies have periods of benefit limited to several weeks or a few months. However, while de novo combination treatment is also preferable, in principle, for patients with chronic hepatitis B, several considerations suggest that de novo combination treatment, with its extra costs and potential extra toxicities, may not be necessary for all hepatitis B patients. The lower/slower emergence of drug-resistant mutants in hepatitis B patients, coupled with the generally slower progression of chronic hepatitis B to endstage complications, the non-progressive (or slowly progressive) liver disease in some patients, and the spontaneous resolution of HBV infection to a minimally replicative state (via HBeAg seroconversion) in a proportion of patients (including some patients with drug-resistant HBV strains) all suggest that, in contrast to the situation with HIV patients, not all hepatitis B patients will require de novo combination treatment regimens to achieve satisfactory clinical outcomes. Additionally, due to the potential regeneration of lost hepatocytes, the clinical (i.e., functional) consequences of resistance-related viral

breakthrough are arguably more reversible in hepatitis B patients than in CD4-depleted HIV patients. This is almost certainly true for the vast majority of hepatitis B patients with non-cirrhotic compensated liver disease, if viral breakthrough and resistance-related liver injury are detected early and appropriate adjustments are made in the antiviral regimen. In contrast, during episodes of viral breakthrough in HIV patients it appears that there is likely to be a lasting decline in immune function due to loss of memory CD4 lymphocytes, which are not fully regenerable. Nonetheless, it should be noted that virologic breakthroughs in hepatitis B patients can be clinically severe, if the patient experiences a severe immune-mediated "flare" in hepatic disease activity with the viral breakthrough or if the patient has underlying cirrhosis and progresses rapidly to hepatic failure.

The rest of this chapter will discuss the status of current anti-HBV therapy and observations of clinically related resistance for each of the currently available anti-HBV agents, and potential treatment strategies for minimizing HBV resistance. The goal is to use these observations, together with consideration of the patients' stage of disease and prognosis for disease progression, to establish an approach toward further optimization of antiviral therapy for various hepatitis B patient populations.

4 Current Antiviral Treatment Options for Hepatitis B Patients and Associated Resistance Observations

There are currently six regulatory-approved antiviral treatment options for patients with chronic hepatitis B: two interferon products, interferon alpha-2b (Intron-A™) and pegylated interferon alpha-2a (Pegasys™); three nucleoside analogs, lamivudine (Epivir-HBV™, Zeffix™), entecavir (Baraclude™), and telbivudine (Tyzeka™, Sebivo™); and one nucleotide analog, adefovir dipivoxil (Hepsera™). Additionally, two nucleotides (tenofovir and ANA380) and two nucleosides (emtricitabine and clevudine) are currently in Phase II–III of clinical testing for hepatitis B.

The large-scale Phase III trial data for all of the currently approved anti-HBV agents support the key treatment concept that inhibition of HBV replication, reflected by substantial and prolonged reduction in serum HBV DNA levels, during the immune clearance phase of HBV infection (i.e., in patients with moderate to high HBV DNA levels, elevated aminotransferases, and necroinflammatory liver damage) is associated with clinical benefits such as decreased liver inflammation, normalized serum ALT levels, and enhanced rates of HBeAg loss/seroconversion compared to no treatment or to placebo treatment. Additionally, a large randomized study of lamivudine vs. placebo, in hepatitis B patients with compensated cirrhosis and active HBV replication, indicated that nucleoside antiviral therapy could reduce patients' progression to clinically decompensated cirrhosis and perhaps reduce the development of hepatocellular carcinoma (17). Treatment with the currently available agents can afford satisfactory disease management for many or perhaps most non-cirrhotic hepatitis B patients, in many cases for several years or more, especially with the newer agents. But in view of the long (10–50 years) evolution of liver disease in HBV chronic carriers there is a continuing need for improved antiviral agents or treatment regimens to further optimize durable response rates and long-term patient outcomes. The rest of this chapter will focus on observations of resistance to the currently available anti-HBV nucleosides and nucleotides, and the implications for further optimization of clinical management of various hepatitis B patient subpopulations. Intrinsic resistance to interferon's beneficial antiviral and immunomodulatory effects, and possible interferon-related selection of viral subpopulations during treatment, will not be discussed further here.

Detailed information on the HBV genomic mutations associated with reduced susceptibility to each of the four current anti-HBV nucleosides/tides is given in an accompanying chapter by Dr. Stephen Locarnini (*The Hepatitis B Virus and Antiviral Drug Resistance: Causes, Patterns, and Mechanisms*). In discussing clinical aspects of HBV drug resistance, it is useful to distinguish among several terms used in the context of discussions of HBV resistance. In the HBV clinical arena the term "genotypic resistance" is often used to denote the detectable presence, in plasma or serum, of HBV strains with mutations that confer reduced drug susceptibility in vitro and/or that have been previously implicated in clinically significant drug resistance. In the context of hepatitis B clinical observations, the term "virologic breakthrough" connotes the presence of recrudescent serum HBV DNA levels after an initial response. In line with this concept, presently there is an evolving expert consensus that virologic breakthrough should be analytically defined as a persistent $1 \log_{10}$ or greater increase in HBV DNA level from a patient's nadir value while on continuous antiviral treatment, after an initial response of at least a $1 \log_{10}$ reduction from the patient's pre-treatment HBV DNA value. In the virology laboratory, the term "phenotypic resistance" connotes an observation of reduced drug susceptibility for a mutant HIV strain or mutant HBV strain (n.b., HBV cannot be propagated in vitro but drug sensitivity can be assessed in transfection assays and in stably HBV-transfected cell lines). In the hepatitis B clinical arena the term "clinical resistance" (or "clinically significant" resistance) usually connotes the presence of viral breakthrough with drug-resistant viral strains together with the findings of clinical disease exacerbation such as elevated serum aminotransferase levels or other clinical or laboratory signs of recrudescent liver disease, in a patient previously thought to be responding to antiviral therapy.

4.1 Lamivudine Resistance

Published clinical experience with lamivudine, from extensive Phase II–IV trials, is instructive with regard to a number of fundamental clinical features of HBV drug resistance. Lamivudine was the first directly acting HBV antiviral agent and was developed at a time when the only other proven treatment option was interferon, to which many patients in the lamivudine clinical trials had previously failed to respond. Prior to trials in hepatitis B patients lamivudine had been tested in HIV patients, and it was known that the M184 codon was the principal HIV mutational hotspot for lamivudine resistance. It was also known, from DNA sequence data, that the HBV Pol/RT had a sequence homologous to the sequence in HIV codon 184; this homologous motif in the HBV Pol/RT is called the "YMDD motif" and is centered on the methionine codon at amino acid position 204 in the HBV Pol/RT. Thus, despite the lack of an in vitro propagation system for HBV and the lack of any clinical data from hepatitis B patients at that time, it was predicted that substitutions at the YMDD locus would be the principal culprit for lamivudine resistance in hepatitis B patients. Although no viral breakthrough was detected in Phase I of the hepatitis B trials with lamivudine (with 1–2 months' treatment), two reports during Phase II hepatitis B trials, and subsequent Phase III trial data, confirmed that most lamivudine resistance in hepatitis B patients is mediated by the emergence of HBV strains with substitutions of valine or isoleucine for the methionine residue at HBV Pol/RT codon 204, the so-called "YMDD mutations" now denoted as M204V and M204I (16, 18–20). In addition, it was found that many or most lamivudine-resistant patients with YMDD-mutant HBV strains, particularly the M204V strains, had a concomitant secondary mutation comprising a substitution of leucine for methionine at HBV Pol/RT codon 180 (the L180M mutation). Subsequently, other secondary HBV Pol/RT mutations were described in patients with lamivudine resistance, as reviewed in the accompanying chapter by Dr. Locarnini. The frequency and functional significance of these other secondary HBV Pol/RT mutations in lamivudine-treated hepatitis B patients has not been fully elucidated; overall it appears that the vast preponderance of clinically significant HBV resistance in lamivudine recipients is due to the common emergence of YMDD-mutant HBV strains, and the clinical significance of the unresolved secondary mutations may be minimal.

The clinical consequences of lamivudine-resistant (YMDD-mutant) HBV strains were delineated in numerous sponsored clinical trials of lamivudine and in investigator-initiated studies, at a time when no salvage therapy was available for patients with lamivudine resistance other than interferon (n.b. many patients had previously failed interferon therapy). As noted earlier, large Phase III–IV clinical trials established that 14–32% of hepatitis B patients receiving lamivudine for 1 year developed HBV genotypic resistance, i.e., PCR-detectable HBV strains with YMDD-associated resistance mutations (14–16, 21–24). Perhaps surprisingly, it was found that the clinical importance of these YMDD-mutant HBV strains was variable, with regard to the impact on serum HBV DNA levels and clinical efficacy outcomes. Although most patients lost appreciable degrees of treatment response, a partial efficacy benefit remained observable in most patients for many months or for several years after the development of detectable YMDD-mutant HBV strains (16, 24, 25). Despite a noticeable degree of viral breakthrough after the development of YMDD-mutant HBV strains in most (but not all) patients, lamivudine recipients with detectable YMDD-mutant HBV tended to maintain partially reduced HBV DNA levels (averaging about $0.5–1.0 \log_{10}$ below pretreatment values) and serum ALT levels tended to remain improved compared to pretreatment values (except for a minority of patients with disease flares that were breakthrough-associated, as discussed below), for observation periods of up to 3 years in the absence of other treatment (16, 24, 25). Also, histologic responses were partially maintained in most lamivudine-resistant patients for a period of time, although longer-term (3-year) data indicated an eventual return of appreciable liver inflammation in many patients (26). On the other hand, one of the more important negative impacts of genotypic HBV resistance was that treatment-related HBeAg loss/seroconversion reverted to a low rate after YMDD-mutant HBV were detected, so that rates of HBeAg loss/seroconversion in lamivudine recipients with YMDD-mutant HBV did not differ from rates of HBeAg loss/seroconversion observed with placebo treatment in the same trials (14, 15, 15, 16, 16, 21, 22, 27).

The clinical observations in hepatitis B patients with lamivudine resistance, mentioned above, were consistent with the rather axiomatic notion that viral strains with resistance-associated mutations in the active domain of the viral polymerase tend to be at least partially replication deficient compared to wild-type strains – though the presence of putative "compensatory" secondary mutations in some patients' YMDD-mutant HBV strains, and the return of serum HBV DNA levels to pretreatment values in some patients, certainly suggest that such an inference should be considered with caution. More importantly, an additional "downside" in the early clinical observations regarding lamivudine resistance was the finding that some patients experienced severe disease "flares" in association with viral breakthrough, indicated by marked aminotransferase elevations, sometimes with biochemical and clinical signs of hepatic insufficiency. Such severe resistance-associated disease flares occasionally progressed rapidly to liver failure or death, while other patients recovered with HBeAg seroconversion and long-term disease remissions (16, 18–20, 28–30). Severe resistance-associated disease flares are sporadic and are essentially unpredictable. An important feature of such events, for patient management is that the ALT elevations and other signs of hepatic injury in such patients rarely (if ever) occur at the time of initial viral breakthrough. Instead, ALT elevations and other flare manifestations typically occur 3–6 months after initial serum HBV DNA breakthrough, an observation that supports pre-emptive adjustment in antiviral therapy at the time of recrudescent HBV DNA levels to avoid clinically severe disease flares, as discussed further.

Overall, lamivudine has proven to be a moderately effective and safe antiviral treatment option for patients with chronic hepatitis B. However, with about 50% of lamivudine recipients having detectable YMDD-mutant HBV after 3 years of treatment, the cumulative incidence of lamivudine resistance is often cited as a key reason for no longer recommending lamivudine as first-line treatment when better treatment options are now available (8, 31). Perhaps overlooked in the reviews of cumulative lamivudine resistance is the fact that, after 3 or 4 years of lamivudine treatment in clinical trials, more than 50% of patients had HBeAg-seroconverted, including an appreciable (ca. 20–30%) proportion of the patients who had developed YMDD-mutant HBV strains during the clinical trials, again suggesting that not all patients with lamivudine resistance will progress to poor outcomes (16, 25–27).

To counter the high cumulative resistance with lamivudine monotherapy, lamivudine has been tested and continues to be tested in combination regimens with other anti-HBV agents, and some clinical experts have been reporting good results using lamivudine as primary therapy in association with proactive use of add-on adefovir therapy for patients showing evidence of, or at risk for, viral breakthrough (32–35). Today, although lamivudine continues to be the globally most-prescribed antiviral agent for hepatitis B, it appears likely that prolonged use of lamivudine monotherapy will decline in the future, but lamivudine will probably continue to be used as a component of hepatitis B antiviral regimens for many years due to its excellent safety profile and relatively low cost. In regard to the latter, it is worth noting that lamivudine became generically available in China in 2006, and the costs of lamivudine therapy are expected to decline further as lamivudine becomes increasingly available from generic suppliers worldwide in the coming years.

4.2 Adefovir Resistance

Adefovir dipivoxil (Hepsera™) was found to have negligible HBV resistance in the 48-week Phase III trials in HBeAg-positive and HBeAg-negative patients with chronic hepatitis B (35, 36). Subsequently, it was found that two key HBV Pol/RT mutations (N236T and Y181V) confer reduced HBV susceptibility in vitro and are associated with HBV DNA breakthrough in hepatitis B patients treated with prolonged adefovir monotherapy (37–39). Additional details regarding adefovir-associated HBV Pol/RT mutations can be found in the accompanying chapter by Dr. Locarnini. Data on long-term resistance in HBeAg-positive hepatitis B patients from the adefovir Phase III trials are incomplete, due to treatment misrandomizations in the second year of the large GS437 Phase III adefovir trial in HBeAg-positive patients, which resulted in the premature termination of trial participation for most patients. Longer-term data on 65 HBeAg-positive patients, treated with adefovir beyond Week 48, indicate that 16 of 64 HBeAg-positive patients (ca. 25%) developed HBV strains with detectable adefovir resistance mutations after a median total duration of 235 weeks (ca. 4½ years) of adefovir treatment (39). Long-term follow-up of Phase III patients with HBeAg-negative chronic hepatitis B, from the GS438 trial, indicated that after 5 years of adefovir 29% of patients had developed adefovir resistance mutations (39). Perhaps more importantly, recent data have consistently indicated that the rate of emergence of HBV resistance to adefovir monotherapy is distinctly higher in patients with pre-existing lamivudine resistance, with 2-year adefovir resistance rates ranging 20% or more in this patient population (40–43).

Intrinsic HBV resistance to adefovir has also been described. Patients carrying HBV strains with an I233V variant substitution in HBV Pol/RT were reported to exhibit non-response to adefovir therapy (44). The I233V HBV polymerase substitution is thought to exist spontaneously in about 1–2% of HBV carriers. Such patients were reported to be responsive to entecavir therapy (45). A later report, however, described four patients with I233V HBV polymerase substitutions and good responses to adefovir, so the issue of pre-existing (i.e., "primary") resistance to adefovir remains controversial (46).

Compared to lamivudine, relatively little data are available regarding longer-term clinical outcomes in hepatitis B patients with adefovir resistance. Although cases of clinically severe viral breakthrough on adefovir have been reported, little clinical data have been reported, regarding salvage treatment of patients with adefovir resistance. Adefovir-resistant HBV strains, at least those with the N236T mutation, are thought to be susceptible to salvage treatment with lamivudine and other nucleosides, which may preclude the opportunity to gain longer-term "natural history" data regarding clinical consequences in patients with adefovir resistance.

4.3 Entecavir Resistance

The recently completed Phase III registration trials of entecavir (Baraclude™) indicated that, like adefovir, resistance to entecavir appeared to be negligible in the first year (48 weeks) of treatment, in HBeAg-positive and HBeAg-negative patients with chronic hepatitis B (47–49). With 96–144 weeks' entecavir treatment, occasional cases of entecavir resistance have been reported, but the overall incidence in the first 3 years is reported to be 1% or less in treatment-naïve-patients (50–52). However, the current resistance data for entecavir are difficult to interpret, since a number of first-year patients are apparently not included in the data analyses for subsequent years. In any case, with 2- and 3-year data available on some entecavir recipients, it can be surmised that HBV resistance continues to appear to be relatively low, at least in those without pre-existing YMDD-mutant HBV strains. In contrast, in separate studies entecavir resistance was observed in 1.6% of lamivudine-resistant patients by week 48, and increased appreciably during 2–3 years of treatment; consequently, entecavir monotherapy is nor recommended as the preferred first-line salvage option for patients with lamivudine-resistant HBV strains (52). Instead, adefovir or possibly tenofovir appear to be preferable for salvage treatment of lamivudine-resistant patients, preferably as add-on therapy with lamivudine rather than as a sequential monotherapy switch, to reduce the chances for sequential evolution of nucleotide (adefovir or tenofovir) resistance in such lamivudine-resistant patients (33, 34, 50, 52).

The genotypic basis of HBV resistance to entecavir is the presence of YMDD mutations (M204V/I), and/or the L180M mutation, together with mutations at any of three HBV Pol/RT codons (T184, S202, or M250) (50–52). In laboratory studies, some mutations in the latter three codons were associated with better HBV DNA replication in vitro (in transfection assays), and correlated with the mutations found at these positions in HBV DNA amplified from patient sera, while other mutations at these three positions showed less replication competence in vitro and were not commonly found in clinical samples (53).

At present there are no appreciable data of longer-term clinical outcome published for patients with entecavir resistance, for whom nucleotide salvage treatment (e.g., with adefovir or tenofovir) is likely to be effective, though clinical data are needed in this regard (52).

4.4 Telbivudine Resistance

In vitro, HBV constructs with the M204I mutation, or with the M204V + L180M double mutation, show reduced susceptibility to telbivudine (Tyzeka™, Sebivo™), although the shift in in vitro susceptibility for these HBV constructs is not as large for telbivudine as it is for lamivudine (54, 55). Interestingly, telbivudine was found to be fully active in vitro against HBV constructs with the M204V mutation alone. Data from patients with lamivudine resistance suggest that the L180M "upstream" mutation arises secondarily, perhaps as a compensatory mutation, after an initial M204V or M204I mutation (20, 52). The in vitro data therefore predicted that, while M204I mutants might emerge in some patients during prolonged telbivudine treatment, the emergence of M204V single mutants or M204V + L180M HBV double mutants (which are the most common YMDD variants on lamivudine therapy) should be low during telbivudine therapy due to the sensitivity of M204V single-mutant HBV strains to telbivudine. This prediction from laboratory data has held true to date, in the first- and second-year data from the global Phase III telbivudine trial (54–57). In this large trial, 5.0% of HBeAg-positive telbivudine recipients and 2.3% of HBeAg-negative telbivudine recipients showed a 1-log or greater HBV DNA breakthrough at 1 year with detectable telbivudine-resistant HBV strains. In both patient populations (HBeAg-positive and HBeAg-negative), the resistance rates for telbivudine were substantially below the resistance rates observed in the lamivudine-treated control group (55–57). Telbivudine resistance increased cumulatively at 2 years of treatment in the Phase III global trial, toward 20% in HBeAg-positive patients and 8% in HBeAg-negative patients, but in both the HBeAg-positive and HBeAg-negative patient populations telbivdine resistance remained significantly below the resistance rates observed in the lamivudine-treated control groups.

In all cases of telbivudine resistance with viral breakthrough in the global Phase III trial, HBV strains carrying the M204I mutation were found; one patient also had co-detectable M204V + L180M mutations (54–57). No telbivudine recipients' HBV DNA had the M204V mutation or the M204V/L180M double mutation without a detectable M204I mutation, confirming that the M204I mutation is the principal telbivudine resistance mutation, and also confirming the relative blockade of M204V-mediated resistance in telbivudine recipients predicted from the preclinical virologic data described above. As for lamivudine, the clinical correlates for M204I-mediated viral resistance were variable in the data from the Phase III study. Over half of the telbivudine recipients with viral breakthrough still had normal ALT levels at the 1-year timepoint (55). HBeAg seroconversion was observed in at least two telbivudine recipients who had developed viral breakthrough with M204I-mutant HBV (54, 57).

HBV DNA sequencing analyses, using sera from telbivudine recipients with 1-year HBV DNA levels ≥ 3 $\log_{10}$ copies/mL in the global Phase III trial, with or without evidence of viral breakthrough, indicated the sporadic presence of other detectable HBV Pol/RT mutations in some patients (55, 57, 58). The secondary mutations L80I/V, L180M, A181T and L229W/V were detected sporadically, in a total of 7% of telbivudine-treated patients, but these HBV polymerase mutations were not associated with viral breakthrough without concomitant detection of the M204I substitution (55, 58).

As for the two other regulatory-approved nucleosides (lamivudine and entecavir), based on laboratory studies with various HBV genomic constructs, patients with telbivudine-resistant HBV strains appear likely to respond to treatment with nucleotides such as adefovir or tenofovir; pilot data in this regard were recently reported (59).

5 Cross-Resistance Issues for Current Anti-HBV Agents

Newer agents such as adefovir, entecavir, and telbivudine are associated with significantly lower emergence of HBV resistance compared to lamivudine – and, in the case of entecavir and telbivudine, with better efficacy than lamivudine in head-to-head trials. These newer agents offer many patients the chance for years-long suppression of HBV replication and consequent abrogation of progression of HBV-associated liver disease. Nonetheless, it appears likely that, due to imperfect efficacy with regard to incomplete suppression of HBV replication and persistence of HBV in the liver, no single antiviral agent for hepatitis B, used as a monotherapy, can be expected to be adequate for managing the preponderance of hepatitis B patients for the duration of their life expectancies. Therefore the best treatment strategies, yet to be determined, will probably use combination regimens and sequential treatment strategies, possibly involving sequential combinations of antiviral agents, with patient management based on viral load monitoring to maximize treatment efficacy and minimize viral resistance.

A key limitation of the current antiviral armamentarium for hepatitis B is the presence of potential HBV cross-resistance within the two major classes of HBV Pol/RT inhibitors, i.e., nucleosides and nucleotides. HBV strains with YMDD mutations (M204V and/or M204I) show reduced susceptibility in vitro, not just to lamivudine, but also to telbivudine and entecavir, as discussed above and in the accompanying chapter by Prof. Locarnini, though there may be clinically important differences with regard to the specifics of shifts in susceptibility for these agents with regard to each type of YMDD mutation. For example, it is potentially interesting that the major source of lost susceptibility for telbivudine is the presence of an M204I mutation while, in contrast, entecavir reportedly shows more appreciable loss of susceptibility with the M204V mutation (53, 54). Similarly, within the nucleotide class of HBV inhibitors, the adefovir-associated resistance mutations, such as N236T and A181V/T, may also confer reduced susceptibility to other nucleotide analogs such as tenofovir and possibly ANA380, although the array of HBV resistance genotypes for the latter agents are yet to be elucidated in large clinical trials.

A disturbing consequence of the limited, class-related array of primary HBV resistance mutations is the potential evolution of multi-drug resistance in patients treated with prolonged nucleoside and nucleotide therapy. Several patients with lamivudine resistance, treated sequentially with lamivudine followed by a switch to adefovir monotherapy, or treated with add-on adefovir therapy in combination with lamivudine, have been documented as having developed HBV strains with resistance mutations to both lamivudine and adefovir (52, 60–62). Due to genotypic cross-resistance within the nucleoside class (re: YMDD mutations) and within the nucleotide class (re: N236T and possibly Y181V mutations), such patients with dual lamivudine and adefovir resistance, although still rare to date, may have "burned through" their current treatment options (other than interferon), since treatment with other nucleosides or nucleotides may be ineffective or only partially effective (52).

Another key HBV cross-resistance issue is that the virologic and clinical correlates of A181V/T/S substitutions need to be examined in greater detail, since A181 substitutions have been proposed as potentially conferring cross resistance between nucleosides and nucleotides, as discussed in the accompanying chapter by Prof. Locarnini. In this regard, there may be distinctions among the various individual anti-HBV nucleosides and nucleotides with regard to the incidence of selecting A181 mutants and the virologic and clinical consequences of the specific A181 mutants selected (A181V, A181T, or A181S). Although A181 mutants have been reported as secondary mutants in occasional lamivudine recipients, such mutants do not appear to be a major cause of HBV DNA breakthrough and clinically significant resistance for lamivudine. In contrast, aside from N236T mutants adefovir preferentially selects primarily A181V mutant HBV strains in hepatitis B patients, and patients with A181V strains often exhibit potentially significant viral breakthrough with A181V mutants despite a limited (less than tenfold) shift in in vitro susceptibility for such mutants to adefovir (38). Conversely, recent sequencing analyses of HBV DNA amplified from telbivudine recipients with residual low-level HBV DNA indicated that A181T substitutions (but not A181V) could be detected occasionally in telbivudine-treated patients, but in the absence of a detectable M204I mutation no telbivudine recipients with the A181T substitution developed HBV DNA breakthrough (54, 55). Thus, adefovir, a nucleotide, and telbivudine, a nucleoside, preferentially select different A181 mutants (A181V vs. A181T, respectively), with apparently different virologic and clinical consequences. In the data available to date the A181T mutants in telbivudine recipients are not associated with clinically appreciable viral breakthrough, in contrast to the A181V mutants observed in adefovir recipients. Since the virologic and clinical correlates of A181 variants may be different for A181V, A181S, and A181T substitutions, it is not presently clear whether A181 substitutions will be broadly important as clinically significant cross-resistance mutations between the nucleoside and nucleotide classes of HBV Pol/RT inhibitors. Further data are needed, from clinical trials utilizing currently available and investigational anti-HBV nucleosides and nucleotides, and from trials of combination regimens of nucleosides and nucleotides.

6 Optimizing Antiviral Therapy for Hepatitis B Patients: Potential Treatment Strategies for Minimizing the Clinical Impact of Antiviral Resistance

In devising treatment strategies to minimize the emergence and clinical impact of HBV resistance, two fundamental observations regarding patients with drug-resistant HBV strains are important. First, longitudinal studies of patients with lamivudine resistance indicated that recrudescence of signs of liver disease correlated with quantitative changes in serum HBV DNA levels, and not with any particular HBV resistance genotype (63). This observation seems likely to prevail for patients with resistance to other anti-HBV agents, as well, since most resistance-associated HBV Pol-RT mutations are conservative with regard to amino acid changes in the overlapping HBsAg reading frame and the resistance mutations typically do not produce changes in immunologically important domains of HBsAg. The notion that progression of liver disease in patients with drug-resistant HBV strains is related to the degree of ongoing HBV replication is also consistent with the quantitative association between HBV DNA levels and disease progression reported from epidemiologic studies of HBV carriers and clinical studies of hepatitis B patients, as cited above (3–5, 9–13).

The second key observation is that patients who achieve non-detectable or very low serum HBV DNA levels during the first 6–12 months of nucleoside/tide treatment have lower resistance rates and better efficacy outcomes compared to patients who have residual HBV DNA levels greater than 3 or 4 $\log_{10}$ copies/mL after 6 months' antiviral treatment (56, 64–66).

The two observations described above support an essential strategy in hepatitis B treatment of maximizing HBV DNA suppression early in treatment, e.g., in the first 6 months, to minimize subsequent resistance emergence, followed by periodic monitoring of serum HBV DNA levels, with appropriate adjustments in treatment when needed to maintain maximal suppression of HBV replication – preferably to maintain nondetectable serum HBV DNA levels, or at least below 3 $\log_{10}$ copies/mL (52, 56, 65, 67).

It is now appropriate to return to the potential role of combination antiviral regimens for the management of hepatitis B patients. While de novo combination treatment is preferable from a purely virologic perspective, prospective trials of de novo combination treatments (double nucleoside/tide treatment, or nucleoside plus interferon) in hepatitis B patients have not shown a consistent and compelling efficacy benefit for the tested combination regimens compared to the monotherapy control arms. Four large Phase III trials of interferon or peg-interferon plus lamivudine failed to show compelling benefit for the combination arms over the monotherapy arms (21, 22, 68, 69). Three trials of interferon with lamivudine in HBeAg-positive patients suggested a potential for enhanced HBeAg clearance on the combination arm, but other efficacy achievements (e.g., histologic response, ALT normalization) for the combination arms were unimpressive and were sometimes better for the monotherapy arms (21, 69, 70). With regard to clinical testing of double nucleoside/tide combination regimens, two Phase II studies of de novo combination treatment in treatment-naïve patients – with lamivudine plus adefovir, or lamivudine plus telbivudine – failed to show compelling efficacy benefits for double nucleoside/tide de novo combination treatment over the concurrent monotherapy control arms after 52 weeks of treatment (65, 71). However, these Phase II studies of double nucleoside/tide de novo combination therapy were of modest scope, viral response kinetics were not examined in detail, and controlled observations were limited to 1-year time periods, during which the resistance rates on the monotherapy arms were expectedly low. Two other Phase II studies suggested better early virologic response kinetics for the combinations of adefovir plus emtricitabine, or adefovir plus lamivudine, compared to adefovir alone (72, 73). However, these results are probably not generalizable for other double nucleioside/ tide combination regimens as they may derive from the known inconsistency in adefovir's antiviral effect, evident in a number of studies (5, 41, 73, 74). Finally a randomized trial of telbivudine monotherapy vs. adefovir monotherapy vs. a randomized deferred assignment of add-on adefovir plus telbivudine combination treatment (the latter beginning 6 months after initiation of treatment with adefovir monotherapy), in treatment-naïve HBeAg-positive patients, demonstrated that telbivudine monotherapy has greater and more consistent anti-HBV potency than adefovir monotherapy; but at 1 year, the efficacy of the deferred adefoir/telbivudine combination treatment was not better than telbivudine alone – although, as in some of the other trials, there was a suggestion that the combination treatment might reduce subsequent viral resistance with longer treatment (72).

Despite the non-compelling efficacy results in studies conducted to date of de novo combination therapy in treatment-naïve patients, most experts believe that, with larger and longer studies, the already-low HBV resistance rates observed with current "second-generation" anti-HBV nucleosides/tides (adefovir, entecavir, telbivudine) could be further reduced with de novo combination treatments, especially combination regimens with potent agents having complementary resistance profiles (e.g., potent nucleoside plus potent nucleotide).

In contrast to non-compelling results for anti-HBV combination therapies in treatment-naive patients, most studies of adefovir treatment of HBV infection in lamivudine-resistant patients have suggested that it is preferable to add on the adefovir salvage treatment and continue the lamivudine regimen, rather than switch to adefovir monotherapy (32–34, 52). Such salvage combination regimens, comprising a nucleoside and a nucleotide with complementary resistance profiles, appear to afford a lower risk for subsequent development of adefovir resistance and multidrug resistance, i.e., lamivudine plus adefovir resistance.

Considering the data reviewed in this chapter, it seems reasonable to infer that the most interesting new clinical trials for treatment-naïve hepatitis B patients with compensated liver disease will be randomized comparisons of two alternate "combination therapy" treatment strategies utilizing the newer, more potent nucleosides and nucleotides, i.e., de novo combination regimens, versus regimens that begin with a potent nucleoside/tide monotherapy and incorporate early treatment intensification (e.g., add-on of a second nucleoside/ tide agent or interferon, 3–6 months after the start of treatment) for patients with suboptimal early virologic responses. Based on the data reviewed above, suboptimal responses could be defined as persisting HBV DNA levels $>3 \log_{10}$ genome copies/mL after 24 weeks of antiviral therapy. Such trials will need to be large and perhaps of longer duration (e.g., 2–3 years), and they will require much resource and commitment – due to the goal of demonstrating statistically significant improvements in already-low rates of HBV resistance and virologic failure with the newer anti-HBV agents. Prospective trials of this type will be the only way to sort-out the real value, in a practical world, of de novo combination treatment vs. treatment intensification strategies, for the many millions of chronic hepatitis B patients worldwide.

Until anti-HBV therapy is more eradicative, and healthcare reimbursement for antiviral therapy is more universal, an important practical question is: which hepatitis B patients need evaluation of de novo combination treatment strategies most urgently? Clinical considerations suggest that the patient groups most likely to benefit from combination therapies are those who have lower disease resolution rates and higher risks for progression to endstage liver disease. Patients with cirrhosis and active HBV replication, patients with HBeAg-negative hepatitis B (with pre-core/core mutant HBV infection), and patients with HIV co-infection or other forms of immunodebilitation are less likely to experience durable disease remissions, spontaneously or with antiviral treatment, and are therefore more likely to need long-term "maintenance" antiviral therapy to achieve prolonged treatment-related suppression of HBV replication. Also, in hepatitis B patients with advanced cirrhosis and active HBV replication, who urgently need effective antiviral therapy to avoid progressive clinical decompensation, resistance-related viral breakthrough may have greater clinical consequences, with rapid progression to liver failure after virologic breakthrough in some patients (30). Consequently, patients with advanced cirrhosis are also good candidates for evaluation of de novo combination treatment strategies.

The key reason for difference in the HBV vs. HIV arenas, regarding the adoption of de novo combination treatment as the preferred strategy, should now be evident from the data reviewed in this chapter: relatively durable responses to antiviral monotherapies, e.g., viral suppression to PCR-nondetectable levels for a year or more, are common in the HBV patients but are essentially unheard of in HIV patients, presumably due to the biologic disease differences listed above in Table 1. In this regard it is important to be cognizant of the reality that reimbursement for antiviral therapy is presently limited in regions where hepatitis B is endemic, and many hepatitis B patients pay for their own care. Consequently the value of de novo combination regimens for hepatitis B patients will need to be proven in adequate sized clinical trials before such regimens can be expected to be widely adopted in the hepatitis B arena.

In conclusion, several issues need comment. Because HIV is usually transmitted horizontally, by sexual contact, and because HIV antivirals have been widely used in developed nations, drug-resistant HIV strains are commonly transmitted and currently account for perhaps 20% of new HIV infections in the U.S. In this regard, multi-resistant HBV are also a potential threat and have been reported in several patients. However, it appears unlikely that transmission of drug-resistant HBV strains will be a proportionally large problem, for the following reasons:, (a) the most common mode of HBV acquisition, globally, is perinatal, not sexual; (b) HBV infection transitions to the inactive carrier state in many patients (spontaneously, or with antiviral treatment); (c) universal HBV vaccination is increasingly successful in reducing the hepatitis B disease burden worldwide; and (d) partners and family members of hepatitis B patients can be effectively vaccinated. These considerations comprise major differences with the HIV arena. However, the expanding issue of multidrug resistance is urgent in the HIV arena and, due to the common signature resistance mutations within the nucleoside and nucleotide classes, there is a pressing need for additional classes of anti-HBV agents, with novel mechanisms of action and/or with novel genotypic resistance profiles, to combat the potential for an increasing prevalence of multi-drug resistant HBV in the presently large population of HBV-infected patients worldwide.

The current anti-HBV armamentarium, together with novel additional agents and data-supported new treatment strategies (de novo combination regimens and/or treatment intensification strategies), will allow prolonged treatment of the great majority of patients with chronic hepatitis B. However, to substantially curtail HBV-associated morbidity and mortality in the current population of 300–400 million chronic HBV carriers, improved HBV screening programs and improved healthcare coverage will also be needed. In the long run, while advances in antiviral therapy and healthcare delivery can reduce the worldwide morbidity and mortality burden associated with chronic HBV infection, continued emphasis on universal HBV vaccination is the ultimate solution to the global prevalence of HBV infection and its associated disease burden.

References

1. Walensky, R. P., et al. The survival benefit of AIDS treatment in the United States. J Infect Dis 2006; 194: 11–19
2. Vermund, S. H. Millions of lives saved with potent antiretroviral drugs in the United States: a celebration, with challenges. J Infect Dis 2006; 194: 1–5
3. Yim, H. J. and A. S.-F. Lok. Natural history of chronic hepatitis B virus infection: what we knew in 1981 and what we know in 2005. Hepatology 2006; 43(2, suppl 1): S173–S181
4. McMahon, B. J. Epidemiology and natural history of hepatitis B. Semin Liver Dis 2005; 25(suppl 1): 3–8
5. Hoofnagle, J. H., et al. Management of hepatitis B: summary of a clinical research workshop. Hepatology 2007; 45(4): 1056–1075
6. Korenman, J., et al. Long-term remission of chronic hepatitis B after alpha-interferon therapy. Ann Intern Med 1991; 114(8): 629–634
7. Lok, A. S. and B. J. McMahon. Practice Guidelines Committee of the American Association for the Study of Liver Diseases: chronic hepatitis B. Hepatology 2001; 34(6): 1225–1241
8. Lok, A. S. and B. J. McMahon. Chronic hepatitis B. Hepatology 2007; 45(2): 507–539
9. Chen, C. J., et al. Risk of hepatocellular carcinoma across a biological gradient of serum hepatitis B virus DNA level. JAMA 2006; 295(1): 65–73
10. Chen, G., et al. Past HBV viral load as predictor of mortality and morbidity from HCC and chronic liver disease in a prospective study. Am J Gastroenterol 2006; 101(8): 1797–1803
11. Yuan, H. J., et al. The relationship between HBV DNA levels and cirrhosis-related complications in Chinese with chronic hepatitis B. J Viral Hepat 2005; 12(4): 373–379
12. Ohata, K., et al. High viral load is a risk factor for hepatocellular carcinoma in patients with chronic hepatitis B virus infection. J Gastroenterol Hepatol 2004; 19: 670–675
13. Yuen, M. F., et al. Prognostic determinants for chronic hepatitis B in Asians: therapeutic implications. Gut 2005; 54(11): 1610–1614
14. Lai, C.-L., et al. A one-year trial of lamivudine for chronic hepatitis B. N Engl J Med 1998; 339: 61–68
15. Dienstag, J. L., et al. Lamivudine as initial treatment for chronic hepatitis B in patients from the United States. N Engl J Med 1999; 341: 1256–1263
16. Lai, C.-L., et al. Prevalence and clinical correlates of YMDD variants during lamivudine therapy for patients with chronic hepatitis B. Clin Infect Dis 2003; 36(6): 687–696
17. Liaw, Y.-F., et al. Lamivudine for patients with chronic hepatitis B and advanced liver disease. N Engl J Med 2004; 351: 1521–1531
18. Bartholomew, M., et al. Hepatitis B virus resistance to lamivudine given for recurrent infection after orthotopic liver transplantation. Lancet 1997; 349: 20–22
19. Ling, R., et al. Selection of mutations in the hepatitis B virus polymerase during therapy of transplant recipients with lamivudine. Hepatology 1996; 24: 711–713

20. Allen, M., et al. Identification and characterization of mutations in hepatitis B virus resistant to lamivudine. Hepatology 1998; 27(6): 1670–1677

21. Schalm, S. W., et al. Lamivudine and alpha-interferon combination treatment of patients with chronic hepatitis B: a randomised trial. Gut 2000; 46: 562–568

22. Schiff, E. R., et al. Lamivudine and 24 weeks of lamivudine/interferon combination therapy for hepatitis B e-antigen positive chronic hepatitis B in interferon non-responders. J Hepatol 2003; 38: 818–826

23. Tassopoulos, N. C., et al. Efficacy of lamivudine in patients with hepatitis B e antigen-negative/hepatitis B virus DNA-positive (pre-core mutant) chronic hepatitis B. Hepatology 1999; 29: 889–896

24. Dienstag, J., et al. Long-term lamivudine therapy in hepatitis B: monitoring of serum HBV DNA and ALT levels in patients with and without YMDD-variant HBV. Abstracts of the N.I.H. Workshop on Management of Hepatitis B, 2000: p. 98

25. Lok, A. S.-F. Perspective: chronic hepatitis B. N Engl J Med 2002; 346(22): 1682–1683

26. Dienstag, J. L., et al. Histological outcome during long-term lamivudine therapy. Gastroenterology 2003; 124: 105–117

27. Perrillo, R. P., et al. Predictors of HBeAg loss after lamivudine treatment for chronic hepatitis B. Hepatology 2002; 36(1): 186–194

28. Lok, A. S., et al. Long-term safety of lamivudine treatment in patients with chronic hepatitis B. Gastroenterology 2003; 125(6): 1714–1722

29. Liaw, Y. F., et al. Acute exacerbation and hepatitis B virus clearance after emergence of YMDD motif mutation during lamivudine therapy. Hepatology 1999; 30(2): 567–572

30. Tillmann, H. L., et al. Risk factors for selection of YMDD mutants, their consequences in liver transplant recipients, ranging from sudden onset of liver failure to no disease. Hepatology 2000; 32 (4 Pt 2): 376A

31. Keeffe, E. B., et al. A treatment algorithm for the management of chronic hepatitis B virus infection in the United States. Clin Gastroenterol Hepatol 2004; 2: 87–106

32. Lampertico, P., et al. Adefovir rapidly suppresses hepatitis B in HBeAg-negative patents developing genotypic resistance to lamivudine. Hepatology 2005; 42(6): 1414–1419

33. Lampertico, P., et al. A multicenter Italian study of rescue adefovir dipivoxil therapy in lamivudine resistant patients: a 2-year analysis of 604 patients. Hepatology 2006; 42(4 suppl 1): 591A

34. Rapti, I., et al. Adding-on versus switching-to adefovir therapy in lamivudine-resistant HBeAg-negative chronic hepatitis B. Hepatology 2007; 45(2): 307–313

35. Marcellin, P., et al. Adefovir dipivoxil for the treatment of hepatitis B e antigen-positive chronic hepatitis B. N Engl J Med 2003; 348(9): 808–816

36. Hadziyannis, S. J., et al. Adefovir dipivoxil for the treatment of hepatitis B e antigen-negative chronic hepatitis B. N Engl J Med 2003; 348(9): 800–807

37. Angus, P., et al. Resistance to adefovir dipivoxil therapy is associated with the selection of a novel mutation in the HBV polymerase. Gastroenterology 2003; 125: 292–297

38. Borroto-Esoda, K., et al. Meta-analysis across adefovir clinical trials demonstrates the absence of novel adefovir-associated mutations and confirms the role of the rtA181V and rtN236T mutations in the HBV polymerase in association with virologic failure. Hepatology 2006; 44(4 suppl 1): 552A

39. Hepsera™ (adefovir dipivoxil) prescribing information, 2006. Gilead Sciences, Foster City, CA

40. Lee, Y. S., et al. Increased risk of adefovir resistance in patients with lamivudine-resistant chronic hepatitis B after 48 weeks of adefovir dipivoxil monotherapy. Hepatology 2006; 43(6): 1385–1391

41. Fung, S. K., et al. Virologic response and resistance to adefovir in patients with chronic hepatitis B. J Hepatol 2006; 44(2): 283–290

42. Lee, C. H., et al. More frequent and earlier emergence of adefovir (ADV) resistance mutations in lamivudine resistant patients treated with ADV compared to previously reported nucleoside-treatment naïve patients (abstract 1009). Hepatology 2005; 42(4 suppl 1): 593A

43. Yeon, J. E., et al. Resistance to adefovir dipivoxil (ADV) in lamivudine-resistant chronic hepatitis B patients treated with ADV. Gut 2006; 55(10): 1488–1495

44. Schildgen, O., et al. Variant of hepatitis B virus with primary resistance to adefovir. N Engl J Med 2006; 354: 1807–1812

45. Chang, T.-T. and C.-L. Lai. Hepatitis B virus with primary resistance to adefovir (letter). N Engl J Med 2006; 355: 322–323

46. Curtis, M., Y. Zhu, and K. Borroto-Esoda. HBV rtI233V polymerase variant remains sensitive to adefovir. J Hepatol 2007; 46 (suppl 1): 26–27

47. Chang, T. T., et al. A comparison of entecavir and lamivudine for HBeAg-positive chronic hepatitis B. N Engl J Med 2006; 354(10): 1001–1010

48. Lai, C. L., et al. Entecavir versus lamivudine for patients with HBeAg-negative chronic hepatitis B. N Engl J Med 2006; 354(10): 1011–1020

49. Colonno, R. J., et al. Entecavir resistance is rare in nucleoside naïve patients with hepatitis B. Hepatology 2006; 44(6): 1656–1665

50. Colonno, R. J., et al. Assessment at three years shows high barrier to resistance is maintained in entecavir-treated nucleoside naïve patients while resistance emergence increases over time in lamivudine refractory patients. Hepatology 2006; 44(4 suppl 1): 229A–230A

51. Baraclude™ (entecavir) prescribing information, 2007. Bristol Myers Squibb, Wallingford, CT

52. Lok, A. S., et al. Antiviral drug-resistant HBV: standardization of nomenclature and assays and recommendations for management. Hepatology 2007; 46(1): 254–265

53. Tenney, D. J., et al. Only a subset of HBV substitutions at entecavir resistance residues lead to phenotypic resistance and virologic rebound. Hepatology 2006; 44(4 suppl 1): 253A

54. Standring, D. N., et al. HBV resistance determination from the telbivudine GLOBE registration trial. J Hepatol 2006; 44(suppl 2): S191

55. Standring, D. N., et al. Resistance determination in patients experiencing virologic breakthrough following telbivudine or lamivudine therapy in the international GLOBE trial. Digestive Diseases Week (DDW) 2007, Abstracts, #S1781

56. Lai, C.-L., et al. Telbivudine versus lamivudine for patients with chronic hepatitis B: one-year results of a global phase III comparative trial. N Engl J Med 2007; 357: 2576–2588

57. Lai, C. L., et al. Two-year results from the GLOBE trial in patients with hepatitis B: greater clinical and antiviral efficacy for telbivudine (LdT) vs. lamivudine. Hepatology 2006; 44(4 suppl 1): 222A

58. Tyzeka™ (telbivudine) prescribing information, 2006. Idenix Pharmaceuticals; Cambridge, MA

59. Gane, E., et al. Adefovir salvage therapy for virologic breakthrough in telbivudine-treated patients from the GLOBE study. J Hepatol 2007; 46(1): S187

60. Yin, H. J., et al. Evolution of multi-drug resistant hepatitis B virus during sequential therapy. Hepatology 2006; 44(3): 703–712

61. Brunelle, M. N., et al. Susceptibility to antivirals of a human HBV strain with mutations conferring resistance to both lamivudine and adefovir. Hepatology 2005; 41(6): 1391–1398

62. Kwon, S. Y., et al. Emergence of dual-resistance HBV mutations to adefovir dipivoxil and lamivudine in a hepatitis B patient with combination therapy for adefovir resistance. J Hepatol 2006; 44(suppl 2): S273

63. Liu, C.-J., et al. Hepatitis B variants in patients receiving lamivudine treatment with breakthrough hepatitis evaluated by serial viral loads and full-length sequences. Hepatology 2001; 34(3): 583–589

64. Yuen, M. F., et al. Factors associated with hepatitis B virus DNA breakthrough in patients receiving prolonged lamivudine therapy. Hepatology 2001; 34(4 Pt 1): 785–791

65. Lai, C.-L., et al. A one-year phase IIb trial of telbivudine (LdT), lamivudine, and the combination, in patients with chronic hepatitis B. Gastroenterology 2005; 129: 528–536

66. Locarnini, S., et al. Incidence and predictors of emergence of adefovir resistant HBV during four years of adefovir dipivoxil (ADV) therapy for patients with chronic hepatitis B (CHB). J Hepatol 2005; 42(suppl): S17

67. Keeffe, E. B., et al. Report of an international workshop: roadmap for management of patients receiving oral therapy for chronic hepatitis B. Clin Gastroenterol Hepatol 2007; 5(8): 890–897

68. Marcellin, P., et al. Peginterferon alfa-2a alone, lamivudine alone, and the two in combination, in patients with HBeAg-negative chronic hepatitis B. N Engl J Med 2004; 351(12): 1206–1217

69. Lau, G. K., et al. Peginterferon Alfa-2a, lamivudine, and the combination for HBeAg-positive chronic hepatitis B. N Engl J Med 2005; 352(26): 2682–2695

70. Chan, H. L. Y., et al. A randomized, controlled trial of combination theapy for chronic hepatitis B: comparing pegylaed interferon-α2b and lamivudine with lamivudine alone. Ann Intern Med 2005; 142(4): 240–251

71. Sung, J. J. Y., et al. A randomised double-blind phase 2 study of lamivudine compared to lamivudine plus adefovir dipivoxil for treatment-naive patients with chronic hepatitis B: week 52 analysis. J Hepatol 2003; 38: 25–26

72. Lau, G., et al. Randomised, double-blind study comparing adefovir dipivoxil plus emtricitabine combination therapy versus adefovir alone in HBeAg + chronic hepatitis B: efficacy and mechanisms of treatment response. Hepatology 2004; 40(4 suppl 1): 272A

73. Ghany, M., et al. Better virolgic response with lamivudine plus adefovir vs adefovir alone for HBeAg-positive chronic hepatitis B. Hepatology 2005; 42(4 suppl 1): 591A

74. Chan, H. L. Y., et al. Telbivudine versus adefovir in patients with HBeAg-positive chronic hepatitis B: a randomized, trial. Ann Intern Med 2007; 147:745–754

Chapter 73
Antimalarial Drug Resistance: Clinical Perspectives

Philip J. Rosenthal

1 Introduction

Malaria is one of the most important infectious diseases in the world, and the problem appears to be worsening. An important contributor to our continued inability to control malaria is the increasing resistance of malaria parasites to available drugs. New drugs are greatly needed, but the continued use of some agents against which resistance has already developed is inevitable. As we attempt to improve methods for malaria surveillance and control, it is important to standardize methods for the assessment of antimalarial drug resistance. Such efforts include the establishment of standard means of assessing responses to antimalarial treatment, the discrimination of recrudescence due to drug resistance from reinfection after treatment, the characterization of molecular mediators of drug resistance in field isolates, and the establishment of improved systems for the in vitro analysis of the drug susceptibility of field isolates.

2 The Current Malaria Situation

In 1955, the World Health Organization (WHO) announced a program to eradicate malaria. Despite some successes, this program was a disappointment. Over recent decades, morbidity and mortality caused by malaria have increased in many parts of the world, and most of the world's population remains at risk of infection. Overall, the numbers are staggering. Malaria parasites are responsible for hundreds of millions of illnesses each year, and *Plasmodium falciparum*, the most virulent human malaria parasite, is estimated to cause over a million deaths each year (1). Thus, malaria is one of the great infectious disease killers, and it exerts an enormous toll on developing countries throughout the tropics. In particular, falciparum malaria is an overwhelming problem in sub-Saharan Africa. Numerous factors contribute to the persistence of a severe worldwide malaria problem. First, efforts to control mosquito vectors, which have at times shown important successes, have been limited by financial constraints and insecticide resistance. Second, programs to treat and control malaria, especially in highly vulnerable young children and pregnant women, are greatly limited by poverty in most endemic regions. Third, despite important advances, an effective malaria vaccine is not yet available and is unlikely to be available in the near future. Fourth, despite great advances in our understanding of malaria in recent years, our ability to develop new strategies to control the disease is limited by an incomplete understanding of the biology of the parasite and of the host response to infection. Fifth, and most relevant to this chapter, malaria parasites have repeatedly demonstrated the ability to develop resistance to available drugs.

3 History of Antimalarial Therapy and Currently Available Drugs

Although the parasites that cause malaria were only discovered in the late nineteenth century, the disease was well described by ancient civilizations, and has been a major human health problem for at least thousands of years. Notably, malaria played an important role in establishing the concept of antimicrobial therapy, with the use of quinine to treat malaria since 1820 (2). The history of quinine therapy begins with the use of the bark of the cinchona tree to treat fevers in South America. This treatment was discovered by the Spanish in the seventeenth century, and cinchona bark became a standard therapy for malaria in Europe by the end of the century. In 1820, Pelletier and Caventou isolated the active antimalarial alkaloid from cinchona bark, which was named quinine. Purified quinine soon replaced the bark as the standard therapy for malaria, and it remains today an important treatment.

P.J. Rosenthal (✉)
Department of Medicine, San Francisco General Hospital,
University of California, San Francisco, CA, USA
rosnthl@itsa.ucsf.edu

D.L. Mayers (ed.), *Antimicrobial Drug Resistance*,
DOI 10.1007/978-1-60327-595-8_73, © Humana Press, a part of Springer Science+Business Media, LLC 2009

Efforts to synthesize quinine analogs led to the identification of a number of quinolines with antimalarial activity by the 1940s. The most important of these were chloroquine, which became the most widely used antimalarial for the next half-century, and primaquine, which remains the standard therapy to eradicate liver forms of *P. vivax* and *P. ovale*. Amodiaquine, which is similar in structure to chloroquine, showed efficacy similar to that of chloroquine, but its use was limited after rare toxicities were seen with chronic use for chemoprophylaxis. Recently, it has been noted that amodiaquine remains active against many chloroquine-resistant infections, and the drug is now being reconsidered, especially as a component of combination therapies (3). Another related drug, mefloquine, was developed by the U.S. Army to treat chloroquine-resistant malaria in the 1970s, and it is now widely used for treatment and chemoprophylaxis. Quinine remains active against *P. falciparum* in most of the world, but owing to its toxicity and cost, its use is mostly limited to the treatment of severe malaria (4).

Folate antagonists also have a long history as antimalarials. The first important agent was pyrimethamine, introduced in 1950, but this compound suffers from rapid selection of resistance. The combination of pyrimethamine and sulfadoxine (SP or Fansidar) was introduced in the 1970s as a replacement for chloroquine in areas with resistance, and although it too now suffers from resistance, it remains an important therapy in many developing countries, in large part because it is simple to use and cheaper than most other antimalarials. Proguanil, which inhibits the same enzyme as pyrimethamine, is now an important component of new combination regimens.

While the Western world was using cinchona bark to treat malaria, extracts of *Artemisia annua* were already an established therapy in China, perhaps dating back thousands of years (5). The active ingredient of this plant was identified in 1972 and named qinghao or artemisinin (6). A number of artemisin derivatives are extremely potent antimalarials and are now playing a major role in treating drug-resistant malaria. Artemisinins are very rapid acting, but owing to short half-lives their use is commonly followed by late recrudescences of infecting parasites, and so they are best used in combination therapy. Combination artemisinin regimens are now widely advocated for the routine treatment of malaria (7), but their use is limited by relatively high cost.

It is clear that for the treatment of *P. falciparum* infections chloroquine is a failed antimalarial drug in almost all areas, that antifolates are also now failing, and that resistance threatens many other agents. A number of other antimalarial agents are available, many of them highly effective in most instances (4). However, newer agents routinely are limited by much higher cost and/or higher potential for toxicity than older agents (Table 1). Newer agents are also threatened by resistance. For this reason, most experts now advocate combination therapy for all new antimalarial compounds. It is

Table 1 Available antimalarial drugs

Drug	Class	Use	Limitations
Chloroquine	4-Aminoquinoline	Treatment and chemoprophylaxis of sensitive parasites	Widespread resistance
Amodiaquine	4-Aminoquinoline	Treatment of some chloroquine-resistant *P. falciparum*	Resistance, rare severe toxicities
Quinine/quinidine	Quinoline methanol	Treatment of chloroquine-resistant *P. falciparum*, including severe disease	Toxic, fairly expensive
Mefloquine	Quinoline methanol	Treatment and chemoprophylaxis of *P. falciparum*	High cost, toxicity, resistance in some areas
Primaquine	8-Aminoquinoline	Eradication of liver forms of *P. vivax* and *P. ovale*	Dangerous hemolysis with G6PD deficiency
Sulfadoxine/pyrimethamine	Folate antagonist, sulfa combination	Treatment of some chloroquine-resistant *P. falciparum*	Resistance in many areas, rare severe toxicities
Doxycycline	Tetracycline antibiotic	Treatment of *P. falciparum* (in combination regimens); chemoprophylaxis	Slow acting, photosensitivity, gastrointestinal toxicity
Clindamycin	Lincosamide antibiotic	Treatment of *P. falciparum* (in combination regimens)	Slow acting, gastrointestinal toxicity
Halofantrine	Phenanthrene methanol	Treatment of *P. falciparum*	High cost, rare severe toxicity
Artemisinins	Endoperoxides	Treatment of multidrug-resistant *P. falciparum*	High cost, late recrudescence
Atovaquone/proguanil (Malarone)	Quinone/folate antagonist combination	Treatment and chemoprophylaxis of *P. falciparum*	High cost
Artemether/lumefantrine	Artemisinin/phenanthrene methanol combination	Treatment of *P. falciparum*	High cost, inconvenient dosing schedule
Chlorproguanil/dapsone	Folate antagonist, sulfone combination	Treatment of multidrug-resistant *P. falciparum* in Africa	Potential for resistance selection, toxicity with G6PD deficiency

argued that the selective pressure for resistance against any single drug will be high, but that combinations, ideally containing drugs with matched half-lives (or including a potent, rapidly active compound to limit parasite biomass), will prevent the selection of resistance (8). Some combinations of older drugs (e.g., amodiaquine/SP (9–11)) or of older drugs with newer artemisinins (e.g., artesunate/SP (10–12) or artesunate/amodiaquine (13)) may provide "stop-gap" coverage for the treatment of malaria, as we await newer, more highly efficacious regimens. Ideally, new combination regimens should be coformulated, with simple (once-daily) dosing schedules to facilitate effective use in resource-poor settings.

Few combination therapies are yet available as coformulated drugs. SP is a synergistic combination, but resistance to either component is common, and markedly limits drug efficacy, so it is in effect a single drug in terms of resistance selection. However, although it targets the same enzymes, the new combination of chlorproguanil and dapsone (CD, lapdap), is probably not prone to ready selection of resistance in Africa, due to a relatively short half-life, and the fact that the mutations that cause chlorproguanil resistance are rare (14). Thus, lapdap, which was released in 2003, and is inexpensive, may prove to be a key new drug for therapy of uncomplicated malaria in Africa. An even better long-term approach may be the combination of lapdap with artesunate. This coformulated regimen is now under development, but will not be available for some years (14). An available coformulated and very efficacious regimen is artemether/lumefantrine (Coartem), and this drug is increasingly advocated, although it is very expensive and requires twice-daily dosing, which is generally considered a major disadvantage for routine use in developing countries (15). At this point, with continued use of failed drugs in many countries, and the availability of multiple imperfect alternatives, additional clinical research is greatly needed to determine which available drug combinations should be advocated for malaria treatment.

4 History, Mechanisms, and Current Epidemiology of Antimalarial Drug Resistance

The discussions of resistance in this chapter refer to *P. falciparum* except where otherwise noted (Table 2). *P. falciparum* is the most important human malaria parasite, because of its prevalence and potential for severe disease, and it is also the para-

Table 2 Antimalarial drug resistance[a]

Drug	Resistance known ?			Mechanism of resistance	Notes
	In vitro[b]	In vivo[c]	Clinical[d]		
Chloroquine	Yes	Yes	Yes	Mutations in *pfcrt*; ? other genes	Resistance very widespread
Amodiaquine	Yes		Yes	Unknown	Often effective vs. chloroquine-resistant parasites
Quinine	Yes		Yes	Mutations in *pfmdr1*? other genes	Resistance primarily in SE Asia, mostly low-level
Mefloquine	Yes		Yes	Mutations in *pfmdr1*? other genes	Resistance primarily in SE Asia, but seen elsewhere
Primaquine	No		Yes	Unknown	Used only for *P. vivax* and *ovale* (with chloroquine)
Sulfadoxine/ pyrimethamine	Yes	Yes ?	Yes	Mutations in DHFR and DHPS	Resistance widespread in Asia and South America and rapidly increasing in Africa
Doxycycline	No	No	No		Used only in combination regimens and prophylaxis
Clindamycin	No	No	No		Used only in combination regimens only
Halofantrine			Yes	Mutations in *pfmdr1*? other genes	Used rarely
Artemisinins			No		Very short half-life probably prevents selection resistance
Atovaquone/ proguanil			Yes	Mutations in cytochrome *c* oxidoreductase and DHFR	Each component rapidly selects for resistance, but combination apparently does not
Artemether/ lumefantrine			No		Very short half-life of artemether probably prevents selection resistance
Chlorproguanil/ dapsone			Yes	Mutations in DHFR and DHPS	Resistance in S. America and Asia, but not in Africa

[a]Information refers to *P. falciparum* except as indicated
[b]Studies of cultured *P. falciparum* parasites
[c]Studies with animal models of malaria
[d]Field studies of treatment responses in patients with clinical malaria

site with by far the greatest drug resistance problem. Although falciparum malaria is frequently severe and even fatal, the vast majority of episodes are nonetheless uncomplicated, especially in highly endemic areas. Parenteral therapies for severe malaria that have minimal problems with drug resistance in most areas, notably quinine, quinidine, and artemisinins, are available. Thus, our greatest need is not new treatments for severe malaria, but the optimization of therapy for the many millions of episodes of uncomplicated falciparum malaria that occur each year. Without effective therapy, patients with uncomplicated malaria will commonly suffer from recurrent symptoms and/or progression to severe disease. Resistance of *P. vivax* to chloroquine and antifolates has also been noted, as will be discussed below. For the other two human malaria parasites *P. ovale* and *P. malariae*, infections are quite uncommon, and information on resistance is limited.

Antimalarial drug resistance must be appreciated in the context of the complex interaction between malaria parasites and the human host (16). In highly endemic regions, young children experience frequent malaria infections and gradually develop effective antimalarial immunity, as they progress from frequent (often severe) clinical illness to asymptomatic infections, to the fairly effective immunity commonly seen in older children and adults. This immunity is not complete, and individuals of all ages can suffer from malaria, but it has an important impact on antimalarial treatment and on our analysis of drug efficacy. In many cases, immune individuals respond clinically to treatment with drugs against which the infecting parasites are resistant. It is difficult to discriminate partial activity of drugs and host immune effects. Other factors including host genetics, variable pharmacokinetics, and strain-specific virulence may also contribute to this complexity.

Drug resistance was not a major problem in antimalarial therapy for many years. Remarkably, resistance to quinine remains a relatively small problem, although quinine-resistant parasites are seen in Southeast Asia (16). The limited selection of quinine-resistant parasites is probably due to the short half-life and limited use of this quite toxic drug. Resistance has not been reported with artemisinin and its analogs, which have very short half-lives.

Since the 1940s, the most important antimalarial has been chloroquine, which was very heavily used to treat malaria and also for widespread chemoprophylaxis in some areas. Chloroquine was even added to table salt in misguided attempts to eradicate malaria (17); these attempts may have done more to select for resistance than to control the disease. Nonetheless, chloroquine resistance developed only slowly. It was first reported in the late 1950s in both Southeast Asia and South America. Since then, it slowly spread around the malarious world, with spread through much of East Asia and South America through the 1960s,

into the Indian Subcontinent in the 1970s, to east Africa in the late 1970s, and then across Africa through the 1980s (18). This slow progression of resistance suggests that the spontaneous selection of the genetic changes that mediate chloroquine resistance has occurred only rarely, and that resistance has principally been due to the gradual spread of resistance-mediating alleles around the world. This concept is supported by recent molecular advances. It is now clear that chloroquine resistance is principally mediated by mutations in the *pfcrt* gene, which is likely a transporter for chloroquine (18–21). A single mutation, *pfcrt* K76T, is the principal mediator of resistance, but this mutation appears to be stable only in the context of multiple other *pfcrt* mutations. In addition, mutations in another gene, *pfmdr1*, and perhaps others, appear to contribute to the chloroquine resistance phenotype, at least with some parasite strains (22). The requirement for multiple mutations has probably limited the selection of chloroquine resistance, but the selection of resistant parasites probably occurred on a number of occasions, as suggested by the identification of different *pfcrt* mutant haplotypes from Southeast Asia, South America, Africa, and Papua New Guinea (18). Nonetheless, once parasites with the mutant genotype were introduced into a region, they spread rapidly, as the selective pressure of heavy chloroquine use in endemic regions has been great. The result is that nearly the entire malarious world now has levels of chloroquine resistance that are unacceptably high (16). Profound economic constraints and apparent partial activity of chloroquine in highly immune populations have allowed it to remain the standard therapy for malaria in many areas, particularly in Africa, but widespread resistance demands changes to other regimens, as are now widely advocated (7).

Resistance to amodiaquine has not been well studied. The drug fails fairly frequently in many areas, but in locations with widespread resistance, it has much better efficacy against uncomplicated malaria than chloroquine (23). It is generally assumed that amodiaquine resistance follows the mechanisms of chloroquine resistance, but that differences in potency often allow continued clinical effectiveness of amodiaquine against chloroquine-resistant parasites (24).

Resistance to quinine, mefloquine, and halofantrine appears to be linked. Resistance to quinine is uncommon, but seen in Southeast Asia, particularly rural areas of Thailand, which appear to have the most resistant malaria parasites in the world. Quinine resistance is often fairly low grade, such that the drug retains some activity, but its action is delayed or diminished (25). Resistance to mefloquine is also uncommon in most areas, but increased after widespread use in Thailand in the 1990s (26). Despite this problem, the combination of mefloquine and artesunate has shown excellent efficacy in Thailand, and apparently even halted the progression of mefloquine resistance in this area (27). Resistance to halofantrine and the related drug lumefantrine (which is available only in combination with artemether) has been little studied. Resistance to quinine, mefloquine, and halofantrine appears to not be associated with mutations in *pfcrt*, but at least in part due to alterations in another putative transporter, Pgh1 (the product of the *pfmdr1* gene) (22).

Resistance to antifolates generally develops quickly after the introduction of a drug for widespread antimalarial therapy. At present, resistance to the most widely used antifolate combination, SP, is widespread in Asia and South America, and is increasing in Africa, particularly East Africa (16). An unfortunate recent scenario in Africa is that countries are changing their first-line antimalarial therapy from chloroquine to SP, and that this change has quickly been followed by the selection of widespread SP resistance. Resistance to antifolates and sulfas is quite well understood. Mutations in the target enzymes dihydrofolate reductase (DHFR) and dihydropteroate synthase (DHPS) are selected by drug pressure, and increasing levels of resistance are seen with increasing numbers of mutations. A pattern of five mutations strongly predicts resistance to SP, and unfortunately parasites with these mutations are now common in East Africa (28). The critical mutations (roughly in the order of usual acquisition) are DHFR S108N, N51I, and C59R, and DHPS A437G and K540E (29). Selection may be in a stepwise manner, progressing from mutations with little impact on clinical responses to those that mediate high-level resistance (29). However, recent evidence suggests a somewhat different scenario, whereby, in the setting of high-level use of SP in Africa, resistance has been brought on by transfer of both critical DHPS mutations upon a background of the three key DHFR mutations (30). Importantly, different patterns of mutations predict resistance against different antifolates. CD remains active against parasites with the five DHFR/DHPS mutations noted above, and in part for this reason is now advocated as an appropriate new drug for widespread use in Africa (14). However, one additional mutation (I164L), which is already common in Asia and South America, but not Africa, will lead to resistance against CD (31). CD is also somewhat protected from resistance selection by a relatively short half-life, but it remains uncertain whether heavier use of SP and/or CD will facilitate selection of highly resistant parasites.

Atovaquone/proguanil was recently introduced as a highly effective drug for treatment or prophylaxis of malaria, although its use in developing countries is limited by its very high cost (32). The efficacy of atovaquone/proguanil is somewhat surprising, as resistance to proguanil is common, because of DHFR mutations as discussed above, and resistance to atovaquone is selected rapidly, with mutations in the target enzyme cytochrome *c* oxidoreductase. Nonetheless, the drug combination, which has strong antimalarial synergy (33), does not appear to be limited by significant resistance problems, perhaps because of the mechanism of synergy independent of enzyme inhibition (32). However, atovaquone/proguanil resistance has recently been reported (34).

Resistance has not been described for antibiotics with antimalarial activity. These drugs are not used as monotherapy, which might select for resistance, but only as components of combination therapy or for chemoprophylaxis. However, widespread antibiotic use for other indications might be expected to select for resistant malaria parasites. Indeed, as this area has been little studied, it is possible that antibiotic-resistant parasites are now circulating.

Resistance has not yet been noted with the artemisinins, an important new class of antimalarials, perhaps owing to its limited use to date and the very short half-lives of all available agents of this class. It is argued that these drugs rapidly deplete parasite biomass such that, even if parasites are not fully eradicated, brief selective pressure on the small number of remaining organisms is unlikely to select for resistance (8). However, parasites that are relatively resistant to artemisinins can be selected in a mouse model (35), raising concern that resistance to this class may be selected with wider use.

An interesting new finding is the observation that malaria parasites in a community may lose their resistant phenotypes when drug pressure is removed. In Malawi, where SP replaced chloroquine for standard antimalarial therapy about a decade ago, recent studies have shown a dramatic decrease in the prevalence of clinical chloroquine resistance and in the *pfcrt* genotype that mediates resistance (36). These results offer the exciting possibility of returning to established old antimalarials after periods of drug withdrawal, possibly as components of drug combinations. However, loss of chloroquine resistance has not been observed in other areas where the drug has been replaced, and it is not clear whether chloroquine or other "failed" drugs will ever again have practical utility in areas where efficacy was lost.

Resistance of *P. vivax* to chloroquine has increasingly been reported from Asia and South America (37). Resistance is likely infrequent in most areas, and considering that vivax malaria is usually not dangerous, continued use of chloroquine for therapy of this infection is generally advocated. *P. vivax* contains a homolog of *pfcrt*, but chloroquine resistance does not appear to be mediated by mutations in this gene (38). Vivax malaria commonly responds poorly to treatment with SP (39), and recent evidence suggests that resistance is mediated by mutations in the *P. vivax dhfr* gene (40). Primaquine is the only drug available to eradicate the stage of *P. vivax* that chronically infects hepatocytes, and serves as a reservoir for subsequent clinical relapses. Primaquine fails intermittently, but it is not clear whether these failures are due to true drug resistance or pharmacokinetic and pharmacodynamic factors (41).

5 Evaluation of Antimalarial Drug Resistance

5.1 Clinical Assessment of Drug Resistance

The methods of assessment of antimalarial drug resistance differ importantly from those for most other infectious microbes. In vitro assessment of parasite resistance is possible, but this procedure is expensive, time consuming, and technically difficult. Therefore, in vitro assays are used only for laboratory studies and limited population surveys, as will be discussed below. In contrast, clinical assessment of antimalarial drug resistance is relatively straightforward, and so the WHO has recommended this system for the assessment of drug efficacies in different populations (42). Although straightforward, methods for clinical assessment of drug response have not been well standardized. This is a problem, as different methodologies will lead to different results, confusing comparisons between studies. Recently, much effort has gone into standardization of the clinical assessment of antimalarial drug efficacy, and standardized systems have been described by the WHO (42). In assessing drug resistance rates in clinical studies, one must be aware that, as discussed above, some patients will typically appear to respond to therapy even when the infecting parasites are drug resistant. Responses may be short-lived, followed by late recrudescence of resistant parasites, and this outcome can best be assessed by long-term follow-up, with molecular studies to discriminate recrudescent from newly infecting parasites. In addition, patients may respond to therapy against which their parasites are resistant because of the combined effects of a partial drug response and underlying antimalarial immunity, and this outcome appears to be quite common in highly endemic areas.

After treatment, patients may express drug failure by remaining ill and failing to clear parasites from the blood. However, failures commonly are less dramatic, with initial apparent responses followed by eventual reappearance of symptoms and parasitemia. This gradation in antimalarial drug responses led to a WHO scale for grading resistance, ranging from RI (good initial response followed by late recurrence) to RIII (minimal initial response) based primarily on serial measurements of parasitemia after treatment (43). In general, it is felt that the degree of inherent parasite resistance to a drug correlates with the grade of clinical resistance (i.e., more resistant parasites are more likely to cause RIII resistance), but, as discussed above, other factors, most notably host immunity, also impact on treatment responses. More recently, it has been suggested that the RI–RIII parasitological scale is not adequate to judge clinical responses. Indeed, the parasitological assessment is likely the most accurate gauge of drug resistance, but it may be less useful for policy makers who are most interested in clinical outcomes. On the basis of these concerns, revised guidelines for assessing drug responses in clinical studies incorporated clinical measures of outcome, ranging from adequate clinical response (ACR) to late treatment failure (LTF) to early treatment failure (ETF) (44). A typical system for the use of both the parasitological and clinical schemes for monitoring resistance is described in a previous report (45). Most recently, the pendulum has swung back, with concern that the clinical measures did not include an adequate assessment of parasite responses to treatment, and so the newest WHO guidelines incorporate both parasitological and clinical grading scales (44) (Table 3). Recent frequent changes in systems for measuring antimalarial drug resistance have been confusing, but it is likely that the newest, more inclusive scale will not undergo significant additional changes in the near future. In addition to standard measures of treatment outcome, secondary outcomes of value include fever clearance time, hematological response, and prevalence of gametocytemia after treatment. These outcomes should not be used to quantify resistance, but offer finer comparisons of different regimens.

A challenge with the clinical assessment of antimalarial drug resistance is to determine whether a late clinical recurrence is due to recrudescence of the parasites that caused the initial infection (true failure) or reinfection with a new strain after treatment. The latter possibility is very common in highly endemic areas. One method of avoiding this concern is to conduct clinical trials in controlled settings where malaria transmission has been eliminated. Such an approach was advocated in older WHO recommendations (42). This approach is possible in some tropical cities (e.g., Bangkok),

Table 3 Treatment outcome classification system for clinical assessment of antimalarial drug efficacy[a]

Outcome category	Criteria
Early treatment failure (ETF)	• Danger signs or severe malaria on days 1–3, in the presence of parasitemia • Parasitemia on day 2 more than on day 0, irrespective of temperature or fever history • Parasitemia on day 3 with temperature ≥38.0°C • Parasitemia on day 3 ≥25% of count on day 0
Late clinical failure (LCF)	• Danger signs or severe malaria after day 3, in the presence of parasitemia • Parasitemia after day 3 with temperature ≥38.0°C or fever in the last 48 h
Late parasitological failure (LPF)	• Parasitemia on day 28 or 42 with temperature <38.0°C and no fever in last 48 h
Adequate clinical and parasitological response (ACPR)	• Absence of parasitemia on last day irrespective of temperature or fever history without meeting any of the criteria for ETF, LCF, or LPF

[a]Adapted from (42)

as patients present commonly after infection in rural areas, but they are very unlikely to be reinfected if they remain in the urban setting through the course of evaluation. Conducting such trials is impractical in Africa and many other areas, however, as transmission is common in cities, and long-term hospitalization in adequately protected environments is not economically feasible.

The traditional means of avoiding the problem of distinguishing recrudescence from reinfection in highly endemic areas has been to conduct trials with follow-up after treatment for only 1–2 weeks. It is argued that few clinical recurrences that occur within 2 weeks will be due to new infections, and so all recurrences can be considered true drug failures. This approach is relatively inexpensive, but flawed. First, some early recurrences may be due to newly infecting parasites. Second, it fails to appreciate the fact that many failures present with recurrent symptoms and parasitemia much longer than 2 weeks after therapy. Third, 2-week outcomes do not necessarily predict longer-term outcomes; owing to differing pharmacokinetic properties and other features, two drugs with similar outcomes after 2 weeks may have very different long-term efficacies. An improved means of conducting drug efficacy trials has recently come about, with the establishment of molecular "fingerprinting" techniques that effectively discriminate different parasite isolates, and thereby allow us to distinguish recrudescence from reinfection. In highly endemic areas, where most studies have taken place, parasites are highly diverse. Thus, the likelihood of chance reinfection with the same strain after treatment is very low. Simple molecular methods involve the amplification of certain highly polymorphic *P. falciparum* genes (most commonly merozoite surface protein-1, merozoite surface protein-2, and/or glutamate-rich protein), nested amplification of regions that are polymorphic in sequence and size, and then comparison of the profiles of isolates obtained before and after treatment (46). These techniques have been validated to effectively distinguish new and recrudescent infections in some areas (47). Related methods utilize single-strand conformational polymorphism fingerprinting, which offers more accuracy in distinguishing parasite alleles, but is more difficult than routine procedures (48). Genotyping throughput can be increased, albeit at increased cost, with real-time polymerase chain reaction (PCR) techniques (49). Alternative methods involve evaluation of microsatellite markers, which has the benefit of assessment of neutral markers, presumably not influenced by immunologic selection, as are antigens such as the merozoite surface proteins (50). However, microsatellite methods have to date been used principally to evaluate parasite population diversity (51), rather than to discriminate strains collected before and after treatment, and so at present the technique best validated for the discrimination of recrudescent and new infecting isolates is the characterization of one or more polymorphic antigens.

5.2 Requirements for Clinical Drug Efficacy Studies

Evaluations of antimalarial drug efficacy and resistance have suffered from disparate methodologies, but there is a growing consensus regarding optimal approaches. A detailed and updated monograph on methods for monitoring antimalarial drug efficacy has recently been published by the WHO (42). WHO methods are focused on simple systems for the surveillance of resistance in developing countries, but optimal methods for research studies, in which resources are less constrained, differ relatively little, except as follows. First, optimal studies should ideally be randomized, blinded comparisons of regimens. Second, studies should include sample size calculations based on hypothesis testing. Third, follow-up after therapy should be for at least 28 days (WHO guidelines allow 14-day follow-up in areas of high transmission), for the reasons discussed above. Fourth, studies should include molecular genotyping to distinguish recrudescence from reinfection after therapy. Indeed, it can be argued that all surveillance, even in resource-poor settings, should include molecular discrimination of recrudescence and new infections, as the added cost of this molecular approach is relatively small, and the added information generated is significant. Fifth, ideal studies might include assessment of blood levels of drugs over the course of therapy, to consider the contribution of pharmacokinetics in outcomes, although consideration of this last factor is currently not practical for most research groups. With these caveats, it is prudent for all studies to follow new guidelines as much as possible, so that the comparison of results from different studies is straightforward. When methods vary, it is useful to report subgroup analyses, to expedite comparisons between studies. Specific concerns regarding the design of clinical assessments of antimalarial drug resistance are as follows.

The clinical assessment and follow-up of patients must be rigorous. Clinical evaluation for malaria is relatively simple, requiring only routine examination skills, a thermometer, and evaluation of blood smears. Some authorities advocate inclusion only of patients that present with a documented fever (42), but considering the intermittent nature of malarial fevers it may be reasonable to allow either fever or history of fever, with parasitemia, as an inclusion criterion for a drug efficacy trial. Clinical trials to monitor drug resistance should include only individuals with uncomplicated malaria, by far the most common presentation of the disease. Standardized criteria are available to eliminate patients with "danger signs" for progression to severe disease or existing evidence of complicated malaria (42, 52). Such patients should be treated promptly, but their outcomes are complex, and not appropriate for study in a simple drug-efficacy trial. Some studies evaluate the clearance of parasites from asymptomatic individuals; this may be of value for a new compound, where trials against asymptomatic parasitemia might precede full efficacy analysis, but for routine resistance monitoring assessment should be of those with symptomatic, uncomplicated malaria. Adequate attention must be paid to sample size such that useful information can be generated, but unnecessary expense avoided (42). Patients must be adequately followed up, often necessitating travel to a patient's home to continue assessment weeks after the initial presentation. Studies with follow-up rates below 80–90% are suspect, as important bias may have been introduced. Once patients are enrolled, all study therapy should be directly observed, ideally in a randomized, blinded comparison of relevant therapies. Quality control is essential for a high-quality clinical study. The reliability of blood smear readings is best assured by including duplicate assessments.

The age and appropriate inclusion criteria of study participants must be decided upon. In areas of low endemicity, malaria occurs infrequently in all ages, antimalarial immunity is roughly similar in all groups, and the choice of age can be determined on the basis of convenience. However, in high-endemicity areas, children develop antimalarial immunity from repeated infections over the first few years of life, and so the choice of age group significantly impacts on outcomes. Typically, in areas with drug resistance, older children and adults respond considerably better than young children, as their underlying immunity allows the control of some infections with drug-resistant parasites. For this reason, many authorities advocate testing of children only under age 5 (generally age 6 months to 5 years) for routine assessments of drug efficacy and resistance. Of course, a study can include older individuals if appropriate for other reasons, but then stratify results to allow the comparison of under-five outcomes across different studies. Inclusion criteria should include fever (or recent history of fever), *P. falciparum* monoinfection, ability to maintain follow-up, and informed consent. Typical exclusion criteria for a drug efficacy study are evidence of severe malaria or "danger signs" (inability to drink or breastfeed, repeated vomiting, recent convulsions, lethargy or unconsciousness, inability to sit or stand up (52)), evidence of another significant illness, malnutrition, mixed infection (including malaria species other than *P. falciparum*), and a history of hypersensitivity to a study drug (42). A history of prior antimalarial drug use is generally not considered an exclusion criterion, as prior drug use is very common in many areas, and methods of ascertaining information on prior drug use are unreliable. Information on prior drug use can be helpful, however, and so serum drug level testing or simpler qualitative urine tests can be included if available (42).

Laboratory diagnosis of malaria must be sound. The standard means of diagnosing malaria is the presence of parasites on a thick blood smear in a patient with symptoms consistent with malaria (principally fever at clinic presentation or a history of recent fever). Thick blood smears are routine in malaria-endemic regions and expertise in reading them is widely available. However, high standards for microscopy are mandatory, and best provided by the participation of experienced microscopists and the confirmation of results by second readings of slides. Additional methods for the molecular diagnosis of malaria are now available, including PCR amplification of parasite DNA and enzymatic and immunologic rapid tests (53, 54). However, PCR results, although offering increased sensitivity and the opportunity to distinguish parasite species, have not been well correlated with clinical outcomes. Indeed, in highly endemic areas the high specificity of PCR can be a drawback, as individuals with asymptomatic infections may be falsely labeled as suffering from acute malaria. Rapid tests show promise, but at present also have concerns regarding sensitivity and specificity such that they are not routinely used in drug efficacy trials. Rather, simple microscopy, with rigorous attention to accuracy in slide reading, is the laboratory cornerstone of a high-quality drug efficacy study.

A specific cut-off for the parasitemia that is diagnostic of clinical malaria must be chosen. Parasitemia is typically measured as the number of parasites per leukocyte on a thick blood smear, assuming a total leukocyte count of 8,000 cells/µl. This is clearly a rough estimate, as leukocyte counts vary greatly, but allows the simple low-cost approximation of parasitemias. If improved means of counting are available, they can be incorporated into clinical studies. Typically, studies in highly endemic areas, such as most of Africa, use low cut-offs for parasitemia for inclusion in clinical trials of up to 2,000 parasites/µl. The justification for these cut-offs is that low-level parasitemias are fairly likely to be asymptomatic, and so febrile patients with such parasitemias may well be ill from another cause. However, parasitemia cut-offs have not been standardized. High cut-offs for parasitemia are sometimes included, to diminish the likelihood that study patients will progress to severe malaria, although the correlation between parasitemia and severity of malaria is poor. Considering these factors and differences in immunity in different areas, current WHO recommendations for parasitemia inclusion criteria are 1,000–100,000 asexual parasites per microliter for areas of low to moderate transmission and 2,000–200,000 asexual parasites per microliter for areas of high transmission (42).

The length of time over which follow-up occurs after treatment is critical in a malaria drug efficacy trial. As noted above, failures after treatment with an inadequate drug may be apparent early, but it is also common for recurrences due to drug failure to present only after a number of weeks. Therefore, it is now clear that all drug efficacy trials should extend follow-up beyond 2 weeks (55). Extending the length of studies adds to the difficulty of maintaining follow-up; a system to pursue patients who do not return to the study clinic for follow up is essential. Another challenge has been discriminating between recurrence due to recrudescence of inadequately treated parasites and reinfection with a new strain after therapy. As noted above, robust molecular techniques are now available for this discrimination, and standardization of methodology is ongoing. The appropriate length of follow-up differs among drugs, but since many antimalarials have long half-lives, it is appropriate to use long follow-up for all tested regimens. There is no standard length of trials, but it seems reasonable to follow patients for at least 4 weeks, and the benefits of extended follow-up probably diminish markedly after 6 weeks.

The discussion above is most appropriate for studies of drug efficacy and resistance in *P. falciparum* infections, but these clinical methods should also be appropriate for *P. vivax*. However, *P. vivax* has an additional feature of relevance to therapy. Unlike *P. falciparum*, *P. vivax* (and *P. ovale*) has a chronic liver (hypnozoite) stage which does not cause disease, but is not eradicated by most available drugs, and so is a reservoir for parasites that can subsequently infect erythrocytes, leading to recurrences after therapy. These infections after adequate eradication of erythrocytic parasites are not due to resistance, but to the progression from hypnozoites to erythrocytic parasites after treatment, and they are referred to as relapses. Relapses usually occur within weeks to months after the initial treatment. Relapses are prevented by treating *P. vivax* infections with primaquine in addition to the schizonticidal agent (usually chloroquine). Without primaquine therapy, it is not possible to distinguish recrudescence due to drug failure from relapse. In addition, failures of primaquine in the eradication of liver stages have been reported (41), but in these cases it has been difficult to asses the relative contributions of chloroquine failure against erythrocytic parasites and primaquine inactivity against hypnozoites.

5.3 Interpretation of Results of Clinical Drug Efficacy Studies

The results of clinical studies must be interpreted with caution, as multiple assumptions are made in analyzing data (e.g., in determining length of follow-up and in distinguishing recrudescence from reinfection), and, as noted above, even in the setting of high-level resistance many patients in endemic areas will appear to respond to therapy. Nonetheless, these studies provide the best available means of assessing drug efficacy. In addition, if consistent methods are maintained, these studies are an excellent means of providing comparisons between locations and serial surveillance at individual locations. It remains unclear, however, just how control programs should act upon specific results. Traditionally, programs have been slow to change treatment policies due

to financial constraints, limitations of alternative therapies, and the inherently slow pace of bureaucratic change. Thus, even now most African countries recommend chloroquine as first-line therapy for malaria, although available data suggest that chloroquine resistance is now very prevalent in nearly all of sub-Saharan Africa. The WHO has attempted to quantify recommendations for changing therapy policy, although their recommendations are intended to be only advisory. Older WHO guidelines stated that a "grace period" existed when failure rates were 0–4% for a particular therapy; an "alert" was sounded when resistance was 5–14%; "action" was recommended when rates were 15–24%; and "change" was advocated when resistance topped 25% (42). The most recent recommendations, based on the newest outcome classification scheme (Table 3), state that policy change should be implemented for Adequate Clinical and Parasitological Response rates of less than 75% (total failure rate over 25%) or Adequate Clinical Response rates under 85% (clinical failure rate over 15%). These recommendations do not clearly specify study details leading to failure percentages, but if one considers long-term (28- or 42-day) outcomes, it is likely that, for nearly all of Africa, it is already appropriate to eliminate chloroquine, and in a number of areas also appropriate to eliminate SP as first-line therapy for malaria. Many countries in Africa and elsewhere are now moving to reconsider malaria treatment policy, and a number of countries have changed policy from chloroquine, often to artemisinin-containing regimens, very recently. However, implementation can be expected to be slow because of financial and infrastructure constraints, and it remains a great challenge to implement needed changes before resistance levels are dangerously high.

5.4 In vtro Assessment of Antimalarial Drug Efficacy

A culture system for *P. falciparum* was developed in the 1970s (56). This system requires human erythrocytes and serum (or serum substitute) and is widely used in research laboratories. Simple in vitro systems have been devised to determine the IC_{50}s of drugs and new candidate antimalarials against cultured parasites. In vitro systems are of great value in assessing responses of parasites to drugs in the laboratory setting. They are of no utility in the management of individual patients, as they are too expensive, time consuming, and erratic to offer useful information to the clinician. However, in vitro tests can complement the clinical testing methods described above to assess the epidemiology of drug resistance in a particular setting. As they are fairly expensive and can require complex equipment, in vitro systems are not widely available in malaria-endemic settings, but where available they have provided useful information. However, broader use of in vitro tests to assess the epidemiology of resistance in field settings will require better standardization of methodologies. In particular, laboratory cut-offs for sensitive vs. resistant parasites are not straightforward. Indeed, it may be impossible to set uniform cut-offs, as done for bacteria, as the degree of biochemical resistance must be interpreted in light of the relative antimalarial immunity of a population when considering its value for predicting clinical outcomes.

The oldest and simplest in vitro field test for antimalarial drug resistance is the "microtest" (57). For this test, blood samples from infected humans are placed in short-term culture in the presence of serial dilutions of test antimalarials. Culture medium is not required, as samples remain in anticoagulated blood. After approximately 1 day, parasite cultures are evaluated microscopically to assess parasite maturation. Since only ring-forms circulate, the presence of multinucleated schizonts is indicative of parasite growth, and an absence of schizonts compared to controls indicates an antiparasitic effect. Curves of percent control schizonts over concentration can be used to determine IC_{50}s. The microtest is limited in that adaptation of parasites to culture is problematic, such that many assessments will fail owing to lack of growth of parasites; for this reason, the parallel assessment of control (untreated) parasites is essential. However, the microtest benefits from relatively little need for expensive equipment, so it is quite suitable for field settings. In a warm climate, only a candle jar is adequate for culture, although facilities for sterile technique, sterile microplates, and incubators to maintain constant temperature of experiments are optimal.

The microtest can be improved with additions that are appropriate for some field settings. Most commonly, the visual inspection of culture smears has been replaced by the quantitative assessment of the uptake of a labeled metabolite (usually [^{3}H]hypoxanthine), following a standard protocol (58). This test, known as the isotopic semimicrotest, requires one expensive piece of equipment, a scintillation spectrometer, but has proven to be robust in some field settings (59). In vitro microtests can also incorporate the washing of cells at the initiation of the experiment. Cultures are then maintained in standard culture medium (56). This technique eliminates host serum, and therefore the contribution of host immunity to drug response, so offers perhaps the best test of true parasite resistance. However, the use of in vitro tests to measure responses of field isolates to drugs remains a specialized procedure available at only a small number of centers in developing countries.

5.5 Molecular Assessment of Antimalarial Drug Resistance

It is now possible to use simple molecular techniques to identify mutations in infecting malaria parasites that predict resis-

tance to two important drugs, chloroquine and SP. Molecular assays may allow surveillance with simple molecular tests to provide spot analyses of resistance in individual locations or populations. Such procedures are not yet routine components of malaria control programs anywhere, but evaluation of mutations predicting chloroquine resistance was recently helpful in determining the best means of treating a malaria epidemic in Mali (60). In the case of chloroquine, the *pfcrt* K76T mutation predicts resistance, and in the case of SP the presence of a series of mutations in *dhfr* and *dhps* likewise predicts resistance. Simple methods have been developed to amplify the genes of interest from blood or, most commonly, blood spots that have been dried on filter paper. In most protocols, a nested amplification is followed by mutation-specific restriction endonuclease digestion, and the size of digestion fragments indicates the presence or absence of the mutation of interest (20, 61). These assays are quite simple, but a number of factors must be considered in interpreting results.

First, as noted in the above sections, the predictive value of tests of parasite resistance must be considered in light of the contribution of antimalarial immunity to treatment outcomes. Thus, specific mutations may have different significance in different populations. For example, infection with a parasite containing the *pfcrt* K76T mutation will likely lead to a very high risk of treatment failure in a malaria-naive individual, but in a highly immune population, many patients infected with mutant parasites will respond to therapy, at least in the short term. Thus, at a number of sites in Mali, the K76T mutation was about 3 times more prevalent than the 14-day chloroquine treatment failure (20). In Uganda, where the 14-day clinical failure rate for chloroquine was 47%, 100% of tested isolates contained the resistance-mediating mutation (62). Other sites have seen similarly high prevalences of the K76T mutation (18). One group has proposed a "genotype failure index", to correlate prevalences of mutant genotypes with clinical outcomes. At a number of sites in Africa, a genotype failure index of about 2 has been seen, predicting that two or more times as many mutant genotypes as clinical failures may be seen (63, 64).

Second, tests of molecular predictors of drug resistance in highly endemic areas must take into account the possibility of mixed infections. Patients are commonly infected with multiple strains. Not uncommonly, both sensitive and resistant genotypes will be present in a single infection. Routine assays can easily identify both strains. Typically, one would assume that a mixed infection will act as a resistant infection, as mutant parasites will grow out under drug pressure.

Third, molecular tests must take great care to avoid contaminations that confound results. PCR-based assays are quite simple and, considering surveillance choices, fairly inexpensive. However, owing to the high sensitivity of PCR, there is a great risk of inaccurate results due to contamination of samples with other parasite DNA. As assays move from the basic laboratory bench to the clinical laboratory or the field, great care must be taken to avoid contamination of samples and to include appropriate positive and negative controls in all experiments.

6 New Directions in Assessment of Antimalarial Drug Resistance

It appears that, after a period of flux, consensus has been reached regarding appropriate means of assessing clinical responses to antimalarial drugs (42). The most recent WHO guidelines support assessment of both clinical and parasitological responses to therapy. These guidelines also support extending follow-up beyond the traditional 14-day period, with the use of molecular genotyping to distinguish recrudescence from reinfection. It is likely that these clinical systems will remain the gold standard for assessment of responses to therapy, and therefore for analysis of drug resistance, for some time to come.

It seems unlikely that the importance of in vitro testing in assessing drug resistance will change in the near future. Such testing will remain valuable at specialized centers that have necessary infrastructure and that have optimized systems to allow correlation between in vitro sensitivity results and the local field situation. However, such systems will remain unavailable in most malaria-endemic regions.

Laboratory systems for the identification of resistance-mediating mutations should have increasing utility. In recent years, simple systems for the identification of relevant mutations have been developed (20, 61). These require rather simple equipment, and so are quite appropriate for use in laboratory settings in developing countries. In addition, these assessments can readily be performed after collection and storage of samples on filter paper, so samples can easily be transported as necessary to ensure that adequate infrastructure is available for testing. The great advantage of genotype studies for resistance is that they are quick and relatively inexpensive, potentially providing policy makers rapid feedback to assess the epidemiology of drug resistance in regions of interest. These molecular tests will not directly provide clinically relevant quantitative data, as prevalences of clinical resistance will be lower than those of resistance-mediating mutations. However, algorithms can be created to allow rough correlation of genotypic and clinical results. In one case, such a system has already had practical utility, as rapid genotype evaluations of parasite strains causing an outbreak in Mali guided therapeutic decisions (60). Genotyping to detect resistance is most developed for the identification of mutations that predict resistance to chloroquine and SP. The use of this system is limited by the understanding that chloroquine resistance is already so common in most areas to render these assessments moot. However, in areas with relatively little resistance (e.g., parts of West Africa, Central America, and the Caribbean), serial testing for the prevalence of resistance-mediating mutations seems an appropriate means of assessing the progression of chloroquine resistance. Mutations predicting antifolate resistance can also now be assessed quite easily. These tests will be valuable to assess progression of SP resistance, especially in Africa, where this drug is increasingly used. In addition, with the release of CD in 2003, surveillance for additional mutations that predict resistance to CD will be important.

7 New Directions in Antimalarial Chemotherapy

The bad news, as discussed in this chapter, is that antimalarial drug resistance is an enormous and growing problem. The good news is that new antimalarial drugs are on the horizon. New agents under testing include analogs of existing antimalarial classes of drugs and new classes, many directed against novel targets (65, 66). Importantly, antimalarial drug discovery and development has recently been energized by a growing consensus, among governments, nongovernmental organizations, and some large corporations, that the development of new drugs for diseases of the developing world is an international responsibility. This new consensus has spawned public–private partnerships, notably the Medicines for Malaria Venture, that are now providing much increased resources for antimalarial drug discovery and development (67). Considering these changes, it seems likely that multiple new drugs will be available to treat malaria over the next few decades. Most likely, new drugs will be released as components of combination therapies, to limit the selection of resistant parasites. Nonetheless, drug resistance remains a major concern. At present, and for the foreseeable future, it remains critical to maintain standardized systems for the assessment of antimalarial drug resistance and to perform serial surveillance of populations at risk to best direct our limited malaria treatment resources.

Addendum for Rosenthal chapter
Important changes since the original writing of this chapter include: 1) endorsement of artemisinin-based combination therapies for uncomplicated falciparum malaria in nearly all endemic countries; 2) the availability of multiple co-formulated artemisinin-based regimens, including artemether-lumefantrine, artesunate-amodiaquine, artesunate-mefloquine, and dihydroartemisinin-piperaquine, each of which has demonstrated excellent efficacy in a number of randomized trials; 3) increased international support that has lessened barriers for the implementation of new antimalarial therapies; 4) increased attention to the use of drugs to prevent malaria in endemic settings, in particular as intermittent preventive therapy for infants and pregnant women; 5) discontinuation of development of one new combination therapy, chlorproguanil-dapsone, due to unacceptable hemologic toxicity; 6) early evidence for possible resistance to artemisinins, with identification of isolates with decreased in vitro sensitivity and demonstration of

delayed parasite clearance after artesunate therapy in Southeast Asia; 7) the optimization of newer methods to assess in vitro antimalarial drug sensitivity without use of radioactive reagents; 8) evidence for additional polymorphisms and alterations in gene copy number potentially mediating resistance to different drugs; and 9) recent establishment of the Worldwide Antimalarial Resistance Network, which will work to standardize and catalogue drug resistance information.

Acknowledgments   The author's research is supported by the National Institutes of Health, the Medicines for Malaria Venture, and the Doris Duke Charitable Foundation, for which he is a Distinguished Clinical Scientist. A critical review of this chapter by Sarah Staedke was greatly appreciated.

References

1. Breman JG. The ears of the hippopotamus: manifestations, determinants, and estimates of the malaria burden. Am J Trop Med Hyg 2001;64(suppl):1–11.
2. Meshnick SR and Dobson MJ. The history of antimalarial drugs. In: Rosenthal PJ, ed. Antimalarial Chemotherapy: Mechanisms of Action, Resistance, and New Directions in Drug Discovery. Totowa, NJ: Humana Press, 2001, pp 15–25.
3. Olliaro P, Nevill C, LeBras J, Ringwald P, Mussano P, Garner P and Brasseur P. Systematic review of amodiaquine treatment in uncomplicated malaria. Lancet 1996;348:1196–201.
4. White NJ. The treatment of malaria. N Engl J Med 1996;335: 800–6.
5. Meshnick SR. Artemisinin and its derivatives. In: Rosenthal PJ, ed. Antimalarial Chemotherapy: Mechanisms of Action, Resistance, and New Directions in Drug Discovery. Totowa, NJ: Humana Press, 2001, pp 191–201.
6. Klayman DL. Qinghaosu (artemisinin): an antimalarial drug from China. Science 1985;228:1049–55.
7. White NJ, Nosten F, Looareesuwan S, Watkins WM, Marsh K, Snow RW, Kokwaro G, Ouma J, Hien TT, Molyneux ME, Taylor TE, Newbold CI, Ruebush TK, II, Danis M, Greenwood BM, Anderson RM and Olliaro P. Averting a malaria disaster. Lancet 1999;353:1965–7.
8. White NJ and Pongtavornpinyo W. The de novo selection of drug-resistant malaria parasites. Proc R Soc Lond B Biol Sci 2003; 270:545–54.
9. Staedke SG, Kamya MR, Dorsey G, Gasasira A, Ndeezi G, Charlebois ED and Rosenthal PJ. Amodiaquine, sulfadoxine/ pyrimethamine, and combination therapy for treatment of uncomplicated falciparum malaria in Kampala, Uganda: a randomised trial. Lancet 2001;358:368–74.
10. Dorsey G, Njama D, Kamya MR, Cattamanchi A, Kyabayinze D, Staedke SG, Gasasira A and Rosenthal PJ. Sulfadoxine/pyrimethamine alone or with amodiaquine or artesunate for treatment of uncomplicated malaria: a longitudinal randomised trial. Lancet 2002;360:2031–8.
11. Rwagacondo CE, Niyitegeka F, Sarushi J, Karema C, Mugisha V, Dujardin JC, Van Overmeir C, van den Ende J and D'Alessandro U. Efficacy of amodiaquine alone and combined with sulfadoxine-pyrimethamine and of sulfadoxine pyrimethamine combined with artesunate. Am J Trop Med Hyg 2003;68:743–7.
12. von Seidlein L, Milligan P, Pinder M, Bojang K, Anyalebechi C, Gosling R, Coleman R, Ude JI, Sadiq A, Duraisingh M, Warhurst D, Alloueche A, Targett G, McAdam K, Greenwood B, Walraven G, Olliaro P and Doherty T. Efficacy of artesunate plus pyrimethamine-sulphadoxine for uncomplicated malaria in Gambian children: a double-blind, randomised, controlled trial. Lancet 2000;355:352–7.
13. Adjuik M, Agnamey P, Babiker A, Borrmann S, Brasseur P, Cisse M, Cobelens F, Diallo S, Faucher JF, Garner P, Gikunda S, Kremsner PG, Krishna S, Lell B, Loolpapit M, Matsiegui PB, Missinou MA, Mwanza J, Ntoumi F, Olliaro P, Osimbo P, Rezbach P, Some E and Taylor WR. Amodiaquine-artesunate versus amodiaquine for uncomplicated Plasmodium falciparum malaria in African children: a randomised, multicentre trial. Lancet 2002;359:1365–72.
14. Lang T and Greenwood B. The development of Lapdap, an affordable new treatment for malaria. Lancet Infect Dis 2003;3:162–7.
15. Lefevre G, Looareesuwan S, Treeprasertsuk S, Krudsood S, Silachamroon U, Gathmann I, Mull R and Bakshi R. A clinical and pharmacokinetic trial of six doses of artemether-lumefantrine for multidrug-resistant Plasmodium falciparum malaria in Thailand. Am J Trop Med Hyg 2001;64:247–56.
16. Wongsrichanalai C, Pickard AL, Wernsdorfer WH and Meshnick SR. Epidemiology of drug-resistant malaria. Lancet Infect Dis 2002; 2:209–18.
17. Hall SA and Wilks NE. A trial of chloroquine-medicated salt for malaria suppression in Uganda. Am J Trop Med Hyg 1967; 16:429–42.
18. Wellems TE and Plowe CV. Chloroquine-resistant malaria. J Infect Dis 2001;184:770–6.
19. Fidock DA, Nomura T, Talley AK, Cooper RA, Dzekunov SM, Ferdig MT, Ursos LM, Sidhu AB, Naude B, Deitsch KW, Su XZ, Wootton JC, Roepe PD and Wellems TE. Mutations in the P. falciparum digestive vacuole transmembrane protein PfCRT and evidence for their role in chloroquine resistance. Mol Cell 2000;6:861–71.
20. Djimde A, Doumbo OK, Cortese JF, Kayentao K, Doumbo S, Diourte Y, Dicko A, Su XZ, Nomura T, Fidock DA, Wellems TE, Plowe CV and Coulibaly D. A molecular marker for chloroquine-resistant falciparum malaria. N Engl J Med 2001;344:257–63.
21. Sidhu AB, Verdier-Pinard D and Fidock DA. Chloroquine resistance in Plasmodium falciparum malaria parasites conferred by pfcrt mutations. Science 2002;298:210–3.
22. Reed MB, Saliba KJ, Caruana SR, Kirk K and Cowman AF. Pgh1 modulates sensitivity and resistance to multiple antimalarials in Plasmodium falciparum. Nature 2000;403:906–9.
23. Brasseur P, Guiguemde R, Diallo S, Guiyedi V, Kombila M, Ringwald P and Olliaro P. Amodiaquine remains effective for treating uncomplicated malaria in west and central Africa. Trans R Soc Trop Med Hyg 1999;93:645–50.
24. Dorsey G, Fidock DA, Wellems TE and Rosenthal PJ. Mechanisms of quinoline resistance. In: Rosenthal PJ, ed. Antimalarial Chemotherapy: Mechanisms of Action, Resistance, and New Directions in Drug Discovery. Totowa, NJ: Humana Press, 2001, pp 153–72.
25. Pukrittayakamee S, Supanaranond W, Looareesuwan S, Vanijanonta S and White NJ. Quinine in severe falciparum malaria: evidence of declining efficacy in Thailand. Trans R Soc Trop Med Hyg 1994;88:324–7.
26. Nosten F, ter Kuile F, Chongsuphajaisiddhi T, Luxemburger C, Webster HK, Edstein M, Phaipun L, Thew KL and White NJ. Mefloquine-resistant falciparum malaria on the Thai-Burmese border. Lancet 1991;337:1140–3.
27. Nosten F, van Vugt M, Price R, Luxemburger C, Thway KL, Brockman A, McGready R, ter Kuile F, Looareesuwan S and White NJ. Effects of artesunate-mefloquine combination on incidence of Plasmodium falciparum malaria and mefloquine resistance in western Thailand: a prospective study. Lancet 2000;356: 297–302.
28. Sibley CH, Hyde JE, Sims PF, Plowe CV, Kublin JG, Mberu EK, Cowman AF, Winstanley PA, Watkins WM and Nzila AM.

Pyrimethamine-sulfadoxine resistance in *Plasmodium falciparum*: what next? Trends Parasitol 2001;17:582–8.

29. Plowe CV. Folate antagonists and mechanisms of resistance. In: Rosenthal PJ, ed. Antimalarial Chemotherapy: Mechanisms of Action, Resistance, and New Directions in Drug Discovery. Totowa, NJ: Humana Press, 2001, pp 173–90.

30. Roper C, Pearce R, Bredenkamp B, Gumede J, Drakeley C, Mosha F, Chandramohan D and Sharp B. Antifolate antimalarial resistance in southeast Africa: a population-based analysis. Lancet 2003;361:1174–81.

31. Peterson DS, Milhous WK and Wellems TE. Molecular basis of differential resistance to cycloguanil and pyrimethamine in *Plasmodium falciparum* malaria. Proc Natl Acad Sci U S A 1990;87:3018–22.

32. Vaidya AB. Atovaquone-proguanil combination. In: Rosenthal PJ, ed. Antimalarial Chemotherapy: Mechanisms of Action, Resistance, and New Directions in Drug Discovery. Totowa, NJ: Humana Press, 2001, pp 203–18.

33. Canfield CJ, Pudney M and Gutteridge WE. Interactions of atovaquone with other antimalarial drugs against *Plasmodium falciparum* in vitro. Exp Parasitol 1995;80:373–81.

34. Fivelman QL, Butcher GA, Adagu IS, Warhurst DC and Pasvol G. Malarone treatment failure and in vitro confirmation of resistance of *Plasmodium falciparum* isolate from Lagos, Nigeria. Malar J 2002;1:1.

35. Peters W and Robinson BL. The chemotherapy of rodent malaria. LVI. Studies on the development of resistance to natural and synthetic endoperoxides. Ann Trop Med Parasitol 1999;93:325–9.

36. Kublin JG, Cortese JF, Njunju EM, Mukadam RA, Wirima JJ, Kazembe PN, Djimde AA, Kouriba B, Taylor TE and Plowe CV. Reemergence of chloroquine-sensitive *Plasmodium falciparum* malaria after cessation of chloroquine use in Malawi. J Infect Dis 2003;187:1870–5.

37. Murphy GS, Basri H, Purnomo, Andersen EM, Bangs MJ, Mount DL, Gorden J, Lal AA, Purwokusumo AR, Harjosuwarno S, et al. Vivax malaria resistant to treatment and prophylaxis with chloroquine. Lancet 1993;341:96–100.

38. Nomura T, Carlton JM, Baird JK, del Portillo HA, Fryauff DJ, Rathore D, Fidock DA, Su X, Collins WE, McCutchan TF, Wootton JC and Wellems TE. Evidence for different mechanisms of chloroquine resistance in 2 Plasmodium species that cause human malaria. J Infect Dis 2001;183:1653–61.

39. Pukrittayakamee S, Chantra A, Simpson JA, Vanijanonta S, Clemens R, Looareesuwan S and White NJ. Therapeutic responses to different antimalarial drugs in vivax malaria. Antimicrob Agents Chemother 2000;44:1680–5.

40. Imwong M, Pukrittayakamee S, Renia L, Letourneur F, Charlieu JP, Leartsakulpanich U, Looareesuwan S, White NJ and Snounou G. Novel point mutations in the dihydrofolate reductase gene of Plasmodium vivax: evidence for sequential selection by drug pressure. Antimicrob Agents Chemother 2003;47:1514–21.

41. Smoak BL, DeFraites RF, Magill AJ, Kain KC and Wellde BT. Plasmodium vivax infections in U.S. Army troops: failure of primaquine to prevent relapse in studies from Somalia. Am J Trop Med Hyg 1997;56:231–4.

42. World Health Organization. Assessment and Monitoring of Antimalarial Drug Efficacy for the Treatment of Uncomplicated Falciparum Malaria. Geneva: World Health Organization, 2003.

43. Rieckmann KH. Monitoring the response of malaria infections to treatment. Bull World Health Organ 1990;68:759–60.

44. World Health Organization. Assessment of Therapeutic Efficacy of Antimalarial Drugs for Uncomplicated Falciparum Malaria in Areas with Intense Transmission. Geneva: World Health Organization, 1996.

45. Dorsey G, Kamya MR, Ndeezi G, Babirye JN, Phares CR, Olson JE, Katabira ET and Rosenthal PJ. Predictors of chloroquine

treatment failure in children and adults with falciparum malaria in Kampala, Uganda. Am J Trop Med Hyg 2000;62:686–92.

46. Viriyakosol S, Siripoon N, Petcharapirat C, Petcharapirat P, Jarra W, Thaithong S, Brown KN and Snounou G. Genotyping of *Plasmodium falciparum* isolates by the polymerase chain reaction and potential uses in epidemiological studies. Bull World Health Organ 1995;73:85–95.

47. Cattamanchi A, Kyabayinze D, Hubbard A, Kamya MR, Rosenthal PJ and Dorsey G. Distinguishing recrudescence from reinfection in a longitudinal antimalarial drug efficacy study: comparison of results based on genotyping of MSP-1, MSP-2, and GLURP. Am J Trop Med Hyg 2003;68:133–9.

48. Ohrt C, Mirabelli-Primdahl L, Looareesuwan S, Wilairatana P, Walsh D and Kain KC. Determination of failure of treatment of *Plasmodium falciparum* infection by using polymerase chain reaction single-strand conformational polymorphism fingerprinting. Clin Infect Dis 1999;28:847–52.

49. Cheesman SJ, de Roode JC, Read AF and Carter R. Real-time quantitative PCR for analysis of genetically mixed infections of malaria parasites: technique validation and applications. Mol Biochem Parasitol 2003;131:83–91.

50. Ferdig MT and Su XZ. Microsatellite markers and genetic mapping in *Plasmodium falciparum*. Parasitol Today 2000;16:307–12.

51. Anderson TJ, Haubold B, Williams JT, Estrada-Franco JG, Richardson L, Mollinedo R, Bockarie M, Mokili J, Mharakurwa S, French N, Whitworth J, Velez ID, Brockman AH, Nosten F, Ferreira MU and Day KP. Microsatellite markers reveal a spectrum of population structures in the malaria parasite *Plasmodium falciparum*. Mol Biol Evol 2000;17:1467–82.

52. Warrell DA, Molyneux ME and Beales PF. Severe and complicated malaria. Trans R Soc Trop Med Hyg 1990;84(suppl 2):1–65.

53. Guthmann JP, Ruiz A, Priotto G, Kiguli J, Bonte L and Legros D. Validity, reliability and ease of use in the field of five rapid tests for the diagnosis of *Plasmodium falciparum* malaria in Uganda. Trans R Soc Trop Med Hyg 2002;96:254–7.

54. Craig MH, Bredenkamp BL, Williams CH, Rossouw EJ, Kelly VJ, Kleinschmidt I, Martineau A and Henry GF. Field and laboratory comparative evaluation of ten rapid malaria diagnostic tests. Trans R Soc Trop Med Hyg 2002;96:258–65.

55. White NJ. The assessment of antimalarial drug efficacy. Trends Parasitol 2002;18:458–64.

56. Jensen JB. In vitro culture of *Plasmodium* parasites. In: Doolan DL, ed. Malaria Methods and Protocols. Totowa, NJ: Humana Press, 2002, pp 477–88.

57. Rieckmann KH, Campbell GH, Sax LJ and Mrema JE. Drug sensitivity of *Plasmodium falciparum*. An in-vitro microtechnique. Lancet 1978;1:22–3.

58. Desjardins RE, Canfield CJ, Haynes JD and Chulay JD. Quantitative assessment of antimalarial activity in vitro by a semiautomated microdilution technique. Antimicrob Agents Chemother 1979;16:710–8.

59. Ringwald P, Bickii J and Basco LK. In vitro activity of antimalarials against clinical isolates of *Plasmodium falciparum* in Yaounde, Cameroon. Am J Trop Med Hyg 1996;55:254–8.

60. Djimde A, Doumbo OK, Steketee RW and Plowe CV. Application of a molecular marker for surveillance of chloroquine-resistant falciparum malaria. Lancet 2001;358:890–1.

61. Duraisingh MT, Curtis J and Warhurst DC. *Plasmodium falciparum*: detection of polymorphisms in the dihydrofolate reductase and dihydropteroate synthetase genes by PCR and restriction digestion. Exp Parasitol 1998;89:1–8.

62. Dorsey G, Kamya MR, Singh A and Rosenthal PJ. Polymorphisms in the *Plasmodium falciparum* pfcrt and pfmdr-1 genes and clinical response to chloroquine in Kampala, Uganda. J Infect Dis 2001;183:1417–20.

63. Kublin JG, Dzinjalamala FK, Kamwendo DD, Malkin EM, Cortese JF, Martino LM, Mukadam RA, Rogerson SJ, Lescano AG, Molyneux ME, Winstanley PA, Chimpeni P, Taylor TE and Plowe CV. Molecular markers for failure of sulfadoxine-pyrimethamine and chlorproguanil-dapsone treatment of *Plasmodium falciparum* malaria. J Infect Dis 2002;185:380–8.

64. Kyabayinze D, Cattamanchi A, Kamya MR, Rosenthal PJ and Dorsey G. Validation of a simplified method for using molecular markers to predict sulfadoxine-pyrimethamine treatment failure in African children with falciparum malaria. Am J Trop Med Hyg 2003;69:247–52.

65. Ridley RG. Medical need, scientific opportunity and the drive for antimalarial drugs. Nature 2002;415:686–93.

66. Rosenthal PJ. Antimalarial drug discovery: old and new approaches. J Exp Biol 2003;206:3735–44.

67. Nwaka S and Ridley RG. Virtual drug discovery and development for neglected diseases through public–private partnerships. Nat Rev Drug Discov 2003;2:919–28.

Chapter 74
Diagnosis and Treatment of Metronidazole-Resistant *Trichomonas vaginalis* Infection

Sarah L. Cudmore and Gary E. Garber

1 *Trichomonas vaginalis*

Trichomonas vaginalis is one of four protozoan species of the family Trichomonadidae known to parasitize humans. Members of this family are characterized by their variable morphology, being spheroid or ovoid in form in axenic culture, but assuming an ameboid shape on contact with other cells (4, 101). Trichomonads reproduce by longitudinal binary fission and lack a cystic stage, although large, round "pseudocysts" have been known to form under unfavorable conditions. All Trichomonadidae possess five anterior flagella, four of which are free moving. The fifth recumbent flagellum is anchored along the organism as a part of the undulating membrane. This membrane extends along at least half the length of the organism, and is supported by a noncontractile costa. Motility, described as "bobbing" or "quivering", is characteristic of this family of organisms (38, 39).

T. vaginalis is the only trichomond known to cause disease in humans. It is the causative agent of the sexually transmitted disease (STD) trichomoniasis. *T. tenax*, usually found in the mouth, has been implicated in respiratory infection but its pathogenicity has never been confirmed (20). *Pentatrichomonas hominis* (104) and *Trichomitus fecalis* have generally been isolated from the lower gastrointestinal tract. However, to date only one case of *T. fecalis* has been confirmed, leaving its identity as a human parasite in question (14).

Nutritionally, *T. vaginalis* is a fastidious organism. Lacking pathways for de novo synthesis of purines (32), pyrimidines (33), fatty acids, and sterols (5), the protozoan relies on salvage pathways to provide the necessary components of lipid and nucleotide metabolism. Amino acid synthesis and conversion is also thought to be limited. Carbohydrates are the preferred source of energy for metabolism. However, metabolic pathways for using amino acids, especially arginine, threonine, and leucine, as energy sources also exist (98), and energy generation using arginine probably takes place even if carbohydrates are available (62).

Energy metabolism takes place in the cytoplasm (for amino acids and carbohydrate glycolysis) and in an organelle called the hydrogenosome (for adenosine triphosphate (ATP) production via substrate-level phosphorylation). The hydrogenosome is analogous in structure and function to the mitochondrion in higher eukaryotes, although it lacks cristae and cytochromes (43, 61). In the hydrogenosome, pyruvate is decarboxylated by an enzyme called pyruvate:ferredoxin oxidoreductase (PFOR). Ferredoxin serves as a terminal electron acceptor for PFOR, eventually leading to the production of acetate (45). The fermentative metabolic processes of *T. vaginalis* also lead to the production of H_2, CO_2, lactate, and glycerol, the proportions of which vary depending on whether the organism grows in the presence or absence of oxygen (69).

A microaerophilic organism, *T. vaginalis* grows well under anaerobic conditions; however, some strains can tolerate oxygen well enough to be grown in ambient air. Optimum conditions are generally considered to be at 37°C in moist air with 5% CO_2 for growth in both axenic and tissue culture (this microaerophilic environment is similar to that found in the human vagina). Interestingly, *T. vaginalis* aerotolerance has often been found to reflect a particular strain's susceptibility to metronidazole, the drug most commonly used to treat trichomoniasis (86).

2 Epidemiology

2.1 Prevalence and Transmission

With 180 million people infected annually, trichomoniasis is the most common nonviral STD worldwide (28). It is ubiquitous, being found in all races and cultures, but is especially prevalent among the underprivileged. It is estimated that at least 5 million new cases emerge in the United States yearly, many in lower-income African Americans (42). Globally, *T. vaginalis* infection is most prevalent in Africa

G.E. Garber (✉)
Division of Infectious Diseases, Ottawa Hospital,
General Campus, Ottawa, ON, Canada
ggarber@ohri.ca

D.L. Mayers (ed.), *Antimicrobial Drug Resistance*,
DOI 10.1007/978-1-60327-595-8_74, © Humana Press, a part of Springer Science+Business Media, LLC 2009

and Asia, with infection rates reaching 40–60% in some populations (22).

Trichomoniasis has long been considered a disease of women, but the disease can also cause significant morbidity in men. Previous studies had shown that less than 5% of the cases of non-gonococcal urethritis are attributable to *T. vaginalis* (52). However, a recent decline in the rates of chlamydial infection in the United States has been accompanied by an apparent increase in the frequency of *T. vaginalis* infection. Up to 17% of male patients with non-gonococcal, non-chlamydial urethritis are now confirmed to be suffering from trichomoniasis (72). It is not yet clear, however, whether this trend represents a bona fide increase in the rate of trichomoniasis, or an improvement in diagnosis of the disease.

The prevalence of *T. vaginalis* infection in women has been found to vary significantly among different populations. Studies have shown that the rate of infection in women attending family planning clinics is about 5% (91). Reports from STD clinics indicate that anywhere from 1% to 40% of female patients are identified with trichomoniasis (64). The highest rates of infection are found in sex trade workers and women incarcerated in correctional facilities, where 50–75% of these groups are infected with *T. vaginalis* (91).

The rate of transmission of *T. vaginalis* differs between sexes. Studies have shown that 15–70% of men who have contact with an infected female partner will develop infection (106, 108). Women exposed to the parasite via an infected male partner have a 65–100% chance of developing trichomoniasis (36, 108). *T. vaginalis* has been found to be able to survive for short periods of time outside of a host if sufficient moisture is maintained. Viable specimens have been obtained from body fluids (urine, semen, and vaginal exudates) 3–6 h after being emitted from the body (27, 107). Live trichomonads have also been isolated from warm, damp washcloths 24 h after incubation (42), and from insufficiently chlorinated swimming pool water for up to 48 h (46). However, there have been no confirmed cases of trichomoniasis caused by exposure to contaminated objects.

2.2 Association with Human Immunodeficiency Virus and Other STDs

Patients with trichomoniasis are at an increased risk of contracting other STDs. This can be due to lifestyle risk factors (i.e., poverty or promiscuity), but may also be a reflection of the fact that *T. vaginalis* cytotoxicity towards urogenital tract epithelial cells (and the increase in vaginal pH commonly seen in infections of women) helps to create an advantageous niche for other sexually transmitted infectious organisms (76). It is also possible that a pre-existing STD could increase the likelihood of developing a trichomonal infection upon exposure to the parasite. One clinical study showed that over 9% of cases of trichomoniasis were accompanied by at least one other STD. *Chlamydia trachomatis* and human papillomavirus (HPV) were the organisms most commonly associated with *T. vaginalis* infection (30).

Similar to other STDs, *T. vaginalis* infection increases the risk of contracting the human immunodeficiency virus (HIV) two- to sixfold (8, 35, 56, 95). Reasons for increased risk include (1) damage to the mucosal surface facilitating viral penetration and (2) an increased number of immune cells at the genital mucosa enabling infection of these cells by HIV (35). Given that *T. vaginalis* and HIV are endemic in similar areas of the world, this means that prevention of trichomoniasis could be an important step in reducing global HIV/AIDS rates.

3 Clinical Aspects

3.1 Trichomoniasis in Men

Trichomoniasis in men is usually an asymptomatic carrier state. When symptomatic infection does occur, it presents as a mild urethritis. Clinical symptoms are similar to non-gonococcal urethritis and include small amounts of clear or purulent discharge, and discomfort or a burning sensation during urination or after sexual intercourse. Rare cases of acute male trichomoniasis are characterized by more severe manifestations of urethral symptoms (49).

The incubation period for *T. vaginalis* infection in men is usually less than 10 days, although longer incubation periods do occur (49). Spontaneous resolution of both inapparent and symptomatic infection is common. One study showed that 70% of untreated, symptomatic men had cleared the parasite within 2 weeks (106). However, it has also been found that some cases of persistent non-gonococcal urethritis, particularly those that have responded poorly to antibiotic therapy, may in fact be caused by resilient or resistant strains of *T. vaginalis*.

Prostatitis is the most common complication associated with trichomoniasis. Balanoposthitis, epidydimitis, and other inflammations of the external genitalia are also frequently seen. There is also evidence linking persistent *T. vaginalis* infection to urethral disease and infertility (48).

3.2 Trichomoniasis in Women

Unlike infection in men, trichomoniasis in women is usually persistent. Incubation periods range from 4 to 28 days (42). Establishment of symptomatic infection usually involves a rise in the normal vaginal pH of 4.0–4.5 to a pH of 5.0 or higher (some of the virulence factors of *T. vaginalis* have been found to be inhibited at normal vaginal pH) (84). This rise in pH is probably attributable to a concomitant decrease in acid-producing vaginal *Lactobacillus*, although the mechanism by which lactobacilli are inhibited or eliminated has not yet been elucidated. The symptoms of trichomoniasis are known to worsen during menses. This is likely a reflection of the fact that iron is an important mediator of many of the parasite's metabolic and pathogenic pathways (particularly cellular adherence) (59). Nearly all cases of urogenital trichomoniasis are found in women of reproductive age, but it is not known if this is due to the unsuitability of the vaginal environment in premenarche and postmenopausal women, or is simply a reflection of the parasite's niche as an STD.

Asymptomatic infection rates range from 10 to 50%, but about 30% of women with an inapparent infection will develop symptomatic trichomoniasis within 6 months (88). Symptomatic infection is rated as mild, acute, or chronic. Chronic infection generally shows a similar clinical presentation to the mild form of the disease, but lasts for an extended period (i.e., years) and/or shows antibiotic resistance. Mild *T. vaginalis* infection is characterized by pruritus, dyspareunia, and sometimes dysuria. Small amounts of mucopurulent vaginal secretion are often present. Acute trichomoniasis usually presents with vulval and vaginal erythema, and 2% of cases show characteristic small hemorrhagic spots on the vagina and cervix, known as strawberry cervix (31, 109). Use of a coloscope will increase the diagnosis of a strawberry cervix to about 90% of patients with acute symptoms (109). Copious discharge is often yellow or green in color, malodorous, and mixed with mucus (31, 109).

T. vaginalis infection has been implicated as a cause of cervical erosion and in the development of cervical cancer, although carcinogenicity likely can be related to high rates of coinfection with HPV (93). Other complications associated with trichomoniasis arise when the parasite invades tissues outside the vagina. Skene's and Bartholin's glands are often infected, and ascending infection has been associated with endometritis and infertility (30). *T. vaginalis* infection can be especially hazardous for pregnant women, predisposing them to premature rupture of the placental membrane, premature labor, and low-birth-weight babies (89, 109).

3.3 Diagnosis

Diagnosis of trichomoniasis is difficult to make on the basis of clinical presentation alone. The high frequency of asymptomatic infection contributes greatly to underdiagnosis of the disease. In addition, the symptoms of *T. vaginalis* infection are often similar to those found in bacterial urogenital infection. As previously mentioned, symptomatic trichomoniasis in men presents as non-gonococcal urethritis. Many symptoms associated with trichomonal infection in women are also common to bacterial vaginosis. For example, in STDs with bacterial etiology, vaginal pH is elevated in 90% of cases (90, 100) and a positive "whiff" test, the presence of a fishy odor when vaginal exudate is mixed with 10% potassium hydroxide, may be present (as in 50% of trichomoniasis cases) (12, 90). Finally, as coinfection with other STDs is not uncommon, it is important that specific tests for trichomoniasis be undertaken to prevent misdiagnosis and inappropriate treatment.

Diagnosis of *T. vaginalis* in women is usually performed after sampling vaginal exudates from the posterior fornix with a sterile cotton-tipped applicator. For men, a fresh semen sample is preferred, although urine is also frequently used. If a sufficient number of trichomonal cells are present (at least 10^4/mL), immediate diagnosis may be possible by microscopic examination of a wet mount. *T. vaginalis* cells are similar in size to leukocytes, but can be identified by their characteristic motility (26, 82). Unfortunately, the reliability of this test is highly variable, and its sensitivity has been quoted in the literature as anywhere from 40 to 90% (75). Additionally, if the test is not performed immediately, specimens are usually kept moist in physiological saline or transport medium, and although this does not (in the short term) affect the viability of trichomonads, it does have a profound negative effect on their motility (81).

The gold standard for diagnosis of trichomoniasis is cultivation of the organisms in axenic medium. Diamond's TYM (trypticase–yeast extract–maltose) supplemented with serum and antibiotics to prevent growth of bacteria and yeast has been found to yield consistently good results. Vaginal specimens can be inoculated into medium immediately or after storage in saline, and growth of motile trichomonads confirms a positive diagnosis. The sensitivity of this test is generally considered to be about 95% (51). Diagnosis of *T. vaginalis* via cultivation also has the advantage that cultivated trichomonads can be maintained for further testing (i.e., antibiotic susceptibility). The disadvantage of this technique is that trichomonads do not grow quickly, and a minimum of 3 days should be allowed before rendering a negative diagnosis (87).

A number of fixed staining techniques have also been employed in the diagnosis of trichomoniasis. These include Giemsa (73), acridine orange (34), and the Papanicolaou (Pap) smear (79) among others. Unfortunately *T. vaginalis* cells often lose their characteristic shape on fixation. Studies on the diagnostic utility of the Pap smear have shown its sensitivity to be about 95% (105). Unfortunately, there is a high frequency of false-positive results (probably due to the similarity in size and shape of *T. vaginalis* and leukocytes). Between 20 and 30% of uninfected women will be falsely diagnosed as having trichomoniasis (103).

A number of immunological methods have also been examined for their efficacy in diagnosing *T. vaginalis* infection. Several blood tests for parasite antibodies were evaluated (including agglutination (97), complement fixation (35, 41), indirect immunofluorescence (47) and enzyme-linked immunosorbent assay (ELISA) (96)), but results were generally disappointing. As with many serological tests, the assays were often not sensitive enough to detect low antibody levels present early in infection or during asymptomatic infection. Conversely, there is a high false-positive rate, likely reflecting that trichomonal antibody is often present (although diminishing in titer) for over a year after resolution of infection (37).

Promising diagnostic techniques have emerged more recently with the development of monoclonal antibodies to *T. vaginalis*. Assays utilizing monoclonal antibodies have been found to be extremely specific (often better than 99%), with a very low rate of false-positive results (51). In addition, these tests can be performed on small amounts of vaginal exudate and, if used in conjunction with culture techniques, can result in extremely sensitive and specific diagnosis of trichomoniasis. Monoclonal antibody-based techniques also have the advantage that the tests are not time sensitive like the wet mount (above). Direct fluorescence antibody staining (DFA) (51) and direct enzyme-linked immunoassay (EIA) (111) are microscopic techniques that have been found to be much more sensitive than the wet mount, although somewhat less sensitive than culture. The advantage of these techniques is that they can be performed rapidly (in less than a day) as opposed to waiting 3–7 days for culture diagnosis. The disadvantage is the potential expense involved. Although only a light microscope is needed for the EIA assay, the DFA technique requires a more costly fluorescence unit. In addition, the high degree of specificity of these tests is based on their use by a trained microscopist, and may suffer if performed by less experienced personnel. Finally, the latex agglutination test is another assay designed for the rapid diagnosis of trichomoniasis. This test can be performed without a microscope in about 5 min, and has been shown to be as sensitive as culturing (10).

Nucleic acid-based techniques such as in situ hybridization and polymerase chain reaction (PCR) have also shown very high specificity in diagnosing *T. vaginalis* infection. For in situ hybridization, for example, very few false-positive results were reported and no cross-reactivity with other vaginal flora was found. Unfortunately, at least 10^4 organisms per sample are required to ensure an accurate result, a condition not always met in asymptomatic cases of trichomoniasis (78). Assessment of PCR probing has shown it to be as accurate as culture in diagnosing *T. vaginalis* infection (92). Unfortunately, the expense involved in using PCR as a diagnostic tool may limit its usefulness.

Finally, it should be noted that isolation of trichomonads to confirm infection in males is often unsuccessful. It is hypothesized that this is because certain aspects of the male genitalia (e.g., an oxidative environment (2), zinc in prostatic fluid (50)) create an inhibitory milieu in which parasite numbers are greatly limited. In the absence of sensitive tests, it is important to assume that any male partner of an infected woman likely harbors the parasite himself. Concurrent treatment of the sexual partner(s) to prevent reinfection is essential.

3.4 Treatment

Metronidazole has been the drug of choice for the treatment of *T. vaginalis* infection since its development in 1959. Derived from the *Streptomyces* spp. antibiotic azomycin, metronidazole (α-hydroxyethyl-2-methyl-5-nitroimidazole) is a member of the nitroimidazole family of prodrugs whose metabolic products have been found to effectively eliminate infection by a number of protozoa and Gram-negative bacteria (16). Although other members of this family, including nimorazole, ornidazole, secnidazole, and tinidazole, are used throughout the world for the treatment of trichomoniasis, until recently metronidazole was the only nitroimidazole approved for use in North America.

Infants who contract *T. vaginalis* during vaginal delivery from an infected mother usually do not require treatment because infection generally resolves within a few weeks as the infant's (maternal) estrogen levels wane. However, if infection becomes symptomatic or progresses past the sixth week of life, metronidazole is generally administered. Treatment is often a single 50 mg/kg dose, or a 10–30 mg/kg dose daily for 5–8 days (65). Canadian guidelines recommend a dose of 15–20 mg/kg, divided into three doses daily for 7 days, or a single dose of 40 mg/kg (to a maximum of 2 g) for the treatment of trichomoniasis in children.

Oral metronidazole is the treatment of choice for trichomoniasis in adults. The recommended regimens are 250 mg three times a day for 7 days, 500 mg twice a day for 7 days, or a single 2-g dose. The single dose treatment is preferred, as compliance is better than with multiple doses, and the overall amount of drug taken is reduced. However, the incidence and severity of side effects does increase slightly with the larger dosage. Metronidazole can also be administered intravenously. This method is often utilized when patients show some intolerance to the drug, as side effects tend to be less severe than with oral treatment. Intravenous metronidazole is administered in a dosage of 500 mg to 2 g over 20 min (65).

A number of topical intravaginal preparations have been used to alleviate the symptoms of trichomoniasis in women. These medications include clotrimazole, nonoxynol-9, and povidone-iodine creams and gels, arsenical pessaries, and both cream and insert metronidazole preparations. There are no topical treatments for trichomoniasis in men.

The usefulness of non-nitroimidazole vaginal creams and inserts as a cure is doubtful, and no studies have shown definitive proof of efficacy. However, these treatments are effective for relief of symptoms. The exception is hamycin, a drug related to amphotericin B. Currently in use in India as a topical treatment for trichomoniasis, hamycin has been found to effectively eliminate infection with both metronidazole-sensitive and -resistant strains of *T. vaginalis*. However, both clinical trials and in vitro testing on tissue culture have shown that the level of toxicity displayed by the drug toward eukaryotic cells makes it a poor choice of treatment (68).

Vaginal administration of metronidazole has been shown to be relatively ineffective as a cure, eliminating infection in only about 20% of cases (3, 44). This is probably due to the fact that trichomonads are not always confined to the vagina, frequently invading Skene's, Bartholin's, and other glands, as well as the urethra (30). As such, a topical vaginal medication is inadequate in completely eliminating infection. However, in cases of recalcitrant *T. vaginalis* infection, vaginal preparations are often added to the treatment regimen to increase the chances of effecting a cure, and because of their comparatively lower risk of side effects (compared to oral administration) (3, 18).

Metronidazole regimens are generally well tolerated, and side effects are rarely of a severity that would necessitate discontinuation of metronidazole therapy. Common side effects include nausea and vomiting, headache, insomnia, dizziness, drowsiness, and rash. Patients taking oral metronidazole have also complained of dry mouth and metallic taste during the course of treatment. More serious side effects such as peripheral neuropathy, palpitation, confusion, eosinophilia, and leukopenia are rare, and seem to be associated with the nitroimidazole family. Cessation of therapy leads to mitigation of side effects, and no long-term adverse events have been identified in humans (64).

Cure rates for oral and intravenous metronidazole therapy of trichomoniasis range from 85 to 95% on the first course of treatment. This rate increases if sexual partner(s) are treated simultaneously to prevent reinfection (65). Partner treatment is highly recommended given the frequency of asymptomatic *T. vaginalis* infection.

4 Metronidazole Resistance

4.1 Mechanisms

Metronidazole enters *T. vaginalis* via passive diffusion and is activated in the hydrogenosome. Within this organelle, the drug competes with hydrogenase (the terminal enzyme of pyruvate decarboxylation) for ferredoxin-bound electrons.

The reduction of metronidazole results in the production of toxic metabolites via the formation of nitro radicals (24, 63). The target of these nitro radicals is hypothesized to be DNA, where transient binding of the active drug leads to disruption and breakage of chromosomal strands, and rapid cell death (within 5 h) (40). The DNA of *T. vaginalis* contains about 71% adenine and thymine residues, and these AT-rich regions are proposed to be both the site of metronidazole activity and the reason for the drug's specificity (23). It is also possible that metronidazole metabolites target and disrupt proteins and protein trafficking (53), but research to validate this is lacking.

Metronidazole resistance is classified as aerobic or anaerobic. Aerobic resistance is a result of impaired oxygen-scavenging mechanisms that lead to a decrease in the metabolism of metronidazole due to oxygen competition for ferredoxin-bound electrons. Increased oxygen concentration and reduction via ferredoxin leads to (1) a decrease in the amount of metronidazole being reduced and less production of active metabolites and (2) the oxidation of metronidazole metabolites back into prodrug by oxygen and oxygen radicals, or futile cycling (83). Decreased ferredoxin activity has also been implicated in aerobic resistance (99), although oxygen-scavenging deficiency alone may be responsible (58). Since metronidazole enters *T. vaginalis* through passive diffusion, reduced metabolism of the drug into its active form will result in less overall trafficking into the cell, and lower efficacy. Aerobic resistance is responsible for nearly all cases of resistant trichomoniasis.

Anaerobic resistance develops when hydrogenosomal proteins involved in the reduction of metronidazole are downregulated or absent. Studies have shown that the transcription of ferredoxin, PFOR, and hydrogenase is drastically reduced or completely eliminated in highly resistant strains (54, 57). Anaerobic resistant *T. vaginalis* strains often have modified hydrogenosomes that are significantly smaller than those found in metronidazole-sensitive trichomonads, presumably reflecting their decreased activity (57). Unlike aerobically resistant trichomonads, which use oxygen to detoxify metronidazole, anaerobically resistant *T. vaginalis* is extremely sensitive to oxygen and may survive only in an anaerobic environment. It is hypothesized that this is because PFOR and hydrogenase have roles in protecting the trichomonad from reactive oxygen radicals. In addition, *T. vaginalis* possesses hydrogenosomal oxidase- and peroxidase-reducing enzymes that help protect the parasite from cell damage due to toxic oxygen species (25). Reduction of hydrogenosomal function may lead to a downregulation in the activity of enzymes that protect *T. vaginalis* from oxygen stress. The extreme sensitivity of anaerobically resistant *T. vaginalis* to oxygen likely explains why such strains are rarely involved in disease, as the urogenital environments of men and women are aerobic and microaerophilic, respectively.

4.2 Diagnosis of Resistance

Infection with metronidazole-resistant *T. vaginalis* is generally suspected when two standard courses of treatment fail to cure, and noncompliance and reinfection can be ruled out. Current estimates are that 5–10% of cases of trichomoniasis will be caused by parasites with some degree of resistance to metronidazole (84). Low or moderately resistant trichomonads are the cause of most recalcitrant infections, although highly resistant organisms have also been isolated from clinical samples.

Metronidazole susceptibility tests for *T. vaginalis* are similar to drug susceptibility assays for other microorganisms. A number of samples of axenic medium containing a range of metronidazole concentrations are prepared. The trichomonal isolate is then inoculated into each drug-medium sample and incubated, for at least 48 h. Metronidazole susceptibility can then be assessed by calculating the minimum inhibitory concentration (MIC) and/or minimum lethal concentration (MLC) of drug for the organism. Inhibitory and lethal concentrations are obtained by observing the parasites for motility after the incubation period. The samples containing immobile trichomonads are then inoculated into fresh drug-free medium, incubated (again for at least 48 h), and re-examined for live cells. The MIC is the lowest metronidazole concentration at which nonmotile parasites survived (i.e., proliferated after the second inoculation). The MLC is the lowest concentration at which all trichomonads were killed (i.e., no growth on secondary inoculation).

In vitro metronidazole susceptibility testing is usually performed under aerobic conditions. This is partly because aerobic testing better reflects the environment in which *T. vaginalis* infection is found, and partly because anaerobic testing does not always accurately reflect clinical presentation (77). In addition, MIC and MLC values can be over 5 times higher in aerobic testing compared to anaerobic (22), thereby allowing better discrimination of the resistance results.

Currently, there is no standard in vitro assay for the determination of *T. vaginalis* susceptibility to metronidazole. Different researchers favor various techniques, under different conditions (aerobic vs. anaerobic), to calculate different results (MIC vs. MLC). A survey of the literature on aerobic susceptibility testing shows that a strain of *T. vaginalis* having an MIC lower than 10 μg/mL, or an MLC lower than 50 μg/mL is generally considered metronidazole susceptible. A trichomonad with an MLC of >400 μg/mL (MIC of >50 μg/mL) would represent a highly drug-resistant strain of the parasite. Unfortunately, there is no direct correlation between the results of in vitro susceptibility assays and recommended dosages for clinical metronidazole treatment (67). However, in vitro testing does reflect the general level of sus-

ceptibility of a clinical isolate to metronidazole, and can be useful in determining a continuing course of therapy if primary treatment fails (66). Susceptibility testing is not routinely available in most diagnostic laboratories.

4.3 Treatment

Infection caused by metronidazole-resistant *T. vaginalis* can often be cured with increased doses of the drug and an extended course of therapy. Not surprisingly, there is a greater rate of adverse events associated with an increased (often double) treatment dose. In an attempt to limit side effects, treatment of refractory infection often combines oral and vaginal metronidazole therapy, or involves intravenous administration of the drug (29). Some success has also been reported in a combination of standard metronidazole treatment and arsenical or clotrimazole pessaries, or zinc sulfate or betadine douches (13, 66, 102). Although evidence as to the efficacy of these therapies as cures is somewhat anecdotal, it is known that the treatments do ameliorate the symptoms of acute trichomoniasis.

Cases of highly drug-resistant *T. vaginalis* infection are difficult to resolve, as very high doses of metronidazole are toxic to the patient. With no alternatives to nitroimidazole drugs available, patients suffering from recalcitrant trichomoniasis are sometimes resigned to recurrent infection, relying on palliative measures to control symptoms. Fortunately such cases are infrequent. Overall, the cure rate for refractory trichomoniasis is 80% for the first course of extended/combined therapy, assuming patient compliance and no re-exposure (80).

5 Alternative Treatments

There are very few therapeutic alternatives for the treatment of *T. vaginalis* infection. The 5-nitroimidazole family of drugs represents the only therapies currently proven to safely and effectively treat trichomoniasis. Of the nitroimidazoles, metronidazole and tinidazole have superior trichomonicidal activity, with most studies showing tinidazole to have a cure rate equal to that of metronidazole, but being effective at a slightly lower dosage (1.5 g single dose) (71, 80). More recently, a nitroimidazole designated EU11100 was synthesized. This drug was shown to be both less toxic than metronidazole and effective at a lower concentration, but to date no clinical trials have been published (21).

An intravaginal preparation, paramomycin, has had some successful trials, including curing at least one patient with recalcitrant trichomoniasis. Unfortunately, as was the case with hamycin (mentioned previously), the side effects were severe, including pain and ulceration of the genital mucosa, making it unlikely that paramomycin is a viable treatment alternative (85).

Aromatic diamidines, which bind at AT-rich sites in the minor groove of DNA, are currently under investigation for anti-trichomonal activity. These synthetic dicationic drugs have a broad spectrum of activity against protozoan parasites. In vitro tests have shown some compounds to be effective against both metronidazole-sensitive and -resistant strains of *T. vaginalis*, implying a different mode of action from nitroimidazoles (17).

A number of compounds containing nitro groups similar to nitroimidazoles have been investigated for activity against *T. vaginalis*. Nitazoxanide is a 5-nitrothiazolyl proven to be active against a broad spectrum of parasites in vitro. The drug was shown to exhibit trichomonicidal activity against both metronidazole-sensitive and -resistant strains. In addition, the drug has been shown to have low toxicity (at least in vitro) (1). Analysis of the nitrothiazole derivative, niridazole, has shown it to possess multiple modes of action that contribute to broad-spectrum antimicrobial activity. Although specific mechanisms of action have not yet been elucidated, both metronidazole-sensitive and -resistant strains of *T. vaginalis* were found to be inhibited by the drug (110). Sulfimidazole possesses two functional groups: a sulfonamide and a 5-nitroimidazole. In vitro testing has shown the drug to be effective against both aerobic and anaerobic bacteria, and metronidazole-sensitive and -resistant *T. vaginalis*. It should be noted however, that MLCs for resistant trichomonads were approximately 5 times more than those for sensitive strains, potentially reflecting *T. vaginalis* resistance to the activity of the 5-nitroimidazole group (70).

Disulfiram, a drug used to treat alcoholism, and its metabolite ditiocarb have shown trichomonicidal activity against both metronidazole-sensitive and -resistant strains of *T. vaginalis*. This is interesting since metronidazole can induce reactions similar to those of disulfiram, specifically nausea and vomiting, if taken with alcohol (6).

Although preliminary in vitro research has been conducted on the trichomonicidal activity of a large number of drugs, testing rarely proceeds to clinical trials. With rates of metronidazole-resistant *T. vaginalis* infection on the rise, it is imperative that alternative therapies become available.

6 Infection Prevention

Infection control of sexually transmitted trichomoniasis is the same as for other STDs. Condoms are effective in preventing the spread of disease, and reduced transmission has been shown in women using either oral (hormonal) or prophylactic vaginal (i.e., nonoxynol-9) contraception (7).

As *T. vaginalis* parasites can be passed from mother to newborn during vaginal birth, pregnant women should be treated to prevent perinatal infection. Previously there have been concerns about metronidazole teratogenicity, based on studies showing mutagenicity in bacteria and carcinogenicity in mice (15, 60). This led to the reluctance to treat pregnant women, or to limiting treatment to the second or third trimester. Several meta-analyses have shown, however, that children born to mothers treated with metronidazole showed no increase in birth defects compared to controls (11, 19, 94). Additionally, there is a proven association between trichomoniasis and pregnancy complications such as preterm labor and low-birth-weight infants. As such, the current standard of care dictates metronidazole treatment for trichomoniasis as soon as possible (in the second trimester).

Currently, there is no vaccine available against *T. vaginalis* infection. However, the existence of a successful vaccination model in mice (74), as well as a vaccine already commercially available for prevention of related *Tritrichomonas foetus* infection in cattle (9, 55), gives hope that eventually the disease will be preventable. Given the relationship between trichomoniasis and other STDs, especially HIV, the development of a vaccine would be an excellent step in preventing morbidity and mortality due to this and other sexually transmitted infections.

References

1. Ackers, J. P. (1990) Immunologic aspects of human trichomoniasis, in *Trichomonads parasitic in humans* (Honigberg, B. M., ed.), Springer, New York, NY, pp. 36–52.
2. Alderete, J. F. and Provenzano, D. (1997) The vagina has reducing environment sufficient for activation of *Trichomonas vaginalis* cysteine proteinases. *Genitourin. Med.* **73**, 291–296.
3. Alper, M. M., Barwin, B. N., McLean, W. M., McGilveray, I. J., and Sved, S. (1985) Systemic absorption of metronidazole by the vaginal route. *Obstet. Gynecol.* **65**(6), 781–784.
4. Arroyo, R., Gonzalez-Robles, A., Martinez-Palomo, A., and Alderete, J. F. (1993) Signalling of *Trichomonas vaginalis* for amoeboid transformation and adhesion synthesis follows cytoadherence. *Mol. Microbiol.* **7**, 299–309.
5. Beach, D. H., Holz, G. G. Jr., Singh, B. N., and Lindmark, D. G. (1990) Fatty acid and sterol metabolism of *Trichomonas vaginalis* and *Tritrichomonas foetus. Mol. Biochem. Parasitol.* **38**, 175–190.
6. Bouma, M., Snowdon, J. D., Fairlamb, A. H., and Ackers, J. P. (1998) Activity of disulfiram ((bis)diethylthiocarbamoyl)disulphide) and didiocarb (diethyldithiocarbamate) against metronidazole sensitive and resistant *Trichomonas vaginalis* and *Tritrichomonas foetus. J. Antimicrob. Chemother.* **42**, 817–820.
7. Bramley, M. and Kinghorn, G. (1979) Do oral contraceptives inhibit *Trichomonas vaginalis? Sex. Transm. Dis.* **6**, 261–263.
8. Cameron, D. E. and Padian, N. S. (1990) Sexual transmission of HIV and the epidemiology of other sexually transmitted diseases. *AIDS* **4**(Suppl 1), S99–S103.

9. Campero, C. M., Hirst, R. G., Ladds, P. W., Vaughn, J. A., Emery, D. L., and Watson, D. L. (1990) Measurement of antibody in serum and genital fluids of bulls with ELISA after vaccination and challenge with *Tritrichomonas foetus*. *Aust. Vet. J.* **67**(5), 175–178.

10. Carney, J. A., Unadkat, P., Yule, A., et al. (1988) A rapid agglutination test for the diagnosis of *Trichomonas vaginalis* infection. *J. Clin. Pathol.* **41**, 806–808.

11. Caro-Paton, T., Carvajal, A., Diego, I. M., Martin-Arias, L. H., Requejo, A. A., and Pinilla, E. R. (1997) Is metronidazole teratogenic? A meta-analysis. *Br. J. Clin. Pharmacol.* **44**, 179–182.

12. Chen, K. C., Amsel, R., Eschenbach, D. A., and Holmes, K. K. (1982) Biochemical diagnosis of vaginitis: determination of diamines in vaginal fluid. *J. Infect. Dis.* **145**, 337–345.

13. Chen, M. Y., Smith, N. A., Fox, E. F., Bingham, J. S., and Barlow, D. (2001) Acetarsol pessaries in the treatment of metronidazole-resistant *Trichomonas vaginalis*. *Int. J. STD AIDS* **10**, 277–280.

14. Cleveland, L. R. (1928) *Tritrichomonas fecalis* nov. sp. of man; its ability to grow and multiply indefinitely in faeces diluted with tap water and in frogs and tadpoles. *Am. J. Hyg.* **8**, 232–255.

15. Conner, T. H., Stoeckel, M., Evrard, J., and Legator, M. S. (1977) The contribution of metronidazole and two metabolites to the mutagenic activity detected in the urine in treated humans and mice. *Cancer Res.* **37**, 629–633.

16. Cosar, C. and Julou, L. (1959) Activity of 1-(2-hydroxyethyl)-2-methyl-5-nitroimidazole (8823 RP) against experimental *Trichomonas vaginalis* infection. *Ann. Inst. Pasteur.* **96**, 238–241.

17. Crowell, A. L., Stephens, C. E., Kumar, A., Boykin, D. W., and Secor, W. E. (2004) Activities of dicationic compounds against *Trichomonas vaginalis*. *Antimicrob. Agents Chemother.* **48**(9), 3602–3605.

18. Cunningham, F. E., Kraus, D. M., Brubaker, L., and Fischer, J. H. (1994) Pharmacokinetics of intravaginal metronidazole gel. *J. Clin. Pharmacol.* **34**, 1060–1065.

19. Czeizel, A. E. and Rockenbauer, M. (1998) A population based case – control teratologic study of oral metronidazole treatment during pregnancy. *Br. J. Obstet. Gynecol.* **105**, 322–327.

20. Dobell, C. C. (1939) The common flagellate of the human mouth, *Trichomonas tenax* (O.F.M.): its discovery and its nomenclature. *Parasitology* **31**, 13–146.

21. Dubini, F., Riviera, L., Cocuzza, C., and Bellotti, M. G. (1992) Antibacterial, antimycotic, and trichomonicidal activity of a new nitroimidazole (EU 11100). *J. Chemother.* **4**(6), 342–346.

22. Dunne, R. L., Dunne, L. A., Upcroft, P., O'Donoghue, P. J., and Upcroft, J. A. (2003) Drug resistance in the sexually transmitted parasitic protozoan *Trichomonas vaginalis*. *Cell Res.* **13**(4), 239–249.

23. Edwards, D. I. (1980) Mechanisms of selective toxicity of metronidazole and other nitroimidazole drugs. *Br. J. Vener. Dis.* **56**, 285–290.

24. Edwards, D. I. (1993) Nitroimidazole drugs – action and resistance mechanisms. I. Mechanisms of action. *J. Antimicrob. Chemother.* **31**, 9–20.

25. Ellis, J. E., Yartlett, N., Cole, D., Humphreys, M. J., and Lloyd, D. (1994) Antioxidant defences in the microaerophilic protozoan *Trichomonas vaginalis*: comparison of metronidazole-resistant and sensitive strains. *Microbiology* **140**, 2489–2494.

26. Fouts, A. C. and Kraus, S. J. (1980) *Trichomonas vaginalis*: a re-evaluation of its clinical presentation and laboratory diagnosis. *J. Infect. Dis.* **141**, 137–143.

27. Gallai, Z. and Sylvestre, L. (1966) The present status of urogential trichomoniasis: a general review of the literature. *Appl. Ther.* **8**, 773–778.

28. Gerbase, A. C., Rowley, J. T., Heymann, D. H., Berkeley, S. B. F., and Piot, P. (1998) Global prevalence and incidence estimates of selected curable STDs. *Sex. Transm. Dis.* **74**(Suppl 1), S12–S16.

29. Grossman, J. H. and Galask, R. P. (1990) Persistent vaginitis caused by metronidazole resistant *Trichomonas*. *Obstet. Gynecol.* **76**, 521–522.

30. Gupta, P. K. and Frost, J. K. (1990) Cytopathology and histopathology of the female genital tract in *T. vaginalis* infection, in *Trichomonads parasitic in humans* (Honigberg, B. M., ed.), Springer, New York, NY, pp. 274–290.

31. Heine, P. and MacGregor, J. A. (1993) *Trichomonas vaginalis*: a re-emerging pathogen. *Clin. Obstet. Gynecol.* **36**, 137–144.

32. Heyworth, P. G., Gutteridge, W. E., and Ginger, C. D. (1982) Purine metabolism in *Trichomonas vaginalis*. *FEBS Lett.* **141**, 106–110.

33. Heyworth, P. G., Gutteridge, W. E., and Ginger, C. D. (1982) Pyrimadine metabolism in *Trichomonas vaginalis*. *FEBS Lett.* **176**, 55–60.

34. Hipp, S. S., Kirkwood, M. W., and Hassan, H. A. (1979) Screening for *Trichomonas vaginalis* infection by use of acridine orange fluorescent microscopy. *Sex. Transm. Dis.* **6**, 235–238.

35. Hoffmann, B., Kazanawska, W., Kilczewski, W., and Krach, J. (1963) Serologic diagnosis of *Trichomonas* infection. *Med. Dosw. Mikrobiol.* **15**, 91–99.

36. Honigberg, B. M. (1978) Trichomonads of importance in human medicine, in *Parasitic protozoa*, vol. 2 (Krieger, J. P., ed.), Academic, New York, NY, pp. 275.

37. Honigberg, B. M. (1987) Immunology of trichomonads, with emphasis on *Trichomonas vaginalis*: a review. *Acta Univ. Carol. Biol.* **30**, 321–336.

38. Honigberg, B. M. and King, V. M. (1964) Structure of *Trichomonas vaginalis* Donne. *J. Parasitol.* **50**, 34–364.

39. Honigberg, B. M. and Brugerolle, G. (1990) Structure, in *Trichomonads parasitic in humans* (Honigberg, B. M., ed.), Springer, New York, NY, pp 5–35.

40. Ings, R. M., McFadzean, J. A., and Ormerod, W. E. (1974) The mode of action of metronidazole in *Trichomonas vaginalis* and other micro-organisms. *Biochem. Pharmacol.* **23**, 1421–1429.

41. Jaakmees, H. P., Teras, J. K., Roigas, E. M., Nigeson, U. K., and Tompel, H. J. (1966) Complement fixing antibodies in the blood sera of men infested with *Trichomonas vaginalis*. *Wiad. Parazytol.* **12**, 378–384.

42. Jirovec, O. and Petru, M. (1968) *Trichomonas vaginalis* and trichomoniasis. *Adv. Parasitol.* **6**, 117–188.

43. Johnson, P. J., Lahti, C. J., and Bradley, P. J. (1993) Biogenesis of the hydrogenosome in the anaerobic protest *Trichomonas vaginalis*. *J. Parasitol.* **79**, 644–670.

44. Kane, P. O., McFadzean, J. A., and Squires, S. (1961) Absorption and excretion of metronidazole. Part II. Studies on primary failures. *Br. J. Vener. Dis.* **37**, 276–277.

45. Kerscher, L. and Oesterhelt, D. (1982) Pyruvate-ferredoxin oxidoreductase – new findings on an ancient enzyme. *Trends Biochem. Sci.* **7**, 371–374.

46. Kozlowska, D. and Wichrowska, B. (1976) The effect of chlorine and its compounds used for disinfection on *Trichomonas vaginalis*. *Wiad. Parazytol.* **22**, 433–435.

47. Kramar, J. and Kucera, K. (1966) Immunofluorescence demonstration of antibodies in urogenital trichomoniasis. *J. Hyg. Epidemiol. Microbiol. Immunol.* **10**, 85–88.

48. Krieger, J. N. (1984) Prostatitis syndromes: pathophysiology, differential diagnosis, and treatment. *Sex. Transm. Dis.* **11**, 100–112.

49. Krieger, J. N. (1990) Epidemiology and clinical manifestations of urogenital trichomoniasis in men, in *Trichomonads parasitic in humans* (Honigberg, B. M., ed.), Springer, New York, NY, pp 235–245.

50. Krieger, J. N. and Rein, M. F. (1982) Zinc sensitivities of *Trichomonas vaginalis*: in vitro studies and clinical implications. *J. Infect. Dis.* **146**, 341–345.

51. Krieger, J. N., Tam, M. R., Stevenes, C. E., Nielsen, I. O., Hale, J., Kiviat, N. B., and Holmes, K. K. (1988) Diagnosis of trichomoniasis: comparison of conventional wet-mount examination with cytologic studies, cultures, and monoclonal antibody staining of direct specimens. *JAMA* **259**, 1223–1227.

52. Krieger, J. N., Jenny, C., Verdon, M., et al. (1993) Clinical manifestations of trichomoniasis in men. *Ann. Intern. Med.* **188**, 844–849.

53. Kulda, J. (1999) Trichomonads, hydrogenosomes, and drug resistance. *Int. J. Parasitol.* **29**, 199–212.

54. Kulda, J., Tachezy, J., and Czerasovova, A. (1993) *In vitro* induces anaerobic resistance to metronidazole in *Trichomonas vaginalis. J. Eukaryot. Microbiol.* **40**, 262–269.

55. Kvasnicka, W. G., Hanks, D., Huang, J. C., Hall, M. R., Sandblom, D., Chu, H. J., Chavez, L., and Acree, W. M. (1992) Clinical evaluation of the efficacy of inoculating cattle with a vaccine containing *Tritrichomonas foetus. Am. J. Vet. Res.* **53**(11), 2023–2027.

56. Laga, M., Manoka, A. T., Kivuvu, M., Malele, B., Tuliza, M., Nzila, N., Goeman, J. B., Batter, F. V., Alary, M., et al. (1993) Non-ulcerative sexually transmitted diseases as risk factors to HIV-1 transmission in women: results from a cohort study. *AIDS* **7**, 95–102.

57. Land, K. M., Clemens, D. L., and Johnson, P. J. (2001) Loss of multiple hydrogenosomal proteins associated with organelle metabolism and high-level drug resistance in trichomonads. *Exp. Parasitol.* **97**, 102–110.

58. Land, K. M., Delgadillo-Correa, M. J., Tachezy, J., Nanacova, S., Hseih, C. L., Sutak, R., and Johnson, P. J. (2004) Targeted gene replacement of a ferredoxin gene in *Trichomonas vaginalis* does not lead to metronidazole resistance. *Mol. Microbiol.* **51**(1), 115–120.

59. Lehker, M. W., Arroyo, R., and Aldrete, J. F. (1991) The regulation by iron of the synthesis of adhesins and cytoadherence levels in the protozoan parasite *Trichomonas vaginalis. J. Exp. Med.* **171**, 2165–2170.

60. Lindmark, D. G. and Muller, M. (1976) Antitrichomonad action, mutagenicity, and reduction of metronidazole and other nitroimidazoles. *Antimicrob. Agents Chemother.* **10**, 476–482.

61. Lindmark, D. G., Muller, M., and Shio, H. (1975) Hydrogenosomes in *Trichomonas vaginalis. J. Parasitol.* **61**, 522–554.

62. Linstead, D. and Cranshaw, M. A. (1983) The pathway of arginine catabolism in the parasitic flagellate *Trichomonas vaginalis. Mol. Biochem. Parasitol.* **8**, 241–252.

63. Lloyd, D. and Kristensen, B. (1985) Metronidazole inhibition of hydrogen production in vivo in drug- sensitive and -resistant strains of *Trichomonas vaginalis. J. Gen. Microbiol.* **131**, 849–853.

64. Lossick, J. G. (1990) Epidemiology of urogenital trichomoniasis Therapy of urogenital trichomoniasis, in *Trichomonads parasitic in humans* (Honigberg, B. M., ed.), Springer, New York, NY, pp. 324–341.

65. Lossick, J. G. (1990) Treatment of sexually transmitted diseases. *Rev. Infect. Dis.* **12**(Suppl 6), S665–S681.

66. Lossick, J. G. and Kent, H. L. (1991) Trichomoniasis: trends in diagnosis and management. *Am. J. Obstet. Gynecol.* **165**(4), 1217–1222.

67. Lossick, J. G., Muller, M., and Gorrell, T. E. (1986) *In vitro* drug susceptibility and doses of metronidazole required for cure in cases of refractory vaginal trichomoniasis. *J. Infect. Dis.* **153**, 948–955.

68. Lushbaugh, W. B., Cleary, J. D., and Finley, R. W. (1995) Cytotoxicity of hamycin for *Trichomonas vaginalis*, HeLa and BHK-21. *J. Antimicrob. Chemother.* **36**, 795–802.

69. Mack, S. R. and Muller, M. (1980) End products of carbohydrate metabolism in *Trichomonas vaginalis. Comp. Biochem. Physiol.* **67**, 213–216.

70. Malagoli, M., Ross, T., Baggio, A., Zandomeneghi, G., Zanca, A., Casolari, C., and Castelli, M. (2002) *In vitro* study of chemotherapeutic activity of sulphimidazole on some sensitive and metronida-

zole resistant *Trichomonas vaginalis* strains. *Pharmacol. Res.* **46**, 469–472.

71. Malla, N., Gupta, I., Sokhey, C., Sehgal, R., Ganguly, N. K., and Mahajan, R. J. (1988) *In vitro* evaluation of metronidazole and tinidazole on strains of *Trichomonas vaginalis. Indian J. Med. Microbiol.* **6**, 297–301.

72. Martin, D. H. and Bowie, W. R. (1999) Urethritis in males, in *Sexually transmitted disease*, 3rd ed. (Holmes, K. K., Mardh, P. A., Sparling, P. F., and Weisner, P. J., eds.) McGraw-Hill, New York, NY, pp. 833–845.

73. Mason, P. R., Super, H., and Fripp, P. J. (1976) Comparison of four techniques for the routine diagnosis of *Trichomonas vaginalis* infection. *J. Clin. Pathol.* **29**, 154–157.

74. McGrory, T. and Garber, G. E. (1992) Mouse intravaginal infection with *Trichomonas vaginalis* and role of *Lactobacillus acidophilus* in sustaining infection. *Infect. Immun.* **60**(6), 2375–2379.

75. McMillan, A. (1990) Laboratory diagnostic methods and cryopreservation of trichomonads, in *Trichomonads parasitic in humans* (Honigberg, B. M., ed.), Springer, New York, NY, pp 297–310.

76. Meysick, K. and Garber, G. E. (1995) *Trichomonas vaginalis. Curr. Opin. Infect. Dis.* **8**, 22–25.

77. Muller, M. (1986) Reductive activation of nitroimidazoles in anaerobic microorganisms. *Biochem. Pharmacol.* **35**, 37–41.

78. Muresu, R., Rubino, S., Rizzu, P., Baldini, A., Colombo, M., and Capuccinelli, P. (1994) A new method for identification of *Trichomonas vaginalis* by fluorescent DNA in-situ hybridization. *J. Clin. Microbiol.* **32**, 1018–1022.

79. Nagesha, C. W., Ananthakrishna, N. C., and Sulochana, P. (1970) Clinical and laboratory studies on vaginal trichomoniasis. *Am. J. Obstet. Gynecol.* **106**, 933–935.

80. Narcisi, E. M. and Secor, W. E. (1996) In vitro effect of tinidazole and furazolidone on metronidazole-resistant *Trichomonas vaginalis. Antimicrob. Agents Chemother.* **40**(5), 1121–1125.

81. Nielson, R. (1969) *Trichomonas vaginalis* I: survival in solid Stuart's medium. *Br. J. Vener. Dis.* **45**, 328–331.

82. O'Connor, B. H. and Adler, M. W. (1979) Current approaches to the diagnosis and reporting of trichomoniasis and candidosis. *Br. J. Vener. Dis.* **55**, 52–57.

83. Perez-Reyes, E., Kalyanaraman, B., and Mason, R. P. (1980) The reductive metabolism of metronidazole and ronidazole by aerobic liver microsomes. *Mol. Pharmacol.* **17**, 239–244.

84. Petrin, D., Delgaty, K., Bhatt, R., and Garber, G. E. (1998) Clinical and microbiological aspects of *Trichomonas vaginalis. Clin. Micrbiol. Rev.* **11**(2), 300–317.

85. Poppe, W. A. J. (2001) Nitroimidazole resistant vaginal trichomoniasis treated with paramomycin. *Eur. J. Obstet. Gynecol. Reprod. Biol.* **96**, 119–120.

86. Rasoloson, D., Tomkova, E., Cammack, R., Kulda, J., and Tachezy, J. (2001) Metronidazole resistant strains of *Trichomonas vaginalis* display increased sensitivity to oxygen. *Parasitology* **123**(1), 45–56.

87. Rayner, C. F. A. (1968) Comparison of culture media for the growth of *Trichomonas vaginalis. Br. J. Vener. Dis.* **44**, 63–66.

88. Rein, M. F. (1977) Trichomoniasis in VD clinic women. Paper presented at the Annual Meeting of the American Public Health Association, Washington DC, November 1.

89. Rein, M. F. and Chapel, T. A. (1975) Trichomoniasis, candidiasis, and the minor venereal diseases. *Clin. Obstet. Gynecol.* **18**, 73–88.

90. Rein, M. F. and Holmes, K. K. (1983) "Nonspecific vaginitis" vulvovaginal candidiasis and trichomoniasis: clinical features, diagnosis, and management, in *Current clinical topics in infectious diseases*, vol. 4 (Remington, J. S. and Swartz, M. N., eds.) McGraw-Hill, New York, NY, pp. 281–315.

91. Rein, M. F. and Muller, M. (1999) *Trichomonas vaginalis* and trichomiasis, in *Sexually transmitted disease*, 3rd ed. (Holmes, K. K., Mardh, P. A., Sparling, P. F., and Weisner, P. J., eds.) McGraw-Hill, New York, NY, pp. 481–492.

92. Riley, D. E., Roberts, M. C., Takayama, T., and Krieger, J. N. (1992) Development of a polymerase chain reaction-based diagnosis of *Trichomonas vaginalis*. *J. Clin. Microbiol.* **30**, 465–472.

93. Rodgerson, E. B. (1972) Vulvovaginal papillomas and *Trichomonas vaginalis*. *Obstet. Gynecol.* **40**, 327–333.

94. Rosa, F. W., Baum, C., and Shaw, M. (1987) Pregnancy outcomes after first-trimester vaginitis drug therapy. *Obstet. Gynecol.* **69**(5), 751–755.

95. Sorvillo, F. and Kerndt, P. (1998) *Trichomonas vaginalis* and amplification of HIV-1 transmission. *Lancet* **351**, 213–214.

96. Street, D. A., Taylor-Robinson, D., Ackers, J. P., Hanna, N. F., and McMillan, A. (1982) Evaluation of an enzyme-linked immunosorbent assay for the detection of antibody to *Trichomonas vaginalis* in sera and vaginal secretions. *Br. J. Vener. Dis.* **58**, 330–333.

97. Teras, J. K., Jaakmees, H. P., Nigeson, U. K., Roigas, E. M., and Tompel, H. J. (1966) Dependence of serologic reactions on the serotypes of *Trichomonas vaginalis*. *Wiad. Parazytol.* **12**, 364–369.

98. Tsukahara, T. (1961) Respiratory metabolism of *Trichomonas vaginalis*. *Jpn. J. Microbiol.* **5**, 157–169.

99. Vidakovic, M., Crossnoe, C. R., Neidre, C., Kim, K., Krause, K. L., and Germanas, J. P. (2003) Reactivity of reduced [2Fe-2S] ferredoxins parallel host susceptibility to nitroimidazoles. *Antimicrob. Agents Chemother.* **47**(1), 302–308.

100. Vontver, L. A. and Eschenbach, D. A. (1981) The role of *Gardnerella vaginalis* in nonpesific vaginitis. *Clin. Obstet. Gynecol.* **24**, 439–460.

101. Warton, A. and Honigberg, B. M. (1979) Structure of trichomonads as revealed by scanning electron microscopy. *J. Protozool.* **26**, 5–62.

102. Watson, P. G. and Pattman, R. S. (1996) Arsenical pessaries in the successful elimination of metronidazole-resistant *Trichomonas vaginalis*. *Int. J. STD AIDS* **10**, 277–280.

103. Weinberger, M. W. and Harger, J. H. (1993) Accuracy of the Papanicolaou smear in the diagnosis of asymptomatic infection with *Trichomonas vaginalis*. *Obstet. Gynecol.* **82**, 425–429.

104. Wenrich, D. H. and Saxe, L. H. (1950) *Trichomonas microti*, n. sp. (Protozoa, Mastigophora). *J. Parasitol.* **36**, 261–269.

105. Werness, B. A. (1989) Cytopathology of sexually transmitted diseases. *Clin. Lab. Med.* **9**, 559.

106. Weston, T. E. and Nicol, C. S. (1963) Natural history of trichomonal infection in males. *Br. J. Vener. Dis.* **39**, 251–257.

107. Whittington, M. J. (1951) The survival of *Trichononas vaginalis* at temperatures below 37°C. *J. Hyg.* **49**, 400–409.

108. Whittington, M. J. (1957) Epidemiology of *Trichomonas vaginalis* infections in the light of improved diagnostic methods. *Br. J. Vener. Dis.* **33**, 80–91.

109. Wolner-Hanssen, P., Krieger, J. N., Stevens, C. E., Kiviat, N. B., Koutsky, L., Critchlow, T., DeRouen, T., Hillier, S., and Holmes, K. K. (1989) Clinical manifestations of vaginal trichomoniasis. *JAMA* **261**(4), 571–576.

110. Yarlett, N., Rowlands, C. C., Yarlett, N. C., Evans, J. C., and Lloyd, D. (1987) Reduction of niridazole by metronidazole resistant and susceptible strains of *Trichomonas vaginalis*. *Parasitology* **94**, 93–99.

111. Yule, A., Gellan, M. C. A., Driel, J. D., et al. (1987) Detection of *Trichomonas vaginalis* antigen in women by enzyme immunoassay. *J. Clin. Pathol.* **40**, 566–568.

Chapter 75
Drug Resistance in *Leishmania*: Clinical Perspectives

Shyam Sundar and Madhukar Rai

1 Overview

Leishmaniasis comprises a group of diverse clinico-pathological entities, caused by the obligate intracellular parasite of the genus *Leishmania*. It occurs in 88 countries in the tropical and temperate regions, 72 of them developing or least developed. Two million cases occur annually, 1–1.5 million of cutaneous leishmaniasis (CL) and its variations, and 500,000 of visceral leishmaniasis (VL). About 350 million people are at risk, with an overall prevalence of 12 million (1). There is gross underreporting of the cases from the endemic region, and there has been a progressive increase in the cases of leishmaniasis and it is being reported from newer areas. Although the distribution of *Leishmania* is limited by the distribution of sandfly vectors, human leishmaniasis is on the increase worldwide. This has been attributed to massive rural–urban migration, widespread deforestation, and agro-industrial projects that are bringing nonimmune dwellers to rural endemic areas. Manmade projects such as dams and irrigation systems have also contributed to the spread of the disease (2).

2 Epidemiology

Ninety per cent of the annual global burden of VL cases occurs in India, Nepal, Bangladesh, and Brazil (1, 3). In these countries, VL is endemic and epidemics are quiet frequent, which lead to considerable mortality, and is a public health problem. Population migration leads to an epidemic scale of the disease in nonimmune areas. An epidemic of VL in Western Upper Nile, southern Sudan, led to about 100,000 deaths among the 280,000 population in this area, and is an example of the devastating nature of the disease if it is transmitted in a nonimmune population (4). In India, about 100,000 cases of VL are estimated to occur annually. Out of these, the state of Bihar accounts for more than 90% of cases (3). Similarly, 90% of all cases of CL occur in Afghanistan, Brazil, Peru, Saudi Arabia, and Syria, while 90% of all cases of mucocutaneous leishmaniasis (MCL) occur in Bolivia, Brazil, and Peru (5).

The emerging HIV/VL coinfection is locked in a vicious circle of mutual reinforcement. The risk of VL among AIDS patients increases by 100–1,000 times in endemic areas, while VL accelerates the onset of AIDS in HIV-infected people. HIV/VL coinfection is being increasingly reported from various parts of the world. At present, although it is being reported from more than 35 countries, most of these cases are from southwestern Europe (6, 7). However, the spread of HIV pandemic to suburban and rural areas of the world, especially in endemic areas of VL, is threatening to make the situation grim. Furthermore, it will urbanize the VL infection, which is essentially a disease of the rural population. Leishmaniasis is caused by at least 20 species of *Leishmania* and is transmitted by about 30 species of the sand fly (1, 8). The varied reservoir hosts, including domestic and/or wild animals, rodents, and human, as well as diverse clinical manifestations are indicative of great epidemiological diversity of the disease. Basically, leishmaniasis represents two ecoepidemiological forms: (1) anthroponotic and (2) zoonotic.

Most forms of leishmaniasis are zoonotic, human beings affected only secondarily, but two species of *Leishmania* can maintain arthroponotic, human–human cycle (9). These species are *L. donovani*, the species responsible for VL in the Indian subcontinent and East Africa, and *L. tropica*, which is responsible for CL in the Old World. However, female sand flies of genus *Phlebotomus* in the Old World and *Lutzomyia* in the New World are the only proven vectors responsible for transmission of disease (10). Consequently, geographical distribution of *Leishmania* is mainly determined by that of sand fly vectors (11–13). The sand fly lives in dark and damp places, and thrives on organic wastes. Poor waste disposal and sanitation are an important factor

S. Sundar (✉)
Professor, Department of Medicine, Institute of Medical Sciences,
Banaras Hindu University, Varanasi, India
shyam_vns@satyam.net.in, shyams@sancharnet.in

D.L. Mayers (ed.), *Antimicrobial Drug Resistance*,
DOI 10.1007/978-1-60327-595-8_75, © Humana Press, a part of Springer Science+Business Media, LLC 2009

for the breeding of sand flies. Because of their small size (2–3 mm), they can penetrate mosquito nets, which need to be impregnated with insecticide to prevent their bite. Another peculiarity of the vector is that they are more active during evenings and nights. Understanding of the vector biology in different areas is vital for vector control and control of leishmaniasis (14).

The epidemiology of leishmaniasis is changing owing to the widespread migration of population and ecological changes induced by developmental activities. Another important factor responsible for the changing profile of leishmaniasis is emerging HIV/VL coinfection. In southwestern Europe, it has created an artificial anthroponotic cycle of transmission, owing to transmission of amastigotes by infected syringes (15). There has been a considerable change in the epidemiological profile of leishmaniasis in these countries. Until 1985, when the first case of Mediterranean HIV/VL coinfection was reported (16), 90% of patients consisted of children under the age of 15 years, whereas now adults constitute >75%, and out of these 50–60% are cases of HIV/VL coinfection. In this region, *L. infantum* has emerged as the third most common opportunistic infection in HIV-infected patients. Moreover, the spreading pandemic of HIV has the potential to change the epidemiology of the disease elsewhere also (6). The overlap in rural and periurban transmission of leishmania with urban and periurban transmission of HIV infection, especially in endemic areas of India and Brazil, can make the situation explosive, with rural transmission of HIV and urbanization of VL.

The sand fly inoculates the promastigote form of the parasite into the skin of the host. In the human host, these are taken up by macrophages or the dendritic cells, where they transform into aflagellar amastigotes. The future course of infection and the type of disease produced depend upon the species of *Leishmania* and the immune response mounted by the host. The clinical syndrome can manifest in any of three different forms: (1) visceral leishmaniasis, (2) cutaneous leishmaniasis, and (3) mucocutaneous leishmaniasis.

Visceral leishmaniasis, also known as "Kala-azar", is the systemic and most severe form, characterized by prolonged and irregular fever often associated with rigor and chills, splenomegaly, lymphadenopathy, hepatomegaly, pancytopenia, progressive anemia, and weight loss. If untreated, VL is uniformly fatal. It is typically caused by the *L. donovani* complex, which includes three species: *L. donovani* (Indian subcontinent and East Africa), *L. infantum* (Mediterranean basin) and *L. chagasi* (Latin America). Leishmaniasis is also emerging as an important opportunistic infection in AIDS patients, and in HIV/VL coinfection the clinical manifestations are atypical and diverse. These, coupled with poor sensitivity of immunological tests in these patients, pose considerable diagnostic difficulties. Patients with VL may develop a chronic form of dermal leishmaniasis characterized by indurated nodules or depigmented macules, and is called post Kala-azar dermal leishmaniasis (PKDL) (17). PKDL is quite common (occurring in >50% patients with VL) in Sudan, and may occur concurrently with VL (17, 18). In the Indian subcontinent it occurs only in a small proportion of patients, 6 months to several years after an episode of VL (19). Spontaneous healing occurs in most patients in Sudan; however, in India treatment is considered necessary. Treatment of PKDL is difficult and requires prolonged courses of antileishmanial drugs irrespective of the geographical location. Patients with PKDL serve as an important reservoir of infection, and VL outbreaks have been linked to PKDL (20).

Cutaneous leishmaniasis is a major health problem in some countries (21–25). In the Old World, it is caused by *Leishmania major*, and manifests as a papule, which enlarges and ulcerates producing painless ulcer with raised and indurated margin. Most patients have 1–2 lesions, which heal spontaneously, but occasionally lesions may be multiple and disabling with disfiguring scars, which create lifelong aesthetic as well as social stigma. *L. tropica* may cause persistent, spreading scarring lesions associated with exaggerated cellular hypersensitivity (leishmaniasis recidivans or lupoid leishmaniasis), and is a difficult problem to treat (26).

In the New World, CL is produced by *L. mexicana*, and the lesions are benign and self-healing, but the sores on sites such as legs and pinna tend to heal slowly, while those on the face may be cosmetically disfiguring (27). Diffuse cutaneous leishmaniasis (DCL), a rare syndrome produced by *L. aetheopica* and *L. amazonensis*, develops because of defective antigen-specific cell-mediated response (28, 29). The lesions are chronic, disseminated, and nonulcerative. They never heal spontaneously, and relapses following treatments are quite frequent. MCL (espundia) produces extensive destructive lesion of nasopharyngeal mucosa. The disfiguring lesions lead to mutilation of the face. It is commonly caused by *Leishmania* species of the New World, such as *L. braziliensis*, *L. panamensis*, and *L. guyanensis*, but mucosal lesions have also been reported in the Old World due to *L. donovani*, *L. major*, and *L. infantum* in immunosuppressed patients (30, 31).

Usually, each species is true to type; but occasionally a dermatotropic species (e.g., *L. tropica*) may cause visceral disease, or the viscerotropic *L. infantum* may cause self-healing skin lesions (32). Viscerotropic and dermatotropic strains of *L. infantum* can be distinguished by isoenzyme analysis. But this distinction breaks down in the face of HIV coinfection, in which many hitherto unknown zymodemes have been identified.

L. braziliensis has, almost uniquely, the capacity to produce secondary mucosal lesions of the nose and mouth. But the joker in the pack is *L. donovani*, which causes chronic post-Kala-azar dermal leishmaniasis (PKDL) in patients recovered from VL, a bizarre condition suggesting either a change in parasite tropism or compartmental immunity.

3 Treatment of Leishmaniasis and Drug Resistance

The treatment options for leishmaniasis are limited and far from satisfactory. For more than 60 years, treatment of leishmaniasis has centered on pentavalent antimonials (Sb^v) in every endemic region of the world. It needs to be given parentrally and is potentially toxic. There has been emergence of Sb^v resistance in the hyperendemic areas of North Bihar in India, where up to 60% patients fail to respond to Sb^v treatment (33, 34). Failure of the drug is attributed to its widespread misuse in this anthroponotic focus with intense transmission (35). Similar potential of resistance exists in East Africa, especially in Sudan, another anthroponotic focus of VL with intense transmission, where poverty, illiteracy, and poor healthcare facilities portend the misuse of drug and consequent emergence of resistance (35). Resistance seems to be a feature of intensive transmission of anthroponotic *L. donovani*, as the epidemic turns endemic in foci where Sb^v has been used as the solo drug for long periods, often with poor supervision and compliance (36). In other parts of the world, Sb^v continues to be effective (37, 38). The HIV/VL coinfected patients are another potential source for the emergence of drug resistance (6, 39). These patients have a high parasite burden and weak immune response. They respond slowly to treatment and have high relapse rates (39, 40). Secondary resistance is quite common in relapsing patients. Furthermore, the reports of transmission of the infection via needle-sharing in HIV/VL coinfected patients in southern Europe threatens to convert an apparently zoonotic disease into the anthroponotic form (6, 41, 42).

After widespread Sb^v failure in Bihar, pentamidine isethionate was used as a second-line drug for these refractory patients; nearly 100% cure rate was achieved, and in spite of being toxic it was used for nearly two decades (43). Its most dreaded toxic effect was insulin-dependent diabetes mellitus in a significant proportion of patients (44). In later studies, a decline in the efficacy from 100 to ~70% was noticed. In the face of increasing unresponsiveness, and the associated serious toxicity, pentamidine fell into disrepute and its use is almost abandoned (45, 46).

For the antimony-refractory patients, amphotericin B was reintroduced in the early 1990s in India. Amphotericin B induces very high cure rates, and resistance is not seen with this drug (47, 48). With lipid formulations of amphotericin B, toxic effects of conventional amphotericin B is eliminated to varying extents depending on the type of formulation used (49), and 1–5 days' treatment is possible in India, as the total dose of the drug can be administered over a short duration, though even with low doses high cure rates are seen in the Indian disease (50–52); however, elsewhere a higher dose administered over a longer period is recommended (53–55). Miltefosine is a newly developed, highly effective oral drug for treatment of leishmaniasis (56). However, it has a long half-life of nearly a week, and therefore there is a built-in potential for development of resistance to it, and in HIV/VL coinfected patients cure rates with miltefosine seem to be no better than with other drugs: in 39 HIV patients with leishmaniasis failing on standard treatment, response was achieved in 25 patients (65%), including 16 patients (43%) with parasitological cure. Repeated responses after relapses and tolerability of long treatment indicate its potential for development of optimized dosage schemes (H. Sindermann, personal communication). However, its solo use in coinfected patients could encourage the appearance of resistance.

3.1 History of Geographical Spread of Resistance

In most parts of the world, about 98–99% previously untreated patients with VL respond well to Sb^v, the recommended first-line treatment. However, the endemic region for VL in North Bihar, India, has the unique distinction of being the only region in the world from where widespread primary failure to Sb^v has been reported (33, 57). Like elsewhere in the world, in India too Sb^v has been the drug to treat VL for several decades. Till the late 1970s, a small daily dose (10 mg/kg; 600 mg maximum) for short duration (6–10 days) was considered adequate, when unconfirmed reports suggested 30% treatment failure with this regimen from four districts most severely effected: Muzaffarpur, Samastipur, Vaishali, and Sitamarhi (58). An expert committee revised the recommendations to use Sb^v in two 10-day courses with an interval of 10 days (59), and improvements in cure rates (99%) were noted (60). However, only a few years later, another study noted 86% cure rates with this regimen (61). In 1984, a WHO expert committee recommended that pentavalent antimony be used in doses of 20 mg/kg/day up to a maximum of 850 mg for 20 days, and the repetition of a similar regimen for 20 days in cases of treatment failures (62). Four years later, Thakur et al. evaluated the WHO recommendations and reported that 20 days' treatment with 20 mg/kg/day (maximum 850 mg) cured only 81% of patients; however, on extending the treatment for 40 days, 97% of patients could be cured (63). Three years later, the same group noted a further decline in cure rate to 71% after 20 days' treatment, and recommended an extended duration of treatment in nonresponders (64). Jha et al. (65) found that extending the therapy for 30 days could cure only 64% patients in a hyperendemic district of Bihar. From these findings it became clear that antimony refractoriness was on ascendancy, but the reports were sketchy and not under strictly controlled conditions. In two studies carried out under strictly supervised treatment schedules, we observed that only about one-third of the patients could be cured with the currently prevailing regimen (33, 34). The incidence of primary unresponsiveness was 52%, whereas 8% of the patients relapsed. Incidentally, only 2% of the patients from the neighboring state of (Eastern) Uttar Pradesh (UP) failed in the treatment (33). Thus, it was reconfirmed that a high level of Sb^v unresponsiveness exists in Bihar, though the drug continues to be effective in other areas. There are reports of antimony resistance spreading to the Terai regions of Nepal, especially from the district adjoining the hyperendemic areas of Bihar, where up to 30% of the patients seems to be unresponsive, though in Eastern Nepal a 90% cure rate has been reported (66). Owing to the anthroponotic nature of transmission in the Indian subcontinent, antileishmanial drugs are likely to meet a similar fate as that of antimony and there is an urgent need to find ways to protect these drugs before we lose them.

HIV/VL coinfected patients respond poorly to Sb^v, as the drug needs an intact immune system to be effective, and the response is not as good as in immunocompetent patients. Initial parasitological cure with Sb^v could be as low as 37% (67), and eventually most of the initially cured patients tend to relapse. These relapsing patients may provide a human reservoir for resistant *Leishmania* with consequent emergence of primary resistance.

The response is not as predictable in patients with CL, because there is considerable variation in sensitivity to Sb^v among primary isolates from untreated patients with cutaneous leishmaniasis, which correlates with patients' response to treatment (68). Primary resistance is quite uncommon, but resistance develops in patients with VL, CL, and MCL who have relapsed. Chances of response to further courses of antimonials diminish once there is a relapse after the initial Sb^v treatment (69).

3.2 Clinical Significance of and Epidemiological Reasons for Drug Resistance

The reason for the emergence of resistance is the widespread misuse of the drug, as Sb^v is freely available in India and is easily accessible over the counter. Most patients (73%) first consult unqualified quacks who might not use the drug appropriately (36). It has been a common practice to start with a small dose and gradually build up the dose over a week. Drug-free intervals are given on the belief that it will prevent renal toxicity. Many a times, the daily dose of drug is split into two injections, given twice daily. These practices presumably expose the parasites to drug pressure, leading to progressive tolerance of the parasite to Sb^v. It has been observed that only a minority (26%) was treated according to the prescribed guidelines, and irregular use and incomplete treatments were common occurrences (36). These facts point to the mishandling of antileishmanial drugs in Bihar, which is a significant contributor to the development of drug resistance (57). Further, recent experiments with intramacrophageal Sb^v sensitivity assays suggest that the refractoriness to Sb^v in Bihar is due to emergence of drug-resistant strains, as clinical isolates from unresponsive patients needed 3 and 5 times greater concentration of Sb^v to achieve similar leishmanicidal activity (ED_{50} and ED_{90}, respectively) than those isolates from Sb^v-responsive patients (70). *Leishmania* do not develop resistance to Sb^v spontaneously, unless they are subjected to drug pressure. In an experimental model, the parasite that was maintained *in vitro* passage in NNN media and posterior passage in hamster did not lose sensitivity to Sb^v (71). However, resistance can be induced in the promastigote by repeated *in vitro* passage of the parasite with stepwise increase in concentration of Sb^v in the culture media (72). The *in vitro* sensitivity also decreases progressively in relapsing patients (73). There are clear indications that Sb^v resistance is a consequence of the exposure to a subtherapeutic dose of Sb^v. Though the *in vitro* data suggest that increasing the dose of Sb^v could overcome the unresponsiveness to a great extent, unfortunately even the current doses produce unacceptable toxicity, and further increase in the quantity of the drug will seriously jeopardize the safety of the patients (70).

In human-to-human (anthroponotic) transmission such as in the Indian and African subcontinents, once Sb^v resistance gets established, it spreads exponentially and organisms sensitive to the drug get eliminated quickly, whereas the drug-resistant parasites continue to circulate in the community. There are no reports of either primary resistance or decline in the efficacy of Sb^v from other endemic foci of VL with canine reservoirs such as in Brazil and southern Europe. It seems that the primary resistance emerges where man is the reservoir of infection, transmission is anthroponotic and intense, and there is a large biomass of parasite.

Unlike VL, there is considerable variation in response to Sb^v in patients with CL and MCL. CL represents a wide variety of clinical diseases produced by different species of *Leishmania*, with variable response to Sb^v. There is no single therapeutic option for all forms of CL. The therapeutic principle of CL is guided by the natural history of sores, the causative species, the possibility of mucosal dissemination, and the cosmetic and functional implications. Moreover, the fact that most CL heals spontaneously over 3–18 months complicates the rationale of drug use. Depending upon the species of the parasite, different clinical forms, and the cellular immune system of the host, a wide range of therapeutic options are available, which includes chemotherapy, cryotherapy, topical and systemic paromomycin, systemic and intralesional pentavalent antimonials, pentamidine, amphotericin B, several other antifungal agents, and immunotherapy. In the multiplicity of therapeutic options, there are some guiding principles. Since most Old World CL heal spontaneously, an expectant approach is justified, as spontaneous healing is associated with the development of protective immunity. Therapy is indicated for lesions on cosmetically important sites such as the face, disabling sites such as joints, and where healing of lesions tend to be slow, such as legs and pinna. Therapy is also indicated in the extensive disease. A detailed account of treatment for CL is beyond the scope of the present review, but recently strains resistant to Sb^v have been reported that were treated successfully with a combination of allopurinol and Sb^v (74).

In New World CL, Sb^v in doses of 20 mg/kg/day failed to cure 10% of patients. Moderate Sb^v resistance exists in nature, and therefore some *Leishmania* strains are innately less susceptible to Sb^v. Drug sensitivity decreases considerably after suboptimal treatment (68, 75), and in association with a host factor that determines a total cure or partial response and subsequent relapse, the relapsing cases lead to secondary unresponsiveness, resulting in total resistance to Sb^v.

3.3 Laboratory Diagnosis of Resistance

In clinical practice, testing susceptibility of the parasite to antileishmanial drug is rarely done. However, the emergence of resistance to antimonials and the potential for development of resistance to the already scarce alternative drugs necessitate drug sensitivity studies to be introduced in clinics. These are also needed to monitor the epidemiology of drug resistance in the community, and to devise strategies and guidelines for the therapeutic component of a control program. It can also be helpful in studying the mechanism of resistance, and in the screening of newer, effective antileishmanial drugs.

Promastigotes, the flagellar forms of *Leishmania*, have been used to study drug sensitivity as well as screening for newer antileishmanial compounds (72, 76, 77). Promastigotes are maintained on Schneider's insect media. Promastigotes (10^5/ml) in the logarithmic growth phase are added to serial dilution of the drug in 96-well microtiter plates and incu-

bated at 22–25°C for 2–7 days until the late log phase (10^7 parasites/ml). The growth of the parasite is monitored by cell counting. To determine the ED$_{50}$, the parasite counts are plotted against drug concentration, and ED$_{50}$ values are extrapolated from the graph. Promastigote assay has the advantage of ease of culture, speed of test, and ease of quantification (78, 79), but has a major drawback that the results do not necessarily correlate with its *in vivo* antileishmanial activity (70). Promastigotes differ from the intracellular aflagellar form found in the mammalian host with respect to sensitivity to various drugs, being less sensitive to Sb^v and more to pentamidine as well as having different bioenergetics (80, 81).

The sensitivity of the intracellular amastigote form was studied *in vitro* using a host cell model (82, 83). In this model, amastigotes were maintained in any of the following cell lines; (1) mouse peritoneal monocyte macrophage (84), (2) human peripheral blood monocyte-macrophage cell line (85), and (3) dog sarcoma and hamster peritoneal cell lines (86). These methods are standard for *in vitro* assessment of drug resistance and the results correlate with the clinical response; however, these are technically demanding and expensive. The percentage of infected macrophage in each assay can be determined directly by looking under an inverted microscope or after harvesting the cell with methanol and staining with Geimsa stain, before counting microscopically. The infection can also be quantified by flow cytometry techniques using lipophosphoglycan (LPG) monoclonal antibody probes (87), which has the advantage of analyzing a large number of cells rapidly. This system clearly correlates with the clinical outcome unlike in the promastigotes in which very little correlation is seen.

The ability to culture axenic amastigotes *in vitro* allows assessment of drug sensitivity and has the advantage of being rapid and as easy as the promastigote assay, with the advantages of the morphological and biochemical characteristics of the amastigote stage (76, 88). However, clinical significance of this system needs to be evaluated before being put to use, as it remains to be seen whether *in vitro* drug sensitivity assays will reflect the outcome in clinics. The drug sensitivity can also be studied in relevant animal models; BALB/c mice for *L. infantum* and Golden hamster for *L. donovani*.

Drug sensitivity assays, using either parasite culture *in vitro* or animal inoculation, are cumbersome, time consuming, and expensive and may not eventually be applied to clinics. Evolution of a quick, simple, and cheap assay is needed if it is to be applied meaningfully to clinical practice. There have been various attempts to develop molecular probes using mutants developed in the laboratory. Unfortunately, none of these hybridizes in clinical isolates from nonresponsive patients (89). Recently, in isolates from Sb^v refractory patients we identified a novel 1.254-kb gene whose locus is on chromosome 9 (89). From this DNA sequence, primers designed to amplify 900 bp were used in PCR with nuclear

DNA isolated from the unresponsive and responsive isolates, and it led to strong amplification in all eight unresponsive isolates. The responsive isolate showed a very faint PCR product, which could be attributed to the fact that amplification increases the copy number of the sequence in drug-unresponsive isolates, although the same is present in wild-type, responsive isolates at a low frequency. Transfection experiments established that this isolated fragment confers antimony resistance to wild-type *Leishmania* species. Whether this recently identified gene sequence can be used as a probe in the clinic to identify antimony-resistant clinical isolates on the Indian subcontinent remains to be established.

3.4 Mechanism of Drug Resistance

Understanding the mechanism of drug resistance is crucial for preventing, monitoring, and reverting it. Unfortunately, little is known about the mechanism underlying the drug resistance as seen in human VL. However, there has been some insight into the possible mechanisms of resistance and characterization of probes for its detection using resistant mutants developed in the laboratories largely applying drug pressure.

After administration, pentavalent antimonials are converted into trivalent compounds for its antileishmanial effect. The reduction of pentavalent to trivalent compound takes place either in macrophages (90) or in the parasite (91). In the latter case, loss of reductase activity of the parasite may lead to resistance. This is supported by the observation that Sb^v-resistant *L. donovani* amastigotes lose their reductase activity (91). Molecular studies have identified an ATP-binding cassette (ABC) transporter system, P-glycoprotein A (PGPA), involved in the metal resistance (92, 93). PGPA is a member of the multidrug-resistance protein family, whose substrate includes organic anions and drugs conjugated to glutathione, glucoroate, or sulfate. *Leishmania* contain glutathione as well as trypanothione (TSH) formed by conjugation of glutathione with spermidine. Transport experiments using radioactive conjugates clearly show that PGPA recognizes and actively transports the metal conjugates (93, 94). Thus, PGPA might be conferring resistance either through efflux from *Leishmania* (93) or by sequestering metal thiol conjugates into a vacuole (94, 95). A laboratory-generated multidrug-resistance (MDR) *Leishmania tropica* line overexpressing a P-glycoprotein-like transporter displayed significant cross-resistance to miltefosine (96). Defective uptake of miltefosine by resistant *L. donovani* (97) lines appeared to be through point mutations on a plasma membrane amino-phospholipid translocase (98).

Although an increased level of TSH has been reported from most of resistant mutant amplification, expression of PGPA is not a universal phenomenon (99, 100). It has been shown than increase in TSH may be mediated by gsh-1 amplification (glutamylcysteine synthtase) and/or ornithine decarboxylase (ODC) overexpressions (101, 102). Moreover, butathione sulfoxemine (BSO), a specific inhibitor of gsh, can reverse resistance to Sb^v in *Leishmania* (103). Most of these observations have come from resistant laboratory strains of *Leishmania*. The gene, recently identified in some of our antimony-unresponsive isolates (see above), clearly seems to be involved in conferring resistance to the parasites; however, the exact mechanism by which it produces resistance remains to be elucidated (89). The amplified sequence in clinical isolates did not hybridize with the PGPA gene or with the multidrug resistance gene (mdr), suggesting involvement of some other mechanism of drug resistance in these strains. Another 7-kb DNA fragment has also been identified, which was able to restore Sb^v reduction activity in mutants to near-wild-type levels (104).

The absence of proper understanding of the mechanism of drug resistance in *Leishmania*, as well as the molecular basis thereof, is a major hurdle in the development of molecular probes that may prove handy in monitoring the evolution and spread of drug resistance in leishmania parasites, and in selecting a drug for treatment of patients in regions with drug resistance.

3.5 Treatment Alternatives

Pentavalent Antimonials: Sb^v has been the only drug used for leishmaniasis for several decades irrespective of the clinical syndrome, region, or species of parasites, and still remains the most important drug. Further, in most parts of the world where leishmaniasis is endemic, access and affordability to a drug is a big issue. Recent studies in various parts of the world have established equivalence (in terms of safety and efficacy) of generic Sb^v to the branded product, which costs several times more (105–107). Thus, the emergence of antimony resistance means that the only affordable drug becomes unavailable to the suffering poor masses of the endemic regions of these developing regions.

Pentamidine: Pentamidine was the first drug to be used for patients refractory to Sb^v (43). This drug is associated with serious adverse events such as insulin-dependent diabetes mellitus, shock, hypoglycemia, and death in a significant proportion of patients. The declining efficacy, resistance, and the serious toxicity associated with the drug and the availability of better alternatives such as amphotericin B led to complete abandonment of this drug for VL (45, 46, 108, 109). However, it has been used to good effect in treatment of both Old and New World CL and MCL. Fewer ejections over short periods result in a high cure rate with minimum toxicity. In French Guyana, in CL caused by *L. guyanensis*, 89%

of cases were cured with two injections (4 mg/kg) given 48 h apart, and 80% of remaining patients were cured by a second course (110). In this dose, the adverse effects were minimum. In Colombian CL, four doses of 2 mg/kg of pentamidine on alternate days cured 84% patients, and four injections of 3 mg/kg cured 94% (111). Its efficacy has also been demonstrated in Brazilian CL (112, 113) and MCL (114).

Amphotericin B: It is a polyene antibiotic, and remains the only viable alternative for Sb^v-resistant cases with VL. It is the most effective antileishmanial drug that induces a high cure rate. At doses of 0.75–1 mg/kg for 15 infusions on alternate days, it cures more than 97% of patients of the Indian VL. It has been used extensively in Bihar, with uniformly good results (48, 108). Occasional relapses (<1%) might occur with amphotericin B, which can be treated successfully with the same drug. Indeed, amphotericin B has been recommended as a first-line drug by Indian National Expert Committee for Sb^v-refractory regions of VL. Though there are reports of secondary resistance in HIV/VL coinfected patients who receive repeated courses of amphotericin B (115), primary resistance to the drug is unknown (116). However, its major drawbacks include the requirement of infusion, which necessitates prolonged hospitalization of up to 5–6 weeks and frequent adverse events requiring close monitoring. These include infusion reactions in the form of increase in fever with rigor and chills and thrombophlebitis; occasionally, serious adverse events such as hypokalemia, thrombocytopenia, myocarditis and even death might occur (49).

Lipid formulations of amphotericin B: In these formulations, the deoxycholate of conventional amphotericin B is replaced by other lipids that mask amphotericin B from susceptible tissues, thereby reducing toxicity. Lipid-associated amphotericin B (AmBisome, Abelcet, Amphotec) has been one of the most remarkable developments in the chemotherapy for leishmaniasis, and offers an important alternative for patients refractory to other antileishmanial agents. The adverse effects of conventional amphotericin B can be circumvented by its use without compromising the efficacy of the drug. It is possible to deliver high doses of the drug over a short period. The dose requirement varies from region to region; while in the Indian subcontinent a small dose induces high cure rates (52, 117), a higher dose in needed for the Mediterranean region and Brazil (53). Safety of liposomal amphotericin B permits administration of the total dose requirement in a single infusion (50, 118). However, prohibitively high cost makes these compounds unaffordable in VL-endemic countries. Though these formulations are widely used in HIV/VL coinfected patients in Europe.

Paromomycin (aminosidine): It is an aminoglycoside antibiotic, and its antileishmanial activity, which is comparable to pentavalent antimonials, was described several decades ago. Its clinical development has been bumpy, and it is not yet registered in any country for the treatment of leishmaniasis. Its efficacy has been demonstrated both in Africa (119) and in India (120, 121). After the results of the ongoing pivotal phase III multimember trial in India are available, the drug could be registered for the treatment of VL, and could provide a suitable alternative to Sb^v, as its safety profile appears to be superior to most antileishmanial drugs in use. Topical preparations of paromomycin, a soft paraffin-based ointment containing 15% of paromomycin and 12% methyl-benzethonium chloride (MBCL), are effective against both Old World as well as New World CL. (122, 123).

Miltefosine: It is an alkyl phospholipid developed as an antitumor agent, and has excellent antileishmanial activity. It is the first orally effective antileishmanial drug, and has undergone extensive trial against VL in Bihar. It has been uniformly effective in both naive as well as Sb^v-refractory patients. In all clinical studies, a cure rate of ≥94% has been found consistently with this drug (56, 124). Miltefosine has been approved in India for treatment of VL at a daily dose of 50–100 mg (~2.5 mg/kg) for 4 weeks. This drug has mild gastrointestinal adverse events such as vomiting and diarrhea in 40 and 20% patients, respectively. The exact mechanism of its antileishmanial activity is yet to be identified. Miltefosine has a median long-terminal half-life of 154 h, which could encourage development of clinical resistance, and the best way to use this drug would be to use it in a combination multidrug therapy. Preliminary results from Columbia suggest its efficacy in CL (125). It is an important antileishmanial drug; however, there are certain major limitations. Therapeutic window for this drug is narrow, and it is teratogenic and abortafacient, which means the drug cannot be used in pregnancy, and women with child-bearing potential must observe contraception for the duration of treatment and for an additional 2 months. Further, rapid therapeutic response coupled with unsupervised treatment can severely affect compliance, and bring a premature end to this very important arsenal against leishmania.

Sitamaquine (WR 6026), a primaquine analog is another orally administrable antileishmanial compound that has been on the horizon for several years, but its clinical development has been very slow. In a preliminary dose escalation phase I trial in Kenya, at the highest dose, 1 mg/kg/day for 4 weeks, four of eight (50%) patients were cured (126). Recently, from Brazil, the report of a phase 2, open-label trial has appeared, and highest cure rate (67%) was achieved with 1.5 mg/kg cohort after a 28-day treatment. Methemoglobinemia, though not treatment limiting, was a common side effect. In three patients, two with 2.0 mg/kg and the only patient treated with 3.25 mg/kg, nephropathy developed. The most surprising element of this study was the lack of linear correlation in response to the dose of the drug used and cure rates (127). Relatively poor efficacy compounded with nephrotoxicity suggests that this drug cannot be used as monotherapy in

Brazilian VL. Allopurinol does not have antileishmanial activity of its own. It is a purine analog, which interferes with ribonucleic acid synthesis. It is effective *in vitro*, but it seems that *Leishmania* are capable of scavenging purines *in vivo* (81). Against certain species of *Leishmania*, it acts synergistically with antimonials *in vitro*; however, its efficacy remains to be established in well-designed, controlled clinical trials, though there are reports of its efficacy in combination with Sb^v or alone for Old World as well as New World CL, and in a few Sb^v-unresponsive VL patients (74, 128–130).

Azole-like ketaconazole and triazoles, intraconazole, and fluconazole have antileishmanial effects (131). These drugs either do not have antileishmanial activity across the board or are not as potent as amphotericin B, but they have the potential to be tried in combination will other drugs. In a well-designed study in patients with CL in Saudi Arabia, fluconazole returned a cure rate of 79% compared to 34% with placebo (132). An interesting study from Peru using imiquimod, an immunomodulator used to treat cervical warts and that has been shown to activate macrophage killing of *Leishmania* species, reported 90% cure rate with topical imiquimod plus meglumine antimonate therapy in patients with cutaneous leishmaniasis who had previously not responded to meglumine antimonate therapy. All patients responded well to this combination therapy (133).

3.5.1 Combination Therapy

In view of the emergence of parasites resistant to antileishmanial drugs such as Sb^v and pentamidine, a change in the strategy to treat leishmaniasis is urgently needed. Combination therapy with multiple drugs similar to those employed in tuberculosis, HIV, or leprosy appears to be an important approach worth considering. A potent drug with a short half-life, which will bring down the parasite load quickly to a level below which new mutants are less likely to emerge, in combination with a drug with long half-life, which will kill the remaining parasite and prevent recrudescence and relapse, could be the ideal strategy. This strategy could help shorten the duration of treatment as well. However, the biggest handicap in this strategy is that there are not enough antileishmanial drugs available to be used in combination. However, several new antileishmanial drugs are at various stages of clinical development and are likely to be available for clinical use soon. One such drug, miltefosine, has already been registered for treatment in India, and it will be tested in other parts of world. Paromomycin and sitamaquine are other drugs in the pipeline. Careful *in vitro* and animal studies for synergism as well as safety could lead to clinical studies. Safety and efficacy of single-dose liposomal amphotericin B also offer numerous possibilities of combining this regimen with other drugs, though the high cost of this formulation

remains the biggest bottleneck. Miltefosine, with its long half-life, ideally should only be used in combination, lest drug resistance should quickly emerge. However, potential combinations have to be established in well-designed clinical trials before eventually being deployed in field.

The resistance of parasite to antileishmanial drugs has been studied in the laboratory for several decades, but knowledge of drug resistance has come largely through monitoring relapse and treatment failure in patients. However, this method is not ideal to monitor drug resistance. The availability of genetic markers and molecular tools for the resistant strain would have greatly facilitated the process, but unfortunately none is available for leishmania. Thus, the setting up of reference laboratories in endemic areas capable of testing drug sensitivity will facilitate identification of resistant strains. In the absence of this facility, it has been suggested that in areas of anthroponotic VL, as soon as the relapse rate increases by more than 3% to a standard drug, combination therapy should be introduced (35). Combination therapy also appears to be the remedy for HIV-coinfected patients, for relapse is the rule in this situation.

3.6 Infection Control Measures

The epidemiology of different forms of leishmaniasis is quite diverse, with different ecological characteristics, different species of sand fly, and different reservoir hosts. Consequently, control strategies need to be tailored to the epidemiological characteristics of the disease. It is impossible to device a single control strategy. However, for any form of leishmaniasis, whether anthroponotic or zoonotic, early case detection and effective treatment will limit the disease-related morbidity and mortality. In anthroponotic foci, it also provides an effective control measure by reducing the reservoirs of infection. Access to antileishmanial drugs is an important issue, and availability of antileishmanial drugs in the endemic areas needs to be ensured, which along with tools for early diagnosis can effectively reduce the disease burden and thus transmission, more so in anthroponotic foci. It could also prove to be an important strategy to prevent emergence of drug resistance. Intense surveillance including active case detection and health education to raise the level of awareness among exposed population and promote community control measures are important for both vector and human reservoir control. Vector control measures with residual insecticide spray can effectively control the disease in anthroponotic foci of VL. A classic example of the efficacy of this strategy is the near disappearance of VL cases in India in the 1960s when insecticides were used extensively as a part of the National Malaria Eradication Programme. Personal protection against sand fly bite may be possible using pyrethroid-impregnated bed nets/sheets/curtains (134, 135) and dog collars in zoonotic foci (136–138).

For zoonotic leishmaniasis, vector control through residual insecticide spraying of houses and animal shelters is restricted to the domestic and peridomestic areas such as Central and South America (*Lutzomyia longipalpis*). Regarding reservoir control, dogs being the main domestic reservoir, humane destruction of infected dogs, identified after annual screening of blood samples by serology, may be a way to control the disease. Nevertheless, the strategy of elimination is not satisfactory, as it provides only a transient effect, and there is always a concern over delay between sampling, diagnosis, and culling of dogs. More effective diagnostic tools may allow culling without delay. In the absence of a reliable tool for detecting infected dogs, dogs may be treated with insecticides, or topical insecticide could be applied, which will protect them from infection as well as prevent sand flies from biting the dogs. Another ingenious method tried has been applying deltamethrin-treated collar to dogs (136, 138). It gives long-term protection against sand fly bite. However, these modalities of disease control, notwithstanding their limitation, are rarely used comprehensively in underdeveloped or developing countries where the disease is endemic.

Vaccination against different forms of leishmaniasis is a viable alternative for the control of the disease. Autoclaved whole parasites with BCG with or without alum have been tested in randomized clinical trials in Iran and Sudan against CL and VL, respectively; however, they failed to provide adequate protection (139, 140). Now recombinant vaccines are being tested for both CL and VL. However, successful vaccination against leishmaniasis still remains a distant reality.

References

1. Desjeux P. Human leishmaniases: epidemiology and public health aspects. World Health Stat Q 1992; 45:267–75.
2. Desjeux P. The increase in risk factors for leishmaniasis worldwide. Trans R Soc Trop Med Hyg 2001; 95:239–43.
3. Bora D. Epidemiology of visceral leishmaniasis in India. Natl Med J India 1999; 12:62–8.
4. Seaman J, Mercer AJ, Sondorp E. The epidemic of visceral leishmaniasis in western Upper Nile, southern Sudan: course and impact from 1984 to 1994. Int J Epidemiol 1996; 25:862–71.
5. Richens J. Genital manifestations of tropical diseases. Sex Transm Infect 2004; 80:12–7.
6. Alvar J, Canavate C, Gutierrez-Solar B, et al. Leishmania and human immunodeficiency virus coinfection: the first 10 years. Clin Microbiol Rev 1997; 10:298–319.
7. Desjeux P, Alvar J. Leishmania/HIV co-infections: epidemiology in Europe. Ann Trop Med Parasitol 2003; 97 Suppl 1:3–15.
8. Killick-Kendrick R. Phlebotomine vectors of the leishmaniases: a review. Med Vet Entomol 1990; 4:1–24.
9. Magill AJ. Epidemiology of the leishmaniases. Dermatol Clin 1995; 13:505–23.
10. Leishmaniasis. Lancet 1968; 2:203–4.
11. Leng YJ, Zhang LM. Check list and geographical distribution of phlebotomine sandflies in China. Ann Trop Med Parasitol 1993; 87:83–94.
12. Morsy TA, el-Missiry AG, Kamel AM, Fayad ME, el-Sharkawy IM. Distribution of *Phlebotomus* species in the Nile Delta, Egypt. J Egypt Soc Parasitol 1990; 20:589–97.
13. Dedet J, Pratlong F. Taxonomy of *Leishmania* and geographical distribution of leishmaniasis. Ann Dermatol Venereol 2000; 127:421–4.
14. Dye C. The logic of visceral leishmaniasis control. Am J Trop Med Hyg 1996; 55:125–30.
15. Desjeux P, Piot B, O'Neill K, Meert JP. Co-infections of leishmania/HIV in south Europe. Med Trop (Mars) 2001; 61:187–93.
16. de la Loma A, Alvar J, Martinez Galiano E, Blazquez J, Alcala Munoz A, Najera R. Leishmaniasis or AIDS? Trans R Soc Trop Med Hyg 1985; 79:421–2.
17. Zijlstra EE, Musa AM, Khalil EA, el-Hassan IM, el-Hassan AM. Post-kala-azar dermal leishmaniasis. Lancet Infect Dis 2003; 3:87–98.
18. Zijlstra EE, el-Hassan AM, Ismael A. Endemic kala-azar in eastern Sudan: post-kala-azar dermal leishmaniasis. Am J Trop Med Hyg 1995; 52:299–305.
19. Thakur CP, Kumar K. Post kala-azar dermal leishmaniasis: a neglected aspect of kala-azar control programmes. Ann Trop Med Parasitol 1992; 86:355–9.
20. Addy M, Nandy A. Ten years of kala-azar in west Bengal, Part I. Did post-kala-azar dermal leishmaniasis initiate the outbreak in 24-Parganas? Bull World Health Organ 1992; 70:341–6.
21. Abdalla RE, Sherif H. Epidemic of cutaneous leishmaniasis in Northern Sudan. Ann Trop Med Parasitol 1978; 72:349–52.
22. Reyburn H, Rowland M, Mohsen M, Khan B, Davies C. The prolonged epidemic of anthroponotic cutaneous leishmaniasis in Kabul, Afghanistan: 'bringing down the neighbourhood'. Trans R Soc Trop Med Hyg 2003; 97:170–6.
23. Aguilar CM, Fernandez E, de Fernandez R, Deane LM. Study of an outbreak of cutaneous leishmaniasis in Venezuela. The role of domestic animals. Mem Inst Oswaldo Cruz 1984; 79:181–95.
24. Follador I, Araujo C, Cardoso MA, et al. Outbreak of American cutaneous leishmaniasis in Canoa, Santo Amaro, Bahia, Brazil. Rev Soc Bras Med Trop 1999; 32:497–503.
25. Sharifi I, Fekri AR, Aflatonian MR, Nadim A, Nikian Y, Kamesipour A. Cutaneous leishmaniasis in primary school children in the south-eastern Iranian city of Bam, 1994–95. Bull World Health Organ 1998; 76:289–93.
26. Gunduz K, Afsar S, Ayhan S, et al. Recidivans cutaneous leishmaniasis unresponsive to liposomal amphotericin B (AmBisome). J Eur Acad Dermatol Venereol 2000; 14:11–3.
27. Grimaldi G, Jr., Tesh RB, McMahon-Pratt D. A review of the geographic distribution and epidemiology of leishmaniasis in the New World. Am J Trop Med Hyg 1989; 41:687–725.
28. Barral A, Costa JM, Bittencourt AL, Barral-Netto M, Carvalho EM. Polar and subpolar diffuse cutaneous leishmaniasis in Brazil: clinical and immunopathologic aspects. Int J Dermatol 1995; 34:474–9.
29. Akuffo HO, Fehniger TE, Britton S. Differential recognition of *Leishmania aethiopica* antigens by lymphocytes from patients with local and diffuse cutaneous leishmaniasis. Evidence for antigen-induced immune suppression. J Immunol 1988; 141:2461–6.
30. Oliveira-Neto MP, Mattos M, Pirmez C, et al. Mucosal leishmaniasis ("espundia") responsive to low dose of *N*-methyl glucamine (Glucantime) in Rio de Janeiro, Brazil. Rev Inst Med Trop Sao Paulo 2000; 42:321–5.
31. Larson EE, Marsden PD. The origin of espundia. Trans R Soc Trop Med Hyg 1987; 81:880.
32. Magill AJ, Grogl M, Gasser RA, Jr., Sun W, Oster CN. Visceral infection caused by *Leishmania tropica* in veterans of Operation Desert Storm. N Engl J Med 1993; 328:1383–7.

33. Sundar S, More DK, Singh MK, et al. Failure of pentavalent antimony in visceral leishmaniasis in India: report from the center of the Indian epidemic. Clin Infect Dis 2000; 31:1104–7.

34. Sundar S, Singh VP, Sharma S, Makharia MK, Murray HW. Response to interferon-gamma plus pentavalent antimony in Indian visceral leishmaniasis. J Infect Dis 1997; 176:1117–9.

35. Bryceson A. A policy for leishmaniasis with respect to the prevention and control of drug resistance. Trop Med Int Health 2001; 6:928–34.

36. Sundar S, Thakur BB, Tandon AK, et al. Clinicoepidemiological study of drug resistance in Indian kala-azar. BMJ 1994; 308:307.

37. Berman JD. Human leishmaniasis: clinical, diagnostic, and chemotherapeutic developments in the last 10 years. Clin Infect Dis 1997; 24:684–703.

38. Herwaldt BL, Berman JD. Recommendations for treating leishmaniasis with sodium stibogluconate (Pentostam) and review of pertinent clinical studies. Am J Trop Med Hyg 1992; 46:296–306.

39. Laguna F, Videla S, Jimenez-Mejias ME, et al. Amphotericin B lipid complex versus meglumine antimoniate in the treatment of visceral leishmaniasis in patients infected with HIV: a randomized pilot study. J Antimicrob Chemother 2003; 52:464–8.

40. Russo R, Nigro LC, Minniti S, et al. Visceral leishmaniasis in HIV infected patients: treatment with high dose liposomal amphotericin B (AmBisome). J Infect 1996; 32:133–7.

41. Alvar J, Gutierrez-Solar B, Pachon I, et al. AIDS and *Leishmania infantum*. New approaches for a new epidemiological problem. Clin Dermatol 1996; 14:541–6.

42. Molina R, Gradoni L, Alvar J. HIV and the transmission of Leishmania. Ann Trop Med Parasitol 2003; 97 Suppl 1:29–45.

43. Jha TK. Evaluation of diamidine compound (pentamidine isethionate) in the treatment resistant cases of kala-azar occurring in North Bihar, India. Trans R Soc Trop Med Hyg 1983; 77:167–70.

44. Jha TK, Sharma VK. Pentamidine-induced diabetes mellitus. Trans R Soc Trop Med Hyg 1984; 78:252–3.

45. Jha SN, Singh NK, Jha TK. Changing response to diamidine compounds in cases of kala-azar unresponsive to antimonial. J Assoc Physicians India 1991; 39:314–6.

46. Thakur CP, Kumar M, Pandey AK. Comparison of regimes of treatment of antimony-resistant kala-azar patients: a randomized study. Am J Trop Med Hyg 1991; 45:435–41.

47. Mishra M, Singh MP, Choudhury D, Singh VP, Khan AB. Amphotericin B for second-line treatment of Indian kala-azar. Lancet 1991; 337:926.

48. Thakur CP, Singh RK, Hassan SM, Kumar R, Narain S, Kumar A. Amphotericin B deoxycholate treatment of visceral leishmaniasis with newer modes of administration and precautions: a study of 938 cases. Trans R Soc Trop Med Hyg 1999; 93:319–23.

49. Sundar S, Mehta H, Suresh AV, Singh SP, Rai M, Murray HW. Amphotericin B treatment for Indian visceral leishmaniasis: conventional versus lipid formulations. Clin Infect Dis 2004; 38:377–83.

50. Sundar S, Jha TK, Thakur CP, Mishra M, Singh VP, Buffels R. Single-dose liposomal amphotericin B in the treatment of visceral leishmaniasis in India: a multicenter study. Clin Infect Dis 2003; 37:800–4.

51. Sundar S, Agrawal G, Rai M, Makharia MK, Murray HW. Treatment of Indian visceral leishmaniasis with single or daily infusions of low dose liposomal amphotericin B: randomised trial. BMJ 2001; 323:419–22.

52. Sundar S, Agrawal NK, Sinha PR, Horwith GS, Murray HW. Short-course, low-dose amphotericin B lipid complex therapy for visceral leishmaniasis unresponsive to antimony. Ann Intern Med 1997; 127:133–7.

53. Berman JD. U.S Food and Drug Administration approval of AmBisome (liposomal amphotericin B) for treatment of visceral leishmaniasis. Clin Infect Dis 1999; 28:49–51.

54. Davidson RN, di Martino L, Gradoni L, et al. Short-course treatment of visceral leishmaniasis with liposomal amphotericin B (AmBisome). Clin Infect Dis 1996; 22:938–43.

55. Seaman J, Boer C, Wilkinson R, et al. Liposomal amphotericin B (AmBisome) in the treatment of complicated kala-azar under field conditions. Clin Infect Dis 1995; 21:188–93.

56. Sundar S, Jha TK, Thakur CP, et al. Oral miltefosine for Indian visceral leishmaniasis. N Engl J Med 2002; 347:1739–46.

57. Sundar S. Drug resistance in Indian visceral leishmaniasis. Trop Med Int Health 2001; 6:849–54.

58. Peters W. The treatment of kala-azar – new approaches to an old problem. Indian J Med Res 1981; 73 Suppl:1–18.

59. Anonymous. Proceedings of the Meeting of an Expert Group on Kala-azar held at Indian Council of Medical Research Headquarters on 9 September, 1977, New Delhi. Indian Council of Medical Research, New Delhi 1977.

60. Aikat BK, Sahaya S, Pathania AG, et al. Clinical profile of cases of kala-azar in Bihar. Indian J Med Res 1979; 70:563–70.

61. Thakur CP, Kumar M, Singh SK, et al. Comparison of regimens of treatment with sodium stibogluconate in kala-azar. Br Med J (Clin Res Ed) 1984; 288:895–7.

62. The leishmaniases. Report of a WHO Expert Committee. World Health Organ Tech Rep Ser 1984; 701:1–140.

63. Thakur CP, Kumar M, Kumar P, Mishra BN, Pandey AK. Rationalisation of regimens of treatment of kala-azar with sodium stibogluconate in India: a randomised study. Br Med J (Clin Res Ed) 1988; 296:1557–61.

64. Thakur CP, Kumar M, Pandey AK. Evaluation of efficacy of longer durations of therapy of fresh cases of kala-azar with sodium stibogluconate. Indian J Med Res 1991; 93:103–10.

65. Jha T, Singh N, Jha S. Therapeutic use of sodium stibogluconate in kala-alar from some hyperendemic districts of N. Bihar, India (Abstract). J Assoc Physicians India 1992; 40:868.

66. Rijal S, Chappuis F, Singh R, et al. Treatment of kala-azar in south-eastern Nepal: decreasing efficacy of sodium stibogluconate and need for a policy to limit further decline. Trans R Soc Trop Med Hyg 2003; 97(3):350–4.

67. Laguna F, Videla S, Jimenez-Mejias ME, et al. Amphotericin B lipid complex versus meglumine antimoniate in the treatment of visceral leishmaniasis in patients infected with HIV: a randomized pilot study. J Antimicrob Chemother 2003; 52(3):464–8.

68. Berman JD, Chulay JD, Hendricks LD, Oster CN. Susceptibility of clinically sensitive and resistant Leishmania to pentavalent antimony in vitro. Am J Trop Med Hyg 1982; 31:459–65.

69. Bryceson AD, Chulay JD, Ho M, et al. Visceral leishmaniasis unresponsive to antimonial drugs. I. Clinical and immunological studies. Trans R Soc Trop Med Hyg 1985; 79:700–4.

70. Lira R, Sundar S, Makharia A, et al. Evidence that the high incidence of treatment failures in Indian kala-azar is due to the emergence of antimony-resistant strains of *Leishmania donovani*. J Infect Dis 1999; 180:564–7.

71. Carrio J, Portus M. In vitro susceptibility to pentavalent antimony in *Leishmania infantum* strains is not modified during in vitro or in vivo passages but is modified after host treatment with meglumine antimoniate. BMC Pharmacol 2002; 2:11.

72. Bhattacharyya A, Mukherjee M, Duttagupta S. Studies on stibanate unresponsive isolates of *Leishmania donovani*. J Biosci 2002; 27:503–8.

73. Faraut-Gambarelli F, Piarroux R, Deniau M, et al. In vitro and in vivo resistance of *Leishmania infantum* to meglumine antimoniate: a study of 37 strains collected from patients with visceral leishmaniasis. Antimicrob Agents Chemother 1997; 41:827–30.

74. Momeni AZ, Reiszadae MR, Aminjavaheri M. Treatment of cutaneous leishmaniasis with a combination of allopurinol and low-dose meglumine antimoniate. Int J Dermatol 2002; 41: 441–3.

75. Grogl M, Thomason TN, Franke ED. Drug resistance in leishmaniasis: its implication in systemic chemotherapy of cutaneous and mucocutaneous disease. Am J Trop Med Hyg 1992; 47:117–26.

76. Sereno D, Lemesre JL. Axenically cultured amastigote forms as an in vitro model for investigation of antileishmanial agents. Antimicrob Agents Chemother 1997; 41:972–6.

77. Jackson JE, Tally JD, Tang DB. An in vitro micromethod for drug sensitivity testing of Leishmania. Am J Trop Med Hyg 1989; 41:318–30.

78. Bodley AL, McGarry MW, Shapiro TA. Drug cytotoxicity assay for African trypanosomes and *Leishmania* species. J Infect Dis 1995; 172:1157–9.

79. Jackson JE, Tally JD, Ellis WY, et al. Quantitative in vitro drug potency and drug susceptibility evaluation of *Leishmania* ssp. from patients unresponsive to pentavalent antimony therapy. Am J Trop Med Hyg 1990; 43:464 80.

80. Bates PA, Robertson CD, Tetley L, Coombs GH. Axenic cultivation and characterization of *Leishmania mexicana* amastigote-like forms. Parasitology 1992; 105 (Pt 2):193–202.

81. Berman JD. Chemotherapy for leishmaniasis: biochemical mechanisms, clinical efficacy, and future strategies. Rev Infect Dis 1988; 10:560–86.

82. Chang KP, Nacy CA, Pearson RD. Intracellular parasitism of macrophages in leishmaniasis: in vitro systems and their applications. Methods Enzymol 1986; 132:603–26.

83. Neal RA, Croft SL. An in-vitro system for determining the activity of compounds against the intracellular amastigote form of *Leishmania donovani*. J Antimicrob Chemother 1984; 14:463–75.

84. Gaspar R, Opperdoes FR, Preat V, Roland M. Drug targeting with polyalkylcyanoacrylate nanoparticles: in vitro activity of primaquine-loaded nanoparticles against intracellular *Leishmania donovani*. Ann Trop Med Parasitol 1992; 86:41–9

85. Abok K, Cadenas E, Brunk U. An experimental model system for leishmaniasis. Effects of porphyrin-compounds and menadione on Leishmania parasites engulfed by cultured macrophages. APMIS 1988; 96:543 51.

86. Mattock NM, Peters W. The experimental chemotherapy of leishmaniasis. I: Techniques for the study of drug action in tissue culture. Ann Trop Med Parasitol 1975; 69:349–57.

87. Di Giorgio C, Ridoux O, Delmas F, Azas N, Gasquet M, Timon-David P. Flow cytometric detection of Leishmania parasites in human monocyte-derived macrophages: application to antileishmanial-drug testing. Antimicrob Agents Chemother 2000; 44:3074–8.

88. Ephros M, Bitnun A, Shaked P, Waldman E, Zilberstein D. Stage-specific activity of pentavalent antimony against *Leishmania donovani* axenic amastigotes. Antimicrob Agents Chemother 1999; 43:278–82.

89. Singh N, Singh RT, Sundar S. Novel mechanism of drug resistance in kala-azar field isolates. J Infect Dis 2003; 188:600–7.

90. Frezard F, Demicheli C, Ferreira CS, Costa MA. Glutathione-induced conversion of pentavalent antimony to trivalent antimony in meglumine antimoniate. Antimicrob Agents Chemother 2001; 45:913–6.

91. Shaked-Mishan P, Ulrich N, Ephros M, Zilberstein D. Novel intracellular SbV reducing activity correlates with antimony susceptibility in *Leishmania donovani*. J Biol Chem 2001; 276:3971–6.

92. Ouellette M, Legare D, Haimeur A, Grondin K, Roy G, Brochu C, Papadopoulou B. ABC transporters in Leishmania and their role in drug resistance. Drug Resist Updat 1998; 1:43–48.

93. Perez-Victoria JM, Di Pietro A, Barron D, Ravelo AG, Castanys S, Gamarro F. Multidrug resistance phenotype mediated by the P-glycoprotein-like transporter in Leishmania: a search for reversal agents. Curr Drug Targets 2002; 3:311–33.

94. Legare D, Richard D, Mukhopadhyay R, et al. The Leishmania ATP-binding cassette protein PGPA is an intracellular metal-thiol transporter ATPase. J Biol Chem 2001; 276:26301–7.

95. Dey S, Ouellette M, Lightbody J, Papadopoulou B, Rosen BP. An ATP-dependent As(III)-glutathione transport system in membrane vesicles of *Leishmania tarentolae*. Proc Natl Acad Sci U S A 1996; 93:2192–7.

96. Perez-Victoria JM, Perez-Victoria FJ, Parodi-Talice A, et al. Alkyl-lysophospholipid resistance in multidrug-resistant *Leishmania tropica* and chemosensitization by a novel P-glycoprotein-like transporter modulator. Antimicrob Agents Chemother 2001; 45:2468–74.

97. Perez-Victoria FJ, Castanys S, Gamarro F. *Leishmania donovani* resistance to miltefosine involves a defective inward translocation of the drug. Antimicrob Agents Chemother 2003; 47:2397–403.

98. Perez-Victoria FJ, Gamarro F, Ouellette M, Castanys S. Functional cloning of the miltefosine transporter. A novel P-type phospholipid translocase from Leishmania involved in drug resistance. J Biol Chem 2003; 278:49965–71.

99. Haimeur A, Brochu C, Genest P, Papadopoulou B, Ouellette M. Amplification of the ABC transporter gene PGPA and increased trypanothione levels in potassium antimonyl tartrate (SbIII) resistant *Leishmania tarentolae*. Mol Biochem Parasitol 2000; 108:131 5.

100. Legare D, Papadopoulou B, Roy G, et al. Efflux systems and increased trypanothione levels in arsenite-resistant Leishmania. Exp Parasitol 1997; 87:275–82.

101. Haimeur A, Guimond C, Pilote S, et al. Elevated levels of polyamines and trypanothione resulting from overexpression of the ornithine decarboxylase gene in arsenite-resistant Leishmania. Mol Microbiol 1999; 34:726–35.

102. Grondin K, Haimeur A, Mukhopadhyay R, Rosen BP, Ouellette M. Co-amplification of the gamma-glutamylcysteine synthetase gene gsh1 and of the ABC transporter gene pgpA in arsenite-resistant *Leishmania tarentolae*. EMBO J 1997; 16:3057–65.

103. Carter KC, Sundar S, Spickett C, Pereira OC, Mullen AB. The in vivo susceptibility of *Leishmania donovani* to sodium stibogluconate is drug specific and can be reversed by inhibiting glutathione biosynthesis. Antimicrob Agents Chemother 2003; 47:1529–35.

104. Zilberstein D, Ephros M. Clinical and laboratory aspects of leishmania chemotherapy in the ear of drug resistance. In: Seed J, ed. World Class Parasites, Vol. 4. London: Kluwer, 2002, pp 115–136.

105. Veeken H, Ritmeijer K, Seaman J, Davidson R. A randomized comparison of branded sodium stibogluconate and generic sodium stibogluconate for the treatment of visceral leishmaniasis under field conditions in Sudan. Trop Med Int Health 2000; 5:312–7.

106. Moore E, O'Flaherty D, Heuvelmans H, et al. Comparison of generic and proprietary sodium stibogluconate for the treatment of visceral leishmaniasis in Kenya. Bull World Health Organ 2001; 79:388–93.

107. Ritmeijer K, Veeken H, Melaku Y, et al. Ethiopian visceral leishmaniasis: generic and proprietary sodium stibogluconate are equivalent; HIV co-infected patients have a poor outcome. Trans R Soc Trop Med Hyg 2001; 95:668–72.

108. Mishra M, Biswas UK, Jha DN, Khan AB. Amphotericin versus pentamidine in antimony-unresponsive kala-azar. Lancet 1992; 340:1256–7.

109. Sundar S. Treatment of visceral leishmaniasis. Med Microbiol Immunol (Berl) 2001; 190:89–92.

110. Nacher M, Carme B, Sainte Marie D, et al. Influence of clinical presentation on the efficacy of a short course of pentamidine in the treatment of cutaneous leishmaniasis in French Guiana. Ann Trop Med Parasitol 2001; 95:331–6.

111. Soto J, Buffet P, Grogl M, Berman J. Successful treatment of Colombian cutaneous leishmaniasis with four injections of pentamidine. Am J Trop Med Hyg 1994; 50:107–11.

112. Correia D, Macedo VO, Carvalho EM, et al. Comparative study of meglumine antimoniate, pentamidine isethionate and aminosidine sulfate in the treatment of primary skin lesions caused

by Leishmania (Viannia) braziliensis. Rev Soc Bras Med Trop 1996; 29:447–53.

113. de Paula CD, Sampaio JH, Cardoso DR, Sampaio RN. A comparative study between the efficacy of pentamidine isothionate given in three doses for one week and N-methil-glucamine in a dose of 20 mg SbV/day for 20 days to treat cutaneous leishmaniasis. Rev Soc Bras Med Trop 2003; 36:365–71.

114. Amato V, Amato J, Nicodemo A, Uip D, Amato-Neto V, Duarte M. Treatment of mucocutaneous leishmaniasis with pentamidine isothionate. Ann Dermatol Venereol 1998; 125:492–5.

115. Di Giorgio C, Faraut-Gambarelli F, Imbert A, Minodier P, Gasquet M, Dumon H. Flow cytometric assessment of amphotericin B susceptibility in Leishmania infantum isolates from patients with visceral leishmaniasis. J Antimicrob Chemother 1999; 44:71–6.

116. Durand R, Paul M, Pratlong F, et al. Leishmania infantum: lack of parasite resistance to amphotericin B in a clinically resistant visceral leishmaniasis. Antimicrob Agents Chemother 1998; 42:2141–3.

117. Sundar S, Jha TK, Thakur CP, Mishra M, Singh VR, Buffels R. Low-dose liposomal amphotericin B in refractory Indian visceral leishmaniasis: a multicenter study. Am J Trop Med Hyg 2002; 66:143–6.

118. Thakur CP. A single high dose treatment of kala-azar with Ambisome (amphotericin B lipid complex): a pilot study. Int J Antimicrob Agents 2001; 17:67–70.

119. Chunge CN, Owate J, Pamba HO, Donno L. Treatment of visceral leishmaniasis in Kenya by aminosidine alone or combined with sodium stibogluconate. Trans R Soc Trop Med Hyg 1990; 84:221–5.

120. Jha TK, Olliaro P, Thakur CP, et al. Randomised controlled trial of aminosidine (paromomycin) v sodium stibogluconate for treating visceral leishmaniasis in North Bihar, India. BMJ 1998; 316:1200–5.

121. Thakur CP, Kanyok TP, Pandey AK, et al. A prospective randomized, comparative, open-label trial of the safety and efficacy of paromomycin (aminosidine) plus sodium stibogluconate versus sodium stibogluconate alone for the treatment of visceral leishmaniasis. Trans R Soc Trop Med Hyg 2000; 94:429–31.

122. el-On J, Halevy S, Grunwald MH, Weinrauch L. Topical treatment of Old World cutaneous leishmaniasis caused by Leishmania major: a double-blind control study. J Am Acad Dermatol 1992; 27:227–31.

123. Krause G, Kroeger A. Topical treatment of American cutaneous leishmaniasis with paromomycin and methylbenzethonium chloride: a clinical study under field conditions in Ecuador. Trans R Soc Trop Med Hyg 1994; 88:92–4.

124. Bhattacharya SK, Jha TK, Sundar S, et al. Efficacy and tolerability of miltefosine for childhood visceral leishmaniasis in India. Clin Infect Dis 2004; 38:217–21.

125. Soto J, Toledo J, Gutierrez P, et al. Treatment of American cutaneous leishmaniasis with miltefosine, an oral agent. Clin Infect Dis 2001; 33:E57–61.

126. Sherwood JA, Gachihi GS, Muigai RK, et al. Phase 2 efficacy trial of an oral 8-aminoquinoline (WR6026) for treatment of visceral leishmaniasis. Clin Infect Dis 1994; 19:1034–9.

127. Dietze R, Carvalho SF, Valli LC, et al. Phase 2 trial of WR6026, an orally administered 8-aminoquinoline, in the treatment of visceral leishmaniasis caused by Leishmania chagasi. Am J Trop Med Hyg 2001; 65:685–9.

128. Martinez S, Marr JJ. Allopurinol in the treatment of American cutaneous leishmaniasis. N Engl J Med 1992; 326:741–4.

129. Momeni AZ, Aminjavaheri M. Successful treatment of non-healing cases of cutaneous leishmaniasis, using a combination of meglumine antimoniate plus allopurinol. Eur J Dermatol 2003; 13:40–3.

130. Chunge CN, Gachihi G, Muigai R, et al. Visceral leishmaniasis unresponsive to antimonial drugs. III. Successful treatment using a combination of sodium stibogluconate plus allopurinol. Trans R Soc Trop Med Hyg 1985; 79:715–8.

131. Croft SL, Yardley V. Chemotherapy of leishmaniasis. Curr Pharm Des 2002; 8:319–42.

132. Alrajhi AA, Ibrahim EA, De Vol EB, Khairat M, Faris RM, Maguire JH. Fluconazole for the treatment of cutaneous leishmaniasis caused by Leishmania major. N Engl J Med 2002; 346:891–5.

133. Arevalo I, Ward B, Miller R, et al. Successful treatment of drug-resistant cutaneous leishmaniasis in humans by use of imiquimod, an immunomodulator. Clin Infect Dis 2001; 33:1847–51.

134. Reyburn H, Ashford R, Mohsen M, Hewitt S, Rowland M. A randomized controlled trial of insecticide-treated bednets and chaddars or top sheets, and residual spraying of interior rooms for the prevention of cutaneous leishmaniasis in Kabul, Afghanistan. Trans R Soc Trop Med Hyg 2000; 94:361–6.

135. Elnaiem DA, Elnahas AM, Aboud MA. Protective efficacy of lambdacyhalothrin-impregnated bednets against Phlebotomus orientalis, the vector of visceral leishmaniasis in Sudan. Med Vet Entomol 1999; 13:310–4.

136. Reithinger R, Coleman PG, Alexander B, Vieira EP, Assis G, Davies CR. Are insecticide-impregnated dog collars a feasible alternative to dog culling as a strategy for controlling canine visceral leishmaniasis in Brazil? Int J Parasitol 2004; 34:55–62.

137. Maroli M, Mizzon V, Siragusa C, D'Oorazi A, Gradoni L. Evidence for an impact on the incidence of canine leishmaniasis by the mass use of deltamethrin-impregnated dog collars in southern Italy. Med Vet Entomol 2001; 15:358–63.

138. Halbig P, Hodjati MH, Mazloumi-Gavgani AS, Mohite H, Davies CR. Further evidence that deltamethrin-impregnated collars protect domestic dogs from sandfly bites. Med Vet Entomol 2000; 14:223–6.

139. Sharifi I, FeKri AR, Aflatonian MR, et al. Randomised vaccine trial of single dose of killed Leishmania major plus BCG against anthroponotic cutaneous leishmaniasis in Bam, Iran. Lancet 1998; 351:1540–3.

140. Khalil EA, El Hassan AM, Zijlstra EE, et al. Autoclaved Leishmania major vaccine for prevention of visceral leishmaniasis: a randomised, double-blind, BCG-controlled trial in Sudan. Lancet 2000; 356:1565–9.

Chapter 76
Human African Trypanosomiasis

Jacques Pépin and Honoré Méda

1 Overview

Human African trypanosomiasis (HAT) is caused by two subspecies of trypanosomes, *Trypanosoma brucei gambiense* and *T.b. rhodesiense*. Clinically, the disease is characterized by an early stage during which patients report non-specific symptoms such as fever and malaise, and trypanosomes are found in the blood or in lymph node aspirates. While in the case of *T.b. rhodesiense* this early stage develops within days of the infective bite and rapidly progresses over days or weeks to a severe disease, patients with *T. b. gambiense* HAT can remain asymptomatic for months or years, or have only intermittent fever. Eventually, when the disease progresses to the late stage with involvement of the central nervous system (CNS), the patients develop somnolence, constant headaches, behavior changes or other neurological symptoms, and trypanosomes are now found in the cerebrospinal fluid (CSF). If untreated, this is ultimately fatal within a few months.

HAT is endemic only in sub-Saharan Africa between latitudes 15° north and 15° south, corresponding to the distribution of its vector (1, 2). *T.b. gambiense* HAT is endemic in western and central Africa and *T.b. rhodesiense* HAT in eastern and southern Africa. Uganda is the only country where both subspecies are present. The disease re-emerged in several countries in the 1990s, following the breakdown of control programs so that the distribution of sleeping sickness nowadays parallels that of wars that have recently devastated parts of Africa, with the highest incidences occurring in the Democratic Republic of Congo (DRC), Angola, and Sudan. The total number of cases is estimated to be ≈100,000 per year, with at least one-third of them remaining undetected and untreated (2). In 2000, WHO estimated that the burden of HAT corresponded to 66,000 deaths per year and 2.05 million disability-adjusted life-years lost (3). The highest incidence is seen in DRC, where 20–25,000 cases

are reported annually; given the breakdown of its health system, the true incidence could be at least twice as high (4). DRC is followed by Angola (≈12,000 cases), southern Sudan (several thousands), Congo-Brazzaville and Central African Republic (≈1,000 cases) while the incidence is much lower in Gabon, Cameroon, and Equatorial Guinea. In West Africa, the disease has disappeared from several countries for ecologic reasons, but a few hundred cases are diagnosed each year in Côte d'Ivoire, Guinea, and Nigeria. In East Africa, an epidemic of Rhodesian HAT in the historical Busoga focus of southeastern Uganda has been much reduced by tsetse fly trapping and case finding and only a few hundreds cases are now reported (5). There remains, however, Gambian HAT in the northwest of the country. Only residual *T.b. rhodesiense* HAT endemicity occurs elsewhere in eastern and southern Africa, with ≈200 reported cases per year in Tanzania, and fewer cases in Zambia, Kenya, Malawi, and Mozambique. Each year, a few dozen cases of *T.b. rhodesiense* trypanosomiasis are diagnosed in tourists who visited the game parks of East and Southern Africa (6), while ≈20 cases of *T.b. gambiense* HAT are diagnosed in Africans who have migrated outside the endemic areas (7). The determinants of the epidemiology of *T.b. gambiense* HAT are: (a) the long duration (months to years) of infection in human hosts with intermittent parasitemia; (b) man-fly contact and infection rates among the tsetse vector; (c) and the impact of active case finding (1). In contrast, *T.b. rhodesiense* trypanosomiasis is a zoonosis and to some extent an occupational disease, with game animals and cattle harboring the parasite and sustaining the sporadic human disease (1). Interhuman spread occurs during epidemics but generally this subspecies offers less potential for large-scale spread because of its acute nature. So far, there is no evidence of an interaction between HAT and HIV infection, but this would need to be examined again now that HIV has spread to rural areas (8).

The overwhelming majority of cases of both *T.b. gambiense* and *T.b. rhodesienese* African trypanosomiasis are diagnosed and treated in rural African hospitals with only the most basic laboratory back-up. The diagnosis is generally

J. Pépin (✉)
Center for International Health, University of Sherbrooke, QC, Canada
jacques.pepin@usherbrooke.ca

D.L. Mayers (ed.), *Antimicrobial Drug Resistance*,
DOI 10.1007/978-1-60327-595-8_76, © Humana Press, a part of Springer Science+Business Media, LLC 2009

made by the documentation of trypanosomes in the unstained lymph node aspirate or wet smear of blood or CSF or in a Giemsa-stained thick smear of blood. More sensitive techniques such as the miniature anion-exchange centrifugation technique, the hematocrit centrifugation technique for an examination of the buffy coat or the quantitative buffy coat technique using acridine orange stain are rarely used. The kit for in vitro isolation (KIVI) and the polymerase chain reaction remain research tools unlikely to be used in the field in the near future (9, 10). As the disease progresses, it becomes more difficult to find parasites in blood and lymph nodes, and it is more likely that only the CSF reveals trypanosomes. Disease staging is usually made through the CSF white cell count (WCC): patients with a CSF WCC of 1–5/mm^3 are considered to be in early stage while those with a CSF WCC $\geq$6/mm^3 are considered to be in late stage. A sensitive but only moderately specific serological assay, the card agglutination test for trypanosomes, can be used in case-finding surveys to identify suspects in whose specimens trypanosomes are looked for.

Most currently recommended drugs have been used for more than a half-century: suramin (a polysulfonated naphthylamine), melarsoprol (a trivalent arsenical) and pentamidine (a diamidine) (11). Eflornithine, a selective and irreversible suicide inhibitor of ornithine decarboxylase (ODC) (one of the limiting steps in polyamines biosynthesis), is the only new drug approved for human use since the end of World War II. Nifurtimox, a drug used in the treatment of American trypanosomiasis, cures at most half the patients at the price of substantial toxicity, and can not be recommended. To select the best treatment for a patient in whom trypanosomes have been found, two questions must be answered: is it *T.b. gambiense* or *T.b. rhodesiense*, and is the patient in early stage or late stage? The first question is easily addressed by geographic considerations. To answer the second, a lumbar puncture (LP) must always be performed. For early-stage Gambian HAT, pentamidine (4 mg/kg IM for 7 days) is the treatment of first choice, and suramin is thought to be less effective. For late-stage *T.b. gambiense* trypanosomiasis, eflornithine (100 mg/kg IV for 14 days) or melarsoprol (2.2 mg/kg IV for 10 days) are equally effective ($\approx$95%), but the latter is more toxic (5% mortality, compared to 2% with eflornithine). Oral eflornithine is less effective than IV eflornithine, due to its 55% bioavailability and the osmotic diarrhea it induces if more than 75 mg/kg every 6 h is given. For patients with *T.b. rhodesiense* trypanosomiasis, early-stage cases should be treated with suramin (pentamidine is ineffective) and late-stage cases need to be given melarsoprol (eflornithine is ineffective) (2). Despite the lack of controlled trials, most authorities recommend that patients with *T.b. rhodesiense* trypanosomiasis should initially be given a small dose of melarsoprol which is progressively increased thereafter (2). The most dreaded complication of melarsoprol treatment is reactive encephalopathy (4–8%, 15% if the CSF WBC is >100/mm^3) which develops abruptly with grand mal seizures, coma, sometimes pulmonary edema, and a case-fatality rate of 50% within a day or two. It is thought that melarsoprol-induced encephalopathy is caused by an immune reaction triggered by the release of trypanosome antigens, rather than a direct toxicity of the arsenical drug. Prednisolone reduces by two-thirds the risk of encephalopathy without increasing the risk of treatment failure (12–14). Melarsoprol-induced encephalopathy is more common in Rhodesian (5–18%) than in Gambian HAT and mortality during treatment is higher (3–12%) (11).

After treatment, Gambian HAT patients need to be followed up for 2 years with LPs every 6 months (every 3 months during the first year post-treatment for *T.b. rhodesiense* patients). The presence of trypanosomes in the CSF is a clear-cut evidence of a relapse, or treatment failure; however, most relapses are diagnosed only on the basis of an abnormal CSF WCC. Patients should be considered as having post-melarsoprol (or post-eflornithine) relapses if their CSF WCC is greater than 50/mm^3 and higher than the previous determination, or if it is 20–49/mm^3 and higher than the previous one with attendant recurrence of symptoms. When in doubt, the LP should be repeated after 1–2 months. The trend in the CSF WCC is more important than the absolute value since many genuinely cured patients have somewhat elevated CSF WCC 6 months after treatment. After pentamidine or suramin treatment of early-stage HAT, the cut-off for diagnosing a relapse is lower (since the CSF WCC was normal to start with): patients with a CSF WCC greater than 20/mm^3 are considered to be relapsing. Those with borderline results (6–19/mm^3) should be retested earlier than the routine 6-month interval. Rarely, patients having received a prior treatment are found to have trypanosomes in the blood or in a lymph node aspirate at follow-up: most such cases might experience a re-infection with a new strain of trypanosomes rather than a relapse with the original strain.

Measurement of in vitro susceptibility of human-infective trypanosomes to trypanocidal drugs has been carried out only in a few studies, on a limited number of samples. This requires firstly the cultivation of trypanosomes, either through inoculation to a rodent in the field, or cryopreservation of blood or CSF for further analysis in a research laboratory thousands of kilometers away (15). Procyclic trypanosomes can be obtained through the KIVI but this can not be used for determination of drug sensitivity (15). As a result, there is indeed little information concerning laboratory-documented drug resistance in African trypanosomes, and this chapter will rather focus on *treatment failures*, defined with the resources available in African hospitals. We will also review the scanty information available from the bench that enables a better understanding of the mechanisms involved in these treatment failures.

2 Geographic Spread

Because of its low incidence and sporadic occurrence, there have been very few publications allowing an examination of geographical diversity in the frequency of treatment failures after treatment of *T.b. rhodesiense* African trypanosomiasis. In Kenya up to 49% of patients treated with suramin without having had a pre-treatment LP eventually relapsed (16), which underlines that the CSF needs to be examined in all patients, even in those without any neurological symptoms, as suramin is 99.7% protein-bound and therefore has negligible CSF penetration. Similarly disastrous results (64% failure) were obtained in Tanzania on a small number of patients given suramin even though the LP had documented a mildly abnormal $(7–10/mm^3)$ CSF WCC (17). In a small number of Kenyan patients given suramin after LP had shown a normal CSF, 7% relapsed, but in Tanzania 31% (15/49) of similar patients relapsed (16, 17). As reviewed elsewhere, failure rates of 5–10% have been reported after melarsoprol treatment of late-stage *T.b. rhodesiense* trypanosomiais in East Africa (11). The data is obviously too scanty to allow any meaningful conclusion about variation in the rate of treatment failure over time or space.

Because of its higher incidence, there is more information concerning failure rates after treatment of *T.b. gambiense* trypanosomiasis. The failure rate after pentamidine treatment of early-stage Gambian trypanosomiasis documented in Nioki, DRC (where two injections of suramin were also given along with six injections of pentamidine) was identical at 7% among patients treated in 1983–1987 and in those treated in 1988–1992 (18). This mirrors the data from several West African countries in the early 1950s and in the 1960s where the failure rate after pentamidine monotherapy was 7% (11). The failure rate is much higher when pentamidine is used in patients with a slightly abnormal CSF WCC (44% in a recent trial in Uganda) (19), which clearly is a contraindication to the use of pentamidine.

The situation with regard to relapses after melarsoprol treatment of late-stage Gambian trypanosomiasis is more complex and worrying. There are at least three foci where the frequency of post-melarsoprol treatment failures is higher than the 5–8% generally seen elsewhere. In southern Sudan, rates of 18% (unknown location) and 20% (Ibbe) have been reported (20, 21). Not too far from there, a 27% rate of treatment failure has been reported in the Arua focus of NW Uganda (22). Finally, in the M'banza Congo focus of northern Angola, 25% of cases treated with melarsoprol remain parasitologically positive in CSF during treatment or relapse within 1 month (23). It had been mentioned anecdotally that 40% of patients treated with melarsoprol in the early 1970s at the Kimpangu hospital of Zaire relapsed (24). This hospital is located at the border with Angola and many of its patients came from that same Angolan focus. The question is whether rates of treatment failure are indeed going up in these places or merely reflect a long-standing decreased susceptibility to melarsoprol of local strains, which became more obvious when the incidence of the disease shot up. In Angola, it might be the latter scenario. In Uganda and Sudan, there is no published literature about rates of treatment failures prior to these recent reports, and it remains unclear whether the rate of failure increased or has always been that high. In Daloa, Côte d'Ivoire, the failure rate after treatment with melarsoprol was 4% among patients treated in 1986–1992 (25) but there has not been more recent case series. In Nioki, DRC, the frequency of post-melarsoprol relapses remained stable over 20 years (1982–2001), except for an increase in 1996–1998, which was entirely attributable to a much higher rate of failure among patients who received graded dosing of melarsoprol during a clinical trial. It is noteworthy that both in Uganda and northern Angola, graded dosing was also used and one wonders if the high rate of relapses documented in these foci might be merely a consequence of the use of sub-optimal therapeutic regimens.

Among late stage cases of *T.b gambiense* sleeping sickness treated with eflornithine, those from NW Uganda had a much higher rate of treatment failure (27% over 2 years) than those from DR Congo, Congo, and Côte d'Ivoire (3%) (26). This underlines the necessity of a strengthened surveillance system for HAT, in which actuarial rates of treatment failures in large cohorts of patients treated in sentinel centers would be monitored with Kaplan–Meier analyses.

3 Risk Factors for Treatment Failures

With regard to the treatment of early-stage Gambian trypanosomiasis with pentamidine, the main risk factor for treatment failure is having a CSF WCC over $5/mm^3$, indicating CNS involvement. Even among patients with a CSF WCC of $1–5/mm^3$, those at the upper end of this range have a slightly higher risk of treatment failure than those at the lower end (18). There is no difference in the failure rate between men and women but relapse rates tend to be somewhat higher in children (10%) than in adults (7%) (27). Although pentamidine penetrates into the CSF to some extent (28), it is clear that the levels reached in the CSF and in the brain are insufficient to achieve a cure predictably. Thus the problem here is not one of drug resistance, but rather of drug penetration. Similarly, among patients with *T.b. rhodesiense* trypanosomiasis, the main risk factor for failure is having an abnormal CSF WCC to start with, in line with the notion that suramin does not penetrate into the CSF.

For cases of late-stage *T.b. gambiense* trypanosomiasis treated with melarsoprol, studies in Uganda and DRC have shown that the presence of trypanosomes in the CSF and/or in the lymph node aspirate at the moment of the initial diagnosis were independent risk factors for failure of melarsoprol therapy (22, 27). In Nioki, DRC, among 1966 patients treated with melarsoprol between 1982 and 1998, there were two other independent predictors of treatment failure: male sex and residence other than in Baboma/Basengele sub-district. CSF WCC was confounded by CSF trypanosomes and was not by itself associated with treatment failure, in contrast with findings from Uganda (22). The association between CSF trypanosomes and failure of melarsoprol is easy to explain: the pharmacokinetics of melarsoprol have been investigated at last during the last decade and, as later discussed, CSF levels are only a fraction of serum levels, leaving little margin when the parasite is somewhat more resistant than usual. One can only speculate that the same mechanism might apply to trypanosomes in the lymph nodes, as the penetration of melarsorpol in various tissues has never been measured. The vast majority of patients who relapse after a first treatment with melarsoprol, and are treated a second time with melarsoprol, relapse again (11, 22). There is thus a subset of patients whose trypanosomes seem inherently resistant to melarsoprol and who will not be cured by this drug.

There is little information on the risk factors for post-melarsoprol treatment failure in patients with *T.b. rhodesiense* trypanosomiasis. However, in contrast with Gambian HAT, patients who relapse after a first course of melarsoprol are usually cured by a second course of the same drug (11) – perhaps because melarsoprol is then given at the highest dosage of 3.6 mg/kg for 12 injections, with the full dose given from the beginning, in contrast to the slowly increasing dosage recommended (perhaps wrongly so) when the drug is used as a first-line treatment (2). As previously mentioned, there is now evidence from Nioki that a graded dosing of melarsoprol leads to a much higher risk of failure, and this should be avoided. It is clear however that the "new regimen" of 2.16 mg/kg for ten daily injections on consecutive days is as effective as the traditional schemes with 1-week drug-free intervals.

Eflornithine is ineffective in patients with *T.b. rhodesiense* trypanosomiasis, even when administered at twice the normal dosage. It is thus intriguing that a higher failure rate was noted in *T.b. gambiense* patients treated in NW Uganda (26), the only country where both species are present. Strains from NW Uganda have been characterized and only *T.b. gambiense* was found, but two isolates showed reduced susceptibility to eflornithine and one wonders if local strains could have ornithine decarboxylase characteristics which are intermediate between *T.b. rhodesiense* and *T.b. gambiense*. Unfortunately, no HIV serology was obtained; anecdotal reports suggest that HIV co-infected patients do poorly when treated with eflornithine (11), but it seems unlikely that HIV prevalence could have been so much higher in NW Uganda than else-

where to account for these findings. In this multicenter study, the presence of trypanosomes in the lymph node aspirate was also an independent risk factor for treatment failure (hazard ratio [HR] 4.1); this time, a CSF WCC >100/mm^3 was also associated with treatment failure (HR: 3.5) while the presence of CSF trypanosomes was of borderline significance (HR: 1.9) (26). Eflornithine is less effective in children who experience a failure rate two to three times higher than adults (26, 27) and children should thus be given higher doses (125–150 mg/kg every 6 h for 14 days). There is no significant difference in the failure rate between men and women. For new cases, eflornithine clearly needs to be given for 14 days; a 7-day regimen results in a failure rate up to 6 times higher than the standard 14-day course (26). Administration of the drug as 200 mg/kg q12h also led to a higher rate of failure (11): it seems that drug levels need to be maintained continuously above some threshold.

4 Pharmacokinetics and Laboratory Diagnosis of Resistance

Twenty-four hours after the administration of melarsoprol, plasma levels are in the range of 2–4 µg/ml, while CSF levels range from 0.02 to 0.07 µg/ml (29–31). Discrepancies between results obtained with a bioassay and with HPLC indicate that melarsoprol is transformed into metabolites with parasiticidal activity (31). These levels can be compared with in vitro susceptibility. Twelve isolates of *T.b. gambiense* from NW Uganda had a higher minimal inhibitory concentration (MIC) (0.009–0.072 µg/ml) than two isolates from Côte d'Ivoire (0.001–0.018 µg/ml); the higher MIC of 0.072 µg/ml was superior to levels that can be expected in CSF (32). In an attempt to investigate causes of treatment failures in northern Angola, melarsoprol pharmacokinetics was investigated: there was no difference between patients with melarsoprol-refractory HAT and those who responded to melarsoprol (30). Unfortunately, isolates from this focus have not been worked up in the laboratory. Similarly, in Uganda, median melarsoprol concentrations in new cases of HAT and in patients who relapsed following melarsoprol treatment were identical in plasma (24 h after last dose: 1.8 and 1.6 µg/ml respectively) and in CSF (0.023 and 0.025 µg/ml) (15). IC$_{50}$ were measured in *T.b. gambiense* isolates from Côte d'Ivoire and Uganda; they did not differ significantly between those who had relapsed after melarsoprol and those who had been cured with this drug, but overall the IC values were much higher in the isolates from Uganda than in those from Côte d'Ivoire (15). The MIC of a small number of *T. b. rhodesiense* isolates, all from SE Uganda, tested for in vitro susceptibility were lower (0.001–0.007) than those of the strains of *T.b. gambiense* from NW Uganda (33, 34). Isolates of *T.b. rhodesiense* from patients with post-melarsoprol relapses had a tenfold-higher MIC (0.02–0.07 μg/ml) (15).

Thus, combining epidemiological data and in vitro measures, the following can be deduced. To achieve cure of patients with late-stage *T.b. gambiense* or *T.b. rhodesiense* trypanosomiasis, one needs to get drug levels in the CSF (and thus in the CNS) that are substantially higher than the MIC. It is speculative to extend this to trypanosomes but the paradigm in the treatment of bacterial meningitis is that the levels of the antibiotic in the CSF must be 10 times the MIC. Treatment failures after melarsoprol are thus more common in countries where the MIC tends to be higher, as the CSF levels of melarsoprol are not predictably several-fold higher than the MIC. Treatment failures are less common with *T.b. rhodesiense* as the MICs of this subspecies, with a limited distribution, are lower. It seems plausible that the same mechanism of suboptimal tissue penetration must underlie the higher failure rate in patients with trypanosomes in lymph node aspirates, specially considering that investigations made with modern imaging techniques in patients treated in industrialized countries have shown that there are important lymphadenopathies not only in the cervical area but in the thorax and the abdomen as well (35). Genetically determined differences in drug metabolism are not involved in variations in rates of treatment failures among countries. The lower efficacy of graded dosing must reflect the delay in obtaining CSF melarsoprol levels that are high enough to achieve a cure. Whether the rate of treatment failure in some areas, and the MIC_{90} of local strains, are actually going up remains unclear. A number of factors might have contributed to slowing down the emergence of melarsoprol-resistant strains: the drug is used only for the treatment of trypanosomiasis, patients have been probably over-treated for decades (36), and patients with post-melarsoprol relapses, who tend to have trypanosomes only in the CSF and not in the blood, are presumably not very infectious.

The same paradigm can explain treatment failures after treatment of early-stage *T.b. gambiense* HAT with pentamidine or of *T.b. rhodesiense* HAT with suramin. Suramin has a half-life of 44–54 days, with plasma levels of over 100 μg/ml for several weeks (37), but is 99.7% protein-bound and its CSF penetration is negligible (38). In patients with African trypanosomiasis treated with ten IM injections of the dimesylate salt of pentamidine, the median half-life was 22.4 h after the first dose and 47.1 h after the final dose (28). Renal clearance corresponded to 2.5–5% of plasma clearance. Pentamidine CSF levels are only 0.5–0.8% of plasma levels (28). In such circumstances, as soon as the parasite invades the CNS, perhaps in some cases even before the cell count of CSF obtained by lumbar puncture goes up, drug levels in the CNS are not high enough to achieve a cure predictably. It is worth remembering, as shown 50 years ago, that almost one-third of patients with a lumbar CSF WCC ≤ 3 show a WCC

≥ 10/mm^3, which is frankly abnormal, when CSF is obtained by a cisternal tap (39), and that trypanosomes appear in the CSF from cisternal tap earlier than that obtained by lumbar puncture (39).

Eflornithine has good CNS penetration and mean CSF/plasma ratios were 0.91 in adults and 0.41 in children (40). Its elimination half-life is 3.3 h and 81% of its elimination is through renal clearance as unchanged drug. CSF levels were 17–165 nmol/ml in adults and 5–70 nmol/ml in children (40). Treatment failures occurred only in patients with CSF levels ≤50 nmol/ml (40). Thus despite its good CSF penetration, there is little margin between what is obtained in the CSF and what is needed; the same might also be true for eflornithine levels in lymph nodes. Children experience a higher relapse rate than adults probably because using the same dosage per kg than in adults result in under-dosing due to their higher creatinine clearance. Given that the drug has a 55% bioavailability when given orally, it becomes difficult to get CSF levels that are high enough when this mode of administration is used. The lack of clinical efficacy of eflornithine in patients with *T.b. rhodesiense* trypanosomiasis is not surprising considering that in *T.b. rhodesiense* strains from SE Uganda, the eflornithine MIC (25–50 μg/ml) was much higher than in *T.b. gambiense* isolates from NW Uganda (1.25–6.25 μg/ml) and from Côte d'Ivoire (1.6–6.3 μg/ml) (34, 35). This intrinsic resistance of *T.b. rhodesiense* to eflornithine is thought to be a consequence of shorter half-life and faster turnover of ornithine decarboxylase compared to the *T.b. gambiense* subspecies (41); therapeutic levels can not be achieved in the CSF, even if the dosage is doubled.

5 Mechanisms of Resistance

Suramin inhibits a large number of enzymes but its antitrypanosomal mode of action is unknown. Suramin resistance can be induced in mice by administration of subcurative doses of the drug. The cellular target of pentamidine is unknown but its uptake is carrier-mediated, corresponding to the inosine-insensitive P2 nucleoside transporter which is also the route of entry of arsenicals, and to two other transporters (42, 43). Glycolytic kinases of trypanosomes were initially suggested as primary targets of melarsoprol. Melarsoprol was later shown to interact with thiol groups of several proteins. Interactions between melarsoprol and the parasite-specific glutathione-spermidine conjugate trypanothione might be of more physiological relevance, and trypanothione is required to maintain a reduced environment within the cell, but whether trypanothione is indeed the main target of melarsoprol remains debated. Mutations in the P2 nucleoside transporter lead to decreased uptake of arsenicals (44) and cross-resistance to diamidines due to a decreased uptake of pentamidine (45), but it seems clear that mutations in the TbAT1 gene are not the only factor explaining post-melarsorpol relapses (46). Cross-resistance between melarsoprol and pentamidine has been described in the laboratory (47), but in clinical practice the vast majority of patients who relapse after pentamidine treatment of early-stage *T.b. gambiense* trypanosomiasis are cured by melarsoprol – perhaps because the failure of pentamidine was not due to reduced sensitivity of the parasite, but to unrecognized CNS involvement and insufficient pentamidine levels in this end organ.

The mechanisms underlying treatment failures after eflornithine treatment of *T.b. gambiense* trypanosomiasis have not been investigated but considering the mode of action of the drug and what is known concerning *T.b. rhodesiense*, it would seem likely that some alteration in the dynamics of ornithine decarboxylase might be involved. Differences in levels of *S*-adenosyl-L-methionine, also involved in the synthesis of polyamines, may be responsible for the lower susceptibility of *T.b. rhodesiense* to eflornithine. A greatly enhanced uptake of ornithine was observed in eflornithine-resistant *T.b. brucei*, thus competing with eflornithine for ODC and leading to sufficient biosynthesis of polyamines and of trypanothione. Reduced drug accumulation has also been proposed as a mechanism of resistance.

6 Treatment Alternatives

Patients who relapse after having received pentamidine for early-stage Gambian HAT should be treated with eflornithine or melarsoprol. Patients who relapse after melarsorpol treatment of late-stage *T.b. gambiense* trypanosomiasis should be treated with eflornithine and vice-versa. For the rare patients who relapse after having received melarsoprol once and eflornithine once, a combination of eflornithine and melarsoprol should be given. In a single case report these two drugs were given simultaneously (48). Such patients should probably be given 14 days of IV eflornithine and melarsoprol. Nifurtimox monotherapy is very unsatisfactory; the combination of melarsoprol and nifurtimox (15 mg/kg) might also be considered in relapsing cases, but high toxicity can be expected (19) and this combination has not been tested in patients with post-melarsoprol relapses, among whom the MIC might be higher, offering less potential for synergism.

Patients who relapse after suramin treatment of early-stage treatment of Rhodesian HAT should be treated with melarsoprol. Most patients who relapse after melarsoprol treatment of Rhodesian HAT are cured by a second course of the same drug. They should then be given 12 injections (three series of four daily injections) with the maximal dosage of

3.6 mg/kg for all injections. For the unfortunate patients who relapse a second time, a combination of melarsoprol and nifurtimox might be considered, but this is purely empirical.

7 Disease Control

The control of *T.b. gambiense* trypanosomiasis relies mainly on the identification in and treatment of the human reservoir during case-finding surveys (1). Vector control can be used in high-incidence foci, but this is expensive and difficult to sustain over many years. *T.b. rhodesiense* trypanosomiasis is a zoonosis with a large animal reservoir, the treatment of which (e.g. cattle) is often required. During epidemics, vector control can be considered and has also been used with some success to decrease the risk among tourists who visit the game parks of East Africa (6).

References

1. Pépin J, Méda H (2001). The epidemiology and control of human African trypanosomiasis. Adv Parasitol 49:71–132.
2. World Health Organization (1998). Control and Surveillance of African Trypanosomiasis. WHO Technical Report Series No 881, Geneva.
3. World Health Organization (2000). The World Health Report 2000: Health Systems Improving Performance, Geneva.
4. Ekwanzala M, Pépin J, Khonde N et al. (1996). In the heart of darkness: sleeping sickness in Zaire. Lancet 348:1427–30.
5. Smith DH, Pépin J, Stich A (1998). Human African trypanosomiasis: an emerging public health crisis. Br Med Bull 54:341–55.
6. Jelinek T, Bisoffi Z, Bonazzi L et al. (2002). Cluster of African trypanosomiasis in travelers to Tanzanian national parks. Emerg Infect Dis 8:634.
7. Lejon V, Boelaert M, Jannin J, Moore A, Buscher P (2003). The challenge of *Trypanosoma brucei gambiense* sleeping sickness diagnosis outside Africa. Lancet Infect Dis 3:804–8.
8. Méda HA, Doua F, Laveissière C et al. (1995). Human immunodeficiency virus infection and human African trypanosomiasis: a case-control study in Côte d'Ivoire. Trans R Soc Trop Med Hyg 89:639–43.
9. Truc P, Aerts D, McNamara JJ et al. (1992). Direct isolation of *Trypanosoma brucei* from man and other animals, and its potential value for the diagnosis of Gambian trypanosomiasis. Trans R Soc Trop Med Hyg 86:627–9.
10. Penchenier L, Simo G, Grébaut P, Nkinin S, Laveissière C, Herder S (2000). Diagnosis of human trypanosomiasis, due to *Trypanosoma brucei gambiense* in central Africa, by the polymerase chain reaction. Trans R Soc Trop Med Hyg 94:392–4.
11. Pépin J, Milord F (1994). The treatment of human African trypanosomiasis. Adv Parasitol 33:1–47.
12. Pépin J, Milord F, Guern C et al. (1989). Trial of prednisolone for prevention of melarsoprol-induced encephalopathy in *gambiense* sleeping sickness. Lancet 333:1246–50.
13. Pépin J, Milord F, Khonde N et al. (1995). Risk factors for encephalopathy and mortality during melarsoprol treatment of *T.b. gambiense* sleeping sickness. Trans R Soc Trop Med Hyg 89:92–7.

14. Pépin J, Milord F, Khonde N et al. (1994). *Gambiense trypano-somiasis*: frequency of, and risk factors for, failure of melarsoprol therapy. Trans R Soc Trop Med Hyg 88:447–52.

15. Brun R, Schumacher R, Schmid C, Kunz C, Burri C (2001). The phenomenon of treatment failures in human African trypanosomia-sis. Trop Med Int Health 6:906–14.

16. Wellde BT, Chumo DA, Reardon MJ et al. (1989). Treatment of Rhodesian sleeping sickness in Kenya. Ann Trop Med Parasitol 83 (suppl 1):99–109.

17. Veeken H, Eveling M, Dolmans W (1989). Trypanosomiasis in a rural hospital in Tanzania. A retrospective study of its management and the results of treatment. Trop Geogr Med 41:113–7.

18. Pépin J, Khonde N (1996). Relapses following treatment with early-stage *Trypanosoma brucei gambiense* sleeping sickness with a combination of pentamidine and suramin. Trans R Soc Trop Med Hyg 90:183–6.

19. World Health Organization (2002). Treatment and drug resistance network for sleeping sickness. Report of the 6th steering commit-tee meeting 28–29 May 2002. WHO/CDS/CSR/EPH/2002.20.

20. Olivier G, Legros D (2001). Trypanosomiase humaine africaine: historique de la thérapeutique et de ses échecs. Trop Med Int Health 6:855–863.

21. Moore A, Richer M (2001). Re-emergence of epidemic sleeping sickness in southern Sudan. Trop Med Int Health 6:342–7.

22. Legros D, Evans S, Maiso F, Enyaru JCK, Mbulamberi D (1999). Risk factors for treatment failure after melarsoprol for *Trypanosoma brucei gambiense* trypanosomiasis in Uganda. Trans R Soc Trop Med Hyg 93:439–42.

23. Stanghellini A, Josenando T (2001). The situation of sleeping sick-ness in Angola: a calamity. Trop Med Int Health 6:330–4.

24. Ruppol JF, Burke J (1977). Follow-up des traitements contre la trypanosomiase expérimenté à Kimpangu (République du Zaire). Ann Soc Belg Med Trop 57:481–94.

25. Miézan TW, Djc NN, Doua F, Boa F (2000). Trypanosomose humaine africaine en Côte d'Ivoire: caractéristiques biologiques après traitement. A propos de 812 cas traités dans le foyer de Daloa (Côte d'Ivoire). Bull Soc Pathol Exot 95:362–5.

26. Pépin J, Khonde N, Maiso F et al. (2000). Short-course eflornithine in Gambian trypanosomiasis: a multicentre randomized controlled trial. Bull World Health Organ 78:1284–95.

27. Pépin J, Mpia B, Iloasebe M (2002). *Trypanosoma brucei gam-biense* African trypanosomiasis: differences between men and women in severity of disease and response to treatment. Trans R Soc Trop Med Hyg 96:421–6.

28. Bronner U, Doua F, Ericsson O, Gustafsson LL, Miézan TW, Rais M, Rombo L (1991). Pentamidine concentrations in plasma, whole blood and cerebrospinal fluid during treatment of *Trypanosoma gambiense* infection in Côte d'Ivoire. Trans R Soc Trop Med Hyg 85:608–11.

29. Burri C, Baltz T, Giroud C, Doua F, Welker HA, Brun R (1993). Pharmacokinetic properties of the trypanocidal drug melarsoprol. Chemotherapy 39:225–34.

30. Burri C, Keiser J (2001). Pharmacokinetic investigations in patients from northern Angola refractory to melarsoprol treatment. Trop Med Int Health 6:412–420.

31. Bronner U, Brun R, Doua F et al. (1998). Discrepancy in plasma melarsoprol concentrations between HPLC and bioassay methods in patients with *T. gambiense* sleeping sickness indicates that melarsoprol is metabolized. Trop Med Int Health 3:913–7.

32. Matovu E, Enyaru JCK, Legros D, Schmid C, Seebeck T, Kaminsky R (2001). Melarsoprol refractory *T.b. gambiense* from Omugo, north-western Uganda. Trop Med Int Health 6:407–11.

33. Iten M, Matovu E, Brun R, Kaminsjy R (1995). Innate lack of susceptibility of Ugandan *Trypanosoma brucei rhodesiense* to DL-difluoromethylornithine (DFMO). Trop Med Parasitol 46:190–4.

34. Matovu E, Iten M, Enyary JCK et al. (1997). Susceptibility of Uganda *Trypanosoma brucie rhodesiense* isolated from man and animal reservoirs to diminazene, isometamidium and melarsoprol. Trop Med Int Health 2:13–8.

35. Sahlas DJ, MacLean JD, Janevski J, Detsky AS (2002). Out of Africa. N Engl J Med 347:749–753.

36. Burri C, Nkunku S, Merolle A, Smith T, Blum J, Brun R (2000). Efficacy of a new, concise, schedule for melarsoprol in treatment of sleeping sickness caused by *Trypanosoma brucei gambiense*: a randomised trial. Lancet 355:1419–25.

37. Collins JM, Klecker RW, Yarchoan R et al. (1986). Clinical phar-macokinetics of suramin in patients with HTLV-III/LAV infection. J Clin Pharmacol 26:22–6.

38. Hawking F (1940). Concentration of Bayer 205 (Germanin) in human blood and cerebrospinal fluid after treatment. Trans R Soc Trop Med Hyg 34:37–52.

39. Neujean G, Evens F (1958). Diagnostic et traitement de la maladie du sommeil à *T. gambiense*. Acad R Sci Coloniales 7:33–9.

40. Milord F, Loko L, Ethier L et al. (1993). Eflornithine concentra-tions in serum and cerebrospinal fluid of 63 patients treated for *T.b. gambiense* sleeping sickness. Trans R Soc Trop Med Hyg 87:473–7.

41. Iten M, Mett H, Evans A, Enyaru JCK, Brun R, Kaminsky R (1997). Alterations in ornithine decarboxylase characteristics account for tolerance of *Trypanosoma brucei rhodesiense* to D,L-α-difluromethylornithine. Antimicrob Agents Chemother 41:1922–5.

42. de Koning HP, Jarvis SM (2001). Uptake of pentamidine in *Trypanosoma brucei brucei* is mediated by the P2 adenosine transporter and at least one novel, unrelated transporter. Acta Trop 80:245–50.

43. de Koning HP (2001). Uptake of pentamidine in *Trypanosoma bru-cei brucei* is mediated by three distinct transporters: implications for cross-resistance with arsenicals. Mol Pharmacol 59:586–92.

44. Carter NS, Fairlamb AH (1993). Arsenical resistant trypanosomes lack an unusual adenosine transporter. Nature 361:173–5.

45. Maser P, Sterrlin C, Kralli A, Kaminsky R (1998). A nucleoside transporter from *Trypanosoma brucei* involved in drug resistance. Science 85:242–4.

46. Matovu E, Geiser F, Schneider V et al. (2001). Genetic variants of the TbAT1 adenosine transporter from African trypanosomes in relapse infections following melarsoprol therapy. Mol Biochem Parasitol 117:73–81.

47. Barrett MP, Fairlamb AH (1999). The biochemical basis of arsenical-diamidine cross-resistance in African trypanosomes. Parasitol Today 15:136–40.

48. Simarro P, Asumu PN (1996). Gambian trypanosomiasis and synergism between melarsoprol and eflornithine: First case report. Trans R Soc Trop Med Hyg 90:315.

Chapter 77
Drug Resistance in *Toxoplasma gondii*

Paul F.G. Sims

1 Overview

Toxoplasma gondii is one of the most widely distributed, and thus successful, parasites on earth. It is a protozoan of the phylum Apicomplexa with a particularly broad host range, probably being able to infect any warm blooded animal (1). In such hosts, progress through its asexual replication cycle involves two quite different forms of the parasite: the rapidly proliferating tachyzoite that establishes the initial infection within many different types of host cells and the much more slowly replicating form, the bradyzoite, that maintains infection within a more limited repertoire of cell types, usually throughout the remaining life of the host.

Sexual replication of *T. gondii* occurs only in its definitive host, members of the Felidae or cat family (2, 3). Here, in addition to the products of the asexual cycle, motile male microgametes and female macrogametes are produced in the epithelial cells of the small intestine. After fusion, these develop into thick-walled unsporulated oocysts that are released into the gut and excreted in very large numbers. Sporulation occurs within the environment, outside any host, and generates highly infectious oocysts that contain two sporocysts with four sporozoites within each of them.

Surprisingly, given the widespread distribution of both the parasite and its definitive host, isolates of *T. gondii* are not as genetically heterogeneous as one might expect, predominantly falling into one of three clonal lineages (4). These can be differentiated by the analysis of restriction fragment length polymorphisms within their genomic DNA and are commonly referred to as types I, II and III (5).

Human infection with *T. gondii* occurs in one of two principal ways: consumption of tissue cysts in raw or undercooked meat; or by accidental ingestion of sporulated oocysts from contaminated water, fruit and vegetables (1).

Immunocompetent individuals infected in either of these ways are unlikely to suffer more than mild flu-like symptoms for a week or so and often show no symptoms at all (6). However, the disappearance or absence of symptoms does not equate to the clearance of the parasite from such individuals. Instead it signals the conversion of the tachyzoites to bradyzoites and the development of cysts, generally found within neuromuscular tissues, which mask the large numbers of organisms they contain from attack by the host immune system. It is in this form that the parasite can maintain infection throughout its host's remaining life.

Vertical transmission resulting from congenital infection is another possible route by which the parasite can spread through the human population. This occurs when a mother is infected, for the first time, during pregnancy. Under these circumstances, tachyzoites can cross the placenta, establishing infection of the foetus and possibly giving rise to spontaneous abortion (7). The likelihood of transmission to the foetus is related to the point during pregnancy at which maternal infection occurs, with the greatest risk of transmission associated with infection during the later stages. However, the most severe foetal damage and the highest risk of spontaneous abortion are associated with early infections.

A much smaller but ever growing number of infections arise as a consequence of tissue transplantation. These may result from reactivation of a pre-existing latent infection as a consequence of the immunosupressive treatment associated with tissue transplantation, but more usually occur when a heart or heart–lung from an infected donor is given to a naïve recipient.

With the exception of congenitally acquired infections, the impact of *T. gondii* on a healthy human adult is minimal. However, once infected, most, if not all, individuals retain viable parasites within tissue cysts; a chronic infection that can later become the source of an acute, life-threatening, disease. Thus bradyzoites, periodically released from such cysts, can transform into rapidly dividing tachyzoites. Under normal circumstances, such a recrudescent infection will once again be controlled by the host's immune system. However, if this is compromised in any way, for

P.F.G. Sims (✉)
Manchester Interdisciplinary Biocentre,
University of Manchester, Manchester, UK
p.sims@manchester.ac.uk

D.L. Mayers (ed.), *Antimicrobial Drug Resistance*,
DOI 10.1007/978-1-60327-595-8_77, © Humana Press, a part of Springer Science+Business Media, LLC 2009

instance by HIV infection or immunosuppressive drugs, infection will become acute and, if untreated, fatal. The impact of toxoplasmosis in AIDS patients has, historically, been very significant, with up to 25% reportedly developing toxoplasmic encephalitis (TE) (8) and, although the annual number of deaths ascribed to AIDS in the USA more than halved between 1992 and 1998 because of the successful deployment of highly active antiretroviral therapy, over 300 such deaths in the latter year were still associated with toxoplasmosis (9). Similarly, acute infection has been reported to develop in 57% of heart or heart–lung transplants (10). The increasing use of immunosuppressive therapies associated with transplantation and cancer treatments, and a population whose average age steadily increases, ensures that an ever greater proportion of the human population have compromised immune systems. Thus, the number of individuals currently at severe risk from toxoplasmosis is probably greater than ever before.

2 History, Epidemiology and Clinical Significance of Drug Resistant *T. gondii*

Clinically, acute toxoplasmosis is usually treated with a combination of the antifolate inhibitors, pyrimethamine (Pm) and sulfadiazine (Sdz) although sometimes the former may be replaced with another antifolate, trimethoprim (Tmp), and the latter with the lincosamide antibiotic, clindamycin (Cmn) (11). The drug combinations used for treatment of acute disease are also the usual choice for prophylaxis. However, because none of the inhibitors commonly used for the treatment of primary disease is able to penetrate tissue cysts and thus clear the bradyzoite form of the parasite, lifelong prophylaxis is essential if recrudescent disease is to be prevented in immunosuppressed patients.

Although the general response to treatment is good, 10% of patients may fail to respond within the first 2 weeks (12–14) and three prospective studies report a complete response to therapy in only 18–55% of patients (12, 15, 16). Moreover, a further 10–20% of those who initially respond may relapse during long-term maintenance therapy, irrespective of which of the drug combinations is used (15, 17, 18). The reasons for relapses during prophylaxis are not entirely clear. Many patients suffer unpleasant and sometimes severe side effects (18) and it is likely that a significant proportion can thus be accounted for by non-compliance. However, compliance has been assured in up to 33% of patients relapsing during long-term maintenance therapy (19), demonstrating that acute infections can become established despite the presence of normally active inhibitors. A similar conclusion is suggested by data concerning the success of prophylactic treatment of heart or heart lung transplant patients with Pm (10). Here, 14% of mismatched recipients (seronegative individuals transplanted with an organ from a seropositive donor) suffered toxoplasmosis despite receiving supervised prophylaxis. Although it is conceivable that host factors could account for these prophylactic failures, another possibility is that the parasites responsible for such disease may be drug resistant.

Laboratory studies have demonstrated that strains of *T. gondii* showing significant resistance to a wide range of inhibitors, including those most frequently used in the clinic, can be isolated (20–27). Moreover, exposure to maintenance therapy as parasites periodically cycle between cyst and free-living forms potentially provides almost ideal conditions for the selection of drug resistant variants. Nevertheless, although the potential for the development of drug resistance certainly exists, it has not been a widely recognised clinical problem.

In some respects, the general failure to recognise that drug resistant *T. gondii* may already be causing human disease is surprising. It has been known for more than 10 years that around 10% of all acute AIDS-related cases fail to show any response at all to clinical treatment (12–14) and, recently, the number of bone marrow transplant patients surviving TE has been reported to be as low as 10% (28). In addition to these general observations, a small number of well-documented individual cases have provided rather stronger evidence for the possible involvement of drug resistant parasites in cases of acute human disease. Thus, Willer and Morgello (29) describe several cases of AIDS patients suffering from TE who failed to respond to conventional treatment (using Pm, Sdz or Cmn). Despite such drug treatment, four out of five of these patients were shown, at autopsy, to have active brain lesions containing parasites, leading the authors to describe these as cases of "resistant toxoplasmosis". Similarly, Huber et al. (30) described another compelling case. An HIV-infected patient with a low but detectable titre of anti-toxoplasma antibody in his serum showed no clinical improvement after treatment with Pm + Sdz for 19 days. Since both a CT scan and an increased antibody titre suggested a *T. gondii* infection resistant to this standard therapy, an alternative treatment with Pm + Cmn was initiated. A clinical improvement was noted within 4 days and this was confirmed by a subsequent CT scan. Together, these data strongly suggest that, in some instances, drug resistant infections can arise and, in addition, the last case highlights sulfonamide as the component that may have been compromised.

The uncertainty about the possible involvement of drug resistant *T. gondii* in human disease has recently been removed (31). Consistent with the suggestion made above, this study presents unequivocal data showing that the

T. gondii parasites associated with a fatal human infection were resistant to the sulfonamide constituent of the Pm + Sdz clinical formulation. Although it was sought, no evidence of resistance to Pm was found. The basis of this study was an extensive PCR analysis of parasites associated with cases of human toxoplasmosis. This enabled the identification of a number of different alleles of the *T. gondii dhps* gene, part of a bifunctional unit that encodes two enzymes of the folate biosynthetic pathway, one of which, dihydropteroate synthase (DHPS), is the molecular target of the sulfonamides. When heterologously expressed in *E. coli*, three of the *dhps* alleles identified in this study were found to encode DHPS enzymes that were sensitive to Sdz. These probably represent the type I, II and III allelic variants of this locus. However, another of the alleles, found associated with a fatal human infection, produced a highly Sdz-resistant enzyme although it differed from one of the variants, experimentally shown to encode a drug sensitive enzyme, by only a single amino acid change. Critically, this same amino acid residue was found to be unchanged in any of the other drug sensitive enzymes but it was seen to be the only amino acid difference between one of them and that encoded in a line of *T. gondii* showing high-level laboratory-induced sulfonamide resistance. Furthermore, mutations affecting the equivalent residues in the *dhps* genes of both the human malaria parasite, *Plasmodium falciparum* (32), and the AIDS-related opportunist pathogen *Pneumocystis carinii* (33), have been implicated in sulfonamide resistance.

3 Laboratory Diagnosis of Drug Resistant Infections

Because of the range of rather non-specific symptoms that can arise as a result of *T. gondii* infection, firm diagnosis is almost always dependent upon laboratory testing. Most of the commonly used diagnostic methods involve serological analyses simply designed to detect anti-parasite antibodies. Unfortunately, such tests provide no insight to the drug sensitivity status of any infection that might thus be demonstrated. However, although not as convenient or as reliable, alternative diagnostic methods that rely on direct detection of parasites rather than serology are also available. With some modification these methods can indicate drug sensitivity. For example, it is possible to culture parasites from clinical material and then directly determine the drug sensitivity profile of a particular parasite. However, establishing such cultures from solid tissue or blood samples is both difficult and time-consuming and together these factors effectively preclude the use of cell culture-based methods for routine diagnosis.

PCR-based methods have also been successfully used to demonstrate the presence or absence of parasite DNA in clinical samples, normally by the amplification of genes encoding surface antigens. By targeting, and subsequently determining, the DNA sequence of genes known to be associated with the development of drug resistance, it has been demonstrated that such methodology can rapidly provide the type of information from which the drug resistant status of *T. gondii* parasites can be established (31). Moreover, it has been further shown that such PCR-based methodology can yield important information on parasite genotype using primary samples from a wide range of clinical materials, including peripheral blood, solid tissue, amniotic and cerebrospinal fluids (34). Thus, although subject to problems associated with the potential for contamination and its inability to discriminate between viable and dead parasites, PCR can offer a useable route to the identification of resistant infections for drugs whose molecular targets are known.

As described above and currently implemented (34), the PCR-based method for the diagnosis of drug resistant *T. gondii* infections is of limited utility and needs to be improved significantly. Thus, identification of drug resistance in this way is dependent on the identification of DNA sequence alterations that have previously been causally linked with such resistance. Any novel sequence alteration that might be found could be associated with resistance, but it could equally well represent a DNA sequence polymorphism that has no involvement whatsoever in drug resistance. Coupling the existing PCR procedure to a direct functional analysis of the amplified sequence would enable rapid identification of any resistance allele, whether previously known or novel. Technology of this type could be applied to the analysis of primary clinical samples and would represent a valuable advance in our ability to both quickly diagnose potentially life-threatening infections and to further investigate the origin and prevalence of such parasites.

4 Treatment Alternatives

The antifolate combination of Pm + Sdz is by far the most common treatment for toxoplasmosis. However, as described above, the effectiveness of the latter component can be compromised by an alteration to the drug target. Cmn can be used to replace Sdz in combination with Pm but this formulation is generally reported to be less effective and suffers the disadvantage that it does not prevent *Pneumocystis carinii* pneumonia (35). This is a significant additional benefit that is conferred by Pm + Sdz and which is particularly important in the case of AIDS patients. However, some 40% of such patients are unable to tolerate long-term exposure to the latter combination (16) and, although Cmn is not itself without problems in this respect, this benefit may be more apparent than real.

Because it is a safe inhibitor with no known side effects on the foetus, Spiramycin has found wide acceptance in the treatment of infections acquired during pregnancy, primarily because it is particularly effective in preventing transmission from the mother to the foetus (36). However, this inhibitor is not very effective in the treatment of established foetal infections (37) or for the treatment of toxoplasmosis in the immunosuppressed (38). Moreover, it persists in the tissues for a long time, increasing the likelihood that drug resistant parasites may be selected during treatment. Its wider use in the treatment of toxoplasmosis thus offers little.

All of the inhibitors considered above share a serious defect with respect to their utility against *T. gondii*. None of them is able to cross the wall of tissue cysts and they are thus unable to attack the bradyzoite form of the parasite found there. In contrast, Atovaquone (Atq), an hydroxynapthoquinone, and the macrolide azithromycin (Azi) are both active against encysted parasites as well as the intracellular, tachyzoite form (35, 39, 40). Although both of these drugs have been identified as useful against ocular toxoplasmosis (41, 42), this is again principally because they are better tolerated by patients rather than because of significantly improved performance over the standard Pm + Smz therapy. A similar outcome is seen when either Atq or Azi is deployed against acute TE (43, 44). Even more disappointing is the poor performance of these two inhibitors when used for maintenance therapy. When used in this way, they have been associated with increased relapse rates (43, 45). This is both surprising and very disappointing, since one might expect that being able to access parasites within tissue cysts would provide these inhibitors with a potentially crucial advantage in this role.

The conclusions we can draw concerning possible alternative therapies are thus depressing. None of the clinically useful alternatives to Pm + Sdz offers significantly improved effectiveness although, in general, they are more readily tolerated by patients. In addition, although only Sdz is known to have been clinically compromised by the development of resistant parasites, laboratory experiments have shown that *T. gondii* can become resistant to all of the inhibitors discussed above and it thus seems likely that, in the clinical setting, the development of resistance to these inhibitors will follow any widespread deployment.

5 Infection Control Measures

The work of Aspinall et al. (31) has established that drug resistant forms of *T. gondii* can contribute to human disease. In the light of this result, it is now important to ask how such

strains arise and what proportion of human infections are associated with drug resistant parasites. Given the life cycle of the parasite and, in the case of the immunosuppressed, the need for long-term maintenance therapy, drug resistant *T. gondii* infections could potentially arise in one of two ways. Both infection with parasites that are already drug resistant and the acquisition of drug resistance by previously sensitive parasites in response to prophylactic treatment, are formally possible. It is important to note that these two possibilities have different implications with respect to the likely future development of drug resistant toxoplasmosis as a more widespread clinical problem. Whilst post-infection selection of resistance is likely to have a devastating effect on the individual concerned, its implications for the community at large are minimal since, except for the limited numbers of congenital and transplant associated infections, there is no human to human transmission of *T. gondii*. On the other hand, evidence of infection with already resistant parasites would indicate the presence, within the environment, of parasites with the potential to create large numbers of ongoing drug resistant infections within the human population.

The sulfonamide resistant parasites identified by Aspinall et al. (31) were associated with a fatal congenital infection and the relevant medical records document the seroconversion of the mother during the first trimester. It is also clear from these records that no sulfonamide was used in the treatment of this patient during her pregnancy. It thus seems probable that, in this case, infection was due to a parasite that was already sulfonamide resistant. The very limited data currently available thus suggest that there may indeed be a reservoir of drug resistant parasites within the environment that are already causing human death and disease. Where might this be located and how could such parasites arise?

Ingested tissue cysts or oocysts are by far the most common sources of human infection. Both of these forms of the parasite are ultimately derived from animals kept either on farms, for meat production, or as domestic pets, respectively. It is these animals therefore that constitute the environmental reservoir from which the vast majority of primary infections of humans originate. Unfortunately, because of their low cost and the broad spectrum of microorganisms against which they are active, sulfonamides have been, and still are, widely used in veterinary medicine (46). Their residues can be readily detected in meat from animals reared world-wide (47, 48) and, presumably as a consequence of their usage, resistance to sulfonamides is very commonly seen amongst bacterial isolates from pigs, cattle, dogs and cats (49–51). It is thus entirely possible that sub-optimal drug treatment regimes within the veterinary sector could also have led to the selection of resistant forms of *T. gondii* in just the same way that these other sulfonamide resistant micro-organisms have presumably arisen. Once established in farm or domestic animals, transfer of resistant parasites to the human population would be almost inevitable. Indeed, the observations of Aspinall et al. (31) that are described above, strongly suggest that this may already be happening.

In conclusion, although it seems likely that drug resistant *T. gondii* currently pose some threat to the human population, this is not yet a major problem. However, this may well change and monitoring the presence of resistant parasites, particularly in food products, would thus seem a prudent public health measure.

Acknowledgments The author would like to thank current and past colleagues at UMIST and the University of Manchester, particularly Professor John Hyde and Dr Tanya Aspinall, and staff of the Toxoplasma Reference Unit, Singleton Hospital, Cardiff for their contributions to underpinning research described in this article.

References

1. Tenter, A. M., Heckeroth, A. R. & Weiss, L. M. (2000). *Toxoplasma gondii*: from animals to humans. *Int. J. Parasitol.* **30**, 1217–1258.

2. Dubey, J. P., Miller, N. L. & Frenkel, J. K. (1970). The *Toxoplasma gondii* oocyst from cat feces. *J. Exp. Med.* **132**, 636–662.

3. Dubey, J. P., Miller, N. L. & Frenkel, J. K. (1970). Characterization of the new fecal form of *Toxoplasma gondii*. *J. Parasitol.* **56**, 447–456.

4. Howe, D. K. & Sibley, L. D. (1995). *Toxoplasma gondii* comprises 3 clonal lineages – correlation of parasite genotype with human-disease. *J. Infect. Dis.* **172**, 1561–1566.

5. Howe, D. K., Honore, S., Derouin, F., et al. (1997). Determination of genotypes of *Toxoplasma gondii* strains isolated from patients with toxoplasmosis. *J. Clin. Microbiol.* **35**, 1411–1414.

6. Ho-Yen, D. O. (2001). Infection in the immunocompetent. In: *Toxoplasmosis: a comprehensive clinical guide* (Joynson, D. H. M. & Wreghitt, T. G., eds.), Cambridge University Press, Cambridge, UK, pp. 125–146.

7. Thulliez, P. (2001). Maternal and foetal infection. In *Toxoplasmosis: a comprehensive clinical guide*. (Joynson, D. H. M. & Wreghitt, T. G., eds.), Cambridge University Press, Cambridge, UK, pp. 193–213.

8. Luft, B. J. & Remington, J. S. (1992). Toxoplasmic encephalitis in AIDS. *Clin. Infect. Dis.* **15**, 211–222.

9. Jones, J. L., Sehgal, M. & Maguire, J. H. (2002). Toxoplasmosis-associated deaths among human immunodeficiency virus-infected persons in the United States, 1992–1998. *Clin. Infect. Dis.* **34**, 1161.

10. Couvreur, J., Tournier, G., Sardetfrismand, A., et al. (1992). Heart or heart–lung transplantation and toxoplasmosis. *Presse Med.* **21**, 1569–1574.

11. Joynson, D. H. M. & Wreghitt, T. G. (eds.) (2001). *Toxoplasmosis: a comprehensive clinical guide*. Cambridge University Press, Cambridge, UK.

12. Luft, B. J., Hafner, R., Korzun, A. H., et al. (1993). Toxoplasmic encephalitis in patients with the acquired immunodeficiency syndrome. *N. Engl. J. Med.* **329**, 995–1000.

13. Porter, S. B. & Sande, M. A. (1992). Toxoplasmosis of the central nervous system in the acquired immunodeficiency syndrome. *N. Engl. J. Med.* **327**, 1643–1648.

14. Renold, C., Sugar, A., Chave, J. P., et al. (1992). Toxoplasma encephalitis in patients with the acquired immunodeficiency syndrome. *Medicine (Baltimore)* **71**, 224–239.

15. Katlama, C., De Wit, S., O'Doherty, E., et al. (1996). Pyrimethamine-clindamycin vs. pyrimethamine-sulfadiazine as acute and long-term therapy for toxoplasmic encephalitis in patients with AIDS. *Clin. Infect. Dis.* **22**, 268–275.

16. Dannemann, B., McCutchan, J. A., Israelski, D., et al. (1992). Treatment of toxoplasmic encephalitis in patients with AIDS. A randomized trial comparing pyrimethamine plus clindamycin to pyrimethamine plus sulfadiazine. *Ann. Intern. Med.* **116**, 33–43.

17. Pedrol, E., Gonzalezclemente, J. M., Gatell, J. M., et al. (1990). Central-nervous-system toxoplasmosis in AIDS patients – efficacy of an intermittent maintenance therapy. *AIDS* **4**, 511–517.

18. Leport, C., Tournerie, C., Raguin, G., et al. (1991). Long-term follow-up of patients with AIDS on maintenance therapy for toxoplasmosis. *Eur. J. Clin. Microbiol. Infect. Dis.* **10**, 191–193.

19. Walckenaer, G., Leport, C., Longuet, P., et al. (1994). Recurrence of cerebral toxoplasmosis in 15 AIDS patients. *Ann. Med. Interne.* **145**, 181–184.

20. Sander, J. & Midtvedt, T. (1971). Development of sulphonamide resistance in *Toxoplasma gondi*. *Acta Pathol. Microbiol. Scand. [B] Microbiol. Immunol.* **79**, 531–533.

21. Camps, M., Arrizabalaga, G. & Boothroyd, J. (2002). An rRNA mutation identifies the apicoplast as the target for clindamycin in *Toxoplasma gondii*. *Mol. Microbiol.* **43**, 1309–1318.

22. McFadden, D. C., Camps, M. & Boothroyd, J. C. (2001). Resistance as a tool in the study of old and new drug targets in Toxoplasma. *Drug Resist. Updat.* **4**, 79–84.

23. Pfefferkorn, E. R., Borotz, S. E. & Nothnagel, R. F. (1992). *Toxoplasma gondii* – characterization of a mutant resistant to sulfonamides. *Exp. Parasitol.* **74**, 261–270.

24. Pfefferkorn, E. R., Nothnagel, R. F. & Borotz, S. E. (1992). Parasiticidal effect of clindamycin on *Toxoplasma gondii* grown in cultured-cells and selection of a drug-resistant mutant. *Antimicrob. Agents Chemother.* **36**, 1091–1096.

25. Pfefferkorn, E. R., Borotz, S. E. & Nothnagel, R. F. (1993). Mutants of *Toxoplasma gondii* resistant to atovaquone (566c80) or decoquinate. *J. Parasitol.* **79**, 559–564.

26. Reynolds, M. G., Oh, J. & Roos, D. S. (2001). In vitro generation of novel pyrimethamine resistance mutations in the *Toxoplasma gondii* dihydrofolate reductase. *Antimicrob. Agents Chemother.* **45**, 1271–1277.

27. Pfefferkorn, E. R. & Borotz, S. E. (1994). Comparison of mutants of *Toxoplasma gondii* selected for resistance to azithromycin, spiramycin, or clindamycin. *Antimicrob. Agents Chemother.* **38**, 31–37.

28. Krouwer, H. G. J. & Wijdicks, E. F. M. (2003). Neurologic complications of bone marrow transplantation. *Neurol. Clin.* **21**, 319–352.

29. Willer, J. & Morgello, S. (1993). Therapy-resistant cerebral toxoplasmosis – a clinicopathological study. *J. Neuropathol. Exp. Neurol.* **52**, 271.

30. Huber, W., Bautz, W., Classen, M., et al. (1995). Cerebral toxoplasmosis in AIDS resistant to pyrimethamine and sulfadiazine. *Dtsch. Med. Wochenschr.* **120**, 60–64.

31. Aspinall, T. V., Joynson, D. H. M., Guy, E., et al. (2002). The molecular basis of sulfonamide resistance in *Toxoplasma gondii* and implications for the clinical management of toxoplasmosis. *J. Infect. Dis.* **185**, 1637–1643.

32. Triglia, T., Wang, P., Sims, P. F. G., et al. (1998). Allelic exchange at the endogenous genomic locus in *Plasmodium falciparum* proves the role of dihydropteroate synthase in sulfadoxine-resistant malaria. *EMBO J.* **17**, 3807–3815.

33. Lane, B. R., Ast, J. C., Hossler, P. A., et al. (1997). Dihydropteroate synthase polymorphisms in *Pneumocystis carinii*. *J. Infect. Dis.* **175**, 482–485.

34. Aspinall, T. V., Guy, E. C., Roberts, K. E., et al. (2003). Molecular evidence for multiple *Toxoplasma gondii* infections in individual patients in England and Wales: public health implications. *Int. J. Parasitol.* **33**, 97–103.

35. McCabe, R. E. (2001). Antitoxoplasma chemotherapy. In: *Toxoplasmosis: a comprehensive clinical guide* (Joynson, D. H. M. & Wreghitt, T. G., eds.), Cambridge University Press, Cambridge, UK, pp. 319–359.

36. Couvreur, J., Desmonts, G. & Thulliez, P. (1988). Prophylaxis of congenital toxoplasmosis. Effects of spiramycin on placental infection. *J. Antimicrob. Chemother*. **22**, 193–200.

37. Wong, S. Y. & Remington, J. S. (1994). Toxoplasmosis in pregnancy. *Clin. Infect Dis*. **18**, 853–861.

38. Leport, C., Vilde, J. L., Katlama, C., et al. (1986). Failure of spiramycin to prevent neurotoxoplasmosis in immunosuppressed patients. *JAMA* **255**, 2290.

39. Araujo, F. G., Huskinson-Mark, J., Gutteridge, W. E., et al. (1992). In vitro and in vivo activities of the hydroxynaphthoquinone 566C80 against the cyst form of *Toxoplasma gondii. Antimicrob. Agents Chemother*. **36**, 326–330.

40. Araujo, F. G., Guptill, D. R. & Remington, J. S. (1988). Azithromycin, a macrolide antibiotic with potent activity against *Toxoplasma gondii. Antimicrob. Agents Chemother*. **32**, 755–757.

41. Pearson, P. A., Piracha, A. R., Sen, H. A., et al. (1999). Atovaquone for the treatment of toxoplasma retinochoroiditis in immunocompetent patients. *Ophthalmology* **106**, 148–153.

42. Bosch-Driessen, L. H., Verbraak, F. D., Suttorp-Schulten, M. S. A., et al. (2002). A prospective, randomized trial of pyrimethamine and azithromycin vs pyrimethamine and sulfadiazine for the treatment of ocular toxoplasmosis. *Am. J. Ophthalmol*. **134**, 34–40.

43. Jacobson, J. M., Hafner, R., Remington, J., et al. (2001). Dose-escalation, phase I/II study of azithromycin and pyrimethamine for the treatment of toxoplasmic encephalitis in AIDS. *AIDS* **15**, 583–589.

44. Fung, H. B. & Kirschenbaum, H. L. (1996). Treatment regimens for patients with toxoplasmic encephalitis. *Clin. Ther*. **18**, 1037–1056.

45. Katlama, C., Mouthon, B., Gourdon, D., et al. (1996). Atovaquone as long-term suppressive therapy for toxoplasmic encephalitis in patients with AIDS and multiple drug intolerance. *AIDS* **10**, 1107–1112.

46. Schwarz, S. & Chaslus-Dancla, E. (2001). Use of antimicrobials in veterinary medicine and mechanisms of resistance. *Vet. Res*. **32**, 201–225.

47. Bjurling, P., Baxter, G. A., Caselunghe, M., et al. (2000). Biosensor assay of sulfadiazine and sulfamethazine residues in pork. *Analyst* **125**, 1771–1774.

48. Bermudez-Almada, M. D., Miranda-Vasquez, L., Espinosa-Plascencia, A., et al. (2001). Sulfonamide residues in muscle of pigs slaughtered in the Northwest of Mexico. *Rev. Cient. (Maracaibo)* **11**, 127–132.

49. Lanz, R., Kuhnert, P. & Boerlin, P. (2003). Antimicrobial resistance and resistance gene determinants in clinical *Escherichia coli* from different animal species in Switzerland. *Vet. Microbiol*. **91**, 73–84.

50. Chang, C. F., Yeh, T. M., Chou, C. C., et al. (2002). Antimicrobial susceptibility and plasmid analysis of *Actinobacillus pleuropneumoniae* isolated in Taiwan. *Vet. Microbiol*. **84**, 169–177.

51. Perreten, V. & Boerlin, P. (2003). A new sulfonamide resistance gene (sul3) in *Escherichia coli* is widespread in the pig population of Switzerland. *Antimicrob. Agents Chemother*. **47**, 1169–1172.

Chapter 78
Drug Resistance in the Sheep Nematode Parasite *Haemonchus contortus*, Mechanisms and Clinical Perspectives

Marleen H. Roos

1 Overview

The parasitic nematode *H. contortus*, a sheep intestinal parasite, has caused serious problems in sheep husbandry and thus production losses for a long time. Although estimation of total cost is difficult, in Australia costs of treatment and loss of production in sheep and cattle were estimated to range around USD 300 million annually in 1990 (1) and this has increased during the years as more expensive drugs were needed to battle the resistance. Therefore, ways to try control this parasite have been many, ranging from changes in maintenance (non-invasive) to the use of broad spectrum drugs or anthelmintics (invasive). These anthelmintics are active against several species of intestinal nematode parasites. In the last 50 years, the development of broad-spectrum anthelmintics by pharmaceutical industries has caused their predominant use over other, usually more laborious, methods. Although in the beginning the new anthelmintics were very effective, treatment failures were reported after a few years of use for all the main nematode parasite species. These failures were met with higher drug doses, but the benefit of that was short-lived. Researchers, pharmaceutical industries and farmers had to recognize that these drugs were selecting for parasites that were resistant to the drugs (for a review see (2, 3). *H. contortus* has been mostly used as a model to study the development and mechanisms of anthelmintic resistance because this parasite was often the first to become resistant and it is the most harmful sheep parasite, as it can kill sheep within a few days. Furthermore, its size is relatively large compared to other species and the life cycle can be reproduced in the laboratory using sheep. Therefore, this parasite species will be discussed here in detail.

There are three main groups of broad-spectrum anthelmintics on the market with cross-resistance among the members of the different groups. They are, in chronological sequence of development in the last 50 years of the previous century:

(a) benzimidazoles (BZ), (b) levamisole (LEV), pyrantel and morantel, and (c) avermectins/milbemycins (IVM) (4–6). For *H. contortus*, another drug, closantel, is available. This is because *H. contortus* is a blood feeder (5).

Benzimidazoles were found to bind to beta-tubulin and inhibit the assembly of microtubules (7). There is a differential binding when compared to the host because binding to host beta-tubulin is lower, to the degree that the concentration that affects nematodes does not affect host mammals. The deleterious effect of BZ was first discovered on fungi and benzimidazole resistance (BZR) in fungi was found to be caused by single point mutations dispersed over the beta-tubulin gene (8). One of these mutations was also identified in BZR parasitic nematodes (9, 10) and can be used as a diagnostic tool (11).

Levamisole and pyrantel were found to act as agonists of nicotinic acetylcholine receptors in the parasitic nematodes. Several of these receptors have been characterized in *H. contortus* and other parasitic nematode species, but the mutation(s) causing resistance have so far not been identified. Resistance tests therefore have to rely on faecal egg reduction tests (FERT) or larval development assays (LDA) that are less sensitive than a PCR (12, 13).

Avermectins/milbemycins were found to interfere with the membrane transporters such as P-glycoprotein. Several other membrane transporters have been characterized, but mutation(s) causing resistance have so far not been identified (14, 15). As for LEV, the resistance tests have to rely on FERT and LDA.

Closantel (CLS), a proton ionophore, is effective against blood-feeding parasites such as *H. contortus*. This parasite has developed resistance to this drug, but the mechanism of the resistance is not known (5).

Managing drug resistance in parasitic nematodes is hampered in the first place by the lack of sensitive tests for LEV, IVM and CLS resistance. Since BZR is now widespread and LEV is not in use anymore because of effective dosing problems and CLS only is effective against *H. contortus*, IVM is mostly the drug of choice. As there are no new drugs in the pipeline for the next few years, it is imperative to develop

M.H. Roos (✉)
Director, RoosProjectConsult, Hulshorst, The Netherlands
m.h.roos@planet.nl

sustainable methods to keep sheep husbandry profitable (4). This is more urgent as the development of anthelmintic resistance seems to be the result of selection of resistant genotypes that are already present in the nematode population. New drugs would thus again select for resistant parasites within a few years.

2 History of Geographical Spread

Sheep and cattle husbandry is a means of income worldwide for farmers. They all have serious problems with production losses caused by intestinal helminth parasites (worms). In the second part of the twentieth century, three groups of broad-spectrum drugs were developed. These three groups had different mechanisms of action and for each drug resistance was reported after a few years of use. This was especially the case for sheep worms as sheep are often used for purposes other than food production such as wool. In that case, there are less restrictions on the use of anthelmintics. Furthermore, the sheep worm *H. contortus* can kill sheep within a few days; for cattle no such worm exists. At the end of the twentieth century, *H. contortus* populations existed that were resistant to all modern anthelmintic groups (16, 17).

Initially, drug resistance was probably confined to the farm where the resistance had developed, but by trading sheep resistance was spread to other farms. In the case of BZR, this spread could be analysed as the mechanism of resistance is known to be correlated with a mutation in the beta-tubulin tub-1 gene. Molecular analysis of the chromosome regions around this beta-tubulin gene of *H. contortus* by RFLP has indicated that the DNA sequences of the surrounding regions differed when the resistant parasites came from different countries and regions (18, 19). Although no RFLP differences were found between susceptible populations from the Netherlands and the United Kingdom, resistant populations from the Netherlands, the United Kingdom, Zimbabwe and the U.S.A. were clearly different from each other. In addition, a population from Scotland was identical to the three resistant populations isolated in the Netherlands, but one isolated in south of England was different from all others. This indicates that these beta-tubulin genes, carrying the identical mutation for resistance, were independently selected in the different countries.

Further analysis of the genes involved in BZ resistance indicated that the mutation in beta-tubulin isotype 1 caused the lower level of resistance, and was the first mutation to be selected by BZ. At higher levels of resistance, selection on another beta-tubulin gene was found to be involved isotype 2. These mechanisms were identified in a laboratory-selected population, but also in a field-selected population in the Netherlands. Other unknown mechanisms of resistance were also present at higher levels of resistance (20). In Australia, multiple mechanisms for resistance to IVM were identified and they were dependent on the different selection protocols (21). It is not clear whether the different mechanisms were correlated to the different levels of resistance (22, 23). The geographical spread of these different mechanisms is not clear.

In vitro selection for resistance to all the drugs seems to be possible all over the world, since BZR selection could be carried out on *H. contortus* populations that had never been in contact with the anthelmintic. The same point mutation in β-tubulin isotype 1 was selected after four generations. Beta-tubulin isotype 2 was also found to be involved (9, 20). In vivo selection for LEV resistance from a susceptible population from Zimbabwe that had presumably never been treated with anthelmintic drugs was possible and a very high resistance was identified after six generations (23). Laboratory selection for IVM resistance required eight generations or less (21, 22, 24). These selections appeared to be stable as little or no reversion was found without drug pressure. This seems to be due to the fact that the selected populations are not less fit than the susceptible ones (25). No reversion of resistance to BZ was found after 6 years of LEV use (26). Apparently, mutations coding for resistance to these drugs are present in the genome of all parasite populations tested and can be selected to the degree that no reversion is possible, indicating that no susceptible alleles were left in the population. The gene frequency of the resistance genes in untreated populations is not known as the tests so far are not sensitive enough to detect this.

The genetic polymorphism of *H. contortus* is extensive as indicated by the fact that no effect was visible on the level of the total genetic polymorphism of the parasite populations after selection for anthelmintic resistance (27). This has made it very difficult to detect mutations for resistance to the other drugs.

Anthelmintic resistance, as a result of drug use, has now been identified all over the world. It is to be expected that all nematode parasite populations are able to respond to the drugs with resistance. Therefore, the geographical spread of anthelmintic resistance is more the result of geographical spread of anthelmintics than of resistant parasites.

3 Epidemiology

The life cycle of *H. contortus* determines in a large degree the epidemiology and spread of infections. It starts on the field as the eggs develop via L1 and L2 to the third larval stage or L3 in about a week. Eggs can survive on the field for several weeks when circumstances are not favourable for development. The third larval stage is the infective stage for sheep. The sheep ingest the L3 during grazing as the L3 larvae move to the top of the grass blade. The ingested L3 develop into the L4 and L5 stages in adults in about 20 days in the abomasum. There, they feed on host blood, up to 12 µl per adult worm per day. The adults start to reproduce and the sheep shed the eggs in the faeces on the field. *H. contortus* is a prolific egg layer, up to 10,000 eggs per day, so new infection is constant (28).

The life cycle indicates that closed flocks develop resistance independent from flocks on other farms. Resistance can spread only by selling sheep, carrying resistant worms, to other farmers. It is therefore very important to make sure that newly introduced sheep on the farm do not carry resistant worms. This is carried out by faecal egg counts. If nematode eggs are found, a drug should be used to kill the worms. However, a negative egg count may not prevent the importation of sheep carrying resistant worms. There is a special stage in the life cycle that incites the L3 parasites stop their development to L4 in the sheep. This happens when the conditions on the field are not favourable for growth on the field of the eggs to L3. This inhibited stage happens in moderate zones in the fall where the worms survive the winter in the host; and in dry regions in the spring where they survive the dry summer in the host. It is not clear how this development to the inhibited L3 stage is triggered. During this inhibited stage, the infected sheep do not shed eggs and the inhibited L3 larvae are less sensitive to drugs probably because their metabolism is at a very low level. Therefore, it is difficult to be absolutely sure that a sheep, introduced on the farm, does not carry (resistant) parasites (28).

Climatic circumstances and flock isolation may increase the selection pressure of drugs on the parasites as has been shown by Papadopoulos et al. (29). In general, when a sheep flock is treated only part of the worm population is treated and under selection pressure, since part of the worm population is on the field and will not be treated: the refugia. The presence of refugia diminishes the selection pressure on the worm population. When sheep are treated before the dry summer or the cold winter with temperatures below 0°C, the part of the worm population on the field will be killed by the drought or frost, respectively. In that case, the total worm population is in the sheep and will be under selection pressure. The same is true when sheep, after being treated, are moved to a freshly mowed or clean pasture. As the not-treated worm field population is removed by mowing, there is no dilution with not-treated worms, i.e. no refugia. In these cases, development of resistance can happen after a few generations. Communal grazing, where farmers treat their part of the community of sheep, seems to select to a slower degree for resistance as the refuge is not only on the field but also in the untreated sheep (29).

Although anthelmintic resistance was detectable after a few years of use of the drugs (2, 3), the fact that the sheep usually were treated without moving to a clean pasture afterwards, with the refugia on the field intact, seems to have delayed the development of resistance. Without these refugia, anthelmintic resistance development would probably have been much faster as can also be shown by using models (30, 31).

4 Clinical Significance

H. contortus is a parasite that penetrates the abomasum lining to feed on blood of the host. The clinical signs are anaemia for H. contortus and diarrhoea for other nematode species. Under certain climatic conditions, infections with *H. contortus* can be massive, up to a few thousand adults. This parasite is the only nematode that can kill the host in a few days by causing anaemia. Even older sheep, that usually can handle a moderate infection due to acquired immunity, may die from a massive infection that can break down immunity. Especially, lambs are vulnerable during the first 6 months of their lives as they cannot develop immunity to *H. contortus* during this period (28). Therefore, the clinical significance of drug resistance in *H. contortus* is very high. As outlined in the previous chapter, drug resistance is probably inherent to drug use in *H. contortus*. This is why other, more sustainable and integrated, methods to control the parasites are urgently needed (32).

5 Laboratory Diagnosis

Diagnosis of anthelmintic resistance is usually carried out on the free living parasite stages, the eggs and the L3 larvae (33). Knowledge about the mechanisms of resistance against the specific drugs in the specific parasite species is needed in order to develop specific tests to diagnose anthelmintic resistance. If these could be developed on the basis of PCRs, this would mean tests for each of the above three nematode species and tests for each of the three main groups of anthelmintics. However, only for BZ resistance these tests were developed for a few species (9, 11, 13) as too little is know about the mechanisms of resistance to LEV and IVM. In addition, sheep have usually been treated, alternatingly, with more than one group of anthelmintics, so diagnosis has to always include tests on the three main groups of anthelmintics. Therefore, the laboratory diagnosis has to rely on less-sensitive tests that use (a) counting of eggs in faeces or (b) development of eggs to L3 in vitro, before and after treatment with each of the three groups of anthelmintics. The advantage is that no previous knowledge is required about the nematode species; the disadvantage of these tests is that resistance is usually only diagnosed when 25% of the parasites is already resistant (34).

The first (a) is the faecal egg count reduction test (FECRT). This means that eggs are counted in faeces before and after drug treatment (35). However, it is not clear which parasite species are involved, as eggs are very similar between the species A worm population with a reduction of eggs lower than 95% by the drug is considered resistant. At this stage, the drug is not of much use anymore for *H. contortus*, as it is a prolific egg layer and the infection will soon return to the same level as before treatment. This test is used for all known drugs and all known parasitic nematodes that excrete eggs in the faeces.

The second group consists of in vitro assays on the basis of development of eggs to L3. At this stage, the species can be identified. Either the egg hatch assay (EHA) or larval development assay (LDA) are used to test resistance to the drugs BZ and LEV (23). Freshly acquired eggs are incubated for 2 days with increasing amounts of the drug. The drug concentration at which only half the eggs hatch is calculated. This drug concentration is compared to one determined for a susceptible population and the degree of resistance is found. Both tests have the disadvantage that a considerable part of the worm population may be resistant before the resistance is discovered, especially if the resistance is recessive. For *H. contortus*, a specific test is available based on the fact that this nematode feeds on sheep blood. The resulting anaemia can be monitored with the FAMACHA. The colour of the mucous membrane of the eyes of sheep is diagnostic for the amount of adult worms in the abomasum (36). In this way, the effect of drugs can be measured.

A specific drug test for the resistance to benzimidazoles is available as a specific PCR test could be developed because of the fact that the resistance has been traced to a point mutation(s) in the beta-tubulin genes (9). This test is still in the experimental stage and not commercially available (11). For avermectins and levamisole no such specific tests are available as the exact mechanism or mutations, causing resistance, are not known even after extensive research (33). This may be due to the fact that *H. contortus* is genetically very polymorphic (27) and comparing susceptible and resistant populations does not show a difference even when the genes known to be involved in the mechanism of the drugs are compared (14, 37).

6 Treatment Alternatives and Infection Control Measures

Treatment alternatives have to be sustainable in order to be useful in the long run. As eradication of the parasites seems to be a remote possibility, equilibrium needs to be reached between cost of control and production losses. This means that integrated control is needed, using all possible means like treatment alternatives and infection control measures, to delay the further development of anthelmintic resistance (32, 38, 39). Although the parasite–host interaction are very complex and many varieties unknown, computer modelling studies may be of help as field experiments are very expensive. They could indicate which combination of drugs, vaccines, biological control means and management procedures would delay resistance and still be profitable for the farmer. Strategic drug management was investigated using these models. The first lesson was to treat as little as possible. Furthermore, simultaneous administration of drug from groups with different action mechanisms was shown to delay the drug resistance while alternation had little effect. Furthermore, allowing for refugia, i.e. not treating part of the worm population was shown to delay the development of resistance and leave susceptible worms in the population. (30, 40–42). Another method to delay anthelmintic resistance that has shown promising results is to replace resistant parasites by feeding susceptible worms to the sheep under controlled circumstances (43).

The integration of new drugs with a novel mode of action in sustainable control systems could be very important. The development of cyclooctadepsipeptides looks very promising (44). The anthelmintic efficacy of several plant extracts was tested and a few of those suggest possible utilization by livestock farmers (45–47). Marine bryozoans produce nematicidal alkaloids that look promising (48–50).

A biological method to control the parasitic nematodes has been developed using nematophagus fungus *Duddingtonia flagrans* to kill the nematode eggs on the pasture. It has been tried out under several circumstances in several parts of the world and could be a valuable part of a sustainable control system (51, 52). This method can be used as an alternative for drugs in drug-resistant worm populations (32). In addition, for organic farmers this would be a feasible method.

The enhancement of the immune system of sheep to parasites has been shown to be an effective control method. This can be carried out in several ways. The first way is better feeding of the sheep. Sheep that are fed with protein supplements are less susceptible to worm infections and the immune system was shown to be involved (53–55). The enhanced immunity was also found during the preparturient period of the ewes. Another way is the breeding of sheep for genetic resistance to nematode parasites which was shown to reduce the infection in the sheep and on the field. The mechanism was found to be an enhanced immune reaction to the parasites (56, 57). Modelling techniques predict that parasite evolution, in response to selective breeding for resistance in the host to parasites, is less than the risks arising from other control strategies such as anthelmintics (58). An additional method, involving enhancement of the immunity against nematode parasites, would be the vaccination against the worms. This has been the subject of extensive research using proteins from different parts and stages of the parasites (59, 60). So far, no 100% effective vaccines have been developed. According to the models, a 70% effective vaccine, when part of an integrated control system, could delay the development of anthelmintic resistance (30). However, in recent years a lot of new knowledge has been gathered on the immunobiology of the host–parasite interactions that allow new vaccine strategies to be considered. Functional genomic techniques such as gene expression analysis by microarrays and gene knock-out technologies have potential to provide high throughput and rapid screening methods. These methods will not only have implications for vaccine research, but also provide novel targets for drug development and genetic selection (61–64). It has to be kept in mind, however, that a highly effective vaccine may cause vaccine-driven selection on antigenic variants of the parasite and may render the vaccine less effective (65). Although these results are from bacteria, there is no reason to suppose that this development will not happen in parasitic nematodes.

A successful and sustainable control of parasitic worms will have to rely on the integration of both drug treatments that are very carefully designed and on other infection control measures. The sustainable control systems will be different in the different geographical regions as the climate, geology and the way of small ruminant farming are different. Computer modelling will be of great help and will show the way to improved worm control and a delay in anthelmintic resistance, integrating new control measures.

References

1. Bird J. The antiparasitics market. Anim. Pharmacol. 1991; S7: 1–14.
2. Kaminsky R. Drug resistance in nematodes: a paper tiger or a real problem? Curr. Opin. Infect. Dis. 2003; 16:559–564.
3. Shoop WL. Ivermectin resistance. Parasitol. Today 1993; 7: 154–159.
4. Horton J. Global anthelmintic therapy programs: learning from history. Trends Parasitol. 2003; 19: 405–409.
5. Martin RJ, Robertson AP, Bjorn H. Target sites of anthelmintics. Parasitology 1997; 114: S111–S124.
6. Croft SL. The current status of antiparasitic chemotherapy. Parasitology 1997; 114:S3–S15.
7. Lacey E, Prichard RJ. Interactions of benzimidazoles (BZ) with tubulin from BZ-sensitive and BZ-resistant isolates of *Haemonchus contortus*. Mol. Biochem. Parasitol. 1986; 19:171–181.
8. Koenraadt H, Sommerville SC, Jones AL. Characterization of mutations in the beta-tubulin gene of benomyl-resistant field strains of *Venturia inaequalis* and other pathogenic fungi. Mol. Plant Pathol. 1992; 82:1348–1354.
9. Kwa MSG, Veenstra JG, Roos MH. Benzimidazole resistance in *Haemonchus contortus* is correlated with a conserved mutation at amino acid 200 in beta-tubulin isotype 1. Mol. Biochem. Parasitol. 1994; 63:299–303.
10. Kwa MSG, Veenstra JG, Roos MH. Beta-tubulin genes from the parasitic nematode *Haemonchus contortus* modulate drug resistance in *Caenorhabditis elegans*. J. Mol. Biol. 1995; 246:500–510.
11. Elard L, Cabaret J, Humbert JF. PCR diagnosis of benzimidazole-susceptibility or – resistance in natural populations of the small ruminant parasite *Teledorsagia circumcincta*. Vet. Parasitol. 1999; 80:231–237.
12. Robertson AP, Bjorn HE, Martin RJ. Pyrantel resistance alters nematode nicotinic acetylcholine receptor single-channel properties. Eur. J. Pharmacol. 2000; 94:1–8.
13. Sangster N, Batterham P, Chapman HD, et al. Resistance to antiparasitic drugs: the role of molecular diagnosis. Int. J. Parasitol. 2002; 32:637–653.
14. Yates DM, Portillo V, Wolstenholme AJ. The avermectin receptors of *Haemonchus contortus* and *Caenorhabditis elegans*. Int. J.Parasitol. 2003; 33:1183–1193.
15. Smith JM, Prichard RK. Localization of p-glycoprotein mRNA in the tissues of *Haemonchus contortus* adult worms and its relative abundance in drug-selected and susceptible strains. J. Parasitol. 2002; 88:612–662.
16. Van Wyk JA, Stenson MO, Van der Merwe JS, et al. Anthelmintic resistance in South Africa: surveys indicate an extremely serious situation in sheep and goat farming. Onderstepoort J. Vet. Res.1999; 66:273–284.
17. Chandrawathani P, Waller PJ, Adnan M, Hoglund J. Evolution of high-level, multiple resistance on a sheep farm in Malaysia. Trop. Anim. Health Prod. 2003; 35:17–25.
18. Kwa SG, Veenstra JG, Roos MH. Molecular characterization of β-tubulin genes present in benzimidazole resistant populations of *Haemonchus contortus*. Mol. Biochem. Parasitol. 1993; 60:133–144.
19. Roos MH, Boersema JH, Borgsteede, FHM, et al. Molecular analysis of selection for benzimidazole resistance in the sheep parasite *Haemonchus contortus*. Mol. Biochem. Parasitol. 1990; 43:77–88.
20. Kwa SG, Kooyman FJN, Boersema JH, Roos MH. Effect of selection for benzimidazole resistance in *Haemonchus contortus* on β-tubulin isotype 1 and isotype 2 genes. Biochem. Biophys. Res. Commun. 1993; 191:413–419.
21. Gill JH, Kerr CA, Shoop WL, Lacey E. Evidence of multiple mechanisms of avermectin resistance in *Haemonchus contortus*-comparison of selection protocols. Int. J. Parasitol.1998; 28:738–789.
22. Le Jambre L, Gill JH, Lenane IJ, Lacey E. Characterization of an Avermectin resistant strain of Australian *Haemonchus contortus*. Int. J. Parasitol. 1995; 25:691–698.
23. Hoekstra R, Visser A, Wiley L, et al. Characterization of an acetylcholine receptor gene of *Haemonchus contortus* in relation to levamisole resistance. Mol. Biochem. Parasitol. 1997; 89:179–187.
24. Egerton JR, Suhayda D, Eary CH. Laboratory selection of *Haemonchus contortus* for resistance to ivermectin. J. Parasitol. 1988; 76:614–617.
25. Elard L, Sauve C, Humbert JF. Fitness of benzimidazole-resistant and – susceptible worms of *Teledorsagia circumcincta*, a nematode parasite of small ruminants. Parasitology 1998; 117:571–578.
26. Borgsteede FHM, Duyn SPJ. Lack of reversion of a benzimidazole resistant strain of *Haemonchus contortus* after six years of Levamisole usage. Res. Vet. Sci. 1989; 47:270–272.
27. Otsen M, Hoekstra R, Plas M, et al. Amplified fragment length polymorphism analysis of genetic diversity of *Haemonchus contortus* during selection for drug resistance. Int. J. Parasitol. 2001; 31:1138–1143.
28. Bowman DD, Lynn RC. Georgis' Parasitology for veterinarians. 1995; W.B. Saunders Company, Philadelphia, pp 165–176.
29. Papadopoulos E, Himonas C, Coles GC. Drought and flock isolation mat enhance the development of anthelmintic resistance in nematodes, Vet. Parasitol. 2001; 97:253–259.
30. Barnes EH, Dobson RJ, Barger IA. Worm control and anthelmintic resistance: adventures with a model. Parasitol. Today 1995; 11:56–63.

31. Van Wyk JA. Refugia – overlooked as perhaps the most potent factor concerning the development of anthelmintic resistance. Onderstepoort J. Vet. Res. 2001; 68:55–67.

32. Waller PJ. International approaches to the concept of integrated control of nematode parasite livestock. Int. J. Parasitol. 1999; 29:155–164.

33. Taylor MA, Hunt KR, Goodyear KL. Anthelmintic resistance detection methods. Vet. Parasitol. 2002; 109:29–43.

34. Jackson F. Anthelmintic resistance – the state of the play. Br. Vet. J. 1993; 149:123–138.

35. Coles GC, Bauer C, Borgsteede FHM, et al. World Association for the Advancement of Veterinary Parasitology (WAAVP) methods for the detection of anthelmintic resistance in nematodes of veterinary importance. Vet. Parasitol. 1992; 44:35–44.

36. Van Wyk JA, Bath GF. The FAMACHA system for managing haemonchosin sheep and goats by clinically identifying individual animals for treatment. Vet. Res. 2002; 33:509–529.

37. Hoekstra R, Visser A, Wiley L, et al. Characterization of an acetylcholine receptor gene of *Haemonchus contortus* in relation to levamisole resistance. Mol. Biochem. Parasitol. 1997; 89:179–187.

38. Coles GC. Sustainable use of anthelmintics in grazing animals. Vet. Rec. 2002; 151:165–169.

39. Van Wijk JA, Coles GC, Krecek RC. Can we slow the development of anthelmintic resistance? An electronic debate. Trends Parasitol. 2002; 18:336–337.

40. Leathwich DM, Vlassoff A, Barlow ND. A model for nematodiasis in New Zealand lambs: the effect of drenching regime and grazing management on the development of anthelmintic resistance. Int. J. Parasitol. 1995; 25:1479–1490.

41. Smith G, Grenfell BT, Isham V, Cornell S. Anthelmintic resistance revisited: under-dosing, chemoprofylactic strategies, and mating probabilities. Int. J. Parasitol. 1999; 29:93–94.

42. Hastings IM. Modelling parasite drug resistance: lessons for management and control strategies. Trop. Med. Int. Health 2001; 6:883–890.

43. Bird J, Shulaw WP, Pope WF, Bremer CA. Control of anthelmintic resistant endoparasites in a commercial sheep flock through parasite community replacement. Vet. Parasitol. 2001; 97:219–225.

44. Harder A, Schmitt-Wrede HP, Krucken J, et al. Cyclooctadepsipeptides – an anthelmintically active class of compounds exhibiting a novel mode of action. Int. J. Antimicrob. 2003; 22:318–331.

45. Alawa CB, Adamu AM, Gefu JO, et al. In vitro screening of two Nigerian medicinal plants (*Veronia amygdalina* and *Annona senegalensis*) for anthelmintic activity. Vet. Parasitol. 2003; 113:59–63.

46. Pessoa LM, Morais SM, Bevilaqua CM, Luciano JH. Anthelmintic activity of essential oil of *Ocimum gratissimum Linn.* and eugenol against *Haemonchus contortus*. Vet. Parasitol. 2002; 109:59–63.

47. Paolini V, Bergeaud JP, Grisez C, et al. Effects of condensed tannins on goats experimentally infected with *Haemonchus contortus*. Vet. Parasitol. 2003; 113:253–261.

48. Narkowics CK, Blackman AJ, Lacey E, et al. Convolutindole A and Convolutamine H, new nematicidal brominated alkaloids from the marine bryozoan *Amantha convoluta*. J. Nat. Prod. 2002; 65:938–941.

49. Capon RJ, Skene C, Liu EH, et al. The isolation of novel nematicidal dithiocyanates from an Australian marine sponge, *Oceania* sp. J. Org. Chem. 2001; 66:7765–7769.

50. Vuong D, Capon RJ, Lacey E, et al. Onnamide F: a new nematicide from a southern Australian marine sponge, *Trachycladus laevispirulifer*. J. Nat. Prod. 2001; 64:640–642.

51. Chandrawathani P, Jamnah O, Waller PJ, et al. Nematophagus fungi as a biological control agent for nematode parasites of small ruminants in Malaysia: a special emphasis on *Duddingtonia flagrans*. Vet. Res. 2002; 33:685–696.

52. Larsen M. Biological control of helminths. Int. J. Parasitol. 1999; 29:139–146.

53. Coop RL, Kyriazakis I. Nutrition-parasite interactions. Vet. Parasitol. 1999; 84:187–204.

54. Strain SA, Stear MJ. The influence of protein supplementation on the immune response to *Haemonchus contortus*. Parasite Immunol. 2001; 23:527–531.

55. Kahn LP, Knox MR, Gray GD, et al. Enhancing immunity to nematode parasites in single-bearing Merino ewes through nutrition and genetic selection. Vet. Parasitol. 2003; 112:211–225.

56. Gauly M, Kraus M, Vervelde L, et al. Estimating genetic differences in natural resistance in Rhon and Merinoland sheep following experimental *Haemonchus contortus* infection. Vet. Parasitol. 2002; 106:55–67.

57. Strain SA, Bishop SC, Henderson NG, Kerr A, et al. The genetic control of IgA activity against *Teledorsagia circumcincta* and its association with parasite resistance in naturally infected sheep. Parasitology 2002; 124:545–552.

58. Bishop SC, Stear MJ. Modelling of host genetics and resistance to infectious diseases: understanding and controlling infections. Vet. Parasitol. 2003; 115:147–166.

59. Kox DP, Redmond DL, Newlands GF, et al. The nature and prospects for gut membrane proteins as vaccine candidates for *Haemonchus contortus* and other ruminant trichostrongyloids. Int. J. Parasitol. 2003; 33:1129–1137.

60. Meeusen ET, Piedrafita D. Exploiting natural immunity to helminth parasites for the development of veterinary vaccines. Int. J. Parasitol. 2003; 33:1285–1290.

61. Yatsuda AP, Krijgsveld L, Cornelissen AWC, et al. Comprehensive analysis of the secreted proteins of the parasite *Haemonchus contortus* reveals extensive sequence variation and differential immune recognition, J. Biol. Chem. 2003; 278:16941–16951.

62. Cowman AF, Crabb BS. Functional genomics: identifying drug targets for parasitic diseases. Trends Parasitol. 2003; 19:538–543.

63. Boyle JP, Yoshino TP. Gene manipulation in parasitic helminths. Int. J. Parasitol. 2003; 33:1259–1268.

64. Goeringer UH, Homann M, Lorger M. In vitro selection of high-affinity nucleic acid ligands to parasite target molecules. Int. J. Parasitol. 2003; 33:1309–1317.

65. Mastrantonio P, Spigaglia P, Van Oirschot H, et al. Antigenic variants in *Bordetella pertusisstrains* isolated from vaccinated and unvaccinated children. Microbiology 1999; 145:2069–2075.

Section L
Measurements of Drug Resistance

Chapter 79
In Vitro Performance and Analysis of Combination Anti-infective Evaluations

Robert W. Buckheit and R. Dwayne Lunsford

1 Introduction

The evaluation of the activity of combinations of two or more anti-infective compounds has gained significant prominence in light of the innate ability of many infectious organisms to rapidly acquire drug resistance. Pathogens react to the administration of anti-infective agents by the outgrowth of preexisting infectious clones with resistance-engendering mutations and by the accumulation of new mutations to allow an escape from the suppressive effects of therapeutic drug regimens (1). Resistance emerges through the error-prone mechanisms of the replicative machinery and through the transmission of resistance elements (2, 3), rendering mono-therapeutic drug strategies problematic. Combination chemotherapy significantly decreases the risk that resistance will arise. In addition, a combination chemotherapy may ameliorate toxicity by permitting lower, less toxic, or non-toxic concentrations of synergistic drugs to be utilized.

In convergent combination therapy (4, 5), the drugs used in this combination, target the same functional protein or enzyme and there is the possibility that lower doses of the individual drugs might be used. A specific therapeutic regimen of several drugs that target multiple essential steps in the replication of the organism is sometimes referred to as divergent drug therapy (5). This strategy benefits from the possibility that organisms resistant to one of the drugs in the combination therapy will remain completely sensitive to the others, whereas cross-resistance may emerge when the drugs inhibit the same replication target. In some cases, targeting the same enzyme or protein may still be considered a divergent therapy since the target may include multiple sites for anti-infective action. An example would be the use of nucleoside and nonnucleoside reverse transcriptase inhibitors in the treatment of infection by the human immunodeficiency virus (HIV) (6).

Another advantage of the combination therapy strategies is that multiple infectious organisms can be targeted (7). The prevalence of co-infections involving HIV is increasing (8) and it is critical to understand the effects of the HIV therapeutic agents when used in patients that are also administered agents targeting hepatitis C virus (HCV) or other opportunistic bacterial and fungal infections, including tuberculosis. Similarly, respiratory infections often include both viral and bacterial components (9) and thus it is important to understand the effects of drug interactions on the efficacy and toxicity of the agents targeting the individual agents.

Finally, though most in vitro combination assays involve the evaluation of efficacy, the evaluation and understanding of combined toxicity is of importance as the therapy moves into the clinical stage (10). For both efficacy and toxicity, the dose response curve that is evaluated in vitro must define the drug interactions over a broad checkerboard pattern of drug concentrations. This thorough analysis allows the investigator to define the interactions at multiple drug ratios and identify the dose response areas where different and distinct efficacy and toxicity interaction regions exist. For example, the combination nucleoside strategy of AZT and Ribavirin employed in HIV therapy results in two completely different regions of interaction between the drugs, with a region of extreme synergistic antiviral activity giving way to a region of significant antagonistic antiviral activity (11). Since the combination drug concentrations employed in the in vitro assays can only be truly evaluated at those concentrations that yield less than or equal to the maximal 100% protection as evaluated from replication or growth of the infectious organism, the combination assays often are performed at concentrations which are much lower than those that would be utilized in the clinic and thus are inadequate for truly evaluating toxicity or efficacy effects at high concentrations. Separate assays at appropriate drug concentrations should always be performed to evaluate toxicity effects in parallel with efficacy evaluations.

In the discussion below, the methodology routinely used to define combination anti-infective evaluations is described.

R.W. Buckheit (✉)
ImQuest BioSciences, Inc., Frederick, MD, USA
rbuckheit@imquest.com

D.L. Mayers (ed.), *Antimicrobial Drug Resistance*,
DOI 10.1007/978-1-60327-595-8_79, © Humana Press, a part of Springer Science+Business Media, LLC 2009

Evolving from the early use of isobolograms and the evaluation of combination chemotherapy strategies for use in cancer patients (12, 13), the combination interaction evaluations used in the past two decades for anti-infective research have primarily involved one of the two methods: the three-dimensional surface models as described by Prichard and Shipman (14) and the median dose effect equation developed by Chou and Talalay (15). A detailed discussion of the primary methodology considerations and analysis alternatives for the performance of combination anti-infective assays will be provided, followed by a discussion of assay modifications that should be employed to fully define the effects of a drug combination regimen. The novel variations of the standard combination assays described, provide a greater understanding of the effects of combination therapy in the cellular and tissue environments where the interactions will occur.

From the perspective of effective and efficient drug development it is critical to understand both the benefits and limitations of the assay methodologies used to evaluate drug combination interactions and the meaning of the results that are obtained. For combination assays, the in vitro analyses are reasonably straightforward, though adequate assay repetition must be used in order to truly and quantitatively determine the interaction of multiple chemotherapeutic agents. Translating in vitro data to in vivo utility is difficult in the light of the natural pharmacokinetic variation in drug concentrations that occur in patients, but several pharmacokinetic models have been described that allow a greater understanding of the relevance and predictability of the in vitro results (16–18). It is also important to appreciate how these combination data will be viewed by regulatory agencies prior to clinical testing. From a regulatory viewpoint, it is fair to say that the absence of synergistic toxicity and/or antiviral antagonism should carefully be evaluated and confirmed, as synergistic or additive results will be dependent on the dose and regimen used in the clinic and may not be predictable from in vitro assays (19).

2 Methods

2.1 Definition of the Dose–Response Curve and Selectivity Index for the Drugs Evaluated

Determination of the efficacy and toxicity of drug interactions requires the appropriate cell-based or biochemical/ enzymatic assay and accurate statistical evaluation. The assays utilized for the combination drug evaluations should be chosen carefully based on the proposed use of the drugs in the clinical setting. In some cases, both cell-based and biochemical assays (20, 21) are required to fully understand the combined effects of the drugs. Evaluation in multiple cell types, including fresh and established human cells, may be necessary depending on the target-cell specificity of the infectious organism.

The starting point for all in vitro evaluations of combination drug interactions is the precise determination of the dose response curve for each of the individual agents that will make up the combination therapy in the appropriate assay model. The assay or assays will yield efficacy values at the 25, 50, 90, 95, and 99% level (EC_{25}, EC_{50}, EC_{90}, EC_{95}, and EC_{99}, respectively). It is these efficacy concentrations that will be used in the combination assay methodology to set the correct dose response surface to be evaluated in a checkerboard pattern of drug concentrations. Additionally, it is important to understand the concentrations of the test compound that cause direct cytotoxicity or cytostasis, yielding 25, 50, 90, 95, and 99% inhibition of cell growth (IC_{25}, IC_{50}, IC_{90}, IC_{95}, and IC_{99} concentration values, respectively). Upon definition of the efficacy and toxicity values for a drug across its dose response curve, the selectivity (or therapeutic) index of the drugs can be calculated (SI_{25}, SI_{50}, SI_{90}, SI_{95}, or SI_{99}); the SI is obtained by calculating the ratio of the IC concentration to the EC concentration at a defined level of protection (IC_x/EC_x) where x is defined as the percent level of protection achieved (20).

The evaluation of the interaction of two drugs requires the selection of a dose response curve for each of the test agents that begins at doses below a concentration yielding any biological effect and increasing in concentration until complete inhibition of the replication of the infectious organism is achieved. Once the dose response curves for each individual component of the combination therapy have been defined, the combination of the two drugs in a checkerboard pattern will yield a broad dose–response surface in three dimensions with the drug concentrations forming the x and y axes and the biological effect on the z axis. The individual dose response curves form one part of the complete dose response surface that can be evaluated.

In performing combination assays it is important to recognize that in most in vitro assay systems, the endpoint boundaries range between 0 and 100% inhibition and thus combination drug effects cannot be quantified, where the additive or synergistic interaction of the two compounds would be expected to exceed 100% inhibition. The concentrations of the agents to be tested must carefully be chosen, so that the activity of the two drugs is not evaluated at a large number of points where additive inhibition exceeds 100%. Similarly, the combination interaction cannot be quantified when an antagonistic interaction results in the level of efficacy falling below 0% protection, or where combination toxicity effects result in percent toxicity exceeding 100%. In addition, the interaction of the two drugs may be different at different drug ratios, with the possibility of defining distinct regions of synergy, additivity, and antagonism across the entire dose response surface. In general each of the test compounds will be evaluated over a range of concentrations that yield a progression of activity from 0 through/to 100% with constant incremental increases in drug concentration. The most sensitive measure of compound interactions over the complete dose response surface occurs, when the incremental increases in drug concentrations are small (2- to 3-fold) from tested dose to the next-higher tested dose.

Finally, the design of the combination assay is dependent on how the data will be analyzed at the conclusion of the experiments. For some analyses, such as the original Chou and Talalay methodology (see below), the assay configuration will involve selection of a ratio of the two drugs to be evaluated and the testing of the effects of the drug combination in fixed multiples of that ratio. Recently, it has been recognized that drug interactions must be observed over a very complete dose response surface (22) and so most analyses are performed with a checkerboard of drug concentrations where every possible combination of concentrations of the two drugs are tested together, yielding a complete three-dimensional combination dose response surface. Over the years the methodology employed to define the effects of two compounds used together have dramatically improved. The discussion below provides an overview of the methodology that has been employed when investigators evaluate combination drug efficacy and toxicity.

It should be noted and emphasized here that the greatest problem with the performance of combination assays is overall assay reproducibility. The size of the combination assays can be extremely large (over 450 data points per assay for three-dimensional models such as MacSynergy II) and data are accumulated across multiple microtiter plates, yielding some level of data variability from assay to assay (inter-assay variability) and plate to plate (intra-assay variability). For combination drug analysis, it is thus important to develop and optimize assays with minimal inter- and intra-assay variation (23). Our experience indicates that the overall interpretation (synergy, antagonism, additivity) is highly reproducible. Variability is usually observed in the peak level of synergy or antagonism and in the concentration of each drug that results in the peak of synergy or antagonism. In general, combination assays must be replicated in order to precisely and quantitatively define the interaction of two drugs; in our experience that has meant the repetition of a given drug combination assay, i.e., a minimum of three to five times, before the relative level of synergy and the concentrations employed to achieve maximal synergy can be discussed with confidence. Despite the use of microtiter plate formats, these assays

require a substantial amount of test compounds compared to routine anti-infective evaluations. For high-throughput screening prior to the precise definition of the most potent combinations, the single-plate combination assay formats may be used, especially under conditions in which test compounds or target cells are limiting.

2.2 Analysis of the Interaction of the Drugs Used in Combination

The benefits of combination chemotherapy have long been recognized and experience with the treatment of HIV infection has driven the utility of combination strategies to new levels of development with three to four drugs forming the core of current highly active antiretroviral chemotherapy (HAART) regimens (24, 25). The methodology used to analyze the results of combination testing also has evolved (11, 14, 22, 26–31). A variety of statistical methods have been developed, all with inherent advantages and disadvantages. Over the entire course of preclinical development of an anti-infective agent, each of these evaluation techniques may be best used depending on the type of assay employed. Some algorithms (such as the three-dimensional MacSynergy II programs) are best suited for extremely large sets of data, with many concentrations in replicate over a wide dose response surface, whereas others are well suited for situations in which the number of data points available for analysis may be limited, such as in animal model testing (Chou and Talalay median dose effect equations). The primary problems encountered in developing the models for the evaluation of combination interactions result from the fact that the combination dose responses represent a three-dimensional issue analyzed in two dimensions and from the fact that no agreement on the definition of additive or synergistic interactions has been obtained (22). Fortunately, the increasing use of automation and highly complex analysis performed by personal computers has allowed three-dimensional dose response curves to be easily visualized and evaluated (14, 32)

In simplest terms, a three-dimensional combination drug assay has two independent variables (the concentrations of the two drugs being evaluated) and one dependent variable (the anti-infective activity of the drug combination). The activity of the drug combination can be visualized as a three-dimensional surface with the drug concentrations on the x and y axes and the biological effect of the combination on the z axis. At the zero concentration points for each individual drug, the two-dimensional dose response curve for a single drug can be observed in the three-dimensional dose response surface. Evaluation of this three-dimensional surface and defining in statistical terms how the compounds interact has been accomplished by a variety of methodologies discussed in more detail below.

The basic dose response surface can be evaluated by connecting the 50% inhibitory levels across the dose response surface to create an isobol at the 50% inhibitory value, with the line that is produced representing all combinations of the two drugs that achieve 50% inhibition of the replication of the infectious organism. The isobol, or line of equal elevation, was originally derived from cartography and is simply the contour line representing various levels of inhibition of the organism (33–41). The isobologram is the two-dimensional contour plot that is the result (34, 35, 41). The shape of the contour lines forming the isobologram represent the three-dimensional dose response surface and thus provides the definition of the interaction of the two compounds as synergistic, additive, or antagonistic (26, 37, 42–47). Typically, isobolograms are plotted at the 50% inhibitory concentration; however any fixed inhibition value can be utilized and in most cases multiple isobolograms should be evaluated to understand the interaction of two drugs across the entire surface, since the complete dose response surface may include regions of synergy, additivity, and antagonism.

In the development of the various analysis models, certain statistical principles were utilized as the basic assumptions underlying the evaluation of the data. For example, several of the programs, notably those defined by Chou and Talalay, based their approach on the median-effect principle (15, 48, 49). The Loewe additivity model is the basis of the null reference model (33). Loewe additivity assumes that two drugs should be indistinguishable from each other with respect to antiviral effects in a combination assay. Thus, in this analysis one assumes that if a given concentration of two drugs inhibits replication by a defined amount, any fractional concentration of one drug (Drug A) combined with the complementary fractional concentration of the second drug (Drug B) should inhibit replication by the same amount. Loewe additivity can be expressed as:

$$1 = D_A / (IC_p)_A + D_B / (IC_p)_B$$

where D_A and D_B are equal to the concentrations of Drug A and Drug B in the mixture that elicits p percent effect, and $(IC_p)_A$ and $(IC_p)_B$ are equal to the concentrations of Drug A and Drug B in the combination that elicits the same p percent effect on the replication of an organism.

Prichard and Shipman based their MacSynergy II analysis program (14) on the Bliss Independence null reference model (50). This model is based on statistical probability and assumes that two drugs should act independently to affect virus replication. Thus if Drug A affects the replication of a population of organisms to a defined level, then the addition of Drug B should affect the remaining population of organisms to the level it would have affected in the absence of Drug A. Bliss Independence can be expressed as:

$$Z = X + Y(1-X)$$

where X is equal to the fractional inhibition produced by the dose of Drug A alone and Y is equal to the fractional inhibition achieved by Drug B alone and Z is equal to the predicted fractional inhibition.

Each of these models offers robust mathematical data interpretation. In the sections below, the various methods that may be employed to evaluate in vitro combination testing results will be described in greater experimental detail. Generally, the models that have been developed to evaluate drug combinations include the fractional product method, the multiple dose response curve method, isobolograms, the combination index method, the differential surface analysis method, and parametric surface fitting methods (14, 15, 27, 32, 36, 43, 45, 47, 51–70).

2.2.1 Multiple Dose–Response Curves

The simplest method of interpretation of the effect of a second drug (Drug B) on the activity of a single agent (Drug A) is to evaluate the effect of a single concentration of Drug B on the dose-response curve of Drug A (Fig. 1). This evaluation superimposes the dose response curves of Drug A obtained in the presence of Drug B and increases or decreases in biological activity that are observed as shifts in the dose response curves due to the presence of the second agent. A wide variety of research papers have been published using this simple evaluation of the combination effects of two drugs (54–57) and although the methods do not employ any statistical evaluation of the data that allow confirmation of the precise interaction as additive, synergistic, or antagonistic, the data evaluation does permit simple interpretation of positive or negative effects of the two drugs. Using this methodology, it is impossible to discriminate between slightly synergistic, slightly antagonistic, or additive interactions, although highly synergistic or highly antagonistic definitions are possible. Multiple dose–response curve evaluations are quite simple to perform, especially with a highly sensitive and reproducible assay system, but they obviously suffer from a lack of rigorous and statistics-based data evaluation and the ever-present issue of investigator bias in the interpretation of results.

2.2.2 Isobolograms

The classic method for detecting and characterizing departures from additivity between combinations is the

Fig. 1 A representative example of the antiviral dose–response curve obtained with a single drug (Drug A) alone and with the addition of a single concentration of a second drug (Drug B). The various dose–response curves with increasing concentrations of Drug B may be compared to each other and that obtained with Drug A alone to evaluate the combination drug effect

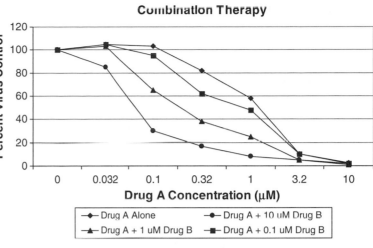

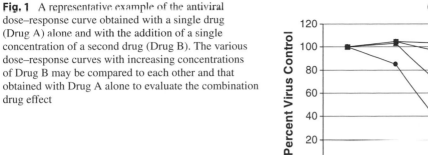

isobologram methodology (Fig. 2) (33, 45, 58–60). This method was originally introduced by Fraser (34, 35). The use of the isobologram technique for analyzing drug combinations was extended by the work of Loewe and Muischnek (33), Loewe (36), and Berenbaum (37) (also see reviews by Gessner (38), Wessinger (39), and Berenbaum (40)). The isobologram is essentially a contour plot of a constant dose response over the dose response surface compared to a plot of the same contour under the assumption of additivity. Thus, for a two-drug combination assay, the isobologram analysis compares the concentrations required to achieve a certain dose response (such as 50% inhibition of replication) to the line of additivity, formed by joining the 50% inhibition concentrations of the two drugs when used alone as calculated experimentally. If the observed isobol falls below the line of additivity, the two drugs interact in a synergistic manner; if they fall above the line of additivity, the drugs are antagonistic. The predominant problem associated with the use of isobolograms to predict drug interaction is data variability. Isobolograms can be used to calculate the predicted interactions of two or three drug combinations.

2.2.3 Combination Index Method

Another widely used and accepted method for the analysis of anti-HIV data is the combination index method of Chou and Talalay (Fig. 3) (15, 27, 32, 61, 62). As originally proposed, the experimental design of the Chou–Talalay method required that the total concentration of two drugs be altered while fixed concentration ratios for the two drugs were maintained. The popularity of this method lies in the fact that relatively few samples are required for computer-based analysis and prediction of the nature of the drug interactions. However, since fixed drug ratios examine only the drug interactions along diagonal lines across the dose–response surface, it is possible the drug ratios chosen by the investigator

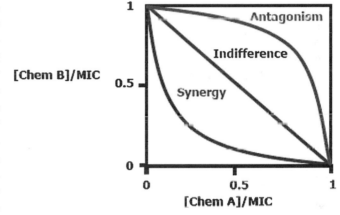

Fig. 2 A representation of the classical isobologram method for the evaluation of compound interactions

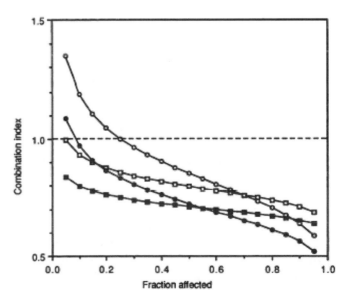

Fig. 3 Representative compound interactions as evaluated by the Chou and Talalay median dose effect equation

do not reveal localized areas of synergism and/or antagonism on the drug dose–response surface plot. This means that several fixed-ratio drug combination experiments must be conducted to examine all diagonal lines across the dose–response surface. Recent adaptations of the combination index model now allow for the analysis of checkerboard patterns of drug concentrations as opposed to fixed ratios. The statistical model of Chou and Talalay is reported to be most useful when data points are limited, such as in animal studies. The limitation of the Chou and Talalay method remains, for the lack of confidence intervals in the statistical analysis of the data.

Through utilization of Monte Carlo mathematical modeling techniques, a probabilistic model, called ComboStat, simulating processes influenced by random factors (e.g., experimental variability associated with repetition of drug-combination studies) was developed (61). Upon application of this mathematical model, statistically relevant confidence intervals have now been assigned to the Combination Index values produced by the Chou-Talalay method. Using this methodology, it is possible to accurately interpret the Chou-Talalay drug-combination index and statistically discriminate between mild synergism/antagonism and additivity. Unfortunately, use of ComboStat, like the original Chou and Talalay program, requires drug combination studies with fixed drug concentration ratios. As mentioned above, this approach only examines drug interactions at diagonal lines across the dose–response surface and local domains of synergism and antagonism can be missed unless all diagonals on the dose–response surface are examined.

2.2.4 Three-Dimensional Surface Analysis

The Prichard and Shipman MacSynergy II model evaluates combination data with assumptions based on same-site or different-site modes of action (14, 63–66). The more rigorous evaluation assumes that the compounds being evaluated act at the same site to inhibit the replication of the infectious organism. The MacSynery II algorithm utilizes the data obtained with each drug alone to calculate the expected level of inhibition of the drug combination at each drug concentration in a checkerboard pattern, generating a three-dimensional surface of expected activity (Fig. 4). The actual data points determined experimentally are derived from the anti-infective assay and are plotted as the Antiviral Surface Plot. The expected activities are subtracted from the experimentally determined values at each data point, resulting in the generation of a three-dimensional Synergy Plot. If the expected and realized activities at each point are identical, a flat plane results indicating that the interaction of the two drugs is additive. If the realized activity is greater than the expected level of activity, positive values are obtained, resulting in regions

extending above the plane. These points represent the drug concentrations at which the activities of the drugs together are greater than that expected, or are synergistic. An antagonistic interaction occurs when the realized level of protection is less than that expected; negative values are plotted three dimensionally as regions extending below the plane. The concentrations of the two compounds yielding maximal synergistic activity can be visualized easily with the Antiviral Contour Plot. MacSynergy II also calculates the volume of the synergy peaks or antagonism depressions and these are used to quantify the amount of synergy or antagonism. The synergy volumes are calculated at the 95, 99, and 99.9% levels of confidence.

2.2.5 Parametric Surface Fitting

Parametric surface fitting is another three-dimensional modeling technique that uses response-surface methodology to fit equations to the experimental data (an example is the COMBO software package) (43, 67–69, 71). Mathematical parameters are used to define the surface as additive, synergistic, or antagonistic. The parametric surface fitting, uses the Loewe additivity equation. Two models have been developed. Unfortunately, both are difficult to utilize and have the inherent problem that the equations were designed to fit a smooth three-dimensional surface, yielding results that are too simplistic for an irregular and complex three-dimensional surface like that obtained from antiviral combination assays.

2.3 Additional Considerations in Design of Combination Drug Evaluations

In addition to choosing the correct assay and an appropriate means of analysis, there are other considerations in developing a combination therapy regimen for clinical testing and use. These considerations are based on the proposed use of the combination therapy, the potential presence of other infections or drugs, the target of the therapy, and the potential for greater than two drugs being utilized. These considerations and their importance will be discussed below.

2.3.1 Combination Efficacy and Combination Toxicity

Evaluation of the combination interactions of two or more compounds should include the evaluation of effects on both anti-infective efficacy and cellular toxicity. In most cases, the drug concentration ranges chosen for the combination

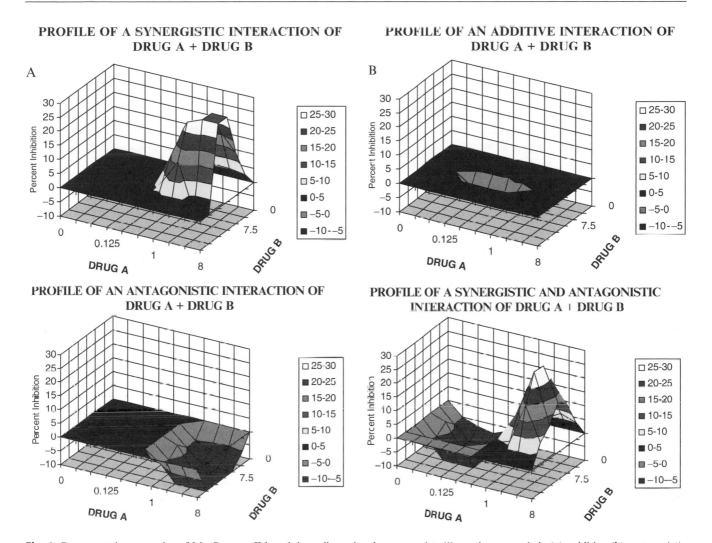

Fig. 4 Representative examples of MacSynergy II based three-dimensional synergy plots illustrating synergistic (**a**), additive (**b**), antagonistic (**c**), or both synergistic and antagonistic (**d**) drug interactions when evaluated in cell-based combination assays

evaluation extends from a low dose with no biological effect through a high dose that yields at or near 100% replication inhibition efficacy. These concentration ranges rarely touch on concentrations that are toxic to the host cells and thus combination toxicity cannot be appropriately evaluated. Thus, in these assays, the toxicity portion of the dose response curve is not observed, although in some cases synergistic toxicity may be observed when significant combination toxicity is present or when the selectivity index for the individual compounds is extremely narrow. Combination toxicity should be evaluated over a dose response curve for the individual compounds that extend from a low concentration with no observed toxic effect on the host cells to a high concentration that results in significant toxic effects. These assays are possible after the complete dose response curves for the individual compounds have been defined. All of the analysis methodologies described above for the evaluation of the combination assays may be used to predict combination toxicity effects. It is possible for anti-infective synergy to be observed that can be explained by a reduction in the

toxicity of the two test compounds when used together. For example, we have shown that the efficacy of ribavirin and interferon-α is synergistically enhanced by the addition of a third compound being developed as an anti-HCV clinical therapeutic; the increased antiviral efficacy of the combination is explained by the action of the third compound in reducing the toxicity of ribavirin, thus enhancing its antiviral interaction and synergistic activity with interferon. Similarly, combinations of anti-HIV NCp7 zinc finger inhibitors with many approved anti-HIV drugs have yielded synergistic anti-HIV activity with the antiviral efficacy derived from the reduced toxicity of the combination of test compounds.

2.3.2 Mutually Exclusive and Mutually Nonexclusive Evaluations

Analysis of combination interactions using some of the available programs, such as MacSynergy II, require the user to determine if the analysis should assume that the drugs inhibit the same or different anti-infective targets. These combination parameters have been defined as mutually exclusive and mutually nonexclusive combinations. As a combination therapy strategy, these two therapeutic regimens have also been described in the literature as convergent (same site) or divergent (different site) anti-infective therapies. In our evaluations we have determined that the choice of analysis options may be even more complex than the simple definition of the target enzyme, protein, or replication pathway. For example, the combination of AZT and ritonavir is a mutually nonexclusive therapy, targeting two different steps in the virus replication cycle and two distinct HIV proteins. However, the combination of the nucleoside RT inhibitor AZT with the nonnucleoside RT inhibitor Sustiva could be evaluated using either the mutually exclusive or mutually nonexclusive equations, since they target the same enzyme (RT) but at completely different sites on the enzyme. In many cases, compounds are evaluated in combination assays before the mechanism of action is known or that compounds may have a primary and a secondary mechanism of action. We have found that the use of the mutually exclusive evaluation equations provides a more robust evaluation of the interaction of the test compounds.

2.3.3 Performance and Evaluation of Three-Drug Combination Assays

With the increasing incidence of transmission of drug-resistant organisms, more than two drugs are often given to patients simultaneously. The numbers of drugs that can and should be used in combination in the clinical setting requires a methodology for evaluating combinations of greater than two test drugs. Prichard and Shipman first described the use of MacSynergy II for evaluating the interaction of three drugs in combination (72). In these assays, the combination dose response surface was evaluated for the two-drug combination of acyclovir and 2-acetylpyridine thiosemicarbazone, generating a dose response surface including 45 data points, each defined in triplicate to allow calculation of the 95% confidence interval for each data point. This dose response surface was replicated five times and each replicate included a single dose of 5-fluoro-deoxyuridine. For each of the five replicate dose response surfaces the activity defined for the two-drug combination was subtracted, yielding the change in activity that resulted from the addition of the third drug. As with the two-drug interaction analysis using MacSynergy II, the synergy volume can be calculated and the concentrations of the drugs that yield synergistic interactions can be directly defined. Using the checkerboard pattern of evaluation, regions of different interactions can also be observed and quantified.

2.3.4 Combination Testing with Resistant Organisms

One of the primary driving forces for the use of combination therapy strategies in the clinic is to suppress the selection and replication of drug-resistant organisms. The component drugs of the combination therapy should each have the capacity to inhibit the replication of viruses that are resistant to the other drugs used in the regimen. In some cases, the drugs used must be able to suppress the replication of resistant viruses that were selected to drugs within the same class of the inhibitor. The in vitro evaluation of the interaction of two or more drugs should be extended to include evaluation of the ability of the combination of drugs to inhibit drug-resistant viruses, especially the variety of multidrug-resistant (MDR) (73) viruses that have begun to circulate in the patient population. With an estimated 10% of new infections involving the transmission of resistant organisms (74, 75), this has become increasingly important for anti-HIV therapy. Therapeutic combinations must be evaluated for inhibition of drug-resistant organisms when searching for drugs for pathogens including 3TC-resistant hepatitis B virus strains, antibiotic-resistant bacteria, and drug-resistant tuberculosis. A number of research reports have demonstrated the ability of a combination of drugs to inhibit a drug-resistant virus to one of the components of the drug regimen. In most cases synergistic or additive antiviral interactions are observed with drug-resistant strains when the test concentration of the drug to which the virus has become resistant is increased relative to the level effective against the wild type. These results would suggest that clinical resistance can be overcome by increasing the dose or by defining and using the highest possible concentration of a drug to essentially sterilize the patient of replicating virus.

2.3.5 Combination Resistance Selection Evaluations

A variety of resistance selection strategies are available to select for the drug- or the antibiotic-resistant organisms. These same strategies can be used to select for viruses or bacteria that are resistant to a combination of drugs either sequentially or in a true combination fashion (Table 1). We have observed that the pattern of resistance engendering mutations changes dramatically when a combination of agents are used in the selection strategy. Resistance selection strategies usually employ a high fixed concentration of the drug used for selection (or combination of drugs) or use the technique of the serial passage of the microbe in the presence of increasing concentrations of the test compound. Since these techniques are routinely employed to select for resistant organisms, the methods do not always provide additional

Table 1 Amino acid changes in virus genome determined by dideoxy sequencing following in vitro drug resistance selection of Compound 1 alone or in combination with Compound 2. The virus passage number sequenced is in *parentheses*

| Compound 2 | Amino acid change (no. of passages in cell culture) with the following Compound 1 | | | |
	None	Calanolide A	Costatolide	Dihydrocostatolide
None	–	T139I	T139I/L100I	L100I
3TC	M184V	M184V/L100I (5)	M184V/L100I (6)	M184V/L100I (5)
Diphenylsulfone	Y181C	V108I (6)	Y188H (6)	ND[a]
E-BPTU	Y181C	K103N/V106I (6)	ND	ND
α-APA	Y181C	ND	K103N (14)	ND
UC10	K101E/Y181C	Y188H (6)	K103N (5)	K103N (5)
TSAO	Y181C	K101E (6)	K101E (6)	K101E (6)
Diarylsulfone	Y181C	Y188H (13)	Y188H (11)	Y188H (8)

data on the relative anti-infective impact of the combination strategy. Techniques have been developed for the passage of the organism in the presence of the drug that are highly standardized with regard to selection pressure (i.e., the EC_{50} or EC_{90} concentration from passage to passage). We have employed a virus transmission sterilization assay with single and multiple drugs to rapidly select for drug-resistant virus strains in the presence of a variety of fixed high concentrations of the test drugs.

2.3.6 Combination Assays to Evaluate Treatment for Multiple Infectious Organisms

Another important consideration in the design of a combination therapy strategy is the effect of the individual drugs on those drugs being used to treat other infectious disease organisms. This is especially important when considering therapies for transplant patients undergoing immunosuppression (neutropenia), immune-compromised AIDS patients, and in situations involving viral and bacterial coinfections. The combination assay strategies discussed in this chapter can be utilized for evaluating the effects of the agents on other indications. For example, an antiviral agent designed to treat HIV infection can be evaluated in anti-bacterial or anti-fungal assays to determine if the addition of the antiviral agent has any positive or negative effect on the efficacy and toxicity of anti-microbial agents. Conversely, anti-microbial agents should be evaluated for their effects on the HIV therapy. Since the drugs may not be active against the target organisms used in the assay (for example, the anti-microbial agent vs. HIV), it is important to utilize therapeutically relevant concentrations of the agent as opposed to trying to define a concentration that is actually active against the non-specific organism. The use of checkerboard drug concentration format for these assays allows the broadest possible dose response surface to be evaluated.

2.4 Special Case: Potentiation and Suppression

In some cases, the two test agents may include one that does not have any detectable activity against the organism being tested or may not be active in the particular assay being employed. In this case, discussions of synergistic and antagonistic interactions of the agents are not completely correct. Combination assays and analysis programs can be performed on these combinations of agents exactly as described above, but the results of the assays should be expressed in terms of potentiation (or enhancement) and suppression (or inhibition) of activity, depending on whether the result was synergistic or antagonistic as defined by the analytical endpoint of the assay. The terms potentiation and suppression are generally correct when discussing combinations of agents active against different organisms. Compounds that have activity in chronic infection models but not in acute infection models against the same organism might be evaluated in potentiation assays with compounds that only exhibit efficacy in the acute infection models. As discussed previously, it is important to carefully choose the drug concentrations to be evaluated so that concentrations are therapeutically relevant, even if a particular drug that is inactive, and that a broad dose response surface is evaluated.

2.4.1 Biological Relevance of the Test System to the Therapeutic Strategy

When considering the effectiveness of a combination therapy, it is critical to select the appropriate system and assay for use in the evaluations. Since most combination therapies will be utilized for the therapeutic treatment of systemic infections, the assays to be utilized should have relevance to the biology of the infection. Thus appropriate cell lines and virus strains should be used and the assay may be modified to more closely mimic the therapeutic environment through the addition of serum proteins and other additives. Combination therapies may also find utility as vaginal or rectal microbicides or for the treatment of wounds or other topical and mucosal infections. In these systems, the cells used for the assays, the isolates chosen for evaluation, and the additives used to mimic the infectious environment will be modified to reflect the therapeutic use of the compound. For some regimens, it is also important to consider the method of formulation of the final product and to perform the combination evaluations under those conditions. For example, the final form of a topical vaginal microbicide often includes excipients that may have therapeutic or toxic effects and that may potentiate or suppress activity of the drug of interest/drug in question (76).

2.4.2 In Vitro Pharmacologic Models and Evaluations

Combination methods have recently been developed to take into account pharmacodynamics of drug exposure (18). In these model systems, the concentrations of the drugs in contact with the cells are continuously modified to approximate the plasma concentrations of the drugs in a human being. Thus rather than culturing cells and virus in the presence of fixed concentrations of the two drugs, in the pharmacodynamic model each drug concentration is fluctuated as it would be in the patient, allowing the investigator to model antiviral and toxic effects more realistically than in tissue culture systems. Though this model is an advancement that can aid in prioritizing combination therapies for clinical use, these methods are very expensive and time consuming and are not practical for routine and high-throughput evaluation of combinations of compounds. In addition, these are still in vitro assays: metabolism of the compounds, generation of metabolites, and interaction with tissues do not occur, and thus they do not completely reflect in vivo use.

3 Virologic Evaluations

3.1 Virus Replication and Functional Cell-Based Assays

The most relevant cell-based assays include clinical strains of virus and fresh human cells. For HIV, assays using fresh human PBMCs, monocyte-macrophages, and dendritic cells, as well as assays with tissues such as cervical explants for microbicide testing, have been developed (6, 20, 77). For a number of other viral agents, a variety of in vitro screening assays involving measurement of cytopathic effects, virus replication, or plaque-formation assays can be performed (78–90). In these cases, the endpoints of the assays are quantitative readouts of the virus production and typically involve the measurement of a viral enzyme, measurement of a viral capsid protein, or measurement of the infectious virus. These values can be entered into the analysis programs defined above as actual raw data values or the values expressed as a percentage of the virus or cell control. Although many of these assays are suitable for high-volume screening, in general the variability in fresh human cell populations requires that many replicates of these assays be performed unless a highly standardized and reproducible infection of the primary cells can be achieved. In addition, the cost of both the assay and the availability of adequate cell numbers or tissues can affect the number of replicates that can be performed.

3.2 Assays Measuring Cytopathic Effects

For anti-infective testing for most organisms, a simple, reproducible, and cost-effective solution to a high-throughput combination of antiviral evaluations is to utilize assays that quantify virus-induced cytopathic effects (CPE) and the ability of test agents to suppress these cytopathic effects (78–90). A number of tetrazolium dyes and other colorimetric reporters can be used to quantify viability in the cell cultures and the differential between the virus and cell controls can be used as the measure of percent protection. These percent protection (or percent cell viability) values can be easily imported directly into the analysis programs and the combination interaction quickly evaluated. One drawback of these assays is that the virus replication is not measured directly, but rather an effect of decreased viral replication is measured (which should, in most cases, be proportional to the level of virus produced). The compound not only has to suppress virus production, but also has to suppress the CPE, which may not be a natural feature of viral infection in the patient. In addition, virus-induced CPE assays routinely use laboratory-derived strains of virus and established human cells that may not accurately mimic infection in patients. Despite these caveats, CPE assays are the assay of choice for high-throughput combination evaluations in the light of their extreme reproducibility (low intra- and inter-assay variability) and low cost. CPE assays are available for nearly all infectious organisms routinely screened in anti-infective development programs. Viral plaque reduction assays are a similar but a more labor-intensive approach since the plaques produced by infection must be microscopically counted, introducing greater cost, variability, and level of assay difficulty than assays using reporter dyes.

3.3 Enzymatic and Biochemical Assays

Biochemical assays that directly quantify the ability of a test compound to inhibit the target enzyme or block binding to a target protein are (in most cases) the simplest and least expensive of the various combination assay formats (20). Biochemical or enzymatic assays effectively reproduce antiviral mechanism of action assays. The read-outs of these assays usually have radioactive, colorimetric, fluorescent, or chemiluminescent endpoints and the values obtained can be compared to a positive and negative control allowing percent inhibition values to be calculated. These values can be directly imported into the programs for analysis of the combination interaction. Although these assays are usually rapid, inexpensive, easy to perform, and extremely reproducible and quantitative, they have several disadvantages. First, they do not take place in the intact cell. These assays do not require the test agents to actually penetrate the cell membrane and accumulate at the site of action. A second issue of biochemical importance is metabolism by the intact cell, such as the phosphorylation required for nucleoside analogs. Antagonistic effects on metabolism would be missed in a biochemical assay. Third, biochemical assays do not provide information on combination toxicity obtained through cell-based assays. Finally, quite often the enzyme that is targeted by one component of the combination therapy is not targeted by the other, and therefore the combination biochemical assay merely informs the investigator whether or not the inactive drug potentiates or interferes with the activity of the active drug in the limited context of the biochemical assay.

3.4 Chronic and Acute Infection Assays

A special case of cell-based assays involves testing of agents in cells that are chronically infected with an infectious organism and that constitutively or latently produce virus. Though most approved antiviral agents target steps that occur early in the infection cycle, assays with chronically or latently infected cells that quantify the effects of test agents on late stages of virus production such as transcription, translation, virus assembly, maturation, and release from the infected cell. The strengths and weaknesses of these cell-based models are identical to those presented above for virus replication-based assays. Though the throughput and reproducibility are much higher than that observed for primary human cell assays, the chronic systems typically require more expensive systems for endpoint detection. In any event, for compounds that target late stages of infection, it is important to test the combination efficacy and toxicity in both acute and chronic infection models in combination with agents that are more than likely active only in the acute infection models. These assays will essentially confirm that the chronic infection inhibitor will not interfere with the acute infection inhibitor and vice versa.

4 Microbiologic Evaluations

The concept of using antimicrobial drugs in combination dates back to the early days of chemotherapy. Combination therapies historically were used either as a means to extend the therapeutic spectrum against diverse genera and organisms of unknown sensitivity or as a means to stem the tide of selection for drug-resistant strains during extended treatment regimens. Representative examples are the well-known combination of trimethoprim and sulfamethoxazole used for multiple bacterial indications (91), multidrug therapy for tuberculosis (92), and eradication of *Helicobacter pylori* in peptic ulcer disease (93). Other examples that fall into the combination category range from the streptogramin-drug Synercid® (a mixture of quinupristin and dalfopristin 30:70 w/w for parenteral administration, Monarch Pharmaceuticals) indicated for vancomycin-resistant *Enterococcus faecium*, to Augmentin® (multiple formulations of amoxicillin and the betalactamase inhibitor clavulanate, GlaxoSmithKline Pharmaceuticals) used primarily for community-acquired pneumonia (CAP), bronchitis, and otitis media. Amoxicillin/clavulanate is unique in that it combines an antibiotic with an inhibitor of a common resistance mechanism (secreted betalactamase).

4.1 Methods to Study Antibiotic Interactions

Several in vitro methods have been devised to measure the interaction between two or more antibiotics in bacterial culture systems. The primary goal of these studies was to determine whether the drugs acted in synergy to increase killing efficiency above that seen with either agent alone, or whether they were antagonistic to each other and thus could have the potential to decrease efficacy and adversely affect clinical outcome. All methods provide either a direct numerical readout such as the fractional inhibitory concentration index (FICI) of a checkerboard test or measurable changes in growth dynamics and viable cell count as seen in time-kill assays from broth cultures.

4.1.1 Checkerboard Testing

This system is an extension of standard broth microdilution methodologies used for the determination of minimum inhibitory concentration (MIC) (94, 95). Presently, no officially recognized checkerboard testing standard exists. However, starting inoculum densities and scoring of bacterial growth at the end of the assays generally follows the MIC microdilution protocols of the Clinical and Laboratory Standards Institute (CLSI; formerly the NCCLS). Checkerboards are simple arrays of serial dilutions of each drug in two dimensions across microtiter plates. Individual MIC values for each drug are determined against the test organism prior to the assay. Starting this drug concentrations are selected such that they bracket the respective MICs by three or four dilutions. After dilution, the plates are incubated and each well is read as for a standard MIC assay. Once wells are scored for growth inhibition, fractional inhibitory concentrations (FICs) are calculated by dividing the MIC of the first drug in combination with the MIC of that drug when used alone. The same process is carried out for the second drug. Both FIC values then are added together to create the fractional inhibitory index (FICI) for the combination. FICI values ≤0.5 indicate synergy whereas values >4.0 indicate antagonism. Values between these two endpoints represent no significant interaction. Since previous literature sources have made claims as to the significance of intermediate FICI values falling between 0.5 and 4.0, the editorial board of the *Journal of Antimicrobial Chemotherapy* in 2003 instituted the requirement that these values be used for manuscript submission and required that intermediate values should be labeled as no interaction (96). These recommendations appear to have broad acceptance in the field.

4.1.2 Time-Kill Testing

Although not as simple to configure as checkerboard arrays, time-kill assays provide both a kinetic readout of bacterial kill rates over the course of the experiment as well as an indication of synergy, antagonism, or indifference after 24 h of antibiotic exposure. These tests are based on the macroscale broth method used for the determination of bactericidal activity as specified by the CLSI (97). Broth cultures are configured with test organism and drugs are added either alone or in combination at fractions or multiples of the MIC (generally ranging from 0.25 to 2 times the MIC) (98). Cultures can be monitored over the course of exposure to examine bacterial growth/kill kinetics and at the end of the assay period for determining synergy, indifference, or antagonism. In this system, White et al. defined synergy as a combination that produced ≥2 $\log_{10}$ reduction in colony-forming units (CFU) compared to the most active of the two drugs when used alone (98). Likewise, ≥100-fold increase in CFU indicated antagonism, whereas <10-fold change indicated indifference.

4.1.3 E-Test Strip

The Epsilometer or E-test strip (AB Biodisk, Solna, Sweden) has been utilized for synergy testing (98). In this configuration, an E-test strip for each drug is placed onto an agar plate inoculated with the test organism. The strips are laid onto the agar surface in a crossed pattern such that the perpendicular intersection of the two strips contact at the precise point on the scale of the individual MIC for each drug. Following incubation, a zone of inhibition radiates out from that point of intersection. The MIC of each drug in combination is read off each scale by noting where the zone of inhibition contacts each strip distal to the point of intersection. FICI values are calculated by the same process as that used for the checkerboard test. Frequent agreement between the E-test, checkerboard, and time-kill assays were found in this study (98), but there was sufficient variability and discordance between the tests to suggest that neither one could be used alone when evaluating new drug combinations. Therefore, when testing new antibacterials or combinations of currently approved drugs for new indications, multiple assays should be performed and compared.

4.2 Combination Testing and Prediction of Clinical Outcome

Despite the availability of testing methods for possible interactions between antibiotics used in combination, the final determination, as with any therapy, is whether or not there is a favorable therapeutic outcome. Few examples of synergistic combination therapy exist in the literature and generally these tend to describe special situations such as therapies for Gram-negative sepsis in neutropenic patients or enterococcal endocarditis (99–101). Even recent guidelines for combination therapy in normal adult community-acquired pneumonia (CAP), where a macrolide-class drug is recommended together with a betalactam, are directed toward increasing spectrum in order to cover atypical organisms rather than for any synergistic pharmacodynamic consideration (102). Investigators must consider the pharmacokinetic properties of the individual agents. Will combining two drugs with vastly different serum half-lives (such as a macrolide and a betalactam) have relevance at the actual site of infection? What about differences in tissue distribution at those sites (103)? One can also argue that static testing methods such as the checkerboard assay have little relevance to the dynamic environment encountered in vivo and that alternative models may be more relevant for predicting clinical outcome (104). At best, assays such as the checkerboard and time-kill can help predict whether any overt antagonism may exist between two antimicrobial drugs and whether the possibility remains for synergism in vivo.

Acknowledgements The authors gratefully acknowledge the assistance of Ms. Karen Watson, M.S. and Ms. Tracy Hartman, M/S. in the preparation and editing of this manuscript.

References

1. Kucers A, Crowe S, Grayson M, Hoy J. The Use of Antibiotics: A Clinical Review of Antibacterial Antifungal and Antiviral Drugs. Rochester, Kent, Great Britain, 1997.
2. Courvalin P. Antimicrobial drug resistance: "prediction is very difficult, especially about the future". Emerg Infect Dis 2005; 11:1503–6.
3. Wainberg MA. The emergence of HIV resistance and new antiretrovirals: are we winning? Drug Resist Updat 2004; 7:163–7.
4. Larder BA, Kellam P, Kemp SD. Convergent combination therapy can select viable multidrug-resistant HIV-1 in vitro. Nature 1993; 365:451–3.
5. Watanabe T, Kamisaki Y, Timmerman H. Convergence and divergence, a concept for explaining drug actions. J Pharmacol Sci 2004; 96:95–100.
6. Buckheit RW, Jr., Hollingshead M, Stinson S, et al. Efficacy, pharmacokinetics, and in vivo antiviral activity of UC781, a highly potent, orally bioavailable nonnucleoside reverse transcriptase inhibitor of HIV type 1. AIDS Res Hum Retroviruses 1997; 13:789–96.
7. Azad RF, Brown-Driver V, Buckheit RW, Jr., Anderson KP. Antiviral activity of a phosphorothioate oligonucleotide complementary to human cytomegalovirus RNA when used in combination with antiviral nucleoside analogs. Antiviral Res 1995; 28.101–11.
8. Brogden K, Guthmiller J. Polymicrobial Diseases. National Animal Disease Center, USDA Agricultural Research Service, Ames, IA, 2002.
9. Bevilacqua S, Rabaud C, May T. [HIV-tuberculosis coinfection]. Ann Med Interne (Paris) 2002; 153:113–8.
10. Bateman DN. Clinical toxicology: clinical science to public health. Clin Exp Pharmacol Physiol 2005; 32:995–8.
11. Spector SA, Kennedy C, McCutchan JA, et al. The antiviral effect of zidovudine and ribavirin in clinical trials and the use of p24 antigen levels as a virologic marker. J Infect Dis 1989; 159:822–8.
12. Frei E, Antman K. Combination chemotherapy, dose and schedule. In: Weichselbaum R, ed. Cancer Medicine. Baltimore, MD: Williams & Wilkins, 1997, pp 817–37.
13. Reynolds CP, Maurer BJ. Evaluating response to antineoplastic drug combinations in tissue culture models. Methods Mol Med 2005; 110:173–83.
14. Prichard MN, Shipman C, Jr. A three-dimensional model to analyze drug–drug interactions. Antiviral Res 1990; 14:181–205.
15. Chou TC, Talalay P. Quantitative analysis of dose–effect relationships: the combined effects of multiple drugs or enzyme inhibitors. Adv Enzyme Regul 1984; 22:27–55.
16. Bilello JA, Bauer G, Dudley MN, Cole GA, Drusano GL. Effect of 2′,3′-didehydro-3′-deoxythymidine in an in vitro hollow-fiber pharmacodynamic model system correlates with results of dose-ranging clinical studies. Antimicrob Agents Chemother 1994; 38: 1386–91.
17. Bilello JA, Bilello PA, Kort JJ, et al. Efficacy of constant infusion of A-77003, an inhibitor of the human immunodeficiency virus type 1 (HIV-1) protease, in limiting acute HIV-1 infection in vitro. Antimicrob Agents Chemother 1995; 39:2523–7.
18. Drusano GL, Prichard M, Bilello PA, Bilello JA. Modeling combinations of antiretroviral agents in vitro with integration of pharmacokinetics: guidance in regimen choice for clinical trial evaluation. Antimicrob Agents Chemother 1996; 40:1143–7.
19. FDA. Antiviral Drug Development: Conducting Virology Studies and Submitting the Data to the Agency.
20. Rice WG, Bader JP. Discovery and in vitro development of AIDS antiviral drugs as biopharmaceuticals. Adv Pharmacol 1995; 33:389–438.
21. Buckheit R. Specialized anti-HIV testing: expediting preclinical drug development. Drug Inf J 1997; 31:13–22.
22. Prichard MN, Shipman C, Jr. Analysis of combinations of antiviral drugs and design of effective multidrug therapies. Antivir Ther 1996; 1:9–20.
23. FDA. Guidance for Industry Bioanalytical Method Validation, 2001.
24. Mocroft A, Vella S, Benfield TL, et al. Changing patterns of mortality across Europe in patients infected with HIV-1. EuroSIDA Study Group. Lancet 1998; 352:1725–30.
25. Palella FJ, Jr., Delancy KM, Moorman AC, et al. Declining morbidity and mortality among patients with advanced human immunodeficiency virus infection. HIV Outpatient Study Investigators. N Engl J Med 1998, 338.853–60.
26. Berenbaum MC. The expected effect of a combination of agents: the general solution. J Theor Biol 1985; 114:413–31.
27. Chou T, Rideout D. Synergism and Antagonism in Chemotherapy. New York: Academic, 1991.
28. Copenhaver T, Lin T, Goldenberg M. Joint Drug Action: A Review. Proceedings of the American Statistical Association, Biopharm Section, 1987, pp 160–164.
29. Greco WR, Bravo G, Parsons JC. The search for synergy: a critical review from a response surface perspective. Pharmacol Rev 1995; 47:331–85.
30. Hall M, Duncan B. Antiviral drug and interferon combinations. In: Field R, ed. Antiviral Agents: The Development and Assessment of Antiviral Chemotherapy. Boca Raton, FL: CRC Press, 1988, pp 29–34.
31. Kodell R, Pounds J. Assisting the toxicity of mixtures of chemicals. In: Krewski C, ed. Statistics in Toxicology. New York: Gordon & Breach, 1991, pp 359–91.
32. Chou J, Chou T. Dose effect analysis with macrocomputers. Amsterdam: Elsevier, 1987.
33. Loewe S, Muischnek H. Kombinations-Wirkungen.1: Mittelilung: hilfsmittle der fragestel-lun. Arch Exp Pathol Pharmacol 1926; 114:313–26.
34. Fraser T. The antagonism between the actions of active substances. BMJ 1872, 485–7.
35. Fraser T. An experimental research on the antagonism between the actions of physostigma and atropia. Proc R Soc Edinb 1870; 7:506–11.
36. Loewe S. The problem of synergism and antagonism of combined drugs. Arzneimittelforschung 1953; 3:285–90.
37. Berenbaum M. Criteria for analyzing interactions between biologically active agents. 1981; 78:90–8.
38. Gessner P. The isobolographic method applied to drug interactions. In: Cohen S, ed. Drug Interactions, Vol. 1974. New York: Raven, 1974, pp 349–62.
39. Wessinger W. Approaches to the study of drug interactions in behavioral pharmacology. Neurosci Behav Rev 1976; 10:103–13.
40. Berenbaum MC. What is synergy? Pharmacol Rev 1989; 41: 93–141.
41. Meadows SL, Gennings C, Carter WH, Jr., Bae DS. Experimental designs for mixtures of chemicals along fixed ratio rays. Environ Health Perspect 2002; 110 Suppl 6:979–83.
42. Galdwin A, Mantel N. The employment of combinations of drugs in the chemotherapy of neoplasia: a review. Cancer Res 1957; 17:635–54.

43. Greco WR, Park HS, Rustum YM. Application of a new approach for the quantitation of drug synergism to the combination of cis-diamminedichloroplatinum and 1-beta-D-arabinofuranosylcytosine. Cancer Res 1990; 50:5318–27.

44. Greco W, Unkelback H-D, Pisch G, et al. Consensus on concepts and terminology for combined action assessment. Arch Complex Environ Stud 1992; 4:65.

45. Poch G. Dose factor of potentiation derived from isoboles. Arzneimittelforschung 1980; 30:2195–6.

46. Prichard M, Shipman C. Letter to the editor in response to J. Suhnel's comment on the paper "A three-dimensional model to analyze drug–drug interactions". Antiviral Res 1992; 384–93.

47. Suhnel J. Comment on the paper: A three-dimensional model to analyze drug–drug interactions. Prichard, M.N. and Shipman, C., Jr. (1990) Antiviral Res 14, 181–206. Antiviral Res 1992; 17:91–8.

48. Chou TC, Talalay P. A simple generalized equation for the analysis of multiple inhibitions of Michaelis–Menten kinetic systems. J Biol Chem 1977; 252:6438–42.

49. Chou T, Talalay P. Analysis of combined drug effects: a new look at a very old problem. Trends Pharmacol Sci 1983; 4:450–4.

50. Bliss C. The toxicity of poisons applied jointly. Ann Appl Biol 1939; 26:385–613.

51. Derwinko B, Lou T, Brown B, Gottlieb J, Freidreich F. Combination chemotherapy in vitro with adriamycin observations of additive, antagonistic and synergistic effects when using two-drug combination on cultured human lymphoma cells. Cancer Biochem Biophys 1976; 1:187–95.

52. Valeriote F, Lin H. Synergistic interaction of anticancer agents: a cellular perspective. Cancer Chemother Rep 1975; 39:895–900.

53. Webb J. Enzyme and Metabolic Inhibitors. Vol. 1. New York: Academic, 1963, pp 33–79, 488–512.

54. Dornsife RE, St Clair MH, Huang AT, et al. Anti-human immunodeficiency virus synergism by zidovudine (3′-azidothymidine) and didanosine (dideoxyinosine) contrasts with their additive inhibition of normal human marrow progenitor cells. Antimicrob Agents Chemother 1991; 35:322–8.

55. Jackson RC. A kinetic model of regulation of the deoxyribonucleoside triphosphate pool composition. Pharmacol Ther 1984; 24:279–301.

56. Johnson JC, Attanasio R. Synergistic inhibition of anatid herpesvirus replication by acyclovir and phosphonocompounds. Intervirology 1987; 28:89–99.

57. Mackay D. An analysis of functional antagonism and synergism. Br J Pharmacol 1981; 73:127–34.

58. Elion G, Singer S, Hitchings G. Antagonists of nucleic acid derivatives. J Biol Chem 1954; 208:477–88.

59. Gennings C, Carter WH, Jr., Campbell ED, et al. Isobolographic characterization of drug interactions incorporating biological variability. J Pharmacol Exp Ther 1990; 252:208–17.

60. Li RC, Schentag JJ, Nix DE. The fractional maximal effect method: a new way to characterize the effect of antibiotic combinations and other nonlinear pharmacodynamic interactions. Antimicrob Agents Chemother 1993; 37:523–31.

61. Belen'kii MS, Schinazi RF. Multiple drug effect analysis with confidence interval. Antiviral Res 1994; 25:1–11.

62. Kong XB, Zhu QY, Ruprecht RM, et al. Synergistic inhibition of human immunodeficiency virus type 1 replication in vitro by two-drug and three-drug combinations of 3′-azido-3′-deoxythymidine, phosphonoformate, and 2′,3′-dideoxythymidine. Antimicrob Agents Chemother 1991; 35:2003–11.

63. Lambert DM, Bartus H, Fernandez AV, et al. Synergistic drug interactions of an HIV-1 protease inhibitor with AZT in different in vitro models of HIV-1 infection. Antiviral Res 1993; 21:327–42.

64. Chong K, Pagano P, Hinshaw R. Bisheteroarylpiperazine reverse transcriptase inhibitor in combination with 3′ azido-3′-deoxythymidine or 2′,3′-dideoxycytidine synergistically inhib-

65. Prichard MN, Prichard LE, Shipman C, Jr. Inhibitors of thymidylate synthase and dihydrofolate reductase potentiate the antiviral effect of acyclovir. Antiviral Res 1993; 20:249–59.

66. Suhnel J. Evaluation of synergism or antagonism for the combined action of antiviral agents. Antiviral Res 1990; 13:23–39.

67. Carter WH, Jr. Relating isobolograms to response surfaces. Toxicology 1995; 105:181–8.

68. Freitas VR, Fraser-Smith EB, Chiu S, Michelson S, Schatzman RC. Efficacy of ganciclovir in combination with zidovudine against cytomegalovirus in vitro and in vivo. Antiviral Res 1993; 21:301–15.

69. Machado SG, Robinson GA. A direct, general approach based on isobolograms for assessing the joint action of drugs in pre-clinical experiments. Stat Med 1994; 13:2289–309.

70. Bauer D. The antiviral and synergistic actions of isatin thiosemicarbazzone and certain phenoxypyrimidines in vaccinia infection in mice. Br J Exp Pathol 1954; 28:105–14.

71. Bunow B, Weinstein J. COMBO: a new approach to the analysis of drug combination in vitro. Ann N Y Acad Sci 1990; 616:490–4.

72. Prichard MN, Prichard LE, Shipman C, Jr. Strategic design and three-dimensional analysis of antiviral drug combinations. Antimicrob Agents Chemother 1993; 37:540–5.

73. Buckheit RW, Jr., White EL, Fliakas-Boltz V, et al. Unique anti-human immunodeficiency virus activities of the nonnucleoside reverse transcriptase inhibitors calanolide A, costatolide, and dihydrocostatolide. Antimicrob Agents Chemother 1999; 43:1827–34.

74. Cane PA. Stability of transmitted drug-resistant HIV-1 species. Curr Opin Infect Dis 2005; 18:537–42.

75. Tozzi V, Corpolongo A, Bellagamba R, Narciso P. Managing patients with sexual transmission of drug-resistant HIV. Sex Health 2005; 2:135–42.

76. Tien D, Schnaare RL, Kang F, et al. In vitro and in vivo characterization of a potential universal placebo designed for use in vaginal microbicide clinical trials. AIDS Res Hum Retroviruses 2005; 21:845–53.

77. Shattock RJ, Griffin GE, Gorodeski GI. In vitro models of mucosal HIV transmission. Nat Med 2000; 6:607–8.

78. Weislow OS, Kiser R, Fine DL, et al. New soluble-formazan assay for HIV-1 cytopathic effects: application to high-flux screening of synthetic and natural products for AIDS-antiviral activity. J Natl Cancer Inst 1989; 81:577–86.

79. Shigeta M, Nakamoto T, Nakahara M, Hiromoto N, Usui T. Horseshoe kidney with retrocaval ureter and ureteropelvic junction obstruction: a case report. Int J Urol 1997; 4:206–8.

80. Huntley CC, Weiss WJ, Gazumyan A, et al. RFI-641, a potent respiratory syncytial virus inhibitor. Antimicrob Agents Chemother 2002; 46:841–7.

81. Appleyard G, Maber HB. A plaque assay for the study of influenza virus inhibitors. J Antimicrob Chemother 1975; 1:49–53.

82. Biron KK, Elion GB. Effect of acyclovir combined with other antiherpetic agents on varicella zoster virus in vitro. Am J Med 1982; 73:54–7.

83. Ouzounov S, Mehta A, Dwek RA, Block TM, Jordan R. The combination of interferon alpha-2b and n-butyl deoxynojirimycin has a greater than additive antiviral effect upon production of infectious bovine viral diarrhea virus (BVDV) in vitro: implications for hepatitis C virus (HCV) therapy. Antiviral Res 2002; 55:425–35.

84. Barnard DL, Hubbard VD, Smee DF, et al. In vitro activity of expanded-spectrum pyridazinyl oxime ethers related to pirodavir: novel capsid-binding inhibitors with potent antipicornavirus activity. Antimicrob Agents Chemother 2004; 48:1766–72.

85. Chiba S, Striker RL, Jr., Benyesh-Melnick M. Microculture plaque assay for human and simian cytomegaloviruses. Appl Microbiol 1972; 23:780–3.

86. Sudo K, Konno K, Yokota T, Shigeta S. A sensitive assay system screening antiviral compounds against herpes simplex virus type 1 and type 2. J Virol Methods 1994; 49:169–78.

87. Mehl JK, Witiak DT, Hamparian VV, Hughes JH. Antiviral activity of antilipidemic compounds on herpes simplex virus type 1. Antimicrob Agents Chemother 1980; 18:269–75.

88. Hosoya M, Shigeta S, Nakamura K, De Clercq E. Inhibitory effect of selected antiviral compounds on measles (SSPE) virus replication in vitro. Antiviral Res 1989; 12:87–97.

89. Palese P, Schulman JL, Bodo G, Meindl P. Inhibition of influenza and parainfluenza virus replication in tissue culture by 2-deoxy-2,3-dehydro-N-trifluoroacetylneuraminic acid (FANA). Virology 1974; 59:490–8.

90. Markland W, McQuaid TJ, Jain J, Kwong AD. Broad-spectrum antiviral activity of the IMP dehydrogenase inhibitor VX-497: a comparison with ribavirin and demonstration of antiviral additivity with alpha interferon. Antimicrob Agents Chemother 2000; 44:859–66.

91. Rubin RH, Swartz MN. Trimethoprim-sulfamethoxazole. N Engl J Med 1980; 303:426–32.

92. ATC/CDC/IDSA. Treatment of tuberculosis. Am J Respir Crit Care Med 2003; 167:603–62.

93. Malfertheiner P, Megraud F, O'Morain C, et al. Current concepts in the management of $Helicobacter\ pylori$ infection – the Maastricht 2 – 2000 Consensus Report. Aliment Pharmacol Ther 2002; 16:167–80.

94. National Committee for Clinical Laboratory Standards. Methods for Dilution Antimicrobial Susceptibility Tests for Bacteria that Grow Aerobically. M7-A6. National Committee for Clinical Laboratory Standards. Wayne, PA, 2003.

95. Eliopoulos G, Moellering R. Antimicrobial combinations. In: Lorian V, ed. Antibiotics in Laboratory Medicine. Baltimore, MD: Williams & Wilkins, 1991, p 60.

96. Odds FC. Synergy, antagonism, and what the chequerboard puts between them. J Antimicrob Chemother 2003; 52:1.

97. National Committee for Clinical Laboratory Standards. Methods for Determining Bactericidal Activity of Antimicrobial Agents. M26-P. National Committee for Clinical Laboratory Standards. Wayne, PA, 1987.

98. White RL, Burgess DS, Manduru M, Bosso JA. Comparison of three different in vitro methods of detecting synergy: time-kill, checkerboard, and E test. Antimicrob Agents Chemother 1996; 40:1914–8.

99. Lau WK, Young LS, Black RE, et al. Comparative efficacy and toxicity of amikacin/carbenicillin versus gentamicin/carbenicillin in leukopenic patients: a randomized prospective trail. Am J Med 1977; 62:959–66.

100. De Jongh CA, Joshi JH, Newman KA, et al. Antibiotic synergism and response in gram-negative bacteremia in granulocytopenic cancer patients. Am J Med 1986; 80:96–100.

101. Weinstein AJ, Moellering RC, Jr. Penicillin and gentamicin therapy for enterococcal infections. JAMA 1973; 223:1030–2.

102. Mandell LA, Bartlett JG, Dowell SF, et al. Update of practice guidelines for the management of community-acquired pneumonia in immunocompetent adults. Clin Infect Dis 2003, 37:1405–33.

103. Muller M, dela Pena A, Derendorf H. Issues in pharmacokinetics and pharmacodynamics of anti-infective agents: distribution in tissue. Antimicrob Agents Chemother 2004; 48:1441–53.

104. Huang V, Rybak MJ. Pharmacodynamics of cefepime alone and in combination with various antimicrobials against methicillin-resistant $Staphylococcus\ aureus$ in an in vitro pharmacodynamic infection model. Antimicrob Agents Chemother 2005; 49:302–8.

Chapter 80
Antimicrobial Susceptibility Testing Methods for Bacterial Pathogens

Fred C. Tenover

1 Introduction

Gone are the days when the antimicrobial susceptibility pattern of a bacterial isolate could be predicted simply on the basis of its species identification. Although *Streptococcus pyogenes* isolates remain susceptible to penicillin, one has to continually ask – for how long? With the discovery of strains of *Staphylococcus aureus* that are highly resistant to vancomycin (1) and strains of *Acinetobacter* species that are pan resistant (2, 3), the role of antimicrobial susceptibility testing in guiding therapy for infectious diseases is becoming more and more important (4). Yet, ironically, many of these novel resistance phenotypes are not easily detected using the automated susceptibility testing methods so prevalent in today's clinical laboratories (5–7). The ability of the clinical laboratory to detect emerging resistance profiles is often directly related to the extra efforts expanded to catch novel resistance mechanisms. Although resistant bacteria were common previously only in intensive care units of hospitals, multidrug resistance has become an issue among strains of community-acquired pathogens such as Salmonella, Shigella, and even *Neisseria gonorrhoeae* (8, 9). To complicate matters even further, resistant organisms that arise in the community are now also spreading into healthcare settings (10, 11). Therefore, it is imperative that changes in resistance patterns of a wide range of bacterial pathogens be monitored continually to ensure optimal treatment both of the individual patients and for maintaining the efficacy of empiric therapy regimens. This chapter will explore the methods used for antimicrobial susceptibility testing of bacterial pathogens.

F.C. Tenover (✉)
Senior Director, Scientific Affairs, Cepheid, Sunnyvale, CA, USA
fred.tenover@cepheid.com

2 Antimicrobial Susceptibility Testing Methods

The two major phenotypic methods of determining the susceptibility of a bacterial isolate to an antimicrobial agent are disk diffusion and minimal inhibitory concentration (MIC) testing. In the United States, approximately 85% of susceptibility test results are produced using automated methods, while the remainder is mostly the result of disk diffusion testing. However, clinical laboratories also utilize a series of screening and confirmation tests to detect subtle resistance mechanisms and ensure the accuracy of antimicrobial susceptibility test reports (Table 1). More recently, molecular methods to detect antimicrobial resistance genes and mutations associated with resistance phenotypes have been introduced into clinical microbiology laboratories. While the most commonly used test is likely the direct detection of methicillin-resistant *Staphylococcus aureus* (MRSA) in nasal samples using real-time polymerase chain reaction (PCR) assays (12), a variety of other testing platforms, including pyrosequencing (13) and peptide–nucleic acid fluorescent in situ hybridization assays (PNA-FISH) (14) are also being introduced in clinical microbiology laboratories.

2.1 Disk Diffusion

The disk diffusion method has one of the more colorful histories among clinical microbiology tests, which includes luminaries in anti-infective research such as Alexander Fleming, John Sherris, and William Kirby; international collaborative studies headed by the highly influential microbiologist Hans Ericsson; and even a U.S. Supreme Court decision (15–17). The method as we now know it consists of placing paper disks saturated with suspected inhibitors of bacterial growth (usually antimicrobial agents) on a lawn of bacteria seeded on the surface of an agar medium, incubating

D.L. Mayers (ed.), *Antimicrobial Drug Resistance*,
DOI 10.1007/978-1-60327-595-8_80, © Humana Press, a part of Springer Science+Business Media, LLC 2009

Table 1 Phenotypic screening and confirmation tests

Test name	Resistance phenotype detected	Organism groups
Aminoglycoside resistance, high level	Loss of synergistic activity with ampicillin, penicillin, and vancomycin	Enterococci
Cefoxitin disk test	*mecA*-Mediated oxacillin resistance	Staphylococci
D-zone test	Inducible clindamycin resistance	Staphylococci, streptococci
Extended spectrum beta-lactamase screening test	Penicillin and cephalosporin resistance	*Escherichia coli*, *Klebsiella* species, *Proteus mirabilis*
Extended spectrum beta-lactamase confirmation test	Penicillin and cephalosporin resistance	*Escherichia coli*, *Klebsiella* species, *Proteus mirabilis*
Nalidixic acid screen	Low level-fluoroquinolone resistance	Salmonella typhi

the plate overnight, and measuring the presence or absence of a zone of inhibition around the disks. In the early 1950s, there was little standardization of the disk content, inoculum size, or incubation conditions among laboratories performing the tests. Often times multiple disks, each with a different concentration of the same antimicrobial agent, were used to assess susceptibility. Ericsson and colleagues developed a standardized single-disk method that was widely used in Scandinavia (18). This served as the basis for an international collaborative study that eventually produced a standardized method. Studies conducted at the University of Washington in the mid-1960s resulted in the technique often referred to as the "Kirby–Bauer method", which was published by Bauer and colleagues in 1966 (19). This method standardized the variables of disk size, inoculum size, temperature, and time of incubation. Results were reported qualitatively as susceptible, intermediate, or resistant. Around this same time, several companies manufactured disks for testing in the United States, but the amount of drug present in the disks varied wildly from lot to lot. The U.S. Food and Drug Administration (FDA) accepted the responsibility for monitoring the content and potency of each lot of disks manufactured in the United States. A challenge to that authority by a disk manufacturer made its way to the U.S. Supreme Court in 1962. In their decision, the Supreme Court not only reaffirmed the responsibility of the FDA to monitor each batch of disks for potency, but noted that manufacturers of antibiotic disks had a legal obligation to describe how the disks were to be used (20). The U.S. Supreme Court recommended the single-disk method of Bauer et al. as the standardized testing method of choice. The rejection rate of antimicrobial disk lots by the FDA dropped from 66% in 1958 to only 5% in 1962. The disk diffusion method described by Bauer et al. has been continually expanded and improved by the National Committee for Clinical Laboratory Standards (now the Clinical and Laboratory Standards Institute (CLSI)) in the United States. Several other international societies (e.g., the British Society for Antimicrobial Chemotherapy and the European Union Committee for Antimicrobial Susceptibility Testing (EUCAST)) have developed similar techniques. Alternative disk-based methods including the Roscoe

NeoSensitabs and the Australian CDM method are also used in some countries. Instruments that measure the zones of inhibition using cameras can speed the process of reading disk diffusion plates. These instruments can also transform the zone diameter readings into approximate MIC values.

2.2 Minimal Inhibitory Concentration Testing

The goal of MIC testing is to provide a quantitative result (in µg/ml) along with a categorical interpretation (susceptible, intermediate, or resistant) that can guide antimicrobial therapy more precisely, particularly for infections in body sites where antimicrobial agents achieve lower concentrations than in serum (e.g., cerebrospinal fluid and bone). MIC testing can be performed by one of several methods including agar dilution, broth microdilution, agar gradient dilution (the Etest method), or by one of several automated methods. Quantitative MIC results are also useful when long-term therapy is required, as for bacterial endocarditis.

2.2.1 Agar Dilution

The agar dilution method involves preparing a series of agar plates containing the antimicrobial agent to be tested in increasing concentrations, usually in doubling dilutions (i.e., 1, 2, 4, 8, 16, 32 µg/ml, etc.). A suspension of the organism to be tested is prepared to equal the turbidity of a 0.5 McFarland standard (approximately 1×10^8 colony forming units (CFU) per ml) and 1–5 µl of this suspension is placed on each of the series of plates with increasing concentrations of the antimicrobial agent using a Steers replicator (approximately 5×10^4 CFU). Thirty different bacterial isolates (plus quality control organisms) can be tested simultaneously on each agar plate. Non-fastidious organisms are incubated at 35°C for 16–18 h usually in ambient air, while fastidious organisms, such as *Streptococcus pneumoniae,* are incubated from 18 to 24 h, typically in a CO_2-enriched atmosphere. The agar dilution method, while laborious owing to the time required to prepare each set of agar plates for each antimicrobial agent to be tested, is often cost effective for laboratories that test large numbers of bacterial isolates against a limited set of antimicrobial agents. The testing medium is usually Mueller–Hinton agar for non-fastidious organisms and Mueller–Hinton agar containing 5% sheep blood for fastidious organisms. The exceptions are *Haemophilus influenzae* isolates, which requires HTM media, and *Neisseria gonorrhoeae*, which requires the GC medium.

2.2.2 Broth Microdilution

Broth microdilution is the standard method used in most reference laboratories in the United States and abroad. The method typically tests twofold dilutions of multiple antimicrobial agents in 96-well disposable plastic trays. The test medium is typically cation adjusted Mueller–Hinton broth, or for fastidious organisms, cation-adjusted Mueller–Hinton broth containing 5% lysed horse blood. A suspension of the organism to be tested is prepared in saline or Mueller–Hinton broth to the turbidity of a 0.5 McFarland standard (approximately 1×10^8 CFU/ml). The suspension is diluted 1:20 in saline, and 1–5 µl of this suspension is transferred to the 96-well tray containing doubling dilutions of the antimicrobial agents to be tested (usually between 8 and 12 antimicrobial agents per tray) using a disposable plastic inoculator (the inoculum size varies with the size of the pins in the inoculator). The final inoculum size is 5×10^5 CFU/ml or 5×10^4 CFU/well.

2.2.3 Automated Susceptibility Testing Methods

A series of commercially available automated and semiautomated methods are available to assist laboratories in testing and reporting the results of antimicrobial susceptibility tests. Most of the methods combine bacterial identification and susceptibility testing reagents in a single panel or card to enhance the speed with which antimicrobial susceptibility testing results can be reported. Many systems also incorporate the software to interpret the results and prepare reports that can be linked readily to laboratory information systems, which in turn deliver the results to the patients' electronic medical record. The goal of the automated methods is to reduce the time necessary to produce accurate identification and susceptibility test results. Indeed, results may be available for some bacterial species in as little as 6 h, versus the 16–18 h often required for disk diffusion testing or standard MIC tests. For staphylococci, the results of oxacillin and vancomycin tests often require prolonged incubation times (usually 24 h) to achieve accurate results. Some systems employ "expert rules" to enhance reporting by recognizing

and flagging unusual results, such as ampicillin-susceptible *Klebsiella pneumoniae*, where the bacterial identification and susceptibility pattern are conflicting with typical results for wild-type *K. pneumoniae* populations, or rare results, such as carbapenem-resistant Enterobacteriaceae or vancomycin-resistant *Staphylococcus aureus*.

Overall, automated systems work well, although they have traditionally shown problems with certain resistance phenotypes including oxacillin-resistant *S. aureus* strains (21) and *Pseudomonas aeruginosa* strains that are resistant to newer β-lactam agents, such as piperacillin (22).

2.2.4 Agar Gradient Dilution

Agar gradient dilution is a proprietary method (called the Etest, AB Biodisk, Solna, Sweden), which incorporates MIC testing into a format similar to the setup of a disk diffusion test. The antimicrobial agent is microencapsulated on the back of a plastic strip and, when placed on the surface of an agar plate, the antimicrobial agent diffuses off the strip into the agar medium in a rapid and predictable fashion forming a gradient. The Etest strip evaluates the inhibitory potential of a single antimicrobial agent over a large range of concentrations. Several Etest strips containing different antimicrobial agents can be arranged on a single agar plate. The Etest method is particularly useful for testing fastidious microorganisms such as campylobacters (23), pneumococci (24), and anaerobic bacteria (25), for which only a limited number of antimicrobial agents need to be tested.

3 Interpretive Guidelines

Once a disk diffusion zone of inhibition has been measured or an MIC for an antimicrobial agent has been determined, and the microbiologist has affirmed that the quality control results indicate that the testing system has performed appropriately, the results of the susceptibility test have to be interpreted. For most antimicrobial agents, the results transmitted to the patient's chart will be "susceptible", "intermediate", or "resistant". If an MIC method was used, the results transmitted may include the quantitative MIC result as well. However, for some antimicrobial agents, such as daptomycin when testing staphylococci, the results transmitted will be either "susceptible" or "non-susceptible". This is because at the time the drug was approved for use by the FDA and when interpretive criteria (i.e., breakpoints) were established by the CLSI, there were inadequate numbers of resistant strains available on which to establish intermediate and resistant breakpoints (26). The lack of interpretive intermediate and resistant breakpoints often poses a challenge for the automated methods which, depending on the system, will either leave the interpretation field blank for a non-susceptible result, or place an "N" or "NS" (for non-susceptible), or an "NI" (for non-interpretable) in the interpretation field – a result that may be confusing to the physician reading the laboratory report. Some microbiology laboratories will override these "non-S, I or R results" and simply report them as resistant to avoid confusing physicians.

The categorical interpretations used for disk diffusion and MIC test results are drawn from one of several standard-setting organizations. In the United States, this is the CLSI. The description of the reference disk diffusion method and the interpretive criteria for antimicrobial agents approved in the United States, and several antimicrobial agents available only outside of the United States, are available in the M2 document (Performance Standards for Antimicrobial Disk Susceptibility Tests). The M2 series is revised every 3 years. The most recent version that was published in 2009 was M2-A10 (27). The agar and broth dilution reference (MIC) methods are described in CLSI document M7 (Methods for Dilution Antimicrobial Susceptibility Tests for Bacteria that Grow Aerobically). The most recent version of this document, also published in 2009, is M7-A8 (28). A separate document containing the interpretive criteria for both disk diffusion and MIC testing, quality control ranges, and methods for preparing and diluting antimicrobial agents is published each year in January (the M100 series). Similar documents are published by the EUCAST (see http://www.srga.org/Eucastwt/bpsetting.htm), the British Society for Antimicrobial Chemotherapy (see http://www.bsac.org.uk/), and other organizations. A new document outlining interpretive criteria for susceptibility tests conducted with infrequently isolated or fastidious bacteria (M45) has recently been published by CLSI (29).

4 Resistance Phenotypes that Require Specialized Testing

4.1 β-Lactam Agents

Resistance to penicillins, cephalosporins, and carbapenems among Gram-negative organisms is usually mediated by β-lactamases, either intrinsic or acquired, that hydrolyze the β-lactam ring of the antimicrobial agent, which detoxifies the drug. Among Gram-positive organisms, in addition to β-lactamases, β-lactam resistance can be mediated by changes in the affinity of the penicillin-binding proteins (PBPs) for the antimicrobial agent. Among staphylococci this is usually mediated by acquisition of a novel PBP (i.e., PBP 2a), while in pneumococci and viridans strepto-

cocci, reduced affinity is usually the result of remodeling of the PBP genes by incorporating foreign DNA to form mosaic genes. β-Lactam resistance in both Gram-positive and Gram-negative organisms poses unique challenges for antimicrobial susceptibility testing methods.

Detection of oxacillin (methicillin) resistance in staphylococci is difficult primarily because oxacillin-resistant strains tend to grow more slowly and often show heteroresistance, i.e., only a fraction of the bacterial population actually manifests the resistance phenotype. Various strategies have been used over the years to increase the likelihood of detecting the resistant subpopulation, including growing the strains at 35°C instead of 37°C, adding 2% NaCl to the testing medium, and incubating the test for a full 24 h (21). More recently, on the basis of studies by Felten et al. (30), Skov et al. (31), Swenson and Tenover (32), and others, CLSI has described a cefoxitin-based disk diffusion test that accurately predicts the presence of the *mecA* gene among both *S. aureus* and coagulase-negative staphylococci. The test can be read in 16–18 h and replaces the use of the oxacillin disk for disk diffusion testing.

Among the Enterobacteriaceae, the major susceptibility testing challenge is to detect the presence of extended-spectrum β-lactamases. These β-lactamases, which are typically encoded by derivatives of bla_{TEM}, bla_{SHV}, and bla_{CTX-M} genes, mediate resistance to aztreonam and third-generation cephalosporins (such as cefotaxime, ceftriaxone, and ceftazidime) (33–35) and, in some cases, fourth-generation cephalosporins (such as cefepime and cefpirome) (36). Since the extended-spectrum β-lactamases (ESBLs) do not hydrolyse all the extended-spectrum cephalosporins at similar rates, some organisms may show resistance to certain cephalosporins but susceptibility to others, even though clinically the latter cephalosporins will not be effective (37, 38). To identify strains of *Escherichia coli*, *K. pneumoniae*, and *Proteus mirabilis* that contain ESBLs, organisms are tested with cefotaxime and ceftazidime, either by disk diffusion or broth microdilution, in the presence and absence of clavulanic acid – a β-lactamase inhibitor. If the zones of inhibition increase by 5 mm or more in the presence of clavulanic acid, or the MICs decrease by three or more doubling dilutions in the presence of clavulanic acid when compared to the results in the absence of clavulanic acid, the strain contains an ESBL (27, 28). Thus, the results for all penicillins, cephalosporins, and aztreonam (but not cefamycins, such as cefoxitin or cefotetan), are reported as resistant. β-Lactam–β-lactamase inhibitor combinations, such as piperacillin–tazobactam, are reported as they test (either susceptible, intermediate, or resistant), since they may still be effective clinically against some ESBL-producing strains of *K. pneumoniae* or *E. coli* (39). Similar strategies to identify plasmid-mediated AmpC β-lactamases using boronic acid have been described (40, 41); however, these tests have not been promulgated by CLSI and currently do not impact the reporting of penicillin or cephalosporin results.

4.2 Macrolides, Azalides, Lincosamides, and Streptogramins

The macrolides, which include agents such as erythromycin and clarithromycin, and the azalides, such as azithromycin, are commonly administered oral drugs used for the treatment of many bacterial respiratory infections and superficial skin infections. Resistance is due to inactivation of drug (mediated by erythromycin esterases or phosphorylases) or to the efflux of the drug out of the cell, or by modification of the site of action (42). The latter mechanism, in which the 23S RNA of the 50S ribosome unit is methylated at a specific adenine residue, which prevents binding of the antimicrobial agent to the ribosome, leads to high-level resistance to macrolides but also affects lincosamides (such as clindamycin) and streptogramins (such as pristinamycin), since all three classes of drugs act by binding to the same site on the bacterial ribosome. The so-called MLS_B-resistance phenotype (for macrolide–lincosamide–streptogramin$_B$) is typically observed in staphylococci and streptococci. Strains of staphylococci and streptococci that test as erythromycin-resistant but clindamycin-susceptible may contain an inducible *erm* gene encoding MLS_B resistance, or an efflux gene such as *msrA* (in staphylococci) or *mefA* (in streptococci). Since mutations in the *erm* genes can lead to clindamycin resistance, and therefore clindamycin treatment failure, it is important to differentiate these two resistance mechanisms in the clinical laboratory to enhance the accuracy of reporting (efflux-mediated resistance cannot mutate to clindamycin resistance). The D-zone test, which is a disk diffusion–based assay, uses an erythromycin disk that is placed 15–25 mm away from a clindamycin disk on an agar plate seeded with a lawn of the test organism (43). Blunting of the zone of inhibition between the erythromycin and clindamycin disks (which forms a "D" shape) indicates the presence of an inducible *erm* gene. A circular zone of inhibition (normal zone) indicates a negative test. If the D-zone test is positive, the results for clindamycin are reported as resistant (44).

4.3 Aminoglycosides

Aminoglycosides are commonly used in conjunction with β-lactam agents (or vancomycin in Gram-positive organisms) to treat serious bacterial infections, such as endocarditis, because the two groups of drugs frequently act synergistically. Resistance to aminoglycosides is typically mediated by enzymes that modify the drug so that uptake into the bacterial cell is impaired (45). However, efflux of drug out of the bacterial cell and permeability barriers to aminoglycosides are also recognized. There are three types of aminoglycoside-modifying enzymes: those that acetylate, adenylate, or phosphorylate the drug. The number of genes encoding variants of these enzymes within each group is remarkably large and diverse. To determine whether there is likely to be synergy between the aminoglycosides (i.e., gentamicin or streptomycin) and a cell wall active agent (either ampicillin or vancomycin) for treating enterococcal infections, special disk diffusion and MIC tests to detect high-level aminoglycoside resistance have been established by CLSI (27, 28). The presence of high-level resistance to either aminoglycoside will negate the likelihood of synergistic activity with a cell wall–active agent.

4.4 Sulfa Drugs and Trimethoprim

Both sulfa drugs and trimethoprim inhibit the enzymatic pathway that synthesizes dihydrofolate. The two drugs are usually tested together in a 19:1 ratio of sulfamethoxazole to trimethoprim (44). Because MIC tests using this combination of drugs often result in trailing end points (i.e., a gradual reduction of growth instead of a clear break between the wells of an MIC plate showing growth and those with no growth), the well showing ≥80% inhibition of growth is usually chosen as the MIC (28).

4.5 Glycopeptides

Glycopeptide resistance can be mediated by a series of genes that effectively remodel the cell wall of an organism by altering the D-alanine-D-alanine binding site of vancomycin to D-alanine-D-lactate or D-alanine-D-serine through introduction of an altered ligase enzyme (e.g., *vanA*). The family of acquired vancomycin resistance genes now includes *vanA*, *vanB*, *vanD*, *vanE*, and *vanG* (46, 47). The *vanA* resistance determinant has been recognized among enterococci (48) and *S. aureus* isolates (49), the latter due to acquisition of Tn *1546* and its variants (50). A second mechanism of resistance noted among glycopeptide-intermediate *S. aureus* (GISA) strains (also called vancomycin intermediate strains or VISAs) is the thickening of the cell wall in conjunction with metabolic changes that make *S. aureus* isolates no longer susceptible to glycopeptides (51–53). While detection of *vanA*-mediated resistance in *S. aureus* has been a challenge for automated MIC methods (54), and in some cases for GISA isolates, GISA isolates have never been detected in the clinical laboratory using disk diffusion (55). Clinical laboratories typically augment their testing for glycopeptide resistance in staphylococci (whether they use an automated susceptibility method or disk diffusion) by inoculating a Brain Heat Infusion agar plate containing 6 μg/ml of vancomycin with approximately 10^6 CFU of the staphylococcal strain to be tested (29). This is a very sensitive method for detecting GISA strains as well as vancomycin-resistant *Staphylococcus aureus* (VRSA).

4.6 Fluoroquinolones

Fluoroquinolones are used widely to treat a variety of infections around the world. Resistance to fluoroquinolones typically arises by alterations in the target enzymes (DNA gyrase and topoisomerase IV) and through changes in drug entry and efflux (56). Recent discovery of plasmid-mediated horizontally transferable genes encoding quinolone resistance (e.g., *qnrA*, *qnrB*, and *qnrS*) perhaps explains some of the rapid emergence of resistance to these drugs (57, 58). Likewise, AAC(6')-Ib-cr, a variant aminoglycoside acetyltransferase capable of modifying ciprofloxacin and reducing its activity, also seems to provide low-level quinolone resistance (59). It appears that low-level resistance to fluoroquinolones (by whatever mechanism) may be responsible for clinical failures when treating *Salmonella typhi* (60) and non-typhoidal Salmonella infections (61). Strains isolated from patients who failed therapy typically show ciprofloxacin MICs that are elevated (0.25–1 μg/ml compared with typical MICs of 0.003–0.06 μg/ml) but still in the susceptible range; however, the nalidixic acid MICs are usually resistant (MIC > 16 μg/ml). Thus, testing nalidixic acid may indicate strains of *S. typhi* that, while still susceptible to fluoroquinolones by in vitro testing, are likely to fail fluoroquinolone therapy (44).

4.7 Oxazolidinones

Oxazolidinones, such as linezolid, have broad activity against many Gram-positive organisms (62). Resistance to the oxazolidinones among staphylococci and enterococci is due to modification of ribosomal RNA often through a G to T substitution at position 2765, or one of several other mutations (63, 64). Detection of resistance to linezolid, particularly among staphylococci, can be difficult by agar-based methods such as disk diffusion and agar gradient dilution, which tend to lack sensitivity to detect some resistant isolates. Studies at the Centers for Disease Control and Prevention (CDC) have indicated that broth-based MIC methods typically have better sensitivity for detecting resistance.

4.8 Lipopetides

Daptomycin is an example of a lipopeptide that is rapidly bactericidal for most Gram-positive bacteria (65–68). Testing daptomycin typically requires the presence of 50 mM Ca^{2+} in the broth or agar medium to achieve accurate results. Disk diffusion testing lacked adequate sensitivity to detect reduced susceptibility to daptomycin in clinical studies. Therefore, the disk diffusion test was withdrawn from the market. However, the agar gradient method was shown to work well (69).

5 Molecular Tests to Detect Resistant Bacteria

5.1 General Considerations

DNA probes and PCR assays have been used for many years to detect antimicrobial resistance genes or mutations associated with resistance in bacterial isolates in research laboratories (70). An extensive list of PCR primers to detect a variety of antimicrobial resistance genes is available (71). Novel molecular assays, such as real-time PCR (72) and pyro-sequencing (13), offer both rapid turnaround times and high sensitivity for identifying antimicrobial resistance genes or mutations associated with resistance in bacterial isolates directly in clinical samples. Such results may be used in conjunction with other rapid technologies, such as PNA-FISH to guide therapy or to decide whether to place a patient in a hospital isolation room (14).

However, there are several caveats associated with using genetic tests to detect resistant organisms. These include lack of expression of resistance genes that are detected, the problem of mixed or normal flora that may contain a resistance gene (such as *vanB* in *Clostridium* species in fecal samples (73)), mutations in target organisms that alter sequences used for PCR primers resulting in false-negative results, and the emergence of novel resistance genes that are not detected by existing genetic assays (71). Each of these can affect the sensitivity or specificity of molecular assays.

5.2 Assays for MRSA and Vancomycin-Resistant Enterococcus (VRE)

The direct detection of MRSA in nasal swabs from patients that are being admitted to a healthcare institution or in patients that will be undergoing a surgical procedure has become a major topic of discussion in the United States (74). The availability of an FDA-cleared amplification-based assay for detection of MRSA (12) has led to a dramatic upswing in the interest of using molecular-based assays for detection of a variety of resistance genes and mutations associated with resistance in clinical laboratories (75, 76). The vancomycin-resistant enterococci, particularly the multiply resistant *E. faecium* isolates which are becoming common in many hospitals, are among other healthcare-associated pathogens that may be monitored using molecular methods (76).

Finally, there is particular interest in rapid detection of mutations associated with resistance to isoniazid, rifampin, and streptomycin in clinical samples containing *Mycobacterium tuberculosis* using novel strategies, such as pyrosequencing (77, 78) Other pyrosequencing assays for mutations associated with bacterial resistance include those for linezolid resistance in enterococci (64) and fluoroquinolone resistance in *Neisseria gonorrhoeae* (79).

6 Conclusions

The goal of antimicrobial susceptibility testing is to provide physicians with data that will assist them in choosing the optimal antimicrobial agent to treat an infection in a patient. Susceptibility testing in most clinical microbiology laboratories represents a combination of phenotypic assays that provide at least qualitative results (susceptible, intermediate, or resistant) for a series of antimicrobial agents, and often quantitative results (MICs) that can guide dosing regimens. Molecular-based tests, such as real-time PCR, may provide rapid information on the presence of MRSA or VRE in patients, which will assist in infection control decisions.

References

1. Chang, S., Sievert, D. M., Hageman, J. C., Boulton, M. L., Tenover, F. C., Downes, F. P., Shah, S., Rudrik, J. T., Pupp, G. R., Brown, W. J., Cardo, D. & Fridkin, S. K. (2003). Infection with vancomycin-resistant *Staphylococcus aureus* containing the vanA resistance gene. *N Engl J Med* **348**, 1342–7.
2. Wang, S. H., Sheng, W. H., Chang, Y. Y., Wang, L. H., Lin, H. C., Chen, M. L., Pan, H. J., Ko, W. J., Chang, S. C. & Lin, F. Y. (2003). Healthcare-associated outbreak due to pan-drug resistant *Acinetobacter baumannii* in a surgical intensive care unit. *J Hosp Infect* **53**, 97–102.
3. Mahgoub, S., Ahmed, J. & Glatt, A. E. (2002). Completely resistant *Acinetobacter baumannii* strains. *Infect Control Hosp Epidemiol* **23**, 477–9.
4. McGowan, J. E., Jr. & Tenover, F. C. (2004). Confronting bacterial resistance in healthcare settings: a crucial role for microbiologists. *Nat Microbiol* **2**, 251–8.
5. Steward, C. D., Mohammed, J. M., Swenson, J. M., Stocker, S. A., Williams, P. P., Gaynes, R. P., McGowan, J. E., Jr. & Tenover, F. C. (2003). Antimicrobial susceptibility testing of carbapenems: multicenter validity testing and accuracy levels of five antimicrobial test methods for detecting resistance in *Enterobacteriaceae* and *Pseudomonas aeruginosa* isolates. *J Clin Microbiol* **41**, 351–8.
6. Tenover, F. C., Kalsi, R. K., Williams, P. P., Carey, R. B., Stocker, S., Lonsway, D., Rasheed, J. K., Biddle, J. W., McGowan, J. E., Jr. & Hanna, B. (2006). Carbapenem resistance in *Klebsiella pneumoniae* not detected by automated susceptibility testing. *Emerg Infect Dis* **12**, 1209–13.
7. Steward, C. D., Stocker, S. A., Swenson, J. M., O'Hara, C. M., Edwards, J. R., Gaynes, R. P., McGowan, J. E., Jr. & Tenover, F. C. (1999). Comparison of agar dilution, disk diffusion, MicroScan, and Vitek antimicrobial susceptibility testing methods to broth microdilution for detection of fluoroquinolone-resistant isolates of the family Enterobacteriaceae. *J Clin Microbiol* **37**, 544–7.
8. Tenover, F. C. & Hughes, J. M. (1996). The challenges of emerging infectious diseases. Development and spread of multiply-resistant bacterial pathogens. *JAMA* **275**, 300–4.
9. Tenover, F. C. & McGowan, J. E., Jr. (1998). Epidemiology and molecular biology of antimicrobial resistance in bacteria. In *Pathology of Emerging Infections 2* (Nelson, A. M. & Horsburgh, C. R., Jr., eds.), pp. 343–59. American Society for Microbiology Press, Washington, DC.
10. Saiman, L., O'Keefe, M., Graham, P. L., III, Wu, F., Said-Salim, B., Kreiswirth, B., LaSala, A., Schlievert, P. M. & Della-Latta, P. (2003). Hospital transmission of community acquired methicillin resistant *Staphylococcus aureus* among postpartum women. *Clin Infect Dis* **37**, 1313–9.
11. Klevens, R. M., Edwards, J. R., Tenover, F. C., McDonald, L. C., Horan, T. & Gaynes, R. (2006). Changes in the epidemiology of methicillin-resistant *Staphylococcus aureus* in intensive care units in US hospitals, 1992–2003. *Clin Infect Dis* **42**, 389–91.
12. Huletsky, A., Lebel, P., Picard, F. J, Bernier, M., Gagnon, M., Boucher, N. & Bergeron, M. G. (2005). Identification of methicillin-resistant *Staphylococcus aureus* carriage in less than 1 hour during a hospital surveillance program. *Clin Infect Dis* **40**, 976–81.
13. Ahmadian, A., Ehn, M. & Hober, S. (2006). Pyrosequencing: history, biochemistry and future. *Clin Chim Acta* **363**, 83–94.
14. Tenover, F. C. (2007). Rapid detection and identification of bacterial pathogens using novel molecular technologies: infection control and beyond. *Clin Infect Dis* **44**, 418–23.
15. Sherris, J. C. (1989). Antimicrobic susceptibility testing. A personal perspective. *Clin Lab Med* **9**, 191–202.
16. Fleming, A. (1929). On the antibacterial action of cultures of a penicillin with a special reference to their use in the isolate of *B. influenzae*. *Br J Exp Pathol* **10**, 226–9.
17. Barry, A. L. (1989). Standardization of antimicrobial susceptibility testing. *Clin Lab Med* **9**, 203–19.
18. Ericsson, H. (1960). The paper disc method for determination of bacterial sensitivity to antibiotics. Studies on the accuracy of the technique. *Scand J Clin Lab Invest* **12**, 408–13.
19. Bauer, A. W., Kirby, W. M., Sherris, J. C. & Turck, M. (1966). Antibiotic susceptibility testing by a standardized single disk method. *Am J Clin Pathol* **45**, 493–6.
20. Federal Register. (1972). Rules and regulations: antibiotic susceptibility discs. *Fed Regist* **37**, 20525.
21. Swenson, J. M., Williams, P. P., Killgore, G., O'Hara, C. M. & Tenover, F. C. (2001). Performance of eight methods, including two new rapid methods, for detection of oxacillin resistance in a challenge set of *Staphylococcus aureus* organisms. *J Clin Microbiol* **39**, 3785–8.
22. Juretschko, S., Labombardi, V. J., Lerner, S. A. & Schreckenberger, P. C. (2007). Accuracy of β-lactam susceptibility testing results for *Pseudomonas aeruginosa* among four automated systems (BD Phoenix, MicroScan WalkAway, Vitek, Vitek 2). *J Clin Microbiol* **45**, 1339–42.
23. Huang, M. B., Baker, C. N., Banerjee, S. & Tenover, F. C. (1992). Accuracy of the E test for determining antimicrobial susceptibilities of staphylococci, enterococci, *Campylobacter jejuni*, and gram-negative bacteria resistant to antimicrobial agents. *J Clin Microbiol* **30**, 3243–8.

24. Jorgensen, J. H., Ferraro, M. J., McElmeel, M. L., Spargo, J., Swenson, J. M. & Tenover, F. C. (1994). Detection of penicillin and extended-spectrum cephalosporin resistance among *Streptococcus pneumoniae* clinical isolates by use of the E test. *J Clin Microbiol* **32**, 159–63.

25. Croco, J. L., Erwin, M. E., Jennings, J. M., Putnam, L. R. & Jones, R. N. (1994). Evaluation of the Etest for antimicrobial spectrum and potency determinations of anaerobes associated with bacterial vaginosis and peritonitis. *Diagn Microbiol Infect Dis* **20**, 213–9.

26. Clinical and Laboratory Standards Institute. (2005). *Performance Standards for Antimicrobial Susceptibility Testing: Fifteenth Informational Supplement.* CLSI, Document M100-S15, CLSI, Wayne, PA.

27. Clinical and Laboratory Standards Institute. (2009). *Performance Standards for Antimicrobial Disk Susceptibility Tests; Approved Standard*–Tenth Edition. CLSI Document M2-A10. Clinical and Laboratory Standards Institute, Wayne, PA.

28. Clinical and Laboratory Standards Institute. (2009). *Methods for Dilution Antimicrobial Susceptibility Tests for Bacteria that Grow Aerobically; Approved Standard*–Eighth Edition. CLSI Document M7-A8. Clinical and Laboratory Standards Institute, Wayne, PA.

29. Clinical and Laboratory Standards Institute. (2005). *Methods for Antimicrobial Dilution or Disk Susceptibility Testing of Infrequently Isolated or Fastidious Bacteria; Proposed Standard*, CLSI Document M45-P. CLSI, Wayne, PA.

30. Felten, A., Grandry, B., Lagrange, P. H. & Casin, I. (2002). Evaluation of three techniques for detection of low-level methicillin-resistant *Staphylococcus aureus* (MRSA): a disk diffusion method with cefoxitin and moxalactam, the Vitek 2 system, and the MRSA-screen latex agglutination test. *J Clin Microbiol* **40**, 2766–71.

31. Skov, R., Smyth, R., Clausen, M., Larsen, A. R., Frimodt-Moller, N., Olsson-Liljequist, B. & Kahlmeter, G. (2003). Evaluation of a cefoxitin 30 μg disc on Iso-Sensitest agar for detection of methicillin-resistant *Staphylococcus aureus*. *J Antimicrob Chemother* **52**, 204–207.

32. Swenson, J. M. & Tenover, F. C. (2005). Results of disk diffusion testing with cefoxitin correlate with presence of mecA in *Staphylococcus* spp. *J Clin Microbiol* **43**, 3818–23.

33. Bush, K. (2001). New β-lactamases in gram-negative bacteria: diversity and impact on the selection of antimicrobial therapy. *Clin Infect Dis* **32**, 1085–9.

34. Bush, K., Jacoby, G. A. & Medeiros, A. A. (1995). A functional classification scheme for beta-lactamases and its correlation with molecular structure. *Antimicrob Agents Chemother* **39**, 1211–33.

35. Bonnet, R. (2004). Growing group of extended-spectrum beta-lactamases: the CTX-M enzymes. *Antimicrob Agents Chemother* **48**, 1–14.

36. Bradford, P. A. (2001). Extended-spectrum beta-lactamases in the 21st century: characterization, epidemiology, and detection of this important resistance threat. *Clin Microbiol Rev* **14**, 933–51.

37. Paterson, D. L., Ko, W. C., Von Gottberg, A., Mohapatra, S., Casellas, J. M., Goossens, H., Mulazimoglu, L., Trenholme, G., Klugman, K. P., Bonomo, R. A., Rice, L. B., Wagener, M. M., McCormack, J. G. & Yu, V. L. (2004). Antibiotic therapy for *Klebsiella pneumoniae* bacteremia: implications of production of extended-spectrum beta-lactamases. *Clin Infect Dis* **39**, 31–7.

38. Paterson, D. L., Ko, W. C., Von Gottberg, A., Mohapatra, S., Casellas, J. M., Goossens, H., Mulazimoglu, L., Trenholme, G., Klugman, K. P., Bonomo, R. A., Rice, L. B., Wagener, M. M., McCormack, J. G. & Yu, V. L. (2004). International prospective study of *Klebsiella pneumoniae* bacteremia: implications of extended-spectrum beta-lactamase production in nosocomial infections. *Ann Intern Med* **140**, 26–32.

39. Rice, L. B., Carias, L. L. & Shlaes, D. M. (1994). In vivo efficacies of beta-lactam-beta-lactamase inhibitor combinations against

a TEM-26-producing strain of *Klebsiella pneumoniae*. *Antimicrob Agents Chemother* **38**, 2663–4.

40. Coudron, P. E. (2005). Inhibitor-based methods for detection of plasmid-mediated AmpC beta-lactamases in *Klebsiella* spp., *Escherichia coli*, and *Proteus mirabilis*. *J Clin Microbiol* **43**, 4163–7.

41. Yagi, T., Wachino, J., Kurokawa, H., Suzuki, S., Yamane, K., Doi, Y., Shibata, N., Kato, H., Shibayama, K. & Arakawa, Y. (2005). Practical methods using boronic acid compounds for identification of class C beta-lactamase-producing *Klebsiella pneumoniae* and *Escherichia coli*. *J Clin Microbiol* **43**, 2551–8.

42. Roberts, M. C. & Sutcliffe, J. (2005). Macrolide, lincosamide, streptogramin, ketolide, and oxazolidinone resistance. In *Frontiers in Antimicrobial Resistance. A Tribute to Stuart B. Levy* (White, D. G., Alekshun, M. N. & McDermott, P. F., eds.), pp. 66–84. ASM, Washington, DC.

43. Steward, C. D., Raney, P. M., Morrell, A. K., Williams, P. P., McDougal, L. K., Jevitt, L., McGowan, J. E., Jr. & Tenover, F. C. (2005). Testing for induction of clindamycin resistance in erythromycin-resistant isolates of *Staphylococcus aureus*. *J Clin Microbiol* **43**, 1716–21.

44. Clinical and Laboratory Standards Institute. (2007). *Performance Standards for Antimicrobial Susceptibility Testing: Seventeenth Informational Supplement.* CLSI, Document M100-S17, CLSI, Wayne, PA.

45. Shaw, K. J., Rather, P. N., Hare, R. S. & Miller, G. H. (1993). Molecular genetics of aminoglycoside resistance genes and familial relationships of the aminoglycoside-modifying enzymes. *Microbiol Rev* **57**, 138–63.

46. Depardieu, F., Bonora, M. G., Reynolds, P. E. & Courvalin, P. (2003). The *vanG* glycopeptide resistance operon from *Enterococcus faecalis* revisited. *Mol Microbiol* **50**, 931–48.

47. Courvalin, P. (2005). Genetics of glycopeptide resistance in gram-positive pathogens. *Int J Med Microbiol* **294**, 479–86.

48. Perichon, B., Casadewall, B., Reynolds, P. & Courvalin, P. (2000). Glycopeptide-resistant *Enterococcus faecium* BM4416 is a VanD-type strain with an impaired D-alanine: D-alanine ligase. *Antimicrob Agents Chemother* **44**, 1346–8.

49. Weigel, L. M., Clewell, D. B., Gill, S. R., Clark, N. C., McDougal, L. K., Flannagan, S. E., Kolonay, J. F., Shetty, J., Killgore, G. E. & Tenover, F. C. (2003). Genetic analysis of a high-level vancomycin-resistant isolate of *Staphylococcus aureus*. *Science* **302**, 1569–71.

50. Clark, N. C., Weigel, L. M., Patel, J. B. & Tenover, F. C. (2005). Comparison of Tn1546-like elements in vancomycin-resistant *Staphylococcus aureus* isolates from Michigan and Pennsylvania. *Antimicrob Agents Chemother* **49**, 470–2.

51. Hiramatsu, K. (1998). Vancomycin resistance in staphylococci. *Drug Resist Updat* **1**, 135–150.

52. Cui, L., Ma, X., Sato, K., Okuma, K., Tenover, F. C., Mamizuka, E. M., Gemmell, C. G., Kim, M. N., Ploy, M. C., El-Solh, N., Ferraz, V. & Hiramatsu, K. (2003). Cell wall thickening is a common feature of vancomycin resistance in *Staphylococcus aureus*. *J Clin Microbiol* **41**, 5–14.

53. Hanaki, H., Kuwahara-Arai, K., Boyle-Vavra, S., Daum, R. S., Labischinski, H. & Hiramatsu, K. (1998). Activated cell-wall synthesis is associated with vancomycin resistance in methicillin-resistant *Staphylococcus aureus* clinical strains Mu3 and Mu50. *J Antimicrob Chemother* **42**, 199–209.

54. Tenover, F. C., Weigel, L. M., Appelbaum, P. C., McDougal, L. K., Chaitram, J., McAllister, S., Clark, N., Killgore, G., O'Hara, C. M., Jevitt, L., Patel, J. B. & Bozdogan, B. (2004). Vancomycin-resistant *Staphylococcus aureus* isolate from a patient in Pennsylvania. *Antimicrob Agents Chemother* **48**, 275–80.

55. Tenover, F. C., Lancaster, M. V., Hill, B. C., Steward, C. D., Stocker, S. A., Hancock, G. A., O'Hara, C. M., Clark, N. C. & Hiramatsu, K. (1998). Characterization of staphylococci with reduced susceptibilities to vancomycin and other glycopeptides. *J Clin Microbiol* **36**, 1020–27.

56. Hooper, D. C. (2001). Emerging mechanisms of fluoroquinolone resistance. *Emerg Infect Dis* **7**, 337–41.

57. Jacoby, G. A., Chow, N. & Waites, K. B. (2003). Prevalence of plasmid-mediated quinolone resistance. *Antimicrob Agents Chemother* **47**, 559–62.

58. Jacoby, G. A., Walsh, K. E., Mills, D. M., Walker, V. J., Oh, H., Robicsek, A. & Hooper, D. C. (2006). qnrB, another plasmid-mediated gene for quinolone resistance. *Antimicrob Agents Chemother* **50**, 1178–82.

59. Robicsek, A., Strahilevitz, J., Jacoby, G. A., Macielag, M., Abbanat, D., Park, C. H., Bush, K. & Hooper, D. C. (2006). Fluoroquinolone-modifying enzyme: a new adaptation of a common aminoglycoside acetyltransferase. *Nat Med* **12**, 83–8.

60. Crump, J. A., Barrett, T. J., Nelson, J. T. & Angulo, F. J. (2003). Reevaluating fluoroquinolone breakpoints for *Salmonella enterica* serotype Typhi and for non-Typhi salmonellae. *Clin Infect Dis* **37**, 75–81.

61. Gay, K., Robicsek, A., Strahilevitz, J., Park, C. H., Jacoby, G., Barrett, T. J., Medalla, F., Chiller, T. M. & Hooper, D. C. (2006). Plasmid-mediated quinolone resistance in non-Typhi serotypes of *Salmonella enterica*. *Clin Infect Dis* **43**, 297–304.

62. Chien, J. W., Kucia, M. L. & Salata, R. A. (2000). Use of linezolid, an oxazolidinone, in the treatment of multidrug-resistant gram-positive bacterial infections. *Clin Infect Dis* **30**, 146–51.

63. Pillai, S. K., Sakoulas, G., Wennersten, C., Eliopoulos, G. M., Moellering, R. C., Jr., Ferraro, M. J. & Gold, H. S. (2002). Linezolid resistance in *Staphylococcus aureus*: characterization and stability of resistant phenotype. *J Infect Dis* **186**, 1603–7.

64. Sinclair, A., Arnold, C. & Woodford, N. (2003). Rapid detection and estimation by pyrosequencing of 23S rRNA genes with a single nucleotide polymorphism conferring linezolid resistance in enterococci. *Antimicrob Agents Chemother* **47**, 3620–2.

65. Arbeit, R. D., Maki, D., Tally, F. P., Campanaro, E. & Eisenstein, B. I. (2004). The safety and efficacy of daptomycin for the treatment of complicated skin and skin-structure infections. *Clin Infect Dis* **38**, 1673–81.

66. Fowler, V. G., Jr., Boucher, H. W., Corey, G. R., Abrutyn, E., Karchmer, A. W., Rupp, M. E., Levine, D. P., Chambers, H. F., Tally, F. P., Vigliani, G. A., Cabell, C. H., Link, A. S., DeMeyer, I., Filler, S. G., Zervos, M., Cook, P., Parsonnet, J., Bernstein, J. M., Price, C. S., Forrest, G. N., Fatkenheuer, G., Gareca, M., Rehm, S. J., Brodt, H. R., Tice, A. & Cosgrove, S. E. (2006). Daptomycin versus standard therapy for bacteremia and endocarditis caused by *Staphylococcus aureus*. *N Engl J Med* **355**, 653–65.

67. Steenbergen, J. N., Alder, J., Thorne, G. M. & Tally, F. P. (2005). Daptomycin: a lipopeptide antibiotic for the treatment of serious Gram-positive infections. *J Antimicrob Chemother* **55**, 283–8.

68. Tally, F. P., Zeckel, M., Wasilewski, M. M., Carini, C., Berman, C. L., Drusano, G. L. & Oleson, F. B., Jr. (1999). Daptomycin: a novel agent for Gram-positive infections. *Expert Opin Investig Drugs* **8**, 1223–38.

69. Jevitt, L. A., Thorne, G. M., Traczewski, M. M., Jones, R. N., McGowan, J. E., Jr., Tenover, F. C. & Brown, S. D. (2006). Multicenter evaluation of the Etest and disk diffusion methods for differentiating daptomycin-susceptible from non-daptomycin-susceptible *Staphylococcus aureus* isolates. *J Clin Microbiol* **44**, 3098–104.

70. Tenover, F. C. (1986). Studies of antimicrobial resistance genes using DNA probes. *Antimicrob Agents Chemother* **29**, 721–5.

71. Tenover, F. C. & Rasheed, J. K. (2003). Detection and characterization of antimicrobial resistance genes in bacteria. In *Manual of Clinical Microbiology*, Eighth edition. (Murray, P. R., Baron, E. J., Jorgensen, J. H., Pfaller, M. A. & Yolken, R. H., eds.). ASM, Washington, DC.

72. Espy, M. J., Uhl, J. R., Sloan, L. M., Buckwalter, S. P., Jones, M. F., Vetter, E. A., Yao, J. D., Wengenack, N. L., Rosenblatt, J. E., Cockerill, F. R., III & Smith, T. F. (2006). Real-time PCR in clinical microbiology: applications for routine laboratory testing. *Clin Microbiol Rev* **19**, 165–256.

73. Ballard, S. A., Grabsch, E. A., Johnson, P. D. & Grayson, M. L. (2005). Comparison of three PCR primer sets for identification of vanB gene carriage in feces and correlation with carriage of vancomycin-resistant enterococci: interference by *vanB* containing anaerobic bacilli. *Antimicrob Agents Chemother* **49**, 77–81.

74. Talbot, T. R. (2007). Two studies feed the debate on active surveillance for methicillin-resistant *Staphylococcus aureus* and vancomycin-resistant enterococci carriage: to screen or not to screen? *J Infect Dis* **195**, 314–7.

75. Wren, M. W., Carder, C., Coen, P. G., Gant, V. & Wilson, A. P. (2006). Rapid molecular detection of methicillin-resistant *Staphylococcus aureus*. *J Clin Microbiol* **44**, 1604–5.

76. Sloan, L. M., Uhl, J. R., Vetter, E. A., Schleck, C. D., Harmsen, W. S., Manahan, J., Thompson, R. L., Rosenblatt, J. E. & Cockerill, F. R., III. (2004). Comparison of the Roche LightCycler vanA/vanB detection assay and culture for detection of vancomycin-resistant enterococci from perianal swabs. *J Clin Microbiol* **42**, 2636–43.

77. Arnold, C., Westland, L., Mowat, G., Underwood, A., Magee, J. & Gharbia, S. (2005). Single-nucleotide polymorphism-based differentiation and drug resistance detection in *Mycobacterium tuberculosis* from isolates or directly from sputum. *Clin Microbiol Infect* **11**, 122–30.

78. Zhao, J. R., Bai, Y. J., Wang, Y., Zhang, Q. H., Luo, M. & Yan, X. J. (2005). Development of a pyrosequencing approach for rapid screening of rifampin, isoniazid and ethambutol-resistant *Mycobacterium tuberculosis*. *Int J Tuberc Lung Dis* **9**, 328–32.

79. Lindback, E., Unemo, M., Akhras, M., Gharizadeh, B., Fredlund, H., Pourmand, N. & Wretlind, B. (2006). Pyrosequencing of the DNA gyrase gene in *Neisseria* species: effective indicator of ciprofloxacin resistance in *Neisseria gonorrhoeae*. *APMIS* **114**, 837–41.

Chapter 81
Drug Resistance Assays for *Mycobacterium tuberculosis*

Leonid Heifets and Gerard Cangelosi

1 Drug Resistant Tuberculosis as a Public Health Problem

The introduction of antimicrobial therapy of tuberculosis during the second half of the last century was a turning point in the millennium-old history of this disease. However, the problem of drug resistance emerged, and with it, two levels of concern. First, such resistance not only poses a public health threat to successful control of TB epidemics, but it also complicates the approach to treatment of individual patients. In previous reviews we have addressed the history of research and evolution of views based on these studies regarding the usefulness of drug susceptibility testing (1, 2). Historically, most skepticism regarding the need for drug susceptibility testing was related to the period before introduction of rifampin (RMP) and pyrazinamide (PZA). It often referred to the inability of laboratories to provide test results rapidly enough for the information to be used to adjust treatment regimens in a timely manner. In 1990, the American Thoracic Society (ATS) and the CDC published the following statement, "Given the low prevalence of drug-resistant *Mycobacterium tuberculosis* (MTBC) in most parts of the United States, the cost of routine testing of all initial isolates is difficult to justify" (3).

Severe outbreaks of drug-resistant tuberculosis in the US in the late 1980s and early 1990s challenged this attitude, and testing of initial isolates for drug susceptibility became mandatory, with emphasis on prompt reporting (4). Drastic measures that were required to address emergence of drug-resistant tuberculosis, which had arisen at least in part, as a result of the initial faulty conclusion that routine susceptibility was not necessary, amounted to billions of dollars. Ironically, the earlier testing of all initial isolates in

the US to detect patients with drug resistance would have cost only approximately $1 million annually, and the emergence of resistance might have been dampened or delayed. Unfortunately, this lesson did not change attitudes outside the US, and the importance and cost-effectiveness of drug susceptibility testing for detection of primary drug resistance is still under-appreciated in many countries with high rates of drug resistance, particularly in those which can economically afford to implement this measure.

With the introduction of the DOTS (directly observed therapy short-course) strategy in 1994–1995 by the WHO/IUTLD, new arguments were initiated; this time in connection with elements of this strategy. One of the components of this strategy is the detection of new infected patients through direct smear examination (without culture isolation), and this approach was justified for two reasons: (1) most countries cannot afford any other diagnostic test, and (2) this inexpensive tool would allow detection of the most infectious patients. Subsequently, in some documents referring to the role of the patients with negative smears as sources of infection, the descriptor "less infectious" was mysteriously replaced with "not infectious." It is now clearly established that at best, smear examination can detect only 50% of culture-positive adult patients with pulmonary tuberculosis (5). According to this report, even if detected (by culture) and treated, these patients become the source of infection for at least 17% of new patients. Focusing on smear examination alone as a sufficient tool for detecting new patients is not only misleading, but also discourages any motivation for planning (technically and financially) more advanced laboratory facilities and services. Moreover, it deprives a growing number of patients with primary drug resistance of the opportunity to detect the resistant nature of their strains so they can receive adequate treatment regimens.

It is now universally recognized that emergence of resistance to anti-tuberculosis drugs is a phenomenon that cannot be avoided (6). Therefore, it is only natural that in many countries prevalence of drug resistance is growing along with greater enrollment of TB patients into

L. Heifets (✉)
Mycobacterial Reference Laboratory, National Jewish Medical and Research Center, Denver, CO, USA
heifetsl@njc.org

D.L. Mayers (ed.), *Antimicrobial Drug Resistance*,
DOI 10.1007/978-1-60327-595-8_81, © Humana Press, a part of Springer Science+Business Media, LLC 2009

treatment programs. This is mostly associated with inefficient control of patient compliance in some areas. Proper implementation of the DOTS strategy was supposed to prevent the spread of drug resistance, and even make it "virtually impossible" for a patient to develop MDR-TB (7). This might have been the case if all (or almost all) patients enrolled in the DOTS program had only pan-susceptible strains. However, a group of authors referring to their experience in Peru stated: "It is not true that DOTS makes it virtually impossible to cause a patient to develop MDR-TB" (8). They demonstrated how patients with initial mono-resistance to RMP or INH develop additional resistance to two other drugs through DOTS treatment, a phenomenon labeled "amplifier effect of short-course therapy."

A global project on drug resistance surveillance provided data indicating "hot spots" and growing prevalence of drug resistance in many areas of the world (9, 10). Quoting data from the first of these reports (9), some authors referred to the median value of 1.4% for primary MDR-TB cases around the world. This implied that primary drug resistance was not an urgent problem, and, therefore, implementation of drug susceptibility testing of initial isolates would not be needed (just as it was earlier in the US "difficult to justify"). In fact, at that time the overall prevalence of primary drug resistance to any drug(s) ranged from 2 to 41% in different countries, with a median of 9.9% and a weighted mean of 18%.

Unfortunately, in the near future, it is unrealistic to anticipate introduction of any laboratory services beyond direct smear examination in countries with very low economic capabilities and without basic infrastructure. Conversely, in many countries with reasonably developed infrastructure and sufficient (though limited) resources, lack of laboratory support for tuberculosis control programs is often not a matter of affordability, but rather underestimation of its importance. For example, all countries listed in the WHO reports as "hot spots" (referring to the prevalence of drug resistance) have necessary infrastructure, means, and experience in laboratory practices (11). Growing prevalence of drug resistance in many countries makes implementation of drug susceptibility testing all the more important, placing it in a new perspective especially for initial clinical isolates. Therefore, the WHO recommends that when resources become available, development of an appropriate laboratory system in countries with growing rates of drug resistance should be among the priorities of national programs (12). In the meantime, epidemiologic surveys systematically conducted to evaluate the dynamics of prevalence of drug resistance in different countries are recommended for identification of problematic areas and proper adjustment of local TB control programs (13).

2 Definitions and Terminology in the Field of Tuberculosis

2.1 Drug-Resistant Strain

The first attempt to establish a consensus and certain standards for drug susceptibility testing of *M. tuberculosis* isolates was made in the early years of antimicrobial therapy of tuberculosis (14, 15). Then, drug-resistant isolate was defined as a strain which is significantly different by a degree of susceptibility from a "wild" strain obtained from a patient never treated with anti-tuberculosis drugs. The isolate is considered "resistant" if it contains more than 1% of bacteria resistant to a given drug (for most drugs). Progress in molecular biology may provide a new definition of drug resistance, and also raise new questions to be addressed, especially considering that resistance to some drugs has more than one genetic mechanism responsible for low and high levels of resistance (16, 17).

2.2 Critical Concentrations

In contrast to other fields of clinical microbiology, drug susceptibility of *M. tuberculosis* is determined by a qualitative test rather than a quantitative assay. In other words, a test with a single drug concentration instead of MIC determination with a series of drug concentrations is the most traditional approach in mycobacteriology. Quantitative tests with a range of drug concentrations for determining MICs are used in this field only for special studies. For routine testing in clinical laboratories, so-called "critical concentrations" of each drug were developed to differentiate between resistant and susceptible, initially for the egg-based Löwenstein–Jensen medium (15), and subsequently for the agar medium (18, 19). Critical concentrations should be calibrated as "halfway" between lowest MICs for resistant strains and highest MICs found for wild susceptible strains. When incorporated into the medium, drugs are partially inactivated in the preparation process, and therefore the critical concentration may not reflect precisely concentrations that are actually interacting with the bacterial inoculum. Therefore, critical concentrations, especially developed for solid media, are not necessarily related to the concentration attainable in vivo and no such correlation should be attempted.

2.3 Direct and Indirect Drug Susceptibility Tests

The direct test is based on inoculation of the drug-containing medium with a raw specimen (usually containing a sufficient number of bacteria as determined by microscopy), whereas indirect test is performed with an isolated pure culture.

2.4 Primary (Initial) Drug Resistance

Resistance to any drug detected in an isolate obtained from a newly diagnosed patient without prior history of antimicrobial therapy, suggesting the probability that such a patient has been infected with a drug-resistant strain.

2.5 Acquired Drug Resistance

Drug resistance detected in an isolate obtained from a patient who has been treated before or is still undergoing treatment with the corresponding antimycobacterial agent(s).

2.6 Multidrug Resistance

Resistance to *both* rifampin (RMP) and isoniazid (INH), with or without resistance to other drugs.

2.7 Poly-resistance

Resistance to any two or more drugs, including RMP or INH, if the isolate is not resistant to both RMP and INH.

2.8 First-Line Drugs

The initial treatment regimen for patients newly diagnosed with tuberculosis is composed from the first-line drugs: isoniazid (INH), rifampin (RMP), pyrazinamide (PZA), and ethambutol (EMB) or streptomycin (SM).

2.9 Second-Line Drugs

All other available anti-tuberculosis drugs represent a back-up for selection in cases of drug-resistance or intolerance to the first-line drugs: ethionamide (ETA), *para*-aminosalicylic acid (PAS), clofazimine (CF), cycloserine (CS), capreomycin (CM), amikacin (AK), kanamycin (KM), moxifloxacin (MX), levofloxacin (LF).

3 Empiric Approach for Detecting Patients with Drug Resistance

Drug susceptibility testing of initial culture isolates, and even culture isolation in all newly diagnosed patients, are not carried out in the majority of countries with high TB prevalence. Instead, quite often the initial step in detecting patients with drug-resistant tuberculosis is based on suspicion derived from the patient's failure to respond to standard treatment regimen. At best, such a suspicion arises only after completion of the intensive phase of therapy (2–3 months from the beginning), and more often only after 6–8 months or longer of unsuccessful therapy. Only then, such a non-responding patient is selected for performance of culture isolation and drug susceptibility testing – usually to the first-line drugs (INH, RMP, EMB or SM, PZA) only – which takes several months. Subsequent testing with second-line drugs (if MDR is detected) would require at least two more months, and perhaps the need to forward the isolate to a reference laboratory capable of performing tests with second-line drugs. As a result, the patient may have been without proper therapy for a year or more, even in places where the second-line drugs are available and where limited laboratory services can be utilized.

Failure to respond to the initial course of therapy may be related to the fact that the patient has had undetected primary resistance to one or more of the administered drugs (including MDR). In such a case, delay in administering an adequate treatment regimen not only compromises the patient's therapy, but may result in development of acquired resistance to other drugs in the initial treatment regimen, a phenomenon labeled "amplifier effect of short-course therapy" (11). In addition, this type of patient becomes a source of infection with a multidrug-resistant strain for a prolonged period of time. In other words, this empiric approach for detecting patients with drug-resistant strains can be dangerous for individual patients and costly for the community. In fact, management of patients with multidrug-resistant tuberculosis, even if their number is still small, can be much more costly than implementing drug susceptibility testing for the initial isolates from all new patients in a community.

4 Drug Susceptibility Tests Using Egg-Based Culture Medium

Historically, three methods based on cultivation of *M. tuberculosis* on starch-free Löwenstein–Jensen medium have been proposed: (1) the proportion method, (2) the resistance ratio (RR) method, and (3) the absolute concentration method (14, 15). Each of these methods can be used as either a direct or indirect test.

Table 1 Critical concentrations (µg/ml) for testing *M. tuberculosis* in solid media

Drug	L–J	7H10 agar	7H11 agar	HSTB agar[a]
Isoniazid	0.2	0.2, 1.0	0.2, 1.0	0.2, 1.0
Rifampin	40.0	1.0	1.0	1.0
Ethambutol	2.0	5.0, 10.0	7.5	12.0
Pyrazinamide	–	–	–	900.0
Streptomycin	4.0	2.0, 10.0	2.0, 4.0	5.0, 10.0
Amikacin	20.0	4.0	6.0	6.0
Kanamycin	20.0	5.0	6.0	6.0
Capreomycin	20.0	10.0	10.0	10.0
Ethionamide	20.0	5.0	10.0	10.0
Cycloserine	–	20.0	60.0	60.0
PAS	0.5	2.0	8.0	8.0
Levofloxacin[a]	–	–	4.0	4.0
Moxifloxacin[a]	–	–	2.0, 4.0	2.0, 4.0

[a]Concentrations in use at the National Jewish Mycobacteriology reference laboratory

The proportion method in its simplified version became the most popular among them. Both drug-free (controls) and drug-containing medium suspensions are coagulated in tubes in a slope position at 85°C for 50 min. This process alone inactivates a substantial proportion of some drugs in addition to their absorption by the medium. Therefore, critical drug concentrations developed for this medium (Table 1) reflect the amounts of drugs added, and not those that remain in the medium to interact with bacteria. Two sets of tubes with drug-containing and drug-free medium are inoculated with a bacterial suspension, 0.1 ml per each slope. The tubes are incubated at 37°C for 1–2 days in a slope position with caps slightly ajar. Afterwards, the caps are tightened, and the tubes are incubated in an upright position. On the 28th day of incubation the colonies are counted to calculate the proportion of colonies grown on drug-containing media to the number of colonies in controls. According to the original description, any proportion that exceeds 1% for INH, RMP and PAS, and 10% for other drugs indicates "resistant," and the results are final. If the proportion is less, then a second reading is required on the 42nd day of cultivation to confirm that the isolate is "susceptible" to the drug in question.

The resistance-ratio (RR) method is perhaps the most accurate, most labor-intensive, and costly among the three methods. The RR is defined as a ratio of MIC for the patient's isolate to the MIC for the drug-susceptible reference strain ($H_{37}Rv$), both tested in the same experiment. MIC determination requires a large number of medium tubes containing a broad range of drug concentrations. For this method, the MIC is defined as the lowest drug concentration in the presence of which the number of colonies is less than 20 after 4 weeks of incubation. RR of two or less is an indication of "susceptible" and eight or greater indicates "resistant."

The absolute concentration method is based on comparison of growth intensity in the presence of critical concentrations

(adjusted for each laboratory) and on drug-free controls. The $H_{37}Rv$ strain is tested in parallel with the same drugs in multiple concentrations for QC of reproducibility. The results are determined after 4 weeks of incubation, or after 5–6 weeks, if growth is insufficient at the 4-week reading. A "susceptible" result is reported if the number of colonies in the presence of drug is less than 20 against more than 100 colonies (up to a confluent growth) grown in drug-free controls.

5 Agar Proportion Method

The major advantage of performing drug susceptibility tests in agar plates is related to the transparency of the medium, which makes it possible to observe the growing colonies at the beginning of their formation. Therefore, final results can be reported within 3 weeks for most isolates, instead of 4–6 weeks or more when using egg-based media. There are at least three types of agar medium that can be used for either direct or indirect test: 7H10, 7H11, and HSTB. Detailed description of their preparation and use can be found in appropriate publications (18–21). These media are made from commercially available 7H10 or 7H11 agar base. The HSTB agar is made from the 7H11 agar base with addition of monosodium phosphate (0.6 g/100 ml of medium) to change the pH of the medium from 6.6 ± 0.2 to 6.2 ± 0.2.

To prepare agar media, the base powder is suspended in distilled water containing glycerol, autoclaved at 121°C for 15 min, and then cooled in a water bath to 52–54°C. Subsequently, an enrichment supplement of 10% is added: OADC (oleate-albumin-dextrose-catalase) for 7H10 or 7H11 medium, and calf or horse serum for HSTB agar. Appropriate drug solutions are added to ensure the necessary critical concentrations (Table 1), and the medium is distributed into agar plates, usually into quadrant plates, approximately 5.0 ml per quadrant. It is now known that some isolates may have genetically predetermined low levels of resistance to INH (22). Therefore, two concentrations of INH shown in Table 1 are needed to distinguish between low and high levels of resistance to this drug. A higher concentration of SM in addition to the critical concentration of this drug (as shown in Table 1) is usually employed in agar media for the purpose of confirmation of resistance in some occasions when the presence of CO_2 may have affected antimicrobial activity of SM.

Two quadrant plates (each with a drug-free quadrant) are needed for a test with four first-line drugs: INH, RMP, EMB, and SM for 7H10 or 7H11 agar. Two HSTB quadrant agar plates can be used for a test with INH, RMP, EMB, and PZA. Four quadrant plates are needed for a test with ten drugs. For a direct test, after the digestion-decontamination procedure, the concentrated sputum is inoculated into plates, 0.1 ml per quadrant. For an indirect test, two sets of plates are used: one inoculated with 10^{-3}-fold and the other with 10^{-5}-fold dilutions of the bacterial suspension adjusted to optical density of the McFarland #1 standard. The plates are incubated at 35–37°C for 3 weeks, protected from light, in an atmosphere of 10% CO_2 for 7H10 and 7H11 agar plates and in a regular incubator (without CO_2) for the HSTB agar. The colonies are counted, and results are reported as a percentage (proportion) on the basis of comparison of the number of colony-forming units (CFU) on drug-containing and drug-free quadrants. The isolate is considered "resistant" if this proportion is 1% or greater for all drugs except PZA. The criterion for PZA is 10%. For 10–15% of isolates growth may not be sufficient at the 3-week reading. Then the plates are re-examined at the 6-week reading; but in such a case only "susceptible" results are considered valid. This is because growth at 6 weeks in drug-containing quadrants may be related to drug degradation during the prolonged incubation period, rather than occurrence of true drug resistance.

6 Drug Susceptibility Testing (Indirect Test) in Liquid Medium

The need for expedited detection of drug resistance was first addressed in the 1980s by developing the drug susceptibility testing procedure (23–25) for the semi-automated Bactec-460 system introduced by Becton Dickinson (Sparks, MD). The liquid medium for this system, 7H12 broth in 12B vials, contains ^{14}C-substrate, consumption of which by the growing bacteria results in release of $^{14}CO_2$ measured by the instrument and expressed as Growth Index (GI). The turnaround time for an indirect test in this system was 9.3 days in our laboratory (26), and overall mean time for primary isolation plus indirect test was 18 days in a cooperative study by five institutions (24). The major disadvantage of this system – the problem of disposal of radioactive materials (12B vials) – stimulated development of new non-radiometric systems.

Three such systems, all fully automated and computerized, are now commercially available: Bactec-960-MGIT (Becton Dickinson Microbiology Systems, Sparks, MD), MB/BacT System (BioMérieux, Durham, NC), and Versa TREK, formerly ESP-II Culture System by Difco (TREK Diagnostic Systems, Westlake, Ohio).

In the Bactec-960 MGIT system, bacterial growth detection is based on consumption of oxygen, which causes the indicator embedded in the bottom of tubes to fluoresce, and the instrument continuously monitors the increase of fluorescence. Comparison of these patterns in drug-containing and drug-free tubes is analyzed by the instrument and automatically reported as "susceptible" or "resistant."

In the MB/BacT system a colorimetric sensor detecting release of CO_2 by the growing bacteria is embedded in the bottom of the vial. Changes in color from dark green to yellow is continuously monitored and reported by the instrument. A "susceptible" result is reported if no color changes occurred in the drug-containing vial or if a positive detection time in this vial is greater than in the drug-free control. A "resistant" result is reported if growth is detected in the drug-containing vial or if the detection time for this vial is shorter than for the drug-free control.

In the Versa TREK system, growth monitoring is based on reduction of pressure in the vials due to consumption of oxygen by the growing bacteria. The conclusion is based on comparison between drug-free controls and drug-containing vials after positive readings have occurred for three consecutive days in the drug-free vial. "Susceptible" is reported if no growth is detected in drug-containing vials, and "resistant" is reported if growth is detected in a drug containing vial at this time-point.

For all four liquid medium systems, critical concentrations have either been developed or suggested for four to five first-line drugs: INH, RMP, EMB, SM, PZA (Table 2). Two concentrations of INH are needed to distinguish between low and high levels of resistance to this drug (22). A lower concentration of EMB (2.5 μg/ml) in the previous insert by Becton Dickinson for the Bactec-460 system appeared to cause false resistance results, and therefore the manufacturer suggested an additional higher concentration of 7.5 μg/ml. Instead, we introduced a concentration of 4.0 μg/ml and, later, 5.0 μg/ml, which appeared to be quite reliable in distinguishing between resistant and susceptible strains. To address the problem of false resistance to PZA, we replaced the concentration of 100.0 μg/ml suggested by the manufacturer with 300.0 μg/ml (1, 29).

Table 2 Critical concentrations (μg/ml) of first-line drugs for testing *M. tuberculosis* in liquid medium systems

Drug	Bactec-460 B-D Insert	Bactec-460 Natl. Jewish	Bactec-960 (MGIT)	VersaTREK	MB/BacT (27)	MB/BacT (28)
Isoniazid	0.1, 0.4	0.1, 0.4	0.1, 0.4	0.1, 0.4	0.09	1.0
Rifampin	2.0	0.5, 2.0	1.0	1.0	0.9	1.0
Ethambutol	2.5, 7.5	5.0	5.0	5.0, 8.0	3.5	2.0
Streptomycin	2.0, 6.0	5.0	1.0, 4.0	–	0.45	1.0
Pyrazinamide	100.0	300.0	100.0	300.0	200.0	50.0

Critical concentrations for the MB/BacT system shown in Table 2 are from two publications and illustrate the diversity in opinions of different authors regarding critical concentrations needed (27, 28). Critical concentrations of various second-line drugs were suggested for the Bactec-460 and Bactec-960 MIGIT systems (1, 30, 31) (Table 3). In addition to these qualitative tests, a quantitative MIC test has been proposed for the Bactec-460 system (Table 4), in which the category "moderately susceptible" corresponds to the critical concentrations in Tables 2 and 3. The critical concentrations listed in the tables reflect the situation at the time of preparation of this paper. However, one should be aware that the manufacturers of liquid medium systems periodically review and change these concentrations according to progress in their evaluation. Up-to-date suggestions are usually listed in the manufacturer's inserts. In addition, some authors have used their own "critical concentrations." Recommendations by the Clinical and Laboratory Standards Institute (formerly NCCLS) (32) may not help to resolve inevitable controversies. Therefore, each laboratory should re-evaluate protocol

suggested by the manufacturer, and, based on appropriate studies, consider different or additional concentrations than those suggested by the manufacturer or various authors.

The validity of results by non-radiometric systems was analyzed in a number of publications on the basis of comparison with the Bactec-460 system and/or with the agar proportion method, both used as reference methods. Unfortunately, even the agar proportion method has been criticized as having improperly calibrated Critical Concentrations (33). As mentioned above, Critical Concentrations for the Bactec-460 system are also far from perfect. Therefore, acceptance of these two systems as reference methods may have relative value. So far, there are no reports in which selected test strains were examined genetically for indication of likelihood of "true" resistance, which could have been especially useful when conflicting results were obtained by compared methods. Nevertheless, a recently published review provides useful information on current literature regarding drug susceptibility testing in the non-radiometric automated liquid medium systems (34). According to this review, each of the available systems provides an opportunity for relatively rapid turnaround time of the indirect drug susceptibility test, although ranges reported by different authors have been broad. Each of these methods has certain advantages and disadvantages. Authors of this review conclude that so far, the MGIT Bactec-960 system appears to be the most reliable option among non-radiometric liquid medium systems, for testing drug susceptibility to first-line antituberculosis drugs in an indirect test.

Table 3 Suggested critical concentrations of second-line drugs for Bactec-460 and Bactec-960 MGIT systems

Drug	In use at Natl. Jewish for Bactec-460 (1, modified)	Suggested for Bactec-460 System (30)	Suggested for Bactec-960 MIGIT System (31)
Ethionamide	2.5	1.25	2.5, 5.0
Kanamycin	5.0	5.0	–
Amikacin	5.0	1.0	1.0
Capreomycin	5.0	1.25	1.25
Levofloxacin	4.0	–	–
Moxifloxacin	4.0	–	0.5, 1.0
Ofloxacin	8.0	2.0	1.0

Table 4 Guidelines in use at the National Jewish Mycobacteriology Laboratory for interpretation of MICs (μg/ml) determined in the Bactec-460 system

Drug	Susceptible	Moderately susceptible (intermediate)	Resistant
Isoniazid	≤0.1	0.4	≥1.6
Rifampin	≤0.5	2.0	≥8.0
Rifabutin	≤0.12	0.25	≥0.5
Ethambutol	≤4.0	8.0	≥16.0
Ethionamide	≤1.25	2.5	≥5.0
Streptomycin	≤2.5	5.0	≥10.0
Amikacin	≤2.5	5.0	≥10.0
Kanamycin	≤2.5	5.0	≥10.0
Capreomycin	≤2.5	5.0	≥10.0
Ofloxacin	≤2.0	4.0	≥8.0
Levofloxacin	≤1.0	2.0	≥4.0
Moxifloxacin	≤1.0	2.0	≥4.0
Cycloserine	≤4.0	8.0	≥16.0
Clofazimine	≤0.12	0.25	≥0.5

7 Molecular Phenotypic and Genotypic Methods

Researchers have long sought ways to speed up the process of gaining prognostic drug susceptibility information as part of laboratory diagnosis of tuberculosis. Although diverse in their scientific underpinnings, new technologies have been divided into two categories, genotypic and phenotypic (2, 35).

Genotypic methods detect bacterial DNA or RNA sequences associated with drug resistance, rather than the resistance phenotype. Most approaches use in vitro DNA amplification such as PCR in combination with diverse methods for detecting specific mutations known to result in drug resistance. Application of this principle to *M. tuberculosis* has been a research goal for many years. Its attraction is the possibility of bypassing the necessity for lengthy cultivation of tubercle bacilli in the laboratory. With the advent of microfluidic "lab-on-a-chip" technologies (36), it may become possible to detect drug-resistant genotypes in point-of-care settings outside of the laboratory.

A persistent obstacle to the application of genotypic approaches is the complexity of the underlying genetics of drug resistance. High-level resistance to most tuberculosis drugs, including INH, can result from diverse mutations in multiple genetic loci, many of which have not been identified (2, 37, 38). A test capable of detecting all known genetic markers of resistance to these drugs would still have less than 100% sensitivity. Low-level resistance represents an additional complexity that is not always addressed in genetic literature.

Although most drug resistance mechanisms are genetically complex, there is an exception to this rule with *M. tuberculosis*. More than 95% of RMP-resistant isolates of *M. tuberculosis* carry point mutations or small deletions/insertions in an 81-base region of the *rpoB* gene coding for the β subunit of DNA-dependent RNA polymerase, or in a smaller region near the 5′ end of the gene. This was established in numerous studies conducted throughout the world (37–40). RMP is a front-line antituberculosis drug, and considered to be a surrogate marker for multi-drug resistance because nearly all MDR TB strains are resistant to RMP (41, 42). It is no surprise that development of genotypic AST methods has focused on this locus.

The first commercial product developed and sold for detection of drug resistant *M. tuberculosis* is INNO-LiPA Rif.TB, the line-probe assay manufactured by Immunogenetics NV. This reverse hybridization test for specific mutations in PCR-amplified *rpoB* sequences offers a user-friendly alternative to DNA sequencing. The INNO-LiPA Rif.TB kit has an oligonucleotide probe specific to the *M. tuberculosis* complex (MTBC), additional probes that recognize relevant segments of the wild-type *rpoB* gene, as well as probes that recognize the most common *rpoB* mutations associated with RMP resistance. The test has generally performed well in trials conducted on isolated bacteria and instrument-positive MGIT cultures (41, 43–45). One of the largest recent studies was conducted on a sample of 1,585 consecutive clinical specimens processed at the New York State Department of Health (44). This sample yielded 70 MGIT cultures that were positive for *M. tuberculosis* by routine methods. The INNO-LiPA Rif.TB test correctly identified 69 of these cultures (98.6%) as containing MTBC. In the same study, a sample of 37 known RMP-susceptible and 64 known RMP-resistant clinical isolates was genotyped by INNO-LiPA Rif.TB, which exhibited 100% specificity and 95.3% sensitivity to RMP resistance relative to standard culture testing. Sequence analysis confirmed that the three RMP-resistant strains not detected by INNO-LiPA Rif.TB, lacked mutations in the targeted *rpoB* regions. The mean time for RMP susceptibility results by INNO-LiPA Rif.TB was reported to be 2 weeks (44).

The INNO-LiPA Rif.TB test was also evaluated for its ability to detect RMP-resistant *M. tuberculosis* directly in processed clinical specimens (46, 47). A recent study in Portugal examined 360 smear-positive respiratory specimens that had been processed by the standard NALC-NaOH method (47). The INNO-LiPA Rif.TB test detected 31 of the 32 culture-confirmed RMP-resistant isolates in the sample set. Overall, it exhibited 96.9% agreement with results obtained much later by use of culture-based susceptibility testing. However, INNO-LiPA Rif.TB was vulnerable to interfering substances and other problems associated with PCR applied directly to patient samples (47).

Additional RMP susceptibility genotyping methods have been designed for clinical laboratory use. These include, but are not limited to, molecular beacons (48), single strand conformation polymorphism (41), DNA chip technologies (49), fluorescent "biprobes" (50), and heteroduplex analysis (51). An excellent recent review (52) should be consulted for additional methods, including FRET-based probes, real-time PCR, and a variety of array-based methods. Typically these tests are reasonably fast and simple to conduct, and they take advantage of the phylogenetic specificity of *rpoB* gene sequences to exclude detection of nontuberculous microorganisms. Nearly all of them require that relevant regions of pathogen DNA be amplified by the polymerase chain reaction (PCR) or equivalent approaches.

In contrast to RMP resistance, genotypic detection of resistance to INH and other drugs is limited by genetic complexity (52–54). In part, for this reason, molecular phenotypic methods have been pursued as alternatives to genotypic approaches. Phenotypic methods measure physiological responses of the pathogens to antibiotic challenge. Culture methods fall into this category. The drug resistance phenotype is detectable regardless of its genetic basis, and high and low-level resistance can be differentiated. New phenotypic technologies use novel molecular or biological indicators that provide information on bacterial physiology more rapidly than is possible when bacterial cell division is measured. The best approaches have some capacity for species-specificity, so that they can be applied directly to raw samples without bacteriological purification of the pathogens (2).

Two new methods; the luciferase reporter phage (LRP) (55–57) and the PhaB (FASTPlaque) test (58, 59), take advantage of the phylogenetic specificity of bacteriophage infection of bacterial cells. Mycobacteriophages are naturally occurring viruses that specifically infect cells of certain *Mycobacterium* species. Detection of such infection in a sample constitutes evidence for the presence of viable *Mycobacterium* cells.

To develop the LRP system (Sequella, Inc., Bethesda, MD), recombinant DNA methods were used to introduce a gene coding for firefly luciferase (*lux*) into the genome of a lysogenic mycobacteriophage, TM4. The engineered phage injects its *lux*-bearing genome into viable mycobacterial cells present in a sample. Luciferase transcribed from the injected *lux* genes catalyzes production of light fueled by ATP. For optimum sensitivity a luminometric instrument is needed to detect luciferase activity. The lysogenic phage used in the LRP assay also infects many nontuberculous mycobacteria, potentially leading to false-positive results. Therefore, a control is added that incorporates the compound p-nitro-β-acetylamino-β-hydroxy propiophenone (NAP), which inhibits growth and LRP infection of *M. tuberculosis* complex strains, but not other mycobacteria. The NAP control confers species specificity with added cost and complexity.

To perform the Biotec BioPhage FAST*Plaque* Assay (Ipswich, UK), excess mycobacteriophage D29 is added to processed sputum. After injection of phage DNA into *M. tuberculosis* cells in the specimen, unabsorbed (extracellular) phages are inactivated using a virucide. D29 is a lytic phage that is specific to MTBC (60, 61), so to use of NAP is not required to achieve specificity. Infection of the phage into *M. tuberculosis* cells is detected by plating the viable intracellular phage along with a lawn of rapidly growing non-virulent indicator host cells (*Mycobacterium smegmatis*). The engineered phage infects the *M. smegmatis* cells, resulting in clearings, or "plaques," on the lawn of *M. smegmatis* colonies. This method is sensitive and inexpensive, but the use of indicator bacteria adds time (an extra day) and considerable complexity to the test. It is necessary to have a microbiology lab and personnel who are trained in aseptic techniques.

A significant rationale for the development of these two phage-based mycobacterial identification tests was their potential utility in rapid phenotypic drug susceptibility testing, and they have been applied to that purpose (55, 56, 58, 59). Mycobacterial cells that are severely inhibited by antibiotics in vitro are not expected to be effectively infected by the phages, and therefore will not yield positive signals in the tests. In an LRP test using a luminometer, it was reported that susceptibility to INH and RMP was determined in 54 h (56). The need for a costly luminometer instrument can be overcome by using Polaroid film to detect luciferase expression (the Bronx Box). However, the relative insensitivity of photographic film increases the test time to 96 h, about the same as the current MGIT method (56). The requirement for NAP controls is a complication associated with the LRP test (57). The FAST *Plaque* test, which uses *M. smegmatis* indicator cells to detect results, also has an AST configuration for RMP resistance (the FAST*Plaque* TB-MDRi test). This test uses a species-specific phage, but the requirement for live indicator bacteria adds complexity. Its performance has been assessed (62–64), and its commercial release is expected in the near future.

Flow cytometry has been proposed as a means to detect phenotypically antibiotic-resistant bacteria. Viable bacteria that survive antibiotic exposure in vitro are detected by virtue of impermeability to fluorescent DNA stains (65) or by their ability to hydrolyze a fluorogenic dye (66). Additional rapid phenotypic tests have been proposed, including DNA probe assessment of precursor rRNA synthesis (67), and various colorimetric assays (68–72). In all cases, bacteria are cultivated in vitro, albeit briefly. Therefore, protection of laboratory personnel is a consideration.

The argument for pursuing phenotypic approaches is their potential to detect resistance to drugs other than RMP. Therefore, it is an unfortunate irony that phenotypic approaches often work best at detecting RMP resistance, which is also amenable to genotypic methods (64). RMP acts rapidly, binding tightly to RNA polymerase and halting RNA synthesis within 3 h of exposure in vitro (67). Other drugs, most notably cell wall synthesis inhibitors such as INH, may take days to exert visible effects. In this regard, genotypic approaches may hold the best promise for molecular drug susceptibility testing. If new isothermal amplifications (73, 74), nanotechnologies (36), and other user-friendly platforms succeed in their promise of bringing DNA detection out of the laboratory, the prospects for broad application of molecular drug susceptibility testing will become brighter.

References

1. Heifets, L. (1991) Drug susceptibility tests in the management of chemotherapy of tuberculosis, in: *Drug Susceptibility in the Chemotherapy of Mycobacterial Infections* (Heifets, L.B., ed.), CRC Press, Boca Raton, FL, pp. 89–121.
2. Heifets, L.B., Cangelosi, G.A. (1999) Drug susceptibility testing of *Mycobacterium tuberculosis*: a neglected problem at the turn of the century. *Int. J. Tuberc. Lung Dis.* **3**(7), 564–581.
3. American Thoracic Society. (1990) Diagnostic standards and classification of tuberculosis. *Am. Rev. Respir. Dis.* **142**(3), 725–735.
4. Tenover, F.C., Crawford, J.T., Heubner, R.E., Geiter, I.J., Horsburg, C.R., Good, R.C. (1993) The resurgence of tuberculosis: is your laboratory ready? *J. Clin. Microbiol.* **31**, 767–770.
5. Behr, M.A., Warren, S.A., Salamon, H., et al. (1999) Transmission of *M. tuberculosis* from patients smear-negative for acid-fast bacilli. *Lancet* **353**, 444–449.
6. Gupta, R. Espinal, M.A., Raviglione, M.C. (2004) Tuberculosis as a major global health problem in 21st century, in: *Tuberculosis and Other Mycobacterial Infections* (Heifets, L., ed.), *Semin. Respir. Crit. Care Med.* **25**(3), 245–253.
7. World Health Organization. (March 24, 1997) TB Treatment Observer. WHO, Geneva.
8. Farmer, P., Bayona, J., Becerra, M., et al. (1998) The dilemma of MDR-TB in the global era. *Int. J. Tuberc. Lung Dis.* **2**, 869–876.
9. Pablos-Mendez, A., Raviglione, M.C., Laszlo, A., et al. (1998) Global surveillance for antituberculosis drugs resistance 1994–1997. *N. Engl. J. Med.* **338**, 1641–1649.
10. Espinal, M.A., Laszlo, A., Simonsen, L., et al. (2001) Global trends in resistance to antituberculosis drugs. *N. Engl. J. Med.* **344**, 1294–1303.
11. World Health Organization. (1998) Atituberculosis Drug Resistance in the World. The WHO/IUTLD Global Project on Antituberculosis Drug Resistance Surveillancein 1994–1997. WHO, Geneva.
12. World Health Organization. (2002) An Expanded DOTS Framework for Effective Tuberculosis Control. WHO/CDS/TB/2002, 297. WHO, Geneva.
13. World Health Organization. (2005) Global Tuberculosis Control: Surveillance, Planning, Financing. WHO/HTM/TB/2005, 349. WHO, Geneva.
14. Canetti, G., Froman, S., Grosset, J., et al. (1963) Mycobacteria: laboratory methods for testing drug sensitivity and resistance. *Bull. World Health Organ.* **29**, 565–578.
15. Canetti, G., Fox, W., Khomenko, A., Mahler, H.T., Menon, M.K., Mitchison, D.A., Rist, M., Smelev, M.A. (1969) Advances in

techniques of testing mycobacterial drug sensitivity and the use of sensitivity tests in tuberculosis control programs. *Bull. World. Health Organ.* **41**, 21–43.

16. Telenti, A. (1997) Genetics of drug resistance in tuberculosis, in: *Tuberculosis* (Iseman, M., Huitt, G., eds.), *Clin. Chest Med.* **18**, 55–64.

17. Takiff, H.E. (2000) The molecular mechanisms of drug resistance, in *M. tuberculosis*, in: *Multi-drug Resistant Tuberculosis* (Bastian, I., Portaels, F., eds.), Kluwer, Dordrecht, the Netherlands, pp.77–114.

18. David, H.L. (1971) Fundamentals of Drug Susceptibility Testing in Tuberculosis. HEW Publication No. 00-2165. CDC, Atlanta, GA.

19. Kent, P.T., Kubica, G.P. (1985) Public Health Mycobacteriology. A Guide for the Level III Laboratory. CDC, Atlanta, GA.

20. Heifets, L., Sanchez, T. (2003/2005) New Agar Medium for Mycobacteria (HSTB). [US Patent No. 6,579,694 B2 and 6,951,733 B2].

21. Heifets, L. (2000) Conventional methods for antimicrobial susceptibility testing of *M. tuberculosis*, in: *Multidrug-Resistant Tuberculosis* (Bastian, I., Portaels, F., eds.), Kluwer, Dordrecht, the Netherlands, pp. 133–143.

22. Madison, B.M., Siddiqi, S.H., Heifets, L., et al (2004) Identification of a *Mycobacterium tuberculosis* strain with stable, low-level resistance to isoniazid. *J. Clin. Microbiol.* **42**(3), 1294–1295.

23. Siddiqi, S.H., Libonati, J.P., Middlebrook, G. (1981) Evaluation of a rapid radiometric method for drug susceptibility testing of *M. tuberculosis*. *J. Clin. Microbiol.* **13**, 908–912.

24. Roberts, G.D., Goodman, N.L., Heifets L., et al. (1983) Evaluation of the BACTEC radiometric method for recovery mycobacteria and drug susceptibility testing of *M. tuberculosis* acid-fast smear-positive specimens. *J. Clin. Microbiol.* **18**, 689–696.

25. Siddiqi, S.H., Hawkins, J.E., Laszlo, A. (1985) Interlaboratory drug susceptibility testing of *M. tuberculosis* by radiometric and two conventional methods. *J. Clin. Microbiol.* **22**, 919–923.

26. Heifets, L.B. (1986) Rapid automated method (BACTEC system) in clinical mycobacteriology. *Semin. Respir. Infect.* **1**, 242–249.

27. Bemer, P., Bodmer, T., Munzinger, J., Perrin, M., Vincent, V., Drugeon, H. (2004) Multicenter evaluation of the MB/BacT system for susceptibility testing of *Mycobacterium tuberculosis*. *J. Clin. Microbiol.* **42**, 1030–1034.

28. Tortoli, E., Mattei, R., Savarino, A., Bartolini, L., Beer, J. (2000) Comparison of *Mycobacterium tuberculosis* susceptibility testing performed with BACTEC 460 TB (Becton Dickinson) and MB/BacT (Organon Teknika) systems. *Diagn. Microbiol. Infect. Dis.* **38**, 83–86.

29. Heifets, L. (2002) Susceptibility testing of *M. tuberculosis* to pyrazinamide. *J. Med. Microbiol.* **51**(1), 11–12.

30. Pfyffer, G.E., Bonato, D.A., Ebrahimzade, A., et al. (1999) Multicenter laboratory validation of susceptibility testing of *M. tuberculosis* against second-line and newer antimicrobial drugs by using the radiometric Bactec-460 technique and the proportion method with solid media. *J. Clin. Microbiol.* **37**(10), 3179–3186.

31. Krüüner, A., Yates, M.D., Drobniewski, F.A. (2006) Evaluation of MGIT 960-bases antimicrobial testing and determination of critical concentrations of first- and second-line antimicrobial drugs with drug-resistant clinical strains of *M. tuberculosis*. *J. Clin. Microbiol.* **44**(3), 811–818.

32. National Committee for Clinical Laboratory Standards. (2003) Susceptibility Testing of Mycobacteria, Nocardia, and Other Aerobic Actinomycetes. Approved Standard M24-A. NCCLS, Wayne, PA.

33. Mitchison, D.A. (1998) Standardisation of sensitivity tests (letter) *Int. J. Tuberc. Lung Dis.* **2**, 69.

34. Piersimoni, C., Olivieri, A., Benacchio, L., Scarparo, C. (2006) Current perspectives on drug susceptibility testing of *M. tuber-*

culosis complex: the automated nonradiometric systems. *J. Clin. Microbiol.* **44**(1), 20–28.

35. Palomino, J.C. (2005) Nonconventional and new methods in the diagnosis of tuberculosis: feasibility and applicability in the field. *Eur. Respir. J.* **26**, 339–350.

36. Jain, K.K. (2003) Nanodiagnostics: application of nanotechnology in molecular diagnostics. *Expert Rev. Mol. Diagn.* **3**, 153–161.

37. Rattan, A., Kalia, A., Ahmad, N. (1998) Multi-drug resistant tuberculosis: molecular perspectives. *Emerg. Infect. Dis.* **4**, 195–209.

38. Somoskovi, A., Parsons, L., Salfinger, M. (2001) The molecular basis of resistance to isoniazid, rifampin, and pyrazinamide in *Mycobacterium tuberculosis*. *Respir. Res.* **2**, 164–168.

39. Chaves, F., Alonso-Sanz, M., Rebollo, M.J., Tercero, J.C., Jiminez, M.S., Noriega, A.R. (2000) *rpoB* mutations as an epidemiological marker of rifampin-resistant *M. tuberculosis*. *Int. J. Tuberc. Lung Dis.* **4**, 765–770.

40. Garcia, L., Alonso-Sanz, M., Rebollo, M.J., Tercero, J.C., Chaves, F. (2001) Mutations in the *rpoB* gene of rifampin-resistant *Mycobacterium tuberculosis* isolates in Spain and their rapid detection by PCR-enzyme-linked immunosorbent assay. *J. Clin. Microbiol.* **39**, 1813–1818.

41. Telenti, A., Honore, N., Bernasconi, C., March, J., Ortega, A., Heym, B., et al. (1997) Genotypic assessment of isoniazid and rifampin resistance in *Mycobacterium tuberculosis*: a blind study at reference laboratory level. *J. Clin. Microbiol.* **35**, 719–723.

42. Watterson, S.A., Wilson, S.M., Yates, M.D., Drobniewski, F.A. (1998) Comparison of three molecular assays for rapid detection of rifampin resistance in *Mycobacterium tuberculosis*. *J. Clin. Microbiol.* **36**, 1969–1973.

43. Rossau, R., Traore, H., De Beenhouwer, H., Mijs, W., Jannes, G., De Rijk, P., et al. (1997) Evaluation of the INNO-LiPA Rif. TB assay, a reverse hybridization assay for the simultaneous detection of *Mycobacterium tuberculosis* complex and its resistance to rifampin. *Antimicrob. Agents Chemother.* **41**, 2093–2098.

44. Somoskovi, A., Song, Q., Mester, J., Tanner, C., Hale, Y.M., Parsons, L.M., et al. (2003) Use of molecular methods to identify the *Mycobacterium tuberculosis* complex (MTBC) and other Mycobacterial species and to detect rifampin resistance in MTBC isolates following growth detection with the BACTEC MGIT 960 system. *J. Clin. Microbiol.* **41**, 2822–2826.

45. Bartfai, Z., Somoskovi, A., Kodmon, C., Szabo, N., Puskas, E., Kosztolanyi, L., et al. (2001) Molecular characterization of rifampin-resistant isolates of *Mycobacterium tuberculosis* from Hungary by DNA sequencing and the line probe assay. *J. Clin. Microbiol.* **39**, 3736–3739.

46. Johansen, I.S., Lundgren, B., Sosnovskaja, A., Thomsen, V.O. (2003) Direct detection of multidrug-resistant *Mycobacterium tuberculosis* in clinical specimens in low- and high-incidence countries by line probe assay. *J. Clin. Microbiol.* **41**, 4454–4456.

47. Viveiros, M., Leandro, C., Rodrigues, L., Almeida, J., Bettencourt, R., Couto, I., et al. (2005) Direct application of the INNO-LiPA Rif.TB line-probe assay for rapid identification of *Mycobacterium tuberculosis* complex strains and detection of rifampin resistance in 360 smear-positive respiratory specimens from an area of high incidence of multidrug-resistant tuberculosis. *J. Clin. Microbiol.* **43**, 4880–4884.

48. El Hajj, H.H., Marras, S.A.E., Tyagi, S., Kramer, F.R., Alland, D. (2001) Detection of rifampin resistance in *Mycobacterium tuberculosis* in a single tube with molecular beacons. *J. Clin. Microbiol.* **39**, 4131–4137.

49. Vernet, G., Jay, C., Rodriguez, M., Troesch, A. (2004) Species differentiation and antibiotic susceptibility testing with DNA microarrays. *J. Appl. Microbiol.* **96**, 59–68.

50. Edwards, K.J., Metherell, L.A., Yates, M., Saunders, N.A. (2001) Detection of rpoB mutations in *Mycobacterium tuberculosis* by biprobe analysis. *J. Clin. Microbiol.* **39**, 3350–3352.

51. Nash, K.A., Gaytan, A., Inderlied, C.B. (1997) Detection of rifampin resistance in *Mycobacterium tuberculosis* by use of a rapid, simple, and effective RNA/RNA mismatch assay. *J. Infect. Dis.* **176**, 533–536.

52. Garcia de Viedma, D. (2003) Rapid detection of resistance in *Mycobacterium tuberculosis*: a review discussing molecular approaches. *Clin. Microbiol. Infect.* **9**, 349–359.

53. Davies, A.P., Billington, O.J., McHugh, T.D., Mitchison, D.A., Gillespie, S.H. (2000) Comparison of phenotypic and genotypic methods for pyrazinamide susceptibility testing with *Mycobacterium tuberculosis*. *J. Clin. Microbiol.* **38**, 3686–3688.

54. Sreevatsan, S., Stockbauer, K.E., Pan, X., Kreiswirth, B.N., Moghazeh, S.L., Jacobs, W.R., Jr., et al. (1997) Ethambutol resistance in *Mycobacterium tuberculosis*: critical role of embB mutations. *Antimicrob. Agents Chemother.* **41**, 1677–1681.

55. Banajee, N., Bobadilla-del-Valle, M., Riska, P.F., Bardarov, S., Jr., Small, P.M., Ponce-de-Leon, A., et al. (2003) Rapid identification and susceptibility testing of *Mycobacterium tuberculosis* from MGIT cultures with luciferase reporter mycobacteriophages. *J. Med. Microbiol.* **52**, 557–561.

56. Hazbon, M.H., Guarin, N., Ferro, B.E., Rodriguez, A.L., Labrada, L.A., Tovar, R., et al. (2003) Photographic and luminometric detection of luciferase reporter phages for drug susceptibility testing of clinical *Mycobacterium tuberculosis* isolates. *J. Clin. Microbiol.* **41**, 4865–4869.

57. Riska, P.F., Jacobs, W.R., Jr., Bloom, B.R., McKitrick, J., Chan, J. (1997) Specific identification of *Mycobacterium tuberculosis* with the luciferase reporter mycobacteriophage: use of *p*-nitro-alpha-acetylamino-beta-hydroxy propiophenone. *J. Clin. Microbiol.* **35**, 3225–3231.

58. Eltringham, I.J., Wilson, S.M., Drobniewski, F.A. (1999) Evaluation of a bacteriophage-based assay (Phage Amplified Biologically Assay) as a rapid screen for resistance to isoniazid, ethambutol, streptomycin, pyrazinamide, and ciprofloxacin among clinical isolates of *Mycobacterium tuberculosis*. *J. Clin. Microbiol.* **37**, 3528–3532.

59. Park, D.J., Drobniewski, F.A., Meyer, A., Wilson, S.M. (2003) Use of a phage-based assay for phenotypic detection of mycobacteria directly from sputum. *J. Clin. Microbiol.* **41**, 680–688.

60. Pearson, R.E., Dickson, J.A., Hamilton, P.T., Little, M.C., Beyer, Jr., W.F. (1997) Mycobacteriophage Specific for the *Mycobacterium tuberculosis* Complex. Becton, Dickinson and Company. [US Patent No. 5,612,182]. Franklin Lakes, NJ, USA.

61. Redmond, W.B., Cater, J.C. (1960) A bacteroiphage specific for *Mycobacterium tuberculosis*, varieties *hominis* and *bovis*. *Am. Rev. Respir. Dis.* **82**, 781–786.

62. Albert, H., Muzzafar, R., Mole, R.J., Trollip, A.P. (2002) Use of the FASTPlaque test for TB diagnosis in low-income countries. *Int. J. Tuberc. Lung Dis.* **6**, 560–561.

63. Albert, H., Trollip, A., Seaman, T., Mole, R.J. (2004) Simple, phage-based (*FASTPlaque*) technology to determine rifampicin resistance of *Mycobacterium tuberculosis* directly from sputum. *Int. J. Tuberc. Lung Dis.* **8**, 1114–1149.

64. Pai, M., Kalantri, S., Pascopella, L., Riley, L.W., Reingold, A.L. (2005) Bacteriophage-based assays for the rapid detection of rifampicin resistance in *Mycobacterium tuberculosis*: a meta-analysis. *J. Infect.* **51**, 175–187.

65. Pina-Vaz, C., Costa-de-Oliveira, S., Rodrigues, A.G. (2005) Safe susceptibility testing of *Mycobacterium tuberculosis* by flow cytometry with the fluorescent nucleic acid stain SYTO 16. *J. Med. Microbiol.* **54**, 77–81.

66. Moore, A.V., Kirk, S.M., Callister, S.M., Mazurek, G.H., Schell, R.F. (1999) Safe determination of susceptibility of *Mycobacterium tuberculosis* to antimycobacterial agents by flow cytometry. *J. Clin. Microbiol.* **37**, 479–483.

67. Cangelosi, G.A., Brabant, W.H., Britschgi, T.B., Wallis, C.K. (1996) Detection of rifampin- and ciprofloxacin-resistant *Mycobacterium tuberculosis* by using species-specific assays for precursor rRNA. *Antimicrob. Agents Chemother.* **40**, 1790–1795.

68. Abate, G., Aseffa, A., Selassie, A., Goshu, S., Fekade, B., WoldeMeskal, D., et al. (2004) Direct colorimetric assay for rapid detection of rifampin-resistant *Mycobacterium tuberculosis*. *J. Clin. Microbiol.* **42**, 871–873.

69. Caviedes, L., Delgado, J., Gilman, R.H. (2002) Tetrazolium microplate assay as a rapid and inexpensive colorimetric method for determination of antibiotic susceptibility of *Mycobacterium tuberculosis*. *J. Clin. Microbiol.* **40**, 1873–1874.

70. Collins, L., Franzblau, S.G. (1997) Microplate alamar blue assay versus BACTEC 460 system for high-throughput screening of compounds against *Mycobacterium tuberculosis* and *Mycobacterium avium*. *Antimicrob. Agents Chemother.* **41**, 1004–1009.

71. Moore, D.A.J., Mendoza, D., Gilman, R.H., Evans, C.A.W., Hollm Delgado, M.G., Guerra, J., et al. (2004) Microscopic observation drug susceptibility assay, a rapid, reliable diagnostic test for multidrug-resistant tuberculosis suitable for use in resource-poor settings. *J. Clin. Microbiol.* **42**, 4432–4437.

72. Syre, H., Valvatne, H., Sandven, P., Grewal, H.M.S. (2006) Evaluation of the nitrate-based colorimetric method for testing the susceptibility of *Mycobacterium tuberculosis* to streptomycin and ethambutol in liquid cultures. *J. Antimicrob. Chemother.* l054.

73. Hara-Kudo, Y, Yoshino, M., Kojima, T., Ikedo, M. (2005) Loop-mediated isothermal amplification for the rapid detection of Salmonella. *FEMS Microbiol. Lett.* **253**, 155–161.

74. Poon, L.L.M., Wong, B.W.Y., Ma, E.H.T., Chan, K.H., Chow, L.M.C., Abeyewickreme, W., et al. (2006) Sensitive and inexpensive molecular test for falciparum malaria: detecting *Plasmodium falciparum* DNA directly from heat-treated blood by loop-mediated isothermal amplification. *Clin. Chem.* **52**, 303–306.

Chapter 82
Fungal Drug Resistance Assays

Sevtap Arikan and John H. Rex

1 The Need for Fungal Drug Resistance Assays

Fungal infections have drawn attention in recent years for several reasons. First, there has been a remarkable increase in the number of patients whose immune system is compromised because of various reasons. As invasive mycoses have emerged as significant causes of morbidity and mortality for this particular patient population, the term "fungal infection" no longer only means a "superficial infection." Second, the number and variety of antifungal agents increased. This is the outcome of the demand for more efficacious and less-toxic antifungal drugs to treat serious infections and the developments in pharmaceutical industry. As a result, several possible therapies exist for some situations (1–7). Third, fungal infections refractory to antifungal therapy because of primary or secondary resistance of the infecting strains to the antifungal agents used for treating these infections, are observed (8–18).

In the era where we have more patients with serious fungal infections, more alternatives to treat these infections, and patients who become or remain resistant to therapy, the best way to optimize the antifungal therapeutic strategies and to predict clinical outcome is to determine the susceptibility profiles of the infecting fungal strains to the antifungal drugs. This great demand thus resulted in the standardization of fungal drug resistance assays and sustained efforts to define their utility.

1.1 Theoretical Limitations on the Correlation of In Vitro Susceptibility with Clinical Outcome

The ultimate goal of routine fungal resistance assays is to predict clinical outcome and permit monitoring and selection of antifungal therapy. The inquiry of to what extent this goal was achieved has been the key question of recent years. A meta-analysis of in vitro–in vivo correlation studies that included patients infected with *Candida*, *Cryptococcus*, or *Histoplasma* and treated with various azoles (fluconazole, itraconazole or ketoconazole) found a clinical success rate of 91% for infections due to isolates susceptible to the antifungal agent used for treatment and a 48% response rate for those infections treated with agents predicted to be resistant (19). Interestingly, these percentages approximated the clinical success rates reported for the treatment of various bacterial infections due to susceptible/resistant strains. On the basis of these data, the concept referred to as the "90–60 rule" has been proposed and states in summary that susceptible isolates respond about 90% of the time and resistant isolates respond about 60% of the time. This conceptual model reminds us that susceptibility assays are helpful in predicting clinical response, but represent only one of the many factors that influence response. Factors such as pharmacokinetic properties of the drug, the immune status of the host, severity of the infection, presence (and removal) of prosthetic devices, and surgical management of the site of infection are all relevant and each, in turn, may be the most powerful factor in a given situation.

Other in vitro–in vivo correlation studies have found only limited correlations between in vitro susceptibility and clinical outcome. For amphotericin B and *Candida*, various in vitro susceptibility testing settings, including CLSI (Clinical and Laboratory Standards Institute, formerly National Committee for Clinical Laboratory Standards-NCCLS) microdilution and Etest methods, and antibiotic medium 3 (AM3) and RPMI 1640 media, have failed to generate MICs that correlated with clinical outcome (20). Similarly, in vitro susceptibility tests could not predict early clinical outcome in

S. Arikan (✉)
Department of Microbiology and Clinical Microbiology, Hacettepe University Medical School, Ankara, Turkey
sevtap.arikan@gmail.com

D.L. Mayers (ed.), *Antimicrobial Drug Resistance*,
DOI 10.1007/978-1-60327-595-8_82, © Humana Press, a part of Springer Science+Business Media, LLC 2009

patients with cryptococcosis, treated with amphotericin B-flucytosine or fluconazole (21). Finally, in vitro–in vivo correlation data for cases with *Aspergillus* infections (22) and for patients treated with echinocandins (23) remain limited.

The differing strength of correlation for different organism–drug combinations may have a variety of causes. In some cases (e.g., *Candida* and the echinocandins), the best interpretation at present is that resistance really is infrequent and most current isolates are basically susceptible to the drug exposures produced by approved therapeutic regimens. In this situation, it is predicted that failures would be distributed without regard for MIC and thus MIC would not correlate with the outcome. Conversely, some situations suggest that the test method appears to be failing in the identification of resistant isolates. This appears to be the case for most organisms and amphotericin B, but this situation is further confounded by the complexity of the effect of host immune function in settings where amphotericin B is used, as well as the general sense that true in vitro resistance to amphotericin B is uncommon. These challenges are not unique to the problem of establishing in vitro–in vivo correlations for fungi, but they are magnified by the smaller clinical datasets typically available for fungal infections.

2 The Currently Used Reference and Alternative Fungal Drug Resistance Assays

2.1 CLSI Reference Broth Dilution Methods

On the basis of multicenter studies that started at the beginning of the 1990s, the CLSI subcommittee on antifungal susceptibility testing standardized reference broth dilution methods for both yeasts (*Candida* spp. and *Cryptococcus neoformans*) (M27-A2) (24) and moulds (*Aspergillus* spp., *Fusarium* spp., *Rhizopus* spp., *Pseudallescheria boydii*, and the mycelial form of *Sporothrix schenckii*) (M38-A) (25). The initial method was a broth macrodilution performed in sterile tubes. Since the data obtained later provided a good correlation between macro- and microdilution assays (26, 27), broth microdilution method performed in sterile, disposable, microdilution plates with 96 U-shaped wells is now more commonly applied, based on its more practical and more cost-effective nature. The major test parameters proposed in CLSI M27-A2 and M38-A documents are summarized in Table 1. Interested readers are encouraged to review the cited CLSI documents for further details of these reference assays.

The relevant MIC ranges (µg/ml) for the quality control (QC) isolates *Candida krusei* ATCC 6258 and *Candida*

parapsilosis ATCC 22019 are shown in Table 2 and the MIC breakpoints for fluconazole, itraconazole, flucytosine, and voriconazole against *Candida* are indicated in Table 3.

The reference CLSI method M38-A does not include the dermatophytes *Microsporum*, *Epidermophyton*, and *Trichophyton*. Some investigators have tested the validity of the method and its modifications for this group of filamentous fungi as well (34–44). A revision to M38-A is under way that incorporates methods for dermatophytes which have been validated in a collaborative multicenter process (43). It is hoped that the availability of a standardized procedure will permit generation of large datasets evaluating the correlation of MIC with clinical outcome for dermatophytic infections.

2.1.1 Current Status and Limitations of the CLSI Broth Dilution Methods

The development of standard assays for testing resistance to antifungal agents has been a remarkable progress of the last decade. These assays are now increasingly and widely used as a routine adjunct for the prediction of clinical outcome and optimization of antifungal therapy. However, certain limitations of these methods still persist.

Amphotericin B Susceptibility Tests

Amphotericin B MICs obtained for *Candida* strains are, in general, distributed in a very narrow range (mostly 0.25–1 µg/ml) and the CLSI method currently fails to separate resistant isolates reliably from the susceptible isolates. Resistant and susceptible isolates have different mean MICs upon repeated testing, but results from single tests are simply not adequate to produce discrimination. This drawback of amphotericin B susceptibility tests appears also to apply to filamentous fungi as well as yeasts. In the efforts to overcome this drawback, various alternatives of the standard method have been studied. Some investigators have found that the use of AM3 instead of RPMI (45) and the application of Etest rather than broth dilution (46) enhance the discrimination of amphotericin B-resistant *Candida*. However, the data obtained in other workers' hands did not support these findings (47) and the issue remains controversial. It also appears that technical issues such as the lot of AM3 used for testing may also produce variation within the results (48).

As an alternative approach, studies using a combination of MIC and minimum lethal concentrations (MLC) have suggested a meaningful correlation between in vitro and clinical resistance for some *Candida* (47) and *Aspergillus* (49) infections treated with amphotericin B. As with the MIC methods, further studies have unfortunately failed to fully support these findings. An analysis of the amphotericin B

Table 1 Test parameters of CLSI M27 A2 (24) and M38 A (25) microdilution methods

Parameters	M27-A2	M38-A
Test medium	RPMI 1640 medium (with L-glutamine and without bicarbonate), with phenol red as a pH indicator, and buffered with MOPS [(3-N-morpholino)propanesulfonic acid)] (pH 7 at 25°C)	
Inoculum preparation	From 24-h-old cultures of *Candida* and 48-h-old cultures of *C. neoformans* at 35°C on Sabouraud dextrose agar	From 7-days-old cultures of *Aspergillus*, *P. boydii*, *Rhizopus*, and *S. schenckii* at 35°C on potato dextrose agar (PDA). *Fusarium* may need to be incubated at 35°C for the first 3 to 4 days and then at 25–28°C until day 7 on PDA
Inoculum density	Adjust the turbidity of the yeast suspension in saline spectrophotometrically at 530 nm to the turbidity of 0.5 McFarland standard (1–5×10^6 cells/ml, ~75–80% transmittance) and then make 1/100 and 1/20 dilutions of this stock suspension, resulting in a final inoculum density of 0.5–2.5×10^3 cells/ml to be used in the test	Conidia/sporangiospores are used as the inoculum. Collect the spores by using sterile saline and probing the colonies with a transfer pipette. Allow the resulting suspension to settle for 3–5 min and use the upper suspension, discarding the settled, hyphal fragments. Adjust the turbidity of the upper suspension spectrophotometrically at 530 nm to ~80–82% transmittance for *Aspergillus* and *S. schenckii* and to ~68–70% for *Fusarium*, *P. boydii*, and *Rhizopus*. Dilute the adjusted inocula 1/50 (2/50 for *P. boydii*) to achieve the final concentration of 0.4–5×10^4 conidia/ml
Final antifungal drug dilutions	Two-fold; often ranges between 64 and 0.125 µg/ml for fluconazole and flucytosine; and between 16 and 0.03 µg/ml for other drugs	Two-fold; often ranges between 16 and 0.03 µg/ml for amphotericin B, itraconazole, and new triazoles
	The use of specific schemes for preparing the dilution series for water-soluble and water-insoluble[a] drugs is recommended in the CLSI document or published literature for optimal accuracy	
Incubation period and temperature	~48 h at 35°C (*Candida*). Evaluate the results after both 24 and 48 h of incubation[b]	~24 h at 35°C (*Rhizopus*)
		~48 h at 35°C (*Aspergillus*, *Fusarium*, and *S. schenckii*)
	~72 h at 35°C (*C. neoformans*)	~72 h at 35°C (*P. boydii*)
MIC reading endpoints[c]	Visual[d] MIC-0 (Amphotericin B)	Visual MIC-0 (Amphotericin B, itraconazole, and other azoles active against moulds – voriconazole, posaconazole, and ravuconazole)
	Visual MIC-2 (Azoles, flucytosine, and novel echinocandins, caspofungin, micafungin, and anidulafungin)	
		Visual MIC-2 and MEC (novel echinocandins, caspofungin, micafungin, and anidulafungin)

MIC-0 minimum inhibitory concentration (µg/ml) that results in complete inhibition of growth; *MIC-2* minimum inhibitory concentration (µg/ml) that inhibits 50% of growth compared to the growth-control well (agitation of the microdilution plates – particularly of drugs that use MIC-2 endpoint – prior to reading is recommended to provide uniform turbidity and eases grading of the growth); *MEC* minimum effective concentration (µg/ml);,minimum concentration of the drug that produces short, aberrant hyphal branchings microscopically. This value is often equivalent to MIC-2 and is macroscopically visualized as a change in the growth pattern; the minimum concentration of the drug that yields granular growth in the well macroscopically (compared to the filamentous growth at growth-control well and at concentrations lower than MEC) is often the MEC value (28)

[a]The solvent is DMSO (dimethyl sulfoxide) for amphotericin B, ketoconazole, itraconazole, posaconazole, ravuconazole, voriconazole, and anidulafungin, and water for fluconazole, flucytosine (5-FC), caspofungin, and micafungin. The diluent for achieving final concentrations is RPMI 1640 for all drugs

[b]Data from some animal experiments suggest that 24-h fluconazole MICs correlate better with clinical outcome compared to 48-h MICs, particularly for *Candida* strains that tend to trail and produce unreliably high MICs at 48 h (29)

[c]Novel echinocandins are not included in the CLSI documents. The suggested MIC reading endpoints and other related information are based on the published literature (28, 30)

[d]As a modification, the MIC results may also be read spectrophotometrically. High levels of agreement between visual and spectrophotometric readings have been detected for MIC-0 of amphotericin B (~97%), and MIC-1 (~92%) and MIC-2 (~88%) of itraconazole (31)

MICs of strains isolated from candidemic patients showed that prediction of clinical amphotericin B resistance was not possible by any of the commonly used in vitro methods (CLSI microdilution, Etest) and test parameters (RPMI 1640 and AM3 as the test media, MIC and MLC as the interpretive criteria) employed so far (20). Overall, the technical problems in the determination of in vitro amphotericin B resistance persist and await further approaches.

Table 2 Relevant MIC (μg/ml)/inhibition zone diameter (mm) ranges obtained by CLSI (a) reference microdilution method (24, 32) and (b) disk diffusion method (33) at 24 and 48 h for quality control (QC) isolates

Isolate	Antifungal drug	Incubation period MIC (μg/ml) 24 h	48 h
(a)			
C. krusei ATCC 6258	Amphotericin B	0.5–2	1–4
	Ketoconazole	0.125–1	0.25–1
	Fluconazole	8–64	16–128
	Itraconazole	0.125–1	0.25–1
	Voriconazole	0.06–0.5	0.125–1
	Posaconazole	0.06–0.5	0.125–1
	Ravuconazole	0.06–0.5	0.25–1
	Flucytosine (5-FC)	4–16	8–32
	Caspofungin	0.125–1	0.5–1
	Anidulafungin	0.03–0.25	0.06–0.5
C. parapsilosis ATCC 22019	Amphotericin B	0.25–2	0.5–4
	Ketoconazole	0.03–0.25	0.06–0.5
	Fluconazole	0.5–4	1–4
	Itraconazole	0.125–0.5	0.125–0.5
	Voriconazole	0.016–0.125	0.03–0.25
	Posaconazole	0.06–0.25	0.06–0.25
	Ravuconazole	0.016–0.125	0.03–0.25
	Flucytosine (5-FC)	0.06–0.25	0.125–0.5
	Caspofungin	0.25–1	0.5–4
	Anidulafungin	1–8	1–8

(b) Isolate	Antifungal drug	Inhibition zone diameter (mm)[a]
C. albicans ATCC 90028	Fluconazole[b]	28–39
	Voriconazole[c]	31–42
C. parapsilosis ATCC 22019	Fluconazole	22–33
	Voriconazole	28–37
C. tropicalis ATCC 750	Fluconazole	26–37
	Voriconazole	–[d]
C. krusei ATCC 6258	Fluconazole	–[d]
	Voriconazole	16–25

[a]At 24 h
[b]25-μg disk content
[c]1-μg disk content
[d]Intensive inter-laboratory variations have been observed. Thus, QC ranges have not been established for these settings

Amphotericin B remains, however, as an important antifungal agent and patient care decisions must still be made with current data. At a pragmatic level, our personal experience to date has been that agar-based methods (e.g., Etest) combined with simultaneous testing of isolates with known levels of resistance have been the most useful approach for estimating the relative susceptibility of a given unknown isolate. We combine this information with the knowledge of genus and species when required to estimate the likelihood that microbiological resistance to amphotericin B is relevant to a current clinical problem.

Table 3 CLSI proposed susceptibility categories of *Candida* strains according to the (a) MIC (μg/ml) interpretive guidelines (24, 50) and (b) inhibition zone diameters (nearest whole millimeter at ~80% inhibition of growth) (33, 50) (There is yet no full consensus for the breakpoints for antifungal drugs not listed in the Table below)

Antifungal agent	Susceptible (S)	Susceptible-dose dependent (S-DD)	Intermediate (I)	Resistant (R)
(a)				
Fluconazole[a]	≤8	16–32[b]	–	≥64
Itraconazole	≤0.125	0.25–0.5[c]	–	≥1
Flucytosine	≤4	–	8–16[d]	≥32
Voriconazole	≤1	2[e]	–	≥4

(b) Antifungal agent	Susceptible (S)	Susceptible-dose dependent (S-DD)	Resistant (R)
Fluconazole (25 μg/disk)	≥19	15–18	≤14
Voriconazole (1 μg/disk)	≥17	14–16	≤13

[a]*C. krusei* is intrinsically resistant to fluconazole and these guidelines should not be used for assessment of fluconazole susceptibility of *C. krusei*
[b]Fluconazole doses of at least 400 mg/day may be required in adults with normal renal function to achieve adequate blood levels for treating infections due to these isolates
[c]Plasma itraconazole concentrations of >0.5 μg/ml may be required for optimal response in treating infections due to these isolates
[d]The clinical meaning of this susceptibility category is not clear
[e]The infections due to these isolates may be appropriately treated in body sites where voriconazole is physiologically concentrated or when it can be used at a high dosage

MIC Breakpoints for the Determination of the Susceptibility Category

Definitive MIC breakpoints are currently available only for fluconazole, itraconazole, flucytosine, and voriconazole against *Candida* (Table 3) (24, 50). There is as yet no full consensus about the breakpoints to be used for *Candida* and other drugs, and yeasts other than *Candida*. Similarly, the MIC breakpoints for moulds are not yet established (25). While this drawback limits the routine use of antifungal susceptibility tests, the relatively high MICs (as compared to the other strains of the same species) in correlation with clinical failure may suggest putative resistance of the infecting strain to the corresponding drug. However, definitive determination of resistance merits further in vitro–in vivo correlation studies and a full consensus about the MIC interpretive guidelines.

Time Required to Finalize the Fungal Resistance Tests

The isolation of the infecting fungus, the growth of the fungus for the fungal resistance assay, and the interpretation of

Table 4 Usual in vitro activity of fluconazole, itraconazole, and voriconazole against various *Candida* species (5)

Species	Fluconazole	Itraconazole	Voriconazole
C. albicans	+++	+++	+++
C. glabrata	+ to ++	+ to ++	++
C. guilliermondii	+++	+++	+++
C. krusei	0	++	++
C. lusitaniae	+++	+++	+++
C. parapsilosis	+++	+++	+++
C. tropicalis	+++	+++	+++

0 = no meaningful activity; + = occasional activity; ++ = moderate activity but resistance is noted; +++ = reliable activity, occasional resistance

the assay take more than 48 h. This time is often even longer for moulds. As a result of this drawback, fungal resistance assays often give the clinician little early guidance in the choice of antifungal therapy for a particular infection. Fortunately, other clues can be applied during the early days of a given infection. Azole susceptibility profiles of *Candida* strains are generally predictable once the species of the isolate is known (Table 4). For example, strains of *C. albicans* are mostly very susceptible, whereas those of *C. glabrata* may be dose-dependent susceptible or resistant at rates varying from one center to other (19, 51). Once antifungal therapy is initiated based on these epidemiological data, the fungal resistance results of the particular infecting strain will then be available and can be used to guide therapy.

2.2 EUCAST Reference Broth Dilution Method

A broth dilution assay for susceptibility testing of fermentative yeasts standardized by European Committee on Antifungal Susceptibility Testing (EUCAST) Subcommittee on Antifungal Susceptibility Testing (AFST) is also available and initially documented in 1999 (52). The assay is similar to the CLSI broth dilution method, except that RPMI 1640 supplemented to 2% glucose (CLSI uses 0.2% glucose), an inoculum density of $1-5 \times 10^5$ cells/ml (haemocytometric adjustment, CLSI uses $0.5-2.5 \times 10^3$ cells/ml, spectrophotometric adjustment), microdilution plates with 96 flat-bottom wells are used (CLSI uses U-shaped wells), and the results are read at 24 h rather than the CLSI-specified time of 48 h. Multicenter evaluation of the EUCAST assay showed that the method yields reproducible results (53) and comparative studies suggest a good correlation (92% agreement rate) between CLSI and EUCAST antifungal susceptibility methods when testing

amphotericin B, flucytosine, fluconazole, and itraconazole against *Candida* spp. (54).

Further studies that compared the fluconazole MICs generated by EUCAST and CLSI methods for *Candida* validated the very good correlation between the two methods. However and notably, the EUCAST MICs were found to be slightly lower than the CLSI MICs (55), especially for isolates with MICs above 2 µg/ml. A comparison of EUCAST and CLSI MICs by using the CLSI MIC breakpoint categorization showed relatively lower rates of agreement between the two methods (78.5 and 58.5% for fluconazole and itraconazole, respectively) (56). MIC breakpoints to be used for EUCAST method and *Candida* have been proposed (http://www.srga.org/eucastwt/MICTAB/index.html). These breakpoints do not provide guidance on interpretation of MICs for *Candida glabrata* or *C. krusei*. For other species, EUCAST subcommittee defines susceptible (S) as an MIC ≤ 2 and resistant (R) as an MIC ≥ 4 µg/ml.

Optimal parameters for antifungal susceptibility testing of *Aspergillus* spp. have also been proposed by EUCAST-AFST. These include the use of RPMI 1640 supplemented to 2% glucose as the test medium, $1-2.5 \times 10^5$ conidia/ml (haemocytometric adjustment) as the inoculum density, 48 h as the incubation period, 35°C as the incubation temperature, and visual reading of MICs at MIC-0 endpoint (57). An overall agreement rate of 92.5% was achieved between the EUCAST standard and the CLSI method when testing posaconazole and voriconazole against *Aspergillus*. Notably, the EUCAST method tended to generate higher MICs as compared to the CLSI method for *Aspergillus* isolates with discrepant results (58). Interpretive breakpoints have not been proposed.

2.3 CLSI Disk Diffusion Method

Following the successful development of standardized broth dilution methods for antifungal susceptibility testing of fungi, the next step was to simplify this approach and make it more attractive for small-volume testing. Disk diffusion has long been a popular and simple technique for susceptibility testing and this methodology has now been adapted by the CLSI to antifungal agents. On the basis of studies of *Candida* vs. fluconazole and voriconazole (59–62), a standardized method (M44-A) for antifungal disk diffusion susceptibility of yeasts, particularly for *Candida* vs. fluconazole and voriconazole is now available (33) and used for antifungal surveillance studies (14). This method employs the basic rules of Kirby-Bauer disk diffusion method. Mueller–Hinton agar supplemented to 2% glucose and 0.5 µg/ml methylene blue dye (pH 7.2–7.4 at room temperature after gelling) is used as the test medium. While the supplementation with glucose provides favorable growth, addition of methylene blue enhances zone edge definition (63). The inoculum density to be used in the test is adjusted in sterile saline to that of 0.5 McFarland standard either visually or spectrophotometrically at 530 nm, yielding a final concentration of $1–5 \times 10^6$ cells/ml. The results are read after incubation of the plates for 18–24 h at 35°C at the inhibition zone diameter to the nearest whole millimeter at ~80% inhibition of growth. The incubation period may be extended to 48 h for isolates which grow insufficiently at 24 h. Disk diffusion interpretive criteria are available for fluconazole and voriconazole vs. *Candida* and are shown in Table 2b.

Although not yet standardized and/or documented, the disk diffusion method is also under investigation for other genus–drug combinations: such as posaconazole vs. *Candida* (64–66); caspofungin vs. *Candida* (67); amphotericin B, flucytosine, and azoles vs. *Geotrichum capitatum* (68); caspofungin and micafungin vs. *Aspergillus* and *Fusarium* (69, 70); posaconazole vs. *Aspergillus*, *Rhizopus*, *Mucor*, *Scedosporium*, and *Fusarium* (71, 72); posaconazole, voriconazole, itraconazole, amphotericin B, and caspofungin vs. *Absidia*, *Aspergillus*, *Alternaria*, *Bipolaris*, *Fusarium*, *Mucor*, *Paecilomyces*, *Rhizopus*, and *Scedosporium* (73); itraconazole, terbinafine, voriconazole, and ravuconazole against *Microsporum* and *Trichophyton* (74); and terbinafine and naftifine vs. *Microsporum*, *Epidermophyton*, and *Trichophyton* (75). The results of these studies, in general, suggest an acceptable degree of correlation between disk diffusion and CLSI reference dilution assays.

Tablet diffusion assay is an agar-based susceptibility testing method which has also been studied in comparison with the CLSI reference disk diffusion assay. This method employs commercially available antifungal tablets (Neo-sensitabs, Rosco Diagnostica, Denmark) instead of disks and have so far yielded acceptable percent agreement rates with reference disk diffusion and microdilution methods when testing fluconazole, voriconazole, itraconazole, and caspofungin against *Candida* or *C. neoformans* (76, 77).

Importantly, reference disk diffusion assays may occasionally yield results that differ from those obtained by broth-based testing (59, 63, 67, 78–80). Some isolates that are susceptible to fluconazole may be categorized as fluconazole-resistant by disk diffusion assay. Disk diffusion assay may also fail to differentiate the fluconazole-resistant isolates from the dose-dependent susceptible ones. Even more importantly, some fluconazole-resistant isolates may be categorized as fluconazole-susceptible by disk diffusion assay. Reference broth dilution assays remain as the gold standard for correct categorization of susceptibility, particularly when the fungal resistance assay is performed for routine purposes and guiding antifungal therapy.

2.4 Colorimetric Broth Dilution Methods

As stated in Table 1, the determination of azole and flucytosine MICs for yeasts demands grading of the amount of growth in comparison with that in growth-control well. Making this assessment requires experience. In order to ease the challenge of grading the results, colorimetric indicators or fluorescent dyes may be used. Colorimetric methods have been employed by commercial assay systems, such as Sensititre YeastOne (Trek Diagnostic Systems Inc., Westlake, Ohio which incorporates Alamar blue as the oxidation–reduction colorimetric indicator) and ASTY panels (Kyokuto Pharmaceutical Industrial Co., Ltd, Tokyo, Japan). Noncommercial products, such as tetrazolium salts have also been used (81, 82).

For situations that do not permit the use of commercially prepared systems, Alamar blue or other colorimetric indicators may also be added in-house to RPMI broth, followed by the application of conventional CLSI microdilution method. The endpoint determination in these methods is mostly based on the visual observation of the color change. Using Alamar blue, blue indicates no growth, purple indicates partial inhibition of growth, and red indicates growth. These results may also be evaluated spectrophotometrically. When tetrazolium salts are used, the color change that reflects metabolic activity may be evaluated spectrophotometrically by measuring the optical density. The yellow tetrazolium salt turns purple when it is cleaved to its formazan derivative.

The commercially available Sensititre YeastOne (Trek Diagnostic Systems Inc., Westlake, Ohio) (68, 83–93) and ASTY panels (94) were compared to the CLSI method for *Candida*, *Aspergillus*, and other clinically significant filamentous fungi by various investigators.

In a study that compared the Sensititre YeastOne panel with CLSI microdilution method for *Candida*, agreement rates of 93, 68, 78, and 80% were attained for amphotericin B, fluconazole, itraconazole, and flucytosine, respectively. These results suggested relatively low rates of correlation, particularly for fluconazole and itraconazole (84). While the agreement rate was found to be low (57%) for itraconazole vs. *Candida* in some other studies as well (85), the results obtained by other investigators did not fully support this finding (86). Some studies, on the other hand, have reported relatively lower agreement rates between Sensititre YeastOne and CLSI method when testing azoles (fluconazole, itraconazole, and voriconazole) against *C. glabrata*, specifically (categorical agreement rates of 34, 68, and 87% for fluconazole, itraconazole, and voriconazole respectively). These results emphasized the need for cautious interpretation of the Sensititre YeastOne results, particularly when testing azoles against *C. glabrata* (89).

Sensititre YeastOne panel has also been explored for its utility in caspofungin susceptibility testing of *Candida*. At the MIC endpoint of complete growth inhibition, the overall agreement rate between Sensititre YeastOne and CLSI reference method was found to be 87% for caspofungin (91).

ASTY panel provided high overall agreement rates of 93 (24 h) and 96% (48 h) for amphotericin B, 5-fluorocytosine (5FC), fluconazole, and itraconazole against *Candida*. Agreement rates were found to range from 90% with itraconazole and flucytosine to 96% with amphotericin B at 24 h and from 92% with itraconazole to 99% with amphotericin B and flucytosine at 48 h (94).

The utility of Sensititre panel/Alamar blue (95, 96) and tetrazolium salts (95, 97) have been investigated also for susceptibility testing of *Aspergillus*. In one of these studies, the use of Alamar blue and reading the results spectrophotometrically yielded comparable results with CLSI method in 94% of the cases for itraconazole and voriconazole, 25% of the cases for flucytosine, and 64% of the cases for amphotericin B (98). In contrast to other results, agreement rates were found to be <66% and >77% for itraconazole and amphotericin B, respectively, at 24 h when the Sensititre method (endpoint: slight growth-MIC-purple for itraconazole, complete inhibition of growth-MIC-blue for amphotericin B) was compared to the CLSI method (endpoint: MIC-0 for both drugs) for *Aspergillus* strains. In the same study, the Sensititre method tended to produce lower MICs compared to the CLSI method and agreement rates varied depending on the MIC endpoint used and the incubation period, yielding more comparable results at 48 h and by using MIC-blue endpoint (96). In other studies that compared Sensititre YeastOne with CLSI M38-A method, overall agreement rates of 93, 90, and 97–99% were obtained for amphotericin B, itraconazole, and voriconazole, respectively, for *Aspergillus* spp. (87, 99).

The agreement between Sensititre YeastOne panel and CLSI microdilution method has been explored in a few studies for filamentous fungi other than *Aspergillus*. In one of these studies, posaconazole was tested by Sensititre YeastOne and CLSI methods against various filamentous fungi, including *Aspergillus*, *Fusarium*, *Rhizopus*, *Absidia*, and *Mucor*. By using the MIC-blue endpoint at 24 h, overall agreement rate within ±1 dilution range was found to be 94% (90). The comparison of these two methods for voriconazole against *Fusarium* spp., *S. apiospermum*, and *Rhizomucor pusillus*, on the other hand, showed percent agreement rates of 97–99% at 48 or 72 h depending on the species (99).

On the other hand, an antifungal susceptibility assay that used the tetrazolium salt 2,3-bis{2-methoxy-4-nitro-5-{(sulfenylamino) carbonyl}-2H-tetrazolium-hydroxide} (XTT) yielded high levels of agreement of >97% for MIC-0 of amphotericin B and 83% for MIC-0, MIC-1, and MIC-2 of itraconazole vs. *Aspergillus*, suggesting potential reliability of this method (100). The XTT assay has been recently used for rapid susceptibility testing of fungi belonging to class Zygomycetes (*Rhizopus*, *Cunninghamella*, *Mucor*, and

Absidia spp.) as well. Percent agreement rates were found to be 93, 76, and 67% for amphotericin B, posaconazole, and voriconazole, respectively. Importantly, the results were achievable as early as 6–12 h after inoculation (101).

Considering all the accumulated data, the only strong conclusion is that the utility of the colorimetric methods varies widely and no one approach has emerged as a consistent leader. While these methods were found to be reliable with high degrees of intra- and interlaboratory reproducibility and acceptable agreement percentages with CLSI reference method in some studies, they failed to provide acceptably comparable results with the CLSI method in others. In some studies, testing itraconazole by using these assays was found to be problematic for both yeasts and moulds. The lack of standardization, particularly in terms of the MIC endpoint and the incubation period to be used, appear to be partly responsible for the poor correlation rates. Thus, using these assays, isolates with discordant results as compared to the reference method may be observed and these need to be evaluated with the reference assay, particularly for routine purposes.

2.5 Etest

Etest (AB BioDisk, Solna, Sweden) method is an agar-based diffusion assay that provides quantitative measure of fungal resistance. It is being studied for both yeasts and moulds although the available data are more extensive for yeast genera. The method uses plastic Etest strips impregnated with a stable concentration gradient of the antimicrobial agent to be tested. Etest strips carrying amphotericin B, ketoconazole, fluconazole, itraconazole, flucytosine, voriconazole, posaconazole, and caspofungin are available.

Except for testing amphotericin B for which antibiotic medium 3 agar may be used (46, 102), the most relevant and commonly used test medium for Etest is RPMI 1640 supplemented to 2% glucose (103). Casitone agar (azoles) (104, 105) and yeast nitrogen base (*C. neoformans*) (106) have been used by some investigators. In addition, similar to that in disk diffusion methodology, Mueller–Hinton agar supplemented with 2% glucose and 0.5 µg/ml methylene blue is also being used for Etest (66, 107, 108) and may produce sharper edges of inhibition ellipse and less intra-elliptic growth when used, particularly, for testing azoles against heavy trailer *Candida* strains.

The inoculum density to be used in the test is adjusted in sterile saline to that of 0.5 McFarland standard either visually or spectrophotometrically at 530 nm, yielding a final concentration of $1–5 \times 10^6$ cells/ml. In accordance with the basic rules of disk diffusion assays, the adjusted inoculum is swabbed onto the agar plate and the Etest strip is placed onto the inoculated medium. The results are read as MICs after incubation of the plates at 35°C for 18–24 and 48 and 72 h (when needed, particularly for *C. neoformans*). The MIC of that particular drug is the concentration designated on the strip at the point where the inhibition ellipse intersects the strip. For azoles and other drugs such as flucytosine that tend to produce partial inhibition, the growth inside the ellipse and the tiny colonies produced near the edge of the ellipse are neglected when reading the MIC value. This provides a reading endpoint that approximates MIC-2 of broth dilution assay and eases the precise determination of MICs particularly of isolates that tend to trail heavily.

The utility of Etest for antifungal susceptibility testing of yeasts (predominantly *Candida* and *C. neoformans*) and filamentous fungi (mostly *Aspergillus* and less extensively *Rhizopus*, *Fusarium*, *Scedosporium*, *Paecilomyces*, and *Acremonium*) has been explored by several investigators. For *Candida*, percent agreement rates of Etest with CLSI reference method were found to be 82–100% for fluconazole (89, 103, 109, 110), 80–95% for itraconazole (89, 109), 91–100% for voriconazole (89, 110, 111), 83–95% for posaconazole (65, 66, 112), and 79–100% for caspofungin (113). Of note and importantly, when the correlation of the susceptibility categories was considered, Etest tended to be less correlated with CLSI method (percent categorical agreement rates of 55, 74, and 76% for fluconazole, itraconazole, and voriconazole, respectively), particularly when testing azoles against *C. glabrata* (89).

For *C. neoformans*, percent agreement rates of Etest with CLSI reference method were found to be 99% for amphotericin B (114), 81% for fluconazole (115), 54% for itraconazole (115), 89% for flucytosine (115), and 94% for voriconazole (114). Etest may ease the discrimination of amphotericin B resistance for both *Candida* and *C. neoformans* regardless of the test medium used (RPMI 1640 supplemented to 2% glucose or antibiotic medium 3) (46, 102, 116).

For *Aspergillus*, percent agreement rates of Etest with CLSI reference method were found to be 89–98% for amphotericin B (87, 117), 67–100% for itraconazole (87, 117, 118), 93–100% for voriconazole (117–119), and 69–80% for caspofungin (30). Less data are available for Etest and other filamentous fungi (*Rhizopus*, *Fusarium*, *Scedosporium*, *Paecilomyces*, and *Acremonium*) (105, 120). For these genera, percent agreement rates were overall high (80 and 96% on Casitone and RPMI-2% glucose agar, respectively) but tended to vary extensively (0–100%) from one genus to other (105).

In some instances, as for testing *Trichosporon asahii*, Etest was found to yield consistently lower MICs with a wider MIC range for amphotericin B, and higher MICs for azoles (fluconazole and itraconazole) when compared to reference microdilution method (121). Similar findings were recorded when testing *C. neoformans* as well; Etest voriconazole MICs were higher than reference microdilution MICs for isolates

that yielded discordant results with the two methods (114). However, such a consistent trend of Etest to increase the MICs for all azoles was not always observed (118).

The performance of the Etest for direct antifungal susceptibility testing of yeasts in positive blood cultures has also been investigated. The results of this study showed that correlation of direct Etest with reference macrodilution method was ≥80% for amphotericin B, flucytosine, and ketoconazole while it was 64–70% for itraconazole (122).

In summary, Etest is a practical method that provides quantitative measure of fungal resistance. The agreement of the method with the reference assay is generally high (79, 89, 103, 111, 118, 123). However, genus-, species- and incubation period-dependent variations in Etest-CLSI reference method percent agreement rates may be observed (27, 89, 96, 105, 119, 124). Standardization of the test parameters and the interpretive reading criteria as well as its correlation with clinical outcome should be addressed.

2.6 Agar Dilution Method

In accordance with its basic principles, agar dilution method employs agar medium plates containing two-fold dilutions of the antifungal agent and inoculated with the suspensions of the fungal strains to be tested. The agar dilution method has so far been explored for amphotericin B, fluconazole, itraconazole, ketoconazole, and flucytosine vs. *Candida* (125, 126), fluconazole vs. *C. neoformans* (127), flucytosine vs. *C. neoformans* (128), amphotericin B, itraconazole, and voriconazole vs. *A. fumigatus* (129), caspofungin vs. *Aspergillus* (130), and terbinafine, naftifine, and itraconazole vs. *Microsporum*, *Epidermophyton*, and *Trichophyton* spp. (75, 131). Agar dilution was also used for testing the antifungal activity of other compounds, such as boric acid (132) and *Melaleuca alternifolia* (tea tree) oil (133) against *Candida*. The method remains unstandardized and labor-intensive and further evaluations are required.

2.7 Determination of Fungicidal Activity

For specific settings, determination of fungicidal activity may provide useful hints of likely clinical outcome. This may be achieved either by determination of the MICs initially, followed by minimum fungicidal (lethal) concentrations (MFC/MLC) on solid media (mostly defined as the least concentration yielding growth of <3 colonies, approximating 99–99.5% killing activity) or by time-kill experiments (134–139). Animal models are also being used for assessment of fungicidal activity. Experimental models of disseminated candidiasis and aspergillosis have proven to be very useful for determination of fungicidal effect. Specifically, the assessment of residual fungal burden in animal models has been shown to be well correlated with the MFC measurements and time-kill results (140).

There is yet no standard procedure for the determination of MFCs. A multicenter study investigated the reproducibility of MFC testing for itraconazole, posaconazole, ravuconazole, voriconazole, and amphotericin B vs. *Aspergillus* spp. In this study, MFC was defined as the lowest drug concentration that yielded <3 colonies which approximated 99–99.5% killing activity and the reproducibility of using four different media (RPMI 1640, RPMI 1640 supplemented to 2% glucose, antibiotic medium 3, and antibiotic medium 3 supplemented to 2% glucose) was investigated. The highest reproducibility (96–100%) was achieved with amphotericin B and the results were good across all the four media. Reproducibility rates were still high but more medium-dependent for azoles (91–98%) (141). Similarly, optimal testing conditions for MFC determinations were investigated for filamentous fungi other than *Aspergillus* as well (142). These studies remain significant as being the initial steps for standardization of MFC testing.

Given these steps towards a standardized MFC method, the utility of the MFC in prediction of clinical outcome should be addressed. A study focusing on the correlation of MFC with clinical outcome has been conducted in candidemic patients treated with amphotericin B. This study found that the strongest predictor for microbiologic failure was 48 h MFC value and an MFC breakpoint of >1 μg/ml (and an MIC breakpoint of ≥1 μg/ml) was proposed (47). However, further supporting data for the correlation of MFC and clinical outcome at various clinical settings are yet lacking and data are needed for amphotericin B as well as other antifungal agents. As is the case with the antibacterial agents, it seems likely that demonstrations of the utility of fungicidal measures will be limited. It may possibly be useful for specific clinical presentations, such as endocarditis, meningitis, septic arthritis, and osteomyelitis, or in existence of poor clinical response to standard, normally effective antifungal therapies in neutropenic patients (140).

For time-kill experiments, the test isolates are exposed to varying concentrations of the drug (for example, ranging from 0.0625 to 16 times the MIC). Samples are then withdrawn at predetermined time points and plated. The viable colony counts on the plates are determined after incubation and the results are plotted as time-kill curves. The method is labor-intensive but provides more detailed information about the pharmacodynamic properties of the drug and whether the killing activity of the antifungal agent for an individual strain is dependent on the concentration (134, 136, 143–146). Similar to MFC testing, no reference method is available for time-kill experiments. Time-kill assay parameters that have been shown to yield reproducible results for *Candida* were proposed by some investigators. These parameters were specified as 10^5 cfu/ml as the inoculum size, RPMI 1640 medium as the test medium for antifungal drugs other than echinocandins (AM3 for echinocandins), 30 μl as the transfer volume, 35°C with agitation as the incubation setting, and ≥99.9% reduction in cfu/ml from the starting inoculum as the endpoint (147).

Overall and conclusively, determination of fungicidal activity by MFC measurements or time-kill assays is yet far from global standardization and awaits further investigations.

2.8 Other Methods: Fully Automated Systems, Flow Cytometry, and Sterol Quantitation

A fully automated commercially available system (VITEK 2 yeast susceptibility test; bioMerieux, Inc.) has recently been developed for antifungal susceptibility testing. VITEK-2 test evaluates the MIC results spectrophotometrically. The system has proven to be in very good agreement with the reference CLSI method (categorical agreement rates of 97.2 and 88.3% at 24 and 48 h, respectively) when testing fluconazole against *Candida*. Importantly, very major errors were very seldom observed (0 and 0.2% at 24 and 48 h, respectively) (148).

The utility of flow cytometric susceptibility tests for rapid determination of fungal resistance of *Candida* (amphotericin B, fluconazole, caspofungin, and flucytosine), *Aspergillus* (amphotericin B, itraconazole, and voriconazole) and *C. neoformans* (amphotericin B and fluconazole) has also been investigated (149). The method employs various membrane potential-sensitive or DNA binding vital dyes (3,3′-dipentyloxacarbocyanine iodide, propidium iodide, acridine orange or FUN1). The decrease or increase in fluorescence intensity of the cells stained with the dye following exposure to the drug is determined. The results are available in 3–8 h. The method appears to be well correlated, in general, with the reference method and Etest (150–155), as well as clinical outcome (156). Flow cytometry provides rapid detection of resistance and has also been proposed as a useful and accurate method for identification of *Candida* strains that are resistant to amphotericin B (157). Despite these advantages, its availability remains limited only to some centers because of the need for a flow cytometer.

Sterol quantitation method that measures cellular ergosterol content rather than growth inhibition has also been investigated as a fungal resistance assay. The method seems to be useful, particularly for *Candida* isolates that exhibit heavy trailing, as these tend to produce unclear visual MIC endpoints for fluconazole and itraconazole at 48 h (158).

3 Indications for Use of Fungal Drug Resistance Assays

Fungal drug resistance assays are used (a) for routine purposes to predict the clinical outcome and optimize antifungal therapy, (b) to provide epidemiological data for the susceptibility profiles and resistance rates of the infecting strains to commonly used drugs at a particular center, and (c) to determine the in vitro antifungal activity of the novel compounds under investigation. Unlike the application for bacteria and antibacterial agents, the use of routine fungal drug resistance assays is indicated only for some fungal strains isolated from clinical samples. These indications are currently more clearly defined for yeasts, particularly for *Candida*, and are listed in Table 5 (19). For filamentous fungi, the relevance and benefit of routine application of these tests are yet poorly defined and require to be warranted by further in vitro–in vivo correlation studies.

4 In Vitro Antifungal Combination Studies

Owing to the low clinical response rates to monotherapy particularly in some opportunistic mycoses, such as aspergillosis, fusariosis, and zygomycosis, as well as the availability of new drugs, antifungal combination studies are now appeal-

ing. The best and most relevant method for testing in vitro interaction of antifungal agents is yet unknown. Although most of the accumulated data on in vitro combination studies used the checkerboard method (based on the determination of fractional inhibitory concentration indices, FICI) (159–165), the relevance of this method is not clear and there are significant problems about its performance, standardization, and interpretation (166). Crossed Etest method (159, 167–169) and time-kill studies (159, 169, 170) are the other methods used for testing in vitro antifungal interactions. Assessments of the antifungal interactions by a fully parametric response surface approach (Greco model) have also been undertaken (171–174), but appear equally difficult to interpret. Many questions yet remain to be resolved for rational use of combination antifungal therapy and standard in vitro methods and animal models followed by clinical trials appear to be the most relevant way of determination of the actual clinical efficacy of antifungal combinations (175–178).

5 Keywords and Conclusions

In the last decade, there has been great progress in standardization and application of fungal resistance assays. However, several issues still remain to be resolved and clarified. While fungal resistance assays currently appear as a significant aid in the prediction of clinical outcome and guiding therapy, the influence of host factors is strong and limits the overall ability of susceptibility testing to completely predict response.

Table 5 Proposed indications for application of *routine* fungal drug resistance assays for clinical isolates (19)

Indication	Antifungal drug to be tested
Invasive infection due to *Candida* spp.	Azoles, particularly fluconazole, and flucytosine
Refractory mucosal infection due to a *Candida* sp. that fails to respond to standard therapy at the standard dose	Azoles, particularly fluconazole
Refractory *C. neoformans* infection that fails to respond to standard therapy at the standard dose[a]	Fluconazole
Any species with a well-known high rate of resistance to any drug or class of drug[a] (e.g., *C. glabrata*-azoles, *C. krusei*-azoles, *C. lusitaniae*-amphotericin B, *Trichosporon* spp.-amphotericin B, *A. terreus*-amphotericin B, *S. apiospermum* and *S. prolificans*-amphotericin B, *H. capsulatum*-fluconazole	Corresponding drug

[a]Owing to the lack of relevant MIC breakpoints for fluconazole vs. *C. neoformans*, amphotericin B vs. any yeast or mould genera, and fluconazole vs. *H. capsulatum*, susceptibility test results of these combinations can provide guidance only by comparison of the MIC results to those of the other strains of the same genus. The interpretation in this case may provide only general guidance. If the MIC of that particular drug is relatively high for that strain when compared to those of the other strains of that genus, this may indicate microbiological resistance

References

1. Arikan S, Rex JH. Lipid-based antifungal agents: current status. Curr Pharm Des 2001;7(5):393–415.
2. Arikan S, Rex JH. New agents for the treatment of systemic fungal infections-current status. Expert Opin Emerg Drugs 2002;7:3–32.
3. Datry A, Thellier M. Echinocandins: a new class of antifungal agents, a new mechanism of action. J Mycologie Medicale 2002;12:S5–S9.
4. Neely MN, Ghannoum MA. The exciting future of antifungal therapy. Eur J Clin Microbiol Infect D 2000;19(12):897–914.
5. Arikan S, Rex JH. Antifungal agents. In: Murray PR, Baron EJ, Jorgensen JH, Landry ML, Pfaller MA, editors. Manual of Clinical Microbiology, 9th edition, vol. 2. Washington, DC: ASM; 2007, pp. 1949–1960.
6. Kwon DS, Mylonakis E. Posaconazole: a new broad-spectrum antifungal agent. Expert Opin Pharmacother 2007;8(8):1167–1178.
7. Aperis G, Mylonakis E. Newer triazole antifungal agents: pharmacology, spectrum, clinical efficacy and limitations. Expert Opin Investig Drugs 2006;15(6):579–602.
8. Alexander BD, Perfect JR. Antifungal resistance trends towards the year 2000: implications for therapy and new approaches. Drugs 1997;54:657–678.

9. Moore CB, Sayers N, Mosquera J, Slaven J, Denning DW. Antifungal drug resistance in *Aspergillus*. J Infect 2000;41(3):203–220.

10. Muller FMC, Weig M, Peter J, Walsh TJ. Azole cross-resistance to ketoconazole, fluconazole, itraconazole and voriconazole in clinical *Candida albicans* isolates from HIV-infected children with oropharyngeal candidosis. J Antimicrob Chemother 2000;46(2):338–341.

11. Canuto MM, Rodero FG. Antifungal drug resistance to azoles and polyenes. Lancet Infect Dis 2002;2(9):550–563.

12. Kontoyiannis DP, Lewis RE. Antifungal drug resistance of pathogenic fungi. Lancet 2002;359(9312):1135–1144.

13. Loeffler J, Stevens DA. Antifungal drug resistance. Clin Infect Dis 2003;36:S31–S41.

14. Pfaller MA, Diekema DJ, Gibbs DL, Newell VA, Meis JF, Gould IM, et al. Results from the ARTEMIS DISK Global Antifungal Surveillance Study, 1997 to 2005: an 8.5-year analysis of susceptibilities of *Candida* species and other yeast species to fluconazole and voriconazole determined by CLSI standardized disk diffusion testing. J Clin Microbiol 2007;45(6):1735–1745.

15. Mellado E, Garcia-Effron G, Alcazar-Fuoli L, Melchers WJG, Verweij PE, Cuenca-Estrella A, et al. A new *Aspergillus fumigatus* resistance mechanism conferring in vitro cross-resistance to azole antifungals involves a combination of cyp51A alterations. Antimicrob Agents Chemother 2007;51(6):1897–1904.

16. Perlin DS. Resistance to echinocandin-class antifungal drugs. Drug Resist Updat 2007;10(3):121–130.

17. Magill SS, Shields C, Sears CL, Choti M, Merz WG. Triazole cross-resistance among *Candida* spp.: case report, occurrence among bloodstream isolates, and implications for antifungal therapy. J Clin Microbiol 2006;44(2):529–535.

18. Rogers TR. Antifungal drug resistance: limited data, dramatic impact? Int J Antimicrob Agents 2006;27:S7–S11.

19. Rex JH, Pfaller MA. Has antifungal susceptibility testing come of age? Clin Infect Dis 2002;35:982–989.

20. Park BJ, Arthington-Skaggs BA, Hajjeh RA, Iqbal N, Ciblak MA, Lee-Yang W, et al. Evaluation of amphotericin B interpretive breakpoints for *Candida* bloodstream isolates by correlation with therapeutic outcome. Antimicrob Agents Chemother 2006;50(4):1287–1292.

21. Dannaoui E, Abdul M, Arpin M, Michel-Nguyen A, Piens MA, Favel A, et al. Results obtained with various antifungal susceptibility testing methods do not predict early clinical outcome in patients with cryptococcosis. Antimicrob Agents Chemother 2006;50(7):2464–2470.

22. Lionakis MS, Lewis RE, Chamilos G, Kontoyiannis DP. *Aspergillus* susceptibility testing in patients with cancer and invasive aspergillosis: difficulties in establishing correlation between in vitro susceptibility data and the outcome of initial amphotericin B therapy. Pharmacotherapy 2005;25(9):1174–1180.

23. Kartsonis N, Killar J, Mixson L, Hoe CM, Sable C, Bartizal K, et al. Caspofungin susceptibility testing of isolates from patients with esophageal candidiasis or invasive candidiasis: relationship of MIC to treatment outcome. Antimicrob Agents Chemother 2005;49(9):3616–3623.

24. National Committee for Clinical Laboratory Standards. Reference method for broth dilution antifungal susceptibility testing of yeasts; Approved standard NCCLS document M27-A2. Wayne, PA: National Committee for Clinical Laboratory Standards; 2002.

25. National Committee for Clinical Laboratory Standards. Reference method for broth dilution antifungal susceptibility testing of filamentous fungi; Approved standard NCCLS document M38-A. Wayne, PA: National Committee for Clinical Laboratory Standards; 2002.

26. Espinel-Ingroff A, Kish CW, Kerkering TM, Fromtling RA, Bartizal K, Galgiani JN, et al. Collaborative comparison of broth macrodilution and microdilution antifungal susceptibility tests. J Clin Microbiol 1992;30:3138–3145.

27. Sewell DL, Pfaller MA, Barry AL. Comparison of broth macrodilution, broth microdilution, and Etest antifungal susceptibility tests for fluconazole. J Clin Microbiol 1994;32:2099–2102.

28. Arikan S, Lozano-Chiu M, Paetznick V, Rex JH. In vitro susceptibility testing methods for caspofungin against *Aspergillus* and *Fusarium* isolates. Antimicrob Agents Chemother 2001;45(1):327–330.

29. Rex JH, Nelson PW, Paetznick VL, Lozano-Chiu M, Espinel-Ingroff A, Anaissie EJ. Optimizing the correlation between results of testing *in vitro* and therapeutic outcome *in vivo* for fluconazole by testing critical isolates in a murine model of invasive candidiasis. Antimicrob Agents Chemother 1998;42:129–134.

30. Espinel-Ingroff A. Evaluation of broth microdilution testing parameters and agar diffusion Etest procedure for testing susceptibilities of *Aspergillus* spp. to caspofungin acetate (MK-0991). J Clin Microbiol 2003;41(1):403–409.

31. Meletiadis J, Mouton JW, Meis JF, Bouman BA, Donnelly PJ, Verweij PE. Comparison of spectrophotometric and visual readings of NCCLS method and evaluation of a colorimetric method based on reduction of a soluble tetrazolium salt, 2,3-bis {2-methoxy-4-nitro-5-[(sulfenylamino) carbonyl]-2H-tetrazolium-hydroxide}, for antifungal susceptibility testing of *Aspergillus* species. J Clin Microbiol 2001;39(12):4256–4263.

32. Barry AL, Pfaller MA, Brown SD, Espinel-Ingroff A, Ghannoum MA, Knapp C, et al. Quality control limits for broth microdilution susceptibility tests of ten antifungal agents. J Clin Microbiol 2000;38(9):3457–3459.

33. National Committee for Clinical Laboratory Standards. Methods for antifungal disk diffusion susceptibility testing of yeasts; Approved Guideline M44-A. Wayne, PA: National Committee for Clinical Laboratory Standards; 2004.

34. Korting HC, Ollert M, Abeck D, The German Colloborative Dermatophyte Drug Susceptibility Study Group. Results of German multicenter study of antimicrobial susceptibilities of *Trichophyton rubrum* and *Trichophyton mentagrophytes* strains causing tinea unguium. Antimicrob Agents Chemother 1995;39:1206–1208.

35. Niewerth M, Splanemann V, Korting HC, Ring J, Abeck D. Antimicrobial susceptibility testing of dermatophytes – comparison of the agar macrodilution and broth microdilution tests. Chemotherapy 1998;44(1):31–35.

36. Norris HA, Elewski BE, Ghannoum MA. Optimal growth conditions for the determination of the antifungal susceptibility of three species of dermatophytes with the use of a microdilution method. J Am Acad Dermatol 1999;40(6 Pt 2):S9–S13.

37. Fernandez-Torres B, Vazquez-Veiga H, Llovo X, Pereiro M, Jr., Guarro J. In vitro susceptibility to itraconazole, clotrimazole, ketoconazole and terbinafine of 100 isolates of *Trichophyton rubrum*. Chemotherapy 2000;46(6):390–394.

38. Jessup CJ, Warner J, Isham N, Hasan I, Ghannoum MA. Antifungal susceptibility testing of dermatophytes: establishing a medium for inducing conidial growth and evaluation of susceptibility of clinical isolates. J Clin Microbiol 2000;38(1):341–344.

39. Barchiesi F, Arzeni D, Camiletti V, Simonetti O, Cellini A, Offidani AM, et al. In vitro activity of posaconazole against clinical isolates of dermatophytes. J Clin Microbiol 2001;39(11):4208–4209.

40. Fernandez-Torres B, Carrillo AJ, Martin E, Del Palacio A, Moore MK, Valverde A, et al. In vitro activities of 10 antifungal drugs against 508 dermatophyte strains. Antimicrob Agents Chemother 2001;45(9):2524–2528.

41. Fernandez-Torres B, Cabanes FJ, Carrillo-Munoz AJ, Esteban A, Inza I, Abarca L, et al. Collaborative evaluation of optimal antifungal susceptibility testing conditions for dermatophytes. J Clin Microbiol 2002;40(11):3999–4003.

42. Mukherjee PK, Leidich SD, Isham N, Leitner I, Ryder NS, Ghannoum MA. Clinical *Trichophyton rubrum* strain exhibiting primary resistance to terbinafine. Antimicrob Agents Chemother 2003;47(1):82–86.

43. Ghannoum MA, Arthington-Skaggs B, Chaturvedi V, Espinel-Ingroff A, Pfaller MA, Rennie R, et al. Interlaboratory study of quality control isolates for a broth microdilution method (modified CLSI M38-A) for testing susceptibilities of dermatophytes to antifungals. J Clin Microbiol 2006;44(12):4353–4356.

44. Barros MED, Santos DDA, Hamdan JS. Evaluation of susceptibility of Trichophyton mentagrophytes and Trichophyton rubrum clinical isolates to antifungal drugs using a modified CLSI microdilution method (M38-A). J Med Microbiol 2007;56(4):514–518.

45. Rex JH, Cooper CR, Jr., Merz WG, Galgiani JN, Anaissie EJ. Detection of amphotericin B-resistant Candida isolates in a broth-based system. Antimicrob Agents Chemother 1995;39:906–909.

46. Wanger A, Mills K, Nelson PW, Rex JH. Comparison of Etest and National Committee for Clinical Laboratory Standards broth macrodilution method for antifungal susceptibility testing: enhanced ability to detect amphotericin B-resistant Candida isolates. Antimicrob Agents Chemother 1995;39:2520–2522.

47. Nguyen MH, Clancy CJ, Yu VL, Yu YV, Morris AJ, Snydman DR, et al. Do in vitro susceptibility data predict the microbiologic response to amphotericin B? Results of a prospective study of patients with Candida fungemia. J Infect Dis 1998;177:425–430.

48. Lozano-Chiu M, Nelson PW, Lancaster M, Pfaller MA, Rex JH. Lot-to-lot variability of antibiotic medium 3 when used for susceptibility testing of Candida isolates to amphotericin B. J Clin Microbiol 1997;35:270–272.

49. Lass-Florl C, Kofler G, Kropshofer G, Hermans J, Kreczy A, Dierich MP, et al. In-vitro testing of susceptibility to amphotericin B is a reliable predictor of clinical outcome in invasive aspergillosis. J Antimicrob Chemother 1998;42(4):497–502.

50. Pfaller MA, Diekema DJ, Rex JH, Espinel-Ingroff A, Johnson EM, Andes D, et al. Correlation of MIC with outcome for Candida species tested against voriconazole: analysis and proposal for interpretive breakpoints. J Clin Microbiol 2006;44(3):819–826.

51. Krcmery V, Barnes AJ. Non-albicans Candida spp. causing fungaemia: pathogenicity and antifungal resistance. J Hosp Infect 2002;50(4):243–260.

52. Subcommittee on Antifungal Susceptibility Testing of the ESCMID European Committee for Antimicrobial Susceptibility Testing, Rodriguez-Tudela JL, Barchiesi F, Bille J, Chryssanthou E, Cuenca-Estrella M, et al. Method for the determination of minimum inhibitory concentration (MIC) by broth dilution of fermentative yeasts. EUCAST Discussion Document E.Dis 7.1. Munich, Germany: European Society for Clinical Microbiology and Infectious Diseases; June 2002.

53. Cuenca-Estrella M, Moore CB, Barchiesi F, Bille J, Chryssanthou E, Denning DW, et al. Multicenter evaluation of the reproducibility of the proposed antifungal susceptibility testing method for fermentative yeasts of the Antifungal Susceptibility Testing Subcommittee of the European Committee on Antimicrobial Susceptibility Testing (AFST-EUCAST). Clin Microbiol Infect 2003;9(6):467–474.

54. Cuenca-Estrella M, Lee-Yang W, Ciblak MA, Arthington-Skaggs BA, Mellado E, Warnock DW, et al. Comparative evaluation of NCCLS M27-A and EUCAST broth microdilution procedures for antifungal susceptibility testing of Candida species. Antimicrob Agents Chemother 2002;46(11):3644–3647.

55. Rodriguez-Tudela JL, Donnelly JP, Pfaller MA, Chryssantou E, Warn P, Denning DW, et al. Statistical analyses of correlation between fluconazole MICs for Candida spp. assessed by standard methods set forth by the European Committee on Antimicrobial Susceptibility Testing (E.Dis. 7.1) and CLSI (M27-A2). J Clin Microbiol 2007;45(1):109–111.

56. Espinel-Ingroff A, Barchiesi F, Cuenca-Estrella M, Pfaller MA, Rinaldi M, Rodriguez-Tudela JL, et al. International and multicenter comparison of EUCAST and CLSI M27-A2 broth micro-

dilution methods for testing susceptibilities of Candida spp. to fluconazole, itraconazole, posaconazole, and voriconazole. J Clin Microbiol 2005;43(8):3884–3889.

57. Lass-Florl C, Cuenca-Estrella M, Denning DW, Rodriguez-Tudela JL. Antifungal susceptibility testing in Aspergillus spp. according to EUCAST methodology. Med Mycol 2006;44:S319–S325.

58. Chryssanthou E, Cuenca-Estrella M. Comparison of the EUCAST-AFST broth dilution method with the CLSI reference broth dilution method (M38-A) for susceptibility testing of posaconazole and voriconazole against Aspergillus spp. Clin Microbiol Infect 2006;12(9):901–904.

59. Barry AL, Pfaller MA, Rennie RP, Fuchs PC, Brown SD. Precision and accuracy of fluconazole susceptibility testing by broth microdilution, Etest, and disk diffusion methods. Antimicrob Agents Chemother 2002;46(6):1781–1784.

60. Hazen KC, Baron EJ, Colombo AL, Girmenia C, Sanchez-Sousa A, del Palacio A, et al. Comparison of the susceptibilities of Candida spp. to fluconazole and voriconazole in a 4-year global evaluation using disk diffusion. J Clin Microbiol 2003;41(12):5623–5632.

61. Kirkpatrick WR, Turner TM, Fothergill AW, McCarthy DI, Redding SW, Rinaldi MG, et al. Fluconazole disk diffusion susceptibility testing of Candida species. J Clin Microbiol 1998;36(11):3429–3432.

62. Meis J, Petrou M, Bille J, Ellis D, Gibbs D. A global evaluation of the susceptibility of Candida species to fluconazole by disk diffusion. Diagn Microbiol Infect Dis 2000;36(4):215–223.

63. Lee S-C, Fung C-P, Lee N, See L-C, Huang J-S, Tsai C-J, et al. Fluconazole disk diffusion test with methylene blue- and glucose-enriched Mueller Hinton agar for determining susceptibility of Candida species. J Clin Microbiol 2001;39:1615–1617.

64. Brown S, Traczewski M. Quality control limits for posaconazole disk susceptibility tests on Mueller–Hinton agar with glucose and methylene blue. J Clin Microbiol 2007;45(1):222–223.

65. Diekema DJ, Messer SA, Hollis RJ, Boyken LB, Tendolkar S, Kroeger J, et al. Evaluation of Etest and disk diffusion methods compared with broth microdilution antifungal susceptibility testing of clinical isolates of Candida spp. against posaconazole. J Clin Microbiol 2007;45(6):1974–1977.

66. Sims CR, Paetznick VL, Rodriguez JR, Chen E, Ostrosky-Zeichner L. Correlation between microdilution, E-test, and disk diffusion methods for antifungal susceptibility testing of posaconazole against Candida spp. J Clin Microbiol 2006;44(6):2105–2108.

67. Lozano-Chiu M, Nelson PW, Paetznick VL, Rex JH. Disk diffusion method for determining susceptibilities of Candida spp. to MK-0991. J Clin Microbiol 1999;37(5):1625–1627.

68. Girmenia C, Pizzarelli G, D'Antonio D, Cristini F, Martino P. In vitro susceptibility testing of Geotrichum capitatum: comparison of the E-test, disk diffusion, and Sensititre colorimetric methods in the NCCLS M27-A2 broth microdilution reference method. Antimicrob Agents Chemother 2003;47(12):3985–3988.

69. Arikan S, Paetznick V, Rex JH. Comparative evaluation of disk diffusion with microdilution assay in susceptibility testing of caspofungin against Aspergillus and Fusarium isolates. Antimicrob Agents Chemother 2002;46(9):3084–3087.

70. Arikan S, Yurdakul P, Hascelik G. Comparison of two methods and three end points in determination of in vitro activity of micafungin against Aspergillus spp. Antimicrob Agents Chemother 2003;47(8):2640–2643.

71. Messer SA, Diekema DJ, Hollis RJ, Boyken LB, Tendolkar S, Kroeger J, et al. Evaluation of disk diffusion and Etest compared to broth microdilution for antifungal susceptibility testing of posaconazole against clinical isolates of filamentous fungi. J Clin Microbiol 2007;45(4):1322–1324.

72. Lopez-Oviedo E, Aller AI, Martin C, Castro C, Ramirez M, Peman JM, et al. Evaluation of disk diffusion method for

determining posaconazole susceptibility of filamentous fungi: comparison with CLSI broth microdilution method. Antimicrob Agents Chemother 2006;50(3):1108–1111.

73. Espinel-Ingroff A, Arthington-Skaggs B, Iqbal N, Ellis D, Pfaller MA, Messer S, et al. Multicenter evaluation of a new disk agar diffusion method for susceptibility testing of filamentous fungi with voriconazole, posaconazole, itraconazole, amphotericin B, and caspofungin. J Clin Microbiol 2007;45(6):1811–1820.

74. Fernandez-Torres B, Carrillo-Munoz A, Inza I, Guarro J. Effect of culture medium on the disk diffusion method for determining antifungal susceptibilities of dermatophytes. Antimicrob Agents Chemother 2006;50(6):2222–2224.

75. Venugopal PV, Venugopal TV. Disk diffusion susceptibility testing of dermatophytes with allylamines. Int J Dermatol 1994;33(10):730–732.

76. Rementeria A, Sanchez-Vargas LO, Villar M, Casals JB, Carrillo-Munoz AJ, Andres CR, et al. Comparison of tablet and disk diffusion methods for fluconazole and voriconazole in vitro activity testing against clinical yeast isolates. J Chemother 2007;19(2):172–177.

77. Espinel-Ingroff A, Canton E, Gibbs D, Wang A. Correlation of Neo-Sensitabs tablet diffusion assay results on three different agar media with CLSI broth microdilution M27-A2 and disk diffusion M44-A results for testing susceptibilities of Candida spp. and Cryptococcus neoformans to amphotericin B, caspofungin, fluconazole, itraconazole, and voriconazole. J Clin Microbiol 2007;45(3):858–864.

78. Matar MJ, Ostrosky Zeichner L, Paetznick VL, Rodriguez JR, Chen E, Rex JH. Correlation between E-test, disk diffusion, and microdilution methods for antifungal susceptibility testing of fluconazole and voriconazole. Antimicrob Agents Chemother 2003;47(5):1647–1651.

79. Morace G, Amato G, Bistoni F, Fadda G, Marone P, Montagna MT, et al. Multicenter comparative evaluation of six commercial systems and the National Committee for Clinical Laboratory Standards M27-A broth microdilution method for fluconazole susceptibility testing of Candida species. J Clin Microbiol 2002;40(8):2953–2958.

80. Sandven P. Detection of fluconazole-resistant Candida strains by a disc diffusion screening test. J Clin Microbiol 1999;37(12):3856–3859.

81. Yang HC, Mikami Y, Yazawa K, Taguchi H, Nishimura K, Miyaji M, et al. Colorimetric MTT assessment of antifungal activity of D0870 against fluconazole-resistant Candida albicans. Mycoses 1998;41(11–12):477–480.

82. Hawser SP, Norris H, Jessup CJ, Ghannoum MA. Comparison of a 2,3-bis(2-methoxy-4-nitro-5-sulfophenyl)-5-[(phenyl-amino) carbonyl]-2H-tetrazolium hydroxide (XTT) colorimetric method with the Standardized National Committee for Clinical Laboratory Standards method of testing clinical yeast isolates for susceptibility to antifungal agents. J Clin Microbiol 1998;36:1450–1452.

83. Pfaller MA, Messer SA, Hollis RJ, Espinel-Ingroff A, Ghannoum MA, Plavan H, et al. Multisite reproducibility of MIC results by the Sensititre (R) YeastOne colorimetric antifungal susceptibility panel. Diagn Microbiol Infect Dis 1998;31(4):543–547.

84. Bernal S, Aller AI, Chavez M, Valverde A, Serrano C, Gutierrez MJ, et al. Comparison of the Sensititre YeastOne colorimetric microdilution panel and the NCCLS broth microdilution method for antifungal susceptibility testing against Candida species. Chemotherapy 2002;48(1):21–25.

85. Chryssanthou E. Trends in antifungal susceptibility among Swedish Candida species bloodstream isolates from 1994 to 1998: comparison of the E-test and the Sensititre YeastOne colorimetric antifungal panel with the NCCLS M27-A reference method. J Clin Microbiol 2001;39(11):4181–4183.

86. Espinel-Ingroff A, Pfaller M, Messer SA, Knapp CC, Killian S, Norris HA, et al. Multicenter comparison of the Sensititre YeastOne colorimetric antifungal panel with the National Committee for Clinical Laboratory Standards M27-A reference method for testing clinical isolates of common and emerging Candida spp., Cryptococcus spp., and other yeasts and yeast-like organisms. J Clin Microbiol 1999;37(3):591–595.

87. Martin-Mazuelos E, Peman J, Valverde A, Chaves M, Serrano MC, Canton E. Comparison of the Sensititre YeastOne colorimetric antifungal panel and Etest with the NCCLS M38-A method to determine the activity of amphotericin B and itraconazole against clinical isolates of Aspergillus spp. J Antimicrob Chemother 2003;52(3):365–370.

88. Pujol I, Capilla J, Fernandez-Torres B, Ortoneda M, Guarro J. Use of the Sensititre colorimetric microdilution panel for antifungal susceptibility testing of dermatophytes. J Clin Microbiol 2002;40(7):2618–2621.

89. Alexander BD, Byrne TC, Smith KL, Hanson KE, Anstrom KJ, Perfect JR, et al. Comparative evaluation of Etest and Sensititre YeastOne panels against the clinical and laboratory standards institute M27-A2 reference broth microdilution method for testing Candida susceptibility to seven antifungal agents. J Clin Microbiol 2007;45(3):698–706.

90. Patel R, Mendrick C, Knapp CC, Grist R, McNicholas PM. Clinical evaluation of the Sensititre YeastOne plate for testing susceptibility of filamentous fungi to posaconazole. J Clin Microbiol 2007;45(6):2000–2001.

91. Canton E, Peman J, Gobernado M, Alvarez E, Baquero F, Cisterna R, et al. Sensititre YeastOne caspofungin susceptibility testing of Candida clinical isolates: correlation with results of NCCLS M27-A2 multicenter study. Antimicrob Agents Chemother 2005;49(4):1604–1607.

92. Espinel-Ingroff A, Pfaller M, Messer SA, Knapp CC, Holliday N, Killian SB. Multicenter comparison of the Sensititre YeastOne colorimetric antifungal panel with the NCCLS M27-A2 reference method for testing new antifungal agents against clinical isolates of Candida spp. J Clin Microbiol 2004;42(2):718–721.

93. Pfaller MA, Espinel-Ingroff A, Jones RN. Clinical evaluation of the Sensititre YeastOne colorimetric antifungal plate for antifungal susceptibility testing of the new triazoles voriconazole, posaconazole, and ravuconazole. J Clin Microbiol 2004;42(10):4577–4580.

94. Pfaller MA, Arikan S, Lozano-Chiu M, Chen YS, Coffman S, Messer SA, et al. Clinical evaluation of the ASTY colorimetric microdilution panel for antifungal susceptibility testing. J Clin Microbiol 1998;36(9):2609–2612.

95. Jahn B, Stuben A, Bhakdi S. Colormetric susceptibilty testing for Aspergillus fumigatus: comparison of menadione-augmented 3-(4,5-dimethyl-2-thiazolyl)-2,5-diphenyl-2H-tetrazolium bromide and Alamar Blue tests. J Clin Microbiol 1996;34:2039–2041.

96. Meletiadis J, Mouton JW, Meis J, Bouman BA, Verweij PE. Comparison of the Etest and the Sensititre colorimetric methods with the NCCLS proposed standard for antifungal susceptibility testing of Aspergillus species. J Clin Microbiol 2002;40(8):2876–2885.

97. Meletiadis J, Mouton JW, Meis J, Bouman BA, Donnelly JP, Verweij PE, et al. Colorimetric assay for antifungal susceptibility testing of Aspergillus species. J Clin Microbiol 2001;39(9):3402–3408.

98. Yamaguchi H, Uchida K, Nagino K, Matsunaga T. Usefulness of a colorimetric method for testing antifungal drug susceptibilities of Aspergillus species to voriconazole. J Infect Chemother 2002;8(4):374–377.

99. Linares MJ, Charriel G, Solis F, Rodriguez F, Ibarra A, Casal M. Susceptibility of filamentous fungi to voriconazole tested by two microdilution methods. J Clin Microbiol 2005;43(1):250–253.

100. Meletiadis J, Mouton JW, Meis JFG, Bouman BA, Donnelly PJ, Verweij PE, et al. Comparison of spectrophotometric and visual readings of NCCLS method and evaluation of a colorimetric method based on reduction of a soluble tetrazolium salt, 2,3-bis {2-methoxy-4-nitro-5-[(sulfenylamino) carbonyl]-2H-tetrazolium-hydroxide}, for antifungal susceptibility testing of *Aspergillus* species. J Clin Microbiol 2001;39(12):4256–4263.

101. Antachopoulos C, Meletiadis J, Roilides E, Sein T, Walsh TJ. Rapid susceptibility testing of medically important zygomycetes by XTT assay. J Clin Microbiol 2006;44(2):553–560.

102. Lozano-Chiu M, Paetznick VL, Ghannoum MA, Rex JH. Detection of resistance to amphotericin B among *Cryptococcus neoformans* clinical isolates: performance of three different media assessed by using E-Test and National Committee for Clinical Laboratory Standards M27-A methodologies. J Clin Microbiol 1998;36:2817–2822.

103. Pfaller MA, Messer SA, Karlsson A, Bolmstrom A. Evaluation of the Etest method for determining fluconazole susceptibilities of 402 clinical yeast isolates by using three different agar media. J Clin Microbiol 1998;36(9):2586–2589.

104. Favel A, Chastin C, Thomet AL, Regli P, Michel-Nguyen A, Penaud A. Evaluation of the E test for antifungal susceptibility testing of *Candida glabrata*. Eur J Clin Microbiol Infect Dis 2000;19(2):146–148.

105. Pfaller MA, Messer SA, Mills K, Bolmstrom A. In vitro susceptibility testing of filamentous fungi: comparison of Etest and reference microdilution methods for determining itraconazole MICs. J Clin Microbiol 2000;38(9):3359–3361.

106. Petrou MA, Shanson DC. Susceptibility of *Cryptococcus neoformans* by the NCCLS microdilution and Etest methods using five defined media. J Antimicrob Chemother 2000;46(5): 815–818.

107. Pfaller MA, Boyken L, Messer SA, Tendolkar S, Hollis RJ, Diekema DJ. Evaluation of the Etest method using Mueller–Hinton agar with glucose and methylene blue for determining amphotericin B MICs for 4,936 clinical isolates of *Candida* species. J Clin Microbiol 2004;42(11):4977–4979.

108. Pfaller MA, Diekema DJ, Boyken L, Messer SA, Tendolkar S, Hollis RJ. Evaluation of the Etest and disk diffusion methods for determining susceptibilities of 235 bloodstream isolates of *Candida glabrata* to fluconazole and voriconazole. J Clin Microbiol 2003;41(5):1875–1880.

109. Colombo AL, Barchiesi F, McGough DA, Rinaldi MG. Comparison of Etest and National Committee for Clinical Laboratory Standards broth macrodilution method for azole antifungal susceptibility testing. J Clin Microbiol 1995;33:535–540.

110. Maxwell MJ, Messer SA, Hollis RJ, Boyken L, Tendolkar S, Diekema DJ, et al. Evaluation of Etest method for determining fluconazole and voriconazole MICs for 279 clinical isolates of *Candida* species infrequently isolated from blood. J Clin Microbiol 2003;41(3):1087–1090.

111. Pfaller MA, Messer SA, Houston A, Mills K, Bolmstrom A, Jones RN. Evaluation of the Etest method for determining voriconazole susceptibilities of 312 clinical isolates of *Candida* species by using three different agar media. J Clin Microbiol 2000;38(10):3715–3717.

112. Pfaller MA, Messer SA, Mills K, Bolmstrom A, Jones RN. Evaluation of Etest method for determining posaconazole MICs for 314 clinical isolates of *Candida* species. J Clin Microbiol 2001;39(11):3952–3954.

113. Pfaller MA, Messer SA, Mills K, Bolmstrom A, Jones RN. Evaluation of Etest method for determining caspofungin (MK-0991) susceptibilities of 726 clinical isolates of *Candida* species. J Clin Microbiol 2001;39(12):4387–4389.

114. Maxwell AJ, Messer SA, Hollis RJ, Diekema DJ, Pfaller MA. Evaluation of Etest method for determining voriconazole and

115. Aller AI, Martin-Mazuelos E, Gutierrez MJ, Bernal S, Chavez N, Recio FJ. Comparison of the Etest and microdilution method for antifungal susceptibility testing of *Cryptococcus neoformans* to four antifungal agents. J Antimicrob Chemother 2000;46(6):997–1000.

116. Peyron F, Favel A, Michel-Nguyen A, Gilly M, Regli P, Bolmstrom A. Improved detection of amphotericin B-resistant isolates of *Candida lusitaniae* by Etest. J Clin Microbiol 2001;39(1):339–342.

117. Guinea J, Pelaez T, Alcala L, Bouza E. Correlation between the E test and the CLSI M-38 A microdilution method to determine the activity of amphotericin B, voriconazole, and itraconazole against clinical isolates of *Aspergillus fumigatus*. Diagn Microbiol Infect Dis 2007;57(3):273–276.

118. Pfaller JB, Messer SA, Hollis RJ, Diekema DJ, Pfaller MA. In vitro susceptibility testing of *Aspergillus* spp.: comparison of Etest and reference microdilution methods for determining voriconazole and itraconazole MICs. J Clin Microbiol 2003;41(3):1126–1129.

119. Espinel-Ingroff A, Rezusta A. E-test method for testing susceptibilities of *Aspergillus* spp. to the new triazoles voriconazole and posaconazole and to established antifungal agents: comparison with NCCLS broth microdilution method. J Clin Microbiol 2002;40(6):2101–2107.

120. Espinel-Ingroff A. Comparison of three commercial assays and a modified disk diffusion assay with two broth microdilution reference assays for testing *Zygomycetes*, *Aspergillus* spp., *Candida* spp., and *Cryptococcus neoformans* with posaconazole and Amphotericin B. J Clin Microbiol 2006;44(10):3616–3622.

121. Arikan S, Hascelik G. Comparison of NCCLS microdilution method and Etest in antifungal susceptibility testing of clinical *Trichosporon asahii* isolates. Diagn Microbiol Infect Dis 2002;43(2):107–111.

122. Chang HC, Chang JJ, Chan SH, Huang AH, Wu TL, Lin MC, et al. Evaluation of Etest for direct antifungal susceptibility testing of yeasts in positive blood cultures. J Clin Microbiol 2001;39(4):1328–1333.

123. Vandenbossche I, Vaneechoutte M, Vandevenne M, De Baere T, Verschraegen G. Susceptibility testing of fluconazole by the NCCLS broth macrodilution method, E-test, and disk diffusion for application in the routine laboratory. J Clin Microbiol 2002;40(3):918–921.

124. Serrano MC, Morilla D, Valverde A, Chavez M, Espinel-Ingroff A, Claro R, et al. Comparison of Etest with modified broth microdilution method for testing susceptibility of *Aspergillus* spp. to voriconazole. J Clin Microbiol 2003;41(11):5270–5272.

125. Tortorano AM, Viviani MA, Barchiesi F, Arzeni D, Rigoni AL, Cogliati M, et al. Comparison of three methods for testing azole susceptibilities of *Candida albicans* strains isolated sequentially from oral cavities of AIDS patients. J Clin Microbiol 1998;36(6):1578–1583.

126. Barchiesi F, Tortorano AM, Di Francesco LF, Cogliati M, Scalise G, Viviani MA. In-vitro activity of five antifungal agents against uncommon clinical isolates of *Candida* spp. J Antimicrob Chemother 1999;43(2):295–299.

127. Kirkpatrick WR, McAtee RK, Revankar SG, Fothergill AW, McCarthy DI, Rinaldi MG, et al. Comparative evaluation of National Committee for Clinical Laboratory Standards broth macrodilution and agar dilution screening methods for testing fluconazole susceptibility of *Cryptococcus neoformans*. J Clin Microbiol 1998;36:1330–1332.

128. Viviani MA, Esposto MC, Cogliati M, Tortorano AM. Flucytosine and cryptococcosis: which in vitro test is the best predictor of outcome? J Chemother 2003;15(2):124–128.

129. Verweij PE, Meusink M, Rijs A, Donnelly JP, Meis J, Denning DW. In-vitro activities of amphotericin B, itraconazole and voriconazole against 150 clinical and environmental *Aspergillus fumigatus* isolates. J Antimicrob Chemother 1998;42(3):389–392.

130. Imhof A, Balajee SA, Marr KA. New methods to assess susceptibilities of *Aspergillus* isolates to caspofungin. J Clin Microbiol 2003;41(12):5683–5688.

131. Mock M, Monod M, Baudraz-Rosselet F, Panizzon RG. Tinea capitis dermatophytes: susceptibility to antifungal drugs tested in vitro and in vivo. Dermatology 1998;197(4):361–367.

132. Otero L, Palacio V, Mendez FJ, Vazquez F. Boric acid susceptibility testing of non-*C-albicans Candida* and *Saccharomyces cerevisiae*: comparison of three methods. Med Mycol 2002;40(3):319–322.

133. Banes-Marshall L, Cawley P, Phillips CA. In vitro activity of *Melaleuca alternifolia* (tea tree) oil against bacterial and *Candida* spp. isolates from clinical specimens. Br J Biomed Sci 2001;58(3):139–145.

134. Ernst EJ, Yodoi K, Roling EE, Klepser ME. Rates and extents of antifungal activities of amphotericin B, flucytosine, fluconazole, and voriconazole against *Candida lusitaniae* determined by microdilution, Etest, and time-kill methods. Antimicrob Agents Chemother 2002;46(2):578–581.

135. Manavathu EK, Cutright JL, Loebenberg D, Chandrasekar PH. A comparative study of the in vitro susceptibilities of clinical and laboratory-selected resistant isolates of *Aspergillus* spp. to amphotericin B, itraconazole, voriconazole and posaconazole (SCH 56592). J Antimicrob Chemother 2000;46(2):229–234.

136. Krishnan S, Manavathu EK, Chandrasekar PH. A comparative study of fungicidal activities of voriconazole and amphotericin B against hyphae of *Aspergillus fumigatus*. J Antimicrob Chemother 2005;55(6):914–920.

137. Barchiesi F, Spreghini E, Tomassetti S, Arzeni D, Giannini D, Scalise G. Comparison of the fungicidal activities of caspofungin and amphotericin B against *Candida glabrata*. Antimicrob Agents Chemother 2005;49(12):4989–4992.

138. Canton E, Peman J, Viudes A, Quindos G, Gobernado M, Espinel-Ingroff A. Minimum fungicidal concentrations of amphotericin B for bloodstream *Candida* species. Diagn Microbiol Infect Dis 2003;45(3):203–206.

139. Ernst EJ, Roling EE, Petzold CR, Keele DJ, Klepser ME. In vitro activity of micafungin (FK-463) against *Candida* spp.: microdilution, time-kill, and postantifungal-effect studies. Antimicrob Agents Chemother 2002;46(12):3846–3853.

140. Pfaller MA, Sheehan DJ, Rex JH. Determination of fungicidal activities against yeasts and molds: lessons learned from bactericidal testing and the need for standardization. Clin Microbiol Rev 2004;17(2):268–280.

141. Espinel-Ingroff A, Fothergill A, Peter J, Rinaldi MG, Walsh TJ. Testing conditions for determination of minimum fungicidal concentrations of new and established antifungal agents for *Aspergillus* spp.: NCCLS Collaborative Study. J Clin Microbiol 2002;40(9):3204–3208.

142. Espinel-Ingroff A, Chaturvedi V, Fothergill A, Rinaldi MG. Optimal testing conditions for determining MICs and minimum fungicidal concentrations of new and established antifungal agents for uncommon molds: NCCLS collaborative study. J Clin Microbiol 2002;40(10):3776–3781.

143. Ernst EJ, Klepser ME, Ernst ME, Messer SA, Pfaller MA. In vitro pharmacodynamic properties of MK-0991 determined by time-kill methods. Diagn Microbiol Infect Dis 1999;33(2):75–80.

144. Burgess DS, Hastings RW, Summers KK, Hardin TC, Rinaldi MG. Pharmacodynamics of fluconazole, itraconazole, and amphotericin B against *Candida albicans*. Diagn Microbiol Infect Dis 2000;36(1):13–18.

145. Klepser ME, Malone D, Lewis RE, Ernst EJ, Pfaller MA. Evaluation of voriconazole pharmacodynamics using time-kill methodology. Antimicrob Agents Chemother 2000;44(7):1917–1920.

146. Toriumi Y, Sugita T, Nakajima M, Matsushima T, Shinoda T. Antifungal pharmacodynamic characteristics of amphotericin B against *Trichosporon asahii*, using time-kill methodology. Microbiol Immunol 2002;46(2):89–93.

147. Klepser ME, Ernst EJ, Lewis RE, Ernst ME, Pfaller MA. Influence of test conditions on antifungal time-kill curve results: proposal for standardized methods. Antimicrob Agents Chemother 1998;42:1207–1212.

148. Pfaller MA, Diekema DJ, Procop GW, Rinaldi MG. Multicenter comparison of the VITEK 2 yeast susceptibility test with the CLSI broth microdilution reference method for testing fluconazole against *Candida* spp. J Clin Microbiol 2007;45(3):796–802.

149. Vale-Silva LA, Buchta V. Antifungal susceptibility testing by flow cytometry: is it the future? Mycoses 2006;49(4):261–273.

150. Joung YH, Kim HR, Lee MK, Park AJ. Fluconazole susceptibility testing of *Candida* species by flow cytometry. J Infection 2007;54(5):504–508.

151. Favel A, Peyron F, De Meo M, Michel-Nguyen A, Carriere J, Chastin C, et al. Amphotericin B susceptibility testing of *Candida lusitaniae* isolates by flow cytofluorometry: comparison with the Etest and the NCCLS broth macrodilution method. J Antimicrob Chemother 1999;43(2):227–232.

152. Ramani R, Chaturvedi V. Flow cytometry antifungal susceptibility testing of pathogenic yeasts other than *Candida albicans* and comparison with the NCCLS broth microdilution test. Antimicrob Agents Chemother 2000;44(10):2752–2758.

153. Ramani R, Gangwar M, Chaturvedi V. Flow cytometry antifungal susceptibility testing of *Aspergillus fumigatus* and comparison of mode of action of voriconazole vis-a-vis amphotericin B and itraconazole. Antimicrob Agents Chemother 2003;47(11):3627–3629.

154. Rudensky B, Broidie E, Yinnon AM, Weitzman T, Paz E, Keller N, et al. Rapid flow-cytometric susceptibility testing of *Candida* species. J Antimicrob Chemother 2005;55(1):106–109.

155. Mitchell M, Hudspeth M, Wright A. Flow cytometry susceptibility testing for the antifungal caspofungin. J Clin Microbiol 2005;43(6):2586–2589.

156. Wenisch C, Moore CB, Krause R, Presterl E, Pichna P, Denning DW. Antifungal susceptibility testing of fluconazole by flow cytometry correlates with clinical outcome. J Clin Microbiol 2001;39(7):2458–2462.

157. Chaturvedi V, Ramani R, Rex JH. Collaborative study of antibiotic medium 3 and flow cytometry for identification of amphotericin B-resistant *Candida* isolates. J Clin Microbiol 2004;42(5):2252–2254.

158. Arthington-Skaggs BA, Lee-Yang W, Ciblak MA, Frade JP, Brandt ME, Hajjeh RA, et al. Comparison of visual and spectrophotometric methods of broth microdilution MIC end point determination and evaluation of a sterol quantitation method for in vitro susceptibility testing of fluconazole and itraconazole against trailing and nontrailing *Candida* isolates. Antimicrob Agents Chemother 2002;46(8):2477–2481.

159. Lewis RE, Diekema DJ, Messer SA, Pfaller MA, Klepser ME. Comparison of Etest, chequerboard dilution and time-kill studies for the detection of synergy or antagonism between antifungal agents tested against *Candida* species. J Antimicrob Chemother 2002;49(2):345–351.

160. Arikan S, Lozano-Chiu M, Paetznick V, Rex JH. In vitro synergy of caspofungin and amphotericin B against *Aspergillus* and *Fusarium* spp. Antimicrob Agents Chemother 2002;46(1):245–247.

161. Velasquez S, Bailey E, Jandourek A. Evaluation of the antifungal activity of amphotericin B in combination with fluconazole, itraconazole, voriconazole or posiconazole against *Candida* species using a checkerboard method. Clin Infect Dis 2000;31(1):266.

162. Dannaoui E, Afeltra J, Meis J, Verweij PE. In vitro suscepti-
     bilities of zygomycetes to combinations of antimicrobial agents.
     Antimicrob Agents Chemother 2002;46(8):2708–2711.

163. Cuenca-Estrella M, Gomez-Lopez A, Buitrago MJ, Mellado E,
     Garcia-Effron G, Rodriguez-Tudela JL. In vitro activities of 10
     combinations of antifungal agents against the multiresistant path-
     ogen *Scopulariopsis brevicaulis*. Antimicrob Agents Chemother
     2006;50(6):2248–2250.

164. Philip A, Odabasi Z, Rodriguez J, Paetznick VL, Chen E, Rex JH,
     et al. In vitro synergy testing of anidulafungin with itraconazole,
     voriconazole, and amphotericin B against *Aspergillus* spp. and
     Fusarium spp. Antimicrob Agents Chemother 2005;49(8):3572–3574.

165. Dannaoui E, Lortholary O, Dromer F. In vitro evaluation of
     double and triple combinations of antifungal drugs against
     Aspergillus fumigatus and *Aspergillus terreus*. Antimicrob Agents
     Chemother 2004;48(3):970–978.

166. Hsieh MH, Yu CM, Yu VL, Chow JW. Synergy assessed by
     checkerboard. A critical analysis. Diagn Microbiol Infect Dis
     1993;16(4):343–349.

167. White RL, Burgess DS, Manduru M, Bosso JA. Comparison
     of three different in vitro methods of detecting synergy: time-
     kill, checkerboard, and E test. Antimicrob Agents Chemother
     1996;40:1914–1918.

168. Kontoyiannis DP, Lewis RE, Sagar N, May G, Prince RA,
     Rolston KVI. Itraconazole-amphotericin B antagonism in
     Aspergillus fumigatus: an E-test-based strategy. Antimicrob
     Agents Chemother 2000;44(10):2915–2918.

169. Canton E, Peman J, Gobernado M, Viudes A, Espinel-Ingroff A.
     Synergistic activities of fluconazole and voriconazole with terbin-
     afine against four *Candida* species determined by checkerboard,
     time-kill, and Etest methods. Antimicrob Agents Chemother
     2005;49(4):1593–1596.

170. Keele DJ, DeLallo VC, Lewis RE, Ernst EJ, Klepser ME.
     Evaluation of amphotericin B and flucytosine in combination against
     Candida albicans and *Cryptococcus neoformans* using time-kill
     methodology. Diagn Microbiol Infect Dis 2001;41(3):121–126.

171. Greco WR, Bravo G, Parsons JC. The search for synergy: a criti-
     cal review from a response surface perspective. Pharmacol Rev
     1995;47(2):331–385.

172. Meletiadis J, Mouton JW, Meis J, Verweij PE. In vitro drug
     interaction modeling of combinations of azoles with terbinafine
     against clinical *Scedospotium prolificans* isolates. Antimicrob
     Agents Chemother 2003;47(1):106–117.

173. Dorsthorst D, Verweij PE, Meis J, Punt NC, Mouton JW. In
     vitro interactions between amphotericin B, itraconazole, and
     flucytosine against 21 clinical *Aspergillus* isolates determined
     by two drug interaction models. Antimicrob Agents Chemother
     2004;48(6):2007–2013.

174. Meletiadis J, Verweij PE, Dorsthorst D, Meis J, Mouton JW.
     Assessing in vitro combinations of antifungal drugs against
     yeasts and filamentous fungi: comparison of different drug inter-
     action models. Med Mycol 2005;43(2):133–152.

175. Dannaoui E, Lortholary O, Dromer F. Methods for antifungal
     combination studies in vitro and in vivo in animal models.
     J Mycologie Medicale 2003;13(2):73–85.

176. Kontoyiannis DP, Lewis RE. Combination chemotherapy for
     invasive fungal infections: what laboratory and clinical studies
     tell us so far. Drug Resist Updat 2003;6(5):257–269.

177. Johnson MD, MacDougall C, Ostrosky-Zeichner L, Perfect JR,
     Rex JH. Combination antifungal therapy. Antimicrob Agents
     Chemother 2004;48:693–715.

178. Mukherjee PK, Sheehan DJ, Hitchcock CA, Ghannoum MA.
     Combination treatment of invasive fungal infections. Clin
     Microbiol Rev 2005;18(1):163–194, CP4.

Chapter 83
Viral Phenotypic Resistance Assays

Neil Parkin

1 Introduction

Phenotypic susceptibility assays are designed to determine the observable susceptibility or resistance of a virus to an antiviral agent. Numerous types of assays have been described. Determination of the susceptibility or resistance to an antiviral agent in cell culture is often reported as the IC_{50} or IC_{90} (concentration of antiviral agent that inhibits viral replication by 50 or 90%, respectively). The IC_{50} or IC_{90} is typically compared to that of a control or reference virus that is assumed to be drug-sensitive, and the results are expressed as a ratio (often referred to as fold change or resistance index) of the experimental virus versus the control (e.g., IC_{50} experimental virus/IC_{50} control virus). Several methodologies have been developed, including the plaque assay and more recently recombinant virus assays (RVAs).

Phenotypic susceptibility assays are used for some viruses in a clinical setting, i.e., to help construct the most active drug regimen for an individual patient's virus. They are also employed in research studies to establish correlations between discrete genotypic changes and drug susceptibility, and in the characterization of cross-resistance patterns for new drugs in pre-clinical and clinical stages of development.

2 Intact Virus Susceptibility Assays

2.1 Plaque Assays

This assay, which was originally developed to study bacteriophages in the late twentieth century (1), catapulted animal virology forward in the early 1950s when the assay was adapted for poliovirus by Dulbecco and Vogt (2–4). The plaque assay is based upon the principle that a single virus particle infection of a single cell in a monolayer culture, overlaid with a semisolid nutrient medium to prevent long-range secondary infection through diffusion, will lead to a local area of cytopathology (the "plaque") after infection, of the immediately surrounding cells. The amount of time required for plaque formation depends on the type of virus, cells, and growth conditions. Plaques are identified visually, often by staining the remaining viable cells. The plaques then appear as clear circles in a stained monolayer of cells (Fig. 1). Alternatively, the monolayer can be stained with an antibody specific for viral antigens, and the plaques (or foci) identified by colorimetric or fluorescence detection methods. The number of "plaque forming units" (pfu) or "focus forming units" (ffu) in a given volume is a measure of the infectious virus titer in a given sample.

The plaque assay can be used to measure drug susceptibility by adding serial dilutions of an anti-viral agent to the growth medium of both the control and test virus infections. A dose response curve (pfu/ml vs. drug concentration) can be generated and the IC_{50} or IC_{90}, or change in IC_{50} or IC_{90} relative to control, can be determined. This "plaque reduction assay" has been utilized to measure drug susceptibility of many virus types, including influenza (5), herpes simplex (HSV) (6), cytomegalovirus (CMV) (7), varicella zoster virus (VZV) (8) and HIV-1 (9). One advantage of plaque assays over other types of infectivity assays is that they provide a visual assessment of viral fitness, as reflected by the size of the plaque. In addition, the presence of a low-level minority species of resistant virus can be detected by virtue of the in vitro selection that occurs during this culture-based assay.

2.2 Virus Yield or Antigen Expression Assays

Similar to plaque reduction assays, the virus yield in the liquid medium of an infected cell culture in the presence of

N. Parkin (✉)
Monogram Biosciences, South San Francisco, CA, USA
nparkin@monogrambio.com

D.L. Mayers (ed.), *Antimicrobial Drug Resistance*,
DOI 10.1007/978-1-60327-595-8_83, © Humana Press, a part of Springer Science+Business Media, LLC 2009

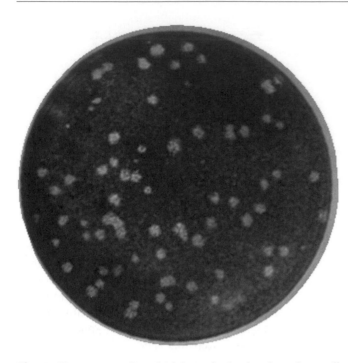

Fig. 1 Plaque assay. Crystal violet stained microtiter plate well showing HSV plaques in Vero cells (image source: http://en.wikipedia. org/wiki/Image:Plaque_assay_macro.jpg)

antiviral drugs can be measured by various techniques, and used to quantitate susceptibility. The quantity of virus in the medium can be determined based on infectivity (e.g., by plaque assay or 50% infectious dose titration), viral antigen production (e.g., by ELISA), cytopathic effect (CPE), or viral nucleic acid production. Virus yield reduction assays have been used to measure drug susceptibility of several viruses including HSV (10–13), influenza virus (5, 14), and CMV (15).

2.3 Limitations of Intact Virus Assays

Plaque reduction and viral spread reduction assays are labor intensive and have limited precision, making them difficult to perform on a large scale for routine clinical use. The assays involve infection with replication competent virus, which undergoes multiple rounds of infection during the assay. In viruses with a high degree of mutagenicity the virus tested in the assay could have altered characteristics compared to those of the patient virus sample. The recovery of infectious virus from clinical specimens is not always reliable and is dependent on titer and fitness, which can vary considerably. Biosafety concerns make large-scale operations involving handling of infectious virus stocks, a logistical obstacle. Finally, some viruses do not form

visible plaques, and others (such as hepatitis C virus) lack an in vitro cell culture system for clinical isolates and thus cannot be studied using plaque or other cell-based assays that rely on infection by intact viruses derived from clinical material.

3 Phenotypic Drug Susceptibility Assays for HIV-1

3.1 Plaque Reduction Assays

Initial measurements of HIV drug susceptibility, including the first description of zidovidine-resistant HIV-1 from infected patients (9), were made using a plaque reduction assay in HeLa cells engineered to express the CD4 receptor (16). Plaques, or foci, of infected cells could be identified and counted, based on the propensity of the infected cells to fuse and form multinucleated syncytia; reduction in focus number in the presence of the drug was used to derive IC_{50} values. Detection of infected cells was simplified by the introduction of a β-galactosidase reporter gene under the control of the HIV-1 LTR (17). Initially, these assays only generated foci or plaques with syncytium-inducing (SI) virus, since HeLa cells naturally express the CXCR4 co-receptor, but not CCR5. Artificial expression of CCR5 in the HeLa/CD4 cells overcame this obstacle (18).

3.2 Peripheral Blood Mononuclear Cell-Based Assays

An alternative method was developed in the early 1990s which used peripheral blood mononuclear cells (PBMC) infected with patient-derived HIV-1, co-cultured with phytohemaglutinin (PHA)-stimulated PBMC from a seronegative donor (19) (Fig. 2). After about 7 days in culture, the supernatant of the culture was collected as the viral stock, which was titered (based on p24 antigen production) on more PHA-stimulated donor PBMC for an additional 7 days. An appropriate dilution of viral stock was added to PHA-stimulated donor PBMC with a known concentration of an anti-HIV agent and grown for a further 7 days. The supernatant was harvested and p24 antigen measured to quantitate virus production and generate susceptibility curves and IC_{50} or IC_{90} values. While this assay was standardized and provided useful phenotypic

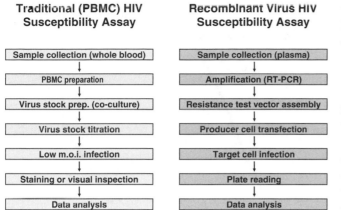

Fig. 2 Comparison of process flow for intact virus (PBMC) and recombinant virus (PhenoSense HIV) assays

drug susceptibility/resistance data, it was cumbersome, imprecise, and slow. In addition, it is possible that the HIV stock derived from latent provirus in infected PBMC did not reflect the strains circulating in the plasma.

3.3 Recombinant Virus Assays

The first recombinant virus assay for HIV generated viable virus by homologous recombination of a reverse transcriptase (RT)-deleted SI viral clone with a PCR-derived pool of RT sequences derived from a patient's proviral DNA samples (20). Recombinant, replication-competent virus was amplified in culture and the virus harvested after 8–10 days, followed by infectivity titration and HeLa CD4+ plaque reduction assay (20) or cell-killing assay using a colorimetric readout (21, 22). This assay represented a major step forward as it eliminated the need for donor PBMC cultures and reduced the potential for selection of virus stocks in culture that might differ from those represented in the original blood sample. However, the turnaround time (3–4 weeks) was still significant. This assay was later modified to measure HIV protease (PR) inhibitor susceptibility, and to amplify viral sequences from plasma instead of proviral DNA, and was commercialized by Virco (Antivirogram) (23).

Significant advances that faciliated the use of phenotypic assays for routine clinical use occurred in the late 1990s. Both VIRalliance and Virologic (now Monogram Biosciences) developed and commercialized rapid HIV phenotypic assays to measure resistance to antiviral drugs. The VIRalliance assay (Phenoscript) (24) involves separate amplification of the gag-PR and the RT regions of HIV

from RNA extracted from patient blood samples. Each PCR product is then separately co-transfected into HeLa cells along with a proprietary plasmid vector. Infections are limited to a single cycle to ensure that the recombinant virus reflects accurately the HIV virus in the patient sample. This is achieved by the deletion of the envelope region from the vector; recombinant virus is pseudotyped with the G-protein of the Vesicular Stomatis virus (VSV-G). For testing of protease inhibitors the transfected producer cells are incubated in the presence of serial dilutions of the drug. The resulting recombinant virus is then used to infect an "indicator cell" containing a LacZ gene under the control of the HIV-1 LTR. For testing of RT inhibitors, virus produced in the absence of the drug is added to cells pre-treated with serial dilutions of the drug. β-galactosidase in infected cells is quantitated using a CPRG-based colorimetric assay.

In the PhenoSense™ phenotypic assay developed by Monogram Biosciences, the patient's PR/RT sequence is amplified as one amplicon and inserted into an indicator gene viral vector, which also contains a luciferase reporter gene, using restriction enzyme digestion and DNA ligation (25) (Fig. 2). Viral stocks are prepared by co-transfecting HEK 293 cells with the test vector DNA and an expression vector that produces the amphotropic murine leukemia virus (aMLV) envelope protein. For testing of protease inhibitors the transfected producer cells are incubated in the presence of serial dilutions of the drug. Pseudotyped viruses harvested from the transfected cells are used to infect fresh HEK293 cells. For testing of RT inhibitors, virus produced in the absence of drug is added to cells pre-treated with serial dilutions of the drug. The production of luciferase is dependent on the completion of a single round of replication (infection, reverse transcription, and integration). Drugs that inhibit viral replication reduce luciferase activity in a dose-dependent manner, allowing the quantitative measurement of HIV viral drug susceptibility/resistance (Fig. 3). The salient distinguishing features of various PR/RT drug susceptibility assays are summarized in Table 1.

The recombinant virus assays described above share some significant drawbacks. Clinically relevant thresholds for the definition of resistance are not known for all drugs (see below). The presence of a minority species of resistant virus(es) may be missed if their relative proportion is below that required for the IC_{50} to shift above the cutoff. The proportion required varies for each drug and mutation pattern. However, both of these limitations (interpretation and detection of minor species) also apply to genotyping assays. Alternative assays, such as "single genome sequencing" or clonal analysis, are too expensive and cumbersome for routine clinical use. Partly to minimize the potential for missing the presence of resistant virus, current recommenda-

Fig. 3 Susceptibility curve (PhenoSense HIV)

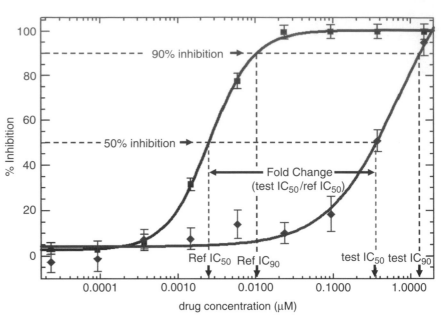

Table 1 Phenotypic assays for HIV PR and RT inhibitor susceptibility

	ACTG/DOD PBMC (19)	Antivirogram (23)	PhenoSense (25)	Phenoscript (24)
Supplier	Various academic labs	Virco, Belgium	Monogram Biosciences, USA	VIRalliance, France
Region of patient virus tested	All	PR 1-99; RT 1-400 Gag variable	PR 1-99; RT 1-305 Gag 418–500	PR 1-99; RT 1-503 Gag variable
Readout	p24 antigen	MTT/cell viability (colorimetric)	Luciferase (luminescent)	β-Galactosidase (colorimetric)
Cells	Donor PBMC	MT-4	HEK 293	P4 HeLa
Virus stock	Replication competent	Replication competent	Replication defective, single cycle	Replication defective, single cycle
Recombinant virus made by	n/a	Homologous recombination	DNA ligation	Homologous recombination
Amplification sensitivity	n/a	>1,000 copies/ml	>500 copies/ml	>1,000 copies/ml
Envelope	Patient HIV env	HIV (HXB2) env	aMLV	VSV-G
TAT	4–6 weeks	3–4 weeks	2 weeks	2–3 weeks
CLIA validated	No	Yes	Yes	Yes

tions emphasize the need to draw the blood sample while the patient is still taking the failing/ineffective drug regimen, to avoid the possibility of archived drug-sensitive virus from outgrowing the resistant variants (26).

Studies that have compared results from different HIV-1 phenotyping assays are limited. Qari et al. tested a panel of 38 samples, many of which were sensitive to all drugs, in the PhenoSense and Antivirogram assays (27). Over 90% of individual results were considered concordant, using a dichotomous scoring system based on susceptibility cutoffs in use at the time of the study. The majority of the discordant results had a fold-change in IC_{50} values close to the cutoff used. Miller et al. used a panel of 28 specimens that included a greater proportion with drug resistance, and compared all three commercially available assays (28). Again, results

were found to concur well in general. The most comprehensive analysis comparing PhenoSense and Antivirogram demonstrated with an improved precision for nucleoside RT inhibitors for PhenoSense (29).

3.3.1 Phenotype Test Interpretation

The interpretation of phenotypic susceptibility assay results is enhanced by relevant thresholds, or "cut-offs," that are intended to define the point above which the utility of a given drug begins to decline. "Clinical cut-offs" based on virologic response data from clinical trials provide the most clinically relevant threshold, but are also most difficult to define. To date, clinical cut-offs for the PhenoSense HIV assay have

Table 2 Phenotypic susceptibility cutoffs (FC)

Drug class	Drug	PhenoSense			Phenoscript			Antivirogram		
		Cutoff	Type[a]	Reference	Cutoff	Type	Reference	Cutoff	Type	Reference
NRTI	Abacavir	4.5	C	(30)	8.0	C	(39)	3.2	C	(40)
	Didanosine	1.3	C	(34)	2.5	C	(39)	2.3	B	(41)
	Lamivudine	3.5	C	(32)	3.0	A	(39)	2.1	B	(41)
	Emtricitabine	3.5	D	(42)				3.7	B	(41)
	Stavudine	1.7	A	(43)	3.0	C	(39)	2.4	B	(41)
	Tenofovir	1.4	C	(35)				2.5	B	(41)
	Zidovudine	1.9	B	(44)	3.5	A	(39)	2.7	B	(41)
NNRTI	Delavirdine	6.2	B	(44)	2.0	A	(39)	7.7	B	(41)
	Efavirenz	3.0	B	(44)	5.0	C	(39)	3.4	B	(41)
	Nevirapine	4.5	B	(44)	2.0	A	(39)	5.2	B	(41)
PI	Atazanavir	2.2	C	(37)				2.0	B	(41)
	Atazanavir/r	5.2	C	(37)	7.0	C	(39)			
	Amprenavir	2.0	B	(44)	2.5	A	(39)	1.8	B	(41)
	Amprenavir/r	4	C	(36)						
	Darunavir/r	10	C	(38)				10	C	(45)
	Indinavir	2.1	B	(44)	2.5	A	(39)	2.1	B	(41)
	Indinavir/r	10	C	(33)	20	C	(39)			
	Lopinavir/r	9	C	(31, 36)	20	C	(39)	10	C	(31)
	Nelfinavir	3.6	B	(44)	2.5	A	(39)	2.3	B	(41)
	Saquinavir	1.7	B	(44)	2.5	A	(39)	1.7	B	(41)
	Saquinavir/r	2.3	C	(36)	11	C	(39)			
	Tipranavir/r	2.0	C	(36)				3.0	C	(46)

[a]A assay/reproducibility cutoff; B biological cutoff; C lower clinical cutoff; D clinical cutoff derived by analogy to critical parameters of lamivudine

been defined for 11 drugs (30–38) and for Phenoscript for 8 drugs (39) (Table 2). In the absence of clinical cut-offs, two alternative types of cut-offs have been used. The "assay" cut-off is defined by the intrinsic variability and technical limits of the assay during repeated testing of patient-derived viruses. The "biological" cut-off is defined by an upper limit of the distribution of susceptibility exhibited by wild-type viruses, for example the mean fold-change + 2 standard deviations (47) or the 99th percentile (44). The clinical relevance of biological cut-offs is limited however, since a higher or lower FC value may be associated with declining virological responses. Importantly, the biological cut-off reflects both natural variation in viral susceptibility and inherent assay variability. Thus, such cutoffs may differ among assays that have different intrinsic variability.

3.3.2 Adaptation of Recombinant Virus Assays to Entry Inhibitors

Enfuvirtide is a synthetic peptide that binds specifically to the gp41 glycoprotein component of the HIV envelope (48). Resistance to enfuvirtide maps to the *env* gene, particularly to certain domains in gp41 (49–51). To monitor the emergence of resistance to enfuvirtide, two of the rapid phenotypic assays (Phenoscript and PhenoSense) originally developed for PR/RT resistance were modified. For Phenoscript, a fragment

of the envelope gene (*env*) spanning gp120 and part of gp41 is amplified and co-transfected with an *env*-deleted provirus vector. Recombinant virus is used to infect cells containing an HIV LTR-β-gal reporter gene and expressing CD4 and one or both of the co-receptors, CCR5 or CXCR4. In the PhenoSense assay, complete gp160 amplicons are transferred to an expression vector, and co-transfected with a luciferase indicator gene vector. Pseudotype virus particles are used to infect cells expressing CD4 and one or both of the co-receptors, CCR5 or CXCR4. Both assays use inhibition of the reporter gene activity to generate IC_{50} or IC_{90} data. Interpretation of the meaning of "decreases in susceptibility" has been hindered by the lack of studies allowing for derivation of a clinical cut-off for enfuvirtide; both assays use a biological cutoff to define a virus as having reduced susceptibility.

3.4 Assays for HIV Fitness and Replication Capacity

Viral fitness is defined as the ability of a virus to reproduce within a defined environment. Mutations that confer drug resistance often reduce viral fitness in the absence of the drug by interfering with one or more critical steps in the replication cycle. Replication capacity (RC) refers to the ability of a virus to replicate in the absence of a drug as compared to that of a wild-type drug sensitive control virus. Several methodologies have been described which determine viral fitness, including replication competent virus growth kinetic assays that compare the efficiency of viral replication of two or more variants in parallel or competitive cultures. Competitive culture assays measure the proportions of competing viruses over time using a variety of techniques including the recombinant marker virus assay (52) and the heteroduplex tracking assay (53). The competition assay is regarded by many as the standard because of its ability to measure the replicative abilities of two viral strains under identical conditions. However, the laborious nature and extended turnaround time of these assays make them impractical for routine clinical use. Recently, rapid single cycle phenotypic susceptibility assays have been adapted to measure RC (Fig. 4). In this case, the reported RC only relates to the portion of the patient sequence transferred to the recombinant virus (i.e., PR and the partial gag and RT sequences included in the amplified fragment), and so the data must be interpreted carefully. Nonetheless there is evidence that if fitness differences are related to changes in PR/RT, the recombinant virus RC assay is a good surrogate of in vivo fitness (54).

Initial studies have shown that there is a wide distribution of RC among the wild-type HIV lacking phenotypic or genotypic resistance (55, 56). In general, drug-resistant HIV has been found to possess reduced RC and in vivo fitness, as demonstrated by the re-appearance of less resistant virus in patients whose antiretroviral therapy is interrupted, concomitant with an increase in viral load and decrease in CD4 cell count (54, 57). However, transmitted multidrug resistant forms of HIV remain resistant for long periods of time even in the absence of drug pressure and with a low viral fitness (58–60), presumably because the reversion rate is

slower than that of the outgrowth of archived drug-sensitive strains, or due to unfavorable (unfit) intermediate forms on the pathway back to a drug-sensitive progenitor (61). The availability of a convenient RC assay and accumulation of large amounts of data has enabled studies correlating the presence of specific resistance-associated mutations with low RC (62–69). Such analyses may facilitate the formulation of treatment strategies designed to force the development of certain mutations which also reduce viral fitness. While the clinical utility of measurements of viral fitness or RC for individual patients is unclear, some reports have indicated a correlation between low RC and preservation of CD4 cell counts (55, 70, 71).

3.5 Determining Co-Receptor Tropism for HIV-1

HIV-1 infection requires interactions between the viral envelope (Env) surface glycoprotein (gp120), the cellular receptor (CD4), and a co-receptor (e.g., CCR5 and/or CXCR4) (72). CCR5, the most commonly used co-receptor, is present on primary T-cells and macrophages; in contrast, CXCR4 is expressed on many cell types, including thymocytes, primary T-cells and macrophages (73). CXCR4-using viruses can induce formation of syncytia when cultured on the CXCR4-bearing MT-2 cell line (SI viruses) (74–78). SI or CXCR4-using viruses are typically found in individuals with advanced disease (79–83). However, it is not clear whether CXCR4 use precedes and causes more rapid disease progression, or is merely the consequence of a change in target cell availability. The recent development of HIV-1 entry inhibitors that target CCR5,

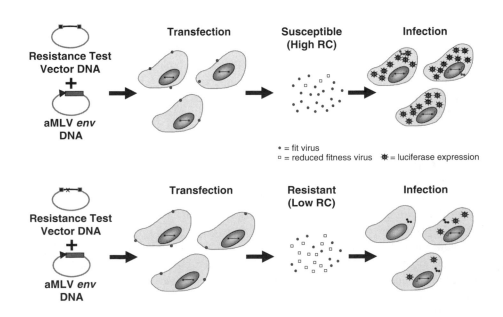

Fig. 4 Replication capacity assay (PhenoSense HIV)

including maraviroc (Pfizer) and vicriviroc (Schering-Plough), has heightened interest in co-receptor usage and assays to measure it (84).

3.5.1 MT-2 Assays

Two standardized MT-2 assay approaches have been described. In one (85) there is a requirement to generate viral stocks from PBMC co-cultures, as described above. These stocks must be titrated and can then be used to infect MT-2 cells. Since MT-2 cells express CXCR4 but not CCR5 (77, 78), only SI (CXCR4-tropic) viruses will be able to infect and induce the formation of syncytia. The assays are typically read 14 days or more after infection. Assessment requires microscopic inspection of individual cultures to determine the presence (SI) or absence (non-SI, or NSI) of syncytia. The second method utilizes direct co-cultivation of patient PBMC with MT-2 cells, followed by microscopic examination (86). Until recently, the MT-2 assay was a common method of determining HIV phenotype in clinical research settings. Early studies utilizing the MT-2 assay established the SI phenotype as an important marker of disease progression (87). Despite these findings, the MT-2 assay has not become a routine clinical monitoring test, owing to the time and labor-dependent nature of the assay process, the lack of ability to directly alter this phenotype by previously available antiretrovirals, the potential drawback that the virus tested is derived from stimulated lymphocytes and not plasma virus and thus may not be representative of circulating virus, and the non-quantitative nature of the assay readout (SI or NSI).

3.5.2 Recombinant Viral Assays for Tropism

Available commercial entry susceptibility assays (see above) have been modified to determine co-receptor tropism (88, 89). Recombinant viruses or reporter pseudotypes are used to infect mammalian cell lines expressing CD4 and either CXCR4 or CCR5. One such high-throughput assay (Trofile™, Monogram Biosciences) (89) has been incorporated into clinical trial protocols for coreceptor inhibitors. This single-cycle assay utilizes luciferase reporter pseudotype viruses and quantitates luciferase activity as relative light units (RLUs) to define infection of U87 cells expressing CD4 and either CXCR4 or CCR5. As a confirmatory step, luciferase production must also be able to be inhibited by an antagonist specific for the coreceptor being tested. This step is particularly relevant when infection levels are low and the result in luciferase activity is close to background levels. The TRT (VirAlliance) assay is similar except that a smaller region of the *env* gene (V1–V3) is amplified, and the readout is based on colorimetric assessment of β-galactosidase activity (88). The two recombinant tropism assays give largely concordant results, with a few notable exceptions of unknown etiology (90).

3.5.3 Comparison of MT-2 and Recombinant Virus Coreceptor Tropism Assays

There are important differences between MT-2 and recombinant virus assays. These assays typically evaluate HIV from distinct compartments; stimulated lymphocytes versus plasma. The MT-2 assay utilizes native virus and recombinant assays evaluate the viral *env* gene. The MT-2 assay permits multiple cycles of replication (and possible amplification of viral subpopulations and/or viral adaptation to culture conditions) while recombinant assays limit replication to a single cycle.

An SI result in an MT-2 assay is an established surrogate for CXCR4 utilization. Currently, only very limited data are available examining the relationship between phenotypes determined by the MT-2 and the Trofile coreceptor tropism assay. However, in one study, 11 individuals with HIV determined to be SI in the MT-2 assay (91) has coreceptor typing performed retrospectively with Trofile and all 11 isolates showed X4 or DM tropism. Interestingly, the luciferase activity in CXCR4 CDs among these 11 SI isolates was not uniform but rather varied over a very broad range. Further studies will be required to determine whether this is clinically meaningful.

In the AIDS Clinical Trials Group 5211 study, the Trofile assay was utilized to select individuals for entry into a clinical trial of vicriviroc (92). MT-2 assays were performed retrospectively among baseline isolates and demonstrated only limited discordance between the two assays (93). Notably, the virus recovery rate among lymphocyte samples processed for the MT-2 assay was low (50%) compared to the proportion of samples successfully phenotyped by the Trofile assay (>90%).

4 Phenotypic Drug Susceptibility Assays for Hepatitis B Virus

Several specific antiviral drugs are now available to combat chronic HBV infection, including pyrimidine analogues (lamivudine) and purine analogues (entecavir, adefovir). As is the case for HIV, the use of these drugs can lead to the emergence of drug-resistant strains, associated with mutations within the polymerase gene ((94), see also the chapter "The Use of Genotypic Assays for Monitoring the Development of Resistance to Antiviral"). With prolonged therapy and continued viral replication, mutations can accumulate and lead to significant cross-resistance between polymerase inhibitors. Thus it may be important to detect and measure HBV drug resistance to manage the therapy of treatment-experienced HBV infected patients.

However, HBV presents unique challenges due to the fact that no cell culture system has been developed which supports replication of intact HBV (e.g., for plaque or viral spread assays). Therefore, assays for measurement of HBV antiviral drug susceptibility rely on several alternative methodologies.

Phenotyping techniques using transient transfections have been applied to study HBV resistance. Site-directed mutagenesis studies using laboratory strains of HBV have been used if a specific mutation is believed to be associated with drug resistance (95, 96). Cell cultures able to support transient HBV replication (e.g., HepG2 or Huh7) are transfected with plasmid vector constructs of the mutated HBV strain. Intracellular genome replication, dependent on the activity of the altered HBV polymerase, in duplicate transfected cultures is compared in the presence and absence of the antiviral drug. Replication was typically monitored by Southern blotting. However, this technique has limited clinical application, due to the cumbersome nature of the readout and questionable relevance of the behavior of individual mutations in a lab strain background. A more relevant approach was developed incorporating PCR amplification of full-length HBV genomes (97). These genomes could be used instead of laboratory generated mutants in transient transfection studies, using Southern blotting or real-time quantitative PCR approaches to monitor replication (98–100). A modified version of one assay has recently been commercialized by VIRalliance (101).

HBV drug susceptibility phenotyping using baculovirus vectors has also been described (102, 103). This technique allows for efficient transduction of recombinant HBV baculoviruses into hepatoma cell lines. Most HBV drug resistant variants have been found to replicate in such a system and to demonstrate the expected drug resistance phenotype. However, the procedure is still too cumbersome for routine use in the clinic.

5 Phenotypic Drug Susceptibility Assays for Hepatitis C Virus

Current treatment of HCV infection is a combination of pegylated interferon and ribavirin. This treatment is only ~50% effective for the subtypes (genotype 1) of HCV most common in North America (104–106). Several new compounds with specific viral targets (primarily the NS3/4A protease or NS5B polymerase) are in development (107, 108). Viral strains resistant to these compounds are likely to emerge with drug treatment, given the error-prone nature of the HCV

RNA-dependent RNA polymerase and high replication rate of HCV in vivo (108–112).

As for HBV, there is no cell culture system available for routine culture of clinical isolates of HCV. Since 1999, most in vitro HCV virology studies have been performed using genotype 1 or 2 subgenomic replicons (113–121) or the single genotype 2a infectious cDNA clone (122–124). Replicons with resistance to virtually every compound tested so far can be selected in vitro, and have been highly informative with respect to determination of the location of sites on the protease or polymerase that interact with the inhibitor, and characterization of cross-resistance (125–136). For example, there appear to be three and possibly four distinct sites where allosteric inhibitors of the NS5B polymerase bind, as determined by the largely non-overlapping sets of mutations selected by the different classes of compound (137). Mutations associated with resistance to NS3/4A protease inhibitors have been detected in HCV from patients treated with the experimental protease inhibitor VX-950 (138).

The development of systems for assessing the drug susceptibility of HCV from patient samples is still in its infancy. Preliminary reports indicate that patient NS5B sequences can be transferred to a luciferase reporter-based replicon vector for susceptibility testing (134, 139–141). The assay format is similar to recombinant assays for HIV-1, in that target sequences are amplified from plasma by RT-PCR, transferred to a viral vector, and transfected into cells treated with the various inhibitors. The key differences include the requirement for in vitro RNA transcription (since the system relies on RNA, not DNA transfection), a cumbersome electroporation step, and the limited number of cell types (derivatives of Huh-7) which are able to support the high level of replication needed for the transient transfection assay format.

Because HCV infection is curable, it is possible that with the advent of more potent antiviral agents used in combination with each other, viral resistance assays will not be needed routinely as they are for HIV-1.

6 Phenotypic Drug Susceptibility Assays for Herpesviruses (HSV, CMV, VZV)

While virus isolation and growth for the clinically important alpha herpesviruses, such as herpes simplex virus (HSV), cytomegalovirus (CMV), and varicella zoster virus (VZV) is technically possible, as for HIV-1 it is wrought with practical obstacles including low reproducibility, long turnaround time, labor intensity, and biosafety concerns. Plaque reduction assays for HSV (6), CMV (7) and VZV (8, 142) are being replaced by recombinant virus systems (143–145), including some which rely on reporter gene readout such as secreted alkaline phosphatase (SEAP) (146). Uncertainty about the clinically meaningful level of resistance is a major issue with the use of these assays (147, 148), as it is for HIV-1.

7 Phenotypic Drug Susceptibility Assays for Influenza Virus

Intact virus phenotypic assays for influenza virus drug susceptibility have mainly been limited to plaque assays, often in Madrin-Darby canine or bovine kidney (MDCK or MDBK) cells. This technique has successfully been used to test drug susceptibility of amantadine, rimantadine, and ribavirin against multiple strains of influenza A and B (149).

The advent of potent neurominidase (NA) inhibitors such as zanamivir and oseltamivir in the mid-1990s provided a new treatment against influenza and also created a renewed interest in antiviral susceptibility assays. Phenotypic assays to measure NA activity in these viruses were developed and are based on an enzymatic assay of virus particle-associated NA, using fluorescent or chemiluminescent NA substrates (150). After virus titration to ensure that the input amount is on the linear portion of the enzyme activity curve, the appropriate dilution of virus and drug are mixed and incubated together after which the fluorescent substrate is added. The reaction is terminated after incubation and the amount of NA-released product is measured (151). The chemiluminescent version of this assay is preferred due to shortened incubation times, but both enzymatic assays are faster than plaque assays. However, since some aspects of NA inhibitor resistance are associated with the hemagglutinin protein (152–155), NA enzyme assays may not completely reflect the inhibitor susceptibility of the intact virus.

Both assays are rapid and reproducible and are used clinically. Given the concern about spread of NA inhibitor resistant influenza viruses, the Neuraminidase Inhibitor Susceptibility Network was established to monitor resistance around the world using the chemiluminescent assay outlined above. Since the introduction of NA inhibitors, detection of resistant viruses has been limited (8 out of 2287 tested), but requires continued surveillance as inhibitor use becomes even more widespread (156).

References

1. d'Herelle F, Smith GH. The Bacteriophage and its Behavior. Baltimore, MD: Williams & Wilkins; 1926.
2. Dulbecco R, Vogt M. Some problems of animal virology as studied by the plaque technique. Cold Spring Harb Symp Quant Biol 1953;18:273–9.
3. Dulbecco R, Vogt M. Plaque formation and isolation of pure lines with poliomyelitis viruses. J Exp Med 1954;99(2):167–82.
4. Dulbecco R, Vogt M. Biological properties of poliomyelitis viruses as studied by the plaque technique. Ann N Y Acad Sci 1955;61(4):790–800.
5. Sidwell RW, Smee DF. In vitro and in vivo assay systems for study of influenza virus inhibitors. Antiviral Res 2000;48(1):1–16.
6. Christophers J, Clayton J, Craske J, et al. Survey of resistance of herpes simplex virus to acyclovir in northwest England. Antimicrob Agents Chemother 1998;42(4):868–72.
7. Landry ML, Stanat S, Biron K, et al. A standardized plaque reduction assay for determination of drug susceptibilities of cytomegalovirus clinical isolates. Antimicrob Agents Chemother 2000;44(3):688–92.
8. Biron KK, Fyfe JA, Noblin JE, Elion GB. Selection and preliminary characterization of acyclovir-resistant mutants of varicella zoster virus. Am J Med 1982;73(1A):383–6.
9. Larder BA, Darby G, Richman DD. HIV with reduced sensitivity to Zidovudine (AZT) isolated during prolonged therapy. Science 1989;243(March 31):1731–4.
10. Drew WL, Miner RC, Marousek GI, Chou S. Maribavir sensitivity of cytomegalovirus isolates resistant to ganciclovir, cidofovir or foscarnet. J Clin Virol 2006;37(2):124–7.
11. Bacon TH, Howard BA, Spender LC, Boyd MR. Activity of penciclovir in antiviral assays against herpes simplex virus. J Antimicrob Chemother 1996;37(2):303–13.
12. Prichard MN, Turk SR, Coleman LA, Engelhardt SL, Shipman C, Jr., Drach JC. A microtiter virus yield reduction assay for the evaluation of antiviral compounds against human cytomegalovirus and herpes simplex virus. J Virol Methods 1990;28(1):101–6.
13. Leary JJ, Wittrock R, Sarisky RT, Weinberg A, Levin MJ. Susceptibilities of herpes simplex viruses to penciclovir and acyclovir in eight cell lines. Antimicrob Agents Chemother 2002;46(3):762–8.
14. McSharry JJ, McDonough AC, Olson BA, Drusano GL. Phenotypic drug susceptibility assay for influenza virus neuraminidase inhibitors. Clin Diagn Lab Immunol 2004;11(1):21–8.
15. Dankner WM, Scholl D, Stanat SC, Martin M, Sonke RL, Spector SA. Rapid antiviral DNA–DNA hybridization assay for human cytomegalovirus. J Virol Methods 1990;28(3):293–8.
16. Chesebro B, Wehrly K. Development of a sensitive quantitative focal assay for human immunodeficiency virus infectivity. J Virol 1988;62(10):3779–88.
17. Kimpton J, Emerman M. Detection of replication-competent and pseudotyped human immunodeficiency virus with a sensitive cell line on the basis of activation of an integrated beta-galactosidase gene. J Virol 1992;66(4):2232–9.
18. Vodicka MA, Goh WC, Wu LI, et al. Indicator cell lines for detection of primary strains of human and simian immunodeficiency viruses. Virology 1997;233(1):193–8.
19. Japour AJ, Mayers DL, Johnson VA, et al. Standardized peripheral blood mononuclear cell culture assay for determination of drug susceptibilities of clinical human immunodeficiency virus type 1 isolates. Antimicrob Agents Chemother 1993;37(5):1095–101.
20. Kellam P, Larder BA. Recombinant virus assay: a rapid, phenotypic assay for assessment of drug susceptibility of human immunodeficiency virus type 1 isolates. Antimicrob Agents Chemother 1994;38(1):23–30.
21. Boucher CAB, Keulen W, Van Bommel T, et al. Human immunodeficiency virus type 1 drug susceptibility determination by using recombinant viruses generated from patient sera tested in a cell-killing assay. Antimicrob Agents Chemother 1996;40(10):2404–9.
22. Pauwels R, Balzarini J, Baba M, et al. Rapid and automated tetrazolium-based colorimetric assay for the detection of anti-HIV compounds. J Virol Methods 1988;20(4):309–21.
23. Hertogs K, De Béthune M-P, Miller V, et al. A rapid method for simultaneous detection of phenotypic resistance to inhibitors of protease and reverse transcriptase in recombinant human

immunodeficiency virus type 1 isolates from patients treated with antiretroviral drugs. Antimicrob Agents Chemother 1998;42(2):269–76.

24. Race E, Dam E, Obry V, Paulous S, Clavel F. Analysis of HIV cross-resistance to protease inhibitors using a rapid single-cycle recombinant virus assay for patients failing on combination therapies. AIDS 1999;13(15):2061–8.

25. Petropoulos CJ, Parkin NT, Limoli KL, et al. A novel phenotypic drug susceptibility assay for human immunodeficiency virus type 1. Antimicrob Agents Chemother 2000;44(4):920–8.

26. Hammer SM, Saag MS, Schechter M, et al. Treatment for adult HIV infection: 2006 recommendations of the International AIDS Society-USA panel. JAMA 2006;296(7):827–43.

27. Qari SH, Respess R, Weinstock H, et al. Comparative analysis of two commercial phenotypic assays for drug susceptibility testing of human immunodeficiency virus type 1. J Clin Microbiol 2002; 40(1):31–5.

28. Miller V, Schuurman R, Clavel F, et al. Comparison of HIV-1 drug susceptibility (phenotype) results reported by three major laboratories. Antivir Ther 2001;6(suppl 1):S129.

29. Zhang J, Rhee SY, Taylor J, Shafer RW. Comparison of the precision and sensitivity of the Antivirogram and PhenoSense HIV drug susceptibility assays. J Acquir Immune Defic Syndr 2005;38(4):439–44.

30. Lanier ER, Hellmann N, Scott J. Determination of a clinically relevant phenotypic resistance "cutoff" for abacavir using the PhenoSense assay. In: 8th Conference on Retroviruses and Opportunistic Infections, 2001 February, Chicago, IL; 2001.

31. Kempf DJ, Isaacson JD, King MS, et al. Analysis of the virologic response with respect to baseline viral phenotype and genotype in protease inhibitor-experienced HIV-1-infected patients receiving lopinavir/ritonavir therapy. Antivir Ther 2002;7(3):165–74.

32. Skowron G, Whitcomb J, Wesley M, et al. Viral load response to the addition of lamivudine correlates with phenotypic susceptibility to lamivudine and the presence of T215Y/F in the absence of M184V. Antivir Ther 1999;4(suppl 1):55–6.

33. Szumiloski J, Wilson H, Jensen E, et al. Relationships between indinavir resistance and virological responses to indinavir-ritonavir-containing regimens in patients with previous protease inhibitor failure. Antivir Ther 2002;7(suppl 1):S127.

34. Flandre P, Chappey C, Marcelin AG, et al. Phenotypic susceptibility to didanosine is associated with antiviral activity in treatment-experienced patients with HIV-1 infection. J Infect Dis 2007;195(3):392–8.

35. Miller MD, Margot N, Lu B, et al. Genotypic and phenotypic predictors of the magnitude of response to tenofovir disoproxil fumarate treatment in antiretroviral-experienced patients. J Infect Dis 2004;189(5):837–46.

36. Coakley EP, Chappey C, Flandre P, et al. Defining lower (L) and upper (U) phenotypic clinical cutoffs (CCO's) for tipranavir (TPV), lopinavir (LPV), saquinavir (SQV) and amprenavir (APV) co-administered with ritonavir (r) within the RESIST Dataset using the PhenoSense Assay. Antivir Ther 2006;11:S81.

37. Coakley EP, Chappey C, Maa JF, et al. Determination of phenotypic clinical cutoffs for atazanavir and atazanavir/ritonavir from AI424-043 and AI424-045. Antivir Ther 2005;10:S8.

38. Coakley EP, Chappey C, Benhamida J, Picchio G, de Béthune M-P. Defining the Upper and Lower Phenotypic Clinical Cut-Offs for Darunavir/r (DRV/r) by the PhenoSense Assay. In: 14th Conference on Retroviruses and Opportunistic Infections, Los Angeles, CA; 2007.

39. Dam E, Obry V, Lecoeur H, et al. Definition of clinically relevant cut-offs for the interpretation of phenotypic data obtained using Phenoscript. Antivir Ther 2001;6(suppl 1):123.

40. Lanier ER, Ait-Khaled M, Scott J, et al. Antiviral efficacy of abacavir in antiretroviral therapy-experienced adults harbouring

41. Verlinden Y, Vermeiren H, Lecocq P, et al. Assessment of the Antivirogram performance over time including a revised definition of biological test cut-off values. Antivir Ther 2005;10:S51.

42. Borroto-Esoda K, Miller M, Petropoulos CJ, Parkin N. A Comparison of the Phenotypic Profiles of Emtricitabine (FTC) and Lamivudine (3TC). In: 44th Interscience Conference on Antimicrobial Agents and Chemotherapeutics, 2004 October 30 – November 2, Washington, DC; 2004.

43. Haubrich R, Keiser P, Kemper C, et al. CCTG 575: a randomized, prospective study of phenotype testing versus standard of care for patients failing antiretroviral therapy. Antivir Ther 2001; 6(suppl 1):63.

44. Parkin NT, Hellmann NS, Whitcomb JM, Kiss L, Chappey C, Petropoulos CJ. Natural variation of drug susceptibility in wild-type human immunodeficiency virus type 1. Antimicrob Agents Chemother 2004;48(2):437–43.

45. De Meyer S, Vangeneugden T, Lefebvre E, et al. Phenotypic and genotypic determinants of resistance to TMC114: pooled analysis of POWER 1, 2 and 3. Antivir Ther 2006;11:S83.

46. Naeger LK, Struble KA. Food and Drug administration analysis of tipranavir clinical resistance in HIV-1-infected treatment-experienced patients. AIDS 2007;21(2):179–85.

47. Harrigan PR, Montaner JS, Wegner SA, et al. World-wide variation in HIV-1 phenotypic susceptibility in untreated individuals: biologically relevant values for resistance testing. AIDS 2001;15(13):1671–7.

48. Greenberg M, Cammack N, Salgo M, Smiley L. HIV fusion and its inhibition in antiretroviral therapy. Rev Med Virol 2004;14(5):321–37.

49. Marcelin AG, Reynes J, Yerly S, et al. Characterization of genotypic determinants in HR-1 and HR-2 gp41 domains in individuals with persistent HIV viraemia under T-20. AIDS 2004;18(9): 1340–2.

50. Wei X, Decker JM, Liu H, et al. Emergence of resistant human immunodeficiency virus type 1 in patients receiving fusion inhibitor (T-20) monotherapy. Antimicrob Agents Chemother 2002;46(6):1896–905.

51. Zollner B, Feucht HH, Schroter M, et al. Primary genotypic resistance of HIV-1 to the fusion inhibitor T-20 in long-term infected patients. AIDS 2001;15(7):935–6.

52. Lu J, Kuritzkes DR. A novel recombinant marker virus assay for comparing the relative fitness of HIV-1 reverse transcriptase variants. J Acquir Immune Defic Syndr 2001;27(1):7–13.

53. Resch W, Parkin N, Stuelke EL, Watkins T, Swanstrom R. A multiple-site-specific heteroduplex tracking assay as a tool for the study of viral population dynamics. Proc Natl Acad Sci U S A 2001;98(1):176–81.

54. Grant RM, Liegler T, Elkin C, et al. Protease Inhibitor Resistant HIV-1 Has Marked Decreased Fitness In Vivo. In: 8th Conference on Retroviruses and Opportunistic Infections, 2001 February, Chicago, IL; 2001.

55. Barbour JD, Hecht FM, Wrin T, et al. Higher CD4+ T cell counts associated with low viral pol replication capacity among treatment-naive adults in early HIV-1 infection. J Infect Dis 2004;190(2):251–6.

56. Bates M, Chappey C, Parkin N. Mutations in p6 Gag Associated with Alterations in Replication Capacity in Drug Sensitive HIV-1 Are Implicated in the Budding Process Mediated by TSG101 and AIP1. In: 11th Conference on Retroviruses and Opportunistic Infections, 2004 February 8–11, San Francisco, CA; 2004.

57. Deeks SG, Wrin T, Liegler T, et al. Virologic and immunologic consequences of discontinuing combination antiretroviral-drug therapy in HIV-infected patients with detectable viremia. N Engl J Med 2001;344(7):472–80.

58. Gandhi RT, Wurcel A, Rosenberg ES, et al. Progressive reversion of human immunodeficiency virus type 1 resistance mutations in vivo after transmission of a multiply drug-resistant virus. Clin Infect Dis 2003;37(12):1693–8.

59. Masquelier B, Capdepont S, Neau D, et al. Virological characterization of an infection with a dual-tropic, multidrug-resistant HIV-1 and further evolution on antiretroviral therapy. AIDS 2007;21(1):103–6.

60. Barbour JD, Hecht FM, Wrin T, et al. Persistence of primary drug resistance among recently HIV-1 infected adults. AIDS 2004;18(12):1683–9.

61. van Maarseveen NM, Wensing AM, de Jong D, et al. Persistence of HIV-1 variants with multiple protease inhibitor (PI)-resistance mutations in the absence of PI therapy can be explained by compensatory fixation. J Infect Dis 2007;195(3):399–409.

62. Martinez-Picado J, Savara AV, Sutton L, D'Aquila RT. Replicative fitness of protease inhibitor-resistant mutants of human immunodeficiency virus type 1. J Virol 1999;73(5):3744–52.

63. Prado JG, Wrin T, Beauchaine J, et al. Amprenavir-resistant HIV-1 exhibits lopinavir cross-resistance and reduced replication capacity. AIDS 2002;16(7):1009–17.

64. Maguire MF, Guinea R, Griffin P, et al. Changes in human immunodeficiency virus type 1 Gag at positions L449 and P453 are linked to I50V protease mutants in vivo and cause reduction of sensitivity to amprenavir and improved viral fitness in vitro. J Virol 2002;76(15):7398–406.

65. Ziermann R, Limoli K, Das K, Arnold E, Petropoulos CJ, Parkin NT. A mutation in human immunodeficiency virus type 1 protease, N88S, that causes in vitro hypersensitivity to amprenavir. J Virol 2000;74(9):4414–9.

66. Resch W, Ziermann R, Parkin N, Gamarnik A, Swanstrom R. Nelfinavir resistant, amprenavir-hypersusceptible strains of human immunodeficiency virus type 1 carrying an N88S mutation in protease have reduced infectivity, reduced replication capacity, and reduced fitness and process the Gag polyprotein precursor aberrantly. J Virol 2002;76(17):8659–66.

67. Deval J, White KL, Miller MD, et al. Mechanistic basis for reduced viral and enzymatic fitness of HIV-1 reverse transcriptase containing both K65R and M184V mutations. J Biol Chem 2004;279(1):509–516.

68. White KL, Margot NA, Wrin T, Petropoulos CJ, Miller MD, Naeger LK. Molecular mechanisms of resistance to human immunodeficiency virus type 1 with reverse transcriptase mutations K65R and K65R + M184V and their effects on enzyme function and viral replication capacity. Antimicrob Agents Chemother 2002;46(11):3437–46.

69. Huang W, Gamarnik A, Limoli K, Petropoulos CJ, Whitcomb JM. Amino acid substitutions at position 190 of human immunodeficiency virus type 1 reverse transcriptase increase susceptibility to delavirdine and impair virus replication. J Virol 2003;77(2):1512–23.

70. Sufka SA, Ferrari G, Gryszowka VE, et al. Prolonged CD4+ cell/virus load discordance during treatment with protease inhibitor-based highly active antiretroviral therapy: immune response and viral control. J Infect Dis 2003;187(7):1027–37.

71. Campbell TB, Schneider K, Wrin T, Petropoulos CJ, Connick E. Relationship between in vitro human immunodeficiency virus type 1 replication rate and virus load in plasma. J Virol 2003;77(22):12105–12.

72. Moser B. Chemokines and HIV: a remarkable synergism. Trends Microbiol 1997;5(3):88–90.

73. Collin M, Illei P, James W, Gordon S. Definition of the range and distribution of human immunodeficiency virus macrophage tropism using PCR-based infectivity measurements. J Gen Virol 1994;75 (Pt 7):1597–603.

74. Tersmette M, de Goede RE, Al BJ, et al. Differential syncytium-inducing capacity of human immunodeficiency virus isolates: frequent detection of syncytium-inducing isolates in patients with acquired immunodeficiency syndrome (AIDS) and AIDS-related complex. J Virol 1988;62(6):2026–32.

75. Fenyo EM, Morfeldt-Manson L, Chiodi F, et al. Distinct replicative and cytopathic characteristics of human immunodeficiency virus isolates. J Virol 1988;62(11):4414–9.

76. Asjo B, Morfeldt-Manson L, Albert J, et al. Replicative capacity of human immunodeficiency virus from patients with varying severity of HIV infection. Lancet 1986;2(8508):660–2.

77. McKnight A, Wilkinson D, Simmons G, et al. Inhibition of human immunodeficiency virus fusion by a monoclonal antibody to a coreceptor (CXCR4) is both cell type and virus strain dependent. J Virol 1997;71(2):1692–6.

78. Chen Z, Zhou P, Ho DD, Landau NR, Marx PA. Genetically divergent strains of simian immunodeficiency virus use CCR5 as a coreceptor for entry. J Virol 1997;71(4):2705–14.

79. Alkhatib G, Combadiere C, Broder CC, et al. CC CKR5: a RANTES, MIP-1alpha, MIP-1beta receptor as a fusion cofactor for macrophage-tropic HIV-1. Science 1996;272(5270):1955–8.

80. Dragic T, Litwin V, Allaway GP, et al. HIV-1 entry into CD4+ cells is mediated by the chemokine receptor CC-CKR-5. Nature 1996;381(6584):667–73.

81. Doranz BJ, Rucker J, Yi Y, et al. A dual-tropic primary HIV-1 isolate that uses fusin and the beta-chemokine receptors CKR-5, CKR-3, and CKR-2b as fusion cofactors. Cell 1996;85(7):1149–58.

82. Deng H, Liu R, Ellmeier W, et al. Identification of a major co-receptor for primary isolates of HIV-1. Nature 1996;381(6584):661–6.

83. Choe H, Farzan M, Sun Y, et al. The beta-chemokine receptors CCR3 and CCR5 facilitate infection by primary HIV-1 isolates. Cell 1996;85(7):1135–48.

84. Schols D. HIV co-receptor inhibitors as novel class of anti-HIV drugs. Antiviral Res 2006;71(2–3):216–26.

85. The ACTG Virology Technical Advisory Committee and the Division of AIDS National Institute of Allergy and Infectious Diseases. The ACTG Virology Manual for HIV laboratories; 1997. Report No. NIH-97-3828.

86. Koot M, Vos AH, Keet RP, et al. HIV-1 biological phenotype in long-term infected individuals evaluated with an MT-2 cocultivation assay. AIDS 1992;6(1):49–54.

87. Koot M, Keet IP, Vos AH, et al. Prognostic value of HIV-1 syncytium-inducing phenotype for rate of CD4+ cell depletion and progression to AIDS. Ann Intern Med 1993;118(9):681–8.

88. Trouplin V, Salvatori F, Cappello F, et al. Determination of coreceptor usage of human immunodeficiency virus type 1 from patient plasma samples by using a recombinant phenotypic assay. J Virol 2001;75(1):251–9.

89. Whitcomb JM, Huang W, Fransen S, et al. Development and characterization of a novel single-cycle recombinant-virus assay to determine human immunodeficiency virus type 1 coreceptor tropism. Antimicrob Agents Chemother 2007;51(2):566–75.

90. Skrabal K, Low AJ, Dong W, et al. Determining human immunodeficiency virus coreceptor use in a clinical setting: degree of correlation between two phenotypic assays and a bioinformatic model. J Clin Microbiol 2007;45(2):279–84.

91. Hendrix CW, Collier AC, Lederman MM, et al. Safety, pharmacokinetics, and antiviral activity of AMD3100, a selective CXCR4 receptor inhibitor, in HIV-1 infection. J Acquir Immune Defic Syndr 2004;37(2):1253–62.

92. Wilkin TJ, Su Z, Kuritzkes DR, et al. HIV Type 1 Chemokine coreceptor use among antiretroviral-experienced patients screened for a clinical trial of a CCR5 Inhibitor: AIDS Clinical Trial Group A5211. Clin Infect Dis 2007;44(4):591–5.

93. Hosoya N, Su Z, Wilkin T, et al. Assessing HIV-1 Tropism in ACTG 5211: A comparison of Assays Using Replication Competent Virus from Peripheral Blood Mononuclear Cells Versus Plasma-Derived Pseudotyped Virions. In: 2nd International Workshop Targeting HIV Entry, Boston, USA; 2006.

94. Shaw T, Bartholomeusz A, Locarnini S. HBV drug resistance: mechanisms, detection and interpretation. J Hepatol 2006;44(3): 593–606.

95. Ladner SK, Miller TJ, King RW. The M539V polymerase variant of human hepatitis B virus demonstrates resistance to 2′-deoxy-3′-thiacytidine and a reduced ability to synthesize viral DNA. Antimicrob Agents Chemother 1998;42(8):2128–31.

96. Chin R, Shaw T, Torresi J, et al. In vitro susceptibilities of wild-type or drug-resistant hepatitis B virus to (−)-beta-d-2,6-diaminopurine dioxolane and 2′-fluoro-5-methyl-beta-l-arabinofuranosyluracil. Antimicrob Agents Chemother 2001;45(9):2495–501.

97. Gunther S, Li BC, Miska S, Kruger DH, Meisel H, Will H. A novel method for efficient amplification of whole hepatitis B virus genomes permits rapid functional analysis and reveals deletion mutants in immunosuppressed patients. J Virol 1995;69(9): 5437–44.

98. Zoulim F. In vitro models for studying hepatitis B virus drug resistance. Semin Liver Dis 2006;26(2):171–80.

99. Durantel D, Brunelle MN, Gros E, et al. Resistance of human hepatitis B virus to reverse transcriptase inhibitors: from genotypic to phenotypic testing. J Clin Virol 2005;34(suppl 1):S34–43.

100. Yang H, Westland C, Xiong S, Delaney WE. In vitro antiviral susceptibility of full-length clinical hepatitis B virus isolates cloned with a novel expression vector. Antiviral Res 2004;61(1): 27–36.

101. Barraud L, Durantel S, Ollivet A, et al. Development of a new high throughput phenotyping test to evaluate the drug susceptibility of HBV strains isolated from patients: Phenoscript-HBV. Antivir Ther 2006;11:S9.

102. Delaney WE, Miller TG, Isom HC. Use of the hepatitis B virus recombinant baculovirus-HepG2 system to study the effects of (−)-beta-2′,3′-dideoxy-3′-thiacytidine on replication of hepatitis B virus and accumulation of covalently closed circular DNA. Antimicrob Agents Chemother 1999;43(8):2017–26.

103. Delaney WE, Edwards R, Colledge D, et al. Cross-resistance testing of antihepadnaviral compounds using novel recombinant baculoviruses which encode drug-resistant strains of hepatitis B virus. Antimicrob Agents Chemother 2001;45(6):1705–13.

104. Jaeckel E, Cornberg M, Wedemeyer H, et al. Treatment of acute hepatitis C with interferon alfa-2b. N Engl J Med 2001;345(20):1452–7.

105. Manns MP, Cornberg M, Wedemeyer H. Current and future treatment of hepatitis C. Indian J Gastroenterol 2001;20(suppl 1): C47–51.

106. Manns MP, McHutchison JG, Gordon SC, et al. Peginterferon alfa-2b plus ribavirin compared with interferon alfa-2b plus ribavirin for initial treatment of chronic hepatitis C: a randomised trial. Lancet 2001;358(9286):958–65.

107. De Francesco R, Migliaccio G. Challenges and successes in developing new therapies for hepatitis C. Nature 2005;436(7053): 953–60.

108. Neyts J. Selective inhibitors of hepatitis C virus replication. Antiviral Res 2006;71(2–3):363–71.

109. Cabot B, Martell M, Esteban JI, et al. Longitudinal evaluation of the structure of replicating and circulating hepatitis C virus quasispecies in nonprogressive chronic hepatitis C patients. J Virol 2001;75(24):12005–13.

110. Martell M, Esteban JI, Quer J, et al. Hepatitis C virus (HCV) circulates as a population of different but closely related genomes: quasispecies nature of HCV genome distribution. J Virol 1992;66(5):3225–9.

111. Neumann AU, Lam NP, Dahari H, et al. Hepatitis C viral dynamics in vivo and the antiviral efficacy of interferon-alpha therapy. Science 1998;282(5386):103–7.

112. Steinhauer DA, Holland JJ. Rapid evolution of RNA viruses. Annu Rev Microbiol 1987;41:409–33.

113. Lohmann V, Korner F, Koch J-O, Herian U, Theilmann L, Bartenschlager R. Replication of subgenomic hepatitis C virus RNAs in a hepatoma cell line. Science 1999;285(5424): 110–3.

114. Blight KJ, Kolykhalov AA, Rice CM. Efficient initiation of HCV RNA replication in cell culture. Science 2000;290(5498): 1972–5.

115. Krieger N, Lohmann V, Bartenschlager R. Enhancement of hepatitis C virus RNA replication by cell culture-adaptive mutations. J Virol 2001;75(10):4614–24.

116. Lohmann V, Korner F, Dobierzewska A, Bartenschlager R. Mutations in hepatitis C virus RNAs conferring cell culture adaptation. J Virol 2001;75(3):1437–49.

117. Blight KJ, McKeating JA, Rice CM. Highly permissive cell lines for subgenomic and genomic hepatitis C virus RNA replication. J Virol 2002;76(24):13001–14.

118. Ikeda M, Yi M, Li K, Lemon SM. Selectable subgenomic and genome-length dicistronic RNAs derived from an infectious molecular clone of the HCV-N strain of hepatitis C virus replicate efficiently in cultured Huh7 cells. J Virol 2002;76(6): 2997–3006.

119. Blight KJ, McKeating JA, Marcotrigiano J, Rice CM. Efficient replication of hepatitis C virus genotype 1a RNAs in cell culture. J Virol 2003;77(5):3181–90.

120. Gu B, Gates AT, Isken O, Behrens SE, Sarisky RT. Replication studies using genotype 1a subgenomic hepatitis C virus replicons. J Virol 2003;77(9):5352–9.

121. Kato T, Date T, Miyamoto M, et al. Efficient replication of the genotype 2a hepatitis C virus subgenomic replicon. Gastroenterology 2003;125(6):1808–17.

122. Wakita T, Pietschmann T, Kato T, et al. Production of infectious hepatitis C virus in tissue culture from a cloned viral genome. Nat Med 2005;11(7):791–6.

123. Zhong J, Gastaminza P, Cheng G, et al. Robust hepatitis C virus infection in vitro. Proc Natl Acad Sci U S A 2005;102(26): 9294–9.

124. Lindenbach BD, Evans MJ, Syder AJ, et al. Complete replication of hepatitis C virus in cell culture. Science 2005;309(5734): 623–6.

125. Lin C, Lin K, Luong YP, et al. In vitro resistance studies of hepatitis C virus serine protease inhibitors, VX-950 and BILN 2061: structural analysis indicates different resistance mechanisms. J Biol Chem 2004;279(17):17508–14.

126. Lu L, Pilot-Matias TJ, Stewart KD, et al. Mutations conferring resistance to a potent hepatitis C virus serine protease inhibitor in vitro. Antimicrob Agents Chemother 2004;48(6):2260–6.

127. Trozzi C, Bartholomew L, Ceccacci A, et al. In vitro selection and characterization of hepatitis C virus serine protease variants resistant to an active-site peptide inhibitor. J Virol 2003;77(6): 3669–79.

128. Nguyen TT, Gates AT, Gutshall LL, et al. Resistance profile of a hepatitis C virus RNA-dependent RNA polymerase benzothiadiazine inhibitor. Antimicrob Agents Chemother 2003;47(11): 3525–30.

129. Migliaccio G, Tomassini JE, Carroll SS, et al. Characterization of resistance to non-obligate chain-terminating ribonucleoside analogs that inhibit hepatitis C virus replication in vitro. J Biol Chem 2003;278(49):49164–70.

130. Tong X, Chase R, Skelton A, Chen T, Wright-Minogue J, Malcolm BA. Identification and analysis of fitness of resistance mutations against the HCV protease inhibitor SCH 503034. Antiviral Res 2006; 28–38.

131. Yi M, Tong X, Skelton A, et al. Mutations conferring resistance to SCH6, a novel hepatitis C virus NS3/4A protease inhibitor: reduced RNA replication fitness and partial rescue by second-site mutations. J Biol Chem 2006; 281(12):8205–8215.

132. Lin C, Gates CA, Rao BG, et al. In vitro studies of cross-resistance mutations against two hepatitis C virus serine protease inhibitors, VX-950 and BILN 2061. J Biol Chem 2005;280(44):36784–91.

133. Le Pogam S, Kang H, Harris SF, et al. Selection and characterization of replicon variants dually resistant to thumb- and palm-binding nonnucleoside polymerase inhibitors of the hepatitis C virus. J Virol 2006;80(12):6146–54.

134. Le Pogam S, Jiang WR, Leveque V, et al. In vitro selected Con1 subgenomic replicons resistant to 2′-C-methyl-cytidine or to R1479 show lack of cross resistance. Virology 2006;351:349–359.

135. Mo H, Lu L, Pilot-Matias T, et al. Mutations conferring resistance to a hepatitis C virus (HCV) RNA-dependent RNA polymerase inhibitor alone or in combination with an HCV serine protease inhibitor in vitro. Antimicrob Agents Chemother 2005;49(10):4305–14.

136. Kukolj G, McGibbon GA, McKercher G, et al. Binding site characterization and resistance to a class of non-nucleoside inhibitors of the hepatitis C virus NS5B polymerase. J Biol Chem 2005;280(47):39260–7.

137. Tomei L, Altamura S, Paonessa G, De Francesco R, Migliaccio G. HCV antiviral resistance: the impact of in vitro studies on the development of antiviral agents targeting the viral NS5B polymerase. Antiviral Chem Chemother 2005;16(4):225–45.

138. Sarrazin C, Kieffer TL, Bartels D, et al. Dynamic hepatitis C virus genotypic and phenotypic changes in patients treated with the protease inhibitor telaprevir. Gastroenterology 2007;132:1767–1777.

139. Ludmerer SW, Graham DJ, Boots E, et al. Replication fitness and NS5B drug sensitivity of diverse hepatitis C virus isolates characterized by using a transient replication assay. Antimicrob Agents Chemother 2005;49(5):2059–69.

140. Tripathi RL, Krishnan P, He Y, et al. Replication efficiency of chimeric replicon containing NS5A-5B genes derived from HCV-infected patient sera. Antiviral Res 2007;73(1):40–9.

141. Penuel E, Han D, Favero K, Lam E, Liu Y, Parkin NT. Development of a rapid phenotypic susceptibility assay for HCV polymerase inhibitors. Antivir Ther 2006;11:S12.

142. Morfin F, Thouvenot D, De Turenne-Tessier M, Lina B, Aymard M, Ooka T. Phenotypic and genetic characterization of thymidine kinase from clinical strains of varicella-zoster virus resistant to acyclovir. Antimicrob Agents Chemother 1999;43(10):2412–6.

143. Bestman-Smith J, Boivin G. Drug resistance patterns of recombinant herpes simplex virus DNA polymerase mutants generated with a set of overlapping cosmids and plasmids. J Virol 2003;77(14):7820–9.

144. Chou S, Waldemer RH, Senters AE, et al. Cytomegalovirus UL97 phosphotransferase mutations that affect susceptibility to ganciclovir. J Infect Dis 2002;185(2):162–9.

145. Kemble G, Duke G, Winter R, Spaete R. Defined large-scale alterations of the human cytomegalovirus genome constructed by cotransfection of overlapping cosmids. J Virol 1996;70(3):2044–8.

146. Chou S, Van Wechel LC, Lichy HM, Marousek GI. Phenotyping of cytomegalovirus drug resistance mutations by using recombinant viruses incorporating a reporter gene. Antimicrob Agents Chemother 2005;49(7):2710–5.

147. Jabs DA, Martin BK, Forman MS, et al. Mutations conferring ganciclovir resistance in a cohort of patients with acquired immunodeficiency syndrome and cytomegalovirus retinitis. J Infect Dis 2001;183(2):333–7.

148. Weinberg A, Leary JJ, Sarisky RT, Levin MJ. Factors that affect in vitro measurement of the susceptibility of herpes simplex virus to nucleoside analogues. J Clin Virol 2007;38(2):139–45.

149. Hayden FG, Cote KM, Douglas RG, Jr. Plaque inhibition assay for drug susceptibility testing of influenza viruses. Antimicrob Agents Chemother 1980;17(5):865–70.

150. Potier M, Mameli L, Belisle M, Dallaire L, Melancon SB. Fluorometric assay of neuraminidase with a sodium (4-methylumbelliferyl-alpha-d-N-acetylneuraminate) substrate. Anal Biochem 1979;94(2):287–96.

151. McKimm-Breschkin J, Trivedi T, Hampson A, et al. Neuraminidase sequence analysis and susceptibilities of influenza virus clinical isolates to zanamivir and oseltamivir. Antimicrob Agents Chemother 2003;47(7):2264–72.

152. Smee DF, Sidwell RW, Morrison AC, et al. Characterization of an influenza A (H3N2) virus resistant to the cyclopentane neuraminidase inhibitor RWJ-270201. Antiviral Res 2001;52(3):251–9.

153. Gubareva LV, Kaiser L, Matrosovich MN, Soo-Hoo Y, Hayden FG. Selection of influenza virus mutants in experimentally infected volunteers treated with oseltamivir. J Infect Dis 2001;183(4):523–31.

154. Blick TJ, Sahasrabudhe A, McDonald M, et al. The interaction of neuraminidase and hemagglutinin mutations in influenza virus in resistance to 4-guanidino-Neu5Ac2en. Virology 1998;246(1):95–103.

155. Bantia S, Ghate AA, Ananth SL, Babu YS, Air GM, Walsh GM. Generation and characterization of a mutant of influenza A virus selected with the neuraminidase inhibitor BCX-140. Antimicrob Agents Chemother 1998;42(4):801–7.

156. Monto AS, McKimm-Breschkin JL, Macken C, et al. Detection of influenza viruses resistant to neuraminidase inhibitors in global surveillance during the first 3 years of their use. Antimicrob Agents Chemother 2006;50(7):2395–402.

Chapter 84
Drug Resistance Assays for Parasites

N.C. Sangster, G.N. Maitland, S. Geerts, Saskia Decuypere, Jean-Claude Dujardin, J.A. Upcroft, P. Upcroft, and M. Duraisingh

1 Introduction

Drug resistance has become an increasingly serious and widespread problem worldwide, impacting across a broad phylogenetic range of important medical and veterinary parasite species. These include parasites from the groups of the Apicomplexa, the flagellates and the helminths. Accurate measurement of resistance is vital for several reasons. In addition to making decisions on effective drug use for parasite control, resistance assays (sometimes called sensitivity assays) are also used to monitor prevalence, severity and dissemination of resistance and to evaluate the impact of control regimes on resistant parasites. In some cases they are used to assist the choice of drugs in clinical situations. A review of the assays currently available and knowledge of the information they provide gives a vital signpost of our current situation across a variety of parasite species and also as a guide in the design of future assays for resistances yet to develop.

Resistance assays consist of various in vivo and in vitro tests. The in vivo tests include various assays with the definitive host species and within experimental host species. There is in an even greater variety of in vitro assays available. These include assays which measure survival of parasites in the presence of drug, phenotypic assays (that measure a mechanism of resistance) and genetic assays (using DNA probes that rely on knowledge of the genetic basis of resistance). The selection of an appropriate assay type and design depends on several factors. One important factor is the prevalence and severity of resistance.

1.1 Establishment, Development and Dispersal of Resistance

Sutherst and Comins (1) describe three components to the genesis of resistance. The first is establishment. This is largely a random event influenced by the population size and diversity and the mutation rate for the gene(s) in question. The second step is development. In this process the use of the selective agent (e.g. the chemical) allows resistance to develop but the prevalence of resistant alleles is too low for resistance to be clinically apparent. In the third step, dispersal, there is further selection and spread of the resistance genes through the wider population of the organisms. At this phase clinical resistance (also termed field resistance) first appears. The processes of development and dispersal are influenced by biology, management and chance events such as linkage disequilibrium and gene dispersal via an intermediate host. These processes are driven by drug selection, reflected in survival and subsequent reproduction of parasites following drug treatment.

1.2 Sensitivity, Specificity and Level of Resistance

Fundamental parameters for all diagnostic assays are their sensitivity and specificity (not to be confused with drug sensitivity). The sensitivity of an assay is defined as the probability that the presence of resistance would be correctly identified, in resistance studies sensitivity is then used to refer to how early or at what level of gene frequency resistance is detected. The sensitivity that is required of an assay depends on the purpose. When resistance is emerging, assays with high sensitivity (e.g. 0.99) are required to detect small increases in prevalence.

Specificity is the probability that a test can correctly identify that resistance is not present. In practice, species identification in resistance assays is often the factor that limits

N.C. Sangster (✉)
School of Animal and Veterinary Sciences, Charles Sturt University, Wagga Wagga, NSW, Australia
nsangster@csu.edu.au

D.L. Mayers (ed.), *Antimicrobial Drug Resistance*,
DOI 10.1007/978-1-60327-595-8_84, © Humana Press, a part of Springer Science+Business Media, LLC 2009

specificity (and sensitivity) and drives the need for simultaneous resistance assays and species identification.

The level of resistance is the degree of resistance in a parasite population. It might be quoted as a percentage of drug efficacy or an EC_{50} on a test (see below).

1.3 Challenges

To be useful, a resistance assay must be able to accurately detect and reflect the frequency of resistance in a population. Various challenges arise in attempting to achieve this aim.

The first important challenge is to be able to detect resistance in the development phase when prevalence of resistant alleles is low but still at a point where further development may be avoided by management. Genetic tests offer the possibility of detecting resistance at this early stage but these require detailed knowledge which is rarely available, especially before resistance is widespread.

Another important challenge is to validate in vitro assays, against the in vivo environment to ensure they provide meaningful clinical data.

Even when good tests are available, the source of the resistant isolates for testing and validation remains an important issue. This is relevant when comparisons of isolates from different geographical regions or between laboratory and field isolates are being made. Resistant lines may be developed in the laboratory by subjecting the parasites to increasingly higher concentrations of drug with each generation, often by in vitro exposure. These isolates are sometimes referred to as 'laboratory' isolates. Possible pitfalls in this approach are that resistant laboratory isolates may differ from field isolates and one field isolate may differ from another, which may lead to the development of inappropriate assays and validation against atypical isolates.

Another challenge is that the nature of resistant populations may differ. For example, some parasitic infections, especially the protozoa that divide asexually, may become near clonal, because all progeny develop from the few survivors of drug treatment. On the other hand, populations of parasitic worms are highly genetically diverse.

Finally, tests have to be available in a timely fashion. There is little point in developing and applying a test for resistance when the prevalence of resistance is greater than 90%.

1.4 Mechanisms of Resistance

A summary of the drug actions and resistance mechanisms of the more important parasites for which resistance is a clinical or field problem appears in Table 1.

2 Assay Methods to Detect Resistance

The general properties of assays follow. Specific assays are listed in Table 2 and some are highlighted in further sections.

2.1 In Vivo Bioassays

2.1.1 In Vivo in Definitive Host

This is the traditional approach to resistance detection and most direct as the data reflects the therapeutic response to a drug. Responses (or efficacy) are usually calculated from numbers of the parasite in a host sampled both before and after the application of treatment. For animal herds, an untreated control group can be compared with an equivalent treated group.

Limitations of this approach include the need for knowledge of efficacy of the drug at the dose rate used in the host species against susceptible and resistant isolates, the cost of maintaining hosts or sampling of patients, the preliminary creation of parasite-free hosts and, in the case of malaria, differentiating between resistance and recrudescence caused by reinfection. An additional concern is the ethics of euthanasia of mammals (say, for worm counts) and the ethics of sampling humans, especially if some individuals remain untreated.

2.1.2 In Vivo in Experimental Hosts

If available, experimental host species can provide greater convenience and cost effectiveness when testing for drug resistance, especially in determining dose–responses. Essential steps in developing such assays are to validate the similarity of the host/parasite relationship between the host and experimental host and the congruence of drug pharmacokinetics.

2.2 In Vitro Assays

2.2.1 Survival (Effect) Assays

In vitro assays have the advantage of being useful to detect resistance without interference by host factors. Generally, they involve exposing individuals of a certain stage of the parasite's life cycle to a set concentration within a range of concentrations of the drug and observing an endpoint, reflecting parasite survival after an appropriate incubation time.

Table 1 Major drug treatments, mode of action and known resistance mechanisms

Parasite and host	Drug/example (abbreviation)	Mode of action	Putative mechanism of resistance
Plasmodium in humans	Aminoquinolones/chloroquine, quinine, mefloquine	Alkalises parasite food vacuoles and prevents lysosomal activity that is essential for haemoglobin degradation	For chloroquine resistance – *Pfcrt* gene – K76T transition has the most consistent correlation with resistance – *Pfmdr1* gene – N86Y transition leading to active efflux pump Mefloquine resistant parasites have multiple copies of *pfmdr1* alleles and a drug efflux phenotype
	Antifolates: Dihydrofolate reductase inhibitors/pyrimethamine proguanil – synergistically with dihydropteroate synthase inhibitors/sulphadoxine, dapsone	Synergistic combinations of antifolates inhibit the utilisation of folate by inhibiting dihydrofolate (dhfr) reductase and dihydropteroate synthase (dhps). Folates are essential for synthesis of pyrimidines and thus DNA	Linked with mutations in *dhfr* and *dhps* *Dhfr* A S108N transition is the initial step rendering the enzyme insusceptible to the drug *Dhps* Transitions S436F, A436F, A437G, K540E, L540E, A581G, A613S, A613T and a mutation at 586 have been reported in resistant parasites
	Sesquiterpenes/artemisinin	Concentrated in RBCs, action may involve damage to the parasite membrane by free radicals or covalent alkylation of proteins. Artemisinin inhibits the Plasmodium SERCA ortholog (2)	Multidrug resistance (drug efflux) like phenomenon
	Diamidines/pentamidine	Accumulation within food vacuole where it binds avidly to ferriprotoporphyrin (FPIX), blocks haemozoin crystallization	
	Tetracyclines/doxycycline	Binds ribosomes to inhibit protein synthesis	
Eimeria in chickens	Ionophores/salinomycin	Act on trophozoite and sporozoite. Opens ion channels in cell membranes leading to collapse of membrane potential and nutrient transport	Unknown
	Sulphonamides/sulphadimidine and trimethoprim	Act on second stage and later schizonts. Act on nucleotide synthesis as p-aminobenzoic acid (PABA) agonists (synergised with dhfr inhibitors) and dhfr inhibitors DNA synthesis (see Sect. 3.1 for details)	Unknown
	Quinolones/decoquinate	Acts on sporozoite. Dihydro-orotate DH inhibitors that prevent synthesis of purines required for DNA replication	
	Pyridones/clopidol Other anticoccidials	Acts on sporozoites through disruption of electron transport Robenidine – interrupts guanine use in DNA synthesis, inhibits oxidative phosphorylation Nicarbazin – energy metabolism in mitochondria Toltrazuril – inhibition of mitochondrial respiration and nuclear pyrimidine in DNA synthesis	
Trypanosoma in ruminants	Phenanthridinium compounds/Isometamidium	Cleavage of kinetoplast DNA – topoisomerase complexes	– Changes in the mitochondrial electrical potential – Nucleoside transporters involved
	Diamidines/diminazene	Binds to kinetoplast DNA and inhibits topoisomerase II and RNA editing (3)	Point mutations in P2 adenosine transporter
	Homidium salts	Interference with: – Glycosomal functions – The function of an unusual AMP binding protein – Trypanothione metabolism – Replication of kinetoplast minicircles (3)	Unknown but may be a change in nucleoside transporters

(continued)

Table 1 (continued)

Parasite and host	Drug/example (abbreviation)	Mode of action	Putative mechanism of resistance
Trypanosoma brucei in humans	Organic arsenical/melarsoprol	Not yet established	Loss of a P2 amino-purine transporter (4, 5) and probably other mechanisms
	Ornithine analogue/eflornithine	Suicide inhibitor of ornithyl decarboxylase (ODC) (6) which is the rate-limiting enzyme for the synthesis of polyamines from ornithine (7)	Unknown but various mechanisms suggested (7)
	Diamidines/pentamidine	Binds to kinetoplast DNA and inhibits topoisomerase thus interfering with kinetoplast replication (8) May cause inhibition of multiple cellular targets (9)	Changes in drug transporters, including the P2 aminopurine transporters and the High Affinity and Low Affinity Pentamidine transporters HAPT1 and LAPT1(4, 5, 10–12)
	Naphthalene derivative/suramin	Target uncertain although has been shown to inhibit many enzymes (13)	Unknown but several mechanisms suggested (7)
Trypansoma cruzi	Nitroimidazole/benznidazole Nitrofuran/nifurtimox	Covalent modification of macromolecules by nitroreduction intermediates (reductive stress) (14) Reduction of the nitro group creates a highly reactive free radical followed by a reactive oxygen species then leads to death (7)	Changes in the enzyme or transporter (7)
Leishmania in humans	Polyene antibiotic/amphotericin B (used as a second-line drug)	Acts preferentially on ergosterol – the predominant sterol in membranes	Resistant parasites showed increased membrane fluidity with changes in lipid composition including an ergosterol precursor
	Pentavalent antimonials/sodium stibogluconate (SbV) Meglumine antimoniate	Activated in vivo. May be associated with inhibition of glycolytic enzymes but also depends on effective host immunity	Depends upon: – Transformation of pentavalent compound to trivalent compound – Formation of a thiol conjugate by unknown conjugase/transferase – Drug extrusion by elevated levels of MRP
	Diamidines/pentamidine	Accumulate within parasites leading to disintegration of the network of kinetoplast DNA and collapse in the mitochondrial membrane potential	Efflux pumps appear to operate in removing cytosolic or membrane-associated drug
	Paromomycin/aminosidine (aminocyclitol-aminoglycoside antibiotic)	Binding to the endoplasmic reticulum may be involved	
	Azoles/itraconazole Ketoconazole Metronidazole	Inhibitors of cytochrome P-450-dependent lanosterol C14 α-demethylase (a step in ergosterol biosynthesis) Itraconazole inhibits an enzymatic activity several steps downstream of squalene synthase in ergosterol biosynthesis	Overexpresion of squalene synthase confers itraconazole resistance
	Nucleoside analogues pyrazolopyrimidines/allopurinol		Differences in the affinity of enzymes of the purine salvage pathway
	Alkyllysophospholipids/miltefosine	Lipid biosynthetic enzymes may represent a target	For miltefosine resistance – Point mutations in a P-type ATPase (15)

Diminazene and Homidium Salts – see *Trypanosoma*

5-Nitroimidazoles, bezimidazoledrugs and substituted acridines – see *Giardia*

Organism	Drug	Mode of action	Mechanism of resistance
Giardia in humans	5-Nitroimidazoles/metronidazole, tinidazole, secnidazole	Prodrug reduced by ferredoxin to active nitro compound in the parasite. Toxicity via depletion of SH groups and DNA strand breaks (16)	Multifactorial – Reduced drug activation through decreased activities of pyruvate:ferredoxin oxidoreductase and/or ferredoxin essential for activation (16) – Drug transport changes (16) – Gene rearrangements (17)
	Benzimidazole drugs/albendazole (ABZ)	Binds tubulin, inhibiting microtubule assembly which is important for the adhesive disk (18)	ABZ-resistant cells have enlarged median bodies suggesting increased microtubule synthesis – No evidence for mutation in *Giardia* tubulin genes (18) – Drug transport changes (membrane blockade or active efflux) – Actively excluded from resistant trophozoites (16)
	Substituted acridine/quinacrine HCl	– Taken up and accumulated – Acts on membrane (16) perhaps by inhibition of the activity of cytoplasmic NADH oxidase (19)	
	Nitrofuran/furazolidone	Reduction of drug by NADH oxidase to toxic nitro radical (19)	
Trichomonas in humans	5-Nitroimidazoles/metronidazole tinidazole	See *Giardia* and (20)	Multifactorial – (Laboratory isolates) down-regulation of hydrogenosome pyruvate:ferredoxin oxidoreductase and ferredoxin transcription – (Clinical isolates) altered drug transport pathways (20)
Entamoeba in humans	Emetine	Unknown	Multidrug resistant transporters involved (21)
	Metronidazole	Prodrug activated by reduction of nitro groups by ferredoxin (22)	Increased superoxide dismutase activity may detoxify active radicals (23)
	Iodoquinol, diloxanide furoate, paromomycin, tetracycline, chloroquine	Tetracycline is presumed to act via inhibition of protein synthesis	
Trichostrongyloids in sheep	Benzimidazole (BZ)/albendazole	Disrupts cellular integrity by specifically binding to parasite tubulin	Selection of alleles of β-tubulin in two steps: (a) Isotype 1 – involving a F200Y transition (F167Y is also implicated) (b) Loss of isotype 2
	Imidazothiazoles and tetrahydropyrimidines/levamisole (LEV)	Cholinergic agonists	Unknown, but may include alterations in receptor subunits, selective expression of subunit genes or modulation of receptor
	Macrocyclic lactones (ML)/ivermectin (IVM)	Opens glutamate-gated Cl− channels on muscles to inhibit pharynx and the somatic musculature	Several candidate genes including *GluCl* receptors
	Salicylanilides/closantel (CLS)	Uncoupling oxidative phosphorylation, lowering cytoplasmic pH and inhibiting glycolysis	
Fasciola in sheep	Salicylanilides/closantel	See Sect. 3.7	
	Benzimidazoles/triclabendazole	Thought to bind to fluke β-tubulin with effects on tegumental synctium and cellular integrity	
Schistosoma in humans	Praziquantel (PZQ)	Putatively acts on voltage-gated Ca^{2+} channels (β subunits) causing increased intracellular $[Ca^{2+}]$ and paralysis	May involve residues at the interface between the α and β domains of the Ca^{2+} channel (24)

[a] Within this table amino acid substitutions are written in the form K76T meaning Lysine is replaced by Threonine at residue number 76

Table 2 Examples of available resistance assays

Parasite and host	Drug/example	In vivo	Survival (dose–response)	Phenotype (site of action)	Genotype
Plasmodium in humans	4-Aminoquinolines/chloroquine	In vivo drug trial with recommended dose rate (defined by WHO in terms of parasite clearance). See text	Inhibition of *P. falciparum* growth and multiplication in presence of antimalarial drug in vitro: 1. WHO microtest: schizont maturation 2. Metabolic endpoint such as isotope incorporation, colorimetric enzyme assays which reflect parasite numbers: – Parasite lactate dehydrogenase – DELI assays – Histidine-rich protein 2 assay 3. Dipsticks based on immunoquantative Plasmodium proteins: – LDH – DELI – Histidine-rich protein 2 assay		AS-PCR and PCR-RFLP – *Pfcrt* base transition causing K76T^n is the most consistent finding Also S72C, M74I, N75E, H97Q, A220S, E271Q, N326S, N326D, I356T, I356L, R371I, R371T – Pfmdr1 gene including substitutions at positions 1034, 1042, 1246
	Antifolate combination: e.g. Pyrimethamine/sulphadoxine				AS-PCR and PCR-RFLP *dhfr* transition S108N plus some of: A16V, S108T C50R, C50I, N51I, C59R, V140L, I164L, *dhps* S436F, A436F, A437G, K540E, L540E, A581G, A613S, A613T and a change at 586
	Mefloquine				1. TC-PCR for increased (e.g. twofold) gene-copy number of the *Pfmdr1* gene 2. *Pfmdr1* substitutions in various alleles, e.g. N86Y, 184, 1034, 1042
Eimeria in poultry	Anticoccidials: – Isometamidium (ISMM)	Feed efficiency trials measuring growth rates of infected birds versus infected and treated birds			
Trypanosoma in ruminants	– Diminazene – Homidium salts	– Test ability of drugs to protect cattle under experimental or natural challenge using parasitaemia as endpoint – 'Block treatment test' of cattle under natural challenge – Test in mice (single or multi-dose test)	– *T. brucei*: incubate metacyclic or bloodstream *T. brucei* in vitro with drugs: survival endpoints used – All trypanosomes: drug incubation followed by Glossina infectivity – Metabolism of the dye Alamar Blue by live cells to generate both a colorimetric and a fluorescent signal (31)		PCR-RFLP *TcoAT1* gene (resistance to diminazene)

Parasite	Drug	In vivo assay	In vitro assay	Other assay / mechanism	PCR-RFLP / molecular markers
Trypanosoma in humans	Antitrypanocidal drugs (Only for isometamidium (ISMM))	In vivo assessment of drug sensitivity in mice; ELISA for isometamidium in combination with parasite detection tests (32)	– Metabolism of the dye Alamar Blue by live cells to generate both a colorimetric and a fluorescent signal (31)	Mitochondrial electrical potential (MEP) assay (33)	PCR-RFLP *TbAT1* gene and other gene(s)
Leishmania in humans	Anti*leishmania* drugs especially pentavalent antimonials (SbV)	BALB/c mice infected with *L. donovani* treated with 1. Miltefosine $ED_{50} = 7.5\,\mu M$ 2. SbV $ED_{50} = 7.6\,\mu g$ SbV/ml (no data published on resistant strains) (34)	Amastigote/macrophage culture assay for SbV resistance; *L. donovani* RF = 3 (35); Also promastigote assay and the axenic amastigote culture assay. See text (34)		
Giardia in humans	5-Nitroimidazoles/ metronidazole tinidazole	Shift of ID_{50} for metronidazole based on parasite numbers in infected mice (36). RF = 2–4	MIC (metronidazole) for survival in culture over 2 days (37); RF = 5–8	Assay for decreased PFOR activity in resistant isolates (38); RF = negative 2–3	Associated chromosome duplications
	Quinacrine	–	ID_{50} 0.2–2.93 μM (39) for susceptible	Drug excluded from resistant trophozoites	
	Benzimidazoles/ albendazole (ABZ)	ID_{50} for ABZ in mice from 9–53 mg/kg (susceptible) (36). RF = 2–10	MIC of 3 μM (susceptible) (37); RF = 4	Drug causes cytoskeleton distortion; resistant trophozoites have enlarged median body but otherwise appear normal	
	Nitrofuran/furazolidone	ED_{50} furazolidone in mice 13.5 mg/kg in mice (susceptible) (40)	ID_{50} 0.3–1.7 μM furazolidone (39)		
	Nitazoxanide		MIC on culture of 12 μM nitazoxanide over 2 days, 50 μM (susceptible) (16); – IC_{50} of 8 μM for nitazoxanide compared with 15 μM for metronidazole (41)		
	Paromomycin	ED_{50} of 7.6 mg/kg (susceptible) (40)			
Trichomonas in humans	Nitroimidazoles/ metronidazole		Aerobic assay over 2 days[b] – metronidazole MIC 25–50 μM (susceptible) (37); RF = 4–8		Down-regulation of hydrogenosome function
Entamoeba in humans	Emetine		IC_{50} for survival in culture >2 μM (42)	Threefold increased expression of *Pgp* in resistant lines (43)	Up-regulation of Pgp mRNA levels
	Metronidazole		MIC in culture of 12.5 μM (susceptible) (37); RF = 2	Increased superoxide dismutase activity in resistant lines (23)	Up-regulation of superoxide dismutase mRNA levels

(continued)

Table 2 (continued)

Parasite and host	Drug/example	In vivo	Survival (dose–response)	Phenotype (site of action)	Genotype
Trichostrongyloids in sheep	Anthelmintics benzimidazole (BZ)	– FECRT[b] <95% efficacy and <90% LCL scored as resistant – Treat and slaughter test	– Larval development assay. [b]RFs for BZ = <70; LEV = >50; IVM = <10) (28)	Radioactive BZ-benzimidazole tubulin binding (BZ)	Benzimidazole – F200Y β-tubulin transition by AS-PCR and pyrosequencing
	levamisole (LEV)		– Egg hatch Assay (LEV)		F167Y is also screened
	Macrocyclic lactones (ML)		– Egg embryonation (BZ) – L3 motility (BZ, MLs)		
	Salicylanilides (SAL)		– Larval paralysis (LEV) – Larval migration assay (SAL) RF = <10		
Fasciola in sheep	Salicylanilides	Rat infection, sheep treat and slaughter trial RF = 2–4			
	Triclabendazole	Treat and slaughter trial RF = >7			
Schistosoma in humans	Schistosomicidal Drugs especially praziquantel (PZQ)	Clinical cure rate	Miracidial morphology (46) and survival analysis in the presence of PZQ	Muscle contraction studies (47) and [45Ca2+]-uptake (48)	Subtracted PCR – overexpressed mRNA coding subunit 1 of the cytochrome c oxidase (49), significance uncertain
		Worm count in treated rodents (44) RF = 3 (45)	RF = 2		

MIC minimum inhibitory concentration; RF resistance factor; PCR polymerase chain reaction; LCL lower confidence limit

[a]Within this table amino acid substations are written in the form K76T meaning Lysine is replaced by Threonine at residue number 76

[b]Assays applied in field for treatment decisions

Examples of end points are maturation, evidence of multiplication, viability or motility, measured by techniques such as parasite enumeration (e.g. visual counting), fluorescent activated cell sorting (FACS) or a feature linked to viability or parasite mass. Where ranges of drug concentrations are employed, a dose–response line can be generated and parameters such as effective dose to kill 50% (ED_{50}) calculated and compared with values from known susceptible parasites. Valid application of in vitro assays relies on co-expression of resistance traits in the life-cycle stages used in vitro and the parasitic stages.

2.2.2 Phenotypic Assay

Phenotype assays are those that measure a resistance phenotype related to the site of resistance. Unlike survival assays, phenotype assays require knowledge of the mechanism of resistance. Some of the types of phenotypes that could lead to resistance are

1. *Alteration or loss of a drug receptor* such as benzimidazole resistance in trichostrongyloids.
2. *Reduced drug levels* through decreased uptake or increased removal (or sequestration) of drug, e.g. mefloquine resistance in *Plasmodium falciparum*.
3. *Reduced concentration of active drug* could occur through decreased drug activation or increased drug metabolism, e.g. metronidazole resistance in *Giardia*.
4. *Alteration of a protein with an action upstream or downstream of the target site* – may result in physiological changes that prevent transduction of the effect, e.g. *Leishmania* resistance to itraconazole.

In parasitology, few of these types of tests are practical. However similar tests are commonly applied in insecticide resistance where detoxifying enzyme activity is a common mechanism of resistance.

2.2.3 Genetic Assay

Genetic tests offer the potential for very sensitive detection of resistance but in order to design and use gene probes, the genetic basis of resistance must be known. Moreover, the mechanisms must be the predominant one for a particular parasite/drug combination.

A number of PCR-based methods have been developed to identify resistance genotypes. The types of assays that are used in this chapter are described below:

1. For single base pair transitions (point mutations) allele-specific PCR (AS-PCR) have been developed. At its simplest, this depends on designing one of the two primers used in the PCR with the 3′ base complementary to one (e.g. resistant) and not the other (e.g. susceptible) allele. An amplification product is obtained only when polymerisation is initiated on both strands (in this case for resistant parasites).
2. PCR-restriction fragment length polymorphism (PCR-RFLP), involves PCR amplification of the region flanking the polymorphism followed by the cleavage of the PCR product with a restriction enzyme that cleaves only the specific (e.g. resistant) allele.
3. PCR-sequence specific oligonucleotide (PCR-SSO) probing involves PCR amplification of the region flanking the polymorphism. The resulting DNA fragments are spotted onto membranes, and resistant sequences are identified by hybridisation with short probes corresponding to resistance sequences (25).
4. Tandem Competitive PCR (TC-PCR) is designed to determine the gene-copy number (26). Tandem-competitive PCR is a refinement of competitive PCR and employs a common competitor molecule containing a tandem array of single copies of competitor sequence for several targets. The copy number of the candidate gene can be compared with a gene with a single copy number from the same parasite. It is especially useful for genes such as multidrug resistance genes (e.g. P-glycoprotein, Pgp).
5. A possible new advance is Fluorogenic PCR assays (FCR) (27). They allow a high throughput analysis of mutation hotspots and are particularly useful in polyclonal infections, allowing for both a real genotyping (which alleles are present in a same parasite) and for a quantification of the different genotypes.

While at present most assay endpoints involve the detection of specific size DNA fragments on agarose gels, future applications may use real-time PCR, melting point analysis or hybridisation (e.g. PCR ELISA) to automate endpoints. Molecular beacons and microarrays may find favour in future applications. Molecular tests also offer the advantage that it may be possible to simultaneously detect resistance and differentiate parasite species.

2.3 Sampling

Correct sampling, including sample size and randomisation, is an important consideration in assays for resistance. Sample size requirements will depend on several factors. In herd animals there is generally an aggregated distribution of parasites between hosts. To overcome possible sampling errors, samples from several animals are used to generate mean values. For instance the faecal egg count reduction test (FECRT) is the most common way to detect clinical resistance in helminths in sheep. Calculations are performed by comparisons of the means derived from faecal egg counts in groups of 10–15 animals each having at least 200 eggs per gram of faeces. If infections are comprised of mixed species then even larger sample sizes are required.

In contrast, in human parasitology we are often concerned with detecting resistance in an individual or a group of individuals. In cases where parasite populations are near clonal fewer samples are required both in terms of parasites and hosts. For example, in malaria sample volumes can be low, ~50 µl (the equivalent of a blood-drop) for molecular analyses such as PCR.

For 'non-clonal' parasite populations the widespread use of molecular diagnosis may be limited by sampling and sample throughput. For example, in order for a molecular assay to be sensitive enough to determine that the prevalence of resistant alleles is less than 1% in the field with 95% confidence, more than 300 alleles have to test negative. With current technology this means more than 150 diploid parasites must be subjected to PCR (28).

A significant dilemma is whether samples should be taken pre-treatment or post-treatment. If samples are pre-treatment they should reflect the true prevalence of resistance. If the samples are post treatment the chances of finding resistant parasites increases and, so too, does the sensitivity of tests.

2.4 Analysis of Data

2.4.1 General

The measurement of resistance is often scored as survival of parasites following a treatment and so parasite numbers (or values that reflect parasite numbers) are commonly recorded. These values are then analysed statistically (e.g. using t tests or F tests) and comparative efficacies generated. Resistance may also be recognised as a reduction in the period of protection that a persistent treatment provides. This provides different types of data and may be amenable to survival analysis.

Resistance assay outputs are quoted as either the proportion of resistant parasites within a population of parasites (population prevalence) or the proportion of regions where resistance is present (e.g. community, farm or shed prevalence). For example, if 25 out of 100 parasites survived a treatment, population prevalence would be 0.25. On the other hand, if 20 out of 50 farms studied have parasite resistance then there would be a farm prevalence of 0.40.

The latter requires categorical results that can be provided either by a breakpoint (e.g. efficacy of treatment less than 90%) or the presence/absence of a gene known to confer resistance.

By measuring the effect against a representative sample of parasites at each concentration over a range of drug

concentrations, such as in an in vitro assay, a plot of response to treatment against dose can be generated. From this the EC_{50} can be calculated. The EC_{50} is the effective concentration or dose of drug that affects 50% of the parasite population. Similar expressions include the ID_{50} (inhibitory dose), LD_{50} (lethal dose), LC_{50} (lethal concentration), and CD_{50} (curative dose). The MIC (minimal inhibitory concentrations) (or MLC, minimum lethal concentration) of a drug is another way to compare isolates. Several of these terms are used in this chapter to describe assay results and are used interchangeably in general descriptions.

The ratio of EC_{50} values between resistant and known susceptible populations of the same species is known as the resistance factor (RF). See Table 1 for known examples of these.

2.4.2 Analysis

Calculations of EC_{50} can be done by converting dose to log dose or ln dose and by plotting these against the response (e.g. % dead) converted to logits or probits. This usually results in a straight line, from which EC_{50} can be read. Modern computer analysis has enabled more accurate curve fitting, as well as automated calculations of EC_{50} and standard errors. Examples include programs such as GraphPad PRISM, and SAS routines. Figure 1 provides an example of a dose–response from an in vitro assay together with calculations of EC_{50} and RF. It also illustrates the shift of the dose–response line to the right in resistant isolates.

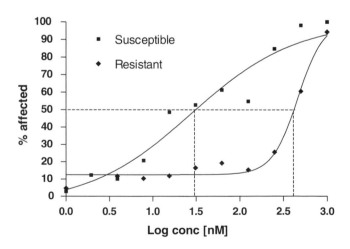

Fig. 1 Concentration/response curves for a larval development assay (LDA) with *Trichostrongylus colubriformis*. Percentage (%) affected refers to failure to develop in the presence of IVM – aglycone. Curves and EC_{50} were plotted and calculated using Graphpad Prism – nonlinear regression (curvefit). EC_{50} for the susceptible isolate was 28 nM (95% confidence interval range of 7–104) and for the resistant isolate was 459 (95% confidence interval range 397–531). The RF is therefore 16.4

2.5 Artefacts

While treatment failure may indicate drug resistance, this is just one cause of treatment failure. Other causes include mis-diagnoses of another mimicking aetiological agent, inappropriate drug choice for the causal parasite, rapid reinfection after treatment and recrudescence of the same infection. Under-dosing through underestimates of body weight or reduced concentration of active drug are other possibilities (29). One example is where the faster metabolism in goats results in poorer efficacy of antiparasitic compounds compared with sheep (30).

3 Parasites

3.1 Plasmodium

Infection of humans with *Plasmodium* parasites, especially *P. falciparum* results in the disease malaria. Drug-resistance in *P. falciparum* (and to a lesser extent *Plasmodium vivax* (50)) to the commonly used antimalarial drugs – chloroquine, pyrimethamine/sulphadoxine and mefloquine – is one of the greatest challenges facing the control of malaria (51, 52). We will focus this section on assays developed to measure drug resistance in *P. falciparum*. These assays are unlikely to be useful in determining the outcome of individual treatment, but are required for surveillance of the prevalence of drug resistance and to assist in the shaping of policies to limit drug resistance.

3.1.1 In Vivo

The presence or absence of parasites following treatment is measured by obtaining patient blood samples at the time of treatment, and then on days 7, 14 and 18 following treatment, and by assessing parasitaemia using light microscopy. Guidelines have been drawn up by the WHO to standardise these assays (53). Therapeutic response is graded as either sensitive, or with three degrees of resistance: RI (parasitaemia clears 25% below the original, but returns within 28 days of the treatment), RII (parasitaemia decreases to between 25 and 75% of the original parasitaemia, but then begins to increase by day 7 following treatment) and RIII (parasitaemia does not decrease to less than 75% of the original parasitaemia).

Because reinfections may occur in the study period a modified set of criteria based on clinical outcome has been proposed: (a) adequate clinical response, (b) early and (c) late treatment failure (54). Genetic typing can add a level of sophistication and help to distinguish between true recrudescence and reinfection but this is time-consuming and expensive (55). Other limitations of in vivo testing include the fact that therapeutic failure could be due to inter-individual differences in drug metabolism in the host, the degree of acquired or innate immunity, and variations in the quality of the drug preparation. Further, in many endemic areas there can be huge logistic difficulties associated with following up patients for 28 days.

3.1.2 Survival: In Vitro

A major advantage in the study of *P. falciparum* is the ability to maintain this parasite in short- and long-term cultures. Short-term culture is useful for drug sensitivity assays and continuous culture within the laboratory (56) has permitted both the study of drug-resistance phenotypes as well as the elucidation of the genetic basis of antimalarial resistance.

Typically in vitro assays start with the newly invaded ring stage of the parasite, which is obtained when a peripheral blood sample is drawn from an infected patient. Fresh *P. falciparum* isolates contain only ring-stage parasites, as other mature stages are sequestered to internal tissues. Parasite growth in each sample is measured in the presence of different amounts of the antimalarial drugs. The simplest method to monitor growth is the measurement of schizont maturation through scoring on microscope slides. Nevertheless, this method is laborious and confounded by subjective decisions on the maturity of the parasites.

More common are the methods based on the completion of a complete parasite life-cycle (57). These assays are suitable for all blood-stage drugs irrespective of their stage of action. Typically, serial dilutions of a drug are made in 96-well plates, to which the parasitised cells are added. These plates are incubated at 37°C for between 48 and 72 h (the longer times permit the analysis of slower-acting and cytostatic drugs such as tetracycline and pyrimethamine). Several methods have been devised to measure growth in these assays. The simplest form is the WHO in vitro microtest (58) based on counting Giemsa-stained parasites by light microscopy. Automated endpoints are ones such as incorporation of radiolabelled metabolic precursors (e.g. [^{3}H] hypoxanthine or isoleucine, as a correlate of growth (59)) or immunoquantitation of the parasite lactate dehydrogenase (LDH) (60) or the Histidine-Rich Protein II (HRPII) (61). The more developed assay is known as the double-site enzyme-linked LDH immunodetection (DELI) assay (62) which uses specific mAbs and an ELISA plate reader as an indirect measure of parasite number and hence growth.

3.1.3 Genetic

Much effort has been focussed on elucidating the genetic basis of resistance to antimalarials in *P. falciparum* (reviewed in (63)). The polymorphisms responsible for resistance are either point mutations or gene amplifications and numerous PCR-based methods have been developed to identify the genetic differences. These include AS-PCR (64), PCR-RFLP (65), PCR-SSO probing (25), and TC-PCR (26).

Although the genetic assays are technically demanding, the samples (blood on filter papers) can be processed at a central facility that possesses the required equipment and technical expertise. A prerequisite for the use of resistance alleles in assays, is the knowledge of associations between the specific allele and resistance. For certain alleles conflicting reports of associations have been obtained, which may reflect epidemiological or methodological differences. Another complicating factor is that in regions of higher transmission, isolates often harbour multiple clones and, consequently, genotypes. Once strong universal associations have been obtained, these methods will prove to be very powerful.

3.1.4 Specimen Collection

The conduct of in vivo tests entails considerable logistics and follow-ups. For in vitro tests, blood samples from infected patients are obtained by venipuncture into tubes with anticoagulants. These samples are then washed and placed into short-term culture assays as soon as possible.

Genetic tests are attractive as they require just a pin-prick of blood, collected onto filter papers. DNA in these samples is stable and can be sent to reference laboratories for processing.

3.1.5 Practical Tests, Clinical Significance and Breakpoints

Choosing which of the available tests to use will depend on the expertise available, as well as the required outcome. Arguably, the degree of in vivo resistance is the type of information likely to influence a change in the drug policy. However, as in vivo tests are logistically difficult to conduct, in vitro assays and genetic tests are gaining support. Once the infrastructure is in place they are easier to conduct and the DELI assay obviates the use of radioactivity. Due to the time required to conduct these assays relative to the speed of disease progression, it is unlikely that these assays will aid in the diagnosis of resistance within individuals. Instead, they are essential in determining the level and prevalence of resistance in the population, which may help to influence policy aimed at maximizing the efficacy of the available antimalarial drugs.

3.1.6 Artefacts

A major confounder of in vivo tests is the presence of immunity, acquired and innate, in certain individuals. Immunity will act to clear resistant parasites as well as sensitive ones, hence leading to underestimations of the level of resistance. In contrast, in areas of high transmission, reinfection with new parasites in the course of a drug treatment can be high. This does not reflect resistant parasites but new infections, leading to overestimates of resistance. Additionally, there may be considerable differences in the metabolism of drugs by different individuals and between populations, as well as differences in the stability and purity of the drugs used in the different trials.

Microscopic methods utilised within the assays are not only laborious, but may also lead to erroneous determinations of parasitaemia as a measure of drug response due to the subjectivity involved in assessing parasitaemia microscopically. Additionally, when dealing with field isolates, many do not grow in culture for reasons other than antimalarial toxicity, and in many cases the rate of reinvasion is much lower than that observed for culture-adapted laboratory isolates, increasing the difficulty in counting parasites.

We also noticed previously a severe 'inoculum effect' in antimalarial testing in vitro (66), emphasizing the need to control the number of red cells, and the parasitaemia at which the drug tests are being set up.

3.2 Eimeria

Coccidiosis caused by several species of the genus *Eimeria* is a major cause of production loss in the chicken industry. Despite resistance being common in several species of *Eimeria* in chickens, drugs such as the ionophores commonly achieve sufficient control in the field.

Diagnosis of resistance is generally performed by infecting groups of birds with suspect resistant *Eimeria* and comparing growth rates and pathology in these birds with those in birds infected with susceptible *Eimeria* in the presence of drug treatment. Resistance in in vivo tests is reported as an anticoccidial index (67) which is calculated using a combination of weight gain, % bird survival, lesion score and oocyst count. Indexes >160 indicate that the isolate is sensitive and those <120 are considered resistant. This approach means diagnosis is delayed to after the point where treatment decisions have already been made.

In order to achieve rapid diagnosis new in vitro tests are essential. The development of such assays would require a significant breakthrough in achieving the in vitro cultivation of the obligate parasitic stages of the life cycle. Understanding the biochemical or genetic mechanisms of resistance to anti-coccidials would also assist in test development and are high priorities for researchers.

3.3 *Trypanosoma (Ruminants)*

Trypanosomosis is a serious disease of domestic and some wild ruminants in Africa and has a major impact on cattle production. The major species which cause disease are *Trypanosoma congolense*, *Trypanosoma vivax* and *Trypanosoma brucei*. Chemotherapy is the principal form of control and widespread use of the phenanthridinium compound isometamidium (ISMM), the diamidine diminazene aceturate and homidium salts, which have been on the market for more than 40 years, has led to resistance (68).

Drug-susceptible isolates are maintained in laboratories where they are used for comparison with field isolates. Investigations into resistance mechanisms have been assisted by the selection in the laboratory of isogenic lines, resistant and susceptible to drugs but with the same genetic background.

3.3.1 In Vivo

Resistance to ISMM can be assessed under natural *Trypanosoma* challenge in the field using the 'block treatment' approach (69). Two groups of infected cattle, one treated with 1 mg/kg ISMM and one untreated control group (each consisting of 30–80 animals) are exposed to natural challenge and tested for the presence of trypanosomes in blood using the phase contrast buffy coat technique (70) every 2 weeks for 3 months. If more than 25% of ISMM-treated cattle become infected within 8 weeks of exposure, drug resistance is strongly suspected (69).

In what is currently an experimental approach, the use of an ELISA for the detection of ISMM in the serum (32) can be combined with the 'block treatment' or individual treatment of ruminants to detect resistant trypanosomes. The presence of trypanosomes in animals with an ISMM serum concentration >0.4 ng/ml suggests that parasites are resistant (71).

It has been shown that longitudinal parasitological field data can be suitably analysed in order to detect problems of resistance to diminazene aceturate (72, 73).

3.3.2 In Vivo (Experimental Animals)

A standardised test is available for the detection of resistance to ISMM or diminazene in experimentally infected mice or cattle (74). The mouse test (preferably using immu-

nosuppressed mice) can only be used for *T. brucei* or *T. congolense* (mice are refractory to *T. vivax*), whereas cattle are susceptible to all three species of trypanosomes. The single dose 1 mg/kg ISMM or 20 mg/kg diminazene test in mice is useful for screening a large number of trypanosome isolates, say, from regional surveys. Two groups of six mice are infected (100,000 trypanosomes inoculated intraperitoneally) and one group is treated 24 h after infection and the other group is left untreated. The multi-dose test in mice includes one control group and at least five treatment groups given discrete doses over the range 0.01–20 mg/kg ISMM or 1–60 mg/kg diminazene. The mice are checked for parasitaemia twice a week for 2 months. Because mouse tests cannot be used to predict the curative dose for ruminants, standardised tests in cattle (or sheep/goats) are necessary to confirm the efficacy of recommended curative doses of trypanocidal drugs in particular circumstances in the field (74).

3.3.3 Survival: In Vitro

In vitro tests using bloodstream or procyclic trypanosomes can be used to detect resistance to the above-mentioned drugs in *T. brucei* and *T. congolense* (31, 75–77). A major disadvantage of these tests is the slow adaptation of the trypanosomes to the culture conditions (78). An alternative approach is the *Glossina* infectivity test (DIGIT) to measure drug resistance in *T. congolense* (79). The main limiting factor for the latter test is the availability of tsetse flies.

3.3.4 Phenotypic Assay

It has been suggested that variations in the mitochondrial electrical potential (MEP) might be the primary factor determining the rate of ISMM accumulation in the trypanosome kinetoplast (33). Initial studies on a limited number of *T. congolense* populations have shown that an increased or a decreased MEP might be a candidate for being a quantitative marker for ISMM susceptibility or resistance, respectively.

3.3.5 Genetic

Some genetic markers are available for the detection of drug resistance in animal trypanosomes. PCR-RFLP tests allow the detection of *T. congolense* and *T. brucei* isolates resistant to ISMM (80, 81) or to diminazene (82). Apparently, more than one resistance mechanism to ISMM exists in *T. congolense* because the PCR-RFLP is not able to detect all strains which are identified as resistant in in vivo tests (80).

3.3.6 Specimen Collection

Blood of animals infected with *T. congolense* or *T. brucei* can be inoculated intraperitoneally into mice (74). In order to minimise selection of sub-populations from the original isolate only two or three passages should occur in mice before carrying out the drug resistance tests. If drug tests cannot be carried out immediately, the trypanosomes should be cryopreserved in liquid nitrogen for later use.

3.3.7 Practical Tests, Clinical Significance and Breakpoints

The most common tests for the detection of trypanocidal drug resistance are the tests in mice or in ruminants. Mouse and cattle tests are generally well correlated in detecting resistance in isolates, but the curative dose cannot be predicted in mice (81).

The major drawback of in vivo tests is their long time course (100 days). Therefore, the in vivo tests are gradually replaced by the molecular tests, which are able to identify drug resistant isolates within a few days.

3.4 Trypanosoma (Humans)

Drug resistance is a major problem in human African trypanosomiasis (HAT) (8, 84) particularly against melarsoprol where treatment failures have increased to up to 30% (85, 86). In order to measure resistance, suspected resistant isolates (87) need to be compared with known sensitive strains in the laboratory. The success of this is limited by the selective pressure on what could be a mixed population isolated for in vitro culturing and *T. b. gambiense*, for example, adapt poorly to culture conditions and achieve low parasitaemia in primary infections of laboratory rodents.

In vivo assessment of drug sensitivity in mice (see Sect. 3.3.2) is still the accepted standard for assessing drug resistance of African trypanosomes. An in vitro method that is reproducible and sensitive is based on the metabolism of the dye Alamar Blue by live cells to generate both a colorimetric and a fluorescent signal (31). Typically 10^4 trypanosomes in 100 μl medium are added to 100 μl of doubling dilutions of the test drug in 96-well plates. After 24 h, the dye is added and incubated for an additional 48 h to yield reliable IC_{50}s.

3.5 Leishmania

Leishmaniasis is caused by several *Leishmania* species, with *L. amazonensis*, *L. donovani*, *L. infantum* and *L. braziliensis* being the most pathogenic. There are cutaneous and visceral forms of disease. Basic treatment of leishmaniasis consists of a first line of pentavalent antimonials (SbV) such as sodium stibogluconate (SSG) and meglumine antimoniate. Alternative treatments are pentamidine, paromomycin (aminosidine) and amphotericin B. A new oral treatment, miltefosine (alkylphosphocholine) has now also been proven to be an effective treatment for visceral leishmaniasis (88).

Clinical unresponsiveness to SSG is being increasingly reported in endemic areas (89). Although immunological, physiological or pharmacological deficiencies in the host might explain the observed variations in clinical response (90). There is also evidence that the development of resistance of the parasite contributes to treatment failure (35, 91–93). SSG seems to have a dual action mode: (a) SSG is converted to SbIII, which in turn has direct leishmanicidal activity (94), and (b) SSG stimulates infected cells to produce microbicidal compounds such as reactive oxygen species and nitric oxide which kill the intracellular parasites (95).

Several mechanisms have been reported for experimentally induced resistance as reviewed by Croft et al. (96) but their role in natural SbV resistance is not straightforward (97). Furthermore, population genetic approaches on natural *Leishmania* populations have suggested that the parasite has a pleiomorphic response to the pressure exerted by the first-line treatment with SSG in natural conditions (98). Therefore, neither a genetic nor a phenotypic assay is as yet available to determine SbV-susceptibility. In vivo and survival assays are currently the only available tools to assess drug activity on a given isolated *Leishmania* strain and there are benefits in using them sequentially. It is important to make comparisons within the same *Leishmania* species, as the susceptibility to a given drug may vary between species (99).

3.5.1 In Vivo (Experimental Animal)

Hamsters and immunodeficient mice are commonly used as laboratory hosts for infection with *Leishmania*, although non-rodent hosts like dogs may give more accurate information on the likely drug activity in humans (100). In vivo assays provide information on host factors such as absorption, metabolism and pharmacokinetics of the drugs, which are not accounted for in the in vitro screens.

Infections can be induced with either amastigotes or promastigotes, although amastigotes give the highest chance of a successful infection. For viscerotropic species, the animals can be inoculated by intrasplenic, intraperitoneal, intravenous or intracardiac routes. Drug activity following treatment is assessed by evaluation of the parasite burdens either by microscopic counting of amastigotes in the spleen or liver impression smears (101) or by limiting dilution culture of infected tissues, a more sensitive method (102, 103). Recently, a real-time PCR assay was developed to improve the detection and quantification of *Leishmania major* in mouse tissue (104). The data are statistically analysed to calculate the dose needed to reduce the parasite load of the treated group to 50% (ED_{50}).

Dermotropic species, on the other hand, are initially inoculated intradermally, thereby mimicking the lower temperature of natural skin infections (105). For cutaneous leishmaniasis, the lesion diameter varies with the species (from a few mm in *L. braziliensis* to a few cm in *L. amazonensis*). Periodic measurement and analysis of the mean lesion diameter following treatment allows for evaluation of drug efficacy.

3.5.2   Survival: In Vitro

Promastigotes

Promastigotes, the vector form of *Leishmania*, can be readily cultured in cell-free media (like GLSH (106)) and is therefore the easiest to use in drug resistance assays. Drug sensitivity is assessed by incubating numbers of logarithmic phase promastigotes with discrete dilutions of drugs over a range of concentrations for 48 h at 26°C. Enzymatic activity (ornithine decarboxylase or acid phosphatase) in the resulting culture correlates to the parasite numbers which then allows for EC_{50} to be determined (107, 108). However, this assay has limited applicability because promastigotes are less susceptible to the SbVs than the intracellular amastigote form. Since *Leishmania* exists naturally the vertebrate host as the amastigote it is more suitable to base drug sensitivity assays on an amastigote-macrophage model.

Amastigote-Macrophage Models

Several coculture models have been reported using a range of different types of host cells, including: (1) a Sticker dog sarcoma cell line (fibroblasts), (2) transformed rodent macrophage cell lines like P388D1 and J774, (3) primary isolated mouse peritoneal macrophages, (4) human monocyte-derived macrophages, (5) human cell lines like U937 and THP-1. The requirements of cell cultures mean this type of assay is clearly limited in its use, because it is costly, time-consuming and technically challenging. Typically, amastigote-infected cells are maintained in a medium with serial dilutions of drug or without drug (control) for 4–7 days, at 37°C for viscerotropic species and at 33–35°C for dermotropic species. Drug activity is then assessed by counting the number of amastigotes/100 host cells in drug-exposed infections or by flow cytometry and compared with the control infections (109). The EC_{50}, is then computed by regression analysis (59, 110). Recent studies question the validity of the in vitro survival models for prognosis of in vivo SSG therapy outcome (111, 112) This is likely due to the stimulating effect of SSG on the infected macrophages, which might be different in vitro, in the absence of any immune components, than in vivo. The value of in vitro SSG susceptibility assays might be further enhanced by including some cytokines to mimic the synergistic effect of the immune system in vivo.

Axenic Amastigote Systems

Promastigotes collected from patients can be transformed to axenic amastigotes by reducing the pH of the medium to 5.5–6.5 and elevating the temperature of cultivation (113). So far, axenic amastigote cultures have been reported for *L. mexicana*, *L. donovani*, *L. major*, *L. amazonensis* and *L. braziliensis*, with some being more amenable to culture than others (114, 115). Axenic amastigotes are seeded at an initial concentration equivalent to early log phase (2×10^5 amastigotes/ml) and allowed to multiply over 3–4 days either in the medium alone (controls) or in the presence of serial dilutions of the drug. The number of amastigotes is then determined by counting or enzymatic assays (116–118) and the EC_{50} is calculated.

Measured resistance in amastigote systems is 3–4 times lower than in amastigote/macrophage systems. This difference might be caused by activation or concentration of the drug within the parasitised macrophage. Because the axenic amastigote assay is technically simpler, low cost, faster and uses the clinically relevant stage of the parasite, it promises to be a useful assay for rapid screening (119).

3.6   Giardia, Trichomonas and Entamoeba

Giardia duodenalis, *Trichomonas vaginalis* and *Entamoeba histolytica* are the most clinically important anaerobic protozoan parasites. Because of their anaerobic metabolism they are all susceptible to metronidazole and other related 5-nitroimidazole drugs such as tinidazole that are used to treat giardiasis and trichomoniasis. However, metronidazole is the only drug approved for the treatment of trichomoniasis in some countries, the only safe treatment for invasive amoebiasis, and the favoured treatment for giardiasis. Albendazole is an alternative for the treatment of giardiasis (22).

3.6.1   In Vivo

There are no in vivo tests in human hosts. However, the ability of axenically cultured *G. duodenalis* to infect and complete its life cycle in suckling mice is well documented (120) and this model has been used to assess drug susceptibilities in vivo for metronidazole, azithromycin and erythromycin at 5–100 mg/kg (121). In most cases the infections spontaneously resolve after about 3 weeks (120). Gerbil and suckling-rat models are also used for giardiasis, the former has the advantage of using adult animals (122). Using isolates from ten infected patients, Lemée et al. (36), infected, treated with metronidazole, and then monitored parasite survival in mice and correlated this with treatment outcomes in the patients. Parasites isolated from three patients in whom treatment with metronidazole failed had ID_{50}s in mice which ranked among the four highest (125–175 mg/kg) of all the ten isolates tested. The ID_{50} in mice of the seven isolates from patients in whom treatment was successful ranged from 31 to 150 mg/kg.

3.6.2 In Vitro

In order to use in vitro tests to estimate the level of susceptibility of G. duodenalis, T. vaginalis and E. histolytica to metronidazole or any other drug, the parasites need to be growing axenically (free of other living organisms). Methods for cultivation of all three parasite species have recently been expertly described (123). However, in spite of their long history of cultivation, fewer than half of G. duodenalis samples can be axenised with some taking months to establish before assays can be performed (16), and establishing E. histolytica axenically is notoriously difficult (124).

Traditionally two choices for assaying in vitro survival of Giardia, Trichomonas and Entamoeba in the presence of drugs have been available: tube assays and microtitre plate assays. A major consideration for Giardia and Entamoeba is the generation of an anaerobic environment. Microtitre plates are problematic due to the variability of the environment created in different laboratories and the need to remove the plates from the anaerobic environment to monitor the assays. Tube assays are cumbersome, time-consuming and prone to variability. A variety of end points (thymidine incorporation (37), uptake of [^{14}C]metronidazole (121), inhibition of adherence (125), live/dead (126)) have been used to report susceptibility including IC_{50} values ranging from 0.06 to 6 µM, ID_{50} values of 1.2 and 9 µM, and minimal lethal concentrations (MLC) after 72 h of 50–100 µM for Giardia, an MLC value of 11.6 µM for the HM-1 strain of E. histolytica and a minimal inhibitory concentration (MIC) of >90 µM after 24 h indicating resistance in anaerobic assays of T. vaginalis (see (22) for references). A proposal to standardise these assays, details the use of the 96-well plates with log2 drug dilutions and the Anaerocult systems from Merck. Plates can be monitored throughout the assay without aerobic exposure (127, 128). This system can also be modified to measure IC_{50} and IC_{90} values (129).

MICs for G. duodenalis (3 days) ranged from 6.3 µM in metronidazole-sensitive isolates to 50 µM for laboratory metronidazole-resistant lines (RF = 8) (37) with metronidazole resistance as high as 20% reported among G. duodenalis isolates (22). MICs (after 2 days) of 3.2 and 25 µM indicated metronidazole-sensitive and highly clinically resistant isolates of T. vaginalis in anaerobic assays, respectively (RF = 7–8) (37). T. vaginalis can also be maintained aerobically for several days and generally exhibits higher MIC values with metronidazole under these conditions (20). Thus the aerobic MICs were 25 and >100 µM for metronidazole-susceptible and highly resistant T. vaginalis (RF = 8). In studies of T. vaginalis in two different female populations 1 of 10 isolates and 4 of 24 isolates had aerobic MIC ≥ 100 µM (J. Upcroft, unpublished data). MICs (1 day) of 12.5–25 µM were found for axenic lines of E. histolytica but there are no confirmed clinical reports of metronidazole-resistant E. histolytica.

3.6.3 Phenotypic Assays

Some effects of anti-giardiasis drugs can be observed microscopically or measured in the laboratory (Table 2). The fluorescent drug quinacrine is visibly excluded from resistant G. duodenalis trophozoites (127). Distortion of Giardia trophozoite cytoskeleton is associated with albendazole (130) and may not occur in resistant individuals. A decrease in the activity of the key metabolic enzyme pyruvate:ferredoxin oxidoreductase (PFOR) can be measured in the laboratory. Decreased PFOR and ferredoxin mRNA levels occur in highly metronidazole-resistant laboratory lines of T. vaginalis (20), increased superoxide dismutase activity occurs in metronidazole-resistant E. histolytica (23) and increased levels of mRNA of P-glycoprotein homologues can be detected in emetine-resistant E. histolytica (43). The relevance of these observations to clinical resistance is unknown.

3.6.4 Genetic

While correlations between genes involved in drug resistance and decreased drug susceptibilities in the anaerobic protozoa have been reported (e.g. down-regulation of hydrogenosome function in T. vaginalis (20), chromosome duplication in G. duodenalis (17), increased superoxide dismutase activity in E. histolytica (23), a threefold increase in P-glycoprotein expression in emetine-resistant trophozoites (21, 43)), no mutational assay is available (Table 2).

3.6.5 Specimen Collection

G. duodenalis samples can be either cysts in stools (purified) or trophozoites from duodenal biopsies introduced directly into the medium (123). Both can be passaged through neonatal mice prior to culture to increase the number of parasites and the chance of establishing a culture (131).

Cysts of *E. histolytica* and the closely related non-pathogenic parasite *E. dispar* can be readily established in xenic or monoxenic culture (123) and assays to determine drug susceptibilities in the presence of bacteria provide a compromise between convenience and accuracy.

T. vaginalis trophozoites are obtained from high vaginal swabs and introduced directly into the medium (123). In our experience it is not difficult to establish 100% of positive *T. vaginalis* samples in axenic culture which may be ready to assay in 1–3 weeks.

While the same medium can be used to culture *G. duodenalis*, *E. histolytica* and *T. vaginalis*, the rates of growth vary greatly. Established cultures of *T. vaginalis* generally require a 10- to 50-µl passage into 5 ml of fresh medium every 2 days, *G. duodenalis* requires 100–200 µl for the same volume every 2 days and *E. histolytica* grows more slowly with a 1 in 4-ml passage needed every 3–4 days.

3.6.6 Practical Tests, Clinical Significance and Breakpoints

Using the in vitro assay systems described above (Sect. 3.5.2) (37) the researcher has a realistic common reference assay for the surveillance of the development of drug resistance in the anaerobic protozoa. Results for *T. vaginalis* resistance using this assay have been returned to a patient within a week (J. Upcroft, unpublished data) but information regarding the resistance status of *G. duodenalis* and *E. histolytica* may take too long to be clinically useful.

If 70 µM is used as an estimate of in vivo (serum) metronidazole concentration after usual, recommended doses (levels in the gut and vagina are likely to be less than this) then laboratory-induced metronidazole-resistant *Giardia* lines which grow in 100 µM metronidazole (132) can be expected to demonstrate clinical resistance in a patient. In the assay system described above, a MIC of 50 µM metronidazole was obtained with highly metronidazole-resistant *Giardia* (37) but clinical breakpoints have not been estimated for *Giardia*.

Similarly with *T. vaginalis*, metronidazole-resistant isolates with MICs of >25 µM (37) or >200 µM in aerobic assays (37) are likely to be resistant in vivo.

Resistance to metronidazole or emetine in *E. histolytica* has been demonstrated in the laboratory (37, 133) but no documented clinically resistant *E. histolytica* has been reported.

3.6.7 Artefacts

Artefacts involved in assaying drug susceptibility in the anaerobic protozoa include: variability in anaerobic environ-

ments generated; the time taken to establish an isolate in culture may result in the selection of organisms not truly representative of the original sample; the end points of the assays observed under the microscope can give rise to variable results; if motility alone is used as an endpoint, not all *Giardia* and *T. vaginalis* strains are equally motile, and pseudopodia of *Entamoeba* trophozoites may not be readily distinguished in live versus dead, rounded up trophozoites. In comparison with the data of Upcroft and Upcroft (133), the aerobic MLC values obtained by Muller et al. (134) on *T. vaginalis* (with aerobic assays conducted in 24-well plates and anaerobic assays carried out in anaerobic jars over 24 h) were 12–150 µM and 360–1,500 µM for metronidazole-susceptible and metronidazole-resistant isolates, respectively; anaerobic MLCs were 3–6 µM and 12–30 µM, respectively.

3.7 Trichostrongyloids

Resistance in the sheep trichostrongyloids is a serious and widespread problem in sheep industries, especially where treatment failures of *Haemonchus contortus* are involved. Not only has resistance occurred to all major anthelmintic classes in several species of parasite, but several isolates are resistant to all major drug classes. The other major species affected include *Trichostrongylus colubriformis* and *Ostertagia circumcincta*. Resistance of nematodes in cattle, horses and humans is appearing but assays are less well developed for these hosts. Further, correlation between in vivo effects of the drugs and in vitro behaviour in resistance tests will be difficult to confirm.

3.7.1 In Vivo

Treat and Slaughter Trials

The traditional, definitive test for resistance involves artificially infecting worm-free sheep with worms, treating them at the manufacturer's recommended dose rates and counting the number of worms surviving at slaughter. By using various control groups (for example untreated and susceptible worm isolates) dose–response curves can be generated and then the ED_{50} and RF calculated. Disadvantages of this method include the difficulty in finding drug-susceptible reference isolates, the creation of worm-free hosts, the ethics of euthanasia of animals and the expense of the procedure. Accordingly it is now only appropriate to perform slaughter trials on sheep when a novel isolation is made because in many cases the relationship and correlations between in vivo and in vitro assays for anthelmintic resistance in sheep parasites have been established (135).

Faecal Egg Count Reduction Trial

Faecal egg count reduction trial (FECRT) is the most common method of diagnosis of anthelmintic resistance in sheep in the field and is used as a treatment decision tool. Protocols are provided in articles by Lyndal-Murphy (136) and Coles et al. (137). Briefly, the test involves the following steps:

1. Select a flock of sheep, 3–6 months old, not treated in the previous 6 weeks (or longer for persistent drugs), with faecal egg counts of >200 epg.
2. Randomly allocate 10–15 animals to each drug treatment class to be tested and 10–15 to be controls. Use coloured markers to identify animals by group. Typically tests include four drug classes plus drug combinations.
3. Dose with liquid anthelmintic based on the manufacturers recommendations for the heaviest animal.
4. Treat each group with the dose of the particular drug as calculated in (3), leaving the controls untreated. Graze the animals together.
5. Return 10–14 days later, collect faecal samples from each animal (labelled by group) and perform individual faecal egg counts by a standard flotation method. Fourteen days is chosen because it is long enough for drugs to exert their effects and for the eggs to be cleared, but not so long that newly ingested larvae will have developed to patency (egg laying).
6. Calculate % reductions compared with controls, using arithmetic group means, but logarithmic error calculations to calculate confidence limits.
7. Anthelmintic resistance is present if efficacy is <95% AND the lower 95% confidence interval is <90%

The data can be complemented by use of culture from eggs to L3 and attribution of eggs in faeces in the same ratio as the genera identified in the L3 cultures.

The advantages of FECRT assays include their simplicity, that it has been widely validated and that the data provided is relevant to field resistance. On the other hand, FECRT can only detect clinical resistance, often not until the frequencies of resistance alleles reach 25% (138). Two visits to the farm are required unless the farmer conducts the treatments and farmers may be reluctant to participate in these tests, especially if sheep are due for slaughter for meat. To a large extent the interpretation of FECRT relies on a correlation between egg counts and worm counts. Some anthelmintics, particularly the macrocyclic lactones, do not kill resistant worms but, do suppress their egg production. Zero egg counts post-treatment that suggest that the worms are drug susceptible may mask cases where worms resume egg production after more than 14 days of treatment. Sensitivity can be improved by using reduced dose rates of drugs, but this approach requires a good knowledge of resistance phenomena. The protocol can be modified for other hosts and, in the

case of horses the calculations can be refined by using individual animal egg counts pre and post treatment (139).

3.7.2 In Vivo (Experimental Animal)

Drug efficacy in guinea pigs (140) and jirds (141) has been used to measure resistance in *T. colubriformis* and *H. contortus*, respectively. Although these techniques are not likely to be used for field detection, they are useful experimental models because several dose rates of drug can be tested more quickly and cheaply than in sheep.

3.7.3 In Vitro

Survival/Development Assays

The best characterised in vitro assay is the larval development assay (LDA) (135). It relies on the development of eggs to L1-L2-L3 in the presence of drugs and has been adapted to a 96-well plate format. Eggs are collected from pooled faecal samples from a farm. Approximately 200 g faeces (collected from the ground after herding the sheep into the corner of a pen for 15 min) are soaked in 200 ml of tap water for at least 30 min and broken up to give a slurry. Eggs are cleaned by sequential sieving, centrifugation on a sucrose gradient and washing. Seventy to one hundred and twenty eggs are pipetted in 10 µl into a pre-prepared plate. The rows of the 96-well plate contain anthelmintics in agar at increasing concentration steps.

Anthelmintic	Approximate concentration range (µM)
Thiabendazole	0.01–10
Levamisole	0.2–20
MBZ plus Levamisole	0.01–10 (MBZ)
	0.2–20 (LEV)
IVM – MS (IVM monosaccharide)	0.005–0.5
IVM – AG (IVM aglycone)	0.01–1

After 7 days of incubation at 25°C the stage of development is scored down a microscope. The concentrations on the plate are arranged so that susceptible isolates hatch at low concentrations in wells coloured green and resistant isolates at high concentrations, coloured red. Results can also be analysed by curve fitting and calculating EC_{50}.

The LDA can be applied to resistance in horse cyathostomes (139) and has several advantages over FECRT. Sample collection is simpler and accomplished in one visit. The tests are repeatable, there is no need to test susceptible isolates and the use of dose–response data plus the use of greater than one hundred eggs/well can provide sensitivity of 95–98%.

The LDA simultaneously assays resistance to the major commercial drugs in a single test.

General disadvantages include that the validity of the assay as a measure of resistance must be confirmed under a range of conditions, trained laboratory staff are required and species identification of larvae is needed. For some parasite species, especially *Ostertagia*, detection of ivermectin resistance in the LDA is not sensitive enough for field use.

Phenotypic Assay

Reduced binding of BZ anthelmintics to worm tubulin is a known resistance phenotype and the binding assays can be performed on a pooled sample of L3 following incubation with isotopically labelled BZ (142). The main drawback of this method is that a radiolabelled drug as well as the skills and equipment to use it are required.

3.7.4 Genetic

While there are a number of research-based tests, only one genetic test is validated for anthelmintic resistance. Benzimidazole resistance is linked to the presence of a predominant allele of the β-tubulin isotype 1 gene containing a F200Y transition (143). This amino acid change is due to a single nucleotide difference.

Although other genetic changes, such as F167Y, may contribute to resistance, this allele appears to be almost universally associated with resistance in sheep nematodes and is therefore an ideal diagnostic feature. Tests have been used for pooled worm samples or single worms for the species *H. contortus* (144) and *O. circumcincta* (145, 146).

An elegant single worm method for AS PCR has been described (146). The reaction uses four primers, two are sense and antisense primers either side of, but at different distances from the site of the single nucleotide difference. Within this nest, is a further sense primer with its 3′ end coinciding with the 'susceptible' base pair, plus an antisense primer complementary to the 3′ end coinciding with 'resistant' base pair. Products are separated by gel electrophoresis. The total product, limited by the outside primers, is the amplification control. Two differently sized products indicate that heterozygous alleles are present and either product alone indicates homozygosity, one size of product for the susceptible, and another for the resistance.

Such tests have further potential if species-specific primers can be designed by taking advantage of species-specific sequences in β-tubulin and to provide simultaneous species and resistance information. Further, if the resistance mechanisms are conserved across the parasite species they may indicate diagnostic tools in horses, cattle and human parasites.

Genetic tests have the potential to detect population prevalence below 1%. Despite knowledge of the genetic mechanism of benzimidazole resistance and the usefulness of the test, the logistics of genetic tests preclude their use in the field. Further, the prevalence of benzimidazole resistance in many countries is so high that diagnosis is no longer useful.

Because current genetic tests provide yes/no answers, the design of tests requires careful thought. Assuming that a genetic test is available, and that it detects a single allele (diploid and autosomal) linked to the resistant phenotype in one species of a parasite, it could be applied to measure the prevalence of resistance in several ways. One would be to collect L3 surviving high drug concentrations on in vitro assay plates (e.g. the LDA) and genotype them individually. Another approach would be to test the population of worms (e.g. eggs or larvae) recovered from a farm or an animal. Using PCR to genotype individual worms would be laborious and expensive hence pooling samples of parasites would have to be considered. Real-time (quantitative) PCR may help to simplify the sampling but would require considerable standardisation (28). For example, a pool of 150 worms would have to test negative for the resistance allele to provide 95% confidence that resistance prevalence was <1%. A useful approach would be to perform three PCRs on different pools of DNA. If no resistant alleles were detected in the pooled DNA from 150, 75 and 30 worms, allele prevalences of <1, 1–2 and 2–5%, respectively, (at confidence level of 95%) would be predicted (147). Such tests would require ideal conditions for both extraction of DNA from all of the worms and PCR-based amplification. A perspective on the developments in the molecular diagnosis of anthelmintic resistance appear in von Samson-Himmelstjerna and Blackhall (148).

3.7.5 Specimen Collection

In Vivo

Because sheep vary considerably in the number of worms that they carry, treatment group sizes need to be 10–15 in order to provide sufficient sampling and power for statistical tests. Clinical samples for FECRT are obtained by collecting 3 g of faeces directly from the rectum of individual sheep on the day of treatment (pre-treatment sample) and 10–14 days after treatment (post-treatment sample). Pre-trial samples should exceed 200 epg.

In Vitro

Sampling for LDAs or egg hatch assays are relatively simple as they use pooled faecal samples. Samples can be cooled to

10°C and air excluded to prevent development during transport. Sealed plastic bags are ideal.

3.7.6 Practical Tests, Clinical Significance and Breakpoints

The most widely used test is the FECRT. Arithmetic group mean of egg counts are used because they indicate potential pasture contamination, are simple to calculate and are conservative estimates of resistance (149). The use of the two criteria (breakpoints) (efficacy <95% and lower confidence intervals <90%) provides a 95% confidence of detecting clinical resistance (137).

For in vitro assays such as the LDA, breakpoints can also be visualised on the colour-coded plates. In addition, the EC_{50} can be calculated by curve fitting and comparing with data available for susceptible isolates. Curve fitting also allows subpopulations to be identified and are useful in the early stages of resistance development.

3.7.7 Artefacts

Despite careful test validation and well-validated sampling frames, assaying resistance remains an inexact science. Apart from the limitations of the tests, mixed species infections that are the norm in the field can interfere with these measurements.

Even in well-controlled laboratory situations, results vary. Apart from the day-to-day variation in results other factors are known to influence resistance levels. Resistance varies over the course of infection (150). Cold storage may also influence resistance (151). There are limitations in the practical application of tests as no universal technique (covering all species and all drugs) is available.

3.8 Fasciola

Reports of resistance to triclabendazole and closantel in the liver fluke *Fasciola hepatica* have come from several countries including Australia, Ireland, Scotland and the Netherlands (152). Internationally, fasciolosis is a very significant disease in farm animals and resistance is a serious impediment to control.

Because of the indirect life cycle (sheep/snail hosts), resistance in flukes is difficult to measure. Generally the treat and slaughter assay involves isolating potentially resistant flukes by treating infected sheep several times with a fasciolicide at the recommended dose rate. Eggs from survivors are hatched in the laboratory and passaged through suitable intermediate host snails in the laboratory. Sheep are divided into groups and infected with metacercariae from the suspected resistant strain and the laboratory-based susceptible strain. Eight weeks after infection half of the sheep are treated with the recommended dose rate of the drug. Animals in other groups are used as controls. Sheep are slaughtered 16 weeks after infection, their livers examined and the numbers of flukes counted. The efficacies of treatment against susceptible and resistant isolates are compared.

Egg count reduction tests are not suitable for flukes because resistance is usually apparent against the immature stages of the fluke, prior to egg-laying.

Some in vitro tests have been described but none developed for routine use. There is potential for using motility of miracidia or hatching of eggs from hosts as an assay for resistance in flukes.

3.9 Schistosoma

Schistosomiasis affects more than 200 million people in 76 countries. These infections are most commonly caused by *S. haematobium*, *S. japonicum*, and *S. mansoni* (153). Although the minor drugs hycanthone, metrifonate and oxamniquine have been used, praziquantel (PZQ) is the drug of choice for treatment for all forms of schistosomiasis (154). Recently, reports of decreased efficacy of PZQ in the field and resistance in laboratory strains of the parasite have appeared. Although other possible causes of treatment failure have not been ruled out, these cases strongly suggest that resistance to PZQ is emerging.

In vivo testing is complicated by the fact that PZQ has a triphasic efficacy profile with the earliest stages of schistosomes being susceptible, followed by progressive insensitivity through to 3–4 weeks after infection and then a gradual regaining of susceptibility at weeks 6–7 after infection (155). In cases of endemic exposure to infection even a drug-susceptible parasite population may contain refractory individuals.

In vivo tests in rodent hosts have been used to test for possible drug resistance (156). Eggs are collected from patients still passing eggs after repeated treatments with an antischistomal drug. Laboratory-reared snails are infected and the cercariae used to infect laboratory rodents (mice or hamsters). Experimental chemotherapy at a range of doses is given to the rodents and by comparing worm counts in control and treated groups an ED_{50} is calculated. This is expensive and slow (approximately 12 weeks), and the correlation between drug sensitivity in mice and the patient is unreliable (144).

In vitro tests include muscle contraction studies (47), miracidial morphology and survival analysis in the presence of drug (46).

Leads to the molecular mechanism of resistance are over-expression of messenger RNA coding for subunit 1 of the mitochondrial enzyme cytochrome *c* oxidase (49) and the knowledge that sensitivity of a Ca^{2+} channel to PZQ depends on residues at the interface between the α and β channel subunits (24).

4 Conclusions

Drug resistance is responsible for parasite control failures in a number of diseases. Costs such as death, debility, reduced capacity to work and production losses are significant and on a global scale. Assays for drug resistance have an essential role in future disease management. Simply, we cannot manage resistance if we cannot measure it.

To be most effective, resistance monitoring should be a routine component of parasitic disease management. This requires accurate assays that are simple, rapid, and can simultaneously test against all relevant available control agents often in several parasite species. The ideal would be an assay that could be performed and interpreted by the patient's (or animals') side. These criteria have proven difficult to meet and drug resistance remains difficult to assay. What we have is a collection of assays, most of which are used in monitoring resistance status and, occasionally, measuring resistance so that decisions on therapy in individuals or herds can be made.

Although some in vivo assays are available there are pressures to develop in vitro and genetic tests. While these latter tests need to be validated against in vivo results they offer the potential advantages of improved speed and sensitivity. We also need to base future tests on better knowledge of resistance mechanisms. Further, we need to understand parasite biology and resistance so that we can design sampling frames to match the mechanism-based tests that will arise.

Acknowledgements Valuable input on tests for human trypanosomes was provided by Harry de Koning, University of Glasgow.

References

1. Sutherst RW, Comins HN. The management of acaricide resistance in the cattle tick, *Boophilus microplus* (Canestrini) (Acari: Ixodidae), in Australia. Bull Entomol Res 1979; 69:519–537.
2. Eckstein-Ludwig U, Webb RJ, van Goethem IDA, et al. Artemisinins target the SERCA of *Plasmodium falciparum*. Nature 2003; 424:957–961.
3. Wang CC. Molecular mechanisms and therapeutic approaches to the treatment of African trypanosomiasis. Annu Rev Pharmacol Toxicol 1995; 35:93–127.
4. Carter NS, Fairlamb AH. Arsenical-resistant trypanosomes lack an unusual adenosine transporter. Nature 1993; 361:173–175.
5. Matovu E, Stewart ML, Geiser F, et al. Mechanisms of arsenical and diamidine uptake and resistance in *Trypanosoma brucei*. Eukaryot Cell 2003; 2:1003–1008.
6. McCann PP, Pegg AE. Ornithine decarboxylase as an enzyme target for therapy. Pharmacol Ther 1992; 54:195–215.
7. De Koning HP. Transporters in African trypanosomes: role in drug action and resistance. Int J Parasitol 2001; 31:511–521.
8. Maser P, Luscher A, Kaminsky R. Drug transport and drug resistance in African trypanosomes. Drug Resist Updat 2003; 6:281–290.
9. Denise H, Barrett MP. Uptake and mode of action of drugs used against sleeping sickness. Biochem Pharmacol 2001; 61:1–5.
10. De Koning HP. Uptake of pentamidine in *Trypanosoma brucei brucei* is mediated by three distinct transporters: implications for cross-resistance with arsenicals. Mol Pharmacol 2001; 59:586–592.
11. Bray PG, Barrett MP, Ward SA, de Koning HP. Pentamidine uptake and resistance in pathogenic protozoa: past, present and future. Trends Parasitol 2003; 19:232–239.
12. De Koning HP, Stewart M, Anderson L, et al. The trypanocide diminazene aceturate is accumulated only through the TbAT1 purine transporter; additional insights in diamidine resistance in African trypanosomes. Antimicrob Agents Chemother 2004; 48:1515–1519.
13. Pepin J, Milord F. The treatment of human African trypanosomiasis. Adv Parasitol 1994; 33:1–47.
14. Urbina JA, Docampo R. Specific chemotherapy of Chagas disease: controversies and advances. Trends Parasitol 2003; 19:495–501.
15. Perez-Victoria FJ, Gamarro F, Ouellette M, Castanys S. Functional cloning of the miltefosine transporter: a novel p-type phospholipid translocase from leishmania involved in drug resistance. J Biol Chem 2003; 278:49965–49971.
16. Wright JM, Dunn LA, Upcroft P, Upcroft JA. Efficacy of antigiardial drugs. Expert Opin Drug Saf 2003; 2:529–541.
17. Chen N, Upcroft JA, Upcroft P. Physical map of a 2 Mb chromosome of the intestinal protozoan parasite *Giardia duodenalis*. Chromosome Res 1994; 2:307–313.
18. Upcroft J, Mitchell R, Chen N, Upcroft P. Albendazole resistance in *Giardia* is correlated with cytoskeletal changes but not with a mutation at amino acid 200 in beta-tubulin. Microb Drug Resist 1996; 2:303–308.
19. Brown DM, Upcroft JA, Upcroft P. A H2O-producing NADH oxidase from the protozoan parasite *Giardia duodenalis*. Eur J Biochem 1996; 241:155–161.
20. Dunne RL, Dunn LA, Upcroft P, et al. Drug resistance in the sexually transmitted protozoan *Trichomonas vaginalis*. Cell Res 2003; 13:239–249.
21. Orozco E, Lopez C, Gomez C, et al. Multidrug resistance in the protozoan parasite *Entamoeba histolytica*. Parasitol Int 2002; 51:353–359.
22. Upcroft P, Upcroft JA. Drug targets and mechanisms of resistance in the anaerobic protozoa. Clin Microbiol Rev 2001; 14:150–164.
23. Samarawickrema NA, Brown DM, Upcroft JA, et al. Involvement of superoxide dismutase and pyruvate: ferredoxin oxidoreductase in mechanisms of metronidazole resistance in *Entamoeba histolytica*. J Antimicrob Chemother 1997; 40:833–840.
24. Kohn AB, Roberts-Misterly JM, Anderson PAV, Greenberg RM. Creation by mutagenesis of a mammalian Ca^{2+} channel [beta] subunit that confers praziquantel sensitivity to a mammalian Ca^{2+} channel. Int J Parasitol 2003; 33:1303–1308.
25. Allbueche A, Silveira H, Conway DJ, et al. High-throughput sequence typing of T-cell epitope polymorphisms in *Plasmodium falciparum* circumsporozoite protein. Mol Biochem Parasitol 2000; 106:273–282.
26. Price RN, Cassar C, Brockman A, et al. The pfmdr1 gene is associated with a multidrug-resistant phenotype in *Plasmodium falciparum* from the western border of Thailand. Antimicrob Agents Chemother 1999; 43:2943–2949.

27. Decuypere S, Elinck E, Van Overmeir C, et al. Pathogen geno-typing in polyclonal infections: application of a fluorogenic polymerase-chain-reaction assay in malaria. J Infect Dis 2003; 188:1245–1249.

28. Sangster NC, Dobson RJ. Anthelmintic resistance. In: Lee DL, ed. The Biology of Nematodes, London: Harwood Academic Publishers, 2002; 531–567.

29. Monteiro AM, Wanyangu SW, Kariuki DP, et al. Pharmaceutical quality of anthelmintics sold in Kenya. Vet Rec 1998; 142:396–398.

30. Hennessy DR. The disposition of antiparasitic drugs in relation to the development of resistance by parasites of livestock. Acta Trop 1994; 56:125–141.

31. Räz B, Iten M, Grether-Buhler Y, et al. The Alamar Blue® assay to determine drug sensitivity of African trypanosomes (*T. b. rhodesiense* and *T. b. gambiense*) in vitro. Acta Trop 1997; 68:139–147.

32. Eisler MC, Elliott CT, Holmes PH. A simple competitive enzyme immunoassay for the detection of the trypanocidal drug isometamidium. Ther Drug Monit 1996; 18:73–79.

33. Peregrine AS, Wells CW, Wilkes JM. Methods for detection of drug resistance in trypanosomes: new developments? ICPTV Newslett 2000; 12–13.

34. Escobar P, Yardley V, Croft SL. Activities of hexadecylphospho-choline (miltefosine), AmBisome, and sodium stibogluconate (Pentostam) against *Leishmania donovani* in immunodeficient scid mice. Antimicrob Agents Chemother 2001; 45:1872–1875.

35. Lira R, Sundar S, Makharia A, et al. Evidence that the high incidence of treatment failures in Indian kala-azar is due to the emergence of antimony-resistant strains of *Leishmania donovani*. J Infect Dis 1999; 180:564–567.

36. Lemee V, Zaharia I, Nevez G, et al. Metronidazole and albendazole susceptibility of 11 clinical isolates of *Giardia duodenalis* from France. J Antimicrob Chemother 2000; 46:819–821.

37. Upcroft JA, Upcroft P. Drug susceptibility testing of anaerobic protozoa. Antimicrob Agents Chemother 2001; 45:1810–1814.

38. Townson SM, Upcroft JA, Upcroft P. Characterisation and purification of pyruvate:ferredoxin oxidoreductase from *Giardia duodenalis*. Mol Biochem Parasitol 1996; 79:183–193.

39. Boreham PF, Phillips RE, Shepherd RW. Heterogeneity in the responses of clones of *Giardia intestinalis* to anti-giardial drugs. Trans R Soc Trop Med Hyg 1987; 81:406–407.

40. Boreham PF, Phillips RE, Shepherd RW. The activity of drugs against *Giardia* intestinalis in neonatal mice. J Antimicrob Chemother 1986; 18:393–398.

41. Adagu IS, Nolder D, Warhurst DC, Rossignol JF. In vitro activity of nitazoxanide and related compounds against isolates of *Giardia intestinalis*, Entamoeba histolytica and *Trichomonas vaginalis*. J Antimicrob Chemother 2002; 49:103–111.

42. Burchard GD, Mirelman D. *Entamoeba histolytica*: virulence potential and sensitivity to metronidazole and emetine of four isolates possessing nonpathogenic zymodemes. Exp Parasitol 1988; 66:231–242.

43. Descoteaux S, Ayala P, Samuelson J, Orozco E. Increase in mRNA of multiple Eh pgp genes encoding P-glycoprotein homologues in emetine-resistant *Entamoeba histolytica* parasites. Gene 1995; 164:179–184.

44. Ismail M, Metwally A, Farghaly A, et al. Characterization of isolates of *Schistosoma mansoni* from Egyptian villagers that tolerate high doses of praziquantel. Am J Trop Med Hyg 1996; 55:214–218.

45. Cioli D, Botros SS, Wheatcroft-Francklow K, et al. Determination of ED50 values for praziquantel in praziquantel-resistant and -susceptible *Schistosoma mansoni* isolates. Int J Parasitol 2004; 34: 979–987.

46. Liang YS, Coles GC, Doenhoff MJ, Southgate VR. In vitro responses of praziquantel-resistant and -susceptible *Schistosoma mansoni* to praziquantel. Int J Parasitol 2001; 31:1227–1235.

47. Ismail M, Botros S, Metwally A, et al. Resistance to praziquantel: direct evidence from *Schistosoma mansoni* isolated from Egyptian villagers. Am J Trop Med Hyg 1999; 60:932–935.

48. William S, Botros S. Validation of sensitivity to praziquantel using *Schistosoma mansoni* worm muscle tension and Ca^{2+}-uptake as possible in vitro correlates to in vivo ED50 determination. Int J Parasitol 2004; 34:971–977.

49. Pereira C, Fallon PG, Cornette J, et al. Alterations in cytochrome-c oxidase expression between praziquantel-resistant and susceptible strains of *Schistosoma mansoni*. Parasitology 1998; 117:63–73.

50. Baird JK, Sustriayu Nalim MF, Basri H, et al. Survey of resistance to chloroquine by *Plasmodium vivax* in Indonesia. Trans R Soc Trop Med Hyg 1996; 90:409–411.

51. Trape JF, Pison G, Preziosi MP, et al. Impact of chloroquine resistance on malaria mortality. C R Acad Sci III 1998; 321:689–697.

52. White NJ, Nosten F, Looareesuwan S, et al. Averting a malaria disaster. Lancet 1999; 353:1965–1967.

53. WHO. Chemotherapy of malaria and resistance to antimalarials. Report of a WHO scientific group. World Health Organ Tech Rep Ser 1973; 529:1–121.

54. WHO. Assessment of therapeutic efficacy of antimalarial drugs for uncomplicated falciparum malaria in areas with intense transmission, vol. II, Geneva, Switzerland: World Health Organization, 1996, 32 pp.

55. Viriyakosol S, Siripoon N, Zhu XP, et al. *Plasmodium falciparum*: selective growth of subpopulations from field samples following in vitro culture, as detected by the polymerase chain reaction. Exp Parasitol 1994; 79:517–525.

56. Trager W, Jensen JB. Human malaria parasites in continuous culture. Science 1976; 193:673–675.

57. Nguyen-Dinh P, Trager W. *Plasmodium falciparum* in vitro determination of chloroquine sensitivity of 3 new strains by a modified 48 hour test. Am J Trop Med Hyg 1980; 29:339–342.

58. Winkler S, Brandts C, Wernsdorfer WH, et al. Drug sensitivity of *Plasmodium falciparum* in Gabon: activity correlations between various antimalarials. Trop Med Parasitol 1994; 45:214–218.

59. Desjardins RE, Canfield CJ, Haynes JD, Chulay JD. Quantitative assessment of antimalarial activity in vitro by a semiautomated microdilution technique. Antimicrob Agents Chemother 1979; 16: 710–718.

60. Piper R, Lebras J, Wentworth L, et al. Immunocapture diagnostic assays for malaria using Plasmodium lactate dehydrogenase (pLDH). Am J Trop Med Hyg 1999; 60:109–118.

61. Noedl H, Wernsdorfer WH, Miller RS, Wongsrichanalai C. Histidine-rich protein II: a novel approach to malaria drug sensitivity testing. Antimicrob Agents Chemother 2002; 46:1658–1664.

62. Druilhe P, Moreno A, Blanc C, et al. A colorimetric in vitro drug sensitivity assay for *Plasmodium falciparum* based on a highly sensitive double-site lactate dehydrogenase antigen-capture enzyme-linked immunosorbent assay. Am J Trop Med Hyg 2001; 64:233–241.

63. Sangster N, Batterham P, Chapman HD, et al. Resistance to antiparasitic drugs: the role of molecular diagnosis. Int J Parasitol 2002; 32:637–653.

64. Adagu IS, Warhurst DC. Allele-specific, nested, one tube PCR: application to Pfmdr1 polymorphisms in Plasmodium falciparum. Parasitology 1999; 119:1–6.

65. Duraisingh MT, Curtis J, Warhurst DC. *Plasmodium falciparum*: detection of polymorphisms in the dihydrofolate reductase and dihydropteroate synthetase genes by PCR and restriction digestion. Exp Parasitol 1998; 89:1–8.

66. Duraisingh MT, Jones P, Sambou I, et al. Inoculum effect leads to overestimation of in vitro resistance for artemisinin derivatives and standard antimalarials: a Gambian field study. Parasitology 1999; 119:435–440.

67. Chapman HD, Shirley MW. Sensitivity of field isolates of *Eimeria* species to monensin and lasalocid in the chicken. Res Vet Sci 1989; 48:114–117.

68. Geerts S, Holmes PH, Diall O, Eisler MC. African bovine trypanosomiasis: the problem of drug resistance. Trends Parasitol 2001; 17:25–28.

69. Eisler MC, McDermott JJ, Mdachi RE, et al. Rapid method for the assessment of trypanocidal drug resistance in the field. In: Proceedings of the 9th Symposium of the International Society for Veterinary Epidemiology and Economics, Nairobi, 2000.

70. Murray M, Murray PK, McIntyre WIM. An improved parasitological technique for the diagnosis of African trypanosomiasis. Trans R Soc Trop Med Hyg 1977; 71:325–326.

71. Eisler MC, Gault EA, Moloo SK, et al. Concentrations of isometamidium in the sera of cattle challenged with drug-resistant *Trypanosoma congolense*. Acta Trop 1997; 63:89–100.

72. Rowlands GJ, Mulatu W, Authie E, et al. Epidemiology of bovine trypanosomiasis in the Ghibe valley, southwest Ethiopia. 2. Factors associated with variations in trypanosome prevalence, incidence of new infections and prevalence of recurrent infections. Acta Trop 1993; 53:135–150.

73. Rowlands GJ. Detecting resistance of trypanocidal infections to diminazene aceturate – a possible field test? ICPTV Newslett 2000; No. 2;8–9

74. Eisler MC, Brandt J, Bauer B, et al. Standardised tests in mice and cattle for the detection of drug resistance in tsetse transmitted trypanosomes of African domestic cattle. Vet Parasitol 2001; 97: 171–182.

75. Gray MA, Kimarua RW, Peregrine AS, Stevenson P. Drug sensitivity screening in vitro of populations of *Trypanosoma congolense* originating from cattle and tsetse flies at Nguruman, Kenya. Acta Trop 1993; 55:1–9.

76. Hirumi H, Hirumi K, Peregrine AS. Axenic culture of *Trypanosoma congolense*: application to the detection of sensitivity levels of bloodstream trypomastigotes to diminazene aceturate, homidium chloride, isometamidium chloride and quinapyramine sulphate. J Protozool Res 1993; 3:52–63.

77. Clausen PH, Pellmann C, Scheer A, et al. Application of in vitro methods for the detection of drug resistance in trypanosome field isolates. ICPTV Newslett 2000; 2:9–12.

78. Geerts S, Holmes PH. Drug management and parasite resistance in bovine trypanosomiasis in Africa. In: (PAAT) RotPAAT, ed. PAAT Technical and Scientific Series, vol. 1, Rome, Italy: Food and Agriculture Organisation of the United Nations, 1998, vii; 31.

79. Clausen PH, Leendertz FH, Blankenburg A, et al. A drug incubation *Glossina* infectivity test (DIGIT) to assess the susceptibility of *Trypanosoma congolense* bloodstream forms to trypanocidal drugs (Xenodiagnosis). Acta Trop 1999; 72:111–117.

80. Delespaux V, Geysen D, Majiwa PAO, Geerts S. Identification of a genetic marker for isometamidium chloride resistance in *T. congolense*. Int J Parasitol 2005; 35:235–243.

81. Afework Y, Maser P, Etschmann B, et al. Rapid identification of isometamidium-resistant stocks of *Trypanosoma b. brucei* by PCR-RFLP. Parasitol Res 2006; 99:253–261.

82. Delespaux V, Chitanga S, Geysen D, et al. SSCP analysis of the P2 purine transporter TcoAT1 gene of *T. congolense* leads to a simple PCR-RFLP test allowing the rapid identification of diminazene resistant stocks. Acta Trop 2006; 100:96–102.

83. Geerts S, Ndung'u JM, Murilla GA, et al. In vivo tests for the detection of resistance to trypanocidal drugs: tests in mice and in ruminants. ICPTV Newslett 2000; 2:6–7.

84. Kaminsky R, Mäser P. Drug resistance in African trypanosomes. Curr Opin Anti-infect Invest Drugs 2000; 2:76–82.

85. Legros D, Evans S, Maiso F, et al. Risk factors for treatment failure after melarsoprol for *Trypanosoma brucei gambiense* trypanosomiasis in Uganda. Trans R Soc Trop Med Hyg 1999; 93: 439–442.

86. Stanghellini A, Josenando T. The situation of sleeping sickness in Angola: a calamity. Trop Med Int Health 2001; 6:330–334.

87. Brun R, Schumacher R, Schmid C, et al. The phenomenon of treatment failures in Human African Trypanosomiasis. Trop Med Int Health 2001; 6:906–914.

88. Jha TK, Sundar S, Thakur CP, et al. Miltefosine, an oral agent, for the treatment of Indian visceral leishmaniasis. N Engl J Med 1999; 341:1795–1800.

89. Sundar S. Drug resistance in Indian visceral leishmaniasis. [Erratum appears in Trop Med Int Health 2002; 7(3):293.] Trop Med Int Health 2002; 7:293–298.

90. Peters BS, Fish D, Golden R, et al. Visceral leishmaniasis in HIV infection and AIDS: clinical features and response to therapy. Q J Med 1990; 77:1101–1111.

91. Faraut-Gambarelli F, Piarroux R, Deniau M, et al. In vitro and in vivo resistance of *Leishmania infantum* to meglumine antimoniate: a study of 37 strains collected from patients with visceral leishmaniasis. Antimicrob Agents Chemother 1997; 41:827–830.

92. Ullman B, Carrero-Valenzuela E, Coons T. *Leishmania donovani*: isolation and characterization of sodium stibogluconate (Pentostam)-resistant cell lines. Exp Parasitol 1989; 69:157–163.

93. Grogl M, Thomason TN, Franke ED. Drug resistance in leishmaniasis: its implication in systemic chemotherapy of cutaneous and mucocutaneous disease. Am J Trop Med Hyg 1992; 47:117–126.

94. Wyllie S, Cunningham ML, Fairlamb AH, Dual action of antimonial drugs on thiol redox metabolism in the human pathogen *Leishmania donovani*. J Biol Chem 2004; 279:39925–39932.

95. Mookerjee BJ, Mookerjee A, Sen P, et al. Sodium antimony gluconate induces generation of reactive oxygen species and nitric oxide via phosphoinositide 3-kinase and mitogen-activated protein kinase activation in *Leishmania donovani*-infected macrophages, Antimicrob Agents Chemother 2006; 50:1788–1797.

96. Croft S L, Sundar S, Fairlamb AH. 2006. Drug resistance in leishmaniasis. Clin Microbiol Rev 2006; 19:111–126.

97. Decuypere S, Yardley V, De Doncker S, et al. A study of the mechanism of natural SbV resistance in Nepalese *Leishmania donovani* isolates based on gene expression analysis. Antimicrob Agents Chemother 2005; 49:4616–4621.

98. Laurent T, Rijal S, Yardley V, et al. Epidemiological dynamics of antimonial resistance in *Leishmania donovani*: genotyping reveals a polyclonal population structure among naturally-resistant clinical isolates from Nepal. Infect Genet Evol 2007; 7:206–212.

99. Croft SL, Yardley V, Kendrick H. Drug sensitivity of *Leishmania* species: some unresolved problems. Trans R Soc Trop Med Hyg 2002; 96:S127–S129.

100. Chapman WL, Jr., Hanson WL, Waits VB, Kinnamon KE. Antileishmanial activity of selected compounds in dogs experimentally infected with *Leishmania donovani*. Rev Inst Med Trop Sao Paulo 1979; 21:189–193.

101. Stauber LA. Characterization of strains of *Leishmania donovani*. Exp Parasitol 1966; 18:1–11.

102. Neal RA, Miles RA. Effect of sodium stibogluconate on infections of *Leishmania enriettii*, with observations on the interaction of drug and immune response. Ann Trop Med Parasitol 1977; 71:21–27.

103. Buffet PA, Sulahian A, Garin YJ, et al. Culture microtitration: a sensitive method for quantifying *Leishmania infantum* in tissues of infected mice. Antimicrob Agents Chemother 1995; 39:2167–2168.

104. Nicolas L, Prina E, Lang T, Milon G. Real-time PCR for detection and quantitation of leishmania in mouse tissues. J Clin Microbiol 2002; 40:1666–1669.

105. Wilson HR, Dieckmann BS, Childs GE. *Leishmania braziliensis* and *Leishmania mexicana*: experimental cutaneous infections in golden hamsters. Exp Parasitol 1979; 47:270–283.

106. Le Ray D, Afchain D, Jadin J, et al. Immunoelectrophoretic diagnosis of visceral leishmaniasis with the use of a hydrosoluble antigenic extract of *Leishmania donovani*. Preliminary results. Ann Soc Belg Med Trop 1973; 53:31–41.

107. Bodley AL, McGarry MW, Shapiro TA. Drug cytotoxicity assay for African trypanosomes and *Leishmania* species. J Infect Dis 1995; 172:1157–1159.

108. Carrio J, de Colmenares M, Riera C, et al. *Leishmania infantum*: stage-specific activity of pentavalent antimony related with the assay conditions. Exp Parasitol 2000; 95:209–214.

109. Di GC, Ridoux O, Delmas F, et al. Flow cytometric detection of *Leishmania* parasites in human monocyte-derived macrophages: application to antileishmanial-drug testing. Antimicrob Agents Chemother 2000; 44:3074–3078.

110. Neal RA, Croft SL. An in vitro system for determining the activity of compounds against the intracellular amastigote form of *Leishmania donovani*. J Antimicrob Chemother 1984; 14:463–476.

111. Yardley V, Ortuño N, Llanos-Cuentas A, et al. American tegumentary leishmaniasis: is antimonial treatment outcome related with parasite drug susceptibility? J Infect Dis. 2006; 194:1168–1175.

112. Rijal S, Yardley V, Chappuis F, et al. Antimonial treatment of visceral leishmaniasis: are current in vitro susceptibility assays adequate for prognosis of in vivo therapy outcome? Microbes Infect 2007; 9:529–535.

113. Zilberstein D, Shapira M. The role of pH and temperature in the development of *Leishmania* parasites. Annu Rev Microbiol 1994; 48:449–470.

114. Doyle PS, Engel JC, Pimenta PF, et al. *Leishmania donovani*: long-term culture of axenic amastigotes at 37 degrees C. Exp Parasitol 1991; 73:326–334.

115. Bates PA, Robertson CD, Tetley L, Coombs GH. Axenic cultivation and characterization of *Leishmania mexicana* amastigote-like forms. Parasitology 1992; 105:193–202.

116. Callahan HL, Portal AC, Devereaux R, Grogl M. An axenic amastigote system for drug screening. Antimicrob Agents Chemother 1997; 41:818–822.

117. Ephros M, Waldman E, Zilberstein D. Pentostam induces resistance to antimony and the preservative chlorocresol in *Leishmania donovani* promastigotes and axenically grown amastigotes. Antimicrob Agents Chemother 1997; 41:1064–1068.

118. Sereno D, Lemesre JL. Use of an enzymatic micromethod to quantify amastigote stage of *Leishmania amazonensis* in vitro. Parasitol Res 1997; 83:401–403.

119. Gupta N, Goyal N, Rastogi AK. In vitro cultivation and characterization of axenic amastigotes of *Leishmania*. Trends Parasitol 2001; 17:150–153.

120. Hill DR, Guerrant RL, Pearson RD, Hewlett EL. *Giardia lamblia* infection of suckling mice. J Infect Dis 1983; 147:217–221.

121. Boreham PF, Upcroft JA. The activity of azithromycin against stocks of *Giardia intestinalis* in vitro and in vivo. Trans R Soc Trop Med Hyg 1991; 85:620–621.

122. Belosevic M, Faubert GM, Maclean JD, et al. *Giardia lamblia* infections in Mongolian gerbils Meriones unguiculatus an animal model. J Infect Dis 1983; 147:222–226.

123. Clark CG, Diamond LS. Methods for cultivation of luminal parasitic protists of clinical importance. Clin Microbiol Rev 2002; 15:329–341.

124. Diamond LS. Axenic cultivation of Entamoeba histolytica: progress and problems. Arch Invest Med (Mex) 1980; 11:47–54.

125. Boreham PF, Phillips RE, Shepherd RW. Altered uptake of metronidazole in vitro by stocks of *Giardia intestinalis* with different drug sensitivities. Trans R Soc Trop Med Hyg 1988; 82:104–106.

126. Pearce DA, Reynoldson JA, Thompson RC. A comparison of two methods for assessing drug sensitivity in *Giardia duodenalis*. Appl Parasitol 1996; 37:111–116.

127. Upcroft JA, Campbell RW, Upcroft P. Quinacrine-resistant *Giardia duodenalis*. Parasitology 1996; 112:309–313.

128. Upcroft JA, Dunn LA, Wright JM et al. P. 5-Nitroimidazole drugs effective against metronidazole-resistant *Trichomonas vaginalis* and *Giardia duodenalis*. Antimicrob Agents Chemother 2006; 50:344–347.

129. Dunn LA, Andrews KT, McCarthy JS, et al. The activity of protease inhibitors against *Giardia duodenalis* and metronidazole-resistant *Trichomonas vaginalis*. Int J Antimicrob Agents 2007; 29:98–102.

130. Chavez B, Cedillo-Rivera R, Martinez-Palomo A. *Giardia lamblia* ultrastructural study of the in vitro effect of benzimidazoles. J Protozool 1992; 39:510–515.

131. Upcroft JA, Upcroft P. Two distinct varieties of *Giardia* in a mixed infection from a single human patient. J Eukaryot Microbiol 1994; 41:189–194.

132. Townson SM, Laqua H, Upcroft P, et al. Induction of metronidazole and furazolidone resistance in *Giardia*. Trans R Soc Trop Med Hyg 1992; 86:521–522.

133. Orozco E, de la Cruz Hernandez F, Rodriguez MA. Isolation and characterization of *Entamoeba histolytica* mutants resistant to emetine. Mol Biochem Parasitol 1985; 15:49–59.

134. Muller M, Meingassner JG, Miller WA, Ledger WJ. Three metronidazole-resistant strains of *Trichomonas vaginalis* from the United States. Am J Obstet Gynecol 1980; 138:808–812.

135. Gill JH, Redwin JM, Van WyK J.A, Lacey E. Avermectin inhibition of larval development in *Haemonchus contortus*: effects of ivermectin resistance. Int J Parasitol 1995; 25:463–470.

136. Lyndal-Murphy M. Anthelmintic resistance in sheep. Australian Standard Diagnostic Techniques for Animal Diseases. Australia: Standing Committee on Agriculture and Resource Management, 1992, pp. 1–17.

137. Coles GC, Bauer C, Borgsteede FHM, et al. World Association for the Advancement of Veterinary Parasitology (W.A.A.V.P.): methods for the detection of anthelmintic resistance in nematodes of veterinary importance. Vet Parasitol 1992; 44:35–44.

138. Martin PJ, Anderson N, Jarrett RG. Detecting benzimidazole resistance with faecal egg count reduction tests and in vitro assays. Aust Vet J 1989; 66:236–240.

139. Pook JF, Power ML, Sangster NC, et al. Evaluation of tests for anthelmintic resistance in cyathostomes. Vet Parasitol 2002; 106:331–343.

140. Kelly JD, Sangster NC, Porter CJ. Use of guinea pigs to assay anthelmintic resistance in ovine isolates of *Trichostrongylus colubriformis*. Res Vet Sci 1981; 30:131–137.

141. Conder GA, Thompson DP, Johnson SS. Demonstration of co-resistance of *Haemonchus contortus* to ivermectin and moxidectin. Vet Rec 1993; 132:651–652.

142. Lacey E, Snowdon KL. A routine diagnostic assay for the detection of benzimidazole resistance in parasitic nematodes using tritiated benzimidazole carbamates. Vet Parasitol 1988; 27:309–324.

143. Kwa MSG, Veenstra JG, Roos MH. Benzimidazole resistance in *Haemonchus contortus* is correlated with a conserved mutation at amino acid 200 in β-tubulin isotype 1. Mol Biochem Parasitol 1994; 63:299–303.

144. Kwa MSG, Veenstra JGH, Van Dijk M, Roos MH. β-Tubulin genes from the parasitic nematode *Haemonchus contortus* modulate drug resistance in *Caenorhabditis elegans*. J Mol Biol 1995; 246:500–510.

145. Elard L, Comes AM, Humbert JF. Sequences of β-tubulin cDNA from benzimidazole-susceptible and -resistant strains of *Teladorsagia circumcincta*, a nematode parasite of small ruminants. Mol Biochem Parasitol 1996; 79:249–253.

146. Elard L, Cabaret J, Humbert JF. PCR diagnosis of benzimidazole-susceptibility or -resistance in natural populations of the small ruminant parasite, *Teladorsagia circumcinta*. Vet Parasitol 1999; 80:231–237.
147. Thrusfield M. Veterinary Epidemiology, 2nd edition, Oxford: Blackwell, 1995.
148. von Samson-Himmelstjerna G, Blackhall, W. Will technology provide solutions for drug resistance in veterinary helminths? Vet Parasitol 2005; 132:223–239.
149. Dash KM, Hall E, Barger IA. The role of arithmetic and geometric mean worm egg counts in faecal egg count reduction tests and in monitoring strategic drenching programs in sheep. Aust Vet J 1988; 65:66–68.
150. Kerboeuf D, Hubert J. Changes in response of *Haemonchus contortus* eggs to the ovicidal activity of thiabendazole during the course of infection. Ann Rech Vet 1987; 18: 365–370.
151. Hendrikx WML. The influence of cryopreservation on a benzimidazole-resistant isolate of *Haemonchus contortus* conditioned for inhibited development. Parasitol Res 1988; 74:569–573.
152. Gassenbeek CPH, Moll L, Cornelissen JBWJ, et al. An experimental study on triclabendazole resistance of *Fasciola hepatica* in sheep. Vet Parasitol 2001; 95:37–43.
153. Magnussen P. Treatment and re-treatment strategies for schistosomiasis control in different epidemiological settings: a review of 10 years' experiences. Acta Trop 2003; 86:243–254.
154. WHO. Prevention and control of schistosomiasis and soil-transmitted helminthiasis. World Health Organ Tech Rep Ser 2002; 912:i–vi, 1–57.
155. Cioli D, Pica-Mattoccia L. Praziquantel. Parasitol Res 2003; 90:S3–S9.
156. Bennett JL, Day T, Liang F, et al. The development of resistance to anthelmintics: a perspective with an emphasis on the antischistosomal drug praziquantel. Exp Parasitol 1997; 87:260–267.

Chapter 85
Genotypic Drug Resistance Assays

A. Huletsky and M.G. Bergeron

1 Introduction

Antimicrobial resistance has become a major public health threat worldwide. Some hospital-acquired pathogens are becoming multiple resistant or totally resistant to antimicrobials. Known examples include vancomycin-resistant *Enterococcus faecium* and *E. faecalis* (VRE), methicillin-resistant *Staphylococcus aureus* (MRSA), vancomycin-intermediate and -resistant *S. aureus* (VISA and VRSA), and extended-spectrum β-lactamases (ESBL) producing Enterobacteriaceae (1). In the community, the prevalence of multidrug resistance in *Streptococcus pneumoniae* is increasing in some countries and includes resistance to β-lactams (intermediate and high-level resistance to penicillin and cross-resistance to cephalosporins), the macrolides and, more recently, the fluoroquinolones (2). Furthermore, virulent strains of MRSA that differ from the hospital strains have emerged in the communities of several countries (3). Another major public health problem is the increasing incidence of multidrug-resistant *Mycobacterium tuberculosis* (4). Physicians practicing in both hospitals and the community must treat infections caused by multiresistant organisms, and new, emerging antimicrobial resistances are becoming more complex to detect (5). With the limited number of antimicrobial agents available to treat the infections caused by multidrug-resistant organisms, the need for rapid and reliable susceptibility testing methods or alternative resistance testing methods for detection of antimicrobial resistance becomes increasingly important. Conventional phenotypic culture-based susceptibility test results are usually obtained in 24–48 h or more after a bacterial culture has been isolated. Moreover, susceptibility tests are not always accurate in difficult-to-detect emerging antimicrobial resistance and often more than one method is needed to obtain an accurate susceptibility profile. The lack of accurate and

timely susceptibility data by the microbiology laboratory has consequences on antibiotic usage and prescription. Patients have to be treated empirically and often with broad-spectrum antibiotics, which results in increased resistance rates and healthcare costs (6). The advances in our understanding of the genetic mechanisms of antimicrobial resistance and the progress in sample preparation, nucleic acid–based amplification, and sensitive nucleic acid detection have allowed the development of genotypic methods for rapid detection of antimicrobial resistance. While most genotypic resistance tests are presently performed with pure bacterial culture which requires at least 18–24 h, it is now possible to identify a microorganism and its resistance to antimicrobial agents directly from clinical specimens in 1 h (7, 8). Some genotypic drug resistance assays are increasingly used in the clinical settings, providing more accurate and rapid resistance testing.

The purpose of this review is to describe the mechanisms of antimicrobial resistance and to present some genotypic drug resistance assays used to detect antimicrobial resistance. Genotypic drug resistance assays that are increasingly used in the clinical microbiology laboratory and their applications in the clinical settings will be further discussed.

2 Mechanisms of Resistance to Antimicrobial Agents

Different strategies have been developed by bacteria to evade the action of the antimicrobial agents. In general, antimicrobial resistance results from (a) production of enzymes that inactivate the antimicrobial agent, (b) acquisition of exogenous resistance genes that are not inhibited by the antimicrobial agent, (c) reduced uptake of the antimicrobial agent, (d) active efflux of the antimicrobial agent, (e) mutation of cellular target genes reducing the binding of the antimicrobial agent, or (f) overproduction of the target of the antimicrobial agent. The major resistance mechanisms for the important antimicrobial classes will be briefly described.

M.G. Bergeron (✉)
Centre de Recherche en Infectiologie of Université Laval,
Québec City, QC, Canada
michel.g.bergeron@crchul.ulaval.ca

D.L. Mayers (ed.), *Antimicrobial Drug Resistance*,
DOI 10.1007/978-1-60327-595-8_85, © Humana Press, a part of Springer Science+Business Media, LLC 2009

2.1 Resistance to Aminoglycosides

The aminoglycosides constitute a large family of antimi-crobials that inhibit the translation process by binding to the bacterial 16S rRNA of the 30S ribosomal subunit. Four mechanisms of resistance to aminoglycosides have been described: (a) alterations in the ribosomal target site (*rrs* gene encoding 16S rRNA and *rpsL* gene encoding the S12 protein) that prevent binding, especially in streptomycin-resistant *M. tuberculosis* (9), (b) decreased cell membrane permeability, (c) expulsion by efflux pumps, and (d) enzy-matic inactivation by aminoglycoside-modifying enzymes (AMEs). Inactivation by AMEs is the most important in terms of frequency and level of resistance (10). Aminoglycosides are modified by three types of enzymes, classified as aminoglycoside phosphotransferases (APHs), aminoglyco-side adenylases (ANTs), and aminoglycoside acetyltrans-ferases (AACs). These enzymes covalently modify specific amino or hydroxyl groups, resulting in aminoglycosides that bind poorly to the target ribosomes. Within each class, there are enzymes with different, specific sites of modification. More than 50 AMEs have been described (10).

2.2 Resistance to β-Lactams

The β-lactams are a structurally diverse group of antimicro-bials that interfere with the synthesis of the bacterial cell wall as a result of their interaction with penicillin-binding proteins (PBPs). Resistance to β-lactam antibiotics can be caused by four different mechanisms: (a) acquisition or hyperexpression of β-lactamases, which is considered the most common resistance mechanism, (b) alteration, overex-pression, or acquisition of PBPs, (c) permeability change in the outer membrane, and (d) active efflux of the antimicro-bial (11). β-Lactamases can be grouped on the basis of either their molecular structure or function. Four different molecu-lar classes of β-lactamases have been defined on the basis of the similarities in amino acid sequences. Classes A, B, and C are serine β-lactamases, whereas class B are metallo-β-lactamases (12).

2.3 Resistance to Glycopeptides

Glycopeptide antibiotics such as vancomycin and teicopla-nin inhibit cell wall synthesis by binding to the terminal D-alanyl-D-alanine of the pentapeptide peptidoglycan pre-cursor molecule. This binding prevents the cross-linking of peptidoglycan precursors necessary for the formation of cell wall. Acquired resistance to vancomycin in Gram-positive

bacteria differs depending on the bacterial species in which they have been described: (a) altered precursor formation in enterococci and staphylococci, (b) mutational cell wall changes in staphylococci, and (c) tolerance in *S. pneumoniae* (1, 13, 14). To date, six gene clusters conferring different glycopeptide resistance phenotypes have been described in enterococci; five are acquired (*vanA*, *vanB*, *vanD*, *vanE*, and *vanG*), while the sixth (*vanC*) is intrinsic to *E. gallinarum*, *E. casseliflavus*, and *E. flavescens* (13). The *vanA*, *vanB*, and *vanD* genes encode D-alanine-D-lactate ligases, whereas the *vanC*, *vanE*, and *vanG* genes encode D-alanine-D-serine ligases. The *vanA* gene has been recently described in dif-ferent glycopeptide-resistant *S. aureus* isolates in the United States (15–17).

2.4 Resistance to Macrolides, Lincosamides, and Streptogramins

Macrolides, lincosamides, and streptogramins (A and B) inhibit protein synthesis by reversibly binding to the pepti-dyl–tRNA binding region of the 50S ribosomal subunit, stimulating dissociation of the peptidyl–tRNA molecule from the ribosome during elongation (18). Three different mechanisms of macrolide, lincosamide, and streptogramin resistance have been described: (a) alterations in the ribo-somal target site by mutations in chromosomal genes (e.g., *rrl* gene encoding 23S rRNA) or mediated by several differ-ent acquired erythromycin ribosomal methylases (*erm*) that methylate the same adenine residue in 23S rRNA resulting in resistance against macrolides, lincosamides, and strepto-gramin B antibiotics (MLS$_B$) (alteration in the target site has not been described for streptogramin A resistance), (b) active efflux of the antimicrobial (e.g., *mef(A)* conferring macrolide resistance, *vga(A)* conferring streptogramin A resistance, and *msr(A)* conferring both macrolide and streptogramin B resistance), and (c) drug inactivation by several different enzymes including esterases (*ere*), phophorylases (*mph*), lyases (*vgb*), and transferases (*vat*) (19, 20).

2.5 Resistance to Quinolones

Quinolones interact with two type-2 topoisomerases, DNA gyrase and topoisomerase IV, both of which are essential for bacterial DNA replication. Inhibition appears to occur by interaction of the drug with a complex composed of DNA and either of these target enzymes. The GyrA and GyrB sub-units of DNA gyrase are respectively homologs with ParC and ParE subunits of topoisomerase IV. Quinolone resistance results mostly from chromosomal mutations in the drug target and alterations of drug access to target enzymes, either by altered permeation mechanism or increased drug efflux (21). Resistance may also be mediated by plasmid-encoded Qnr proteins that protect DNA from quinolone binding, compromising efficacy (22).

2.6 Resistance to Trimethoprim–Sulfamethoxazole

Trimethoprim and sulfonamide are inhibitors of two enzymes (dihydrofolate reductase (DHFR) and dihydropteroic acid synthase (DHPS, respectively) that act sequentially in the formation of tetrahydrofolate (THF). Resistance to trimethoprim can be conferred by promoter mutations leading to overproduction of DHFR, point mutations within the *dhfr* genes, or both mechanisms. More common is the acquisition of low-affinity *dhfr* genes, of which approximatley 20 have been described (23). Resistance to sulfonamides can be caused by point mutations in chromosomal *dhps* genes and by acquisition of different low-affinity *dhps* genes (23).

2.7 Resistance to Tetracyclines

The tetracyclines are a group of bacteriostatic antibiotics that act by binding reversibly to the 16S rRNA near the ribosomal acceptor A site, inhibiting the attachment of aminoacyl-tRNA to this site, thereby preventing the elongation step of protein synthesis (24). Tetracycline resistance is caused by four mechanisms: (a) active efflux which keeps tetracycline out of the cytoplasm, (b) inactivation of the tetracycline molecules, (c) rRNA mutations which prevents tetracycline from binding to the ribosome, and (d) ribosomal protection which prevents tetracycline from binding to the ribosome (25).

2.8 Resistance to Chloramphenicol

Chloramphenicol binds to the 50S ribosomal subunit and inhibits prokaryotic peptidyltranferase. The most common mechanism of resistance to chloramphenicol is the production of chloramphenicol acetyltransferases (CATs) which inactivate the antibiotic. A large number of CAT genes have been reported, and these determinants generally confer high levels of resistance to chloramphenicol (26). Resistance to chloramphenicol can also be caused by target site mutations, permeability barriers, phosphotransferase inactivation, and active efflux (27).

2.9 Resistance to Linezolid

Linezolid, an oxazolidinone antimicrobial, inhibits bacterial protein synthesis by binding to the domain V region of the 23S rRNA (28). Resistance to linezolid is principally mediated by a G2576U single nucleotide mutation in the central region of domain V of one or more alleles of the *rrl* gene encoding 23S rRNA (29). Mutations in the *rplD* gene encoding the riboprotein L4 have also been described (30).

2.10 Resistance to Rifampin

Rifampin acts by binding to the β subunit of the bacterial DNA-dependent RNA polymerase encoded by the *rpoB* gene resulting in transcription inhibition (31). Resistance to rifampin is conferred by chromosomal mutations or short deletions and insertions in the central region of the *rpoB* gene (32).

2.11 Resistance to Isoniazid

Isoniazid is a synthetic antimicrobial agent used for the treatment of infections caused by *M. tuberculosis* complex. The precise mechanism of action is still unclear but the target seems to be inhibition of mycolic acid synthesis (31). Resistance to isoniazid may result from mutations in five different genes: (a) the *katG* gene encoding the catalase-peroxidase, (b) the *inhA* gene encoding an enoyl reductase, (c) the *ahpC* gene encoding an alkyl hydroperoxide reductase subunit, (d) the *kasA* gene encoding a putative β-ketoacyl acyl carrier protein synthase, and (e) the *ndh* gene encoding a NAD deshydrogenase (31–33).

2.12 Resistance to Ethambutol

Ethambutol is a synthetic antituberculosis agent. This compound inhibits outer mycobacterial membrane formation by inhibiting the arabinosyltransferase (31). Resistance to ethambutol often results from mutations in the *embB* encoding the arabinosyltransferase (34).

2.13 Resistance to Pyrazinamide

Pyrazinamide, the pyrazine analog of nicotinamide, is a prodrug for *M. tuberculosis*, which requires conversion to the active pyrazinoic acid by the bacterial pyrazinamidase. Resistance to pyrazinamide is usually caused by mutations in the *pncA* gene encoding the pyrazinamidase or in the putative regulatory region upstream of the gene (20).

3 Methods to Detect Resistance

The clinical microbiology laboratory has the responsibility to provide reliable and accurate susceptibility data of significant bacterial isolates in a time frame that is useful to the clinicians to prescribe the most appropriate antimicrobial agent (least expensive and/or narrower spectrum) for a particular infection, and when possible, to reduce the development of resistance. Determining the antimicrobial susceptibility profile of a pathogen is considered as important as the identification of the pathogen involved in the infection itself. This is becoming even more essential in an era of increasing antimicrobial resistance in which treatment options are limited to newer, more costly antimicrobial agents. The antimicrobial susceptibility of a clinical isolate measured by conventional phenotypic susceptibility methods is presently the parameter provided to clinicians. However, an isolate that is defined as sensitive to an antimicrobial agent is not always treated with success, but most resistant isolates result in treatment failure. Therefore, it is becoming important to develop methods that will allow detection of resistance mechanisms and to better understand which resistance mechanisms are the most difficult to detect (35). During the past years, optimization of conventional susceptibility tests and development of novel phenotypic methods for resistance mechanisms that are difficult to detect have been carried out (36). As an alternative or complement to these phenotypic tests, several genotypic drug resistance assays have been developed and are increasingly used in the clinical microbiology laboratory, offering rapid, accurate, and sensitive methods to detect the presence of antimicrobial resistance.

3.1 Phenotypic Assays/Susceptibility Tests (Culture)

Conventional culture-based susceptibility methods measure the in vitro phenotypic expression of resistance which can be interpreted quantitatively as the minimum inhibitory concentration (MIC) or interpreted qualitatively as sensitive, intermediate, or resistant. MIC is defined as the lowest concentration of an antimicrobial agent that inhibits the visible growth of an organism over a defined interval. Several methods for routine antimicrobial susceptibility testing are used in the clinical microbiology laboratory. The phenotypic resistance can be quantitatively reported as the MIC for dilution methods (broth and agar dilution) and antibiotic gradient diffusion (e.g., Etest), or may be expressed qualitatively with the disk diffusion method (e.g., Bauer–Kirby

disk diffusion). Broth microdilution methods have been adapted to automated instrument-based systems facilitating the reading and interpretation of results. These instruments can provide both species identification and antibiotic susceptibility results within 24–48 h. The systems currently available include the Microscan WalkAway system (Siemens Healthcare Diagnostics, Deerfield, IL, USA), the Vitek and Vitek 2 systems (bioMérieux, Marcy l'Étoile, France), and the Phoenix system (BD Diagnostic Systems, Sparks, MD, USA). Detailed descriptions as well as advantages and limitations of these systems can be found in a recent review (37).

Regardless of the microorganism and antibiotic tested as well as the method used, the results obtained by in vitro antibiotic susceptibility testing can vary greatly depending on the culture medium, inoculums, concentration of the organism tested, and the conditions of incubation (duration, temperature, atmosphere). In North America, the Clinical and Laboratory Standards Institute (CLSI, formerly NCCLS) publications provide up-to-date guidelines on methodologies and standardized control procedures to ensure accuracy and reproducibility within and between laboratories (38, 39). Different national standardized methods may be used outside of North America including those published by the British Society of Antimicrobial Chemotherapy (BSAC) in the United Kingdom and other equivalents in Europe (40) (see Sect. 3.2.4).

3.2 Special Phenotypic Susceptibility Methods

Conventional susceptibility testing methods or automated systems are not reliable for certain fastidious organisms or organisms with difficult-to-detect resistance mechanisms (36). Fastidious organisms (e.g. *Mycobacterium* species, *Streptococcus* species including *S. pneumoniae*, *Haemophilus* species, *N. gonorrhoeae*, and anaerobic bacteria) require special growth media and conditions, and certain organisms with inducible resistance or subtle change in MICs (at or near the breakpoint) (e.g. MRSA, VRE, VISA, and ESBL-producing Enterobacteriaceae) require special phenotypic testing methods for detection of antimicrobial resistance. A complete description of susceptibility test methods used for these fastidious organisms and difficult-to-detect resistance mechanisms can be found in recent reviews (31, 36, 41–43). Some examples of phenotypic methods used for difficult-to-detect resistance are further described.

3.2.1 Detection of Oxacillin Resistance in Staphylococci

At least three different resistance mechanisms contribute to oxacillin resistance in *S. aureus*: (a) production of an additional PBP (PBP 2a, also called PBP 2′) encoded by the chromosomal *mecA* gene, (b) inactivation of the drug by increased production of β-lactamase which results in low level or borderline resistance (BORSA), and (c) production of modified intrinsic PBPs (MOD-SA) with altered affinity for the drug which also results in borderline resistance (43). It is important to differentiate isolates that have *mecA*-positive resistance from isolates that have the two other types of resistance because *mecA* gene confers resistance to all β-lactams and isolates carrying *mecA* are usually multidrug resistant which is not the case for the two other types of resistance. Some isolates carrying *mecA* are either homogeneous or heterogeneous in their expression of resistance. Contrary to isolates with homogeneous resistance, heterogeneous resistance results in MICs that appear to be borderline and can be confused with BORSA or MOD-SA isolates for which MICs are also borderline. BORSA resistance can usually be distinguished from *mecA* resistance by the addition of a β-lactamase inhibitor (e.g., clavulanic acid) to the oxacillin MIC test, which lowers the MIC by two dilutions or more (43). The presence of *mecA*-positive *S. aureus* isolates can be detected simply and reliably by the oxacillin agar screen test (38, 39). Usually, BORSA isolates do not grow on the agar screen plate; however, MOD-SA may grow, depending on the oxacillin MIC of the strain. Several rapid phenotypic methods that detect oxacillin resistance in staphylococci from culture are commercially available. They included latex agglutination tests that detect the presence of PBP 2a: such as the MRSA–Screen test (Denka Seiken Co., Ltd, Tokyo, Japan), the PBP 2′ latex agglutination test (Oxoid Limited, Basingstoke, UK), and the Mastalex-MRSA test (Mast Diagnostics, Bootle, UK). These methods are increasingly used in the clinical microbiology laboratory to detect MRSA.

3.2.2 Detection of Vancomycin Resistance in Enterococci and Staphylococci

Among the six glycopeptide resistance phenotypes described to date in enterococci (13) (see Sect. 2), three are most commonly found in the clinical settings: (a) high-level vancomycin resistance with teicoplanin resistance (VanA phenotype), (b) moderate to high-level vancomycin resistance, usually without teicoplanin resistance (VanB phenotype), and (c) intrinsic low-level resistance associated with *Enterococcus gallinarum*, *E. casseliflavus*, and *E. flavescens* (VanC phenotype) (43). Standard culture-based methods commonly used in clinical laboratories sometimes fail to detect low-level vancomycin resistance (VanB and VanC phenotypes) in certain enterococcal strains (38, 43). The use of the vancomycin agar screening test to detect low-level vancomycin resistance in enterococci is recommended by the CLSI since 1993 (38, 39). However, from an infection control perspective, it is important to distinguish the *vanC*-containing enterococcal species that can grow on the agar screening plate from the clinically important VRE, which include *E. faecalis* and *E. faecium* (38, 43) (see Sect. 3.3.3).

Strains of VISA are difficult to detect using disk diffusion procedures and some automated systems (44). The mechanism of resistance in these strains is still unknown. However, it has been shown that the cooperative effect of cell wall clogging and thickening through alteration of the cell wall metabolic pathway can prevent vancomycin to reach its target (45, 46). Laboratories that routinely use disk diffusion or an automated system for staphylococcal susceptibility testing may use vancomycin agar screen tests to screen *S. aureus* isolates for reduced susceptibility to vancomycin (38, 39). The MIC for vancomycin must then be determined with a quantitative method including broth dilution, agar dilution, or agar gradient (Etest). Vancomycin-resistant *S. aureus* (VRSA) strains containing the *vanA* gene are usually detected reliably with the broth microdilution method. However, the use of the vancomycin agar screening test is recommended when other MIC methods have not been validated to detect VRSA (38).

3.2.3 Detection of Enzyme-Mediated Resistance

For many organisms producing enzyme-mediated resistance, it can be quicker and more reliable to detect the enzyme conferring resistance. In the clinical laboratory, these tests are limited for detecting β-lactamase activity (43). Three direct β-lactamase assays, the acidimetric, iodometric, and chromogenic methods, have been used for detection of β-lactamase; however, the chromogenic method is the most reliable. The chromogenic cephalosporin nitrocefin can be used in a test tube, but most laboratories use a paper disk impregnated with the nitrocefin, which is commercially available (e.g., Cefinase, Becton-Dickinson Microbiology Systems, Cockeysville, MD, USA). A color change indicates the destruction of the nitrocefin substrate by a β-lactamase. This test is useful for detecting β-lactamase produced by enterococci, staphylococci, *Bacteroides* sp., *H. influenzae*, *M. catarrhalis*, and *N. gonorrhoeae*.

3.2.4 Clinical Significance of Breakpoints

The goal of antimicrobial susceptibility testing is to predict the clinical outcome by classifying a bacterial strain into clinically relevant categories (i.e., susceptible, intermediate, or resistant) on the basis of established breakpoints based on MIC. A breakpoint for an antibiotic is usually selected as the therapeutic concentration in blood that can be readily achieved with usual dosing regimens, but this is not easily determined. Depending on the approach taken, up to four sources of data can be examined in establishing MIC breakpoints used to interpret antimicrobial susceptibility tests: (a) MIC distributions, (b) pharmacokinetics and pharmacodynamics, (c) clinical and bacteriological response rates, and

(d) zone diameter distributions for disk diffusion methods (47). Breakpoints must be periodically re-evaluated following changes in bacterial resistance, susceptibility test methods, or antibiotic regimens. However, MIC measurements are influenced in vitro by a number of variables including the composition of the test medium, the inoculum size, the duration of incubation, and the presence of resistant subpopulations of the organisms (48). Moreover, the condition tested in vitro for determining MIC cannot mimic other factors that can influence the in vivo antimicrobial activity including sub-MIC effects, postantibiotic effects, protein binding, variations in redox potential at sites of infection, and differences in drug levels in blood and at the site of infection (48). Nevertheless, when the MIC is determined under standardized condition, it provides a convenient reference point for the setting of breakpoints for predicting the efficacy in vivo.

The interpretative breakpoints assigned to an antimicrobial agent can have a significant impact on the prescribing of that drug for empiric therapy by influencing the resistance rates measured at the local, regional, national, or international level (49). In North America, the CLSI has the responsibility to establish breakpoints. However, different countries have established different breakpoints to define resistance (40) (see Sect. 3.1). This difference may be related to different dosages or administration intervals or can result from technical aspects such as different susceptibility test media and test conditions (48). Moreover, some countries may be more or less conservative in determining susceptibility. Therefore, it is sometimes confusing to compare resistance rates among countries if different methods have been used. In Europe, efforts have been made to harmonize susceptibility methods and MIC breakpoints (50).

3.3 Genotypic Assays

Phenotypic methods for susceptibility testing are usually simple, and automated systems have greatly facilitated the susceptibility testing procedures and data analysis (37). Even though incubation time to obtain susceptibility data is reduced to 3–5 h with some automated systems, or shorter (15 min) with special susceptibility tests (e.g. MRSA screen test), all the phenotypic susceptibility methods require bacterial isolation, and hence the results are not available until 2 days or more after a treatment is started. Several of the presently performed susceptibility tests are highly dependant on experimental conditions, and special phenotypic tests must often be performed to obtain an accurate susceptibility profile. Moreover, there is presently no international agreement on susceptibility methods and interpretation of breakpoints in antimicrobial susceptibility testing (see Sects. 3.1 and 3.2.4).

There are several advantages of using genotypic methods for resistance testing compared to conventional susceptibility methods (51): (a) detection of resistance genes is more accurate for detection of isolates with difficult-to-detect resistance profiles (MICs at or near the breakpoint of inducible resistance) since it does not depend on the variable gene expression under laboratory conditions (36); (b) genotypic tests provide resistance profiles rapidly since they can be performed directly from clinical specimens, which is particularly important not only for organisms that cannot be cultured, are not easily cultured, or for slow-growing organisms, but also to choose the most appropriate therapy early in the course of disease before cultures are positive; (c) genotypic tests may diminish the biohazard risk associated with the propagation of a microorganism by culture; (d) genotypic tests are a powerful tool for epidemiological study of antimicrobial resistance in a hospital or the community by providing an immediate insight into the genetic mechanism underlying the resistance phenotype; and (e) genotypic tests can be used as a gold standard for evaluating new, improved susceptibility methods for testing clinical isolates with difficult-to-detect resistance profiles.

With the progress in the understanding of antimicrobial resistance mechanisms and the increasing number of resistance gene sequences available in public databases (52), several genotypic assays have been developed for detection of bacterial genes and mutations associated with resistance. Table 1 lists the common antibiotic resistance genes for which genotypic resistance assays have been developed. Some recent reviews provide more details on several genotypic resistance assays (51, 273–275). Some genotypic assays are commercially available but most of them can be used in life science research only; they cannot be used for diagnostic applications (Table 2). Indeed, there are presently few commercialized genotypic resistance tests approved by the US Food and Drug Administration (FDA) for diagnostic applications (see Sect. 3.3.2).

Most genotypic resistance assays developed rely on amplification of a DNA segment containing a part of or the entire resistance gene, or the part of an intrinsic bacterial gene harboring the mutations associated with resistance. Amplification techniques used for genotypic testing include nucleic acid target amplification (e.g., polymerase chain reaction (PCR), strand displacement amplification, self-sustaining sequence replication, transcription-mediated amplification, nucleic-acid sequence–based amplification (NASBA)), probe amplification (e.g., ligase chain reaction and Qβ replicase amplification), and signal amplification (e.g., branched-probe (bDNA) assay) (275). The amplification product or amplicon can be detected by different methods; the most common are gel electrophoresis methods, probe hybridization assays, restriction fragment length polymorphism (RFLP) analysis, or DNA

Table 1 Common resistance genes detected by genotypic methods

Antimicrobial agent	Gene (reference)
Aminoglycosides	*aac(3)-Ia* (53–55), *aac(3)-Ib* (54), *aac(3)-IIa* (53, 54), *aac(3)-IIb* (54), *aac(6′)-aph(2″)* (56–64), *aac(6′)-IIa* (54), *aac(6′)-Ib* (55, 65), *ant(2″)-Ia* (55, 66), *ant(4′)-Ia* (57, 60, 62–64, 67), *aph(3′)-Ia* (55), *aph(3′)-IIIa* (55–57, 60, 62–64, 67, 68), *aph(3′)-VIa* (55, 69)
Streptomycin	*rpsL*[a] (70–74), *rrs*[a] (72, 73, 75), *ant(3″)-Ia* (76), *ant(6)-Ia* (57, 76)
β-Lactams	blaOXA-type (77–81), blaSHV-type (77, 82–86), blaTEM-type (77, 80, 83, 87–89), blaCTX-M-type (81, 83, 84, 90–94), blaAmpC-type (78, 95–98), blaIMP (81, 88, 99–106), blaVIM (78, 81, 102, 104, 105, 107, 108), *blaZ* (57, 109), *mecA* (56, 57, 109–151), SCC*mec/orfX* junction (8), *pbp1a*[a] (152–154), *pbp2b*[a] (152, 153, 155–158), *pbp2x*[a] (152, 153)
Macrolides, lincosamides, streptogramin B	*erm(A)* (57–59, 68, 159, 160), *erm(B)* (57, 58, 68, 159–161), *erm(C)* (57–59, 68, 162)
Macrolides, streptogramin B	*msr(A)* (57, 58, 159, 162)
Macrolides	*mef(A)* (57, 68, 161, 163)
Streptogramin A	*vga(A)* (164, 165), *vga(B)* (164), *vat(A)* (57, 59, 164), *vat(B)* (57, 59, 164–166), *vat(C)* (57, 59, 164), *vat(D)* (57, 164–168), *vat(E)* (57, 164, 168)
Streptogramin B	*vgb(A)* (57, 164, 167), *vgb(B)* (57, 164)
Linezolid	*rrl*[a] (169–171)
Quinolones	*gyrA*[a] (56, 71, 72, 110, 172–199), *gyrB*[a] (56, 71, 72, 174, 176, 178, 179, 183, 185, 186, 190, 192, 193, 198), *parC*[a] *(grlA)* (56, 110, 172, 174–176, 179, 182–186, 190–194, 196, 198, 200, 201), *parE*[a] *(grlB)* (56, 110, 174–176, 179, 183–186, 190–193, 198)
Chloramphenicol	*cat1* (66), *cat2* (66), *catP* (57, 202), *catQ* (57, 202), *cat*$_{pC194}$ (57, 68, 202), *cat*$_{pC221}$ (57, 202), *florR* (66, 80, 88)
Ethambutol	*embB*[a] (71, 73, 74, 203–206)
Pyrazinamide	*pncA*[a] (71, 74, 199, 207–210)
Rifampin	*rpoB*[a] (56, 71–74, 205, 210–237)
Isoniazid	*katG*[a] (71, 72, 74, 205, 216, 218, 230, 231, 233–241), *inhA*[a] (73, 217, 218, 230–233, 236, 239, 241)
Vancomycin	*vanA* (57, 242–255), *vanB* (57, 242–246, 248–250, 252–255), *vanC* (57, 242, 243, 245, 246, 249, 250), *vanD* (57, 250, 252, 256), *vanE* (57, 252, 257), *vanG* (57, 252, 258)
Tetracycline	*tet(B)* (88, 259–262), *tet(K)* (57, 59, 259–261, 263, 264), *tet(L)* (259, 261, 263, 264), *tet(M)* (57, 59, 68, 259–265), *tet(O)* (259–265)
Sulfonamides	*sul1* (66, 88, 266–268), *sul2* (66, 88, 267, 268), *sul3* (267, 268)
Trimethoprim	*dhfrIa* (23, 66, 88, 268–270), *dhfrIb* (23, 88, 269, 270), *dhfrV* (23, 268–270), *dhfrVI* (23, 269, 270), *dhfrVII* (23, 268–270), *dhfrVIII* (23, 269–271), *dhfrXII* (268–270), *dhfrXV* (272), *dhfrXVII* (268)

[a]Nucleotide mutations conferring resistance are usually detected in these genes

sequencing (275). PCR amplification is the most commonly used nucleic acid amplification technique for the detection of antimicrobial resistance genes. However, the combination of PCR amplification with post-PCR amplicon detection called "conventional PCR" has found limited acceptance for diagnostic laboratory testing due to the time-consuming nature of these post-PCR detection approaches and the problem of carry-over contaminations (276). The real-time PCR technology has found wider acceptance for PCR genotypic resistance methods in routine microbiology laboratories because this closed-tube amplification process, which is monitored in real time by using fluorescence techniques, is fast owing to ultrarapid thermal cycling and easy to perform, while the risk of carryover is minimized (277). A variety of real-time PCR assays have been developed for detection of antibiotic resistance genes and mutations (Table 1).

However, real-time PCR technology is limited by the number of genetic targets that can be simultaneously detected because of the restricted number of fluorophores that can be discriminated by the optical detection systems. The microarray technology is one of the most promising tools that allow detection of the multiple genes and mutations associated with

resistance in a single assay. Microarrays are capable of analyzing hundreds to thousands of different targets simultaneously in a relatively short period of time (56). It also offers the possibility of multiple hybridization on oligonucleotide probes either directly extracted from a specimen or, more often, generated by an amplification step. Several oligonucleotide microarrays, combined or not with multiplex amplification, have been developed to detect multiple antibiotic resistance genes and mutations (56, 57, 87, 88, 110, 159, 172–175, 207, 211–219, 278, 279) (Table 1). In the next section, some genotypic resistance assays that are increasingly used in the clinical microbiology laboratories are further described.

3.3.1 Genotypic Detection of Drug-Resistant *Mycobacterium tuberculosis*

The increasing incidence of multidrug-resistant tuberculosis (MDR-TB) is a serious global health problem causing an important rise in morbidity and mortality (4). The rapid identification of MDR-TB is essential to improve TB treatment, prevention, and control (280). However, because

Table 2. Commercial genotypic resistance drug assays

Antimicrobial agent and gene	Organism	Molecular method	Manufacturer
Glycopeptides			
$vanA + vanB + vanB2/3$	Enterococci[c]	Real-time PCR	LightCycler VRE (Roche)
$vanA + vanB$	Enterococci[c]	Real-time PCR	BD GeneOhm VanR[b] (BD Diagnostics-GeneOhm)
$vanA + vanB$	Enterococci[c]	Real-time PCR	Xpert $vanA/vanB$[b] (Cepheid)
$vanA + vanB$	Enterococci[c] + S. aureus[c]	DNA probe-based hybridization	$vanA/vanB$ EVIGENE (AdvanDX)
$vanA + vanB + vanC1 + vanC2/C3$ + 23S rDNA[d]	E. faecalis + E. faecium + E. gallinarum + E. casseliflavus	PCR-based reverse hybridization DNA strip assay	GenoType Enterococcus (Hain Lifescience)
β-Lactams			
$mecA$	Staphylococci[c]	Real-time PCR	LightCycler MRSA (Roche)
$mecA$	S. aureus[c]	Real-time PCR	Onar MRSA screen (Minerva Biolabs)
$mecA$	Staphylococci[c]	DNA probe-based hybridization	$mecA$ EVIGENE (AdvanDX)
$mecA$	S. aureus[c]	Real-time PCR	LightCycler SeptiFast MecA Test[b] (Roche)
$mecA$ + 23S rDNA[d]	S. aureus + S. epidermidis	PCR-based reverse hybridization DNA strip assay	GenoType MRSA (Hain Lifescience)
$mecA$ + 23S rDNA[d]	S. aureus + S. haemolyticus + S. epidermidis + S. hominis + S. warneri + S. simulans		GenoType Staphylococcus (Hain LifeScience)
$orfX$[d]/SCCmec	S. aureus	PCR-based reverse hybridization DNA strip assay	GenoType MRSA Direct[b], GenoQuick MRSA[b] (Hain Lifescience)
$orfX$[d]/SCCmec	S. aureus	Real-time PCR	BD GeneOhm MRSA[a, b] (BD Diagnostics-GeneOhm)
$orfX$[d]/SCCmec + nuc[d]	S. aureus	Real-time PCR	BD GeneOhm StaphSR[a] (BD Diagnostics-GeneOhm)
$orfX$[d]/SCCmec	S. aureus	Real-time PCR	Xpert MRSA[a, b] (Cepheid)
$orfX$[d]/SCCmec + $mecA$ + spa[d]	S. aureus	Real-time PCR	Xpert MRSA/SA SSTI[a, b], Xpert MRSA/SA BC[a] (Cepheid)
$bla_{VIM} + bla_{IMP}$	Enterobacteriaceae[c] + P. aeruginosa[c] + Acinetobacter spp.[c]	PCR-ELISA	hyplex MBL ID (BAG Health Care)
$bla_{TEM} + bla_{SHV} + bla_{CTX-M} + bla_{OXA}$	ESBL-producing bacteria[c]	PCR-ELISA	hyplex ESBL ID (BAG Health Care)
Mupirocin			
$mupA$	S. aureus[c]	DNA probe-based hybridization	$mupA$ EVIGENE (AdvanDX)
β-Lactams + glycopeptides			
$mecA + vanA + vanB + vanC1 + vanC2/C3$ + 23S rDNA[d]	Streptococci + staphylococci + enterococci	PCR-based reverse hybridization DNA strip assay	GenoType BC grampositive (Hain Lifescience)
$orfX$[d]/SCCmec + $mecA + vanA + vanB + nuc$[d] + tuf[d] + ddl[d]	Staphylococci + E. faecalis + E. faecium	PCR-Liquid array	MVPlex (Genaco Biomedical Products/QIAGEN)
β-Lactams + mupirocin			
$mecA + mupA$	S. aureus + S. epidermidis + S. haemolyticus	PCR-ELISA	hyplex StaphyloResist plus (BAG Health Care)
β-Lactams + aminoglycosides + macrolides + lincosamides + streptogramins + tetracyclines			
$mecA + aacA/aphD + ermA + ermC + tetK + tetM + nuc$[d] + tuf[d]	S. aureus + S. epidermidis + S. haemolyticus + S. hominis + S. lugdunensis + S. simulans	PCR-Liquid array	StaphPlex (QIAGEN)
Glycopeptides + aminoglycosides			
$vanA + vanB + aacA/aphD$	E. faecium + E. faecalis	PCR-ELISA	hyplex EnteroResist (BAG Health Care)
Rifampin			
$rpoB$ mutations + 16S-23S rDNA spacer region[d]	M. tuberculosis complex	PCR-based reverse hybridization line probe assay	INNO-LiPA Rif.TB (Innogenetics)
Rifampin + isoniazid			
$rpoB$ and $katG$ mutations + 23S rDNA[d]	M. tuberculosis complex	PCR-based reverse hybridization DNA strip assay	GenoType MTBDR (Hain Lifescience)

[a]U.S. FDA approved

[b]This assay is performed directly from clinical specimens without previous culture

[c]Bacterial identification is not provided with this test

[d]This gene is used for bacterial identification

M. tuberculosis is slow growing, identification and determination of the susceptibility profile of this organism can take several weeks. In the last few years, broth-based methods, either manual or fully automated, have allowed accelerated culture of mycobacteria and the availability of antibiogram. Nevertheless, conventional susceptibility testing methods may still take a few weeks after the primary culture results are available. Reviews of susceptibility methods for mycobacteria were recently published (31, 281–283). Advances in our understanding of the genetic mechanisms of drug resistance in *M. tuberculosis* have made possible the development of several different rapid genotypic drug resistance assays (32). Most molecular methods for detecting resistance are based on determining the presence/absence of the mutations associated with resistance (Table 1). A few years ago, genotypic assays were mostly developed for detection of rifampin resistance because the genetic basis of rifampin resistance in *M. tuberculosis* is simple and well characterized, being caused by specific mutations in the *rpoB* gene in more than 95% of rifampin-resistant TB (32) (see Sect. 2). Moreover, resistance to rifampin can often be used as a marker of MDR-TB, since more than 90% of rifampin-resistant TB are also resistant to isoniazid (32). However, in the past few years, molecular methods have been developed to detect mutations in most known target genes including *rpoB*, *katG*, *embB*, *pncA*, *gyrA*, *gyrB*, *rrs*, and *rpsL* (Table 1). Several different molecular methods have been used to detect these mutations including DNA sequencing, PCR-single-strand conformation polymorphism, PCR-restriction fragment length polymorphism, heteroduplex analysis, RNA/RNA mismatch assay, multiplex allele-specific PCR, linear signal amplification, real-time PCR using different types of fluorescent probes, and hybridization on strips, in microplates, and on arrays; most of these methods have recently been reviewed (20, 273, 284–287). Two molecular assays, namely, INNO-LiPA Rif.TB (Innogenetics, Gent, Belgium) and Genotype MTBDR (Hain LifeScience, Nehren, Germany), are commercially available for detection of rifampin resistance (detecting mutations in *rpoB*) and both rifampin and isoniazid resistance (detecting mutations in both *rpoB* and *katG*), respectively (Table 2). These assays are based on a multiplex amplification in combination with reverse hybridization to identify either wild-type sequence or specific mutations. A systematic meta-analysis of studies that have evaluated the diagnosis accuracy of LiPA for detection of rifampin resistance in diverse geographic areas has revealed that, when applied to isolates, LiPA had sensitivities greater than 95% and close to 100% specificity, whereas when applied directly to clinical specimens, LiPA had 100% specificity and sensitivity that ranged between 80 and 100% (288). Genotype MTBDR has also been evaluated in a recent study for detection of mutations conferring resistance to rifampin and isoniazid in clinical *M. tuberculosis* isolates. Compared to

conventional susceptibility testing, the sensitivity and specificity were 99 and 100% for rifampin resistance and 88.4 and 100% for isoniazid resistance, respectively (289). The use of molecular methods to detect resistance markers in mycobacteria is an area of great potential benefit to the clinical mycobacteriology laboratory allowing diagnosis of MDR-TB just a few days after sample collection. However, with the exception of molecular detection of rifampin resistance, the correlation between phenotypic and genotypic resistance testing is not always accurate because resistance to every antituberculous drugs is still not fully known.

3.3.2 Genotypic Detection of Oxacillin Resistance in Staphylococci

Despite improvement and development of phenotypic methods to detect oxacillin resistance (see Sect. 3.2.1), molecular detection of the *mecA* gene is now considered the "gold standard" for detection of oxacillin resistance in *S. aureus*, as it does not depend on the variable expression of the PBP 2a (290). Numerous molecular-based tests have been developed to increase the sensitivity, specificity, and speed for MRSA detection. Most of these methods detect an *S. aureus*-specific gene and/or *mecA* (109, 111–134). Some of these molecular methods have been used to detect MRSA directly from a variety of clinical specimens including cerebrospinal and peritoneal fluids, endotracheal aspirates, and blood or blood cultures (114, 135–142). More recently, a number of real-time PCR assays have also been developed to identify MRSA isolates (143–147), and some have been used to identify MRSA directly from blood cultures (148, 149).

Because of the increasing prevalence of MRSA worldwide, the prevention and control of MRSA spread remains a major challenge (291). Active surveillance cultures for identification of MRSA carriers is one of the most common and effective measures to prevent the spread of MRSA in healthcare facilities (292, 293). However, despite improvement and development of novel susceptibility testing methods for detecting MRSA from screening samples, it takes at least 48–72 h to identify MRSA (see Sect. 3.2.1). During the past years, efforts have been made to develop novel genotypic approaches for rapid detection of MRSA. Although detection of an *S. aureus*-specific gene and *mecA* can be used to identify MRSA from pure cultures or directly from sterile specimens such as blood (see above), this approach cannot be applied for detection of MRSA from nonsterile specimens such as nasal screening specimens containing a mixed flora of CoNS and *S. aureus*, because both can carry *mecA* (294). Recently, novel strategies using real-time PCR have been developed to rapidly identify MRSA from nonsterile screening specimens. One approach used an MRSA-selective overnight broth enrichment prior to real-time PCR for identification of

MRSA from screening swabs, obviating the need for subculture on agar media, but this method still needs an overnight broth culture step (150). Another assay combined immunomagnetic enrichment in *S. aureus* and real-time quantitative triplex qPCR, measuring simultaneously *mecA* and *femA* from both *S. aureus* and *S. epidermidis* (295). This quantitative approach allows discrimination of the measured *mecA* signal and identification of MRSA from screening specimens in about 6 h after sample collection. Another real-time PCR assay using a novel strategy, which is based on our increasing knowledge of the genetic elements containing *mecA*, has recently been developed in our laboratory for detection of MRSA directly from nasal screening swabs (8). The *mecA* gene is carried by a novel mobile genetic element, designated staphylococcal cassette chromosome *mec* (SCC*mec*), inserted near the chromosomal origin of replication (296). Five distinct types of SCC*mec* (I, II, III, IV, and V) have been described (297, 298). The novel real-time PCR assay developed by our group for rapid detection of MRSA comprises five primers specific to the right extremity sequences of the different staphylococcal cassette chromosome *mec* (SCC*mec*) containing *mecA*, including three new genotypes that we recently characterized (8). These five primers are used in combination with a primer specific to the *S. aureus* chromosomal *orfX* gene sequence located at the right of the SCC*mec* integration site, thereby providing a link between *mecA* and *S. aureus*. By linking *mecA* to *S. aureus*, this PCR test allows the detection of MRSA directly from clinical specimens containing a mixture of staphylococci without previous isolation or enrichment of the bacteria, thereby reducing the number of sample preparation steps and time to results. This new PCR assay was combined with a rapid and simple DNA extraction method that we also have developed, allowing detection of MRSA directly from nasal swab specimens in approximately 1 h. This assay has been evaluated during an MRSA surveillance program for screening of nasal MRSA carriers on 331 nasal specimens (7). The sensitivity and the specificity of this PCR assay were 100 and 96%, respectively, whereas the positive and negative predictive values were 95.3 and 100%, respectively. On the basis of our initial research, a commercial version of this assay, which requires little hands-on time and fits easily into any laboratory's routine, has been cleared by the FDA (BD GeneOhm MRSA, BD Diagnostics-GeneOhm, Québec, Canada). The performance of this commercial test has recently been evaluated using 288 nasal samples (299). The diagnostic values of this test were 91.7% sensitivity, 93.5% specificity, 82.5% positive predictive value, and 97.1% negative predictive value. By providing an immediate (~1 h) detection of MRSA carriers, this test should facilitate and intensify surveillance of MRSA carriers in healthcare settings and should help control the spread of MRSA.

3.3.3 Genotypic Detection of Glycopeptide Resistance in Enterococci and Staphylcocci

Most conventional phenotypic susceptibility methods can detect accurately high-level vancomycin resistance in enterococci (VanA and VanD phenotypes); however, detection of low-level vancomycin resistance (VanB, VanC, VanE, and VanG phenotypes) and differentiation between different Van types are difficult by phenotypic methods (see Sect. 3.2.2). Numerous amplification or probe hybridization assays have been developed to detect the various *van* genes conferring glycopeptide resistance in enterococci (242–249, 300, 301) (Table 1). Some molecular assays detecting the most common *van* genes (*vanA*, *vanB*, and *vanC*) are commercially available (Table 2). Recently, a multiplex PCR for detection of the six types of glycopeptide resistance genes (*vanA*, *vanB*, *VanC*, *vanD*, *vanE*, and *vanG*) was developed (250). This multiplex PCR also contained primers specific to *E. faecium*, *E. faecalis*, *S. aureus*, and *S. epidermidis*, allowing detection of both glycopeptide-resistant enterococci and the newly described vancomycin-resistant *S. aureus* containing *vanA*. With the recent emergence of *vanA*-containing *S. aureus*, other groups have developed real-time PCR assays for detection of vancomycin-resistant *S. aureus* (251). However, new alleles of *van* genes were recently described, emphasizing the need for more universal *van* gene primers in the future (252, 302, 303).

Because VRE (including *E. faecalis* and *E. faecium*) have become increasingly important pathogens within the healthcare settings, great emphasis has been placed on rapid detection of VRE-colonized patients. Prompt detection of the carrier state is recommended for preventing the transmission of these organisms (292, 304). However, despite development of various selective culture media and novel susceptibility testing methods for detecting VRE from screening samples (see Sect. 3.2.2), it still takes more than 48 h to identify VRE (305). From the six different glycopeptide resistance genes described in VRE, *vanA* and *vanB* are the most prevalent and clinically important from an infection control perspective because of the transmissibility of these genes. Since *vanA* and *vanB* are generally associated with *E. faecalis* and *E. faecium*, different PCR assays, including gel-based PCR assays and real-time PCR assays, have been developed to detect these two resistance genes directly from fecal specimens without the need to include PCR primers specific to these two bacterial species (253–255, 306, 307). However, bacterial species other than *E. faecalis* and *E. faecium* have been noted to contain these genes, but they are found infrequently (15–17, 252, 308–328). The first real-time PCR assay developed for *vanA* and *vanB* detection was first used for detection of these genes from isolated colonies (329), and then applied for detection of these genes directly from rectal swabs (253). The sensitivity of this PCR assay for *vanA* and *vanB* detection directly from rectal specimens was very low (45%) because of a high level of PCR inhibition (55%) of the rectal swab specimens. This was a result of the poor performance of the commercial DNA extraction kit used in this study to remove PCR inhibitors (253). A commercial version of this real-time PCR assay is now available for research use only (LightCycler VRE detection, Roche Diagnostics, Indianapolis, IN, USA) (Table 2). The performance of this commercial assay was evaluated for direct detection of VRE from 894 perianal stool swabs using another commercial nucleic acid extraction kit prior to PCR (306). The sensitivity and the specificity of this PCR assay were 100 and 97%, respectively, whereas the positive and negative predictive values were 42 and 100%, respectively. The turnaround time for this assay including nucleic acid extraction was 3.5 h. Our group has also developed a real-time PCR assay combined with a rapid DNA extraction procedure for detection of *vanA* and *vanB* directly from rectal swabs in less than 1 h. This assay has been evaluated during two independent surveillance programs for screening of VRE carriers using 101 and 62 rectal swabs (330, 331). The sensitivity of our PCR assay was 100% and the specificity ranged from 96.8 to 98%, whereas the positive predictive value ranged from 70 to 92.3% and the negative predictive value was 100%. These studies have shown that when real-time PCR assays for detection of *vanA* and *vanB* are combined with an appropriate sample preparation step to remove PCR inhibitors, they can detect VRE carriers rapidly and accurately. This suggests that genotypic assays could have important implication for the implementation of effective measures to control the spread of VRE.

3.3.4 Potential Artifacts of Genotypic Resistance Testing

There are some potential artifacts of genotypic resistance testing to determine the resistance profile of a microorganism. For example, the presence of a resistance gene may not be always indicative of a resistant bacterium and does not necessarily lead to treatment failure, because the level of expression may be low. For example, the development of resistance by β-lactamase production among members of *Enterobacteriaceae* depends on the mode and level of expression (332). However, the presence of a gene can be indicative of the potential to develop resistance. For example, in a recent study of antimicrobial resistance in *S. aureus* it had been shown that the presence of *mecA* did not necessarily result in oxacillin resistance phenotype; however, oxacillin-susceptible *S. aureus* isolates carrying this gene were easily selected for resistance expression by exposure to increasing antibiotic concentrations, suggesting that, at least for certain resistance genes, the presence of a gene is sufficient for a bacterium to

eventually become resistant to the drug (58, 109). Another limitation of the resistance testing is that the absence of a gene coding for a resistance to a drug does not always mean that the bacterium is susceptible to that drug because resistance testing identifies only genes or mutations that have been characterized and other unknown resistance mechanisms may exist. Therefore, continuously updated epidemiological studies of resistant bacteria based on susceptibility testing and study of novel resistance mechanisms would help to develop genotypic tests for detection of the new types of resistance that undoubtely will arise in bacteria in the future.

4 The Future of Genotypic Drug Resistance Detection

During the past decade, there has been enormous progress in the development of genotypic drug resistance assays that provide more accurate and rapid antimicrobial resistance testing. Genotypic drug resistance assays are increasingly used in the clinical microbiology laboratories, especially for detection of antimicrobial resistance in microorganisms that grow slowly, such as multidrug-resistant *M. tuberculosis,* or for rapid detection of difficult-to-detect resistance mechanisms such as those found in MRSA and VRE. With the increasing prevalence of multidrug-resistant pathogens, there is an urgent need for novel rapid genotypic diagnostic tests for the detection of resistant pathogens without the need of the time-consuming culture-based systems. To be useful for physicians, future genotypic diagnostic tests for detection of antimicrobial-resistant pathogens will have to detect and identify rapidly (in less than 1 h) all possible causative pathogens for a specific infection or syndrome (e.g., meningitis, nosocomial pneumonia, septicemia, etc.) as well as the associated genes or mutations conferring resistance to potentially useful therapeutic agents.

Nucleotide sequences of several conserved genetic targets for bacterial identification and antimicrobial resistance genes and mutations for detection of resistance are available in public databases (52). However, the development of genotypic tests that will allow sensitive detection of multiple pathogens, as well as multiple antimicrobial resistance genes and mutations, directly from clinical specimens will pose major challenges. DNA microarrays will certainly provide an essential multidetection technology, but conventional DNA microarrays are presently not sensitive enough to detect the small numbers of bacterial cells found in clinical samples. The use of multiplex PCR for amplification of different target genes combined with detection on DNA microarrays of capture probes represents one of the most powerful strategies and is being increasingly used (see Sect. 3.3). However, sensitive multiplex PCR is restricted to a limited number of PCR primers because of uncontrollable primer–primer interactions. New technologies allowing both PCR amplification and multidetection on the microarray have been developed and should help to solve the challenge of sensitive multidetection on microarray. Recent advances in these solid-phase PCR technologies have shown that is possible to detect as low as 100–1,000 copies of genomic bacterial DNA (333, 334).

The development of ultrasensitive biosensors for nucleic acid analysis is another promising tool that could obviate the need for multiplex target amplification in the future (335, 336). For example, a new sensitive detection technology of unamplified genomic DNA based on colorimetric scatter of gold nanoparticle probes on microarray has been developed and used for the rapid detection of *mecA* in MRSA DNA derived from $<10^5$ cells (337). More recently, an innovative new biosensor, which is based on the different conformations adopted by a cationic polythiophene when electrostatically bound to nucleic acid and on the efficient and fast energy transfer between the resulting fluorescent polythiophene/double strand-DNA complex and neighboring fluorescent-labeled DNA probes, has been reported. This molecular system allowed the detection of as few as five copies of the DNA target extracted from clinical specimens in 5 min. Extension of such new transduction methods for applications in microarray devices offers significant potential for high sensitivity without amplification (338).

An important challenge posed by the development of sensitive nucleic acid detection technologies remains the development of rapid, simple, and efficient methods for microbial nucleic acid extraction from a variety of clinical specimens. An optimal specimen preparation must efficiently release the nucleic acid from the microorganims, preserve the integrity of the nucleic acid target, remove or neutralize clinical specimens substances that are frequently present in clinical specimens that inhibit amplification and/or detection of nucleic acids, and concentrate the target nucleic acids into an aqueous solution suitable for amplification and/or detection. Over the past decade, a variety of nucleic acid extraction procedures and commercial reagents and kits have been used in molecular diagnostics (339, 340). Today, most molecular diagnostic microbiology laboratories use commercially available prepackaged, extraction kits, or reagents for extraction of nucleic acids (DNA and/or RNA). These commercial systems for nucleic acid extraction and purification are either manual or automated and are often based on nucleic acid capture technologies using, for example, magnetic beads or silica matrix (341). Automation should help to provide rapid, cost-effective, and consistent results.

The most appropriate source of clinical specimens will also be critical for the development of genotypic tests for the detection of antimicrobial-resistant pathogens (342). Moreover, the appropriate specimen volume (especially when the number of infectious organisms per test volume is small), the choice of specimen collection device, and transport storage conditions that will stabilize microbial and more particularly nucleic acids will also be essential. Currently, most commercially available sample collection and transport devices are developed and validated exclusively for standard culture-based diagnostic microbiology. However, over the past few years several manufacturers have developed sample collection and transport systems that are compatible and validated with genotypic assays (339).

Finally, the next generation of genotypic tests for detection of antimicrobial-resistant pathogens should be fully automated with integrated sample preparation and nucleic acid detection with biosensing elements leading to point-of-care diagnostics. Indeed, several point-of-care diagnostics devices are currently in development that can identify a variety of nucleic acid targets from multiple types of samples in under an hour (343). Recent advances in nanotechnology and microfluidic or "lab-on-a-chip" systems should revolutionize the detection of antimicrobial-resistant pathogens in the future (344–350).

Acknowledgements This work was supported by a grant from the Canadian Institutes for Health Research (CIHR) and by a grant from Genome Canada and Génome Québec.

References

1. Walsh FM, Amyes SG. Microbiology and drug resistance mechanisms of fully resistant pathogens. Curr Opin Microbiol 2004;7:439–444.
2. Low DE. The era of antimicrobial resistance-implications for the clinical laboratory. Clin Microbiol Infect 2002;8 Suppl 3:9–20; discussion 33–25.
3. Vandenesch F, Naimi T, Enright MC, et al. Community-acquired methicillin-resistant *Staphylococcus aureus* carrying Panton-Valentine leukocidin genes: worldwide emergence. Emerg Infect Dis 2003;9:978–984.
4. World Health Organization. Anti-tuberculosis drug resistance in the world: third global report/The WHO/IUATLD global project on anti-tuberculosis drug resistance surveillance, 1999–2002. The World Health Organization/International Union Against Tuberculosis Drug Resistance Surveillance, Geneva, 2004.
5. McGowan JE, Jr., Tenover FC. Confronting bacterial resistance in healthcare settings: a crucial role for microbiologists. Nat Rev Microbiol 2004;2:251–258.
6. Bergeron MG, Ouellette M. Preventing antibiotic resistance using rapid DNA-based diagnostic tests. Infect Control Hosp Epidemiol 1998;19:560–564.
7. Huletsky A, Lebel P, Picard FJ, et al. Identification of methicillin-resistant *Staphylococcus aureus* carriage in less than 1 hour during a hospital surveillance program. Clin Infect Dis 2005;40:976–981.
8. Huletsky A, Giroux R, Rossbach V, et al. New real-time PCR assay for rapid detection of methicillin-resistant *Staphylococcus aureus* directly from specimens containing a mixture of staphylococci. J Clin Microbiol 2004;42:1875–1884.

9. Musser JM. Antimicrobial agent resistance in mycobacteria: molecular genetic insights. Clin Microbiol Rev 1995;8:496–514.

10. Azucena E, Mobashery S. Aminoglycoside-modifying enzymes: mechanisms of catalytic processes and inhibition. Drug Resist Updat 2001;4:106–117.

11. Amyes SG. Resistance to beta-lactams-the permutations. J Chemother 2003;15:525–535.

12. Bush K, Jacoby GA, Medeiros AA. A functional classification scheme for beta-lactamases and its correlation with molecular structure. Antimicrob Agents Chemother 1995;39:1211–1233.

13. Courvalin P. Genetics of glycopeptide resistance in gram-positive pathogens. Int J Med Microbiol 2005;294:479–486.

14. Henriques Normark B, Normark S. Antibiotic tolerance in pneumococci. Clin Microbiol Infect 2002;8:613–622.

15. Centers for Disease Control and Prevention. Vancomycin-resistant *Staphylococcus aureus* – New York. MMWR Morb Mortal Wkly Rep 2004;53:322–323.

16. Centers for Disease Control and Prevention. Vancomycin-resistant *Staphylococcus aureus* – Pennsylvania. MMWR Morb Mortal Wkly Rep 2002;51:902–903.

17. Centers for Disease Control and Prevention. *Staphylococcus aureus* resistant to vancomycin – United States. MMWR Morb Mortal Wkly Rep 2002;51:565–567.

18. Di Giambattista M, Chinali G, Cocito C. The molecular basis of the inhibitory activities of type A and type B synergimycins and related antibiotics on ribosomes. J Antimicrob Chemother 1989;24:485–507.

19. Roberts MC, Sutcliffe J, Courvalin P, Jensen LB, Rood J, Seppala H. Nomenclature for macrolide and macrolide-lincosa mide-streptogramin B resistance determinants. Antimicrob Agents Chemother 1999;43.2823–2830.

20. Jalava J, Marttila H. Application of molecular genetic methods in macrolide, lincosamide and streptogramin resistance diagnostics and in detection of drug-resistant *Mycobacterium tuberculosis*. APMIS 2004;112:838–855.

21. Hooper DC. Mechanisms of fluoroquinolone resistance. Drug Resist Updat 1999;2:38–55.

22. Nordmann P, Poirel L. Emergence of plasmid-mediated resistance to quinolones in *Enterobacteriaceae*. J Antimicrob Chemother 2005;56:463–469.

23. Huovinen P, Sundstrom L, Swedberg G, Skold O. Trimethoprim and sulfonamide resistance. Antimicrob Agents Chemother 1995;39:279–289.

24. Schnappinger D, Hillen W. Tetracyclines: antibiotic action, uptake, and resistance mechanisms. Arch Microbiol 1996;165:359–369.

25. Chopra I, Roberts M. Tetracycline antibiotics: mode of action, applications, molecular biology, and epidemiology of bacterial resistance. Microbiol Mol Biol Rev 2001;65:232–260.

26. Murray IA, Shaw WV. O-Acetyltransferases for chloramphenicol and other natural products. Antimicrob Agents Chemother 1997;41:1–6.

27. Schwarz S, Kehrenberg C, Doublet B, Cloeckaert A. Molecular basis of bacterial resistance to chloramphenicol and florfenicol. FEMS Microbiol Rev 2004;28:519–542.

28. Matassova NB, Rodnina MV, Endermann R, et al. Ribosomal RNA is the target for oxazolidinones, a novel class of translational inhibitors. RNA 1999;5:939–946.

29. Meka VG, Gold HS, Cooke A, et al. Reversion to susceptibility in a linezolid-resistant clinical isolate of *Staphylococcus aureus*. J Antimicrob Chemother 2004;54:818–820.

30. Wolter N, Smith AM, Farrell DJ, et al. Novel mechanism of resistance to oxazolidinones, macrolides, and chloramphenicol in ribosomal protein L4 of the *pneumococcus*. Antimicrob Agents Chemother 2005;49:3554–3557.

31. Inderlied CB, Pfyffer GE. Susceptibility test methods: mycobacteria. In: Murray PR, Baron EJ, Jorgensen JH, Pfaller MA, Yolken RH, eds. Manual of Clinical Microbiology, 8th edition, Washington, DC: ASM, 2003, pp. 1149–1177.

32. Ramaswamy S, Musser JM. Molecular genetic basis of antimicrobial agent resistance in *Mycobacterium tuberculosis*: 1998 update. Tuber Lung Dis 1998;79:3–29.

33. Lee AS, Teo AS, Wong SY. Novel mutations in *ndh* in isoniazid-resistant *Mycobacterium tuberculosis* isolates. Antimicrob Agents Chemother 2001;45:2157–2159.

34. Telenti A, Philipp WJ, Sreevatsan S, et al. The *emb* operon, a gene cluster of *Mycobacterium tuberculosis* involved in resistance to ethambutol. Nat Med 1997;3:567–570.

35. Shima SM, Donahoe LW. Bacterial resistance: how to detect three types. MLO Med Lab Obs 2004;36:12–16.

36. Jorgensen JH, Ferraro MJ. Antimicrobial susceptibility testing: special needs for fastidious organisms and difficult-to-detect resistance mechanisms. Clin Infect Dis 2000;30:799–808.

37. Evangelista AT, Truant AL. Rapid systems and instruments for antimicrobial susceptibility. In: Truant AL, ed. Manual of Commercial Methods in Clinical Microbiology. Washington, DC: ASM, 2002, pp. 413–428.

38. Clinical and Laboratory Standards Institute. Performance standards for antimicrobial susceptibility testing; sixteenth informational supplement. CLSI document M100-S15. Wayne, PA, USA; 2006.

39. Clinical and Laboratory Standards Institute. Methods for dilution antimicrobial susceptibility tests for bacteria that grow aerobically; Approved standard, 7th edition. CLSI document M7-A7. Wayne, PA, USA; 2006.

40. Ferraro MJ. Should we reevaluate antibiotic breakpoints? Clin Infect Dis 2001;33 Suppl 3:S227 S229.

41. Hindler JF, Swenson JM. Susceptibility test methods: Fastidious bacteria. In: Murray PR, Baron EJ, Jorgensen JH, Pfaller MA, Yolken RH, eds. Manual of Clinical Microbiology, 8th edition, Washington, DC: ASM, 2003, pp. 1128–1140.

42. Citron DM, Hecht DW. Susceptibility test methods: anaerobic bacteria. In: Murray PR, Baron EJ, Jorgensen JH, Pfaller MA, Yolken RH, eds. Manual of Clinical Microbiology, 8th edition, Washington, DC: ASM, 2003, pp. 1141–1148.

43. Swenson JM, Hindler JF, Jorgensen JH. Special phenotypic methods for detecting antibacterial resistance. In: Murray PR, Baron EJ, Jorgensen JH, Pfaller MA, Yolken RH, eds. Manual of Clinical Microbiology, 8th edition, Washington, DC: ASM, 2003, pp. 1178–1195.

44. Tenover FC, Lancaster MV, Hill BC, et al. Characterization of staphylococci with reduced susceptibilities to vancomycin and other glycopeptides. J Clin Microbiol 1998;36:1020–1027.

45. Cui L, Iwamoto A, Lian JQ, et al. Novel mechanism of antibiotic resistance originating in vancomycin-intermediate *Staphylococcus aureus*. Antimicrob Agents Chemother 2006;50:428–438.

46. Cui L, Lian JQ, Neoh HM, Reyes E, Hiramatsu K. DNA microarray-based identification of genes associated with glycopeptide resistance in *Staphylococcus aureus*. Antimicrob Agents Chemother 2005;49:3404–3413.

47. Turnidge JD, Ferraro MJ, Jorgensen JH. Susceptibility test methods: general consideration. In: Murray PR, Baron EJ, Jorgensen JH, Pfaller MA, Yolken RH, eds. Manual of Clinical Microbiology, 8th edition, Washington, DC: ASM, 2003, pp. 1102–1107.

48. Jorgensen JH, Ferraro MJ. Antimicrobial susceptibility testing: general principles and contemporary practices. Clin Infect Dis 1998;26:973–980.

49. Jorgensen JH. Who defines resistance? The clinical and economic impact of antimicrobial susceptibility testing breakpoints. Semin Pediatr Infect Dis 2004;15:105–108.

50. Kahlmeter G, Brown DF, Goldstein FW, et al. European harmonization of MIC breakpoints for antimicrobial susceptibility testing of bacteria. J Antimicrob Chemother 2003;52:145–148.

51. Rasheed JK, Tenover FC. Detection and characterization of antimicrobial resistance genes in bacteria. In: Murray PR, Baron EJ, Jorgensen JH, Pfaller MA, Yolken RH, eds. Manual of Clinical Microbiology, 8th edition, Washington, DC: ASM, 2003, pp. 1196–1212.

52. Benson DA, Karsch-Mizrachi I, Lipman DJ, Ostell J, Wheeler DL. GenBank. Nucleic Acids Res Suppl 2005;33:D34–D38.

53. Noppe-Leclercq I, Wallet F, Haentjens S, Courcol R, Simonet M. PCR detection of aminoglycoside resistance genes: a rapid molecular typing method for *Acinetobacter baumannii*. Res Microbiol 1999;150:317–322.

54. Miller GH, Sabatelli FJ, Hare RS, et al. The most frequent aminoglycoside resistance mechanisms – changes with time and geographic area: a reflection of aminoglycoside usage patterns? Aminoglycoside Resistance Study Groups. Clin Infect Dis 1997;24 Suppl 1:S46–S62.

55. Seward RJ, Lambert T, Towner KJ. Molecular epidemiology of aminoglycoside resistance in *Acinetobacter* spp. J Med Microbiol 1998;47:455–462.

56. Vernet G, Jay C, Rodrigue M, Troesch A. Species differentiation and antibiotic susceptibility testing with DNA microarrays. J Appl Microbiol 2004;96:59–68.

57. Perreten V, Vorlet-Fawer L, Slickers P, Ehricht R, Kuhnert P, Frey J. Microarray-based detection of 90 antibiotic resistance genes of gram-positive bacteria. J Clin Microbiol 2005;43:2291–2302.

58. Martineau F, Picard FJ, Lansac N, et al. Correlation between the resistance genotype determined by multiplex PCR assays and the antibiotic susceptibility patterns of *Staphylococcus aureus* and *Staphylococcus epidermidis*. Antimicrob Agents Chemother 2000;44:231–238.

59. Strommenger B, Kettlitz C, Werner G, Witte W. Multiplex PCR assay for simultaneous detection of nine clinically relevant antibiotic resistance genes in *Staphylococcus aureus*. J Clin Microbiol 2003;41:4089–4094.

60. Klingenberg C, Sundsfjord A, Ronnestad A, Mikalsen J, Gaustad P, Flaegstad T. Phenotypic and genotypic aminoglycoside resistance in blood culture isolates of coagulase-negative staphylococci from a single neonatal intensive care unit, 1989–2000. J Antimicrob Chemother 2004;54:889–896.

61. Kao SJ, You I, Clewell DB, et al. Detection of the high-level aminoglycoside resistance gene *aph(2″)-Ib* in *Enterococcus faecium*. Antimicrob Agents Chemother 2000;44:2876–2879.

62. Choi SM, Kim SH, Kim HJ, et al. Multiplex PCR for the detection of genes encoding aminoglycoside modifying enzymes and methicillin resistance among *Staphylococcus* species. J Korean Med Sci 2003;18:631–636.

63. Ardic N, Sareyyupoglu B, Ozyurt M, Haznedaroglu T, Ilga U. Investigation of aminoglycoside modifying enzyme genes in methicillin-resistant staphylococci. Microbiol Res 2006;161:49–54.

64. Vanhoof R, Godard C, Content J, Nyssen HJ, Hannecart-Pokorni E. Detection by polymerase chain reaction of genes encoding aminoglycoside-modifying enzymes in methicillin-resistant *Staphylococcus aureus* isolates of epidemic phage types. Belgian Study Group of Hospital Infections (GDEPIH/GOSPIZ). J Med Microbiol 1994;41:282–290.

65. Ploy MC, Giamarellou H, Bourlioux P, Courvalin P, Lambert T. Detection of *aac(6′)-I* genes in amikacin-resistant *Acinetobacter* spp. by PCR. Antimicrob Agents Chemother 1994;38:2925–2928.

66. Randall LP, Cooles SW, Osborn MK, Piddock LJ, Woodward MJ. Antibiotic resistance genes, integrons and multiple antibiotic resistance in thirty-five serotypes of *Salmonella enterica* isolated from humans and animals in the UK. J Antimicrob Chemother 2004;53:208–216.

67. Vakulenko SB, Donabedian SM, Voskresenskiy AM, Zervos MJ, Lerner SA, Chow JW. Multiplex PCR for detection of aminoglyco-side resistance genes in enterococci. Antimicrob Agents Chemother 2003;47:1423–1426.

68. Cerda Zolezzi PC, Laplana LM, Calvo CR, Cepero PG, Erazo MC, Gómez-Lus R. Molecular basis of resistance to macrolides and other antibiotics in commensal viridans group streptococci and *Gemella* spp. and transfer of resistance genes to *Streptococcus pneumoniae*. Antimicrob Agents Chemother 2004;48:3462–3467.

69. Vila J, Ruiz J, Navia M, et al. Spread of amikacin resistance in *Acinetobacter baumannii* strains isolated in Spain due to an epidemic strain. J Clin Microbiol 1999;37:758–761.

70. Mieskes KT, Rusch-Gerdes S, Truffot-Pernot C, et al. Rapid, simple, and culture-independent detection of *rpsL* codon 43 mutations that are highly predictive of streptomycin resistance in *Mycobacterium tuberculosis*. Am J Trop Med Hyg 2000;63:56–60.

71. Shi R, Otomo K, Yamada H, Tatsumi T, Sugawara I. Temperature-mediated heteroduplex analysis for the detection of drug-resistant gene mutations in clinical isolates of *Mycobacterium tuberculosis* by denaturing HPLC, SURVEYOR nuclease. Microbes Infect 2006;8:128–135.

72. Siddiqi N, Shamim M, Hussain S, et al. Molecular characterization of multidrug-resistant isolates of *Mycobacterium tuberculosis* from patients in North India. Antimicrob Agents Chemother 2002;46:443–450.

73. Mokrousov I, Bhanu NV, Suffys PN, et al. Multicenter evaluation of reverse line blot assay for detection of drug resistance in *Mycobacterium tuberculosis* clinical isolates. J Microbiol Methods 2004;57:323–335.

74. Cooksey RC, Morlock GP, Holloway BP, Limor J, Hepburn M. Temperature-mediated heteroduplex analysis performed by using denaturing high-performance liquid chromatography to identify sequence polymorphisms in *Mycobacterium tuberculosis* complex organisms. J Clin Microbiol 2002;40:1610–1616.

75. Meier A, Kirschner P, Bange FC, Vogel U, Bottger EC. Genetic alterations in streptomycin-resistant *Mycobacterium tuberculosis*: mapping of mutations conferring resistance. Antimicrob Agents Chemother 1994;38:228–233.

76. Kobayashi N, Alam M, Nishimoto Y, Urasawa S, Uehara N, Watanabe N. Distribution of aminoglycoside resistance genes in recent clinical isolates of *Enterococcus faecalis*, *Enterococcus faecium* and *Enterococcus avium*. Epidemiol Infect 2001;126:197–204.

77. Colom K, Perez J, Alonso R, Fernandez-Aranguiz A, Larino E, Cisterna R. Simple and reliable multiplex PCR assay for detection of bla_{TEM}, bla_{SHV} and bla_{OXA-1} genes in *Enterobacteriaceae*. FEMS Microbiol Lett 2003;223:147–151.

78. Shin KS, Han K, Lee J, et al. Imipenem-resistant *Achromobacter xylosoxidans* carrying bla_{VIM-2}-containing class 1 integron. Diagn Microbiol Infect Dis 2005;53:215–220.

79. Da Silva GJ, Quinteira S, Bertolo E, et al. Long-term dissemination of an OXA-40 carbapenemase-producing *Acinetobacter baumannii* clone in the Iberian Peninsula. J Antimicrob Chemother 2004;54:255–258.

80. Güerri ML, Aladueña A, Echeíta A, Rotger R. Detection of integrons and antibiotic-resistance genes in *Salmonella enterica* serovar Typhimurium isolates with resistance to ampicillin and variable susceptibility to amoxicillin-clavulanate. Int J Antimicrob Agent 2004;24:327–333.

81. van Loon HJ, Box ATA, Verhoef J, Fluit AC. Evaluation of genetic determinants involved in β-lactam- and multiresistance in a surgical ICU. Int J Antimicrob Agents 2004;24:130–134.

82. Neonakis IK, Scoulica EV, Dimitriou SK, Gikas AI, Tselentis YJ. Molecular epidemiology of extended-spectrum beta-lactamases produced by clinical isolates in a university hospital in Greece: detection of SHV-5 in *Pseudomonas aeruginosa* and prevalence of SHV-12. Microb Drug Resist 2003;9:161–165.

83. Paterson DL, Hujer KM, Hujer AM, et al. Extended-spectrum beta-lactamases in *Klebsiella pneumoniae* bloodstream isolates from s

even countries: dominance and widespread prevalence of SHV- and CTX-M-type beta-lactamases. Antimicrob Agents Chemother 2003;47:3554–3560.

84. Chia JH, Chu C, Su LH, et al. Development of a multiplex PCR and SHV melting-curve mutation detection system for detection of some SHV and CTX-M beta-lactamases of *Escherichia coli*, *Klebsiella pneumoniae*, and *Enterobacter cloacae* in Taiwan. J Clin Microbiol 2005;43:4486–4491.

85. Rasheed JK, Jay C, Metchock B, et al. Evolution of extended-spectrum beta-lactam resistance (SHV-8) in a strain of *Escherichia coli* during multiple episodes of bacteremia. Antimicrob Agents Chemother 1997;41:647–653.

86. Nuesch-Inderbinen MT, Hachler H, Kayser FH. Detection of genes coding for extended-spectrum SHV beta-lactamases in clinical isolates by a molecular genetic method, and comparison with the E test. Eur J Clin Microbiol Infect Dis 1996;15:398–402.

87. Grimm V, Ezaki S, Susa M, Knabbe C, Schmid RD, Bachmann TT. Use of DNA microarrays for rapid genotyping of TEM beta-lactamases that confer resistance. J Clin Microbiol 2004;42: 3766–3774.

88. van Hoek AH, Scholtens IM, Cloeckaert A, Aarts HJ. Detection of antibiotic resistance genes in different *Salmonella* serovars by oligonucleotide microarray analysis. J Microbiol Methods 2005;62:13–23.

89. Alonso R, Fernandez-Aranguiz A, Colom K, Cisterna R. Non-radioactive PCR-SSCP with a single PCR step for detection of inhibitor resistant beta-lactamases in *Escherichia coli*. J Microbiol Methods 2002;50:85–90.

90. Woodford N, Fagan EJ, Ellington MJ. Multiplex PCR for rapid detection of genes encoding CTX-M extended-spectrum β-lactamases. J Antimicrob Chemother 2006;57:154–155.

91. Xu L, Ensor V, Gossain S, Nye K, Hawkey P. Rapid and simple detection of bla_{CTX-M} genes by multiplex PCR assay. J Med Microbiol 2005;54:1183–1187.

92. Pitout JD, Hossain A, Hanson ND. Phenotypic and molecular detection of CTX-M-beta-lactamases produced by *Escherichia coli* and *Klebsiella spp*. J Clin Microbiol 2004;42:5715–5721.

93. Pallecchi L, Malossi M, Mantella A, et al. Detection of CTX-M-Type β-lactamase genes in fecal *Escherichia coli* isolates from healthy children in Bolivia and Peru. Antimicrob Agents Chemother 2006;48:4556–4561.

94. Mushtaq S, Woodford N, Potz N, Livermore DM. Detection of CTX-M-15 extended-spectrum beta-lactamase in the United Kingdom. J Antimicrob Chemother 2003;52:528–529.

95. Yan JJ, Hong CY, Ko WC, et al. Dissemination of bla_{CMY-2} among *Escherichia coli* isolates from food animals, retail ground meats, and humans in southern Taiwan. Antimicrob Agents Chemother 2004;48:1353–1356.

96. Corvec S, Caroff N, Espaze E, Marraillac J, Drugeon H, Reynaud A. Comparison of two RT-PCR methods for quantifying *ampC* specific transcripts in *Escherichia coli* strains. FEMS Microbiol Lett 2003;228:187–191.

97. Pérez-Pérez FJ, Hanson ND. Detection of plasmid-mediated *ampC* β-lactamase genes in clinical isolates by using multiplex PCR. J Clin Microbiol 2002;40:2153–2162.

98. Zhang YL, Li JT, Zhao MW. Detection of *ampC* in *Enterobacter cloacae* in China. Int J Antimicrob Agents 2001;18:365–371.

99. Hirakata Y, Izumikawa K, Yamaguchi T, et al. Rapid detection and evaluation of clinical characteristics of emerging multiple-drug-resistant gram-negative rods carrying the metallo-beta-lactamase gene bla_{IMP}. Antimicrob Agents Chemother 1998;42:2006–2011.

100. Senda K, Arakawa Y, Ichiyama S, et al. PCR detection of metallo-beta-lactamase gene (bla_{IMP}) in gram-negative rods resistant to broad-spectrum β-lactams. J Clin Microbiol 1996;34:2909–2913.

101. Yan JJ, Ko WC, Chuang CL, Wu JJ. Metallo-beta-lactamase-producing *Enterobacteriaceae* isolates in a university hospital in

Taiwan: prevalence of IMP-8 in *Enterobacter cloacae* and first identification of VIM-2 in *Citrobacter freundii*. J Antimicrob Chemother 2002;50:503–511.

102. Wang CX, Mi ZH. IMP-1 metallo-beta-lactamase-producing *Pseudomonas aeruginosa* in a university hospital in the People's Republic of China. J Antimicrob Chemother 2004;54:1159–1160.

103. Shibata N, Doi Y, Yamane K, et al. PCR typing of genetic determinants for metallo-beta-lactamases and integrases carried by gram-negative bacteria isolated in Japan, with focus on the class 3 integron. J Clin Microbiol 2003;41:5407–5413.

104. Toleman MA, Biedenbach D, Bennett DM, Jones RN, Walsh TR. Italian metallo-beta-lactamases: a national problem? Report from the SENTRY Antimicrobial Surveillance Programme. J Antimicrob Chemother 2005;55:61–70.

105. Lee K, Ha GY, Shin BM, et al. Metallo-beta-lactamase-producing Gram-negative bacilli in Korean Nationwide Surveillance of Antimicrobial Resistance group hospitals in 2003: continued prevalence of VIM-producing *Pseudomonas* spp. and increase of IMP-producing *Acinetobacter* spp. Diagn Microbiol Infect Dis 2004;50:51–58.

106. Pitout JD, Gregson DB, Poirel L, McClure JA, Le P, Church DL. Detection of *Pseudomonas aeruginosa* producing metallo-beta-lactamases in a large centralized laboratory. J Clin Microbiol 2005;43:3129–3135.

107. Yan JJ, Hsueh PR, Ko WC, et al. Metallo-beta-lactamases in clinical *Pseudomonas* isolates in Taiwan and identification of VIM-3, a novel variant of the VIM-2 enzyme. Antimicrob Agents Chemother 2001;45:2224–2228.

108. Fiett J, Baraniak A, Mrowka A, et al. Molecular epidemiology of acquired-metallo-beta-lactamase-producing bacteria in Poland. Antimicrob Agents Chemother 2006;50:880–886.

109. Martineau F, Picard FJ, Grenier L, Roy PH, Ouellette M, Bergeron MG. Multiplex PCR assays for the detection of clinically relevant antibiotic resistance genes in staphylococci isolated from patients infected after cardiac surgery. The ESPRIT Trial. J Antimicrob Chemother 2000;46:527–534.

110. Nagaoka T, Horii T, Satoh T, et al. Use of a three-dimensional microarray system for detection of levofloxacin resistance and the *mecA* gene in *Staphylococcus aureus*. J Clin Microbiol 2005;43:5187–5194.

111. Schmitz FJ, Mackenzie CR, Hofmann B, et al. Specific information concerning taxonomy, pathogenicity and methicillin resistance of staphylococci obtained by a multiplex PCR. J Med Microbiol 1997;46:773–778.

112. Zambardi G, Reverdy ME, Bland S, Bes M, Freney J, Fleurette J. Laboratory diagnosis of oxacillin resistance in *Staphylococcus aureus* by a multiplex-polymerase chain reaction assay. Diagn Microbiol Infect Dis 1994;19:25–31.

113. Kobayashi N, Wu H, Kojima K, et al. Detection of *mecA*, *femA*, and *femB* genes in clinical strains of staphylococci using polymerase chain reaction. Epidemiol Infect 1994;113:259–266.

114. Mason WJ, Blevins JS, Beenken K, Wibowo N, Ojha N, Smeltzer MS. Multiplex PCR protocol for the diagnosis of staphylococcal infection. J Clin Microbiol 2001;39:3332–3338.

115. Tsuji H, Tsuru T, Okuzumi K. Detection of methicillin-resistant *Staphylococcus aureus* in donor eye preservation media by polymerase chain reaction. Jpn J Ophthalmol 1998;42:352–356.

116. Skov RL, Pallesen LV, Poulsen RL, Espersen F. Evaluation of a new 3-h hybridization method for detecting the *mecA* gene in *Staphylococcus aureus* and comparison with existing genotypic and phenotypic susceptibility testing methods. J Antimicrob Chemother 1999;43:467–475.

117. Olsson-Liljequist B, Larsson P, Ringertz S, Lofdahl S. Use of a DNA hybridization method to verify results of screening for

methicillin resistance in staphylococci. Eur J Clin Microbiol Infect Dis 1993;12:527–533.

118. Archer GL, Pennell E. Detection of methicillin resistance in staphylococci by using a DNA probe. Antimicrob Agents Chemother 1990;34:1720–1724.

119. Jonas D, Grundmann H, Hartung D, Daschner FD, Towner KJ. Evaluation of the *mecA femB* duplex polymerase chain reaction for detection of methicillin-resistant *Staphylococcus aureus*. Eur J Clin Microbiol Infect Dis 1999;18:643–647.

120. Rothschild CB, Triscott MX, Bowden DW, Doellgast G. A microtiter plate assay using cascade amplification for detection of nonisotopically labeled DNA. Anal Biochem 1995;225:64–72.

121. Towner KJ, Talbot DC, Curran R, Webster CA, Humphreys H. Development and evaluation of a PCR-based immunoassay for the rapid detection of methicillin-resistant *Staphylococcus aureus*. J Med Microbiol 1998;47:607–613.

122. Ubukata K, Nakagami S, Nitta A, et al. Rapid detection of the *mecA* gene in methicillin-resistant staphylococci by enzymatic detection of polymerase chain reaction products. J Clin Microbiol 1992;30:1728–1733.

123. Hamels S, Gala JL, Dufour S, Vannuffel P, Zammatteo N, Remacle J. Consensus PCR and microarray for diagnosis of the genus *Staphylococcus*, species, and methicillin resistance. BioTechniques 2001;31:1364–1366, 1368, 1370–1372.

124. Kolbert CP, Arruda J, Varga-Delmore P, et al. Branched-DNA assay for detection of the *mecA* gene in oxacillin-resistant and oxacillin-sensitive staphylococci. J Clin Microbiol 1998;36:2640–2644.

125. Levi K, Bailey C, Bennett A, Marsh P, Cardy DL, Towner KJ. Evaluation of an isothermal signal amplification method for rapid detection of methicillin-resistant *Staphylococcus aureus* from patient-screening swabs. J Clin Microbiol 2003;41:3187–3191.

126. Fong WK, Modrusan Z, McNevin JP, Marostenmaki J, Zin B, Bekkaoui F. Rapid solid-phase immunoassay for detection of methicillin-resistant *Staphylococcus aureus* using cycling probe technology. J Clin Microbiol 2000;38:2525–2529.

127. Kearns AM, Seiders PR, Wheeler J, Freeman R, Steward M. Rapid detection of methicillin-resistant staphylococci by multiplex PCR. J Hosp Infect 1999;43:33–37.

128. Vannuffel P, Gigi J, Ezzedine H, et al. Specific detection of methicillin-resistant *Staphylococcus* species by multiplex PCR. J Clin Microbiol 1995;33:2864–2867.

129. Sakoulas G, Gold HS, Venkataraman L, DeGirolami PC, Eliopoulos GM, Qian Q. Methicillin-resistant *Staphylococcus aureus*: comparison of susceptibility testing methods and analysis of *mecA*-positive susceptible strains. J Clin Microbiol 2001;39:3946–3951.

130. Smyth RW, Kahlmeter G, Olsson Liljequist B, Hoffman B. Methods for identifying methicillin resistance in *Staphylococcus aureus*. J Hosp Infect 2001;48:103–107.

131. Petersson AC, Miorner H. Species-specific identification of methicillin resistance in staphylococci. Eur J Clin Microbiol Infect Dis 1995;14:206–211.

132. Salisbury SM, Sabatini LM, Spiegel CA. Identification of methicillin-resistant staphylococci by multiplex polymerase chain reaction assay. Am J Clin Pathol 1997;107:368–373.

133. Cuny C, Salmenlinna S, Witte W. Evaluation of a reverse hybridization blot test for detection of oxacillin-resistant *Staphylococcus aureus*. Eur J Clin Microbiol Infect Dis 2001;20:906–907.

134. Siripornmongcolchai T, Chomvarin C, Chaicumpar K, Limpaiboon T, Wongkhum C. Evaluation of different primers for detecting *mecA* gene by PCR in comparison with phenotypic methods for discrimination of methicillin-resistant *Staphylococcus aureus*. Southeast Asian J Trop Med Public Health 2002;33:758–763.

135. Lem P, Spiegelman J, Toye B, Ramotar K. Direct detection of *mecA*, *nuc* and 16S rRNA genes in BacT/Alert blood culture bottles. Diagn Microbiol Infect Dis 2001;41:165–168.

136. Carroll KC, Leonard RB, Newcomb-Gayman PL, Hillyard DR. Rapid detection of the staphylococcal *mecA* gene from BACTEC blood culture bottles by the polymerase chain reaction. Am J Clin Pathol 1996;106:600–605.

137. Jaffe RI, Lane JD, Albury SV, Niemeyer DM. Rapid extraction from and direct identification in clinical samples of methicillin-resistant staphylococci using the PCR. J Clin Microbiol 2000;38:3407–3412.

138. Hallin M, Maes N, Byl B, Jacobs F, De Gheldre Y, Struelens MJ. Clinical impact of a PCR assay for identification of *Staphylococcus aureus* and determination of methicillin resistance directly from blood cultures. J Clin Microbiol 2003;41:3942–3944.

139. Maes N, Magdalena J, Rottiers S, De Gheldre Y, Struelens MJ. Evaluation of a triplex PCR assay to discriminate *Staphylococcus aureus* from coagulase-negative staphylococci and determine methicillin resistance from blood cultures. J Clin Microbiol 2002;40:1514–1517.

140. Schmitz FJ, Steiert M, Hofmann B, et al. Detection of staphylococcal genes directly from cerebrospinal and peritoneal fluid samples using a multiplex polymerase chain reaction. Eur J Clin Microbiol Infect Dis 1998;17:272–274.

141. Vannuffel P, Laterre PF, Bouyer M, et al. Rapid and specific molecular identification of methicillin-resistant *Staphylococcus aureus* in endotracheal aspirates from mechanically ventilated patients. J Clin Microbiol 1998;36:2366–2368.

142. Kitagawa Y, Ueda M, Ando N, et al. Rapid diagnosis of methicillin-resistant *Staphylococcus aureus* bacteremia by nested polymerase chain reaction. Ann Surg 1996;224:665–671.

143. Grisold AJ, Leitner E, Muhlbauer G, Marth E, Kessler HH. Detection of methicillin-resistant *Staphylococcus aureus* and simultaneous confirmation by automated nucleic acid extraction and real-time PCR. J Clin Microbiol 2002;40:2392–2397.

144. Rohrer S, Tschierske M, Zbinden R, Berger-Bachi B. Improved methods for detection of methicillin-resistant *Staphylococcus aureus*. Eur J Clin Microbiol Infect Dis 2001;20:267–270.

145. Elsayed S, Chow BL, Hamilton NL, Gregson DB, Pitout JD, Church DL. Development and validation of a molecular beacon probe-based real-time polymerase chain reaction assay for rapid detection of methicillin resistance in *Staphylococcus aureus*. Arch Pathol Lab Med 2003;127:845–849.

146. Reischl U, Linde HJ, Metz M, Leppmeier B, Lehn N. Rapid identification of methicillin-resistant *Staphylococcus aureus* and simultaneous species confirmation using real-time fluorescence PCR. J Clin Microbiol 2000;38:2429–2433.

147. Killgore GE, Holloway B, Tenover FC. A 5′ nuclease PCR (TaqMan) high-throughput assay for detection of the *mecA* gene in staphylococci. J Clin Microbiol 2000;38:2516–2519.

148. Tan TY, Corden S, Barnes R, Cookson B. Rapid identification of methicillin-resistant *Staphylococcus aureus* from positive blood cultures by real-time fluorescence PCR. J Clin Microbiol 2001;39:4529–4531.

149. Shrestha NK, Tuohy MJ, Hall GS, Isada CM, Procop GW. Rapid identification of *Staphylococcus aureus* and the *mecA* gene from BacT/ALERT blood culture bottles by using the LightCycler system. J Clin Microbiol 2002;40:2659–2661.

150. Fang H, Hedin G. Rapid screening and identification of methicillin-resistant *Staphylococcus aureus* from clinical samples by selective-broth and real-time PCR assay. J Clin Microbiol 2003;41:2894–2899.

151. Murakami K, Minamide W, Wada K, Nakamura E, Teraoka H, Watanabe S. Identification of methicillin-resistant strains of staphylococci by polymerase chain reaction. J Clin Microbiol 1991;29:2240–2244.

152. Nagai K, Shibasaki Y, Hasegawa K, et al. Evaluation of PCR primers to screen for *Streptococcus pneumoniae* isolates and beta-lactam resistance, and to detect common macrolide resistance determinants. J Antimicrob Chemother 2001;48:915–918.

153. Jalal H, Organji S, Reynolds J, Bennett D, O'Mason E, Jr., Millar MR. Determination of penicillin susceptibility of *Streptococcus pneumoniae* using the polymerase chain reaction. Mol Pathol 1997;50:45–50.

154. du Plessis M, Smith AM, Klugman KP. Application of *pbp1A* PCR in identification of penicillin-resistant *Streptococcus pneumoniae*. J Clin Microbiol 1999;37:628–632.

155. Ubukata K, Asahi Y, Yamane A, Konno M. Combinational detection of autolysin and penicillin-binding protein 2B genes of *Streptococcus pneumoniae* by PCR. J Clin Microbiol 1996;34:592–596.

156. du Plessis M, Smith AM, Klugman KP. Rapid detection of penicillin-resistant *Streptococcus pneumoniae* in cerebrospinal fluid by a seminested-PCR strategy. J Clin Microbiol 1998;36:453–457.

157. Beall B, Facklam RR, Jackson DM, Starling HH. Rapid screening for penicillin susceptibility of systemic pneumococcal isolates by restriction enzyme profiling of the *pbp2B* gene. J Clin Microbiol 1998;36:2359–2362.

158. O'Neill AM, Gillespie SH, Whiting GC. Detection of penicillin susceptibility in *Streptococcus pneumoniae* by *pbp2b* PCR-restriction fragment length polymorphism analysis. J Clin Microbiol 1999;37:157–160.

159. Volokhov D, Chizhikov V, Chumakov K, Rasooly A. Microarray analysis of erythromycin resistance determinants. J Appl Microbiol 2003;95:787–798.

160. Sutcliffe J, Grebe T, Tait-Kamradt A, Wondrack L. Detection of erythromycin-resistant determinants by PCR. Antimicrob Agents Chemother 1996;40:2562–2566.

161. Amezaga MR, McKenzie H. Molecular epidemiology of macrolide resistance in β-haemolytic streptococci of Lancefield groups A, B, C and G and evidence for a new *mef* element in group G streptococci that carries allelic variants of *mef* and *msr(D)*. J Antimicrob Chemother 2006;57:443–449.

162. Shortridge VD, Flamm RK, Ramer N, Beyer J, Tanaka SK. Novel mechanism of macrolide resistance in *Streptococcus pneumoniae*. Diagn Microbiol Infect Dis 1996;26:73–78.

163. Clancy J, Petitpas J, Dib-Hajj F, et al. Molecular cloning and functional analysis of a novel macrolide-resistance determinant, *mefA*, from *Streptococcus pyogenes*. Mol Microbiol 1996;22:867–879.

164. Haroche J, Morvan A, Davi M, Allignet J, Bimet F, El Solh N. Clonal diversity among streptogramin A-resistant *Staphylococcus aureus* isolates collected in French hospitals. J Clin Microbiol 2003;41:586–591.

165. Robredo B, Singh KV, Torres C, Murray BE. Streptogramin resistance and shared pulsed-field gel electrophoresis patterns in *vanA*-containing *Enterococcus faecium* and *Enterococcus hirae* isolated from humans and animals in Spain. Microb Drug Resist 2000;6:305–311.

166. Allignet J, el Solh N. Diversity among the gram-positive acetyltransferases inactivating streptogramin A and structurally related compounds and characterization of a new staphylococcal determinant, *vatB*. Antimicrob Agents Chemother 1995;39:2027–2036.

167. Jensen LB, Hammerum AM, Aerestrup FM, van den Bogaard AE, Stobberingh EE. Occurrence of *satA* and *vgb* genes in streptogramin-resistant *Enterococcus faecium* isolates of animal and human origins in The Netherlands. Antimicrob Agents Chemother 1998;42:3330–3331.

168. Werner G, Klare I, Heier H, et al. Quinupristin/dalfopristin-resistant enterococci of the *satA* (*vatD*) and *satG* (*vatE*) genotypes from different ecological origins in Germany. Microb Drug Resist 2000;6:37–47.

169. Werner G, Strommenger B, Klare I, Witte W. Molecular detection of linezolid resistance in *Enterococcus faecium* and *Enterococcus faecalis* by use of 5' nuclease real-time PCR compared to a modified classical approach. J Clin Microbiol 2004;42:5327–5331.

170. Woodford N, Tysall L, Auckland C, et al. Detection of oxazolidinone-resistant *Enterococcus faecalis* and *Enterococcus faecium* strains by real-time PCR and PCR-restriction fragment length polymorphism analysis. J Clin Microbiol 2002;40:4298–4300.

171. Sinclair A, Arnold C, Woodford N. Rapid detection and estimation by pyrosequencing of 23S rRNA genes with a single nucleotide polymorphism conferring linezolid resistance in enterococci. Antimicrob Agents Chemother 2003;47:3620–3622.

172. Booth SA, Drebot MA, Martin IE, Ng LK. Design of oligonucleotide arrays to detect point mutations: molecular typing of antibiotic resistant strains of *Neisseria gonorrhoeae* and hantavirus infected deer mice. Mol Cell Probes 2003;17:77–84.

173. Yu X, Susa M, Knabbe C, Schmid RD, Bachmann TT. Development and validation of a diagnostic DNA microarray to detect quinolone-resistant *Escherichia coli* among clinical isolates. J Clin Microbiol 2004;42:4083–4091.

174. Couzinet S, Yugueros J, Barras C, et al. Evaluation of a high-density oligonucleotide array for characterization of *grlA*, *grlB*, *gyrA* and *gyrB* mutations in fluoroquinolone resistant *Staphylococcus aureus* isolates. J Microbiol Methods 2005;60:275–279.

175. Davies TA, Goldschmidt R. Screening of large numbers of *Streptococcus pneumoniae* isolates for mutations associated with fluoroquinolone resistance using an oligonucleotide probe assay. FEMS Microbiol Lett 2002;217:219–224.

176. Pan XS, Ambler J, Mehtar S, Fisher LM. Involvement of topoisomerase IV and DNA gyrase as ciprofloxacin targets in *Streptococcus pneumoniae*. Antimicrob Agents Chemother 1996;40:2321–2326.

177. Cheng AF, Yew WW, Chan EW, Chin ML, Hui MM, Chan RC. Multiplex PCR amplimer conformation analysis for rapid detection of *gyrA* mutations in fluoroquinolone-resistant *Mycobacterium tuberculosis* clinical isolates. Antimicrob Agents Chemother 2004;48:596–601.

178. Dauendorffer JN, Guillemin I, Aubry A, et al. Identification of mycobacterial species by PCR sequencing of quinolone resistance-determining regions of DNA gyrase genes. J Clin Microbiol 2003;41:1311–1315.

179. Takahashi H, Kikuchi T, Shoji S, et al. Characterization of *gyrA*, *gyrB*, *grlA* and *grlB* mutations in fluoroquinolone-resistant clinical isolates of *Staphylococcus aureus*. J Antimicrob Chemother 1998;41:49–57.

180. Weigel LM, Steward CD, Tenover FC. *gyrA* mutations associated with fluoroquinolone resistance in eight species of *Enterobacteriaceae*. Antimicrob Agents Chemother 1998;42:2661–2667.

181. Ozeki S, Deguchi T, Yasuda M, et al. Development of a rapid assay for detecting *gyrA* mutations in *Escherichia coli* and determination of incidence of *gyrA* mutations in clinical strains isolated from patients with complicated urinary tract infections. J Clin Microbiol 1997;35:2315–2319.

182. Qiang YZ, Qin T, Fu W, Cheng WP, Li YS, Yi G. Use of a rapid mismatch PCR method to detect *gyrA* and *parC* mutations in ciprofloxacin-resistant clinical isolates of *Escherichia coli*. J Antimicrob Chemother 2002;49:549–552.

183. Bachoual R, Tankovic J, Soussy CJ. Analysis of the mutations involved in fluoroquinolone resistance of in vivo and in vitro mutants of *Escherichia coli*. Microb Drug Resist 1998;4:271–276.

184. Walker RA, Saunders N, Lawson AJ, et al. Use of a LightCycler *gyrA* mutation assay for rapid identification of mutations confer-

ring decreased susceptibility to ciprofloxacin in multiresistant *Salmonella enterica* serotype Typhimurium DT104 isolates. J Clin Microbiol 2001;39:1443–1448.

185. Ling JM, Chan EW, Lam AW, Cheng AF. Mutations in topoisomerase genes of fluoroquinolone-resistant salmonellae in Hong Kong. Antimicrob Agents Chemother 2003;47:3567–3573.

186. Giraud E, Brisabois A, Martel JL, Chaslus-Dancla E. Comparative studies of mutations in animal isolates and experimental in vitro- and in vivo-selected mutants of *Salmonella* spp. suggest a counterselection of highly fluoroquinolone-resistant strains in the field. Antimicrob Agents Chemother 1999;43:2131–2137.

187. Zirnstein G, Li Y, Swaminathan B, Angulo F. Ciprofloxacin resistance in *Campylobacter jejuni* isolates: detection of *gyrA* resistance mutations by mismatch amplification mutation assay PCR and DNA sequence analysis. J Clin Microbiol 1999;37:3276–3280.

188. Wilson DL, Abner SR, Newman TC, Mansfield LS, Linz JE. Identification of ciprofloxacin-resistant *Campylobacter jejuni* by use of a fluorogenic PCR assay. J Clin Microbiol 2000;38:3971–3978.

189. Beckmann L, Muller M, Luber P, Schrader C, Bartelt E, Klein G. Analysis of *gyrA* mutations in quinolone-resistant and -susceptible *Campylobacter jejuni* isolates from retail poultry and human clinical isolates by non-radioactive single-strand conformation polymorphism analysis and DNA sequencing. J Appl Microbiol 2004;96:1040–1047.

190. Ip M, Chau SS, Chi F, Qi A, Lai RW. Rapid screening of fluoroquinolone resistance determinants in *Streptococcus pneumoniae* by PCR-restriction fragment length polymorphism and single-strand conformational polymorphism. J Clin Microbiol 2006;44:970–975.

191. Alonso R, Morales G, Escalante R, Campanario E, Sastre L, Martinez-Beltran JL. An extended PCR-RFLP assay for detection of *parC*, *parE* and *gyrA* mutations in fluoroquinolone-resistant *Streptococcus pneumoniae*. J Antimicrob Chemother 2004;53:682–683.

192. Morrissey I, Farrell DJ, Bakker S, Buckridge S, Felmingham D. Molecular characterization and antimicrobial susceptibility of fluoroquinolone-resistant or -susceptible *Streptococcus pneumoniae* from Hong Kong. Antimicrob Agents Chemother 2003;47:1433–1435.

193. Pestova E, Beyer R, Cianciotto NP, Noskin GA, Peterson LR. Contribution of topoisomerase IV and DNA gyrase mutations in *Streptococcus pneumoniae* to resistance to novel fluoroquinolones. Antimicrob Agents Chemother 1999;43:2000–2004.

194. Shigemura K, Shirakawa T, Okada H, et al. Rapid detection of *gyrA* and *parC* mutations in fluoroquinolone-resistant *Neisseria gonorrhoeae* by denaturing high-performance liquid chromatography. J Microbiol Methods 2004;59:415–421.

195. Sultan Z, Nahar S, Wretlind B, Lindback E, Rahman M. Comparison of mismatch amplification mutation assay with DNA sequencing for characterization of fluoroquinolone resistance in *Neisseria gonorrhoeae*. J Clin Microbiol 2004;42:591–594.

196. Tanaka M, Nakayama H, Haraoka M, Saika T. Antimicrobial resistance of *Neisseria gonorrhoeae* and high prevalence of ciprofloxacin-resistant isolates in Japan, 1993 to 1998. J Clin Microbiol 2000;38:521–525.

197. Li Z, Yokoi S, Kawamura Y, Maeda S, Ezaki T, Deguchi T. Rapid detection of quinolone resistance-associated *gyrA* mutations in *Neisseria gonorrhoeae* with a LightCycler. J Infect Chemother 2002;8:145–150.

198. Lee JK, Lee YS, Park YK, Kim BS. Alterations in the GyrA and GyrB subunits of topoisomerase II and the ParC and ParE subunits of topoisomerase IV in ciprofloxacin-resistant clinical isolates of *Pseudomonas aeruginosa*. Int J Antimicrob Agents 2005;25:290–295.

199. Lee AS, Tang LL, Lim IH, Wong SY. Characterization of pyrazinamide and ofloxacin resistance among drug resistant *Mycobacterium tuberculosis* isolates from Singapore. Int J Infect Dis 2002;6:48–51.

200. Lapierre P, Huletsky A, Fortin V, et al. Real-time PCR assay for detection of fluoroquinolone resistance associated with *grlA* mutations in *Staphylococcus aureus*. J Clin Microbiol 2003;41:3246–3251.

201. Decousser JW, Methlouthi I, Pina P, Collignon A, Allouch P. New real-time PCR assay using locked nucleic acid probes to assess prevalence of ParC mutations in fluoroquinolone-susceptible *Streptococcus pneumoniae* isolates from France. Antimicrob Agents Chemother 2006;50:1594–1598.

202. Trieu-Cuot P, de Cespedes G, Bentorcha F, Delbos F, Gaspar E, Horaud T. Study of heterogeneity of chloramphenicol acetyltransferase (CAT) genes in streptococci and enterococci by polymerase chain reaction: characterization of a new CAT determinant. Antimicrob Agents Chemother 1993;37:2593–2598.

203. Mokrousov I, Narvskaya O, Limeschenko E, Otten T, Vyshnevskiy B. Detection of ethambutol-resistant *Mycobacterium tuberculosis* strains by multiplex allele-specific PCR assay targeting *embB306* mutations. J Clin Microbiol 2002;40:1617–1620.

204. Ahmad S, Mokaddas E, Jaber AA. Rapid detection of ethambutol-resistant *Mycobacterium tuberculosis* strains by PCR-RFLP targeting *embB* codons 306 and 497 and *iniA* codon 501 mutations. Mol Cell Probes 2004;18:299–306.

205. Wada T, Maeda S, Tamaru A, Imai S, Hase A, Kobayashi K. Dual-probe assay for rapid detection of drug-resistant *Mycobacterium tuberculosis* by real-time PCR. J Clin Microbiol 2004;42:5277–5285.

206. Johnson R, Jordaan AM, Pretorius L, et al. Ethambutol resistance testing by mutation detection. Int J Tuberc Lung Dis 2006;10:68–73.

207. Denkin S, Volokhov D, Chizhikov V, Zhang Y. Microarray-based *pncA* genotyping of pyrazinamide-resistant strains of *Mycobacterium tuberculosis*. J Med Microbiol 2005;54:1127–1131.

208. Suzuki Y, Suzuki A, Tamaru A, Katsukawa C, Oda H. Rapid detection of pyrazinamide-resistant *Mycobacterium tuberculosis* by a PCR-based in vitro system. J Clin Microbiol 2002;40:501–507.

209. McCammon MT, Gillette JS, Thomas DP, et al. Detection by denaturing gradient gel electrophoresis of *pncA* mutations associated with pyrazinamide resistance in *Mycobacterium tuberculosis* isolates from the United States-Mexico border region. Antimicrob Agents Chemother 2005;49:2210–2217.

210. Liu YP, Behr MA, Small PM, Kurn N. Genotypic determination of *Mycobacterium tuberculosis* antibiotic resistance using a novel mutation detection method, the branch migration inhibition *M. tuberculosis* antibiotic resistance test. J Clin Microbiol 2000;38:3656–3662.

211. Mikhailovich V, Lapa S, Gryadunov D, et al. Identification of rifampin-resistant *Mycobacterium tuberculosis* strains by hybridization, PCR, and ligase detection reaction on oligonucleotide microchips. J Clin Microbiol 2001;39:2531–2540.

212. Yue J, Shi W, Xie J, et al. Detection of rifampin-resistant *Mycobacterium tuberculosis* strains by using a specialized oligonucleotide microarray. Diagn Microbiol Infect Dis 2004;48:47–54.

213. Deng JY, Zhang XE, Lu HB, et al. Multiplex detection of mutations in clinical isolates of rifampin-resistant *Mycobacterium tuberculosis* by short oligonucleotide ligation assay on DNA chips. J Clin Microbiol 2004;42:4850–4852.

214. Bi LJ, Zhou YF, Zhang XE, Deng JY, Wen JK, Zhang ZP. Construction and characterization of different MutS fusion proteins as recognition elements of DNA chip for detection of DNA mutations. Biosens Bioelectron 2005;21:135–144.

215. Sougakoff W, Rodrigue M, Truffot-Pernot C, et al. Use of a high-density DNA probe array for detecting mutations involved in rifampicin resistance in *Mycobacterium tuberculosis*. Clin Microbiol Infect 2004;10:289–294.

216. Tang X, Morris SL, Langone JJ, Bockstahler LE. Microarray and allele specific PCR detection of point mutations in *Mycobacterium tuberculosis* genes associated with drug resistance. J Microbiol Methods 2005;63:318–330.

217. Aragon LM, Navarro F, Heiser V, Garrigo M, Espanol M, Coll P. Rapid detection of specific gene mutations associated with isoniazid or rifampicin resistance in *Mycobacterium tuberculosis* clinical isolates using non-fluorescent low-density DNA microarrays. J Antimicrob Chemother 2006;57:825–831.

218. Kim SY, Park YJ, Song E, et al. Evaluation of the CombiChip Mycobacteria Drug-Resistance detection DNA chip for identifying mutations associated with resistance to isoniazid and rifampin in *Mycobacterium tuberculosis*. Diagn Microbiol Infect Dis 2006;54:203–210.

219. Head SR, Parikh K, Rogers YH, Bishai W, Goelet P, Boyce-Jacino MT. Solid-phase sequence scanning for drug resistance detection in tuberculosis. Mol Cell Probes 1999;13:81–87.

220. Kapur V, Li LL, Hamrick MR, et al. Rapid *Mycobacterium* species assignment and unambiguous identification of mutations associated with antimicrobial resistance in *Mycobacterium tuberculosis* by automated DNA sequencing. Arch Pathol Lab Med 1995;119:131–138.

221. Scarpellini P, Braglia S, Carrera P, et al. Detection of rifampin resistance in *Mycobacterium tuberculosis* by double gradient-denaturing gradient gel electrophoresis. Antimicrob Agents Chemother 1999;43:2550–2554.

222. Nash KA, Gaytan A, Inderlied CB. Detection of rifampin resistance in *Mycobacterium tuberculosis* by use of a rapid, simple, and specific RNA/RNA mismatch assay. J Infect Dis 1997;176:533–536.

223. Thomas GA, Williams DL, Soper SA. Capillary electrophoresis-based heteroduplex analysis with a universal heteroduplex generator for detection of point mutations associated with rifampin resistance in tuberculosis. Clin Chem 2001;47:1195–1203.

224. Garcia L, Alonso Sanz M, Rebollo MJ, Tercero JC, Chaves F. Mutations in the *rpoB* gene of rifampin-resistant *Mycobacterium tuberculosis* isolates in Spain and their rapid detection by PCR-enzyme-linked immunosorbent assay. J Clin Microbiol 2001;39:1813–1818.

225. El-Hajj HH, Marras SA, Tyagi S, Kramer FR, Alland D. Detection of rifampin resistance in *Mycobacterium tuberculosis* in a single tube with molecular beacons. J Clin Microbiol 2001;39:4131–4137.

226. Fan XY, Hu ZY, Xu FH, Yan ZQ, Guo SQ, Li ZM. Rapid detection of *rpoB* gene mutations in rifampin-resistant *Mycobacterium tuberculosis* isolates in shanghai by using the amplification refractory mutation system. J Clin Microbiol 2003;41:993–997.

227. Williams DL, Spring L, Gillis TP, Salfinger M, Persing DH. Evaluation of a polymerase chain reaction-based universal heteroduplex generator assay for direct detection of rifampin susceptibility of *Mycobacterium tuberculosis* from sputum specimens. Clin Infect Dis 1998;26:446–450.

228. Carvalho WS, Spindola de Miranda S, Costa KM, et al. Low-stringency single-specific-primer PCR as a tool for detection of mutations in the *rpoB* gene of rifampin-resistant *Mycobacterium tuberculosis*. J Clin Microbiol 2003;41:3384–3386.

229. Iwamoto T, Sonobe T. Peptide nucleic acid-mediated competitive PCR clamping for detection of rifampin-resistant *Mycobacterium tuberculosis*. Antimicrob Agents Chemother 2004;48:4023–4026.

230. Ruiz M, Torres MJ, Llanos AC, Arroyo A, Palomares JC, Aznar J. Direct detection of rifampin- and isoniazid-resistant *Mycobacterium tuberculosis* in auramine-rhodamine-positive sputum specimens by real-time PCR. J Clin Microbiol 2004;42:1585–1589.

231. Espasa M, Gonzalez-Martin J, Alcaide F, et al. Direct detection in clinical samples of multiple gene mutations causing resistance of *Mycobacterium tuberculosis* to isoniazid and rifampicin using fluorogenic probes. J Antimicrob Chemother 2005;55:860–865.

232. Park YK, Shin S, Ryu S, et al. Comparison of drug resistance genotypes between Beijing and non-Beijing family strains of *Mycobacterium tuberculosis* in Korea. J Microbiol Methods 2005;63:165–172.

233. Nikolayevsky V, Brown T, Balabanova Y, Ruddy M, Fedorin I, Drobniewski F. Detection of mutations associated with isoniazid and rifampin resistance in *Mycobacterium tuberculosis* isolates from Samara Region, Russian Federation. J Clin Microbiol 2004;42:4498–4502.

234. Arnold C, Westland L, Mowat G, Underwood A, Magee J, Gharbia S. Single-nucleotide polymorphism-based differentiation and drug resistance detection in *Mycobacterium tuberculosis* from isolates or directly from sputum. Clin Microbiol Infect 2005;11:122–130.

235. Bockstahler LE, Li Z, Nguyen NY, et al. Peptide nucleic acid probe detection of mutations in *Mycobacterium tuberculosis* genes associated with drug resistance. BioTechniques 2002;32:508–510, 512, 514.

236. Telenti A, Honore N, Bernasconi C, et al. Genotypic assessment of isoniazid and rifampin resistance in *Mycobacterium tuberculosis*: a blind study at reference laboratory level. J Clin Microbiol 1997;35:719–723.

237. Cooksey RC, Holloway BP, Oldenburg MC, Listenbee S, Miller CW. Evaluation of the invader assay, a linear signal amplification method, for identification of mutations associated with resistance to rifampin and isoniazid in *Mycobacterium tuberculosis*. Antimicrob Agents Chemother 2000;44:1296–1301.

238. Leung ET, Kam KM, Chiu A, et al. Detection of *katG* Ser315Thr substitution in respiratory specimens from patients with isoniazid-resistant *Mycobacterium tuberculosis* using PCR-RFLP. J Med Microbiol 2003;52:999–1003.

239. Herrera-Leon L, Molinas T, Saiz P, Saez Nieto JA, Jimenez MS. New multiplex PCR for rapid detection of isoniazid-resistant *Mycobacterium tuberculosis* clinical isolates. Antimicrob Agents Chemother 2005;49:144–147.

240. Parsons LM, Salfinger M, Clobridge A, et al. Phenotypic and molecular characterization of *Mycobacterium tuberculosis* isolates resistant to both isoniazid and ethambutol. Antimicrob Agents Chemother 2005;49:2218–2225.

241. Zhang M, Yue J, Yang YP, et al. Detection of mutations associated with isoniazid resistance in *Mycobacterium tuberculosis* isolates from China. J Clin Microbiol 2005;43:5477–5482.

242. Dutka-Malen S, Evers S, Courvalin P. Detection of glycopeptide resistance genotypes and identification to the species level of clinically relevant enterococci by PCR. J Clin Microbiol 1995;33:24–27.

243. Miele A, Bandera M, Goldstein BP. Use of primers selective for vancomycin resistance genes to determine *van* genotype in enterococci and to study gene organization in VanA isolates. Antimicrob Agents Chemother 1995;39:1772–1778.

244. Jayaratne P, Rutherford C. Detection of clinically relevant genotypes of vancomycin-resistant enterococci in nosocomial surveillance specimens by PCR. J Clin Microbiol 1999;37:2090–2092.

245. Bell JM, Paton JC, Turnidge J. Emergence of vancomycin-resistant enterococci in Australia: phenotypic and genotypic characteristics of isolates. J Clin Microbiol 1998;36:2187–2190.

246. Patel R, Uhl JR, Kohner P, Hopkins MK, Cockerill FR, III. Multiplex PCR detection of *vanA*, *vanB*, *vanC-1*, and *vanC-2/3* genes in enterococci. J Clin Microbiol 1997;35:703–707.

247. Dutka-Malen S, Leclercq R, Coutant V, Duval J, Courvalin P. Phenotypic and genotypic heterogeneity of glycopeptide resistance determinants in gram-positive bacteria. Antimicrob Agents Chemother 1990;34:1875–1879.

248. Modrusan Z, Marlowe C, Wheeler D, Pirseyedi M, Bryan RN. Detection of vancomycin resistant genes *vanA* and *vanB* by cycling probe technology. Mol Cell Probes 1999;13:223–231.

249. Poulsen RL, Pallesen LV, Frimodt-Moller N, Espersen F. Detection of clinical vancomycin-resistant enterococci in Denmark by multiplex PCR and sandwich hybridization. APMIS 1999;107:404–412.

250. Depardieu F, Perichon B, Courvalin P. Detection of the *van* alphabet and identification of enterococci and staphylococci at the species level by multiplex PCR. J Clin Microbiol 2004;42:5857–5860.

251. Sinsimer D, Leekha S, Park S, et al. Use of a multiplex molecular beacon platform for rapid detection of methicillin and vancomycin resistance in *Staphylococcus aureus*. J Clin Microbiol 2005;43:4585–4591.

252. Domingo MC, Huletsky A, Giroux R, et al. High prevalence of glycopeptide resistance genes *vanB*, *vanD*, and *vanG* not associated with enterococci in human fecal flora. Antimicrob Agents Chemother 2005;49:4784–4786.

253. Palladino S, Kay ID, Flexman JP, et al. Rapid detection of *vanA* and *vanB* genes directly from clinical specimens and enrichment broths by real-time multiplex PCR assay. J Clin Microbiol 2003;41:2483–2486.

254. Paule SM, Trick WE, Tenover FC, et al. Comparison of PCR assay to culture for surveillance detection of vancomycin-resistant enterococci. J Clin Microbiol 2003;41:4805–4807.

255. Petrich AK, Luinstra KE, Groves D, Chernesky MA, Mahony JB. Direct detection of *vanA* and *vanB* genes in clinical specimens for rapid identification of vancomycin resistant enterococci (VRE) using multiplex PCR. Mol Cell Probes 1999;13:275–281.

256. Perichon B, Reynolds P, Courvalin P. *VanD*-type glycopeptide-resistant *Enterococcus faecium* BM4339. Antimicrob Agents Chemother 1997;41:2016–2018.

257. Fines M, Perichon B, Reynolds P, Sahm DF, Courvalin P. *vanE*, a new type of acquired glycopeptide resistance in *Enterococcus faecalis* BM4405. Antimicrob Agents Chemother 1999;43:2161–2164.

258. McKessar SJ, Berry AM, Bell JM, Turnidge JD, Paton JC. Genetic characterization of *vanG*, a novel vancomycin resistance locus of *Enterococcus faecalis*. Antimicrob Agents Chemother 2000;44:3224–3228.

259. Bryan A, Shapir N, Sadowsky MJ. Frequency and distribution of tetracycline resistance genes in genetically diverse, nonselected, and nonclinical *Escherichia coli* strains isolated from diverse human and animal sources. Appl Environ Microbiol 2004;70:2503–2507.

260. Fluit AC, Florijn A, Verhoef J, Milatovic D. Presence of tetracycline resistance determinants and susceptibility to tigecycline and minocycline. Antimicrob Agents Chemother 2005;49:1636–1638.

261. Call DR, Bakko MK, Krug MJ, Roberts MC. Identifying antimicrobial resistance genes with DNA microarrays. Antimicrob Agents Chemother 2003;47:3290–3295.

262. Aminov RI, Chee-Sanford JC, Garrigues N, Mehboob A, Mackie RI. Detection of tetracycline resistance genes by PCR methods. Methods Mol Biol 2004;268:3–13.

263. Nishimoto Y, Kobayashi N, Alam MM, Ishino M, Uehara N, Watanabe N. Analysis of the prevalence of tetracycline resistance genes in clinical isolates of *Enterococcus faecalis* and *Enterococcus faecium* in a Japanese hospital. Microb Drug Resist 2005;11:146–153.

264. Aarestrup FM, Agerso Y, Gerner-Smidt P, Madsen M, Jensen LB. Comparison of antimicrobial resistance phenotypes and resistance genes in *Enterococcus faecalis* and *Enterococcus faecium* from humans in the community, broilers, and pigs in Denmark. Diagn Microbiol Infect Dis 2000;37:127–137.

265. Olsvik B, Olsen I, Tenover FC. Detection of *tet(M)* and *tet(O)* using the polymerase chain reaction in bacteria isolated from patients with periodontal disease. Oral Microbiol Immunol 1995;10:87–92.

266. Guerra B, Soto SM, Arguelles JM, Mendoza MC. Multidrug resistance is mediated by large plasmids carrying a class 1 integron in the emergent *Salmonella enterica* serotype [4,5,12:i:–]. Antimicrob Agents Chemother 2001;45:1305–1308.

267. Grape M, Sundstrom L, Kronvall G. Sulphonamide resistance gene *sul3* found in *Escherichia coli* isolates from human sources. J Antimicrob Chemother 2003;52:1022–1024.

268. Blahna MT, Zalewski CA, Reuer J, Kahlmeter G, Foxman B, Marrs CF. The role of horizontal gene transfer in the spread of trimethoprim-sulfamethoxazole resistance among uropathogenic *Escherichia coli* in Europe and Canada. J Antimicrob Chemother 2006;57:666–672.

269. Adrian PV, Klugman KP, Amyes SG. Prevalence of trimethoprim resistant dihydrofolate reductase genes identified with oligonucleotide probes in plasmids from isolates of commensal faecal flora. J Antimicrob Chemother 1995;35:497–508.

270. Adrian PV, Thomson CJ, Klugman KP, Amyes SG. Prevalence and genetic location of non-transferable trimethoprim resistant dihydrofolate reductase genes in South African commensal faecal isolates. Epidemiol Infect 1995;115:255–267.

271. Sundstrom L, Jansson C, Bremer K, Heikkila E, Olsson-Liljequist B, Skold O. A new *dhfrVIII* trimethoprim-resistance gene, flanked by IS*26*, whose product is remote from other dihydrofolate reductases in parsimony analysis. Gene 1995;154:7–14.

272. Adrian PV, du Plessis M, Klugman KP, Amyes SG. New trimethoprim-resistant dihydrofolate reductase cassette, *dfrXV*, inserted in a class 1 integron. Antimicrob Agents Chemother 1998;42:2221–2224.

273. Fluit AC, Visser MR, Schmitz FJ. Molecular detection of antimicrobial resistance. Clin Microbiol Rev 2001;14:836–871.

274. Tenover FC, Rasheed JK. Detection of antimicrobial resistance genes and mutations with antimicrobial resistance in microorganism. In: Persing DH, Tenover FC, Versalovic J, et al., eds. Molecular Microbiology. Diagnostic Principles and Practices. Washington, DC: ASM, 2004, pp. 391–406.

275. Cockerill FR, III. Genetic methods for assessing antimicrobial resistance. Antimicrob Agents Chemother 1999;43:199–212.

276. Cockerill FR, III. Application of rapid-cycle real-time polymerase chain reaction for diagnostic testing in the clinical microbiology laboratory. Arch Pathol Lab Med 2003;127:1112–1120.

277. Wilhelm J, Pingoud A. Real-time polymerase chain reaction. ChemBioChem 2003;4:1120–1128.

278. Frye JG, Jesse T, Long F, et al. DNA microarray detection of antimicrobial resistance genes in diverse bacteria. Int J Antimicrob Agents 2006;27:138–151.

279. Gryadunov D, Mikhailovich V, Lapa S, et al. Evaluation of hybridisation on oligonucleotide microarrays for analysis of drug-resistant *Mycobacterium tuberculosis*. Clin Microbiol Infect 2005;11:531–539.

280. Shinnick TM, Iademarco MF, Ridderhof JC. National plan for reliable tuberculosis laboratory services using a systems approach. Recommendations from CDC and the association of public health laboratories task force on tuberculosis laboratory services. MMWR Recomm Rep 2005;54:1–12.

281. Piersimoni C, Olivieri A, Benacchio L, Scarparo C. Current perspectives on drug susceptibility testing of *Mycobacterium tuberculosis* complex: the automated nonradiometric systems. J Clin Microbiol 2006;44:20–28.

282. Roberts GD, Hall L, Wolk DM. Mycobacteria. In: Truant A, ed. Manual of Commercial Methods in Clinical Microbiology. Washington, DC: ASM, 2002, pp. 256–273.

283. Kim SJ. Drug-susceptibility testing in tuberculosis: methods and reliability of results. Eur Respir J 2005;25:564–569.

284. Garcia de Viedma D. Rapid detection of resistance in *Mycobacterium tuberculosis*: a review discussing molecular approaches. Clin Microbiol Infect 2003;9:349–359.

285. Marttila HJ, Soini H. Molecular detection of resistance to antituberculous therapy. Clin Lab Med 2003;23:823–841.

286. Soini H, Musser JM. Molecular diagnosis of mycobacteria. Clin Chem 2001;47:809–814.

287. Shamputa IC, Rigouts And L, Portaels F. Molecular genetic methods for diagnosis and antibiotic resistance detection of mycobacteria from clinical specimens. APMIS 2004;112:728–752.

288. Morgan M, Kalantri S, Flores L, Pai M. A commercial line probe assay for the rapid detection of rifampicin resistance in *Mycobacterium tuberculosis*: a systematic review and meta-analysis. BMC Infect Dis 2005;5:62.

289. Hillemann D, Weizenegger M, Kubica T, Richter E, Niemann S. Use of the genotype MTBDR assay for rapid detection of rifampin and isoniazid resistance in *Mycobacterium tuberculosis* complex isolates. J Clin Microbiol 2005;43:3699–3703.

290. Chambers HF. Methicillin resistance in staphylococci: molecular and biochemical basis and clinical implications. Clin Microbiol Rev 1997;10:781–791.

291. Barrett SP, Mummery RV, Chattopadhyay B. Trying to control MRSA causes more problems than it solves. J Hosp Infect 1998;39:85–93.

292. Muto CA, Jernigan JA, Ostrowsky BE, et al. SHEA guideline for preventing nosocomial transmission of multidrug-resistant strains of *Staphylococcus aureus* and *Enterococcus*. Infect Control Hosp Epidemiol 2003;24:362–386.

293. Revised guidelines for the control of methicillin-resistant *Staphylococcus aureus* infection in hospitals. British Society for Antimicrobial Chemotherapy, Hospital Infection Society and the Infection Control Nurses Association. J Hosp Infect 1998;39:253–290.

294. Aires De Sousa M, Santos Sanches I, Ferro ML, De Lencastre H. Epidemiological study of staphylococcal colonization and cross-infection in two West African Hospitals. Microb Drug Resist 2000;6:133–141.

295. François P, Pittet D, Bento M, et al. Rapid detection of methicillin-resistant *Staphylococcus aureus* directly from sterile or nonsterile clinical samples by a new molecular assay. J Clin Microbiol 2003;41:254–260.

296. Kuroda M, Ohta T, Uchiyama I, et al. Whole genome sequencing of meticillin-resistant *Staphylococcus aureus*. Lancet 2001;357:1225–1240.

297. Ito T, Okuma K, Ma XX, Yuzawa H, Hiramatsu K. Insights on antibiotic resistance of *Staphylococcus aureus* from its whole genome: genomic island SCC. Drug Resist Updat 2003;6:41–52.

298. Ito T, Ma XX, Takeuchi F, Okuma K, Yuzawa H, Hiramatsu K. Novel type V staphylococcal cassette chromosome *mec* driven by a novel cassette chromosome recombinase, *ccrC*. Antimicrob Agents Chemother 2004;48:2637–2651.

299. Warren DK, Liao RS, Merz LR, Eveland M, Dunne WM, Jr. Detection of methicillin-resistant *Staphylococcus aureus* directly from nasal swab specimens by a real-time PCR assay. J Clin Microbiol 2004;42:5578–5581.

300. Kilic A, Baysallar M, Bahar G, Kucukkaraaslan A, Cilli F, Doganci L. Evaluation of the EVIGENE VRE detection kit for detection of *vanA* and *vanB* genes in vancomycin-resistant enterococci. J Med Microbiol 2005;54:347–350.

301. Appleman MD, Citron DM, Kwok R. Evaluation of the Velogene genomic assay for detection of *vanA* and *vanB* genes in vancomycin-resistant Enterococcus species. J Clin Microbiol 2004;42:1751–1752.

302. Boyd DA, Kibsey P, Roscoe D, Mulvey MR. *Enterococcus faecium* N03-0072 carries a new VanD-type vancomycin resistance determinant: characterization of the *VanD5* operon. J Antimicrob Chemother 2004;54:680–683.

303. Boyd DA, Du T, Hizon R, et al. VanG-type vancomycin-resistant *Enterococcus faecalis* strains isolated in Canada. Antimicrob Agents Chemother 2006;50:2217–2221.

304. US Department of Health and Human Services – Public Health Service. Recommendations for preventing the spread of vancomycin resistance. Recommendations of the Hospital Infection Control Practices Advisory Committee (HICPAC). MMWR Recomm Rep 1995;44:1–13.

305. Brown DF, Walpole E. Evaluation of selective and enrichment media for isolation of glycopeptide-resistant enterococci from faecal specimens. J Antimicrob Chemother 2003;51:289–296.

306. Sloan LM, Uhl JR, Vetter EA, et al. Comparison of the Roche LightCycler *vanA/vanB* detection assay and culture for detection of vancomycin-resistant enterococci from perianal swabs. J Clin Microbiol 2004;42:2636–2643.

307. Diekema DJ, Dodgson KJ, Sigurdardottir B, Pfaller MA. Rapid detection of antimicrobial-resistant organism carriage: an unmet clinical need. J Clin Microbiol 2004;42:2879–2883.

308. Arthur M, Courvalin P. Genetics and mechanisms of glycopeptide resistance in enterococci. Antimicrob Agents Chemother 1993;37:1563–1571.

309. Cercenado E, Unal S, Eliopoulos CT, et al. Characterization of vancomycin resistance in *Enterococcus durans*. J Antimicrob Chemother 1995;36:821–825.

310. Chang S, Sievert DM, Hageman JC, et al. Infection with vancomycin-resistant *Staphylococcus aureus* containing the *vanA* resistance gene. N Engl J Med 2003;348:1342–1347.

311. Dutka-Malen S, Blaimont B, Wauters G, Courvalin P. Emergence of high-level resistance to glycopeptides in *Enterococcus gallinarum* and *Enterococcus casseliflavus*. Antimicrob Agents Chemother 1994;38:1675–1677.

312. Gonzalez-Zorn B, Courvalin P. *vanA*-mediated high level glycopeptide resistance in MRSA. Lancet Infect Dis 2003;3:67–68.

313. Leclercq R, Dutka-Malen S, Brisson-Noel A, et al. Resistance of enterococci to aminoglycosides and glycopeptides. Clin Infect Dis 1992;15:495–501.

314. Ligozzi M, Lo Cascio G, Fontana R. *vanA* gene cluster in a vancomycin-resistant clinical isolate of *Bacillus circulans*. Antimicrob Agents Chemother 1998;42:2055–2059.

315. Mevius D, Devriese L, Butaye P, Vandamme P, Verschure M, Veldman K. Isolation of glycopeptide resistant *Streptococcus gallolyticus* strains with *vanA*, *vanB*, and both *vanA* and *vanB* genotypes from faecal samples of veal calves in The Netherlands. J Antimicrob Chemother 1998;42:275–276.

316. Power EG, Abdulla YH, Talsania HG, Spice W, Aathithan S, French GL. *vanA* genes in vancomycin-resistant clinical isolates of *Oerskovia turbata* and *Arcanobacterium* (*Corynebacterium*) *haemolyticum*. J Antimicrob Chemother 1995;36:595–606.

317. Poyart C, Pierre C, Quesne G, Pron B, Berche P, Trieu-Cuot P. Emergence of vancomycin resistance in the genus *Streptococcus*: characterization of a *vanB* transferable determinant in *Streptococcus bovis*. Antimicrob Agents Chemother 1997;41:24–29.

318. Rosato A, Pierre J, Billot-Klein D, Buu-Hoi A, Gutmann L. Inducible and constitutive expression of resistance to glycopeptides and vancomycin dependence in glycopeptide-resistant *Enterococcus avium*. Antimicrob Agents Chemother 1995;39:830–833.

319. Stinear TP, Olden DC, Johnson PD, Davies JK, Grayson ML. Enterococcal *vanB* resistance locus in anaerobic bacteria in human faeces. Lancet 2001;357:855–856.

320. Torres C, Reguera JA, Sanmartin MJ, Perez-Diaz JC, Baquero F. vanA-mediated vancomycin-resistant Enterococcus spp. in sewage. J Antimicrob Chemother 1994;33:553–561.

321. Domingo MC, Huletsky A, Bernal A, et al. Characterization of a Tn5382-like transposon containing the vanB2 gene cluster in a Clostridium strain isolated from human faeces. J Antimicrob Chemother 2005;55:466–474.

322. Liassine N, Frei R, Jan I, Auckenthaler R. Characterization of glycopeptide-resistant enterococci from a Swiss hospital. J Clin Microbiol 1998;36:1853–1858.

323. Dahl KH, Sundsfjord A. Transferable vanB2 Tn5382-containing elements in fecal streptococcal strains from veal calves. Antimicrob Agents Chemother 2003;47:2579–2583.

324. Fontana R, Ligozzi M, Pedrotti C, Padovani EM, Cornaglia G. Vancomycin-resistant Bacillus circulans carrying the vanA gene responsible for vancomycin resistance in enterococci. Eur J Clin Microbiol Infect Dis 1997;16:473–474.

325. Patel R. Enterococcal-type glycopeptide resistance genes in non-enterococcal organisms. FEMS Microbiol Lett 2000;185:1–7.

326. Launay A, Ballard SA, Johnson PD, Grayson ML, Lambert T. Transfer of vancomycin resistance transposon Tn1549 from Clostridium symbiosum to Enterococcus spp. in the gut of gnotobiotic mice. Antimicrob Agents Chemother 2006;50:1054–1062.

327. Ballard SA, Pertile KK, Lim M, Johnson PD, Grayson ML. Molecular characterization of vanB elements in naturally occurring gut anaerobes. Antimicrob Agents Chemother 2005;49:1688–1694.

328. Ballard SA, Grabsch EA, Johnson PD, Grayson ML. Comparison of three PCR primer sets for identification of vanB gene carriage in feces and correlation with carriage of vancomycin-resistant enterococci: interference by vanB-containing anaerobic bacilli. Antimicrob Agents Chemother 2005;49:77–81.

329. Palladino S, Kay ID, Costa AM, Lambert EJ, Flexman JP. Real-time PCR for the rapid detection of vanA and vanB genes. Diagn Microbiol Infect Dis 2003;45:81–84.

330. Huletsky A, Lebel P, Leclerc B, et al. Rapid detection of vancomycin-resistant enterococci directly from rectal swabs by real-time PCR using the Smart Cycler®. 41th Interscience Conference on Antimicrobial Agents and Chemotherapy, Chicago, IL, 2001; Abstract 1195.

331. Huletsky A, Ferraro MJ, Leclerc B, et al. Less than one-hour detection of vancomycin-resistant enterococci directly from fecal specimens by real-time PCR using the Smart Cycler®. 12th European Congress of Clinical Microbiology and Infectious Diseases, Milan, Italy, 2002; Abstract P718.

332. Livermore DM. Clinical significance of beta-lactamase induction and stable derepression in gram-negative rods. Eur J Clin Microbiol 1987;6:439–445.

333. Pemov A, Modi H, Chandler DP, Bavykin S. DNA analysis with multiplex microarray-enhanced PCR. Nucleic Acids Res 2005;33:e11.

334. Westin L, Miller C, Vollmer D, et al. Antimicrobial resistance and bacterial identification utilizing a microelectronic chip array. J Clin Microbiol 2001;39:1097–1104.

335. Piunno PA, Krull UJ. Trends in the development of nucleic acid biosensors for medical diagnostics. Anal Bioanal Chem 2005;381:1004–1011.

336. Vercoutere W, Akeson M. Biosensors for DNA sequence detection. Curr Opin Chem Biol 2002;6:816–822.

337. Storhoff JJ, Lucas AD, Garimella V, Bao YP, Muller UR. Homogeneous detection of unamplified genomic DNA sequences based on colorimetric scatter of gold nanoparticle probes. Nat Biotechnol 2004;22:883–887.

338. Ho HA, Dore K, Boissinot M, et al. Direct molecular detection of nucleic acids by fluorescence signal amplification. J Am Chem Soc 2005;127:12673–12676.

339. Picard FJ, Bergeron MG. Rapid molecular theranostics in infectious diseases. Drug Discov Today 2002;7:1092–1101.

340. Wolk D, Mitchell S, Patel R. Principles of molecular microbiology testing methods. Infect Dis Clin North Am 2001;15:1157–1204.

341. Jungkind D, Kessler HH. Molecular methods for diagnosis of infectious diseases. In: Truant AL, ed. Manual of Commercial Methods in Clinical Microbiology. Washington, DC: ASM, 2002, pp. 306–323.

342. Raoult D, Fournier PE, Drancourt M. What does the future hold for clinical microbiology? Nat Rev Microbiol 2004;2:151–159.

343. Holland CA, Kiechle FL. Point-of-care molecular diagnostic systems-past, present and future. Curr Opin Microbiol 2005;8:504–509.

344. Liu RH, Yang J, Lenigk R, Bonanno J, Grodzinski P. Self-contained, fully integrated biochip for sample preparation, polymerase chain reaction amplification, and DNA microarray detection. Anal Chem 2004;76:1824–1831.

345. Anderson RC, Su X, Bogdan GJ, Fenton J. A miniature integrated device for automated multistep genetic assays. Nucleic Acids Res 2000;28:e60.

346. Walt DR. Chemistry. Miniature analytical methods for medical diagnostics. Science 2005;308:217–219.

347. Kricka LJ, Park JY, Li SF, Fortina P. Miniaturized detection technology in molecular diagnostics. Expert Rev Mol Diagn 2005;5:549–559.

348. Mothershed EA, Whitney AM. Nucleic acid-based methods for the detection of bacterial pathogens: present and future considerations for the clinical laboratory. Clin Chim Acta 2006;363:206–220.

349. Peytavi R, Raymond FR, Gagne D, et al. Microfluidic device for rapid (<15 min) automated microarray hybridization. Clin Chem 2005;51:1836–1844.

350. Bissonnette L, Bergeron MG. Next revolution in the molecular theranostics of infectious diseases: microfabricated systems for personalized medicine. Expert Rev Mol Diagn 2006;6:433–450.

Chapter 86

The Use of Genotypic Assays for Monitoring the Development of Resistance to Antiviral Therapy for HIV-1 Infection and Other Chronic Viral Diseases

Jorge L. Martinez-Cajas, Marco Petrella, and Mark A. Wainberg

1 Introduction

The routine introduction of genotypic drug resistance assays in the clinical microbiology setting represents a significant milestone in treatment of HIV-1 infection. These laboratory methods permit characterization of specific changes in the genomic nucleotide sequence of viral isolates in comparison to an HIV-1 reference strain to monitor the development of resistance to antiretroviral therapy (1, 2). With genotypic testing, mutations that emerge spontaneously as a result of error-prone viral replication and/or that are selected by drug pressure in the HIV-1 polymerase (*pol*) or envelope (*env*) genes are commonly detected by automated techniques based on the Sanger method for dideoxy-terminator nucleotide sequencing (1) or, alternatively, with hybridization tests such as the line probe assay (LiPA) that monitor point mutations at codons known to be important for resistance to specific antiretroviral agents (ARVs) (1, 3, 4). The effective utilization of genotypic drug resistance assays for HIV-1 infection also requires expert clinical interpretation of often complex mutational patterns. This task has been greatly facilitated by the use of several computerized algorithms that have been specifically designed for HIV-1 genotypic analysis (5–7).

Resistance-conferring mutations that encode single or multiple amino acid substitutions in the reverse transcriptase (RT) or protease (PR) enzymes or the heptad repeat 1 (HR-1) domain of gp41 in the HIV-1 envelope have been shown to be directly responsible for diminished susceptibility to the inhibitors of these viral targets and may, therefore, be viewed as important molecular markers that are predictive of drug resistance (8). The prognostic value of genotypic resistance testing in improving virological outcomes to antiretroviral therapy for HIV-1 infection has been docu-mented in several prospective and retrospective clinical studies, including comparisons against standard of care (9–12). In addition, health economics analyses from the CPCRA 046 (13) and VIRADAPT (14) studies have con-firmed the benefit conferred by genotypic resistance testing when used for guiding therapy choice decisions in patients who experienced virological failure on an initial antiretro-viral regimen. In CPCRA 046, patients receiving standard antiretroviral therapy regimens were randomly assigned to one of two study groups in which therapeutic decisions were determined by clinical judgment alone or, alterna-tively, using genotypic antiretroviral resistance testing (GART) as an adjunct to clinical judgment (9). With GART, 34% of patients were reported to achieve a successful viro-logical response compared to 22% of patients in whom therapy choice decisions were based entirely on physician clinical judgment (9–12). Similar results have also been reported from the VIRADAPT study (10), in which 32% of patients assigned to the drug resistance genotyping (DRG) group responded satisfactorily to antiretroviral therapy compared to a response rate of 14% in patients without DRG (10, 13).

The benefit conferred by HIV-1 genotyping in treatment-experienced patients has also been further corroborated by the Havana trial (15). In this study, a significantly greater proportion of patients in whom genotyping was used to guide therapy choice decisions achieved undetectable plasma viremia (i.e., HIV-1 RNA <400 copies/mL) after 24 weeks of therapy as compared to patients managed in accordance with the standard of care alone (15). Additionally, the use of expert advice to assist with treatment decisions was also shown to be associated with improved virological response, especially in patients who had experienced a second viro-logical failure (15). Thus, the results from CPCRA 046, VIRADAPT, and Havana, as well as those from other related studies conducted in settings that more closely reflect cur-rent clinical practice (16), support the use of genotypic drug resistance assays and expert advice as important interven-tions to improve the sustained effectiveness of antiretroviral therapy in patients with HIV-1 infection.

M.A. Wainberg (✉)
McGill University AIDS Centre, Jewish General Hospital,
Montréal, QC, Canada
mark.wainberg@mcgill.ca

D.L. Mayers (ed.), *Antimicrobial Drug Resistance*,
DOI 10.1007/978-1-60327-595-8_86, © Humana Press, a part of Springer Science+Business Media, LLC 2009

The scope of utilization of genotypic drug resistance assays is increasing and this technology is also being used, albeit on a more limited basis, to monitor resistance to antiviral drugs used for the treatment of hepatitis B (HBV) infection as well as a limited number of other chronic viral diseases associated with certain herpes viruses, e.g., cytomegalovirus (CMV) (1, 2, 17). Although antiviral drugs have also recently become available for some other viral infections such as influenza, the routine use of genotypic drug resistance tests may not be equally practical or feasible in all situations (1). Interestingly, molecular genotyping of validated tumor molecular markers, akin to drug resistance testing for HIV-1 infection, may also be of value in the future to help predict the development of resistance to novel targeted anticancer drugs (18). For example, genotypic surveillance of the Bcr-Abl/c-kit tumor marker in chronic myelogenous leukemia (CML) may be used to detect resistance to targeted anticancer drugs such as Gleevec (imatinib mesylate, STI571) that are now used to treat this disease (19). This therapeutic strategy could be advantageous with respect to the selection of alternate courses of therapy in patients with CML who have become refractory to treatment with Gleevec and, therefore, may also result in improved therapeutic outcomes compared to patients in whom genotypic drug resistance testing was not used for guidance of chemotherapy (18).

In this review, genotypic drug resistance associated with antiviral therapy for HIV-1 infection and other chronic viral diseases will be discussed.

2 Genotypic Drug Resistance in HIV-1 Infection

The development of resistance to antiretroviral agents (ARVs) is largely thought to be a consequence of incompletely suppressive regimens and, moreover, constitutes a serious limitation in regard to the sustained effectiveness of these drugs for the treatment of HIV-1 infection (20–23). HIV-1 variants that harbor resistance mutations to drugs from any of the currently approved classes of antiretroviral agents including the recently introduced fusion inhibitor, enfuvirtide (T-20), may precede the initiation of therapy because of spontaneous mutagenesis or transmission of drug-resistant viruses and are subsequently selected by antiretroviral therapy (8, 24). Genotypic analysis has shown that prolonged exposure to combination therapy is associated with complex and often overlapping patterns of resistance-conferring mutations commensurate with increasing levels of resistance and, for that matter, cross-resistance to some of the antiretroviral drugs comprising the

therapeutic regimen. In general, multiple drug mutations to any single or combination of ARVs need to be selected in order to produce clinical resistance to most ARVs. However, this is not the case for a limited number of nucleoside analog reverse transcriptase inhibitors (NRTIs) such as lamivudine (3TC) and a closely related compound, emtricitabine (FTC), and also for most non-nucleoside inhibitors (NNRTIs) of HIV-1 reverse transcriptase (RT). These compounds possess relatively low genetic barriers for the development of drug resistance compared to the protease inhibitors (PIs), and can often experience substantial loss of antiviral activity following the appearance of a single primary drug resistance mutation in RT (25–29). Table 1 shows most HIV-1 drug resistance mutations that are usually associated with antiretroviral therapy.

3 Nucleoside Analog Reverse Transcriptase Inhibitors

Unlike ARVs from other drug classes, NRTIs are administered to patients as precursor compounds that are phosphorylated to their active triphosphate form by host cellular kinases (30, 31). NRTIs mimic the naturally occurring deoxynucleotide triphosphates (dNTPs) and can effectively compete with these intracellular substrates for binding to RT and incorporation into proviral DNA. However, NRTIs lack a 3′ hydroxyl group that is necessary for DNA polymerization, and therefore the antiviral activity of these compounds results from their ability to cause chain termination of nascent viral DNA strands (30, 32–34).

Mutations associated with drug resistance have been reported in response to the use of any single NRTI (8). However, not all drugs elicit the same mutagenic response, and consequently resistance patterns and sensitivity must be considered on an individual drug basis. For example, resistance to 3TC develops quickly both in vitro (27, 29) and in patients treated with 3TC-containing regimens (35, 36). High-level resistance to this nucleoside analog (i.e., 500- to 1,000-fold increase in IC_{50}) is mediated by a single mutation that encodes substitution of a methionine amino acid residue for either isoleucine (M184I) or, more commonly, valine (M184V) at position 184 in HIV-1 RT (29, 37–39). Moreover, a novel mutational pattern in RT consisting of V118I alone or in association with E44A/D has also been shown to confer moderate phenotypic resistance (i.e., threefold to fourfold increase in IC_{50}) to 3TC in the absence of M184V (40, 41). Increased prevalence of both V118I and E44A/D is associated with long-term ZDV/d4T usage.

In contrast to these findings with 3TC, resistance to zidovudine (ZDV) and other NRTIs may become clinically

Table 1 Common antiretroviral drug resistance mutations

Nucleoside (tide) reverse transcriptase inhibitor (NRTI) mutations associated with HIV drug resistance		
NRTI		
Abacavir	K65R, L74V, Y115F, M184V	
Didanosine	K65R, L74V	
Lamivudine/emtricitabine	K65R, M184V	
Stavudine	M41L, D67N, K70R, L210W, T215YF, K219KE	
Tenofovir	K65R, K70E	
Zidovudine	M41L, D67N, K70R, L210W, T215YF, K219KE	
TAMs	M41L, D67N, K70R, L210W, T215YF, K219KE	Affect all NRTIs
69 Insertion	TAMs plus T69X+X or XX	Affect all NRTIs
151 Complex	A62V, V75I, F77L, F116Y and Q151M	Affect all NRTIs except tenofovir

Non-nucleoside (tide) reverse transcriptase inhibitor (NNRTI) mutations associated with HIV drug resistance	
NNRTI	
Delavirdine	K103N, V106AM, Y181C, Y188L, P236L
Efavirenz	K103N, V106AM, V108I, Y181C, Y188L, G190SA, P225H
Nevirapine	K103N, V106AM, V108I, Y181CI, Y188CLH, G190A

Protease inhibitor (PI) resistance mutations according to the IAS-US A panel for antiretroviral drug resistance

	Cross-resistance mutation		Unique mutations	
PI	Major	Minor	Major	Minor
Saquinavir	L90M, G48V	10IRV, 24I, 54VL, 62V, 71VT, 73S, 77I, 82AFTS, 84V		
Indinavir/RTV	46IL, 82AFT, 84V	10IRV, 20MR, 24I, 32I, 36I, 54V, 71VT, 73SA, 77I, 90M		
Nelfinavir	90M	10FIRV, L24I, M36I, M46IL, A71VT, G73S, V77I, V82AFTS, I84V, N88DS	30N	
Fosamprenavir/RTV	I50V	L10FIRV, V32I, M46IL, I47V, I54LVM, G73S, V82AFST, L90M		
Lopinavir/RTV	V32I, I47VA, V82AFTS	L10FIRV, K20MR, L24I, L33F, M46IL, I50V, F53L, I54VLAMTS, A71VT, G73S, I84V, I90M		L63P
Atazanavir	I84V, N88S,	L10IFVC, K20RMITV, L24I, V32I, L33IFV, M36ILV, M46IL, G48V, F53LY, I54, LVMTA, I62V, A71VITL, G73CSTA, V82ATFI, L90M	I50L	G16E, E34Q, D60E, I64LMV, I93LM
Tipranavir	L33F, V82LT, I84V	L10V, K20MR, E35G, M36I, K43T, M46L, I47V, I54AMV, L90M		I13V, Q58E, H69K, T74P, N83D
Darunavir	I50V, I54ML, I84V	V11I, V32I, L33F, I47V, G73S,	L76V	V11I, L89V

important only about 6 months after initiation of therapy (42, 43). Furthermore, prolonged exposure to ZDV is characterized by a stepwise accumulation of resistance mutations, referred to as thymidine analog mutations (TAMs), that can result in progressive loss of antiviral activity to this compound. The TAMs comprise a group of six drug resistance mutations (i.e., M41L, D67N, K70R, L210W, T215Y/F, and K219Q) in RT that were initially described in connection with ZDV resistance and have also been implicated in reduced sensitivity to stavudine (d4T) (8, 44–47). In addition, TAMs can also confer moderate levels of resistance to other NRTIs such

as didanosine (ddI) and zalcitabine (ddC), depending on the mutational pattern that is present. However, L74V is the primary resistance-conferring mutation that is selected by ddI, which is responsible for the greatest loss of antiviral activity with this drug (8, 42, 44, 46). Similarly, the selection of various TAMs is also associated with decreased susceptibility to ddC, although, as with ddI, other resistance-conferring mutations (i.e., K65R and T69N) are also important in this regard (8, 42, 45, 46). It is also noteworthy that whereas discriminatory mutations in RT such as M184V confer resistance primarily against the drugs that select them, TAMs, on the other hand, can mediate diminished drug susceptibility against an extended array of unrelated NRTIs (8, 44–47).

Genotypic analysis of viral isolates from patients treated with antiretroviral regimens that included d4T or ZDV has pointed to the existence of two major genetic pathways in regard to the development of resistance to thymidine analogs as evidenced through the detection of differential patterns of TAMs over time (48–51). Initially, each of the M41L and T215Y/F mutations are commonly present in both pathways (50) and they are followed by the stepwise accumulation of other TAMs at positions 210 and 215 (i.e., 41L-210W-215Y pattern) or, alternatively, at positions 67, 70, and 219 (i.e., 67N-70R-219Q/E pattern) (48, 49, 51). Furthermore, the specific sequence of TAM accumulation observed may be dependent on whether ZDV monotherapy or dual NRTI combinations were used for initiation of antiretroviral therapy. Monotherapy with ZDV has been shown to be more commonly associated with the K70R mutation appearing first, leading predominantly to selection of the 67N-70R-219Q/E pattern (48), whereas patients who started treatment with either ZDV/ddI or ZDV/ddC usually initially developed 215Y/F followed by 41 L and 210 W (48). Moreover, the 41L-210W-215Y pattern appears to be more prevalent than 67N-70R-219Q/E (52). The V118I and E44A/D mutations frequently cluster jointly with the 41L-210W-215Y pathway but have only been observed individually in association with the 67N-70R-219Q/E pattern (52). TAMs from the 41L-210W-215Y pathway generally yield higher levels of cross-resistance to other NRTIs when present together with other mutations than do the same number of TAMs from the 67N-70R-219Q/E pathway (52).

Another less frequently observed resistance mutation, K65R, has been shown to be associated with prior treatment with abacavir (ABC)-containing regimens and results in reduced antiviral susceptibility to both ABC and the nucleotide analog reverse transcriptase inhibitor tenofovir (TDF). Hence, resistance to these ARVs can develop independently via genetic pathways involving either the TAMs or K65R as the signature drug resistance mutations (53). K65R is also selected by TDF in vitro (54) and has been observed with low frequency (i.e., 3% of cases) in clinical trials of patients with HIV-1 infection who were treated with a TDF-containing regimen for up to 96 weeks (55).

The simultaneous presence of K65R together with TAMs is very rare in clinical samples. One study found only a negative association of K65R and TAMs (except for Q151M (positive association) and K70R (no association)) (56). Site-directed mutagenesis experiments that introduced both TAMs and K65R into clinical isolates determined a reciprocal antagonistic phenotypic effect. TAMs reduced the resistance conferred by K65R to TDF, ABC, and ddC, and K65R decreased the resistance conferred by TAMs to AZT.

TAMs had no effect on the resistance conferred by K65R against 3TC or FTC, but enhanced the resistance of M184V against each of ABC, ddI, and TDF (56). This finding adds support to the sequential use of AZT and TDF-based NRTI backbones.

Mutational patterns that are associated with broad cross-resistance to multiple NRTIs have also been identified. The Q151 multidrug resistance (MDR) complex is encoded by five mutations in RT: A62V, V75I, F77L, F116Y, and Q151M. These mutations were initially observed in viral isolates from patients with HIV-1 infection who received combination therapy with ZDV plus either ddC or ddI for over 1 year (57, 58). Primary resistance mutations that are usually associated with resistance to ZDV, ddI, or ddC in monotherapy were not present in these isolates. Q151M is the first of these five mutations to develop in vivo and, compared to the other Q151M MDR substitutions, also produces the most resistance to additional NRTIs (57). In addition, it has been shown that a family of insertion mutations between codons 67 and 70 in RT can cause resistance to a variety of NRTIs including ZDV, 3TC, ddI, ddC, and d4T. Usually, these mutations confer resistance to multiple NRTIs when present in a ZDV-resistant background (59, 60). The development of these mutations is also correlated with prior treatment with ZDV/ddI and ZDV/ddC combination therapy regimens. However, the prevalence of the insertion mutations has been reported to be lower than that for the substitutions comprising the Q151M MDR complex (61).

4 Non-nucleoside Reverse Transcriptase Inhibitors

NNRTIs act as noncompetitive antagonists of enzyme activity by binding to a hydrophobic pocket that is located adjacent to the catalytic site of RT (62, 63). NNRTIs reduce the catalytic rate of polymerization without affecting nucleotide binding or nucleotide-induced conformational change (64). These drugs are particularly active at template positions at which the RT enzyme naturally pauses and, moreover, do not appear to influence the competition between dideoxynucleotide triphosphates (ddNTPs) and the naturally occurring dNTPs for insertion into the growing proviral DNA chain (65).

Diminished sensitivity to NNRTIs appears quickly both in tissue culture selection protocols and in patients (25, 62, 63). NNRTIs share a common binding site, and mutations that encode NNRTI resistance are located within the binding pocket that makes drug contact (62–69). This explains the finding that extensive cross-resistance is observed among all currently approved NNRTIs (25, 70, 71). A substitution at codon 181 (i.e., Y181C) is a common mutation that encodes cross-resistance among many NNRTIs (25, 68, 70, 72).

Replacement of Y181 by a serine or histidine also conferred HIV resistance to NNRTIs (73). A mutation at amino acid 236 (i.e., P236L), conferring resistance to a particular class of NNRTIs that include delavirdine, can also diminish resistance to nevirapine and other NNRTIs, particularly if a Y181C mutation is also present in the same virus (74). Y188C and Y188H are other important mutations that can also confer resistance to NNRTIs.

Another drug resistance mutation, namely K103N, is also commonly observed and is responsible for reduced susceptibility to all approved NNRTIs (25, 68, 70, 72). Substitution of K103N results in alteration of interactions between NNRTIs and RT. The K103N mutation shows synergy with Y181C in regard to resistance to NNRTIs, unlike antagonistic interactions involving Y181C and P236L (75).

5 Protease Inhibitors

Drug-resistant viruses have been observed in the case of all PIs developed to date (76–78). In addition, some strains of HIV have displayed cross-resistance to a variety of PIs after either clinical use or in vitro drug exposure (76–78). In general, the patterns of mutations observed with PIs are more complex and extensive than those observed with RT antagonists (8). This involves greater variability as well in temporal patterns of appearance of different mutations and the manner in which different combinations of mutations can give rise to phenotypic resistance. These data suggest that the viral protease (PR) enzyme can adapt more easily than RT to pressures exerted by antiviral drugs. At least 70 mutations in PR have been identified as responsible for resistance to PIs (8, 76–79).

In general, several mutations are necessary in order for PIs to lose activity against HIV-1. Certain mutations within the HIV-1 PR affect the enzyme more than others and can on their own confer resistance to certain PIs (76–78). In particular, D30N and D50L are unique to nelfinavir and atazanavir, respectively. Saquinavir, an early PI, predominantly selects for the mutations L90M and G48V. Amprenavir and fosamprenavir can select for D50V, which can confer some degree of cross-resistance to darunavir (DRV) (80). Regarding lopinavir, PR requires to accumulate at least five mutations to become highly resistance to this drug (81, 82). Recently, the presence of mutation I47A, although uncommon, was shown to result in very high levels of resistant to lopinavir (>100-fold increase in IC_{50}) and hypersusceptibility to saquinavir (83, 84). Unique signature mutations have not been well defined for either tipranavir or darunavir.

A variety of mutations may confer cross-resistance among multiple drugs within the PI family. Cross-resistance mutations can lower the affinities of PIs, but the specific effects of these mutations vary according to each individual PI. As a classical example, the mutations V82F/I84V can contribute to resistance against almost all PIs currently available for therapy. These two positions are located in the β-sheet of the active site cavity of the PR, a structure to which all PIs must bind to inactivate the enzyme. Interestingly, the IAS USA Drug Resistance Mutation Panel considers that mutations at position 82 can affect all PIs in clinical use to date, except DRV (although the resistance profile of DRV is not yet completely determined) (79). Similarly, the I84V mutation affects all PIs in clinical use and is a major mutation for five of them. Despite being located outside the active site, the L90M mutation also affects all PIs except DRV and, on its own, does not contribute to tipranavir (TPV) resistance (79). Extensive reviews on the effect of each resistance mutation on each particular PI go beyond the scope of this chapter and can be found elsewhere (85).

On the other hand, wide arrays of secondary mutations have been observed, which, when combined with primary mutations, can cause increased levels of resistance. Mutations such as L90M and L63P (a common polymorphism) have no discernible effect on binding affinity, but can partially restore PR catalytic activity and hence viral fitness (86). It should be noted that resistance to PIs can also result from mutations within the substrates of the PR enzyme. The gag and gag–pol precursor proteins of HIV can acquire mutations at or close to their cleavage sites, which render them more susceptible to hydrolysis by PR (87–90). Thus, cleavage occurs more efficiently and viral fitness can be restored to some degree. Some of the gag and gag–pol mutations that have been reported in treatment-experienced patients include the p7/p1 mutations A431V, K436R, I437V, and p1/p6-gag mutations L449F/V, P452S-P453L/A (91). At least one of these mutations was detected in 60% of therapy-experienced patients compared to 10% in treatment-naïve patients (91). Nevertheless, the full clinical significance of these cleavage site mutations in regard to PI resistance remains to be elucidated.

6 Fusion Inhibitors (Enfuvirtide, T-20)

Enfuvirtide (T-20) is the first entry in a novel class of antiretroviral agents known as HIV-1 entry inhibitors and has recently been approved for the treatment of HIV-1 infection (78, 92). This compound is a synthetic peptide consisting of 36 amino acids that are homologous to the residues located at positions 127–162 from the C-terminus of the heptad repeat 2 (HR-2) domain in the gp41 transmembrane glycoprotein of the viral envelope. T-20 binds competitively to the HR-1 domain within gp41, thereby preventing interaction with HR-2 and formation of the hairpin-like structure that is required for fusion of the viral and host cell membranes (78, 79, 92, 93).

In the TORO-1 and TORO-2 studies, the addition of T-20 to optimized background therapy consisting of three to five active antiretroviral drugs, which were selected using genotypic drug resistance testing, was shown to result in significant reduction of plasma HIV-1 RNA and CD4 cell count increases compared to optimized background therapy alone in heavily treatment-experienced patients with HIV-1 infection that was resistant to NRTIs, NNRTIs, and PIs (80, 81, 94, 95). The results from additional open-label and controlled clinical trials with this drug have similarly demonstrated improved treatment outcomes for up to 48 weeks in HIV-1 patients who were experiencing virological failure on previous regimens (82, 83, 96, 97). In phase I clinical testing, resistance to T-20 developed rapidly as shown by rebounding plasma HIV-1 RNA after 14 days of monotherapy in four patients receiving an intermediate dose (i.e., 30 mg twice daily) of T-20 (98, 84). Genotypic analysis of cloned virus from these patients showed that resistance to T-20 was produced by substitutions in the highly conserved GIV motif, which comprises a three-amino-acid sequence between residues 36 and 38 within the HR-1 domain that is essential for fusion of viral and cellular membranes to occur. Mutants that harbored a single amino acid substitution in GIV (i.e., G36D, I37V, and V38A/M) were frequently detected (98, 84). G36D and, in particular, V38A both exhibited significant increases in the IC_{50} for T-20 compared to HIV-1 strains with wild-type envelope sequences. In addition, dual mutants that contained G36D together with substitutions at other amino acid residues within HR-1 (i.e., Q32H/R and Q39R) were also observed and were shown to confer reduced susceptibility to T-20 to an extent similar to that produced with G36D by itself (98, 84). Interestingly, variability in the HR-1 domain at positions that are associated with resistance to T-20 has been demonstrated in both subtype B (i.e., residues 37, 39, and 42) and in non-B (i.e., residue 42) HIV-1 strains isolated from T-20-naïve patients (99, 85). However, the major GIV mutants commonly associated with T-20-resistant isolates were not observed in the absence of drug treatment, suggesting that primary genotypic resistance to this drug is uncommon (99, 85). Further study is needed to better understand the long-term implications of these uncommon resistance mutations in HIV-1 patients undergoing therapy with fusion inhibitors.

7 Limitations of Genotype Resistant Testing for Treatment of Infection with HIV-1

Although genotype resistance testing represents an important advance in HIV therapy, it adds complexity to the management of HIV infection, since interpretation of results are not straightforward and clinical correlates do not yet exist for all resistance mutations. The limitations for genotype resistance

tests include inability to detect virus archived in viral reservoirs, insensitivity to viral minority populations (population that are less than 20% of the total viral mixture), and the requirement of a minimum viral load (500–1,000 plasma HIV RNA copies/mL) for detection to be achieved. However, it is generally accepted that genotype is more sensitive for minority populations than phenotype testing. For instance, genotyping can detect sentinel mutations (e.g., M184V) before changes in phenotypic resistance become evident. Importantly, several studies have clearly demonstrated that expert advice adds benefit to results from resistance testing (12, 15, 16, 100–102).

On the other hand, large databases of paired genotype–phenotype assays have allowed the construction of "virtual phenotype" estimators that quantify HIV-1 resistance to ARV drugs on the basis of a statistical prediction of the phenotype for a given genetic sequence. The accuracy of such estimations depends on the frequency of genotypes in the database that match the problem genotype and the variability in drug susceptibility of the phenotypes used to create the predicting pool. Uncommon sequences and those with suboptimal matches will have less accurate predictive value than those that are more frequent and better matched. Although a good correlation of virtual phenotypes with "real phenotypes" has been reported (103, 104) it should be kept in mind that "virtual phenotype" is a probability estimation. Further research is advancing in order for informatic aids to be able to display options of antiretroviral regimens starting from the computerized evaluation of a viral nucleic sequence.

Finally, there is subrepresentation of non-B subtype genetic sequences in current HIV resistance databases that have been used to generate resistance algorithms. Therefore, resistance pathways and mutations may be limited in the interpretation of resistance of non-B subtype clinical isolates. A classical example in subtype C HIV-1 exposed to efavirenz in tissue culture is the emergence of the V106M mutation which was observed to arise in the place of the V106A substitution, more commonly seen with subtype B viruses (105). It is not yet known to what extent natural polymorphisms of different non-B subtypes can lead to different mutation patterns of frequency of individual mutations. For instance, a rapid emergence of K65R has been reported in tissue culture of subtype C HIV-1 in the presence of TDF. A high prevalence of this mutation has also been described in patients in Bostwana taking ddI (106, 107).

8 Hepatitis B Infection

Antiviral treatment of chronic hepatitis B has regained importance since only a small proportion of actively infected patients achieve the desirable outcomes with interferon-based therapy. Also, new data suggests that higher viral loads are associated, at least in Asian populations, with increased risk of developing cirrhosis and hepatocellular carcinoma (108, 109). Hence, suppression of viral load with the use of antiviral drugs in chronic HBV infection emerges as a promising option for reduction of patient morbidity.

Four NRTIs are currently licensed for treatment of chronic HBV infection: lamivudine (3TC), adefovir, entecavir, and telvibudine. They are used either alone or in association with immunotherapy, i.e., interferon α (regular or pegylated), in treatment of HIV/HBV coinfection. All are highly active against HBV and are frequently used together with antiretroviral therapy directed against chronic HIV-1 infection. Other drugs not yet specifically licensed for HBV treatment but have excellent anti-HBV activity are famciclovir, tenofovir, emtricitabine, clevudine, pradefovir, ANA 380, myrcludex, and valtorcitabine.

Lamivudine is a widely utilized antiviral drug often used in initiation of therapy in patients with hepatitis B infection (HBV). In both immune-competent and HIV/AIDS patients with HBV co-infection, the prevalence of lamivudine (3TC)-resistant HBV variants has been reported to be approximately 16–43% after 1 year and up to 70% at 4 years of treatment (110, 111). The rtM204V (previously position M552V) mutation induces a 1,000-fold decrease in susceptibility to lamivudine in vitro in comparison to wild-type HBV (112). Drug-resistant virus can be selected after 6 months of lamivudine therapy in these patients and its presence has been shown to increase with the duration of exposure to this drug (110, 113). As is also the case with HIV-1, genotypic analysis has shown that resistance to lamivudine results principally from either isoleucine (I) or valine (V) amino acid substitutions in place of methionine (M) at position rt204 within the C domain of the highly conserved tyrosine–methionine–aspartate–aspartate (YMDD) motif of the HBV DNA polymerase (1, 110). Compensatory mutations associated with lamivudine resistance (rtV173L, rtL180M) are found in the B domain (114, 115). This mutation and, similarly, the M184V/I substitution in HIV-1 RT are responsible for high-level resistance to lamivudine.

In addition to rtM204I/V, several other mutations in the HBV polymerase gene have been shown to emerge following prolonged exposure to lamivudine and are associated with diminished susceptibility to this drug. Specific patterns of these mutations are used to assign lamivudine-resistant HBV variants to one of two genotypic groups. HBV group I mutants contain lamivudine resistance mutations that are located in both the polymerase B and C domains, which include predominantly the rtL180M (previously L528M) and rtM204I/V (previously M552I/)) substitutions, respectively. Group II viruses, on the other hand, are characterized by the presence of rtM204I in the C domain as the main lamivudine resistance–conferring mutation and have been shown to occur less frequently than their group I counterparts (110).

Resistance to other nucleosides analogs used for the treatment of HBV infection has also been documented. Compounds such as ganciclovir (GCV) and famciclovir (FCV) are potent inhibitors of the HBV polymerase both in vitro and in vivo and, although they appear less effective than lamivudine (1, 113), both these antiviral agents have been used on an investigational basis to treat HBV infection. Genotypic analysis has revealed that the most important resistance-conferring mutations to these drugs are selected outside of the YMDD motif and include the rtV173L (previously V521L), rtP177L (previously P525L), rtL180M (previously L528M/V), T184S (previously T532S), and rtV207I (previously V555I) substitutions in the B domain of the HBV polymerase gene. Furthermore, it has been shown that the rtV207I substitution produces the highest attenuation of antiviral susceptibility to FCV and that both this mutation and rtP177L are associated with cross-resistance to lamivudine (1).

Adefovir dipivoxil (PMEA), a novel antiviral drug from a class of compounds known as nucleotide analog reverse transcriptase inhibitors (NtRTIs) (116), has been licensed for the treatment of chronic hepatitis B (117–119). Resistance to adefovir appears to develop infrequently in vivo, and in two large placebo-controlled trials that included 700 patients with HBV infection (117, 118) treatment with adefovir for 48 weeks did not select for mutations associated with resistance to this compound (120). Substitutions in the conserved domains of HBV polymerase (i.e., rtS119A, rtH133L, rtV214A, and rtH234Q) were infrequently detected as minority species in the clinical isolates of four adefovir-treated patients from these studies. Moreover, these secondary mutations did not confer phenotypic resistance to adefovir and were not associated with the diminished virological response to this drug during the treatment period (120). However, continued exposure to therapeutic levels of adefovir for up to 96 weeks resulted in selection of an adefovir-resistance mutation within the HBV polymerase D domain (i.e., rtN236T) in one patient (121). Other reports from patients receiving 10 mg/d as monotherapy registered 2, 5.9, 18, and 29% of resistant mutants after 2–5 years of treatment (121–123). Clinical isolates that harbored this substitution were shown to have reduced antiviral activity to adefovir in vitro but remained susceptible to lamivudine and entecavir (121). The mutation rtA181V in the B domain of the polymerase has been more recently described, and can confer some loss of susceptibility to lamivudine (123, 124). Also, adefovir resistance has been seen to emerge more frequently in lamivudine-resistant patients than in those without previous lamivudine resistance (10% vs. 0%)(125). However, adefovir resistance is less likely to occur when adefovir is given in addition, rather than as a substitute, for lamivudine (126). Therefore, the addition of adefovir to lamivudine-failing patients has become widely accepted. Importantly, a virus variant carrying the mutation rtI233V, which occurs naturally, appears to have lower susceptibility to adefovir (127). This mutation has not been selected in vitro nor seen in patients experiencing virological breakthrough. In general, these data point to the essentiality of always initiating the therapy of HBV disease with combination therapy.

The nucleoside analog, entecavir, was approved for treatment of HBV infection in 2005. Virologic breakthrough confirmed by genotypic analysis has been seen during phase II and III clinical trials in 5.8% of patients treated by entecavir after lamivudine failure for 1 year, 10% for 2 years, and 25% for 3 years (128–131). The patients reported with resistance to entecavir had two signature lamivudine-resistance mutations in the HBV polymerase, rtL180M and rtM204V, along with the novel mutations rtM250V or rtS202I and rtT184G. The mutation more closely linked to entecavir resistance appears to be rtM250V within a background of lamivudine-resistance mutations (128). To date, primary resistance to entecavir in the absence of previously existing lamivudine resistance has not been reported (128). Also, recent studies indicate that entecavir possesses activity against HIV-1 as well as against HBV and can select for the M184V mutation in HIV-1 (132). This finding may lead to revision of current guidelines of treatment in HIV/HBV coinfected patients.

Emtricitabine (FTC) is an L nucleoside very similar to lamivudine. When administered as monotherapy for HBV infection, it selects for the rtM204I/V (YIDD/YMDD) mutations in the C domain of the HBV polymerase. The rate of YMDD mutations emerging in patients receiving 200 mg of FTC per day has been reported to be 9–13% at week 48 of treatment and 19% at week 96 of treatment (133).

Telbivudine is a potent L-analog and the latest antiviral drug to be approved for treatment of chronic hepatitis B. Resistance was seen in about 5% of patients after 1 year of treatment and is attributable to a rtM204I mutation in the HBV polymerase "YIDD", but this does not seem to be linked to the rtM204V mutation in the "YMDD" motif of the HBV polymerase (134). Telbivudine resistance mutations do not overlap with the entecavir resistance mutations, leaving a full option for patients failing therapy with either of these

agents. Finally, the emergence of resistance to all drugs used to date for the treatment of HBV provides testimony to the need for combination therapy in clinical practice.

9 Herpes Virus Infections: Cytomegalovirus and Herpes Simplex Virus

The incidence of opportunistic infections associated with HIV/AIDS has significantly declined as a result of the introduction of highly active antiretroviral therapy (HAART). However, in certain clinical settings, such as in patients with severe primary combined immunodeficiency (SCID) and patients requiring organ transplantation, the development of cytomegalovirus (CMV) infection remains a serious complication that generally requires the use of antiviral therapy (1, 135). In the pre-HAART era, the rate of resistance to each of the anti-CMV drugs was estimated to be approximately 25% per person-year (136–139).

Regarding human CMV therapy, a diverse array of drugs, which includes acyclovir, gancyclovir (GCV), the oral prodrug of valgancyclovir (a prodrug which is transformed into GCV first pass metabolism), foscarnet (FOS), the nucleotide analog, cidofovir (CDV), and fomivirsen, are used to treat CMV disease (1, 116, 135). These compounds have been shown to suppress viral replication through inhibition of the viral DNA polymerase which is encoded by the CMV UL54 gene. Sequence analysis has demonstrated that mutations in this gene can confer resistance to each of these three drugs. In addition, GCV, like all other nucleoside analogs, needs to be activated to its virologically competent form, GCV-triphosphate. This process initially involves the phosphorylation of GCV to its monophosphate moiety by a viral-encoded phosphotransferase (see Fig. 1). This

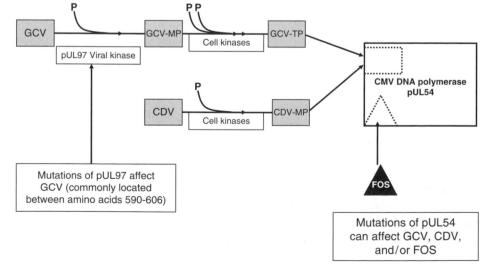

Fig. 1 Anti CMV drugs: mechanisms of action and resistance. (Gancyclovir) GCV needs to be first phophorylated by a viral kinase encoded by the gene UL97. The CMV DNA polymerase, encoded by the gene UL54, can also mutate and potentially cause resistance to CGV, cidofovir (CDV), and foscarnet (FOS)

enzyme is expressed by the UL97 gene. Studies have shown that resistance to GCV can manifest as early as 10 days following initiation of therapy with this drug, and that numerous mutations, many of which are located between amino acid residues 590–606 or at position 460 or 520 (140) in UL97, may contribute to reduced susceptibility to GCV in some immunocompromised patients (135). Similarly, a novel deletion mutant involving an 11-amino-acid sequence between positions 590 and 600 in UL97 has also been identified in GCV-resistant isolates from a patient with SCID (141). In other studies, GCV-associated mutations in UL97 were found to be highly prevalent in viral isolates that displayed varying degrees of resistance to GCV (142). However, sequence analysis of UL97 alone cannot be used to predict the level of resistance to GCV without knowledge of additional genotypic and/or phenotypic information obtained in regard to UL54 (1). During prolonged GCV therapy, UL97 mutations appear early and result in lower-level resistance, whereas UL54 mutations appear later and confer higher-level resistance (142–145).

Recent studies of clinical isolates from AIDS and solid organ transplant patients have documented that the most frequent UL97 mutations present in GCV-resistant mutants were A594V, L595S, M460V, and H520Q (145–147). Other common UL97 mutations related to resistance include C592G and C603W. The mutations associated with the highest rate of increase in GCV resistance have been M460V, C603W, deletion of codons 595–603, H520Q, L595S, A594V, C607Y, and deletion of codon 595 with a change in resistance from 4.9- to 13.3-fold depending on the mutation (140, 148–151). In contrast, mutations C592G, A594T, and E596G, as well as deletion of codon 600, confer a lower decrease in drug susceptibility (140).

The CMV DNA polymerase, which is encoded by the gene pUL54, can also mutate in response to drug pressure and such mutations can potentially affect all currently approved antivirals. Some of the most frequent DNA polymerase mutations causing drug resistance are V715M, V781I, and L802M, which confer resistance to FOS, F412C, L501I/F, and P522S, and result in resistance to GCV and CDV. The mutation A809V, which confers resistance to GCV and FOS; the mutation N408K, which confers resistance to GCV and CDV; and the mutation A834P, which causes resistance to GCV, FOS, and CDV have also been reported (152, 153). Some mutations (A834P, E756K, and V812L and the deletion of codons 981 and 982) can cause resistance to all three of those antivirals (152–154). The effect of combined mutations can be synergistic, as is the case with mutations N408K and A834P. N408K and A834P cause a 4.2- and 5.4-fold increase in resistance against GCV, respectively. When present together, the resulting increase in resistance is 22.7-fold, rendering the virus highly resistant to this drug (153). The mutations L501I and K513N and deletion of codons 981–982 result in

6- to 8-fold decrease in GCV susceptibility, and mutations F412C/V, K513N, and A987G have been associated with a 10- to 18-fold decrease in CDV susceptibility (152, 154, 155). In addition, the substitutions D588N, V715M, E756K, L802M, and T821I can reduce the susceptibility to FOS from 5.5- to 21-fold (152, 154–157).

Fomivirsen (ISIS 2922) is a 21-base oligonucleotide with phosphorothioate linkages that are complementary to human CMV immediate-early 2 (IE2) mRNA. Hence, fomivirsen binds to this complementary CMV mRNA sequence and inhibits translation of several CMV immediate-early proteins (32, 158). Although a resistant virus has been isolated in vitro, the mechanism of resistance was not due to loss of encoded complementarity with the oligonucleotide. To date, no report has been published on fomivirsen resistance in patients (159).

As is also the case with CMV disease, the prevalence of drug-resistant HSV variants is both highest and of greatest concern in immunocompromised hosts (160). It has been reported that up to 30% of allogeneic bone marrow transplant patients may be infected with acyclovir (ACV)-resistant HSV (161) (97). These mutants arise spontaneously and are selected by exposure to antiviral agents. Resistance to ACV and also to related drugs such as penciclovir that are used for the treatment of HSV infection arises predominantly from mutations in the virally encoded thymidine kinase gene (TK). The TK gene product is responsible for the phosphorylation of ACV to ACV-monophosphate, an important initial step that is essential for the activation of nucleoside analogs such as ACV in HSV-infected cells. ACV resistance mutations in TK involve nucleotide additions, deletions, or substitutions that often occur in regions that contain a high density of guanine–cytosine (G–C) sequences and that are thought to be more prone to mutagenesis. Examples of common ACV resistance mutations in TK include repeated nucleotides at codon 92, a frameshift mutation at codon 146 that is detected in the majority of ACV-resistant clinical isolates, an arginine substitution at codon 176 in HSV type 1 or, alternatively, at codon 177 in HSV type 2, and an amino acid substitution at codon 336 that is observed in both clinical and laboratory HSV strains with reduced sensitivity to ACV (161). Furthermore, genotypic studies have shown that TK possesses an unusually high propensity for the development of mutations associated with polymorphisms that do not confer resistance to ACV. These polymorphisms are located throughout the TK gene but do not involve conserved domains or the nucleotide sequences that encode the ATP and nucleoside binding sites within TK. Lastly, mutations in the conserved domains of the HSV DNA polymerase gene have also been shown to be involved in resistance to ACV (161, 162). For example, the L774V substitution in the polymerase conserved region VI has been shown to be associated with diminished susceptibility to both ACV and the pyrophosphate analog foscarnet (163).

10 Future Perspectives

As reviewed here, the application of genotypic resistance testing has proven to be instrumental for the clinical monitoring of antiretroviral drug resistance, and now constitutes an important component of the standard of care for patients with HIV-1 infection in industrialized nations. Furthermore, the results of several studies including CPCRA 046, VIRADAPT, and the Havana trial have confirmed the prognostic value and cost effectiveness of genotypic resistance testing for guidance of therapy in patients who experience virological failure during second or later regimens. In particular, HIV-1 genotyping is an essential strategy for the optimization of combination therapy used in salvage regimens, which include the fusion inhibitor T-20.

However, despite these significant advances, the high cost and complexity associated with genotypic drug resistance assays remain important economic and technological barriers in regard to their wider implementation, especially in resource-poor countries (164). Careful planning and prioritized use of genotyping are essential in order to achieve the best cost–benefit in these circumstances. There are also several other potential applications for genotyping that may represent opportunities for further improvements in therapeutic outcomes for HIV-1 infection. An example concerns the use of genotypic analysis for monitoring polymorphisms in non-B HIV-1 subtypes, which may be important in regard to differential patterns of antiretroviral susceptibility compared to HIV-1 subtype B viruses. For instance, some subtype C HIV-1 variants are known to possess naturally occurring polymorphisms at several RT and PR codons that are implicated in drug resistance (165, 166). Studies have showed that the presence of these polymorphisms did not significantly reduce susceptibility to ARVs nor diminish the effectiveness of an initial antiretroviral therapy regimen for a period of up to 18 months (165, 167). However, it has also been suggested that polymorphisms at resistance positions may facilitate selection of novel pathways in some cases, leading to drug resistance especially with incompletely suppressive antiretroviral regimens (165). This, in turn, may have important clinical implications with respect to the choice and long-term benefit of antiretroviral therapy, which may indeed warrant increased genotypic surveillance, particularly as the worldwide prevalence of non-B HIV-1 infection is increasing rapidly (168). HIV-1-infected pregnant women who have previously received antiretroviral therapy represent another important case in whom genotypic drug resistance testing may be a perinatal strategy for guidance of therapy to prevent HIV transmission to infants (169, 170).

Genotypic monitoring may also be of prognostic value in the clinical management of patients with primary HIV-1 drug resistance. The prevalence of primary HIV-1 drug resistance (RT and PR resistance–associated mutations) in recently infected individuals in Europe (171) and North America (172, 173) has been estimated to be approximately 7 and 20%, respectively. In addition, recent reports suggest that a trend exists towards worldwide transmission of drug-resistant HIV-1 variants in antiretroviral therapy-naïve individuals (174). Of particular interest and concern is the transmission in primary HIV-1 infection of highly resistant and of multidrug resistant (MDR) HIV-1 variants that harbor resistance-conferring mutations to two or three classes of ARVs. Studies have shown that these viruses display in vivo replication competence that is often comparable to that of the drug-sensitive species and, moreover, that they are able to establish persistent infections in the absence of antiretroviral drug pressure (165–177). The use of HIV-1 genotyping in this clinical setting may allow earlier detection of HIV-1 MDR variants and, therefore, increase the likelihood for improved therapeutic outcomes during chronic infection. Furthermore, such testing may help to reduce the overall the spread of HIV-1 drug resistance.

As mentioned previously, the use of interpretative algorithms in conjunction with HIV-1 genotyping has facilitated prediction of drug resistance from the plethora of mutational patterns that are frequently associated with failing antiretroviral regimens. Two types of computer-based algorithms have been developed for analysis of HIV-1 genotypic data: rule-based algorithms and a virtual phenotype (178). Rule-based algorithms are derived from knowledge of in vitro drug susceptibility assays, the relationship between specific resistance-associated mutations and virological responses in HIV-1 infected patients, and expert opinion (179). The virtual phenotype, on the other hand, utilizes databases that correlate various mutational patterns with actual in vitro phenotypic resistance and clinical response in order to infer the level of drug resistance (i.e., sensitive, intermediate, or resistant) to ARVs that is displayed by a viral isolate on the basis of its HIV-1 genotype (178). Discordant results among widely used interpretative algorithms, in which a viral isolate is scored as sensitive by one program and resistant by another, are frequent. This situation constitutes an important limitation of current technology and, moreover, underscores the technical challenges associated with the coding and interpretation of complex patterns of drug resistance mutations.

Several studies have shown that discordance between various algorithms is greatest with NRTIs, with the exception of 3TC, as compared to NNRTIs and most PIs, where the level of disagreement is usually less (180–182). For example, in one study that examined the Stanford University Database (HIV db), Bayer Diagnostics TRUGENE (BDT), and the Virco VirtualPhenotype (VP) HIV-1 genotyping programs, discordant results for interpretation of drug susceptibility to ddI, ddC, d4T, and ABC were reported in excess of 50 and 40% of cases in comparisons between the HIV db and VP and BDT and VP algorithms, respectively (181). In contrast to these findings, concordant scores for 3TC were obtained with all three genotyping programs in more than 90% of the cases studied (181). It has also been suggested that the discordance that exists between algorithms reflects a need for increased clinical validation and better consensus in interpretation of drug resistance data during the development of these tools, especially for some drugs such as NRTIs (180, 181).

In addition, the use of phenotypic drug resistance assays in conjunction with genotyping may be of further predictive value in some situations (179, 183). Unlike genotyping, phenotypic tests represent a more direct method for detection of HIV-1 drug resistance, which is based on changes in the 50% inhibitory concentration (i.e., IC_{50}) for a particular ARV in regard to a viral isolate in comparison with a HIV-1 reference strain (7, 179, 184, 185). However, discordances between genotypic and phenotypic tests are not uncommon and can arise as a result of several circumstances (82, 179, 186). In instances of either genotypic–phenotypic discordance or disagreements between different HIV-1 genotypic interpretative systems, access to expert advice on HIV-1 drug resistance may be invaluable in order to help reduce uncertainty with respect to decisions about a subsequent therapeutic regimen.

Lastly, genotypic drug resistance testing has also been successfully implemented for other chronic viral infections (i.e., HBV, CMV, and HSV) and may also hold promise for guiding therapy choice decisions to improve treatment outcomes for certain types of cancer. The development and future availability of antiviral therapy for additional viral diseases as well as the identification of novel molecular markers for cancer are likely to be key determinants in regard to the extended utilization of genotypic drug resistance assays.

Acknowledgments JLMC and MP equally contributed to the preparation of this review. Research performed by Marco Petrella was in partial fulfillment of the Ph.D. degree, Faculty of Graduate Studies and Research, McGill University, Montreal, Canada. Research performed by Jorge L Martinez-Cajas was funded by the Canadian HIV Trials Network.

References

1. Arens M. Clinically relevant sequence-based genotyping of HBV, HCV, CMV, and HIV. J Clin Virol 2001;22(1):11–29
2. Smith TF. Susceptibility testing. Viral pathogens. Infect Dis Clin North Am 2001;15(4):1263–1294
3. Servais J, Lambert C, Fontaine E, et al. Comparison of DNA sequencing and a line probe assay for detection of human immunodeficiency virus type 1 drug resistance mutations in patients failing highly active antiretroviral therapy. J Clin Microbiol 2001;39(2):454–459
4. Stuyver L, Wyseur A, Rombout A, et al. Line probe assay for rapid detection of drug-selected mutations in the human immunodeficiency virus type 1 reverse transcriptase gene. Antimicrob Agents Chemother 1997;41(2):284–291
5. Hanna GJ, D'Aquila RT. Clinical use of genotypic and phenotypic drug resistance testing to monitor antiretroviral chemotherapy. Clin Infect Dis 2001;32(5):774–782
6. Schmidt B, Korn K, Walter H. Technologies for measuring HIV-1 drug resistance. HIV Clin Trials 2002;3(3):227–236
7. Youree BE, D'Aquila RT. Antiretroviral resistance testing for clinical management. AIDS Rev 2002;4(1):3–12
8. D'Aquila RT, Schapiro JM, Brun-Vezinet F, et al. Drug resistance mutations in HIV-1. Top HIV Med 2003;11(3):92–96
9. Baxter JD, Mayers DL, Wentworth DN, et al. A randomized study of antiretroviral management based on plasma genotypic antiretroviral resistance testing in patients failing therapy. CPCRA 046 Study Team for the Terry Beirn Community Programs for Clinical Research on AIDS. AIDS 2000;14(9):F83–F93
10. Durant J, Clevenbergh P, Halfon P, et al. Drug-resistance genotyping in HIV-1 therapy: the VIRADAPT randomised controlled trial. Lancet 1999;353(9171):2195–2199
11. Meynard JL, Vray M, Morand-Joubert L, et al. Phenotypic or genotypic resistance testing for choosing antiretroviral therapy after treatment failure: a randomized trial. AIDS 2002;16(5):727–736
12. Torre D, Tambini R. Antiretroviral drug resistance testing in patients with HIV-1 infection: a meta-analysis study. HIV Clin Trials 2002;3(1):1–8
13. Weinstein MC, Goldie SJ, Losina E, et al. Use of genotypic resistance testing to guide HIV therapy: clinical impact and cost-effectiveness. Ann Intern Med 2001;134(6):440–450
14. Chaix C, Grenier-Sennelier C, Clevenbergh P, et al. Economic evaluation of drug resistance genotyping for the adaptation of treatment in HIV-infected patients in the VIRADAPT study. J Acquir Immune Defic Syndr 2000;24(3):227–231
15. Tural C, Ruiz L, Holtzer C, et al. Clinical utility of HIV-1 genotyping and expert advice: the Havana trial. AIDS 2002;16(2):209–218
16. Badri SM, Adeyemi OM, Max BE, Zagorski BM, Barker DE. How does expert advice impact genotypic resistance testing in clinical practice? Clin Infect Dis 2003;37(5):708–713
17. Pillay D. Emergence and control of resistance to antiviral drugs in resistance in herpes viruses, hepatitis B virus, and HIV. Commun Dis Public Health 1998;1(1):5–13
18. Petrella M, Montaner J, Batist G, Wainberg MA. The role of surrogate markers in the clinical development of antiretroviral therapy: a model for early evaluation of targeted cancer drugs. Cancer Invest 2004;22(1):149–160
19. Roumiantsev S, Shah NP, Gorre ME, et al. Clinical resistance to the kinase inhibitor STI-571 in chronic myeloid leukemia by mutation of Tyr-253 in the Abl kinase domain P-loop. Proc Natl Acad Sci U S A 2002;99(16):10700–10705
20. Lorenzi P, Opravil M, Hirschel B, et al. Impact of drug resistance mutations on virologic response to salvage therapy. Swiss HIV Cohort Study. AIDS 1999;13(2):F17–F21
21. Quiros-Roldan E, Signorini S, Castelli F, et al. Analysis of HIV-1 mutation patterns in patients failing antiretroviral therapy. J Clin Lab Anal 2001;15(1):43–46
22. Rousseau MN, Vergne L, Montes B, et al. Patterns of resistance mutations to antiretroviral drugs in extensively treated HIV-1-infected patients with failure of highly active antiretroviral therapy. J Acquir Immune Defic Syndr 2001;26(1):36–43
23. Winters MA, Baxter JD, Mayers DL, et al. Frequency of antiretroviral drug resistance mutations in HIV-1 strains from patients failing triple drug regimens. The Terry Beirn Community Programs for Clinical Research on AIDS. Antivir Ther 2000;5(1):57–63
24. Yeni PG, Hammer SM, Carpenter CC, et al. Antiretroviral treatment for adult HIV infection in 2002: updated recommendations of the International AIDS Society-USA Panel. JAMA 2002;288(2):222–235

25. Deeks SG. International perspectives on antiretroviral resistance. Nonnucleoside reverse transcriptase inhibitor resistance. J Acquir Immune Defic Syndr 2001;26 Suppl 1:S25–S33

26. Gao HQ, Boyer PL, Sarafianos SG, Arnold E, Hughes SH. The role of steric hindrance in 3TC resistance of human immunodeficiency virus type-1 reverse transcriptase. J Mol Biol 2000;300(2):403–418

27. Quan Y, Gu Z, Li X, Li Z, Morrow CD, Wainberg MA. Endogenous reverse transcription assays reveal high-level resistance to the triphosphate of (-)2'-dideoxy-3'-thiacytidine by mutated M184V human immunodeficiency virus type 1. J Virol 1996;70(8): 5642–5645

28. Quiros-Roldan E, Airoldi M, Moretti F, et al. Genotype resistance profiles in patients failing an NNRTI-containing regimen, and modifications after stopping NNRTI therapy. J Clin Lab Anal 2002;16(2):76–78

29. Tisdale M, Kemp SD, Parry NR, Larder BA. Rapid in vitro selection of human immunodeficiency virus type 1 resistant to 3'-thiacytidine inhibitors due to a mutation in the YMDD region of reverse transcriptase. Proc Natl Acad Sci U S A 1993;90(12):5653–5656

30. Squires KE. An introduction to nucleoside and nucleotide analogues. Antivir Ther 2001;6 Suppl 3:1–14

31. Stein DS, Moore KH. Phosphorylation of nucleoside analog antiretrovirals: a review for clinicians. Pharmacotherapy 2001;21(1):11–34

32. Anderson KS. Perspectives on the molecular mechanism of inhibition and toxicity of nucleoside analogs that target HIV-1 reverse transcriptase. Biochim Biophys Acta 2002;1587(2–3):296–299

33. Goody RS, Muller B, Restle T. Factors contributing to the inhibition of HIV reverse transcriptase by chain-terminating nucleotides in vitro and in vivo. FEBS Lett 1991;291(1):1–5

34. Mitsuya H, Jarrett RF, Matsukura M, et al. Long-term inhibition of human T-lymphotropic virus type III/lymphadenopathy-associated virus (human immunodeficiency virus) DNA synthesis and RNA expression in T cells protected by 2',3'-dideoxynucleosides in vitro. Proc Natl Acad Sci U S A 1987;84(7):2033–2037

35. Schuurman R, Nijhuis M, van Leeuwen R, et al. Rapid changes in human immunodeficiency virus type 1 RNA load and appearance of drug-resistant virus populations in persons treated with lamivudine (3TC). J Infect Dis 1995;171(6):1411–1419

36. Wainberg MA, Salomon H, Gu Z, et al. Development of HIV-1 resistance to (-)2'-deoxy-3'-thiacytidine in patients with AIDS or advanced AIDS-related complex. AIDS 1995;9(4):351–357

37. Back NK, Nijhuis M, Keulen W, et al. Reduced replication of 3TC-resistant HIV-1 variants in primary cells due to a processivity defect of the reverse transcriptase enzyme. EMBO J 1996;15(15): 4040–4049

38. Boucher CA, Cammack N, Schipper P, et al. High-level resistance to (−) enantiomeric 2'-deoxy-3'-thiacytidine in vitro is due to one amino acid substitution in the catalytic site of human immunodeficiency virus type 1 reverse transcriptase. Antimicrob Agents Chemother 1993;37(10):2231–2234

39. Gao Q, Gu Z, Parniak MA, et al. The same mutation that encodes low-level human immunodeficiency virus type 1 resistance to 2',3'-dideoxyinosine and 2',3'-dideoxycytidine confers high-level resistance to the (−) enantiomer of 2',3'-dideoxy-3'-thiacytidine. Antimicrob Agents Chemother 1993;37(6):1390–1392

40. Hertogs K, Bloor S, De Vroey V, et al. A novel human immunodeficiency virus type 1 reverse transcriptase mutational pattern confers phenotypic lamivudine resistance in the absence of mutation 184V. Antimicrob Agents Chemother 2000;44(3):568–573

41. Romano L, Venturi G, Bloor S, et al. Broad nucleoside-analogue resistance implications for human immunodeficiency virus type 1 reverse-transcriptase mutations at codons 44 and 118. J Infect Dis 2002;185(7):898–904

42. Lange J. A rational approach to the selection and sequencing of nucleoside/nucleotide analogues: a new paradigm. Antivir Ther 2001;6 Suppl 3:45–54

43. Mayers DL. Prevalence and incidence of resistance to zidovudine and other antiretroviral drugs. Am J Med 1997;102(5B):70–75

44. Gotte M, Wainberg MA. Biochemical mechanisms involved in overcoming HIV resistance to nucleoside inhibitors of reverse transcriptase. Drug Resist Updat 2000;3(1):30–38

45. Loveday C. International perspectives on antiretroviral resistance. Nucleoside reverse transcriptase inhibitor resistance. J Acquir Immune Defic Syndr 2001;26 Suppl 1:S10–S24

46. Miller V, Larder BA. Mutational patterns in the HIV genome and cross-resistance following nucleoside and nucleotide analogue drug exposure. Antivir Ther 2001;6 Suppl 3:25–44

47. Soriano V, de Mendoza C. Genetic mechanisms of resistance to NRTI and NNRTI. HIV Clin Trials 2002;3(3):237–248

48. Bocket L, Yazdanpanah Y, Ajana F, et al. Thymidine analogue mutations emergence in antiretroviral-naive patients on triple therapy including either zidovudine or stavudine. In: XII International HIV Drug Resistance Workshop, Cabo del Sol, Los Cabos, Mexico, June 10–14, 2003

49. Flandre P, Descamps D, Joly V, et al. Predictive factors and selection of thymidine analogue mutations by nucleoside reverse transcriptase inhibitors according to initial regimen received. Antivir Ther 2003;8(1):65–72

50. Marcelin A, Wirden M, Delaugerre C, et al. Selection of thymidine analogue mutations by nucleoside reverse transcriptase inhibitors occurs step by step and through two different pathways. Antivir Ther 2002;7:S34, Abstract 40

51. Van Houtte M, Lecocq P, Bacheler L. Prevalence and quantitative phenotypic resistance patterns of specific nucleoside analogue mutation combinations and of mutations 44 and 118 in reverse transcriptase in a large dataset of recent HIV-1 clinical isolates. In: XII International HIV Drug Resistance Workshop, Cabo del Sol, Los Cabos, Mexico, June 10–14, 2003

52. Kuritzkes D, Bassett R, Young R, et al. for ACTG 306 and 370 Protocol Teams. Rate of emergence of thymidine analogue resistance mutations in HIV-1 reverse transcriptase selected by stavudine or zidovudine-based regimens in treatment-naïve patients. Antivir Ther 2002;7:S31, Abstract 36

53. Winston A, Mandalia S, Pillay D, Gazzard B, Pozniak A. The prevalence and determinants of the K65R mutation in HIV-1 reverse transcriptase in tenofovir-naive patients. AIDS 2002;16(15): 2087–2089

54. Wainberg MA, Miller MD, Quan Y, et al. In vitro selection and characterization of HIV-1 with reduced susceptibility to PMPA. Antivir Ther 1999;4(2):87–94

55. Margot NA, Isaacson E, McGowan I, Cheng A, Miller MD. Extended treatment with tenofovir disoproxil fumarate in treatment-experienced HIV-1-infected patients: genotypic, phenotypic, and rebound analyses. J Acquir Immune Defic Syndr 2003;33(1):15–21

56. Parikh UM, Bacheler L, Koontz D, Mellors JW. The K65R mutation in human immunodeficiency virus type 1 reverse transcriptase exhibits bidirectional phenotypic antagonism with thymidine analog mutations. J Virol 2006;80(10):4971–4977

57. Shirasaka T, Kavlick MF, Ueno T, et al. Emergence of human immunodeficiency virus type 1 variants with resistance to multiple dideoxynucleosides in patients receiving therapy with dideoxynucleosides. Proc Natl Acad Sci U S A 1995;92(6):2398–2402

58. Ueno T, Shirasaka T, Mitsuya H. Enzymatic characterization of human immunodeficiency virus type 1 reverse transcriptase resistant to multiple 2',3'-dideoxynucleoside 5'-triphosphates. J Biol Chem 1995;270(40):23605–23611

59. Boyer PL, Sarafianos SG, Arnold E, Hughes SH. Nucleoside analog resistance caused by insertions in the fingers of human immunodeficiency virus type 1 reverse transcriptase involves ATP-mediated excision. J Virol 2002;76(18):9143–9151

60. Larder BA, Bloor S, Kemp SD, et al. A family of insertion mutations between codons 67 and 70 of human immunodeficiency virus

type 1 reverse transcriptase confer multinucleoside analog resistance. Antimicrob Agents Chemother 1999;43(8):1961–1967

61. Van Vaerenbergh K, Van Laethem K, Albert J, et al. Prevalence and characteristics of multinucleoside-resistant human immunodeficiency virus type 1 among European patients receiving combinations of nucleoside analogues. Antimicrob Agents Chemother 2000;44(8):2109–2117

62. Ding J, Das K, Moereels H, et al. Structure of HIV-1 RT/TIBO R 86183 complex reveals similarity in the binding of diverse nonnucleoside inhibitors. Nat Struct Biol 1995;2(5):407–415

63. Wu JC, Warren TC, Adams J, et al. A novel dipyridodiazepinone inhibitor of HIV-1 reverse transcriptase acts through a nonsubstrate binding site. Biochemistry 1991;30(8):2022–2026

64. Spence RA, Kati WM, Anderson KS, Johnson KA. Mechanism of inhibition of HIV-1 reverse transcriptase by nonnucleoside inhibitors. Science 1995;267(5200):988–993

65. Gu Z, Quan Y, Li Z, Arts EJ, Wainberg MA. Effects of nonnucleoside inhibitors of human immunodeficiency virus type 1 in cell-free recombinant reverse transcriptase assays. J Biol Chem 1995;270(52):31046–31051

66. Chong KT, Pagano PJ, Hinshaw RR. Bisheteroarylpiperazine reverse transcriptase inhibitor in combination with 3'-azido 3' deoxythymidine or 2',3'-dideoxycytidine synergistically inhibits human immunodeficiency virus type 1 replication in vitro. Antimicrob Agents Chemother 1994;38(2):288–293

67. Esnouf R, Ren J, Ross C, Jones Y, Stammers D, Stuart D. Mechanism of inhibition of HIV-1 reverse transcriptase by nonnucleoside inhibitors. Nat Struct Biol 1995;2(4):303–308

68. Richman D, Shih CK, Lowy I, et al. Human immunodeficiency virus type 1 mutants resistant to nonnucleoside inhibitors of reverse transcriptase arise in tissue culture. Proc Natl Acad Sci U S A 1991;88(24):11241–11245

69. Vandamme AM, Debyser Z, Pauwels R, et al. Characterization of HIV-1 strains isolated from patients treated with TIBO R82913. AIDS Res Hum Retroviruses 1994;10(1):39–46

70. Byrnes VW, Sardana VV, Schleif WA, et al. Comprehensive mutant enzyme and viral variant assessment of human immunodeficiency virus type 1 reverse transcriptase resistance to nonnucleoside inhibitors. Antimicrob Agents Chemother 1993;37(8):1576–1579

71. Fletcher RS, Arion D, Borkow G, Wainberg MA, Dmitrienko GI, Parniak MA. Synergistic inhibition of HIV-1 reverse transcriptase DNA polymerase activity and virus replication in vitro by combinations of carboxanilide nonnucleoside compounds. Biochemistry 1995;34(32):10106–10112

72. Balzarini J, Karlsson A, Perez-Perez MJ, Camarasa MJ, Tarpley WG, De Clercq E. Treatment of human immunodeficiency virus type 1 (HIV-1)-infected cells with combinations of HIV-1-specific inhibitors results in a different resistance pattern than does treatment with single-drug therapy. J Virol 1993;67(9):5353–5359

73. Sardana VV, Emini EA, Gotlib L, et al. Functional analysis of HIV-1 reverse transcriptase amino acids involved in resistance to multiple nonnucleoside inhibitors. J Biol Chem 1992;267(25):17526–17530

74. Dueweke TJ, Pushkarskaya T, Poppe SM, et al. A mutation in reverse transcriptase of bis(heteroaryl)piperazine-resistant human immunodeficiency virus type 1 that confers increased sensitivity to other nonnucleoside inhibitors. Proc Natl Acad Sci U S A 1993;90(10):4713–4717

75. Nunberg JH, Schleif WA, Boots EJ, et al. Viral resistance to human immunodeficiency virus type 1-specific pyridinone reverse transcriptase inhibitors. J Virol 1991;65(9):4887–4892

76. Condra JH. Virological and clinical implications of resistance to HIV-1 protease inhibitors. Drug Resist Updat 1998;1(5):292–299

77. Deeks SG. Failure of HIV-1 protease inhibitors to fully suppress viral replication. Implications for salvage therapy. Adv Exp Med Biol 1999;458:175–182

78. Murphy RL. New antiretroviral drugs part I: PIs. AIDS Clin Care 1999;11(5):35–37

79. Johnson VA, Brun-Vezinet F, Clotet B, et al. Update of the drug resistance mutations in HIV-1: Fall 2006. Top HIV Med 2006;14(3):125–130

80. De Meyer S, Vangeneugden T, Lefebvre E, et al. Phenotypic and genotypic determinants of resistance to TMC114: pooled analysis of POWER 1, 2 and 3. In: XV International Drug Resistance Workshop, June 13–17, 2006. Sitges, Spain, 2006, Abstract 73

81. Carrillo A, Stewart KD, Sham HL, et al. In vitro selection and characterization of human immunodeficiency virus type 1 variants with increased resistance to ABT-378, a novel protease inhibitor. J Virol 1998;72(9):7532–7541

82. Parkin NT, Chappey C, Petropoulos CJ. Improving lopinavir genotype algorithm through phenotype correlations: novel mutation patterns and amprenavir cross-resistance. AIDS 2003;17(7): 955–961

83. de Mendoza C, Valer L, Bacheler L, Pattery T, Corral A, Soriano V. Prevalence of the HIV-1 protease mutation I47A in clinical practice and association with lopinavir resistance. AIDS 2006;20(7): 1071–1074

84. Kagan RM, Shenderovich MD, Heseltine PN, Ramnarayan K. Structural analysis of an HIV-1 protease I47A mutant resistant to the protease inhibitor lopinavir. Protein Sci 2005;14(7):1870–1878

85. Turner D, Schapiro JM, Brenner BG, Wainberg MA. The influence of protease inhibitor resistance profiles on selection of HIV therapy in treatment-naive patients. Antivir Ther 2004;9(3):301–314

86. Martinez-Picado J, Savara AV, Sutton L, D'Aquila RT. Replicative fitness of protease inhibitor-resistant mutants of human immunodeficiency virus type 1. J Virol 1999;73(5):3744–3752

87. Gatanaga H, Suzuki Y, Tsang H, et al. Amino acid substitutions in Gag protein at non-cleavage sites are indispensable for the development of a high multitude of HIV-1 resistance against protease inhibitors. J Biol Chem 2002;277(8):5952–5961

88. Tamiya S, Mardy S, Kavlick MF, Yoshimura K, Mistuya H. Amino acid insertions near Gag cleavage sites restore the otherwise compromised replication of human immunodeficiency virus type 1 variants resistant to protease inhibitors. J Virol 2004;78(21):12030–12040

89. Doyon L, Croteau G, Thibeault D, Poulin F, Pilote L, Lamarre D. Second locus involved in human immunodeficiency virus type 1 resistance to protease inhibitors. J Virol 1996;70(6): 3763–3769

90. Doyon L, Payant C, Brakier-Gingras L, Lamarre D. Novel Gag-Pol frameshift site in human immunodeficiency virus type 1 variants resistant to protease inhibitors. J Virol 1998;72(7):6146–6150

91. Verheyen J, Litau E, Sing T, et al. Compensatory mutations at the HIV cleavage sites p7/p1 and p1/p6-gag in therapy-naive and therapy-experienced patients. Antivir Ther 2006;11(7):879–887

92. Cervia JS, Smith MA. Enfuvirtide (T-20): a novel human immunodeficiency virus type 1 fusion inhibitor. Clin Infect Dis 2003;37(8):1102–1106

93. Tomaras GD, Greenberg ML. Mechanisms for HIV-1 Entry: current strategies to interfere with this step. Curr Infect Dis Rep 2001;3(1):93–99

94. Lalezari JP, Henry K, O'Hearn M, et al. Enfuvirtide, an HIV-1 fusion inhibitor, for drug-resistant HIV infection in North and South America. N Engl J Med 2003;348(22):2175–2185

95. Lazzarin A, Clotet B, Cooper D, et al. Efficacy of enfuvirtide in patients infected with drug-resistant HIV-1 in Europe and Australia. N Engl J Med 2003;348(22):2186–2195

96. Lalezari JP, DeJesus E, Northfelt DW, et al. A controlled Phase II trial assessing three doses of enfuvirtide (T-20) in combination with abacavir, amprenavir, ritonavir and efavirenz in non-nucleoside reverse transcriptase inhibitor-naive HIV-infected adults. Antivir Ther 2003;8(4):279–287

97. Lalezari JP, Eron JJ, Carlson M, et al. A phase II clinical study of the long-term safety and antiviral activity of enfuvirtide-based antiretroviral therapy. AIDS 2003;17(5):691–698

98. Wei X, Decker JM, Liu H, et al. Emergence of resistant human immunodeficiency virus type 1 in patients receiving fusion inhibitor (T-20) monotherapy. Antimicrob Agents Chemother 2002;46(6):1896–1905

99. Roman F, Gonzalez D, Lambert C, et al. Uncommon mutations at residue positions critical for enfuvirtide (T-20) resistance in enfuvirtide-naive patients infected with subtype B and non-B HIV-1 strains. J Acquir Immune Defic Syndr 2003;33(2):134–139

100. Bossi P, Peytavin G, Ait-Mohand H, et al. GENOPHAR: a randomized study of plasma drug measurements in association with genotypic resistance testing and expert advice to optimize therapy in patients failing antiretroviral therapy. HIV Med 2004;5(5):352–359

101. Clevenbergh P, Bozonnat MC, Kirstetter M, et al. Variable virological outcomes according to the center providing antiretroviral therapy within the PharmAdapt clinical trial. HIV Clin Trials 2003;4(2):84–91

102. Saracino A, Monno L, Locaputo S, et al. Selection of antiretroviral therapy guided by genotypic or phenotypic resistance testing: an open-label, randomized, multicenter study (PhenGen). J Acquir Immune Defic Syndr 2004;37(5):1587–1598

103. Graham N PM, Verbiest W, Harrigan R, Larder B. The virtual phenotype is an independent predictor of clinical response. In: Program and Abstracts of the 8th Conference on Retroviruses and Opportunistic Infections, 4–8 February 2001. Chicago, USA, Abstract 524

104. Larder BA KS, Hertogs K. Quantitative prediction of HIV-1 phenotypic drug resistance from genotypes: the virtual phenotype (VirtualPhenotype). Antiviral Ther 2000;5 Suppl 3:49, Abstract 63

105. Brenner B, Turner D, Oliveira M, et al. A V106M mutation in HIV-1 clade C viruses exposed to efavirenz confers cross-resistance to non-nucleoside reverse transcriptase inhibitors. AIDS 2003;17(1):F1–F5

106. Brenner BG, Oliveira M, Doualla-Bell F, et al. HIV-1 subtype C viruses rapidly develop K65R resistance to tenofovir in cell culture. AIDS 2006;20(9):F9–F13

107. Doualla-Bell F, Avalos A, Brenner B, et al. High prevalence of the K65R mutation in human immunodeficiency virus type 1 subtype C isolates from infected patients in Botswana treated with didanosine-based regimens. Antimicrob Agents Chemother 2006;50(12):4182–4185

108. Chen CJ, Yang HI, Su J, et al. Risk of hepatocellular carcinoma across a biological gradient of serum hepatitis B virus DNA level. JAMA 2006;295(1):65–73

109. Iloeje UH, Yang HI, Su J, Jen CL, You SL, Chen CJ. Predicting cirrhosis risk based on the level of circulating hepatitis B viral load. Gastroenterology 2006;130(3):678–686

110. Nafa S, Ahmed S, Tavan D, et al. Early detection of viral resistance by determination of hepatitis B virus polymerase mutations in patients treated by lamivudine for chronic hepatitis B. Hepatology 2000;32(5):1078–1088

111. Lai CL, Dienstag J, Schiff E, et al. Prevalence and clinical correlates of YMDD variants during lamivudine therapy for patients with chronic hepatitis B. Clin Infect Dis 2003;36(6):687–696

112. Allen MI, Deslauriers M, Andrews CW, et al. Identification and characterization of mutations in hepatitis B virus resistant to lamivudine. Lamivudine Clinical Investigation Group. Hepatology 1998;27(6):1670–1677

113. Papatheodoridis GV, Dimou E, Papadimitropoulos V. Nucleoside analogues for chronic hepatitis B: antiviral efficacy and viral resistance. Am J Gastroenterol 2002;97(7):1618–1628

114. Melegari M, Scaglioni PP, Wands JR. Hepatitis B virus mutants associated with 3TC and famciclovir administration are replication defective. Hepatology 1998;27(2):628–633

115. Delaney WE IV, Yang H, Miller MD, Gibbs CS, Xiong S. Combinations of adefovir with nucleoside analogs produce additive antiviral effects against hepatitis B virus in vitro. Antimicrob Agents Chemother 2004;48(10):3702–3710

116. De Clercq E. Clinical potential of the acyclic nucleoside phosphonates cidofovir, adefovir, and tenofovir in treatment of DNA virus and retrovirus infections. Clin Microbiol Rev 2003;16(4):569–596

117. Hadziyannis SJ, Tassopoulos NC, Heathcote EJ, et al. Adefovir dipivoxil for the treatment of hepatitis B e antigen-negative chronic hepatitis B. N Engl J Med 2003;348(9):800–807

118. Karayiannis P. Hepatitis B virus: old, new and future approaches to antiviral treatment. J Antimicrob Chemother 2003;51(4):761–785

119. Marcellin P, Chang TT, Lim SG, et al. Adefovir dipivoxil for the treatment of hepatitis B e antigen-positive chronic hepatitis B. N Engl J Med 2003;348(9):808–816

120. Westland CE, Yang H, Delaney WE IV, et al. Week 48 resistance surveillance in two phase 3 clinical studies of adefovir dipivoxil for chronic hepatitis B. Hepatology 2003;38(1):96–103

121. Angus P, Vaughan R, Xiong S, et al. Resistance to adefovir dipivoxil therapy associated with the selection of a novel mutation in the HBV polymerase. Gastroenterology 2003;125(2):292–297

122. Brunelle MN, Jacquard AC, Pichoud C, et al. Susceptibility to antivirals of a human HBV strain with mutations conferring resistance to both lamivudine and adefovir. Hepatology 2005;41(6):1391–1398

123. Villeneuve JP, Durantel D, Durantel S, et al. Selection of a hepatitis B virus strain resistant to adefovir in a liver transplantation patient. J Hepatol 2003;39(6):1085–1089

124. Fung SK, Andreone P, Han SH, et al. Adefovir-resistant hepatitis B can be associated with viral rebound and hepatic decompensation. J Hepatol 2005;43(6):937–943

125. Lee YS, Suh DJ, Lim YS, et al. Increased risk of adefovir resistance in patients with lamivudine-resistant chronic hepatitis B after 48 weeks of adefovir dipivoxil monotherapy. Hepatology 2006;43(6):1385–1391

126. Lampertico P, Viganò M, Manenti E, Iavarone M, Lunghi G, Colombo M. Five years of sequential LAM TO LAM+ADV therapy suppresses HBV replication in most HBeAg-negative cirrhotics, preventing decompensation but not hepatocellular carcinoma. J Hepatol 2006;44(S2):S38, Abstract 85

127. Chang TT, Lai CL. Hepatitis B virus with primary resistance to adefovir. N Engl J Med 2006;355(3):322–323; author reply 323

128. Tenney DJ, Levine SM, Rose RE, et al. Clinical emergence of entecavir-resistant hepatitis B virus requires additional substitutions in virus already resistant to lamivudine. Antimicrob Agents Chemother 2004;48(9):3498–3507

129. Chang T-T, Gish RG, Hadziyannis SJ, et al. A Dose-ranging study of the efficacy and tolerability of entecavir in lamivudine-refractory chronic hepatitis B patients. Gastroenterology 2005; 129(4):1198

130. Colonno RJ, Rose RE, Pokornowski K, Baldick CJ, Kleszewski K, Tenney DJ. Assessment at three years show high barrier to resistance is maintained in entecavir-related nucleoside naive patients while resistance emergence increase over time in lamivudine refractory patients. In: AASLD, October 27–31, 2006. Boston, MA, Abstract 110

131. Sherman M, Yurdaydin C, Sollano J, et al. Entecavir for treatment of lamivudine-refractory, HBeAg-positive chronic hepatitis B. Gastroenterology 2006;130(7):2039

132. McMahon M, Jilek B, Brennan T, et al. The anti-hepatitis B drug entecavir inhibits HIV-1 replication and selects HIV-1 variants resistant to antiretroviral drugs. In: 14th conference on retroviruses and opportunistic infections, February 25–28, 2007. Los Angeles, Abstract 136LB

133. Saag MS. Emtricitabine, a new antiretroviral agent with activity against HIV and hepatitis B virus. Clin Infect Dis 2006;42(1):126–131

134. Lai CL, Leung N, Teo EK, et al. A 1-year trial of telbivudine, lamivudine, and the combination in patients with hepatitis B e antigen-positive chronic hepatitis B. Gastroenterology 2005; 129(2):528–536

135. Wolf DG, Yaniv I, Honigman A, Kassis I, Schonfeld T, Ashkenazi S. Early emergence of ganciclovir-resistant human cytomegalovirus strains in children with primary combined immunodeficiency. J Infect Dis 1998;178(2):535 538

136. Cherrington JM, Fuller MD, Lamy PD, et al. In vitro antiviral susceptibilities of isolates from cytomegalovirus retinitis patients receiving first- or second-line cidofovir therapy: relationship to clinical outcome. J Infect Dis 1998;178(6):1821–1815

137. Jabs DA, Enger C, Dunn JP, Forman M. Cytomegalovirus retinitis and viral resistance: ganciclovir resistance. CMV Retinitis and Viral Resistance Study Group. J Infect Dis 1998;177(3): 770–773

138. Jabs DA, Enger C, Forman M, Dunn JP. Incidence of foscarnet resistance and cidofovir resistance in patients treated for cytomegalovirus retinitis. The Cytomegalovirus Retinitis and Viral Resistance Study Group. Antimicrob Agents Chemother 1998;42(9):2240–2244

139. Weinberg A, Jabs DA, Chou S, et al. Mutations conferring foscarnet resistance in a cohort of patients with acquired immunodeficiency syndrome and cytomegalovirus retinitis. J Infect Dis 2003;187(5):777–784

140. Chou S, Waldemer RH, Senters AE, et al. Cytomegalovirus UL97 phosphotransferase mutations that affect susceptibility to ganciclovir. J Infect Dis 2002;185(2):162–169

141. Wolf DG, Yaniv I, Ashkenazi S, Honigman A. Emergence of multiple human cytomegalovirus ganciclovir-resistant mutants with deletions and substitutions within the UL97 gene in a patient with severe combined immunodeficiency. Antimicrob Agents Chemother 2001;45(2):593–595

142. Smith IL, Cherrington JM, Jiles RE, Fuller MD, Freeman WR, Spector SA. High-level resistance of cytomegalovirus to ganciclovir is associated with alterations in both the UL97 and DNA polymerase genes. J Infect Dis 1997;176(1):69–77

143. Erice A, Gil-Roda C, Perez JL, et al. Antiviral susceptibilities and analysis of UL97 and DNA polymerase sequences of clinical cytomegalovirus isolates from immunocompromised patients. J Infect Dis 1997;175(5):1087–1092

144. Jabs DA, Martin BK, Forman MS, et al. Mutations conferring ganciclovir resistance in a cohort of patients with acquired immunodeficiency syndrome and cytomegalovirus retinitis. J Infect Dis 2001;183(2):333–337

145. Jabs DA, Martin BK, Forman MS, et al. Longitudinal observations on mutations conferring ganciclovir resistance in patients with acquired immunodeficiency syndrome and cytomegalovirus retinitis: The Cytomegalovirus and Viral Resistance Study Group Report Number 8. Am J Ophthalmol 2001;132(5): 700–710

146. Boivin G, Gilbert C, Gaudreau A, Greenfield I, Sudlow R, Roberts NA. Rate of emergence of cytomegalovirus (CMV) mutations in leukocytes of patients with acquired immunodeficiency syndrome who are receiving valganciclovir as induction and maintenance therapy for CMV retinitis. J Infect Dis 2001;184(12): 1598–1602

147. Lurain NS, Bhorade SM, Pursell KJ, et al. Analysis and characterization of antiviral drug-resistant cytomegalovirus isolates from solid organ transplant recipients. J Infect Dis 2002;186(6):760–768

148. Baldanti F, Silini E, Sarasini A, et al. A three-nucleotide deletion in the UL97 open reading frame is responsible for the ganciclovir resistance of a human cytomegalovirus clinical isolate. J Virol 1995;69(2):796–800

149. Baldanti F, Underwood MR, Talarico CL, et al. The Cys607→Tyr change in the UL97 phosphotransferase confers ganciclovir resistance to two human cytomegalovirus strains recovered from two immunocompromised patients. Antimicrob Agents Chemother 1998;42(2):444–446

150. Chou S, Erice A, Jordan MC, et al. Analysis of the UL97 phosphotransferase coding sequence in clinical cytomegalovirus isolates and identification of mutations conferring ganciclovir resistance. J Infect Dis 1995;171(3):576–583

151. Hanson MN, Preheim LC, Chou S, Talarico CL, Biron KK, Erice A. Novel mutation in the UL97 gene of a clinical cytomegalovirus strain conferring resistance to ganciclovir. Antimicrob Agents Chemother 1995;39(5):1204–1205

152. Chou S, Lurain NS, Thompson KD, Miner RC, Drew WL. Viral DNA polymerase mutations associated with drug resistance in human cytomegalovirus. J Infect Dis 2003;188(1):32–39

153. Scott GM, Weinberg A, Rawlinson WD, Chou S. Multidrug resistance conferred by novel DNA polymerase mutations in human cytomegalovirus isolates. Antimicrob Agents Chemother 2007;51(1):89 94

154. Cihlar T, Fuller MD, Mulato AS, Cherrington JM. A point mutation in the human cytomegalovirus DNA polymerase gene selected in vitro by cidofovir confers a slow replication phenotype in cell culture. Virology 1998;248(2):382 393

155. Baldanti F, Underwood MR, Stanat SC, et al. Single amino acid changes in the DNA polymerase confer foscarnet resistance and slow-growth phenotype, while mutations in the UL97 encoded phosphotransferase confer ganciclovir resistance in three double-resistant human cytomegalovirus strains recovered from patients with AIDS. J Virol 1996;70(3):1390–1395

156. Chou S, Marousek G, Guentzel S, et al. Evolution of mutations conferring multidrug resistance during prophylaxis and therapy for cytomegalovirus disease. J Infect Dis 1997;176(3):786–789

157. Mousavi-Jazi M, Schloss L, Drew WL, et al. Variations in the cytomegalovirus DNA polymerase and phosphotransferase genes in relation to foscarnet and ganciclovir sensitivity. J Clin Virol 2001;23(1–2):1–15

158. Anderson KP, Fox MC, Brown-Driver V, Martin MJ, Azad RF. Inhibition of human cytomegalovirus immediate-early gene expression by an antisense oligonucleotide complementary to immediate-early RNA. Antimicrob Agents Chemother 1996;40(9):2004–2011

159. Mulamba GB, Hu A, Azad RF, Anderson KP, Coen DM. Human cytomegalovirus mutant with sequence-dependent resistance to the phosphorothioate oligonucleotide fomivirsen (ISIS 2922). Antimicrob Agents Chemother 1998;42(4):971–973

160. Chen Y, Scieux C, Garrait V, et al. Resistant herpes simplex virus type 1 infection: an emerging concern after allogeneic stem cell transplantation. Clin Infect Dis 2000;31(4):927–935

161. Morfin F, Thouvenot D. Herpes simplex virus resistance to antiviral drugs. J Clin Virol 2003;26(1):29–37

162. Chibo D, Druce J, Sasadeusz J, Birch C. Molecular analysis of clinical isolates of acyclovir resistant herpes simplex virus. Antiviral Res 2004;61(2):83–91

163. Hwang YT, Zuccola HJ, Lu Q, Hwang CB. A point mutation within conserved region VI of herpes simplex virus type 1 DNA polymerase confers altered drug sensitivity and enhances replication fidelity. J Virol 2004;78(2):650–657

164. Petrella M, Brenner B, Loemba H, Wainberg MA. HIV drug resistance and implications for the introduction of antiretroviral therapy in resource-poor countries. Drug Resist Updat 2001;4(6): 339–346

165. Holguin A, Soriano V. Resistance to antiretroviral agents in individuals with HIV-1 non-B subtypes. HIV Clin Trials 2002;3(5):403–411

166. Kantor R, Zijenah LS, Shafer RW, et al. HIV-1 subtype C reverse transcriptase and protease genotypes in Zimbabwean patients failing antiretroviral therapy. AIDS Res Hum Retroviruses 2002;18(18):1407–1413

167. Alexander CS, Montessori V, Wynhoven B, et al. Prevalence and response to antiretroviral therapy of non-B subtypes of HIV in antiretroviral-naive individuals in British Columbia. Antivir Ther 2002;7(1):31–35

168. Kantor R, Katzenstein D. Polymorphism in HIV-1 non-subtype B protease and reverse transcriptase and its potential impact on drug susceptibility and drug resistance evolution. AIDS Rev 2003;5(1):25–35

169. Fowler MG. Prevention of perinatal HIV infection. What do we know? Where should future research go? Ann N Y Acad Sci 2000;918:45–52

170. Welles SL, Pitt J, Colgrove R, et al. HIV-1 genotypic zidovudine drug resistance and the risk of maternal – infant transmission in the women and infants transmission study. The Women and Infants Transmission Study Group. AIDS 2000;14(3): 263–271

171. Yerly S, Kaiser L, Race E, Bru JP, Clavel F, Perrin L. Transmission of antiretroviral-drug-resistant HIV-1 variants. Lancet 1999;354(9180):729–733

172. Salomon H, Wainberg MA, Brenner B, et al. Prevalence of HIV-1 resistant to antiretroviral drugs in 81 individuals newly infected by sexual contact or injecting drug use. Investigators of the Quebec Primary Infection Study. AIDS 2000;14(2): F17–F23

173. Simon V, Vanderhoeven J, Hurley A, et al. Evolving patterns of HIV-1 resistance to antiretroviral agents in newly infected individuals. AIDS 2002;16(11):1511–1519

174. Wensing AM, Boucher CA. Worldwide transmission of drug-resistant HIV. AIDS Rev 2003;5(3):140–155

175. Brenner BG, Routy JP, Petrella M, et al. Persistence and fitness of multidrug-resistant human immunodeficiency virus type 1 acquired in primary infection. J Virol 2002;76(4):1753–1761

176. Chan KC, Galli RA, Montaner JS, Harrigan PR. Prolonged retention of drug resistance mutations and rapid disease progression in the absence of therapy after primary HIV infection. AIDS 2003;17(8):1256–1258

177. Simon V, Padte N, Murray D, et al. Infectivity and replication capacity of drug-resistant human immunodeficiency virus type 1 variants isolated during primary infection. J Virol 2003;77(14):7736–7745

178. Sturmer M, Doerr HW, Preiser W. Variety of interpretation systems for human immunodeficiency virus type 1 genotyping: confirmatory information or additional confusion? Curr Drug Targets Infect Disord 2003;3(4):373–382

179. Parkin N, Chappey C, Maroldo L, Bates M, Hellmann NS, Petropoulos CJ. Phenotypic and genotypic HIV-1 drug resistance assays provide complementary information. J Acquir Immune Defic Syndr 2002;31(2):128–136

180. De Luca A, Perno CF. Impact of different HIV resistance interpretation by distinct systems on clinical utility of resistance testing. Curr Opin Infect Dis 2003;16(6):573–580

181. Kijak GH, Rubio AE, Pampuro SE, et al. Discrepant results in the interpretation of HIV-1 drug-resistance genotypic data among widely used algorithms. HIV Med 2003;4(1):72–78

182. Sturmer M, Doerr HW, Staszewski S, Preiser W. Comparison of nine resistance interpretation systems for HIV-1 genotyping. Antivir Ther 2003;8(3):239–244

183. Zazzi M, Romano L, Venturi G, et al. Comparative evaluation of three computerized algorithms for prediction of antiretroviral susceptibility from HIV type 1 genotype. J Antimicrob Chemother 2004;53(2):356–360

184. Demeter L, Haubrich R. International perspectives on antiretroviral resistance. Phenotypic and genotypic resistance assays: methodology, reliability, and interpretations. J Acquir Immune Defic Syndr 2001;26 Suppl 1:S3–S9

185. Dunne AL, Mitchell FM, Coberly SK, et al. Comparison of genotyping and phenotyping methods for determining susceptibility of HIV-1 to antiretroviral drugs. AIDS 2001;15(12): 1471–1475

186. Zolopa AR. Genotype-phenotype discordance: the evolution in our understanding HIV-1 drug resistance. AIDS 2003;17(7): 1077–1078

Chapter 87
Antimicrobial Resistance: An International Public Health Problem

Carlos A. DiazGranados and John E. McGowan Jr.

1 Introduction

Microorganisms resistant to multiple anti-infective agents have increased around the world (1). A few bacterial organisms associated with infections in the healthcare setting now are completely resistant to all commonly employed antimicrobial agents (2). Other multidrug-resistant (MDR) bacteria that previously were frequent only in acute care hospitals recently have been recovered in extended care facilities, ambulatory surgical units, home healthcare, and other healthcare settings (3, 4). Bacterial resistance in community settings is important as well; this is especially true in developing countries (5). Resistance among non-bacterial organisms poses a public health concern as well, as reflected in the widespread occurrence of primary HIV resistance (6), MDR tuberculosis (7), and *Plasmodium falciparum* malaria (8).

These worldwide increases in prevalence of resistance are a concern because they threaten both optimal care of patients with infection and the viability of current healthcare systems (9–12). For example, antibacterial drug resistance has a clear impact on patient mortality and morbidity (13). Of additional concern is the economic impact of such infections (14, 15). In the United States, resistance is especially costly for healthcare systems and for the third-party payers that support such systems (16, 17). Costs would be sizeable as well for countries with nationally based health care programs. The incremental cost of caring for patients infected with resistant organisms has several aspects (13, 18). As the proportion of resistant organisms in a community increases, physicians must substitute from older and usually inexpensive drugs to newer, more expensive agents (19). Such costs in the United States are borne only in part by third-party payers, which often reimburse on the basis of head count, diagnosis-related

groups, or other formulas unrelated to specific services provided to an individual patient. Thus, most costs associated with resistant infections must be absorbed by the healthcare system itself (20). As prevalence of MDR organisms increases, these additional costs will become a greater and greater threat to the financial stability of local, regional, and national healthcare systems, many of which already are struggling to survive.

2 Public Health as a Perspective on Resistance (10)

Public health involves the population as a whole – it focuses on what we as a society do to ensure conditions in which we can be healthy (21, 22). This distinguishes it from the efforts of medical health care, which focus on treatment of illness in individuals (23). This "societal" perspective of public health, fueled by an aim of social good, has a broad perspective encompassing entire populations, whether of towns, cities, countries, or even the entire world (14). As the goal from this perspective is to maximize health for the whole population, a long time frame for evaluation is usually appropriate. Since antimicrobials enhance both prevention and treatment of infections in society, society considers them a valuable resource (24). As resistance diminishes this resource, a societal goal would be to minimize resistance, and therefore to reduce forces that produce resistance (25, 26).

All use of antimicrobials enhances the likelihood of resistance (12). From a societal viewpoint, then, use of antimicrobials for appropriate treatment and prevention of infection would be an appropriate rate of depletion of the value of antimicrobial effectiveness (20, 27). By contrast, overuse or misuse of antimicrobials would be an inappropriately increased depletion of these resources. From other perspectives, this consequence to society often is ignored because the short-term outcome and costs of drug use (for example, for perioperative prophylaxis) can be measured more readily and the

J.E. McGowan Jr. (✉)
Department of Epidemiology, Rollins School of Public Health,
Atlanta, GA, USA
jmcgowa@sph.emory.edu

D.L. Mayers (ed.), *Antimicrobial Drug Resistance*,
DOI 10.1007/978-1-60327-595-8_87, © Humana Press, a part of Springer Science+Business Media, LLC 2009

detrimental effect on long-term usefulness currently is not well quantified for most situations (28).

Costs of resistance from a public health perspective can be summarized as those resulting from treatment of infected patients, those resulting from treatment of patients not infected with resistant organisms, as well as those from antimicrobial use in agriculture, animal breeding, aquaculture, and industry (Table 1).

The impact of antimicrobial resistance includes that of mortality, morbidity, and extra costs in addition to that for patients infected with susceptible strains of the same organism. Thus, impact includes additional mortality, excess use of health care resources (derived from the care of resistant infections, prevention of transmission, maximization of appropriate empiric therapy, and resistance surveillance), excess loss of productivity, and excess "intangible" costs (patient and physician anxiety about treatment failure, added pain, suffering, and inconvenience). Additionally, the antimicrobial drug markets may be affected by patterns of resistance, generally compromising the marketability of older (usually cheaper and narrow-spectrum) drugs and favoring marketability of newer (usually more expensive and broad-spectrum) ones (29).

Table 1 Factors contributing to the public health impact of antimicrobial resistance

Resulting from antimicrobial use in infected patients infected with resistant organism(s)	Added[a] deaths
	Added pain/suffering/inconvenience/anxiety
	Added costs for increased hospital stay: resulting work absence and productivity
	Added costs for antimicrobial drug purchase (use of more expensive agents)
	Added costs for diagnostic and therapeutic procedures dealing with initial treatment and complications
	Added costs for infection control activities
	Loss of markets for old drugs (minus gain in markets for new drugs)
Resulting from antimicrobial use in patients not infected with resistant organism(s)	Added costs for substitution of drug in empiric treatment because resistant organism may be present (usually broader coverage, selecting for new emergence of resistance)
	Added costs for substitution of drug in empiric treatment because resistant organism may be present (usually more expensive)
	Added costs for infection surveillance
	Added anxiety about treatment failure
Resulting from nonhuman antimicrobial use (animals, aquaculture, agriculture, industry, etc.)	Emergence of resistance in human populations by transfer of resistance determinants from non-human settings

[a]Beyond that of similar infection with susceptible organism

2.1 Morbidity and Mortality

Several studies show that the mortality of infections caused by resistant organisms is higher than that of infections caused by susceptible organisms. For example, it is estimated that the mortality of bloodstream infections (BSI) caused by vancomycin-resistant enterococci (VRE) is more than double that of BSI caused by vancomycin-susceptible enterococci (VSE) after adjusting for severity of illness (30). Similarly, the mortality of bacteremia caused by methicillin-resistant *Staphylococcus aureus* (MRSA) is double that of bloodstream invasion due to methicillin-susceptible *Staphylococcus aureus* (MSSA), even after adjusting for severity of illness (31). Increased mortality has also been described for many other infectious diseases, including resistant Gram-negative bacteria (32–34), MDR tuberculosis (35, 36), and chloroquine-resistant malaria (37). Interestingly, the same has not been found for *Streptococcus pneumoniae*, for which antimicrobial resistance has not been clearly shown to increase mortality (38).

Additive mortality is assessed on a societal level by considering the consequences of premature death. The societal cost of a premature death is difficult to quantify. One component that can be approximately quantified is the one associated with loss of productivity (number of productive years lost times average yearly productivity). More difficult to measure is the impact of loss of life on others (including the extra suffering and inconvenience caused to family members and friends), but this has been estimated by the "willingness-to-pay" methodology (20). Some investigators have estimated the cost of a premature death as US\$ 1–3 million (39).

2.2 Added Healthcare Costs

Infections caused by resistant microbes are also associated with added healthcare costs. These costs correspond to all the direct and indirect costs required for patient care (healthcare worker's time, medications, devices, tests, administration, space, utilities, and patient's travel costs) (40). For infections that require hospital admission, these costs have been estimated by comparing total hospital expenditure for patients infected with a resistant organism with that for patients infected with a susceptible strain of the same organism. Some of these studies have attempted to control for confounding introduced by comorbidities, severity of illness, or other variables. The added cost derived from infections with VRE has been estimated between US\$ 27,000 and US\$ 79,589 among patients with similar underlying severity of illness (41, 42). In another study, the cost of dealing with MRSA bacteremia exceeded that for MSSA bacteremia by almost US$ 10,000 per episode, even after controlling for confounding variables (43).

Another method to estimate the added utilization of healthcare resources derived from antimicrobial resistance is by comparing the length of hospital stay (LOS) of patients infected with resistant organisms with stay of patients infected with susceptible strains of the same organisms. LOS was estimated to be significantly longer for patients infected with resistant strains of *Staphylococcus aureus*, *Klebsiella pneumoniae*, *Acinetobacter baumannii*, *Pseudomonas aeruginosa* (44), and *Enterococcus* spp. (45).

Studies of infections for which therapy is mainly administered out of the hospital also show significantly increased costs as a consequence of resistance. For example, treatment of MDR tuberculosis is estimated to be up to 100 times more costly than treatment of susceptible tuberculosis (23).

From healthcare system and societal points of view, the cost generated by resistance surveillance and infection control activities is also attributable to resistance (46). Although recommended by some authorities (47), these expenses are relevant and can be unsustainable in settings of significant resource limitation (48). For example, the surveillance and infection control activities deemed optimal for VRE control were estimated to cost US$ 253,099 during a 2-year period in a single institution in the US (49). These expenditures would be cost effective if they prevent future infections (50). However, they are attributable to resistance because they are the result of the healthcare system awareness of the consequences of infections with VRE. If VRE was not already perceived as a problem, these activities would not be performed.

Antimicrobial resistance creates an additional societal burden by the phenomenon of resistance-induced antimicrobial substitution (19). This occurs in the setting of empiric therapy, in which the physician attempts to maximize the chances of administering an appropriate antibiotic to an infected patient when the antimicrobial susceptibility of the infecting organism is unknown. When prevalence of resistance increases to an antimicrobial in frequent use for empiric therapy, that drug often is dropped in favor of another drug that is still presumed active against the resistant microbe. The second drug is often more expensive, has a broader spectrum, and is more toxic than the initial medication. Moreover,

this switch often is made not only for treating patients with infectious syndromes for which the resistant microbe is considered likely, but also for patients in whom the organism is considered less likely. The antimicrobial substitution generates excess cost because of the use of a more expensive drug, the extra side effects derived from it in individual patients, and the ecologic pressure that favors emergence of resistance to the second agent (19). Unfortunately, studies exploring the cost of resistance-induced antimicrobial substitution are scarce. As an example, it was estimated that treating 150 million patients with malaria using quinine instead of chloroquine as first-line therapy would increase expenditures by US$ 100 million (51).

3 Contrasts Between the Public Health View of Resistance and Other Views

Several different viewpoints can be taken of resistance and its impact (Table 2) (14). These perspectives have many similarities, but also differ in several ways. The view of resistance from the public health perspective described above will be contrasted, in turn, with those of physicians, patients, healthcare businesses (both providers and payers), and drug industry firms.

3.1 Physicians

Physicians and other prescribers focus most on individual patients. The outcome they seek is the absence of disease in persons who have disease at the time of their encounter with the physician (52). The time frame of most encounters is short-term resolution of single episodes, whether or not the patient and physician have a continuing care relationship. From this treatment perspective, loss of effectiveness of a single antimicrobial agent in the presence of more antimicrobials that would adequately treat indications previously served by the now-ineffective drug would be of little or no concern. However, prescribers would be affected by a decline in the

Table 2 Different perspectives on the importance of antimicrobial resistance[a]

	Public ("Society")	Medical	Patient	Healthcare business	Industry
Focus	Population	Individual	Individual	Care group	Potential clients
Outcome	Maximize health	Absence of disease	Absence of disease	Reduce cost of care	Product sales
Time frame	Long	Short	Short	Short	Short, long
Motivation	Social good	Professionalism	Personal well-being	Profit	Profit
Approach	Reduce forces leading to resistance	Treatment	Treatment	Cost containment	Develop new drugs, maintain lifecycle of old drugs

[a]Adapted in part from (14)

number of available drugs to the point that would decrease the likelihood of treatment success (53). If this occurred, they would be greatly alarmed to encounter the absence of current development of new effective agents (54). Thus, the impact of resistance on the prescriber depends greatly on whether other drugs are available for patient treatment (14).

3.2 Patients

The major motivation for patients to participate in the treatment process is their own well-being. The main impact for them is that of morbidity and mortality due to a resistant organism (53). In addition, however, there is a direct economic impact when charges for drugs and services increase as a by-product of the need to treat resistant infections (especially when patients pay retail prices for their health care).

3.3 Healthcare Businesses

For the administrators who control healthcare system financial resources (whether they are systems that provide health services or fiscal agencies that pay for such services for insured or governmental groups), the major impact of resistance is measured in terms of economic consequences. These managers also desire reduction of morbidity and mortality, but look to accomplish this goal with fiscal efficiency (i.e., by least expenditure of increasingly scarce financial resources). Antimicrobials usually provide cost-effective care of patients with infection who are part of their defined client base (20). Occurrence of resistance is of interest to the health business professional only to the degree that it affects or has the potential to affect the enrolled population of the organization. Measures that must be taken to deal with resistance may bring with them incremental costs of drugs as well as diagnostic and therapeutic services. In addition, the institution must fund costs for personnel time, supplies, space, and equipment for institutional programs to deal with resistance (pharmacy and therapeutics committees, antimicrobial use review, practice guidelines, etc.).

3.4 Industry

The focus for pharmaceutical firms, diagnostic instrument manufacturers, and other industry groups providing products for treatment and prevention of infectious diseases (antimicrobial agents, products to stimulate host defenses, vaccines, etc.) is similar in some ways to that of the healthcare business.

In this case, however, the clients of interest are the potential users of their products, both directly (patients) and indirectly (health care systems, governments, etc.). Product sales are the desired outcome, and a short-term view of sales is part of their outlook. However, industry also must take a longer view of the subject and consider the impact of resistance as a potential opportunity for introduction and sales of new products. This leads to a two-sided view of the problem. On one hand, the firms wish to maintain the life of their current antimicrobial products, a goal that is threatened by development of new patterns of antimicrobial resistance pertinent to the product. On the other hand, resistance may make obsolete the product of a competitor, opening up the field for a company's product that may have been less marketable because it cost more or met therapeutic needs less well. In addition, resistance to their own drugs or those of competitors may produce a niche for a new antimicrobial where one was not present before. Thus, the consequences of resistance to these firms depend on the particular situation.

3.5 Summary: A Dramatic Difference in Viewpoints

It is clear, then, that there is a disconnect between the view of antimicrobial use from the perspective of society and that of the other groups considered above (55, 56).

4 Influences on Resistance and Control Strategies

The forces that influence the rates of antimicrobial resistance are several (Fig. 1). The ecologic pressure derived from the use of antimicrobial agents is the main driving force for the emergence of resistance, whereas spread is further facilitated by transmission of resistant organisms, both at the community and hospital levels (57, 58). Thus, attempts to control resistance have embraced many different strategies. Such strategies must focus on efforts at several different levels of responsibility, from provider to international agencies (10). These efforts are similar regardless of the type of infectious disease being controlled (Table 3). However, some of the specific actions required for the control of certain resistant organism may differ from those required to control others. For instance, certain control strategies may apply to the prevention and control of resistant tuberculosis, whereas others may apply for the control of resistance in HIV infection. The next paragraphs expand the contents presented in Table 3 and point out some examples of differing approaches according to the type of infectious disease.

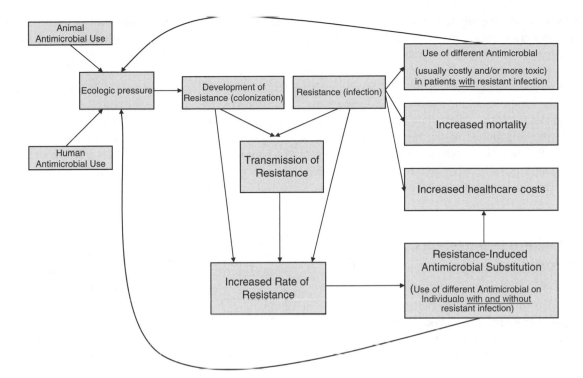

Fig. 1 Forces influencing antimicrobial resistance and its consequences (10)

Table 3 Possible control strategies for controlling resistance, by levels of responsibility within the public health and healthcare systems

Strategy	Provider level	Local health department/hospital level	Regional health department level	National level	International level
Patient education	Conduct	Provide materials	Provide materials	Provide materials	Provide materials
Prescriber education	Educate self	Provide materials	Provide materials	Provide materials	Provide materials
Resistance and antimicrobial use surveillance	Report cases	Resistance and antibiotic use summaries[a]	Resistance and antibiotic use summaries[a]	Resistance and antibiotic use summaries[a]	Resistance and antibiotic use summaries[a]
Treatment	Implement	Community programs	Provide guidelines and resources; ensure drug supply/quality	Provide guidelines and resources; ensure drug supply/quality	Provide guidelines and resources; promote drug supply/quality
Preventing spread	Implement isolation, quarantine, vaccination	Contact tracing, vaccination campaigns	Provide guidelines and resources, vaccination campaigns	Provide guidelines and resources, vaccination campaigns	Provide guidelines and resources
Research	Study individual patients or a group of patients (case reports and case series)	Study effective provision of services	Study effective provision of services	Support local and regional studies; study drug, diagnostic test, and vaccine development	Support national studies; study drug, diagnostic test, and vaccine development

[a]Aggregate and disseminate

4.1 Providers

Regardless of which resistant organisms are of interest, healthcare providers should educate their patients about mechanisms of transmission, behaviors to avoid spread to others, and the importance of compliance with medications to avoid the emergence of resistance (59, 60). If available, educational tools and materials should be used. In order to educate patients, the providers need to be educated and updated themselves. They should be able to judge accurately when a certain antimicrobial is needed and when it is unnecessary, and additionally they should be able to transmit this certainty to an anxious patient. If susceptibility testing is available at the provider level, providers should note cases of public health interest and report these cases to local public health officials. Providers should take the initiative for patient's isolation and quarantine if this is needed according to the type of infection and to the social conditions of the patient. For example, isolation is recommended for a patient with cavitary pulmonary tuberculosis who is admitted to the hospital but not for a patient with HIV infection seen in the outpatient clinic. Providers should always be advocates for the patient's best interests in local, regional, and national policy making (61).

4.2 Local Health Departments and Hospitals

Local health departments and hospitals should participate in education, generating useful tools and disseminating them to providers and patients as well as using them in their own work. They should make available to providers some type of testing for susceptibility in order to facilitate surveillance (60, 62). In the case of tuberculosis, surveillance is performed to facilitate mycobacterial cultures and provide susceptibility testing for some or all culture-positive specimens (63, 64). In the case of HIV infection, genotypic or phenotypic resistance testing is used as part of surveillance in at least some settings (65). The extent of surveillance (number of cases subjected to surveillance of resistance) should be defined by local health departments in consultation with regional and national health departments. In settings with ample resources, surveillance should be done ideally at a patient level, whereas in settings with significant resource limitation, surveillance should be performed at a population level, according to existing priorities (66).

Resistance summaries should be reported to the providers, the community, and the regional health officials on a periodic basis. Local health departments need to promote treatment and prevention in accordance with regional and national guidelines. For tuberculosis, direct observed therapy programs and contact tracing are highly favored (64). For HIV, individual case management as well as community programs should be promoted with the participation of family or social networks to optimize adherence (67–69). Local health departments should also optimize the consistent supply of good-quality medications.

4.3 Regional, National, and International Health Organizations

All of these groups have similar responsibilities in the effort to control resistance (59–61). They should aggregate, sum-

marize, and disseminate surveillance reports (62, 70). Regional and national budgets need to support surveillance, treatment, and prevention activities, as well as guideline development and research initiatives. Similarly, efforts required for the containment of resistance at all levels should be supported by advocacy for political will and initiative as well as appropriate legislation (71, 72).

International agencies should promote the development of comprehensive guidelines. For example, guidelines for management of tuberculosis should ideally assist in the detection and management of individual cases, the prevention of spread, the tracing of contacts, and the regulation of medication manufacturing and distributing practices. National organizations should then translate these guidelines into forms that are appropriate for their level of available resources (see next section). All levels of organizations should incorporate intersector responses to fight poverty and promote a health system that maximizes access to care (59–61). In addition, they should regulate antimicrobial manufacturing and distribution as well as its use in agriculture, aquaculture, and other industries. International agencies should assist national organizations in these endeavors and promote international advocacy and research partnerships.

5 Public Health Perspectives of Antimicrobial Resistance According to Resource Limitation Levels (10)

Since antimicrobial resistance is both a cause and a consequence of resource utilization, forces that drive the emergence and spread of resistance are clearly different according to the different levels of resource limitation. Similarly, the public health consequences and the appropriate public health policy responses are different for each scenario. Table 4 shows a somewhat simplistic categorization of the emergence and spread of resistance, its public health consequences, and the possible responses according to resource limitation levels.

5.1 Settings with Extensive Resources

For comparison purposes, let us suppose that in Utopia there is minimal resource limitation, antimicrobials are always used appropriately, and infection control practices are timely and adequately implemented. In this scenario, some resistance will emerge unavoidably because of the use of antimicrobials, but its spread will be limited as a consequence of good infection control strategies. The excess resistance and

Table 4 Public health perspectives of antimicrobial resistance according to resource limitation levels (10)

Resource limitation level	Extreme resource limitation	Significant to moderate resource limitation	Minimal to moderate resource limitation	Minimal resource limitation
Resource use	Minimal to none	Some (inconsistent and/or insufficient)	Inappropriate (excessive use and poor compliance)	"Perfect" use
Antimicrobial use and consequence	No antimicrobial use – minimal antimicrobial resistance (naturally occurring)	Inconsistent antimicrobial use (interrupted supply), suboptimal dosing, use of counterfeit drugs, nonprescription antimicrobial use – excessive emergence of resistance	Excessive use of antimicrobials (including those not use in humans), use of broad-spectrum rather than narrow-spectrum agents – excessive emergence of resistance	Appropriate (indication and dosing) and consistent (uninterrupted supply) use of good-quality antimicrobials – unavoidable emergence of resistance
Infection control resources use and consequences	No infection control activities but minimal transmission of resistance	Inconsistent and incomplete infection control practices in hospitals and community – excessive transmission of resistance	Inappropriate use of infection control strategies (noncompliance, non-timely use) – excessive transmission of resistance	Appropriate use of isolation practices and other infection control strategies (including vaccines) – minimization of resistance transmission
Public health consequences	Excess mortality due to treatable infections – excessive public health cost	Excess mortality, excess healthcare costs and morbidity due to infection caused by resistant organisms – excessive public health cost	Excess mortality, excess healthcare costs and morbidity due to infection caused by resistant organisms – excessive public health cost	Unavoidable but justifiable emergence of resistance and public health costs
Possible responses	Scale up antimicrobial agents, surveillance, vaccination and infection control strategies (resource availability)	Optimize appropriate and consistent use of good quality antimicrobials Surveillance Prioritize vaccination and infection control practices to decrease transmission	Optimize appropriate antimicrobial use (antibiotic stewardship) Surveillance Optimize infection control practices and vaccination Drug, vaccine and diagnostics development	Drug development Vaccine development Diagnostics development Surveillance
Setting	Extremely poor countries or areas	Mainly developing countries	Mainly developed countries	Nonexisting (Utopia)

costs derived from antimicrobial use are justified since deaths from infection are being prevented by the rational use of antimicrobials. In this scenario, the benefit derived from antibiotic use outweighs the risks of emerging resistance. Resources can also be allocated to optimize active surveillance, and to the development of diagnostic tests, new antimicrobials, and vaccines. Of course, Utopia does not exist.

5.2 Settings with Minimal Resources

In settings in which resource limitation is extreme, antimicrobials are not available, and minimal resistance emerges as a natural phenomenon (73). Since the frequency of resistance is minimal, the frequency of transmission is also minimal. This setting may apply to areas of the world in which native populations are still marginalized and disconnected from civilization (74). In this case, excessive deaths are caused by infections that are treatable with antimicro-

bial agents, and therefore the public health cost for the group is very high. The appropriate response for this scenario is to scale up antimicrobial use while incorporating surveillance, vaccination, and infection control activities at the same time.

5.3 Settings with Significant Resource Limitation

This scenario may predominate in many of the developing countries and some rural and community centers of the developed world. In these settings, antimicrobials are available in some extent, but its use is often inadequate because of interrupted supply, inappropriate dosing, use of counterfeit drugs, and scarcity of regulations regarding antimicrobial purchase (25, 59–61, 75). As a consequence, the emergence of resistance is excessive. Additionally, because of limitations in resources allocated to infection control both at the community and the hospital levels, transmission of resistance is relevant (60). In this scenario, the excess infections caused by antimicrobial-resistant organisms create excessive deaths and healthcare costs. Appropriate public health responses for this scenario include optimization of use and supply of good-quality antimicrobials, active antimicrobial resistance surveillance, and prioritization of vaccination and locally cost-effective infection control practices.

5.4 Settings with Minimal to Moderate Resources

This situation predominates in the developed world and in high-complexity centers in the developing world. In settings such as these, antimicrobials are readily available. However, antimicrobial use is often excessive and the antimicrobials used are frequently expensive and broad spectrum (76, 77). Additionally, antimicrobials are commonly used in animals, agriculture, aquaculture, and industry (78). The ecologic pressure created by the excessive antimicrobial use causes an excessive emergence of resistance. In these settings, significant resources are devoted to infection control practices (14), but these practices are often not followed or are implemented inappropriately. The net effect is again excessive transmission of resistance. The excess infections caused by antimicrobial-resistant organisms create excessive deaths and healthcare costs. Appropriate public health responses for this scenario include optimization of antimicrobial use (antimicrobial stewardship (27)), active antimicrobial resistance and antimicrobial use surveillance, and optimization of vaccination and infection control practices. In this situation, some resources can be invested in drug, diagnostics, and vaccine development.

6 Conclusion: Antimicrobial Resistance in the Era of Globalization: An International Concern for Public Health

Human migration, animal and vector movement, and food markets may facilitate the spread of antimicrobial resistance across almost any geographic or political boundary (23). For example, the strain 23F-1 of *Streptococcus pneumoniae* originally described in Spain rapidly spread to other areas in Europe and Africa, and then to many areas in the Americas and East Asia (5, 23). Resistant *Salmonella* spp. isolates were introduced to Denmark through the importation of boar's meat from Canada (23). Chloroquine resistance in *Plasmodium falciparum* was established in Southeast Asia in the late 1970s, and spread to almost the rest of the world by

the mid-1990s (23). Cases of MDR tuberculosis and extensively drug-resistant (XDR) tuberculosis are geographically widespread (63). This phenomenon creates additional challenges for the global containment of resistance. It demands concerted efforts from multiple health and industry sectors in both developed and developing countries, as well as the strengthening of multinational/international partnerships and regulations. Public health must be in the forefront of these efforts.

References

1. McDonald, L. C. (2006). Trends in antimicrobial resistance in health care-associated pathogens and effect on treatment. *Clin Infect Dis* 42 Suppl 2, S65–S71
2. Paterson, D. L. (2006). The epidemiological profile of infections with multidrug-resistant *Pseudomonas aeruginosa* and *Acinetobacter* species. *Clin Infect Dis* 43 Suppl 2, S43–S48
3. Sun, H. Y., Chen, S. Y., Chang, S. C., Pan, S. C., Su, C. P. & Chen, Y. C. (2006). Community-onset *Escherichia coli* and *Klebsiella pneumoniae* bacteremia: influence of health care exposure on antimicrobial susceptibility. *Diagn Microbiol Infect Dis* 55, 135–141
4. Rozenbaum, R., Silva-Carvalho, M. C., Souza, R. R., Melo, M. C., Gobbi, C. N., Coelho, L. R., Ferreira, R. L., Ferreira-Carvalho, B. T., Schuenck, A. L., Neves, F. M., Silva, L. R. & Figueiredo, A. M. (2006). Molecular characterization of methicillin-resistant *Staphylococcus aureus* disseminated in a home care system. *Infect Control Hosp Epidemiol* 27, 1041–1050
5. Okeke, I. N., Laxminarayan, R., Bhutta, Z. A., Duse, A. G., Jenkins, P., O'Brien, T. F., Pablos-Mendez, A. & Klugman, K. P. (2005). Antimicrobial resistance in developing countries. Part I: recent trends and current status. *Lancet Infect Dis* 5, 481–493
6. Wensing, A. M., van de Vijver, D. A., Angarano, G., Asjo, B., Balotta, C., Boeri, E., Camacho, R., Chaix, M. L., Costagliola, D., De Luca, A., Derdelinckx, I., Grossman, Z., Hamouda, O., Hatzakis, A., Hemmer, R., Hoepelman, A., Horban, A., Korn, K., Kucherer, C., Leitner, T., Loveday, C., MacRae, E., Maljkovic, I., de Mendoza, C., Meyer, L., Nielsen, C., Op de Coul, E. L., Ormaasen, V., Paraskevis, D., Perrin, L., Puchhammer-Stockl, E., Ruiz, L., Salminen, M., Schmit, J. C., Schneider, F., Schuurman, R., Soriano, V., Stanczak, G., Stanojevic, M., Vandamme, A. M., Van Laethem, K., Violin, M., Wilbe, K., Yerly, S., Zazzi, M. & Boucher, C. A. (2005). Prevalence of drug-resistant HIV-1 variants in untreated individuals in Europe: implications for clinical management. *J Infect Dis* 192, 958–966
7. Dye, C., Scheele, S., Dolin, P., Pathania, V. & Raviglione, M. C. (1999). Consensus statement. Global burden of tuberculosis: estimated incidence, prevalence, and mortality by country. WHO Global Surveillance and Monitoring Project. *JAMA* 282, 677–686
8. Olliaro, P. (2005). Drug resistance hampers our capacity to roll back malaria. *Clin Infect Dis* 41 Suppl 4, S247–S257
9. McGowan, J. E., Jr. (2004). Minimizing antimicrobial resistance: the key role of the infectious diseases physician. *Clin Infect Dis* 38, 939–942
10. Diaz Granados CA, Cardo DM, McGowan JE. Jr. Antimicrobial resistance: international control strategies, with a focus on limited-resource settings. Internal J Antimicrob Agents 2008;33:1–9
11. Centers for Disease Control and Prevention. (2006). *Management of Multidrug Resistant Organisms in Healthcare Settings, 2006.* Atlanta, GA: Centers for Disease Control and Prevention, Healthcare

Infection Control Practices Advisory Committee (HICPAC); 73 pp, accessed at http://www.cdc.gov/ncidod/dhqp/pdf/ar/mdroGuideline2006.pdf on December 21

12. Dellit, T. H., Owens, R. C., McGowan, J. E., Jr., Gerding, D. N., Weinstein, R. A., Burke, J. P., Huskins, W. C., Paterson, D. L., Fishman, N. O., Carpenter, C. F., Brennan, P. J., Billeter, M. & Hooton, T. M. (2007). Infectious Diseases Society of America and the Society for Healthcare Epidemiology of America guidelines for developing an institutional program to enhance antimicrobial stewardship. *Clin Infect Dis* 44, 159–177

13. Cosgrove, S. E. (2006). The relationship between antimicrobial resistance and patient outcomes: mortality, length of hospital stay, and health care costs. *Clin Infect Dis* 42 Suppl 2, S82–S89

14. McGowan, J. E., Jr. (2001). Economic impact of antimicrobial resistance. *Emerg Infect Dis* 7, 286–292

15. Howard, D., Cordell, R., McGowan, J. E., Jr., Packard, R. M., Scott, R. D., II & Solomon, S. L. (2001). Measuring the economic costs of antimicrobial resistance in hospital settings: summary of the Centers for Disease Control and Prevention-Emory Workshop. *Clin Infect Dis* 33, 1573–1578

16. Howard, D. H., Scott, R. D., II, Packard, R. & Jones, D. (2003). The global impact of drug resistance. *Clin Infect Dis* 36, S4–S10

17. Wang, Y. C. & Lipsitch, M. (2006). Upgrading antibiotic use within a class: tradeoff between resistance and treatment success. *Proc Natl Acad Sci U S A* 103, 9655–9660

18. Engemann, J. J., Carmeli, Y., Cosgrove, S. E., Fowler, V. G., Bronstein, M. Z., Trivette, S. L., Briggs, J. P., Sexton, D. J. & Kaye, K. S. (2003). Adverse clinical and economic outcomes attributable to methicillin resistance among patients with *Staphylococcus aureus* surgical site infection. *Clin Infect Dis* 36, 592–598

19. Howard, D. H. (2004). Resistance-induced antibiotic substitution. *Health Econ* 13, 585–595

20. Laxminarayan, R., Malani, A. (2007). *Extending the Cure: Policy Responses to the Growing Threat of Antibiotic Resistance*, Resources for the Future, Washington DC 2007

21. Institute of Medicine. (1988). *The Future of Public Health*, National Academy Press, Washington, DC

22. Gerberding, J. L. (2005). Protecting health – the new research imperative. *JAMA* 294, 1403–1406

23. Heymann, D. L. (2006). Resistance to anti-infective drugs and the threat to public health. *Cell* 124, 671–675

24. Levy, S. B. & Marshall, B. (2004). Antibacterial resistance worldwide: causes, challenges and responses. *Nat Med* 10, S122–S129

25. Sarkar, P. & Gould, I. M. (2006). Antimicrobial agents are societal drugs: how should this influence prescribing? *Drugs* 66, 893–901

26. Dowell, S. F. (2004). Antimicrobial resistance: is it really that bad? *Semin Pediatr Infect Dis* 15, 99–104

27. Fishman, N. (2006). Antimicrobial stewardship. *Am J Infect Control* 34, S55–S63; discussion S64–S73

28. Scott, R. D., II, Solomon, S. L. & McGowan, J. E., Jr. (2001). Applying economic principles to health care. *Emerg Infect Dis* 7, 282–285

29. Shlaes, D. M., Projan, S. J. & Edwards, J. E., Jr. (2004). Antibiotic discovery: state of the state. *ASM News* 70, 275–281

30. DiazGranados, C. A., Zimmer, S. M., Klein, M. & Jernigan, J. A. (2005). Comparison of mortality associated with vancomycin-resistant and vancomycin-susceptible enterococcal bloodstream infections: a meta-analysis. *Clin Infect Dis* 41, 327–333

31. Cosgrove, S. E. & Carmeli, Y. (2003). The impact of antimicrobial resistance on health and economic outcomes. *Clin Infect Dis* 36, 1433–1437

32. Cosgrove, S. E., Kaye, K. S., Eliopoulous, G. M. & Carmeli, Y. (2002). Health and economic outcomes of the emergence of third-generation cephalosporin resistance in *Enterobacter* species. *Arch Intern Med* 162, 185–190

33. Tumbarello, M., Spanu, T., Sanguinetti, M., Citton, R., Montuori, E., Leone, F., Fadda, G. & Cauda, R. (2006). Bloodstream infections caused by extended-spectrum-beta-lactamase-producing *Klebsiella pneumoniae*: risk factors, molecular epidemiology, and clinical outcome. *Antimicrob Agents Chemother* 50, 498–504

34. Ramphal, R. & Ambrose, P. G. (2006). Extended-spectrum beta-lactamases and clinical outcomes: current data. *Clin Infect Dis* 42 Suppl 4, S164–S172

35. Frieden, T. R., Munsiff, S. S. & Ahuja, S. D. (2007). Outcomes of multidrug-resistant tuberculosis treatment in HIV-positive patients in New York City, 1990–1997. *Int J Tuberc Lung Dis* 11, 116

36. Gandhi, N. R., Moll, A., Sturm, A. W., Pawinski, R., Govender, T., Lalloo, U., Zeller, K., Andrews, J. & Friedland, G. (2006). Extensively drug-resistant tuberculosis as a cause of death in patients co-infected with tuberculosis and HIV in a rural area of South Africa. *Lancet* 368, 1575–1580

37. Trape, J. F., Pison, G., Preziosi, M. P., Enel, C., Desgrees du Lou, A., Delaunay, V., Samb, B., Lagarde, E., Molez, J. F. & Simondon, F. (1998). Impact of chloroquine resistance on malaria mortality. *C R Acad Sci III* 321, 689–697

38. Moroney, J. F., Fiore, A. E., Harrison, L. H., Patterson, J. E., Farley, M. M., Jorgensen, J. H., Phelan, M., Facklam, R. R., Cetron, M. S., Breiman, R. F., Kolczak, M. & Schuchat, A. (2001). Clinical outcomes of bacteremic pneumococcal pneumonia in the era of antibiotic resistance. *Clin Infect Dis* 33, 797–805

39. Phelps, C. E. (1989). Bug/drug resistance: sometimes less is more. *Med Care* 27, 194–203

40. Meltzer, M. I. (2001). Introduction to health economics for physicians. *Lancet* 358, 993–998

41. Stosor, V., Peterson, L. R., Postelnick, M. & Noskin, G. A. (1998). *Enterococcus faecium* bacteremia – does vancomycin resistance make a difference? *Arch Intern Med* 158, 522–527

42. Song, X., Srinivasan, A., Plaut, D. & Perl, T. M. (2003). Effect of nosocomial vancomycin-resistant enterococcal bacteremia on mortality, length of stay, and costs. *Infect Control Hosp Epidemiol* 24, 251–256

43. Lodise, T. P. & McKinnon, P. S. (2005). Clinical and economic impact of methicillin resistance in patients with *Staphylococcus aureus* bacteremia. *Diagn Microbiol Infect Dis* 52, 113–122

44. Brooklyn Antibiotic Resistance Task Force. (2002). The cost of antibiotic resistance: effect of resistance among *Staphylococcus aureus*, *Klebsiella pneumoniae*, *Acinetobacter baumannii*, and *Pseudmonas aeruginosa* on length of hospital stay. *Infect Control Hosp Epidemiol* 23, 106–108

45. Salgado, C. D. & Farr, B. M. (2003). Outcomes associated with vancomycin-resistant enterococci: a meta-analysis. *Infect Control Hosp Epidemiol* 24, 690–698

46. Howard, D. H. & Scott, R. D., II. (2005). The economic burden of drug resistance. *Clin Infect Dis* 41 Suppl 4, S283–S286

47. Muto, C. A., Jernigan, J. A., Ostrowsky, B. E., Richet, H. M., Jarvis, W. R., Boyce, J. M. & Farr, B. M. (2003). SHEA guideline for preventing nosocomial transmission of multidrug-resistant strains of *Staphylococcus aureus* and enterococcus. *Infect Control Hosp Epidemiol* 24, 362–386

48. Edmond, M. (2003). Cost-effectiveness of perirectal surveillance cultures for controlling vancomycin-resistant Enterococcus. *Infect Control Hosp Epidemiol* 24, 309–310; author reply 310–312

49. Muto, C. A., Giannetta, E. T., Durbin, L. J., Simonton, B. M. & Farr, B. M. (2002). Cost-effectiveness of perirectal surveillance cultures for controlling vancomycin-resistant Enterococcus. *Infect Control Hosp Epidemiol* 23, 429–435

50. Perencevich, E. N., Fisman, D. N., Lipsitch, M., Harris, A. D., Morris, J. G., Jr. & Smith, D. L. (2004). Projected benefits of active surveillance for vancomycin-resistant enterococci in intensive care units. *Clin Infect Dis* 38, 1108–1115

51. Phillips, M. & Phillips-Howard, P. A. (1996). Economic implications of resistance to antimalarial drugs. *Pharmacoeconomics* 10, 225–238

52. Price, D. (2006). Impact of antibiotic restrictions: the physician's perspective. *Clin Microbiol Infect* 12 Suppl 5, 3–9

53. Scott, R. D. II, Solomon, S. L., Cordell, R., Roberts, R. R., Howard, D. & McGowan, J. E. Jr. (2005). Measuring the attributable costs of resistant infections in hospital settings. In: *Antibiotic Optimization: Concepts and Strategies in Clinical Practice* (Owens, R. C. Jr., Ambrose, P. G. & Nightingale, C. H., eds.), pp. 141–179. Marcel Dekker, Inc., New York

54. Talbot, G. H., Bradley, J., Edwards, J. E., Jr., Gilbert, D., Scheld, M. & Bartlett, J. G. (2006). Bad bugs need drugs: an update on the development pipeline from the Antimicrobial Availability Task Force of the Infectious Diseases Society of America. *Clin Infect Dis* 42, 657–668

55. Aiello, A. E., King, N. B. & Foxman, B. (2006). Ethical conflicts in public health research and practice: antimicrobial resistance and the ethics of drug development. *Am J Public Health* 96, 1910–1914

56. Garau, J. (2006). Impact of antibiotic restrictions: the ethical perspective. *Clin Microbiol Infect* 12 Suppl 5, 16–24

57. Struelens, M. J. (2003). Multidisciplinary antimicrobial management teams: the way forward to control antimicrobial resistance in hospitals. *Curr Opin Infect Dis* 16, 305–307

58. Stein, G. E. (2005). Antimicrobial resistance in the hospital setting: impact, trends, and infection control measures. *Pharmacotherapy* 25, 44S–54S

59. Simonsen, G. S., Tapsall, J. W., Allegranzi, B., Talbot, E. A. & Lazzari, S. (2004). The antimicrobial resistance containment and surveillance approach – a public health tool. *Bull World Health Organ* 82, 928–934

60. Okeke, I. N., Klugman, K. P., Bhutta, Z. A., Duse, A. G., Jenkins, P., O'Brien, T. F., Pablos-Mendez, A. & Laxminarayan, R. (2005). Antimicrobial resistance in developing countries. Part II: strategies for containment. *Lancet Infect Dis* 5, 568–580

61. WHO. (2006). Global tuberculosis control. WHO report 2006 (WHO/HTM/TB/2006.361). World Health Organization (WHO)

62. Alliance for Prudent Use of Antibiotics. (2005). Executive summary: global antimicrobial resistance alerts and implications. *Clin Infect Dis* 41 Suppl 4, S221–S223

63. Centers for Disease Control and Prevention. (2006). Emergence of *Mycobacterium tuberculosis* with extensive resistance to second-line drugs – worldwide, 2000–2004. *MMWR Morb Mortal Wkly Rep* 55, 301–305

64. WHO. (2003). Anti-tuberculosis drug resistance in the world. Third global report. Geneva, World Health Organization, 2003 (WHO/HTM/TB/2004.343) WHO/IUATLD Global Project on Anti-tuberculosis Drug Resistance Surveillance

65. World Health Organization. (2006). Antiretroviral therapy for HIV infection in adults and adolescents: Recommendations for a public health approach. Available at http://www.who.int/hiv/pub/guidelines/artadultguidelines.pdf, accessed 14 Feb 2007, vol. 2007

66. Bogaards, J. A. & Goudsmit, J. (2003). Meeting the immense need for HAART in resource-poor settings. *J Antimicrob Chemother* 52, 743–746

67. Kushel, M. B., Colfax, G., Ragland, K., Heineman, A., Palacio, H. & Bangsberg, D. R. (2006). Case management is associated with improved antiretroviral adherence and CD4+ cell counts in homeless and marginally housed individuals with HIV infection. *Clin Infect Dis* 43, 234–242

68. Jones, D. L., Ishii, M., LaPerriere, A., Stanley, H., Antoni, M., Ironson, G., Schneiderman, N., Van Splunteren, F., Cassells, A., Alexander, K., Gousse, Y. P., Vaughn, A., Brondolo, E., Tobin, J. N. & Weiss, S. M. (2003). Influencing medication adherence among women with AIDS. *AIDS Care* 15, 463–474

69. Smith, S. R., Rublein, J. C., Marcus, C., Brock, T. P. & Chesney, M. A. (2003). A medication self-management program to improve adherence to HIV therapy regimens. *Patient Educ Couns* 50, 187–199

70. Levy, S. B. & O'Brien, T. F. (2005). Global antimicrobial resistance alerts and implications. *Clin Infect Dis* 41 Suppl 4, S219–S220

71. Oliver, T. R. (2006). The politics of public health policy. *Annu Rev Public Health* 27, 195–233

72. Metlay, J. P., Powers, J. H., Dudley, M. N., Christiansen, K. & Finch, R. G. (2006). Antimicrobial drug resistance, regulation, and research. *Emerg Infect Dis* 12, 183–190

73. Sato, K., Bartlett, P. C. & Saeed, M. A. (2005). Antimicrobial susceptibility of *Escherichia coli* isolates from dairy farms using organic versus conventional production methods. *J Am Vet Med Assoc* 226, 589–594

74. Blomberg, B., Olsen, B. E., Hinderaker, S. G., Langeland, N., Gasheka, P., Jureen, R., Kvale, G. & Midtvedt, T. (2005). Antimicrobial resistance in urinary bacterial isolates from pregnant women in rural Tanzania: implications for public health. *Scand J Infect Dis* 37, 262–268

75. Mamun, K. Z., Tabassum, S., Shears, P. & Hart, C. A. (2006). A survey of antimicrobial prescribing and dispensing practices in rural Bangladesh. *Mymensingh Med J* 15, 81–84

76. Pelletier, L. L., Jr. (1985). Hospital usage of parenteral antimicrobial agents: a gradated utilization review and cost containment program. *Infect Control* 6, 226–230

77. Fraser, G. L., Stogsdill, P., Dickens, J. D., Jr., Wennberg, D. E., Smith, R. P., Jr. & Prato, B. S. (1997). Antibiotic optimization. An evaluation of patient safety and economic outcomes. *Arch Intern Med* 157, 1689–1694

78. Molbak, K. (2004). Spread of resistant bacteria and resistance genes from animals to humans – the public health consequences. *J Vet Med B Infect Dis Vet Public Health* 51, 364–369

Chapter 88
Hospital Infection Control: Considerations for the Management and Control of Drug-Resistant Organisms

Gonzalo M.L. Bearman and Richard P. Wenzel

1 Introduction

The prevalence of nosocomially acquired, antibiotic-resistant organisms has increased significantly over the last 20 years. Data from the National Nosocomial Infections Surveillance (NNIS) system report published in 2000 revealed an alarming proportion of drug-resistant pathogens (1). The NNIS system data comprise a nonrandom sample of 290 hospitals from 42 states. Monthly reports of nosocomial infections and microbiology data from participating institutions are analyzed. From the sample, in 2000, 52% of all *Staphylococcus aureus* isolates were resistant to methicillin, 25% of enterococci were vancomycin resistant, and 88% of coagulase negative staphylococci were methicillin resistant (1). An increase in drug-resistant staphylococci and enterococci has also been reported in Europe and South America (2–4).

As nosocomial infections with drug-resistant pathogens become increasingly more common and endemic, healthcare systems have taken various infection control measures to limit both their frequency and spread. Three parameters define the prevalence of drug resistant bacteremia: how much enters the institution from outside, how much is selected by antibiotic use and misuse, and how much spreads from person to person (5). The early recognition and isolation of incoming patients harboring resistant pathogens, appropriate antibiotic control programs, and assiduous infection control minimize cross-infection. Within the infection control domain, there may be specific efforts to minimize patient, healthcare worker, and environmental reservoirs, as well as efforts to create meticulous hand hygiene and glove and gown use. In addition, surveillance systems for infection with nosocomial pathogens are essential for establishing endemic rates and for defining outbreaks. Aggressive surveillance for asymptomatic reservoirs may be of value but is not without controversy. Other considerations for an infection control program include hospital design considerations and antibiotic control programs.

2 The Importance of Patient and Healthcare Worker Colonization with Drug-Resistant Pathogens: Reservoirs for Infection

Colonization serves as a significant reservoir of drug-resistant, nosocomial pathogens. Patient colonization by drug-resistant pathogens such as vancomycin-resistant enterococci (VRE) and methicillin-resistant *Staphylococcus aureus* (MRSA) has been well described. Thirty to 50% of healthy adults have nasal colonization with *S. aureus* (6, 7) with 10–20% persistently colonized (both methicillin-susceptible *Staphylococcus aureus* (MSSA) and MRSA isolates can be persistent colonizers). Colonization with MRSA has been well documented in various healthcare settings. It has been reported that 25% of patients admitted to a hospital will become nasally colonized with *S. aureus* (8). This figure varies widely on the basis of different populations and risk factors, and rates as high as 40–60% have been reported in select populations including diabetic patients and HIV-positive patients. Certain populations are predisposed to colonization with *S. aureus* at the time of admission. Dupeyron et al. prospectively analyzed *S. aureus* colonization in a cohort of 551 cirrhotic patients. Screening nasal and rectal swabs were performed within 48 h of admission to the hospital. The investigators reported carriage rates of 19% for MSSA and 16% for MRSA. When comparing nasal carriers vs. non-carriers, the investigators documented a greater frequency of prior MRSA bacteremia and urinary tract infections, respectively, 8.3% vs. 0.8% and 11.4% vs. 0.6%. Additionally, the colonizing MRSA strain matched the invasive strain by pulse field gel electrophoresis (9).

In a different prospective series, however, only 2.7% of the isolates identified as MRSA (10). Using a case–control study and multivariate analysis to determine risk factors for MRSA colonization, independent predictors for colonization with MRSA were prior admission to a nursing home (odds ratio (OR) 16.5) and a prior hospitalization of greater than 5 days' duration within the past year (10).

Surveillance in nursing home settings reveals an increasing prevalence of *S. aureus* colonization. A prospective study in the

G.M.L. Bearman (✉)
Virginia Commonwealth University Medical Center, Richmond, VA, USA
gbearman@mcvh-vcu.edu

D.L. Mayers (ed.), *Antimicrobial Drug Resistance*,
DOI 10.1007/978-1-60327-595-8_88, © Humana Press, a part of Springer Science+Business Media, LLC 2009

Table 1 Summary of selected infection control measures for the management and control of drug-resistant organisms

Infection control measure	Rationale	Comment
Nasal decontamination with mupirocin	Twenty-five percent of patients admitted to a hospital will become nasally colonized with *S. aureus*	In one prospective study, the use of intranasal mupirocin in a surgical cohort was effective in reducing the frequency of *S. aureus* nosocomial infections only in patients previously colonized with *S. aureus*
	Compared with MSSA colonization, both MRSA colonization and MRSA acquisition during hospitalization increased the relative risk of infection	Mupirocin decreased the rate of *S. aureus* infections in hemodialysis patients
Environmental decontamination	The inanimate environment can be contaminated with MRSA, *C. difficile*, VRE and drug-resistant Gram-negative rods. This is a potential reservoir for cross-transmission of nosocomial pathogens via the hands of healthcare workers	All healthcare facilities should develop policies for the terminal and periodic disinfection of patient care areas and environmental services
		This policy should include input from infection control practitioners, industrial hygienists, and environmental services supervisors
Hand hygiene	Hand hygiene is the single most effective method to limit the spread of drug-resistant pathogens and nosocomial infections	Increased accessibility to hand hygiene agents is associated with improved compliance
	Multiple opportunities exist in the hospital environment for the contamination of healthcare workers' hands including direct patient care and contact with environmental surfaces	Medicated hand washing agents are bactericidal (alcohol, chlorhexidine gluconate, triclosan) and effectively reduced bacterial counts on the hands
		Chlorhexidine has the advantage of producing a residual antibacterial effect, thereby limiting hand recontamination until the time of the next hand hygiene episode
		Sustained improvements in hand hygiene compliance should include efforts that stress increased use of accessible, easy-to-use, medicated hand hygiene products, coupled with a hospitalwide, administration-backed, priority hand hygiene campaign
Gloves	Gloves should be worn to prevent healthcare worker exposure to bloodborne pathogens and to prevent contamination of hands with drug-resistant pathogens during patient care activities	Even with proper glove use, hand may become contaminated during the removal of the glove or with micro-tears that allow for microorganism transmission
		Glove use should not be used as a substitute for hand hygiene
Gowns	Several studies have documented colonization of healthcare worker's apparel and instruments during patient care activities without the use of gowns	The use of gloves *and* gowns is the convention for limiting the cross-transmission of nosocomial pathogens; however, the incremental benefit of gown use, in endemic settings, may be minimal
Transmission-based precautions	Transmission-based precautions are for selected patients who are known or suspected to harbor certain infections	Contact precautions are commonly employed for the endemic control of MRSA, VRE, *C. difficile* and multidrug-resistant Gram-negative rods
Airborne precautions Droplet precautions Contact precautions		Contact precautions are typically employed along with other infection control measures during nosocomial outbreaks of drug-resistant infections
Screening for asymptomatic patient colonization with drug-resistant pathogens	Some authorities advocate active surveillance cultures to identify the reservoirs of MRSA and VRE	This measure is controversial
	The goal of active surveillance is to identify every colonized patient so that infection control interventions such as contact isolation and cohorting can be implemented to reduce the risk of nosocomial cross-transmission	The majority of the studies had multiple interventions and major methodological weaknesses. As such, the quality of evidence in many studies was considered weak
		The use of strict isolation practices may have a detrimental impact on the process and quality of patient care
Antibiotic control program	Prolonged antibiotic prophylaxis with cephalosporins was an independent risk factor on logistic regression analysis for infections with cephalosporin-resistant Gram-negative rods	The degree in which antibiotic pressure directly contributes to the cross-transmission of nosocomial infections remains poorly defined
	Enteric VRE colonization has been associated with cephalosporin use	Consideration should be given to antibiotic restriction and control programs in the event of elevated rates of nosocomial drug-resistant pathogens
	MRSA colonization has been associated with fluoroquinolone use	

(continued)

Table 1 (continued)

Infection control measure	Rationale	Comment
Hospital infection surveillance program	The purpose of a hospital infection surveillance program is to define endemic rates, recognize outbreaks, and develop institution-specific antibiograms These data is later applied for the planning and implementation of risk-reduction policies and interventions	For greater effectiveness, infection control surveillance should be both concurrent (during hospitalization) and active (performed by trained, infection control professionals) Both clinical and microbiological data are essential to compile accurate surveillance data

mid-1980s by Scheckler et al. failed to document MRSA colonization in a cohort of community-based nursing homes (11). Another study of community-based nursing homes from the early 1990s revealed 24% of patients with *S. aureus* colonization, while 8.7% of all patients were colonized with MRSA (12). Lee et al. reported *S. aureus* colonization and infection in a 149-bed skilled nursing facility over a 1-year period. In this series, nasal and stool or rectal screening cultures were done on admission and then on a quarterly basis for a year. At the conclusion of the study, 35% of all patients were colonized with *S. aureus* at least once during the period of analysis. Of the positive cultures, 72% were MSSA, 25% MRSA, and 3% were mixed phenotype. Only a minority of patients colonized developed an infection with *S. aureus*. The authors reported no association between MRSA colonization and greater frequency of *S. aureus* infection (13).

MRSA colonization has been studied in the intensive care setting. Garrouste-Orgeas et al. prospectively studied MRSA colonization and infection in a medical-surgical intensive care unit of a tertiary care medical center (14). In this prospective, observational study, cultures were obtained within 48 h of hospitalization, and weekly thereafter. Five percent of all patients were colonized with MRSA at the time of admission, and 4.9% were newly colonized with MRSA during the course of their ICU stay. After multivariate analysis, factors associated with MRSA infection were severity of illness (Hazard Ratio (HR) 1.64), male gender (HR 2.2), and MRSA colonization (HR 3.84). However, MRSA colonization was not associated with increased mortality (14). Overall, 10% of patients in the cohort were colonized with MRSA. A similar rate of MRSA colonization has been documented by other investigators (15).

Cocolonization or coinfection with multidrug-resistant (MDR) pathogens has been reported in several different populations. A point prevalence survey of antimicrobial-resistant pathogens in skilled care facility residents revealed a high rate of MRSA colonization (16). Of the 177 patients surveyed, 24% were colonized with MRSA. Additionally, extended-spectrum β-lactamase (ESBL)-producing organisms were discovered in their patient population, including *Klebsiella pneumoniae* (18%), *Escherichia coli* (15%), and VRE (3.5%). As these patients were asymptomatic, the investigators discovered a large, unrecognized pool of antimicrobial-resistant pathogens in their nursing home population (16). Warren et al. determined the occurrence of cocolonization and coinfection with VRE and MRSA among medical patients in a medical intensive care

unit of a tertiary care medical center. Screening cultures were obtained in adults requiring at least 48 h of intensive care therapy. The study evaluated 878 consecutive patients. Of these, 40% were either colonized or infected with VRE, 4.4% were either colonized or infected with MRSA, and 9.5% had either cocolonization or coinfection with MRSA and VRE. Risk factors for cocolonization or coinfection were increasing age, prior hospitalization within the preceding 6 months, and admission to a long-term care facility (17). In a study of patients at high-risk wards at an urban academic center, almost 30% of patients carrying VRE were cocolonized with MRSA (18).

3 The Impact of Colonization Status on Nosocomial Infections

An association between MRSA colonization and the subsequent development of MRSA nosocomial infections exists. Pujol et al. prospectively analyzed the relationship of MRSA nasal colonization and bacteremia. During a 1-year period in an intensive care unit, nasal swabs were obtained from all patients within 48 h post admission and then weekly. Thirty percent of all patients were nasal *S. aureus* carriers: 17% with MSSA and 13% with MRSA. Bacteremia was observed in 38% of the MRSA carriers and 9.5% of the MSSA carriers. Using Cox-proportional hazards modeling, the relative risk (RR) of *S. aureus* bacteremia was 3.9 when comparing MRSA to MSSA nasal carriers.

Other investigators have confirmed the significance of MRSA colonization and its predilection for subsequent infection. Davis et al. investigated MRSA colonization at hospital admission and its effect on subsequent MRSA infection (19). Nares cultures were obtained on admission on patients admitted to various hospital units, including medical, surgical, and trauma intensive care units. The patients were followed for the study period and then for 1 year thereafter. Nasal colonization with MSSA far exceeded that with MRSA (21% vs. 3.4%). However, 19% of patients with MRSA colonization at admission and 25% with subsequent colonization developed infection with MRSA. Reported infections included line sepsis, bacteremias, as well as skin and soft tissue infections. Compared with MSSA colonization, both MRSA colonization and MRSA acquisition during hospitalization increased the relative risk of infection (RR 13 and RR 12) (19).

Nasal carriage of both MRSA and MSSA has been associated with increased risk of vascular access-related infections in type II diabetic patients on dialysis. In this series, nasal swabs were performed in 208 patients enrolled for long-term hemodialysis between 1996 and 1999 (20). Persistent nasal carriage was defined as two or more positive cultures. Type II diabetic patients had higher MSSA and MRSA carriage rates (54 and 19%) than non-diabetic patients (6%). Overall, 73% of all diabetic patients were colonized nasally with either MRSA or MSSA. Additionally, when compared to non-diabetic hemodialysis patients, the relative risk for vascular-access-associated bloodstream infection was significantly greater (RR 3.19, $P < 0.0001$) (20). Lastly, published data suggest that healthcare workers colonized with drug-resistant pathogens may be associated with cross-transmission and nosocomial infections. Wang et al. investigated a hospital-acquired outbreak of MRSA infection initiated in a surgeon carrier (21). Over a 4-month period, five patients who had undergone open-heart surgery developed surgical wound infections and mediastinitis with MRSA. Investigation by the infection control team led to MRSA nasal screening of all ICU staff and of the surgical team. Pulse field gel electrophoresis technology was employed for isolate typing. Of the five nosocomial MRSA infections, all had the same attending surgeon and 2–3 assistant surgeons. Surveillance cultures of the staff were all negative save for one assistant surgeon, who was present in all the five cases. The typing profile of the surgeon's isolate was identical to that of three of the cases. The remaining two isolates were lost and hence not typed; however, these were presumed to be identical to the others owing to the same antibiogram (21). Other investigators have reported healthcare colonization and its effect on cross-transmission and subsequent MRSA infection and colonization. Boyce et al. reported the spread of MRSA within a hospital. A healthcare worker with chronic sinusitis was the purported source (22). In addition, outbreaks of MRSA infections in a burn unit have implicated nursing staff as sources (23, 24).

4 The Role of Mupirocin for *S. aureus* Nasal Carriage Decolonization

Given the importance of *S. aureus* as a nosocomial pathogen, decolonization of carriers has been attempted in various populations. Early investigations employed both topical and systemic therapy for the eradication of *S. aureus* nasal colonization. In the 1980s, in experimental studies, it was shown that mupirocin was effective in reducing nasal carriage of volunteers with MRSA (25). Subsequently it was shown that mupirocin was active against methicillin-resistant strains of *S. aureus*. (25). In the early 1990s, Darouich et al. as part of a multidisciplinary approach, attempted to control

the spread of MRSA within a spinal cord unit (26). Eleven patients in the spinal cord unit were colonized with MRSA. The sites of colonization varied but included nares, axilla, tracheostomy site, urethra, wounds, and urine. Ten of the colonized patients received a 2-week course of 100 mg of minocycline twice daily and 600 mg of rifampin once daily. The remaining patient was treated for only 1 week with the minocycline/rifampin combination. For those that were nasally colonized, nasal mupirocin ointment was applied twice daily for 5 days. The authors reported eradication of MRSA colonization in 10 of the 11 patients (26).

Subsequent data suggest that for nasal MRSA, mupirocin alone may be sufficient for decolonization. In a 6-month, 2-step prospective study from France, the efficacy of nasal mupirocin for the prevention of *S. aureus* nasal carriage was assessed (27). In the first 4 months, all patients in the surgical intensive care unit (SICU) were cultured without the nasal decontamination protocol. Nasal and surgical wound swabs and tracheal secretions were collected on admission and then once weekly. In the following 2 months, all patients in the SICU were given twice-daily intranasal mupirocin for 1 week. In the comparison, 31.3% of untreated patients and 5.1% of mupirocin-treated patients subsequently acquired nasal *S. aureus* while in the SICU. In addition, nasal carriers were more commonly colonized in the bronchopulmonary tract and surgical wound (62%) than non-nasal carriers (14%). When compared to the nontreatment group, the bronchopulmonary tract infection rate was reduced in the group receiving mupirocin treatment. Thus, in a SICU cohort, the use of prophylactic mupirocin treatment reduced the rate of both MRSA nasal colonization and subsequent MRSA colonization bronchopulmonary infection (27). Additionally, the use of mupirocin has successfully decreased the rates of *S. aureus* infections in dialysis patients, even though most of these isolates were methicillin sensitive (28).

Intranasal mupirocin has been employed to prevent postoperative *S. aureus* infections. Perl et al. conducted a randomized, double-blind, placebo-controlled study to determine the efficacy of mupirocin in both the reduction of surgical site infections and in the prevention of other nosocomial infections (29). A total of 3,864 patients were included in an intention-to-treat analysis, and of these, 891 patients (32.1%) were *S. aureus*-colonized in the anterior nares. The cohort underwent either general, gynecologic, neurologic, or cardiothoracic surgery. At the conclusion of the study, 2.3% of the mupirocin recipients and 2.4% of the placebo recipients had *S. aureus* infections at the surgical site. However, in a subset analysis of *S. aureus* nasal carriers, 4.0% of those that had received mupirocin had nosocomial *S. aureus* infections, compared to 7.7% for those that had received a placebo ($P = 0.02$). Thus, in this analysis, the use of intranasal mupirocin in a surgical cohort was effective in reducing the frequency of *S. aureus* nosocomial infections only in patients previously colonized with *S. aureus*. For patients known to be nasal carriers of *S. aureus*, consideration should be given to the preoperative application of mupirocin.

5 Environmental Contamination

The literature is replete with reports of environmental contamination by drug-resistant pathogens. Although the inanimate environment is not directly responsible for cross-transmission and patient inoculation with nosocomial pathogens, its role as a potential reservoir of nosocomial pathogens should not be overlooked. The environment represents a potential source for hand contamination of the healthcare worker, an important step in the cross-transmission of nosocomial pathogens. It is well documented that patients colonized or infected with drug-resistant pathogens contaminate the inanimate environment. Boyce and colleagues studied the role of contaminated environmental surfaces as reservoirs of MRSA in hospitals by performing a culture survey of inanimate objects in the rooms of patients with MRSA (22). Three hundred and fifty surfaces were sampled from 38 patients either colonized or infected with MRSA. Of these surfaces, 27% were contaminated with MRSA. The most commonly reported contaminated objects included the floor, bed linens, patient gowns, overbed tables, and blood pressure cuffs. Additionally, cultures of gowns and gloves from hospital personnel performing nursing care activities on MRSA-positive wounds or urine revealed a high proportion of gown and glove contamination (65% and 58%, respectively). Of additional importance was the observation that 42% of personnel with no direct patient contact, but with environmental contact, contaminated their gloves with MRSA (22). A similar degree of environmental contamination has been reported in both burn unit and surgical populations (30–34).

Contamination can extend beyond the immediate patient care area. Devine et al. surveyed two acute care hospitals (A and B) in the United Kingdom with a focus on contamination of ward-based computer modules (35). In total, 25 computer terminals were cultured for MRSA. Of these, six (24%) were positive for MRSA. Five of the six positive computer terminal cultures were from Hospital A. The antibiograms of the positive MRSA cultures were similar and resembled the typical hospital strains. Both institutions had similar hand hygiene policies and MRSA control policies. However, the institutional rates of MRSA transmission between hospitals A and B in 1999 were different (1.02 per 100 admissions vs. 0.5 per 100 admissions). Additionally, the infection control team of Hospital B reviewed handwashing compliance regularly with doctors and nurses. This hospital also reported a greater rate of paper towel consumption, a surrogate marker for hand hygiene compliance. Although the direction of transfer is impossible to define from such studies, the data suggest that inanimate reservoirs, such as commonly used computer terminals, have the potential to contaminate the hands of healthcare workers (HCWs). Furthermore, hand hygiene compliance, suggested by a greater rate of paper towel consumption, may be essential in minimizing this risk and is correlated with both a lower frequency of computer terminal contamination and a lesser rate of MRSA transmission within a hospital (35).

Environmental contamination with VRE has also been described. Previous studies have implicated environmental contamination of multiuse inanimate objects with monoclonal VRE outbreaks (36, 37). However, the inanimate environment is likely an important step in endemic cross-transmission of VRE. In the mid-1990s, Bonten et al. investigated VRE colonization of patients and environmental contamination with VRE in a major tertiary care medical center (38). Over a 2-month period, daily cultures from body sites (including rectum, groin, oropharynx, trachea, and stomach) and from environmental surfaces (bedrails, sheets, blood pressure cuff, urinary containers, and enteral feeding tubes) were obtained from ventilated patients admitted to the medical intensive care unit. Additionally, rectal cultures were obtained from all nonventilated patients in the same intensive care unit. The proportion of VRE-colonized patients between ventilated and nonventilated patients varied significantly, 24% vs. 6%, respectively. A total of 1,294 environmental cultures were obtained. Of these, 157 (12%) were VRE positive. The most common sites of VRE contamination were the bedrail, sheets, blood pressure cuff, urine container, and enteral feed tubing. Pulse-field gel electrophoresis of the isolates revealed 20 distinct VRE strains (38). As such, in this tertiary-care medical intensive care unit, VRE colonization was highly endemic and polyclonal.

The importance of environmental contamination as a potential risk factor for VRE acquisition in the medical intensive care unit was further investigated by Martinez et al. (39). Employing a retrospective case–control study conducted on patients in a medical intensive care unit of a tertiary-care medical center, 30 patients with VRE acquisition during their ICU stay were matched with 60 controls. The controls were randomly selected, VRE-negative patients who had been hospitalized in the medical intensive care unit for at least the same number of days as a case patient. Active surveillance for VRE was in place in the ICUs of the study institution with rectal swabs being performed within 48 h of admission and then once weekly. Screening for VRE colonization was performed on 169 patients. Of these, 32 (19%) were colonized on admission and 31 (23%) acquired VRE during their ICU stay. Additionally, a concurrent environmental survey was performed in the medical intensive care unit. Positive samples were collected from light switches, toilet rinser, bathroom faucets, telephones, and IV pumps. Six different PFGE VRE strains were found. Multivariable logistic regression modeling was employed to identify VRE acquisition in hospitalized patients. In addition to the length of stay greater than 1 week prior to ICU admission (OR 18.5), receipt of vancomycin (OR 6.3), and use of quinolones (OR 14.8) prior to ICU admission, patient placement in a contaminated room (OR 81.7) carried the greatest OR for VRE acquisition (39).

VRE environmental contamination has been reported in non-intensive-care settings. Trick at et al. investigated the frequency of VRE environmental contamination in a 146-bed rehabilitation facility (40). Using a cross-sectional study design, rectal cultures were obtained from 74 (80%) patients in the rehabilitation facility. Environmental cultures were obtained from surfaces in 15 patient rooms over five different floors and from common use areas on eight floors. A total of 319 environmental surfaces were sampled. Eighteen percent (13) of the 74 patients were VRE colonized, and 10% (32) of the environmental surfaces were VRE colonized. For samples obtained from patient rooms, contamination was most common on shower seats (33%), bed rails (20%), counters (20%), and bedside commodes (20%). VRE was recovered from blood pressure cuff, glucometer, handrail, washer/dryer knob, and exercise mat. Compared to patients with either unknown VRE colonization status (13%) or who are VRE negative (0%), surface contamination was more common in patients with VRE colonization (24%). Additionally, surfaces were more likely contaminated in a room housing an incontinent patient (40).

Mayer et al. prospectively examined the frequency of environmental VRE contamination, comparing VRE-colonized patients who were either continent or incontinent of stool (41). A total of 30 VRE-colonized patients were analyzed, 15 of whom were incontinent of stool and 15 were continent. Environmental cultures were obtained from the bed rails, bedside table, and call buttons. These were obtained at baseline, and then at 2 and 5 days after environmental disinfection. There was no statistical significance between the two groups in the proportion of patients with at least one VRE-positive environmental culture (60% continent, 73% incontinent) at baseline and after disinfection (60 and 80%). These findings suggest that patients who are enterically colonized with VRE, and are either continent or incontinent of feces, frequently contaminate the environment.

The distribution of drug-resistant pathogens within the hospital is not limited exclusively to intensive care units and to MRSA or VRE. In a study from Germany, up to 20 different environmental samples were surveyed from 190 patients harboring either MRSA, VRE, or MDR Gram-negative rods (MDR GNRs) (42). The samples were obtained from hospitalized patients both in intensive care units and general medical wards. A total of 1,827 samples were obtained in the survey. The proportion of environmental cultures positive for MRSA or VRE was 24.7% compared with 4.9% for MDR GNRs. The most commonly isolated MDR GNR was

P. aeruginosa, S. maltophilia, E. coli, Enterobacter species, and *Serratia* species. Both Gram-positive and Gram-negative pathogens were isolated from bed covers, bed sheets, urinals, infusion pumps, personnel gowns, patient showers, bedside table, floor, door handle, bed rail, chair, respirator, basin fitting, bathroom door, toilet seat, and shower. The degree of environmental contamination did not differ between the intensive care units and the general medical wards (42).

Recently, in an important study by Duckro et al. the role of the environmental hand contamination in the sequence of cross-transmission was empirically observed. The investigators sought to determine the frequency of VRE transmission from contaminated environmental sites to clean sites via the hands of HCWs. Cultures were obtained from the intact skin of 22 patients colonized with VRE and from various environmental sites before and after routine care by 98 HCWs. Cultures were obtained from the hands of the HCWs before and after patient care, and PFGE typing of the isolates was performed. Sixteen (10.6%) of 151 previously culture-negative sites were culture-positive for VRE after contact with HCW hands. Of these 16 VRE transfer sites, 12 were patient body sites (43). In this analysis, VRE was transferred from contaminated sites in the environment or on the patient's intact skin to clean, previously noncontaminated environmental and body sites via the HCW in 10.6% of the opportunities.

These data suggest that the hospital environment is a potentially important reservoir for cross-transmission of drug-resistant pathogens.

As patients colonized with resistant pathogens can contaminate the environment, proper environmental disinfection is an important step for minimizing the risk or cross-transmission. An extensive review of approved disinfectants and environmental cleaning practices is beyond the scope of this chapter. However, several general principles are of note. Terminal cleaning of patient rooms should aim to minimize the persistence of drug-resistant pathogens. Hospital environmental services personnel should clean the bed frame and handrails, mattress, and all other patient-room furniture with an Environmental Protection Agency (EPA)-approved disinfectant and used according to manufacturers' guidelines (44). Suction containers should be removed and prepared for disposal or reprocessing, and all other reusable equipment should be decontaminated using an (EPA)-approved disinfectant. The bathroom in an isolation room should be thoroughly cleaned and disinfected, with particular attention paid to the sink, toilet and door-handle areas. Environmental surfaces with a high degree of patient body and hand contact such as bed rails, doorknobs, bathrooms, light switches, and wall areas should be cleaned with greater frequency and not exclusively at the time of patient discharge. All healthcare facilities should develop policies for the terminal and periodic disinfection of patient care areas and environmental services. This policy should include input from infection control practitioners, industrial hygienists, and environmental services supervisors.

6 Hand Hygiene

Hand hygiene, either by conventional hand washing or disinfection, is the single most effective method to limit the spread of drug-resistant pathogens and nosocomial infections (45). Conceptually, the cross-transmission of nosocomial pathogens is summarized as follows (46):

- Organisms present either on the patient's skin or from the inanimate environment must be transferred to the hands of the healthcare worker.
- Nosocomial pathogens must be capable of surviving on the hand of the healthcare worker.
- Hand hygiene must be either inadequate or omitted.
- The contaminated hands of the healthcare worker must then come into contact with another patient, or with an inanimate surface that will later come into contact with the patient.

The microorganisms of the hand can be divided into *transient flora* and *resident flora* (47). The resident flora is typically of low-virulence pathogens such as *Micrococcus*, coagulase-negative *Staphylococcus*, and *Corynebacterium*. These organisms are difficult to remove by handwashing yet are rarely pathogenic except when introduced to the patient by invasive procedures. Transient flora are acquired largely by contact with either the patient or an inanimate object, are loosely attached to the skin and are easily removed by handwashing (47). These organisms include MRSA, VRE, and MDR GNRs. Additionally, these bacteria are important causes of nosocomial infections.

Numerous studies have shown that multiple opportunities exist in the hospital environment for the contamination of the hands of the healthcare worker. Nosocomial pathogens can be recovered from a variety of patient-care scenarios. Patient contact, including contact with wounds and intact skin, can result in healthcare worker hand contamination (48–59). Areas of high nosocomial pathogen concentration on patient skin include the axillae, trunk, perineum, inguinal region, and hands (51, 53, 54, 56, 58–60). As previously mentioned, the inanimate environment is a source of contamination.

Healthcare workers should practice hand hygiene before and after each patient contact. Methods of hand hygiene include washing with plain soap and water, or using an antibacterial agent such as alcohol, chlorhexidine gluconate, or Triclosan either as detergent washes or as waterless hand-rubs. Conventional soap and water may have various shortcomings and barriers to compliance. Although soap and water can remove loosely adherent transient skin, these agents have minimal antimicrobial activity (46). For effective bacterial reduction, a 30 s hand rub is recommended, but unfortunately, this length of hand washing is rarely practiced. In addition, several studies have demonstrated that handwashing with both plain soap and water can result in skin irritation, dryness, and, paradoxically, an increase in microbial counts on the skin (61–65). Medicated hand washing agents are bactericidal (alcohol, chlorhexidine gluconate, triclosan) and effectively reduce bacterial counts on the hands. Moreover, chlorhexidine has the advantage of producing a residual antibacterial effect, thereby limiting hand recontamination until the time of the next hand hygiene episode (66).

At least one study supports the effectiveness of chlorhexidine as a hand antiseptic agent with regard to infection control endpoints. Doebbling et al. compared different hand hygiene agents with the end result of hand hygiene compliance observation and the reduction of nosocomial infections in an intensive care unit setting (67). During an 8-month period, a prospective multiple crossover trial was conducted in three intensive care units. The trial involved 1,894 adult patients exposed to alternate months of either chlorhexidine or 60% alcohol solution with the optional use of a nonmedicated soap. A greater frequency of nosocomial infections was seen with the combination of alcohol and soap compared to the chlorhexidine hand hygiene agent (202 vs. 152). However, during periods of chlorhexidine use, there was a decrease in the rate of nosocomial infections and an increase in the observed frequency of hand hygiene compliance, coupled with a volume of chlorhexidine consumption that exceeded that of the alcohol-based agent. The difference in nosocomial infections may have been partly due to increased compliance with hand hygiene practices. Regardless, owing to their bactericidal properties, medicated hand hygiene agents, including chlorhexidine, alcohol, and Triclosan, should be highly considered, especially in environments with elevated rates of drug-resistant pathogens.

Unfortunately, data on healthcare worker hand hygiene practice are discouraging. The reasons for poor compliance are multiple and have been studied by numerous investigators. Observational studies of hand hygiene compliance report compliance rates of 5–81% (68–100). Factors cited that may influence poor adherence with hand hygiene include insufficient time, understaffing, patient overcrowding, lack of knowledge of hand hygiene guidelines, skepticism about hand washing efficacy, inconvenient location of sinks and hand disinfectants, and lack of hand hygiene promotion by the institution (46).

In the intensive care units, where critically ill patients are particularly susceptible to nosocomial infections, hand hygiene is poor. A British study performed a detailed survey of hand hygiene practices in 16 intensive care units (47).

Additionally, 381 (non-nurse) healthcare professionals were observed for hand hygiene compliance. Compliance with hand hygiene and proper glove use ranged from 9 to 25%. Survey responses suggested that poor compliance with hand hygiene in the ICU was secondary to multiple issues including ineffective communication of infection control recommendations, insufficient promotion of hand antisepsis, and a deficiency of infection control education (47). Poor compliance with hand hygiene was similarly observed by Kaplan et al. in a tertiary-care American hospital (101). Physician compliance with hand hygiene was 19%, while compliance by the nursing staff was 63%. Greater compliance with hand hygiene was observed among the nursing staff with a 1:1 bed to sink ratio than those with a greater bed to sink ratio (76% vs. 51%) (101).

Efforts to improve hand hygiene both in the ICUs and throughout the hospital likely require simultaneous interventions on multiple levels. In a study by Bischoff et al., where alcohol-based hand sanitizers were introduced to an intensive care unit, the greatest increment in hand hygiene compliance was observed when the hand sanitizer to healthcare worker ratio went from 1:4 to 1:1, thereby underscoring the importance of accessibility (102). As such, the CDC now suggests promoting alcohol-based hand sanitizer access both by bedside dispensers and healthcare worker pocket-sized dispensers (46). Pittet and colleagues improved overall compliance with hand hygiene by implementing a hospitalwide program with special emphasis on bedside alcohol-based hand disinfection. The campaign ran from December 1994 to December 1997 and consisted primarily of hand hygiene promotion through large, conspicuous posters promoting hand hygiene throughout patient care areas. The project was supported and heavily promoted by senior hospital management. Additionally, alcohol-based hand-rub solutions were distributed in large amounts, mounted on beds/walls, and given to HCWs to encourage packet carriage for convenience of use. During this time frame, seven institutionwide hand hygiene observational surveys were performed twice yearly. Additional measures included monitoring nosocomial infection rates, the rate of MRSA infections, and overall consumption of handrub disinfectant. In this 3-year study, 20,000 opportunities for hand hygiene were observed. Compliance with hand hygiene improved from a baseline of 44% in 1994 to 66% in 1997. Of note, hand hygiene improved markedly among nursing staff but remained poor among physicians. Additionally, over the study period, the overall prevalence of nosocomial infections decreased from 16.9% to 9.9%, MRSA transmission rates decreased from 2.16 to 0.93 episodes per 10,000 patient days, and the consumption of alcohol-based hand-rub increased from 3.5L to 15.4L per 1,000 patient days (103). Unfortunately, as multiple interventions were employed simultaneously, the relative effect of each component was difficult to properly assess. Thus, although the most efficient

and effective means for sustained improvements in hand hygiene compliance have yet to be defined, measures should at least include efforts that stress increased use of accessible, easy-to-use, medicated hand hygiene products, coupled with a hospitalwide, administration-supported, high-priority hand hygiene educational and promotional campaign.

7 The Use of Gloves and Gowns to Limit Cross-Transmission of Nosocomial Pathogens

Gloves should be worn to prevent exposure of the healthcare worker to bloodborne pathogens and to prevent contamination of hands with drug-resistant pathogens during patient care activities. Nevertheless, even with proper glove use, hands may become contaminated during the removal of the glove or with micro-tears that allow for microorganism transmission (104). Glove use should not be a substitute for hand hygiene. The promotion of glove use may increase compliance with hand hygiene protocols. A recent study by Kim and colleagues observed the rate of hand disinfection with glove use and patient isolation (105). In this prospective, observational study, hand hygiene and glove use compliance were observed and measured in two intensive care units of a tertiary-care hospital. Over 40h of observation, 589 opportunities for hand disinfection were noted. Overall hand hygiene compliance was 22%. The investigators found a statistically significant positive association between glove use and subsequent hand disinfection (RR 3.9, 95%CI 2.5–6.0). Isolation precautions did not significantly increase hand hygiene compliance. For infection control purposes, glove use should be promoted as a means of limiting hand contamination with drug-resistant pathogens such as MRSA and VRE. Additionally, glove use and hand hygiene should be promoted concurrently.

8 Gowns

Gowns have been used as part of contact precaution protocols to limit the spread of nosocomial pathogens. Several studies have documented colonization of the apparel and instruments of the HCWs without the use of gowns during patient care activities (106–108). One study by Boyce et al. demonstrated the efficacy of disposable gowns in the prevention of clothing contamination of HCWs (22, 109). Srinivasen et al. prospectively measured the effect of gown and glove use in a 16-bed medical intensive care unit of a tertiary-care medical center. Over a 3-month period, all admissions to a medical ICU were screened for VRE by perirectal swab. Patients who were culture-positive for VRE were isolated by hospital policy, requiring the use of gown and glove for patient care. For the following 3 months, precautions were changed to glove use alone. The VRE acquisition rate was 1.8 cases per 100 patient days at risk in the gown/glove group and 3.78 per 100 patient days during glove use alone ($P = 0.04$)

Not all studies, however, support the routine use of gowns for infection control measures. In addition, with regard to the endpoint of colonization and cross-transmission, there may be little incremental benefit to gown use over proper glove use and hand hygiene alone. Pelke et al. studied the effect of gowning in a neonatal intensive care unit over an 8-month time frame employing alternating 2-month gowning and non-gowning cycles. The outcomes of interest were colonization patterns, necrotizing enterocolitis, respiratory syncytial virus, other nosocomial infections, mortality, and handwashing. The investigators failed to document any significant difference between the gowning and non-gowning cohorts with respect to the rates of bacterial colonization, infection type, or mortality. In addition, no significant difference in hand hygiene practice was observed (110).

Other investigators have compared gown use in addition to gloves and the effect on nosocomial transmission of VRE. Slaughter et al. compared the universal gloving vs. universal gown and glove use on the acquisition of VRE in a medical intensive care unit. This prospective study involved 181 consecutive admissions. Half of the 16-bed ICU was designated for universal gown and glove use during patient care activities, and the other half was for universal gloving for patient care activities. Rectal surveillance cultures were taken daily from patients along with monthly environmental cultures of bed rails, bedside tables, and other common objects in patient rooms. The investigators found no superiority in the universal use of gowns and gloves vs. the use of gloves only in preventing the rectal colonization of VRE in a medical intensive care unit cohort (111). Trick and colleagues compared the impact of routine glove use vs. contact isolation on the transmission of MDR bacteria in a skilled nursing home environment (112). Over an 18-month period, all residents admitted to the skilled care unit of an acute and long-term care unit were randomly allocated to two different contact isolation precautions (gown and glove use) vs. routine glove use during patient care. No differences were observed in the transmission of antimicrobial-resistant bacteria, including MRSA, VRE, and extended-spectrum β-lactamase-producing *K. pneumoniae* and *E. coli* between the two study groups. Of note, greater compliance with proper glove use and hand hygiene was seen in the routine glove use section. Thus, although the use of gloves *and* gowns is the convention for limiting the cross-transmission of nosocomial pathogens, the incremental benefit of gown use, in endemic settings, may be minimal.

9 Transmission-Based Precautions

Transmission-based precautions are for selected patients who are known or suspected to harbor certain infections. These precautions are divided into three categories, reflecting differences in disease transmission. Some diseases may require more than one isolation category. The essential elements of transmission-based precautions are summarized below.

9.1 Airborne Precautions

Airborne precautions are designed to prevent diseases that are transmitted by droplet nuclei or contaminated dust particles. Droplet nuclei, because of their size, can remain suspended in the air for prolonged periods, even after the infected patient has left the room. Agents requiring airborne precautions include *M. tuberculosis*, varicella zoster virus, influenza, and measles virus.

All patients needing airborne precautions should be assigned to a private room with special engineering and ventilation considerations. The door to this room must be closed at all possible times. The isolation room must be maintained at negative pressure in comparison to the surroundings. As such, droplet nuclei are prevented from traveling into the environment. In addition, the air within the isolation room should either be vented to the outside or passed through high-efficiency particle filters (46, 113).

All personnel entering the isolation room are required by federal regulations to don masks for respiratory protection. If a patient must move from the isolation room to another area of the hospital, the patient should be made to wear a mask during the transport. Anyone entering the isolation room to provide care to the patient must wear a special mask called a respirator. These respirator masks are approved by the National Institute for Occupational Safety and Health and are capable of filtering 1-μm particles with an efficiency of 95% (N-95 mask). By regulation, all HCWs must be fit-tested for N-95 masks and must be taught to check for proper fit each time prior to use (46, 113). Rapid airborne isolation of patients with known or suspected MDR *M. tuberculosis*, along with proper N-95 mask use by HCWs, is essential to limit the spread of this pathogen.

9.2 Droplet Precautions

Droplet precautions prevent the transmission of organisms that travel via droplets generated during phonation, sneezing, or coughing, or during invasive respiratory tract procedures.

These particles are not suspended in the air for extended periods and typically do not travel beyond several feet from the patient. Patients who require droplet precautions should be placed in a private room or should be cohorted with a roommate who is infected with the same organism. The door to the room may remain open. Healthcare workers should wear a mask when within 3 ft of the patient. Patients moving about the hospital away from the isolation room should wear a mask. Examples of diseases requiring droplet precautions are meningococcal meningitis, *H. influenza*, influenza, mumps, and German measles (rubella) (114).

9.3 Contact Precautions

Contact precautions prevent spread of organisms from an infected patient through direct (touching the patient) or indirect (touching surfaces or objects that have been in contact with the patient) contact. This type of precaution requires the patient to either be placed in a private room or be cohorted with a roommate with the same. Healthcare workers should don gloves upon entering the room. After patient care or environmental contact, the gloves should be removed and hand hygiene should be performed prior to leaving the room. In addition, the use of protective gowns have been advocated to decrease the risk of healthcare worker garment contamination. Patient care items used for a patient in contact precautions, such as a stethoscopes and blood pressure cuffs, should not be shared with other patients unless they are properly cleaned and disinfected before reuse. Patients should be restricted to the isolation room (114).

Contact precautions are indicated for patients with drug-resistant pathogens such as MRSA, VRE, and MDR GNRs. In addition, contact isolation is recommended for diarrheal illnesses of infectious origin and for infections with *C. difficile*.

10 Measures to Control Nosocomial Outbreak of Drug-Resistant Pathogens

Data published by the CDC report that more than 70% of bacterial pathogens implicated in nosocomial infections are resistant to at least one commonly used anti-infective (115). In addition, current evidence suggests that the proportion of MRSA and VRE attributable to cross-transmission is significant. Transmission of clonal MRSA strains within a healthcare setting has been confirmed by PFGE and has occurred in various healthcare settings including general hospital wards, neonatal intensive care units, and surgical intensive care units (116–126). Similarly, the clonal transmission of

VRE within healthcare settings has been documented via molecular typing (127–136).

There is no one-size-fits-all approach to the control of nosocomial drug-resistant pathogens such as MRSA or VRE. The literature is replete with reports of intervention and programs to limit the spread of drug-resistant pathogens. These examples, occurring in diverse patient populations such as those in hospital wards, intensive care units, and neonatal units, typically involve different combinations of multiple interventions such as surveillance cultures, PFGE typing of isolates, patient isolation, cohorting, gloving, gowning, antibiotic restriction, and healthcare worker decolonization (10, 137–142). The best approach for controlling the nosocomial spread of pathogens such as MRSA or VRE should take into account the frequency of nosocomial transmission, the reservoirs, patient risk factors, and the resources of the healthcare system for implementation of varied infection control measures.

11 Screening for Asymptomatic Patient Colonization with Drug-Resistant Pathogens

As the incidence of both patient infection and colonization with drug-resistant pathogens such as MRSA or VRE has increased, the management of this phenomenon has evolved. Aggressive strategies include screening to detect asymptomatic carriers and the strict use of isolation measures to control spread. Nevertheless, there has been much debate about the rationale and efficacy of this practice to control the endemic spread of potential nosocomial pathogens.

In the latest guidelines by the Society for Healthcare Epidemiology of America (SHEA) for the prevention and spread of antibiotic-resistant pathogens, the use of active surveillance cultures to identify the reservoirs of MRSA and VRE is strongly recommended (143). The ultimate goal of active surveillance is to identify every colonized patient so that infection control interventions such as contact isolation and cohorting can be implemented to reduce the risk of nosocomial cross-transmission. As per the SHEA guidelines, these active surveillance cultures are indicated at the time of hospital admission for patients at high risk for carriage of MRSA and/or VRE (143–148). For patients with ongoing or prolonged hospitalization, or at high risk for VRE or MRSA carriage due to hospital location, underlying comorbidities, and concurrent antibiotic therapy, periodic reculturing is recommended, typically on a weekly basis (117, 134, 149–156). Furthermore, for facilities with high endemic rates of VRE or MRSA, as determined by surveillance of high-risk patients, an institutionwide survey should be conducted so that these patients are identified and placed in either contact isolation or cohorted (143).

However, a recently published review of isolation policies by the British National Health Service highlighted the strong evidence for the effectiveness of different isolation and screening policies for MRSA (157). Data were extracted from articles reporting infection control mechanisms, policies, and interventions for MRSA-related outcomes, including colonization or infection. From 4,382 abstracts, 254 full article appraisals were made, with 46 papers included in the final review. Of the 46 studies, 18 included the use of isolation wards, 9 used nurse cohorting, and 19 involved other isolation policies including multiple combinations of different interventions such as patient cohorting in single or multiple occupancy rooms, strict use of gown, glove, and mask, changes in antibiotic formulary, screening on admission and weekly thereafter, prompt patient discharge, mupirocin for decolonization, hand hygiene education with and without feedback to HCWs, and antibiotic restriction. Although the review concluded that concerted efforts, including isolation, can reduce the rates of MRSA in both endemic and epidemic settings, several other findings were noteworthy. The majority of the studies had multiple interventions and major methodological weaknesses such as lack of measures to prevent bias, the absence of consideration for confounding, and inappropriate statistical analysis. As such, the quality of evidence in many studies was considered weak, many alternative and plausible explanations for the reduction in MRSA could not be excluded, and the role and impact of isolation measures were not assessed by well-designed studies.

At least one recently published, well-designed, prospective study evaluated the efficacy of single room and cohort isolation for MRSA in the intensive care unit setting (158). In this 1-year analysis conducted in the intensive care units of two teaching hospitals, MRSA screening was performed both on admission and then weekly for all patients. During the first 3 months and the last 3 months, all MRSA-positive patients were moved either to a single-occupancy isolation room or cohorted with other MRSA-positive patients. During the middle 6-month period, MRSA-positive patients were not placed in isolation or cohorted unless they were cocolonized with another multiresistant pathogen. Patient characteristics, hand hygiene compliance, and MRSA acquisition rates were similar in the periods when patients were moved and not moved. Using cox-proportional hazard modeling to control for confounders such as gender, age, APACHE II score, antibiotic use, number of intravascular catheters, and colonization pressure, no significant reduction in MRSA acquisition was observed between the two groups (158).

The use of strict isolation practices may have a detrimental impact on the process and quality of patient care. Evans prospectively observed surgical patients in both the intensive care unit and on a general surgical floor. In both the ICU and surgical floor, surgical patients on contact isolation had fewer healthcare worker visits and less contact time overall despite a higher severity of illness as measured by APACHE II

score (159). Stelfox et al. studied the quality of medical care received by patients isolated for MRSA-related infection control precautions using a case–control study design. Although isolated and control patients had similar baseline characteristics, isolated patients were twice as likely as nonisolated patients to experience adverse events during their hospitalization. These adverse events included supportive care measures and process of care measures such as days with incomplete or absent vitals signs, and days without documented nursing and physician progress notes. Additionally, patients on MRSA contact isolation expressed greater dissatisfaction with the quality of their treatment (160). Similarly, Saint and colleagues observed in a prospective cohort study of two in-patient medical services that patients on contact isolation were half as likely to be examined by an attending physician as nonisolated patients (161).

Contact isolation may have a detrimental psychological impact on patients. One cross-sectional, matched case–control study compared contact isolated vs. nonisolated elderly patients (162). The level of depressive and anxiety symptoms exhibited by the contact isolation group exceed that of the non-contact-isolation group. Catalano et al. prospectively studied the impact of contact isolation on anxiety and depression in noncritically ill hospitalized patients (163). Patients on contact isolation for either MRSA or VRE were compared with other hospitalized patients with infectious diseases not requiring isolation. All patients were evaluated with the Hamilton Anxiety and Depression Rating scale at baseline and then later during the hospital course. Although no significant differences in baseline anxiety and depression scores were noted, for patients in contact isolation statistically significant higher scores on both scales were reported later during the course of hospitalization.

Thus, the optimal strategy for control of endemic, resistant pathogens such as MRSA or VRE is yet to be defined. Aggressive measures involving surveillance cultures for colonized patient reservoirs may not effectively reduce the rate of pathogen cross-transmission. Additionally, surveillance cultures with consequent the implantation of isolation measures may have the impact of increased patient depression and anxiety, and may be detrimental to the both the process and quality of care.

12 Antibiotic Control Programs and Surveillance for Nosocomial Infections

The implications of widespread antibiotic use, including the impact on public health, are beyond the scope of this chapter. The reader is referred to other chapters in this textbook for further information on the topic. Although the degree to which antibiotic pressure directly contributes to the cross-transmission of nosocomial infections remains poorly defined, several studied and observations are worth mentioning. Harbath and colleagues prospectively studied surgical site infections in cardiovascular surgical patients. In this cohort, prolonged antibiotic prophylaxis with cephalosporins was an independent risk factor on logistic regression analysis for infections with cephalosporin-resistant GNRs (164). Additionally, in a prospective, nonrandomized cohort study in a neonatal ICU, a change to a new empiric antibiotic regimen resulted in a decrease in colonization or infection by Gram-negative organisms resistant to the standard or prior empiric regimen (165). Donskey and colleagues showed that enteric VRE colonization was significantly associated with colonization pressure, presence of feeding tube, and cephalosporin use (166). Similarly, MRSA colonization has been associated with antibiotic use. A significant risk factor for prolonged MRSA colonization, as defined by multivariate regression analysis, was fluoroquinolone use (167). Additionally, using an ecologic study design, investigators from Belgium reported a direct association between fluoroquinolone use and MRSA infections (168). Consideration should be given to antibiotic restriction and control programs in the event of elevated rates of nosocomial drug-resistant pathogens.

The purpose of a surveillance program is to define and track the rates of endemic and epidemic nosocomial infections. Endemic rates are best defined by surveillance over an extended time frame, typically greater than 1 year. Outbreaks are defined as infection rates in excess of the endemic rate. For greater effectiveness, infection control surveillance should be both concurrent (during hospitalization) and active (performed by trained, infection-control professionals). As such, both clinical and microbiological data are essential to compile accurate surveillance data.

In hospitals with limited resources, effort should be concentrated on units at high risk for nosocomial infections. Frequently, owing to limited resources, active surveillance is focused exclusively on high-risk populations such as those in intensive care units, burn units, high-risk surgical procedures, and bone marrow transplant recipients. As real-time or continuous surveillance is a time-consuming activity, requires detailed work over a period of time to produce beneficial results, and is subject to budgetary constraints, care should be taken in the selection of surveillance populations to benefit most from this type of program. This is essential for both the identification and control of drug-resistant pathogens.

Lastly, laboratory-based surveillance is also important for the detection and control of drug-resistant pathogens. This type of surveillance serves to monitor the culture results and antimicrobial susceptibility patterns. This may also include culture results of isolates representing colonization. Unlike concurrent active surveillance, laboratory surveillance can more readily be performed on a housewide basis and does not require a bedside, clinical review. This process results in

the publishing of institution-specific antibiograms and aids in the detection of emerging antimicrobial resistance patterns, but is not sensitive in differentiating between infecting and colonizing pathogens. Ultimately, the purpose of hospital infections surveillance programs is to define endemic rates, recognize outbreaks, and obtain data of value in recognizing the extent and cause of the infections. These data are later applied for the planning and implementation of risk-reduction policies and interventions.

13 Conclusion

The prevalence of hospital-acquired, antibiotic-resistant pathogens has increased significantly over the last 20 years. Hospital infection control programs are seen as increasingly important for the control of antibiotic-resistant organisms. Strategies to control the spread of hospital-acquired infections by drug-resistant pathogens are multiple. The patient, healthcare worker, and the environment are reservoirs for drug-resistant pathogens. For high-risk patients colonized with MRSA, such as surgical candidates and those in intensive care units, decolonization with nasal mupirocin should be considered. Patients colonized with resistant pathogens such as MRSA, VRE, and drug-resistant GNRs can contaminate the environment. As such, all healthcare facilities should develop policies for the terminal and periodic disinfection of patient care areas and environmental services. Cross-transmission of nosocomial pathogens by the hands of healthcare workers has been well documented. Meticulous hand hygiene should be practiced with medicated hand-washing agents (alcohol, chlorhexidine gluconate, Triclosan) that are bactericidal and effectively reduce bacterial counts on the hands. Measures to promote hand hygiene compliance should include efforts that stress increased use of accessible, easy-to-use, medicated hand hygiene products, coupled with a hospitalwide, administration-backed, high-priority hand hygiene campaign. Glove use is beneficial in limiting the contamination of healthcare workers' hands but is not a substitute for hand hygiene. Concerns about the contamination of personnel clothing with nosocomial pathogens has led to the use of gowns for patients in contact isolation. The incremental benefit of gowns and glove use may be minimal. Transmission-based precautions are useful for the control of nosocomial infections and include contact, airborne, and droplet precautions. Aggressive surveillance for asymptomatic reservoirs may be of value but is not without controversy, including questions about efficacy and effect on the quality of care. Other considerations for an infection control program include antibiotic control programs and surveillance systems for infections with nosocomial pathogens. This type of surveillance is essential for establishing endemic rates, defining outbreaks, and developing institution-specific antibiograms. In the end, the purpose of a hospital infections surveillance program is to define endemic rates, recognize outbreaks, and obtain data of value in recognizing the extent and cause of the infections. This data is later applied for the planning and implementation of risk-reduction policies and interventions.

Acknowledgments I am indebted to Ms. Kari McLaughlin for her invaluable assistance in the preparation of this manuscript.

References

1. National Nosocomial Infections Surveillance (NNIS) system report, data summary from January 1992–April 2000, issued June 2000. American Journal of Infection Control. 2000;28:429

2. Reacher M, Shah A, Livermore D, et al. Bacteraemia and antibiotic resistance of its pathogens reported in England and Wales between 1990 and 1998: trend analysis. British Medical Journal. 2000;320:213

3. Diekema D, Pfaller M, Jones R, et al. Trends in antimicrobial susceptibility of bacterial pathogens isolated from patients with bloodstream infections in the USA, Canada and Latin America. International Journal of Antimicrobial Agents. 2000;13:257

4. Kresken M, Hafner D. Drug resistance among clinical isolates of frequently encountered bacterial species in central Europe during 1975–1995. Infection. 1999;27 Suppl 2:S2

5. Wong M, Kauffman C, Standiford H, Linden P, Fort G, Fuchs H, et al. Effective suppression of vancomycin-resistant Enterococcus species in asymptomatic gastrointestinal carriers by a novel glycolipodepsipeptide, ramoplanin. Clinical Infectious Diseases. 2001;33:1476

6. Noble W, Valkenburg H, Wolters C. Carriage of Staphylococcus aureus in random samples of a normal population. Journal of Hygiene. 1967;65:567

7. Casewell M, Hill R. The carrier state: methicillin-resistant Staphylococcus aureus. Journal of Antimicrobial Chemotherapy. 1986;18 Suppl A:1

8. Willems FTC. Epidemiology of nasal carriage of Staphylococcus aureus. In: van der Meer JWM, ed. Nasal Carriage of Staphylococcus aureus. A Round-Table Discussion. Amsterdam: Excerpta Medica; 1990:3

9. Dupeyron C, Campillo B, Mangeney N, Bordes M, Richardet J, Leluan G. Carriage of Staphylococcus aureus and of gram-negative bacilli resistant to third-generation cephalosporins in cirrhotic patients: a prospective assessment of hospital-acquired infections. Infection Control and Hospital Epidemiology. 2001;22:427

10. Jernigan J, Clemence M, Stott G, Titus M, Alexander C, Palumbo C, Farr B. Control of methicillin-resistant Staphylococcus aureus at a university hospital: one decade later. Infection Control and Hospital Epidemiology. 1995;16:686–696

11. Sheckler W, Peterson P. Infections and infection control among residents of eight rural Wisconsin nursing homes. Archives of Internal Medicine. 1986;146:1981–1984

12. Hsu C. Serial survey of methicillin-resistant Staphylococcus aureus nasal carriage among residents in a nursing home. Infection Control and Hospital Epidemiology. 1991;12:416–421

13. Lee Y, Cesario T, Gupta G, Flionis L, Tran C, Decker M, Thrupp L. Surveillance of colonization and infection with Staphylococcus aureus susceptible or resistant to methicillin in a community skilled-nursing facility. American Journal of Infection Control. 1997;25:312–321

14. Garrouste-Orgeas M, Timsit J, Kallel H, Ali A, Dumay M, Paoli B, Misset B, Carlet J. Colonization with methicillin-resistant Staphylococcus aureus in ICU patients: morbidity, mortality, and glycopeptide use. Infection Control and Hospital Epidemiology. 2001;22:687

15. Girou E, Pujade G, Legrand P, Cizeau F, Brun-Buisson C. Selective screening of carriers for control of methicillin-resistant Staphylococcus aureus (MRSA) in high-risk hospital areas with a high level of endemic MRSA. Clinical Infectious Diseases. 1999;27:543

16. Trick W, Weinstein R, DeMarais P, Kuehnert M, Tomaska W, Nathan C, et al. Colonization of skilled-care facility residents with antimicrobial-resistant pathogens. Journal of the American Geriatrics Society. 2001;49:270

17. Warren D, Nitin A, Hill C, Fraser V, Kollef M. Occurrence of co-colonization or co infection with vancomycin-resistant enterococci and methicillin-resistant Staphylococcus aureus in a medical intensive care unit. Infection Control and Hospital Epidemiology. 2004;25:99

18. Franchi D, Climo M, Wong A, Edmond M, Wenzel R. Seeking vancomycin resistant Staphylococcus aureus among patients with vancomycin-resistant enterococci. Clinical Infectious Diseases. 1999;29.1566

19. Davis K, Stewart J, Crouch H, Florez C, Hospenthal D. Methicillin-resistant Staphylococcus aureus (MRSA) Nares colonization at hospital admission and its effect on subsequent MRSA infection. Clinical Infectious Diseases. 2004;39:776

20. Saxena An, Panhotra B, Venkateshappa C, Sundaram D, Naguib M, Uzzaman W, Mulhim K. The impact of nasal carriage of methicillin-resistant and methicillin-susceptible Staphylococcus aureus (MRSA & MSSA) on vascular access-related septicemia among patients with type-II diabetes on dialysis. Renal Failure. 2002;24:763

21. Wang J, Chang S, Ko W, Chang Y, Chen M, Pan H, Luh K. A hospital-acquired outbreak of methicillin-resistant Staphylococcus aureus infection initiated by a surgeon carrier. Journal of Hospital Infection. 2001;47:104

22. Boyce J, Potter-Bynoe G, Chenevert C, King T. Environmental contamination due to methicillin-resistant Staphylococcus aureus: possible infection control implications. 1997;18:622

23. Arnow P, Allyn P, Nichols E, Hill D, Pezzlo M, Bartlett R. Control of methicillin-resistant Staphylococcus aureus in a burn unit: role of nurse staffing. Journal of Trauma. 1982;22:954

24. Espersen F, Nielsen P, Lund K, Sylvest B, Jensen K. Hospital-acquired infections in a burn unit caused by an imported strain of Staphylococcus aureus with unusual multi-resistance. Journal of Hygiene. 1982;88:535

25. Reagan D, Doebbeling R, Pfaller M, Sheetz C, Houston A, Hollis F, Wenzel R. Elimination of coincident Staphylococcus aureus nasal and hand carriage with intranasal application of mupirocin calcium ointment. Annals of Internal Medicine. 1991;114:101

26. Darouiche R, Wright C, Hamill R, Koza M, Lewis D, Markowski J. Eradication of colonization by methicillin-resistant Staphylococcus aureus by using oral minocycline–rifampin and topical mupirocin. Antimicrobial Agents and Chemotherapy. 1991;35:1612

27. Talon D, Rouget C, Cailleaux V, Bailly P, Thouverez M, Barale F, Michel-Briand Y. Nasal carriage of Staphylococcus aureus and cross-contamination in a surgical intensive care unit: efficacy of mupirocin ointment. Journal of Hospital Infection. 1995;30:39

28. Herwaldt L. Staphylococcus aureus nasal carriage and surgical-site infections. Surgery. 2003;134:S2

29. Perl T, Cullen J, Wenzel R, Zimmerman B, Pfaller M, Sheppard D, Twombley J, French P, Herwaldt L, et al. Intranasal mupirocin to prevent postoperative Staphylococcus aureus infections. New England Journal of Medicine. 2002;346:1871

30. Crossley K, Landesman B, Zaske D. An outbreak of infections caused by strains of Staphylococcus aureus resistant to

methicillin and aminoglycosides, II: epidemiologic studies. Journal of Infectious Diseases. 1979;139:280

31. Everett E, McNitt T, Rahm A, Stevens B, Peterson H. Epidemiologic investigations of methicillin-resistant *Staphylococcus aureus* in a burn unit. Military Medicine. 1978;143:165

32. Espersen F, Nielsen P, Lund K, Sylvest B, Jensen K. Hospital-acquired infections in a burn unit caused by an imported strain of *Staphylococcus aureus* with unusual multi-resistance. Journal of Hygiene. 1982;88:535

33. Rutala W, Katz E, Sherertz R, Sarubbi F. Environmental study of a methicillin-resistant *Staphylococcus aureus* epidemic in a burn unit. Journal of Clinical Microbiology. 1983;18:683

34. Bartzokas C, Paton J, Gibson M, Graham F, McLoughlin G, Croton R. Control and eradication of methicillin-resistant *Staphylococcus aureus* on a surgical unit. New England Journal of Medicine. 1984;311:1422

35. Devine J, Cooke R, Wright E. Is methicillin-resistant *Staphylococcus aureus* (MRSA) contamination of ward-based computer terminals a surrogate marker for nosocomial MRSA transmission and handwashing compliance? Journal of Hospital Infection. 2001;48:72

36. Livornese L, Dias S, Samel C, et al. Hospital-acquired infection with vancomycin-resistant *Enterococcus faecium* transmitted by electronic thermometers. Annals of Internal Medicine. 1992;117:112

37. Boyce J, Opal S, Chow J, et al. Outbreak of multi-drug-resistant *Enterococcus faecium* with transferable vanB class vancomycin resistance. Journal of Clinical Microbiology. 1994;32:1148

38. Bonten M, Hayden M, Nathan C, van Voorhis J, Matushek M, Slaughter S, Rice T, Weinstein R. Epidemiology of colonization of patients and environment with vancomycin-resistant enterococci. The Lancet. 1996;348:1615

39. Martinez J, Ruthazer R, Hanjosten K, Barefoot L, Snydman D. Role of environmental contamination as a risk factor for acquisition of vancomycin-resistant enterococci in patients treated in a medical intensive care unit. Archives of Internal Medicine. 2003;163:1905

40. Trick W, Temple R, Chen D, Wright M, Solomon S, Peterson L. Patient colonization and environmental contamination by vancomycin-resistant enterococci in a rehabilitation facility. Archives of Physical Medicine Rehabilitation. 2002;83:899

41. Mayer R, Geha R, Helfand M, Hoyen C, Salata R, Donskey C. Role of fecal incontinence in contamination of the environment with vancomycin-resistant *Enterococci*. American Journal of Infection Control. 2003;31:221

42. Lemmen S, Hafner H, Zolldann D, Stanzel S, Lutticken R. Distribution of multi-resistant Gram-negative versus Gram-positive bacteria in the hospital inanimate environment. Journal of Hospital Infection. 2004;56:191

43. Duckro A, Blom D, Lyle E, Weinstein R, Hayden M. Transfer of vancomycin-resistant enterococci via health care worker hands. Archives of Internal Medicine. 2005;165:302

44. APIC Guideline for Selection and Use of Disinfectants. American Journal of Infection Control. 1996;24:313

45. Larson E, and the Association for Professionals in Infection Control and Epidemiology 1992–1993 and 1994 APIC Guidelines Committee. APIC guideline for handwashing and hand antisepsis in health care settings. American Journal of Infection Control. 1995;23:251

46. Centers for Disease Control and Prevention: Guideline for Hand Hygiene in Health-care Settings. Morbidity and Mortality Weekly Report. 2002;51

47. Sproat L, Inglis T. A multicentre survey of hand hygiene practice in intensive care units. Journal of Hospital Infection. 1994;26:137

48. Lowbury E. Gram-negative bacilli on the skin. British Journal of Dermatology. 1969;81 Suppl 1:55

49. Noble W. Distribution of the Micrococcaceae. British Journal of Dermatology. 1969;81 Suppl 1:27

50. McBride M, Duncan W, Bodey G, McBride C. Microbial skin flora of selected cancer patients and hospital personnel. Journal of Clinical Microbiology. 1976;3:14

51. Casewell M. Role of hands in nosocomial gram-negative infection. In: Maiback HI, Aly R, eds. Skin Microbiology: Relevance to Clinical Infection. New York, NY: Springer-Verlag, 1981

52. Larson E, McGinley K, Foglia A, Talbot G, Leyden J. Composition and antimicrobic resistance of skin flora in hospitalized and healthy adults. Journal of Clinical Microbiology. 1986;23:604

53. Ehrenkranz N, Alfonso B. Failure of bland soap handwash to prevent hand transfer of patient bacteria to urethral catheters. Infection Control and Hospital Epidemiology. 1991;12:604

54. Sanderson P, Weissler S. Recovery of coliforms from the hands of nurses and patients: activities leading to contamination. Journal of Hospital Infections. 1992;21:85

55. Coello R, Jimenez J, Garcia M, et al. Prospective study of infection, colonization and carriage of methicillin-resistant *Staphylococcus aureus* in an outbreak affecting 990 patients. European Journal of Microbiology and Infectious Diseases. 1994;13:74

56. Sanford M, Widmer A, Bale M, Jones R, Wenzel R. Efficient detection and long-term persistence of the carriage of methicillin-resistant *Staphylococcus aureus*. Clinical Infectious Diseases. 1994;19:1123

57. Bertone S, Fisher M, Mortensen J. Quantitative skin cultures at potential catheter sites in neonates. Infection Control and Hospital Epidemiology. 1994;15:315

58. Bonten M, Hayden M, Nathan C, VanVoorhis J, et al. Epidemiology of colonization of patients and environment with vancomycin-resistant enterococci. Lancet. 1995;348:1615

59. Larson E, Cronquist A, Whittier S, Lai L, Lyle C, Della Latta P. Differences in skin flora between inpatients and chronically ill patients. Heart Lung. 2000;29:298

60. Polakoff S, Richards I, Parker M, Lidwell O. Nasal and skin carriage of *Staphylococcus aureus* by patients undergoing surgical operation. Journal of Hygiene. 1967;65:559

61. Larson E, Leyden J, McGinley K, Grove G, Talbot G. Physiologic and microbiologic changes in skin related to frequent handwashing. Infection Control. 1986;7:59

62. Meers P, Yeo G. Shedding of bacteria and skin squames after handwashing. Journal of Hygiene. 1978;81:99

63. Winnefeld M, Richard M, Drancourt M, Grobb J. Skin tolerance and effectiveness of two hand decontamination procedures in everyday hospital use. British Journal of Dermatology. 2000;143:546

64. Maki D, Zilz M, Alvarado C. Evaluation of the antibacterial efficacy of four agents for handwashing. In: Nelson JC, Grassi C, eds. Current Chemotherapy and Infectious Disease Proceedings of the 11th International Congress on Chemotherapy and the 19th ICAAC. Washington DC: American Society for Microbiology, 1979

65. Boyce J, Kelliher S, Vallande N. Skin irritation and dryness associated with two hand-hygiene regimens: soap-and-water handwashing versus hand antisepsis with an alcoholic hand gel. Infection Control and Hospital Epidemiology. 2000;21:442

66. Wade J, Casewell M. The evaluation of residual antimicrobial activity on hands and its clinical relevance. Journal of Hospital Infection 1991;18 Supp B:23

67. Doebbeling B, Stanley G, Sheetz C, Pfaller M, Houston A, Annis L, Li N, Wenzel R. Comparative efficacy of alternative hand-washing agents in reducing nosocomial infections in intensive care units. The New England Journal of Medicine. 1992;327:88

68. Pittet D, Hugonnet S, Harbarth S, Mourouga P, Sauvan V, Touveneau S. Effectiveness of a hospital-wide programme to improve compliance with hand hygiene. Lancet. 2000;356:1307

69. Lund S, Jackson J, Leggett J, Hales L, Dworkin R, Gilbert D. Reality of glove use and handwashing in a community hospital. American Journal of Infection Control. 1994;22:352

70. Meengs M, Giles B, Chisholm C, Cordell W, Nelson D. Hand washing frequency in an emergency department. Annals of Emergency Medicine. 1994;23:1307

71. Mayer J, Dubbert P, Miller M, Burkett P, Chapman S. Increasing handwashing in an intensive care unit. Infection Control. 1986;7:259

72. Preston G, Larson E, Stamm W. The effect of private isolation rooms on patient care practices, colonization and infection in an intensive care unit. American Journal of Medicine. 1981;70:641

73. Kaplan L, McGuckin M. Increasing handwashing compliance with more accessible sinks. Infection Control. 1986;7:408

74. Bischoff W, Reynolds T, Sessler C, Edmond M, Wenzel R. Handwashing compliance by health care workers. The impact of introducing an accessible, alcohol-based hand antiseptic. Archives of Internal Medicine. 2000;160:1017

75. Wurtz R, Moye G, Jovanovic B. Handwashing machines, hand-washing compliance, and potential for cross-contamination. American Journal of Infection Control. 1994;22:228

76. Albert R, Condie F. Hand-washing patterns in medical intensive-care units. New England Journal of Medicine. 1981;304:1465

77. Larson E. Compliance with isolation technique. American Journal of Infection Control. 1983,11.221

78. Donowitz L. Handwashing techniques in a pediatric intensive care unit. American Journal of Diseases of Children. 1987;141:683

79. Conly J, Hill S, Ross J, Lertzman J, Louie T. Handwashing practices in an intensive care unit: the effects of an education program and its relationship to infection rates. American Journal of Infection Control. 1989;17:330

80. DeCarvalho M, Lopes J, Pellitteri M. Frequency and duration of handwashing in a neonatal intensive care unit. Pediatric Infectious Diseases Journal. 1989;8:179

81. Graham M. Frequency and duration of handwashing in an intensive care unit. American Journal of Infection Control. 1990;18:77

82. Dubbert P, Dolce J, Richter W, Miller M, Chapman S. Increasing ICU staff handwashing: effects of education and group feedback. Infection Control and Hospital Epidemiology. 1990;11:191

83. Simmons B, Bryant J, Neiman K, Spencer L, Arheart K. The role of handwashing in prevention of endemic intensive care unit infections. Infection Control and Hospital Epidemiology. 1990;11:589

84. Pettinger A, Nettleman M. Epidemiology of isolation precautions. Infection Control and Hospital Epidemiology. 1991;12:303

85. Lohr J, Ingram D. Dudley S, Lawton E, Donowitz L. Hand washing in pediatric ambulatory settings: an inconsistent practice. American Journal of Diseases of Children 1991;145:1198

86. Raju T, Kobler C. Improving handwashing habits in the newborn nurseries. Am J Med Sci. 1991;302:355

87. Larson E, McGinley K, Foglia A, et al. Handwashing practices and resistance and density of bacterial hand flora on two pediatric units in Lima, Peru. American Journal Infection Control. 1992;20:65

88. Zimakoff J, Stormark M, Larsen S. Use of gloves and handwashing behaviour among health care workers in intensive care units. A multicentre investigation in four hospitals in Denmark and Norway. The Journal of Hospital Infection. 1993;24:63–67

89. Pelke S, Ching D, Easa D, Melish M. Gowning does not affect colonization or infection rates in a neonatal intensive care unit. Archives of Pediatric Adolescent Medicine. 1994;148:24

90. Gould D. Nurses' hand decontamination practice: results of a local study. Journal Hospital of Infection. 1994;28:15

91. Shay D, Maloney S, Montecalvo M, et al. Epidemiology and mortality risk of vancomycin-resistant enterococcal bloodstream infections. Journal of Infectious Diseases. 1995;172:993

92. Berg D, Hershow R, Ramirez C. Control of nosocomial infections in an intensive care unit in Guatemala City. Clinical Infectious Diseases. 1995;21:588

93. Tibbals J. Teaching hospital medical staff to handwash. Medical Journal of Australia. 1996;164:395

94. Slaughter S, Hayden M, Nathan C, et al. A comparison of the effect of universal use of gloves and gowns with that of glove use alone on acquisition of vancomycin-resistant enterococci in a medical intensive care unit. Annals of Internal Medicine. 1996;125:448

95. Dorsey S, Cydulka R, Emerman C. Is handwashing teachable?: failure to improve handwashing behavior in an urban emergency department. Academic Emergency Medicine. 1995;3:360

96. Watanakunakorn C, Wang C, Hazy J. An observational study of hand washing and infection control practices by healthcare workers. Infection Control and Hospital Epidemiology. 1998;19:858

97. Avila-Aguero M, UmaZa M, Jimenez A, Faingezicht I, Paris M. Handwashing practices in a tertiary-care, pediatric hospital and the effect on an education program. Clinical Performance of Quality Health Care. 1998;6:70

98. Kirkland K, Weinstein J. Adverse effects on contact isolation. Lancet. 1999;354:1177

99. Maury E, Alzieu M, Baudel J, et al. Availability of an alcohol solution can improve hand disinfection compliance in an intensive care unit. American Journal of Respiratory Critical Care Medicine. 2000;162:324

100. Muto C, Sistrom M, Farr B. Hand hygiene rates unaffected by installation of dispensers of a rapidly acting hand antiseptic. American Journal of Infection Control. 2000;28:273

101. Kaplan L, McGuckin M. Increasing handwashing compliance with more accessible sinks. Infection Control. 1986;7:408

102. Bischoff W, Reynolds T, Sessler C, Edmond M, Wenzel R. Handwashing compliance by health care workers: The impact of introducing an accessible, alcohol-based hand antiseptic. Archives of Internal Medicine. 2000;160:1017

103. Pittet D, Hugonnet S, Harbarth S, Mourouga P, Sauvan V, Touveneau S, Perneger T, and the members of the Infection Control Programme. Effectiveness of a hospital-wide programme to improve compliance with hand hygiene. The Lancet. 2000;356:1307

104. Doebbeling B, Pfaller M, Houston A, et al. Removal of nosocomial pathogens from the contaminated glove: Implications for glove reuse and handwashing. Annals of Internal Medicine. 1988;109:394

105. Kim P, Roghmann M, Perencevich E, Harris A. Rates of hand disinfection associated with glove use, patient isolation, and changes between exposure to various body sites. American Journal of Infection Control. 2003;31:97

106. Zachary K, Bayne P, Morrison V, Ford D, Silver L, Hooper D. Contamination of gowns, gloves, and stethoscopes with vancomycin-resistant enterococci. Infection Control and Hospital Epidemiology. 2001;22:560

107. Boyce J, Potter-Bynoe G, Chenevert C, King T. Environmental contamination due to methicillin-resistant *Staphylococcus aureus*: possible infection control implications. Infection Control and Hospital Epidemiology. 1997;18:622

108. Boyce J, Chenevert C. Isolation gowns prevent health care workers (HCWs) from contamination their clothing, and possibly their hands, with methicillin-resistant *Staphylococcus aureus* (MRSA) and resistant enterococci. Presented at the 8th Annual Meeting of the Society for Healthcare Epidemiology of America. 1998;Orlando, FL. Abstract S74:52

109. Roman R, Smith J, Walker M, et al. Rapid geographic spread of a methicillin-resistant *Staphylococcus aureus* strain. Clinical Infectious Diseases. 1997;25:698

110. Pelke S, Ching D, Easa D, Melish M. Gowning does not affect colonization or infection rate in a neonatal intensive care unit. Archives of Pediatric and Adolescent Medicine. 1994;148:1016

111. Slaughter S, Hayden M, Nathan C, Hu T, Rice T, Voorhis J, Matushek M, Franklin C, Weinstein R. A comparison of the effect of universal use of gloves and gowns with that of glove

use along on acquisition of vancomycin-resistant Enterococci in a medical intensive care unit. Annals of Internal Medicine. 1996;125:448

112. Trick W, Weinstein R, DeMarais P, Tomaska W, Nathan C, McAllister S, et al. Comparison of routine glove use and contact-isolation precautions to prevent transmission of multidrug-resistant bacteria in a long-term care facility. Journal of the American Geriatrics Society. 2004;52:2003

113. Centers for Disease Control and Prevention. Guidelines for preventing the transmission of *Mycobacterium tuberculosis* in health-care facilities. MMWR Morbidity and Mortality Weekly Report. 1994;43:1

114. HICPAC Guidelines. http://www.cdc.gov/ncidod/hip/ISOLAT/Isolat.htm

115. Centers for Disease Control and Prevention. Campaign to Prevent Antimicrobial Resistance in Healthcare Settings: Why a Campaign? Atlanta, GA: Centers for Disease Control and Prevention, 2001

116. Haley R, Cushion N, Tenover F, et al. Eradication of endemic methicillin-resistant *Staphylococcus aureus* infections from a neonatal intensive care unit. Journal of Infectious Diseases. 1995;171:612

117. Jernigan J, Titus M, Groschel D, Getchell-White S, Farr B. Effectiveness of contact isolation during a hospital outbreak of methicillin-resistant *Staphylococcus aureus*. American Journal of Epidemiology. 1996;143:496

118. Salmenlinna S, Lyytikainen O, Kotilainen P, Scotford R, Siren E, Vuopio-Varkila J. Molecular epidemiology of methicillin-resistant *Staphylococcus aureus* in Finland. European Journal of Clinical Microbiology and Infectious Diseases. 2000;19:101

119. Roberts R, de Lancastre A, Eisner W, et al. Molecular epidemiology of methicillin-resistant *Staphylococcus aureus* in 12 New York hospitals: MRSA collaborative group. Journal of Infectious Diseases. 1998;178:164

120. de Lancaster H, Severina E, Roberts R, Kreiswirth B, Tomasz A. Testing the efficacy of a molecular surveillance network: methicillin-resistant *Staphylococcus aureus* (MRSA) and vancomycin-resistant *Enterococcus faecium* (VREF) genotypes in six hospitals in the metropolitan New York City area. Microbial Drug Resistance. 1996;2:343

121. Villari P, Faullo C, Torre I, Nani E. Molecular characterization of methicillin-resistant *Staphylococcus aureus* (MRSA) in a university hospital in Italy. European Journal of Epidemiology. 1998;14:802

122. Diekema D, Pfaller M, Trunidge J, et al. Genetic relatedness of multidrug-resistant, methicillin-resistant *Staphylococcus aureus* bloodstream isolates: SENTRY antimicrobial resistance surveillance centers worldwide. Microbial Drug Resistance. 2000;6:213

123. Vriens M, Fluit A, Troelstra A, Verhoef J, Van Der Werken C. Are MRSA more contagious than MSSA in a surgical intensive care unit? Infection Control and Hospital Epidemiology. 2002;23:491

124. Dominguez M, De Lencastre H, Linare J, Tomasz A. Spread and maintenance of a dominant methicillin-resistant *Staphylococcus aureus* (MRSA) clone during an outbreak of MRSA disease in a spanish hospital. Journal of Clinical Microbiology. 1994;32:2081

125. Embil J, McLeod J, Al-Barrak A, Thompson G, Aoki F, Witwicki E, Stranc M, Kabani A, Nicoll D, Nicolle L. An outbreak of methicillin-resistant *Staphylococcus aureus* on a burn unit: potential role of contaminated hydrotherapy equipment. Burns. 2001;27:681

126. Spindel S, Strausbaugh L, Jacobsen C. Infections caused by *Staphylococcus aureus* in a veteran's affairs nursing home care unit: a 5-year experience. Infection Control and Hospital Epidemiology. 1995;16:217

127. Boyce J, Mermel L, Zervos M, et al. Controlling vancomycin-resistant enterococci. Infection Control and Hospital Epidemiology. 1995;16:634

128. Boyce J, Opal S, Chow J, et al. Outbreak of multi-drug resistant *Enterococci faecium* with transferable vanB class vancomycin resistance. Journal of Clinical Microbiology. 1994;32:1148

129. Clark N, Cooksey B, Hille B, Swenson J, Tenover F. Characterization of glycopeptide-resistant enterococci from U.S. Hospitals. Antimicrobial Agents and Chemotherapy. 1993;37:2311

130. Handwerger S, Raucher B, altarac D, et al. Nosocomial outbreak due to *Enterococcus faecium* highly resistant to vancomycin, penicillin, and gentamicin. Clinical Infectious Diseases. 1993;16:750

131. Livornese L, Dias S, Romanowski B, et al. Hospital-acquired infection with vancomycin-resistant *Enterococcus faecium* transmitted by electronic thermometers. Annals of Internal Medicine. 1992;117:112

132. Kim W, Weinstein R, Hayden M. The changing molecular epidemiology and establishment of endemicity of vancomycin resistance in enterococci at one hospital over a 6-year period. Journal of Infectious Diseases. 1999;179:163

133. Moreno R, Grota P, Crisp C, et al. Clinical and molecular epidemiology of vancomycin-resistant *Enterococcus faecium* during its emergence in a city in Southern Texas. Clinical Infectious Diseases. 1995;21:1234

134. Byers K, Anglim A, Anneski C, et al. A hospital epidemic of vancomycin-resistant enterococcus: risk factors and control. Infection Control and Hospital Epidemiology. 2001;22:140

135. Falk P, Winnike J, Woodmansee C, Desai M, Mayhall G. Outbreak of vancomycin-resistant Enterococci in a burn unit. Infection Control and Hospital Epidemiology. 2000;21:575

136. Montecalvo M, Horowitz H, Gedris C, Carbonaro C, Tenover F, Issah A, Cook P, Wormser G. Outbreak of vancomycin-, ampicillin-, and aminoglycoside-resistant *Enterococcus faecium* bacteremia in an adult oncology unit. Antimicrobial Agents and Chemotherapy. 1994;38:1363

137. Duerden M, Bergeron J, Baker R, Braddom R. Controlling the spread of vancomycin-resistant enterococci with a rehabilitation cohort unit. Archives of Physical Medicine and Rehabilitation. 1997;78:553

138. Farr B. Prevention and control of methicillin-resistant *Staphylococcus aureus* infections. Current Opinion in Infectious Diseases. 2004;17:317

139. Saiman L, Cronquist A, Wu F, Zhou J, Rubenstein D, Eisner W, Kreiswirth B, Della-Latta P. An outbreak of methicillin-resistant *Staphylococcus aureus* in a neonatal intensive care unit. Infection Control and Hospital Epidemiology. 2003;24:317

140. Graham P, Morel A-S, Zhou J, Wu F, Della-Latta P, Rubenstein D, Saiman L. Epidemiology of methicillin-susceptible *Staphylococcus aureus* in the neonatal intensive care unit. Infection Control and Hospital Epidemiology. 2002;23:677

141. Hartstein A, Denny M, Morthland V, LeMonte A, Pfaller M. Control of methicillin-resistant *Staphylococcus aureus* in a hospital and an intensive care unit. Infection Control and Hospital Epidemiology. 1995;16:405

142. Richet H, Wiesel M, Le Gallou F, Andre-Richet B, Espaze E, et al. Methicillin-resistant *Staphylococcus aureus* control in hospitals: the French experience. Infection Control and Hospital Epidemiology. 1996;17:509

143. Muto C, Jernigan J, Ostrowsky B, Richet H, Jarvis W, Boyce J, Farr B. SHEA guideline for preventing nosocomial transmission of multidrug-resistant strains of *Staphylococcus aureus* and *Enterococcus*. Infection Control and Hospital Epidemiology. 2003;24:362

144. Troillet N, Carmeli Y, Samore M, et al. Carriage of methicillin-resistant *Staphylococcus aureus* at hospital admission. Infection Control and Hospital Epidemiology. 1998;19:181

145. Muto C, Cage E, Durbin L, Simonton B, Farr B. The utility of culturing patients on admission transferred from other health care facilities for methicillin-resistant *Staphylococcus aureus* (MRSA). Ninth Annual Meeting of the Society for Health Epidemiology of America. 1999;San Francisco, CA. Abstract M33:67

146. Nouer A, Araujo A, Chebabo A, Cardoso F, Pinto M, Hospital Universitario Universidade Federal do Rio de Janeiro. Control of methicillin-resistant *Staphylococcus aureus* (MRSA) in an intensive care unit after the institution of routine screening. Presented at 42nd General Meeting of the Interscience Conference on Antimicrobial Agents and Chemotherapy. 2002;San Francisco, CA. Abstract K-98

147. Calfee D, Giannetta E, Durbin L, Farr B. The increasing prevalence of MRSA and VRE colonization among patients transferred from primary and secondary health care facilities. Presented at the 11th Annual Meeting of the Society for Healthcare Epidemiology of America. 2001;Toronto, ON, Canada. Abstract 171

148. Muto C, Cage E, Durbin L, Simonton B, Farr B. The utility of culturing patients on admission transferred from other hospitals or nursing homes for vancomycin resistant Enterococcus (VRE). Presented at the 35th Annual Meeting of the Infectious Diseases Society of America. 1998;Denver, CO. Abstract

149. Back N, Linnemann C, Staneck J, Kotagal U. Control of methicillin-resistant *Staphylococcus aureus* in a neonatal intensive-care unit: use of intensive microbiologic surveillance and mupirocin. Infection Control and Hospital Epidemiology. 1996;17:227

150. Calfee D, Farr B. Infection control and cost control in the era of managed care. Infection Control and Hospital Epidemiology. 2002;223:407

151. Rupp M, Marion N, Fey P, et al. Outbreak of vancomycin-resistant *Enterococcus faecium* in a neonatal intensive care unit. Infection Control and Hospital Epidemiology. 2001;22:301

152. Price C, Paule S, Noskin G, Peterson L. Active surveillance reduces vancomycin-resistant enterococci (VRE) bloodstream isolates. Presented at the 39th Annual Meeting of the Infectious Diseases Society of America. 2001;San Francisco, CA. Abstract 212:75

153. Siddiqui A, Harris A, Hebden J, Wilson P, Morris J, Roghmann M. The effect of active surveillance for vancomycin resistant enterococci in high risk units on vancomycin resistant enterococci incidence hospital-wide. American Journal of Infection Control. 2002;30:40

154. Calfee D, Giannetta E, Farr B. Effective control of VRE colonization using CDC recommendations for detection and isolation. Presented at the 38th Annual Meeting of the Infectious Diseases Society of America. 2000;New Orleans, LA. Abstract 21:44

155. Cantey J, Rhoton B, Southgate W, Snyder C. Control of spread of methicillin resistant *Staphylococcus aureus* in a neonatal ICU. Presented at the 12th Annual Meeting of the Society for Healthcare Epidemiology of America. 2002;Salt Lake City, UT. Abstract 36:49

156. Muto C, Giannetta E, Durbin L, Simonton B, Farr B. Cost effectiveness of perirectal surveillance cultures for controlling vancomycin-resistant enterococcus. Infection Control and Hospital Epidemiology. 2002;23:429

157. Cooper B, Medley G, Stone T, Duckworth G, Kibbler C, Lai R, et al. Systematic review of isolation policies in the hospital management of methicillin resistant *Staphylococcus aureus*: a review of the literature with epidemiological and economic modeling. Health Technology Assessment. 2003;7

158. Cepeda J, Whitehouse T, Cooper B, Heails J, Jones K, Kwaku F, et al. Isolation of patients in single rooms or cohorts to reduce spread of MRSA in intensive-care units: prospective two-centre study. The Lancet. 2005;365:295

159. Evans H, Shaffer M, Hughes M, Smith R, Chong T, Raymond D, et al. Contact isolation in surgical patients: A barrier to care? Surgery. 2003;134:180

160. Stelfox H, Bates D, Redelmeier D. Safety of Patients Isolated for Infection Control. JAMA. 2003;290:1899

161. Saint S, Higgins L, Nalamothu B, Chenoweth C, Arbor A. Do physicians examine patients in contact isolation less frequently? A brief report. American Journal of Infection Control. 2003;31:354

162. Tarzi S, Kennedy P, Stone S, Evans M. Methicillin-resistant *Staphylococcus aureus*: psychological impact of hospitalization and isolation in an older adult population. Journal of Hospital Infection. 2001;49:250

163. Catalano G, Houston S, Catalano M, Butera A, Jennings S, Hakala S, et al. Anxiety and depression in hospitalized patients in resistant organism isolation. Southern Medical Journal. 2003;96:141

164. Harbarth S, Samore MH, Lichtenberg D, Carmeli Y. Prolonged antibiotic prophylaxis after cardiovascular surgery and its effects on surgical site infections and antimicrobial resistance. Circulation. 2000;101:2916

165. de Man P, Verhoeven B, Verbrugh H, et al. An antibiotic policy to prevent emergence of resistant bacilli. Lancet. 2000;355:973

166. Donskey C, Chowdhry T, Hecker M, et al. Effect of antibiotic therapy on the density of vancomycin-resistant enterococci in the stool of colonized patients. New England Journal of Medicine. 2000;343:1925

167. Harbarth S, Liassine N, Charan S, et al. Risk factors for persistent carriage of methicillin-resistant *Staphylococcus aureus*. Clinical Infectious Diseases. 2000;31:1380

168. Crowcroft N, Ronveaux O, Monnet D, Mertens R. Methicillin-resistant *Staphylococcus aureus* and antimicrobial use in Belgian hospitals. Infection Control and Hospital Epidemiology. 1999;20:31

Chapter 89
Controlling the Spread of Resistant Pathogens in the Intensive Care Unit

David K. Henderson

1 Overview

As is detailed carefully throughout this text, the issue of antimicrobial resistance has surfaced as a major challenge to modern medicine in the twentieth and twenty-first centuries. The problems presented by burgeoning antimicrobial resistance are magnified in the highly technical environment of the modern intensive care unit (ICU). Modern medicine has allowed practitioners to treat diseases heretofore considered beyond therapy. Nonetheless, some of these aggressive therapies are associated with prolonged periods of profound immunosuppression and require increasingly invasive interventions. Patients in ICU frequently develop nosocomial infections and such infections are often severe, difficult to treat, and at substantial risk for recurrence. With multiple exposures to antimicrobial agents, high levels of microbial colonization with nosocomial pathogens, and prolonged immunosuppression, such patients are at extraordinarily high risk for the development of infection with resistant pathogens (1). Some of the most aggressive, resistant pathogens have become endemic in hospital environments, and many of these pathogens have established residence in ICUs (2–4). Examples of such emerging pathogens are methicillin-resistant Staphylococci – both *Staphylococcus aureus* (MRSA) and coagulase-negative Staphylococci – and the vancomycin-resistant enterococcus (VRE). The subsequent identification of methicillin-resistant Staphylococci that have acquired resistance to vancomycin as a result of transfer of genetic material from the vancomycin-resistant enterococcus (5–7) has made controlling the spread of these organisms in the ICU environment even more important. Additionally, resistant Gram-negative pathogens, such as *Acinetobacter baumannii* (8–12), as well as resistant strains of *Pseudomonas aeruginosa* (9, 13–19) and *Stenotrophomonas maltophilia* (10, 16, 20) can establish endemic residence in

the ICU and can result in clustered infections and unnecessary morbidity and mortality.

This chapter discusses the special issues relating to the ICU and its environment that make antimicrobial resistance a major problem confronting critical care clinicians. The chapter addresses: (1) reservoirs of infection in the ICU; (2) some of the most common and most problematic "infectious syndromes encountered by intensivists; 3) a few of the most perplexing resistant pathogens of special interest to ICU clinicians, and (4) approaches to the prevention of infections caused by these resistant pathogens in the ICU environment.

2 Reservoirs

The nosocomial reservoirs for resistant organisms often vary by the pathogen and the clinical setting. Organisms can be spread from person to person from the hands of healthcare workers. They can be carried chronically in the anterior nares of patients or providers, or in the fecal flora of patients. Staphylococci are often carried on the skin and mucous membranes of staff and patients (21). Staphylococci may colonize several sites on the body, including the face, hands, axillae, and groin; however, their primary reservoir is the epithelium of the anterior nares (22). Patients who are colonized and/or infected with resistant Staphylococci serve as the most likely reservoir for the spread of these organisms within healthcare institutions (23). Studies from as recently as 2 years ago suggest that 30–60% of healthy adults carry *S. aureus* and further suggest that 10–20% of these individuals are chronically colonized (24, 25). Many patients are identified as nasal carriers of *S. aureus* – including the carriage of methicillin-resistant strains – at the time of hospital admission (26, 27). By no means are healthcare workers immune to this phenomenon. Studies suggest that the rate of *S. aureus* carriage among healthcare workers and hospital staff may be quite problematic (28–30), with as many as 6% of healthcare workers carrying methicillin-resistant Staphylococci in their anterior nares in some studies.

D.K. Henderson (✉)
Clinical Center, National Institutes of Health, Bethesda, MD, USA
dkh@nih.gov

D.L. Mayers (ed.), *Antimicrobial Drug Resistance*,
DOI 10.1007/978-1-60327-595-8_89, © Humana Press, a part of Springer Science+Business Media, LLC 2009

The primary route of MRSA transmission within the hospital appears to be from patient to patient, with healthcare workers the likely vector carrying the organisms on their hands. In addition, some studies have suggested that resistant Staphylococci can establish an inanimate environmental reservoir and can persist on contaminated objects in the environment. When these objects are used on subsequent patients, they may serve as vehicles of transmission for the resistant pathogens – either as a result of the patient having direct contact with the contaminated objects or a healthcare worker handling the object and then touching the patient (31–33). Some respected investigators believe that environmental or fomite spread may be substantially underestimated as a potential nosocomial route of transmission of resistant Staphylococci.

2.1 Fecal and Cutaneous Flora

Some pathogens (e.g., *Clostridium difficile, Enterococcus faecium*, resistant Enterobacteriaceae, etc.) can be carried in the fecal flora of both patients and staff. In many instances, these organisms are literally overwhelmed by the remaining fecal flora and cause little problem until some factor causes the organism to gain a selective advantage in the fecal flora (e.g., the administration of antimicrobial agents to which the majority of the fecal flora – and especially the fecal anaerobes – are susceptible, but to which the pathogen is not). Similarly, organisms can be carried as part of the cutaneous flora, causing few problems, until the normal flora are influenced by external forces, such as antimicrobial agents. In the ICU environment, the flora of the hands of healthcare providers represents a major risk for transmission to highly susceptible patients. Resistant organisms may establish either transient or more permanent residence as part of the cutaneous flora of the hands of healthcare workers. In the absence of appropriate hand hygiene, such organisms may be spread with facility from patient to patient. Similarly, patients or visitors may spread such organisms as a result of their carriage of these pathogens.

2.2 The Inanimate Environment

Certain organisms have a proclivity for establishing reservoirs in the inanimate environment in healthcare settings. Many such organisms find moist places in the environment and establish residence. Examples include *Stenotrophomonas maltophilia*, several species of Pseudomonas, *C. difficile*, and several others, including many aerobic Gram-negative rods. These organisms often have extremely limited nutritional requirements and can survive even reasonably harsh conditions in the environment. Such organisms, once established in a reservoir, may cause recurring clustered infections in an ICU environment. In some situations, identifying the reservoir may be extremely difficult (34). The inanimate environment of the ICU contains several loci that can, in the absence of attention to the details of cleaning and infection control, present a formidable problem for detection.

3 Major Infectious Disease Syndromes Commonly Encountered in the ICU

Whereas virtually any infectious syndrome may occur in patients hospitalized in the ICU, several syndromes are worthy of special mention because of the frequency with which they occur as well as the frequency with which these syndromes are associated with resistant pathogens. In particular, to be able to implement strategies to prevent these syndromes, providers must understand the pathogenetic mechanisms responsible for their occurrence. The syndromes I have chosen to highlight as deserving of special attention are device-associated bacteremia, ventilator-associated pneumonia, and sepsis (usually arising from the gastrointestinal tract) in immunosuppressed patients. The intensivist must be particularly attuned to the pathogenetic mechanisms associated with the occurrence of all of these infectious syndromes in the ICU patient population, as well as the factors that increase the likelihood that these infections will be caused by resistant organisms.

Most, if not all, of these syndromes are by-products of medical progress. We are now able to keep patients alive longer (and therefore at risk for these infectious syndromes) through the use of aggressive chemo- and immunotherapies, sophisticated life-support devices, and other invasive diagnostic and therapeutic approaches. Use of each drug or device is associated with increased risks for complications, including infection. Seriously ill patients in the ICU often sustain repeated bouts of infection and are therefore exposed to multiple courses of antibacterial, antiviral, and antifungal agents. With inadequate host defenses and multiple invasive devices in place, these patients are essentially incubators for microbial resistance.

3.1 Device-Associated Bacteremia

The occurrence of device-associated bacteremia in patients hospitalized in an ICU has become extraordinarily commonplace. Microorganisms can reach the circulation via three separate pathways along an intravascular catheter: at the catheter insertion site; along hubs (35, 36), junctions, and connectors; and via intrinsic or extrinsic contamination of the infusion fluid. Insertion site colonization and infection is facilitated by conditions that favor the growth and proliferation of skin flora, thereby facilitating the migration of organisms from the skin surface along the catheter insertion tract. This migration is facilitated by capillary action. Contamination may occur at the time of insertion or days later. This type of contamination will most commonly result in colonization along the external surface of catheter and is facilitated by fibrin sheath/platelet deposition on the external catheter surface and organism-produced biofilm at the catheter surface in the circulatory channel.

The skin flora of hospitalized patients quickly changes during hospitalization. In instances in which resistant pathogens are endemic in the ICU, these organisms often quickly become part of the patient's cutaneous flora. Simply as a result of being present in the ICU environment, the patient's normal skin flora may be replaced by resistant pathogens, including Staphylococci (including MRSA), other pathogens endemic to the ICU, and VRE. The source of these new florae may be the patient, a provider, or the inanimate environment of the ICU.

Similarly, for contamination introduced into the system via the catheter hub, the catheter's junctions and connectors, the resident skin flora are the most common pathogens producing device-associated infection. Again, the source of these organisms may be the patient, a healthcare provider, or the ICU environment. These organisms are introduced into the system at the time the device is being manipulated. This pathway is more likely to produce colonization of the catheter lumen. Because infection is introduced as the device is being manipulated, this route of infection becomes increasingly important as a source of infection as the duration of catheterization increases. The likelihood of contamination and colonization may relate to the design of the device, and also will be facilitated by fibrin sheath production, platelet deposition, and or biofilm development on the catheter surface.

Contamination introduced via the infusion fluid itself occurs less commonly. Such contamination may be intrinsic (i.e., due to contamination during manufacture or processing) or extrinsic (i.e., contamination introduced at the time the fluid is hung or at the time additives are injected into the container).

3.2 Ventilator-Associated Pneumonia

The reservoir for ventilator-associated pneumonia is again most commonly the patient's own oropharyngeal flora. Patients' oral flora change quickly, often in critically ill patients within 24 h of hospitalization, from the normal, primarily anaerobic flora to an oral flora that is predominantly S. aureus and aerobic Gram-negative rods. When the patient is intubated and placed on a ventilator, the risk for pulmonary infection increases dramatically. The endotracheal tube itself contributes to this risk. Direct inoculation through the respiratory apparatus may occur, either as a result of cross-contamination or from breaks in sterile technique.

The inner lumen of an endotracheal tube also rapidly develops a biofilm containing microorganisms (37, 38), such as aerobic Gram-negative rods and S. aureus, at very high concentrations. This biofilm can be inoculated directly into the lower respiratory tract either by ventilatory flow or by inserting suction catheters through the tube and producing infectious emboli (39, 40). Additionally, in the critically ill, supine, ventilated patient, oral secretions pool in the oropharynx and subglottic space above the tracheal tube cuff, forming a reservoir of secretions contaminated with the altered flora (39, 40). Leakage of pooled secretions around the cuff occurs almost uniformly in these patients.

If the patient has a nasotracheal tube or has had a nasogastric tube inserted, the risk of nosocomial sinusitis is increased. In a patient with a substantially altered mental status, such sinus infections often are unsuspected and undiagnosed. Predominant pathogens for these sinus infections are aerobic Gram-negative rods. More importantly, the development of nosocomial sinusitis increases the risk of ventilator-associated pneumonia by a factor of 4 (41).

The positioning of the patient is also associated with risk for ventilator-associated pneumonia. Aspiration of gastric contents occurs 4 times more frequently when the patient is in the supine position than when the head of the patient's bed is elevated at a 45° angle (42). Isolation of the same organisms from the stomach, pharynx, and endobronchial samples occurred in 32% of semirecumbent patients in one study, compared to 68% of patients in the supine position (43). Unfortunately, gastric reflux occurs irrespective of body position in mechanically ventilated patients who have nasogastric tubes.

Often, ventilated patients are placed on histamine-2 receptor blockers to decrease gastric acidity and reduce the risk for gastric hemorrhage. Decreased gastric acidity (which is clearly appropriate for ventilated patients) increases the rate of gastric colonization. Both histamine-2 receptor blockers and sucralfate increase the gastric pH and, therefore, also increase the level of gastric colonization.

Enteral feedings (often administered to such patients) also increase the risk for gastric colonization with Gram-negative bacilli. The use of either continuous or intermittent enteral feeding increases gastric pH and is associated with an 80% risk for Gram-negative colonization of the stomach (44). Conversely, the maintenance of adequate nutritional status is clearly associated with a reduced risk for ventilator-associated pneumonia, and enteral nutrition is clearly the route of choice for these patients. In instances in which patients in the ICU have received multiple courses of empiric and/or therapeutic antimicrobials, the likelihood that the organism colonizing the stomach is a multiresistant pathogen is increased substantially.

3.3 Sepsis in Immunosuppressed Patients in the ICU

Immunosuppressed patients lack many of the normal physical barriers to infection that immunocompetent patients have. Often, the immunosuppressed patient has disorders of skin and/or mucous membrane integrity that serve as portals for entry for pathogens. The normal process of skin desquamation comes to a halt during radiation or chemotherapy, the skin becomes dry, and the normal pH and skin temperature may be lowered. All these changes facilitate colonization with nosocomial pathogens. Again, in instances in which patients in the ICU have been exposed to multiple courses of antimicrobials, the likelihood that the organism colonizing the skin is a multiresistant pathogen (e.g., MRSA, VRE, *Acinetobacter baumannii*) is increased substantially. With respect to the patient's mucous membranes, substantial inflammation (mucositis) is extremely common during chemotherapy or radiation. Following irradiation and/or chemotherapy, the mucous membranes secrete the proinflammatory cytokines interleukin-1 and tumor necrosis factor-alpha (45). Following therapy, patients' mucous membranes experience accelerated apoptosis without cell renewal, ultimately resulting in an ulcerative phase that is perpetuated by interaction among the dead and dying tissues with the local nosocomially acquired oropharyngeal microflora and their products. This ulcerative phase is followed by a healing phase that restores the integrity of the mucous membrane barrier. Similarly, lesions may develop in the patient's gastrointestinal tract, which permit entry of gastrointestinal flora to the circulation. Additionally, the administration of antimicrobials may facilitate colonization of the gut with resistant pathogens. Additional possible portals of entry for resistant nosocomial pathogens include the respiratory tract, the genitourinary tract (particularly if the tract has been instrumented), and a variety of others.

Patients receiving aggressive chemotherapy also develop deficits in both the nonspecific and specific aspects of immunity. With respect to so-called nonspecific immunity, such patients develop granulocytopenia; in addition, the reduced number of granulocytes they have do not work well. With respect to specific immunity, both the cellular and humoral aspects are transiently damaged and dysfunctional. T-cell "help" is deficient and patients on long-term treatment may even develop hypogammaglobulinemia.

For all of these reasons, these patients are at extreme risk for infection. Pathogens causing infections in these patients may originate from the patient's endogenous flora, from the hands of their providers, from the hands of their healthcare providers, from fomites and equipment, from the inanimate healthcare environment, and even from the air. As rough approximations, about 80% of bacterial pathogens causing infection in neutropenic patients originate from patients' endogenous flora, and approximately half of the patients' endogenous microbial flora is acquired nosocomially. For the reasons noted above, the normal flora of the oropharynx, the skin, and the lower gastrointestinal tract are perturbed, and, particularly because of the frequent exposures to broad-spectrum antimicrobials, resistant organisms play an increasingly important role in colonization and infection in this setting. Resistant pathogens frequently encountered in the ICU causing these infections include MRSA, VRE, resistant strains of *Klebsiella/Enterobacter/Serratia*, resistant strains of *Pseudomonas aeruginosa, Stenotrophomonas maltophilia,* and multiresistant strains of *Acinetobacter*, including *A. baumannii*.

4 Resistant Pathogens of Particular Interest to ICU Staff

Certain resistant pathogens are worthy of special mention as particularly problematic for patients hospitalized in the ICU. Whereas virtually all bacterial, viral, and fungal pathogens can present problems for patients hospitalized in the ICU, four bacterial pathogens have emerged as particularly challenging for critical care staff in the past two decades. The pathogens that have emerged as particularly problematic for the ICU are methicillin-resistant Staphylococci, as well as the vancomycin-resistant enterococcus, *Clostridium difficile*, and *Acinetobacter baumannii*. ICU infections associated with each of these pathogens will be discussed in more detail.

4.1 Methicillin-Resistant Staphylococcus aureus

Resistant *S. aureus* organisms are often spread to patients from the hands of healthcare workers; these organisms may be acquired from an infected or colonized patient and then transferred to another patient in instances in which hand hygiene procedures are inadequate to remove the organisms. The ICU environment, with its attendant urgencies and immediacy of care, is an ideal environment for this kind of spread. Thus, over the past three decades, resistant Staphylococci have become predominant pathogens in the

ICU (23). As noted above, resistant Staphylococci can also establish transient residence on objects in the environment and be spread from these objects to patients, often via the healthcare workers' hands (31–33). Since Staphylococci are primarily considered skin and nare colonizers, environmental or fomite spread of resistant Staphylococci may be substantially underestimated as a route of nosocomial transmission.

Resistant Staphylococci, as is the case for the relatively susceptible Staphylococcal organisms, possess essentially the same number of toxins and virulence factors and, hence, are aggressive human pathogens capable of producing significant infections in even immunologically normal patients. In the ICU setting, MRSA are primarily encountered as pathogens causing skin and soft tissue infections, wound infections, device-associated bacteremias, and, somewhat less frequently, pulmonary infection. The propensity for MRSA to cause device-associated bacteremias is well established. Though somewhat controversial, some investigators believe that such infections can be more virulent than other Staphylococcal bacteremias, may be more difficult to treat, and may have more long-term sequelae. Several studies have demonstrated that resistant Staphylococcal infections are associated with prolonged hospitalization and increased costs of hospitalization (46–51).

In terms of treatment of MRSA infections, the critical care practitioner has several options. Antimicrobial selection for MRSA infections should be governed by disease severity, susceptibility patterns, clinical response to therapy, and cost. Current therapeutic options include vancomycin, linezolid, the cyclic lipopeptide, Daptomycin, Syncercid (quinupristin/dalfopristin), and tigecycline. Tigecycline has been used successfully as salvage therapy for instances of linezolid failure (52). In addition, one small series of tigecycline successes when used as primary therapy for deep-seated MRSA infections has been described (53). An occasionally overlooked, but nonetheless important, therapeutic intervention for resistant Staphylococcal infections is assuring adequate drainage of purulent fluid collections.

A major concern on the horizon is the acquisition of further antimicrobial resistance by MRSA. A great deal of concern has been expressed about the development of vancomycin resistance in some isolates of *S. aureus*. *S aureus* isolates possessing intermediate resistance to vancomycin were first isolated from a hospitalized patient in Japan (54). Four subsequent cases were identified in the United States (55–57). Each of these patients had had prior extensive exposure to vancomycin and developed mutant organisms that had substantially thickened cell walls, thereby producing relative resistance to vancomycin. The development of strains that were completely resistant to vancomycin seemed inevitable. Indeed, although the transfer of VanA resistance from VRE to MRSA was first accomplished in a laboratory experiment (58), several clinical isolates of MRSA that have acquired

the enterococcal VanA gene have now been recovered from patients in the US (5–7, 59).

4.2 Vancomycin-Resistant Enterococcus

The Vancomycin-resistant enterococcus (VRE) was first detected in Europe as early as 1987, but its appearance was preceded by substantial resistance to other antimicrobials (e.g., resistances to β-lactam antibiotics, such as ampicillin, as well as extremely high-level resistance to aminoglycosides) among enterococcal isolates. Epidemiologically, these isolates are interesting in that there are substantial geographical differences in the epidemiology when one compares North American and European isolates. Whereas VRE are prevalent in both European livestock and healthy people, it is less of a nosocomial pathogen in Europe. Conversely, VRE is predominantly a healthcare-associated pathogen in the US, for which no community reservoir has been identified. In Europe, VRE is only just now becoming an important healthcare-associated pathogen. Until the past 2 years, the outbreaks of VRE infection that had occurred in European institutions had been sporadic and had been associated with few serious infections. The striking prevalence of vancomycin resistance among enterococcal isolates in Europe is thought to be due to the widespread use of a related glycopeptide compound, avoparcin, as a growth-promoting agent in animal husbandry.

In North America, VRE is a significant nosocomial pathogen. Colonization with VRE is becoming increasingly common in the ICU, especially among chronically ill, critically ill, and immunocompromised patients who have received multiple courses of broad-spectrum antimicrobials. Because the organism can be carried on healthcare workers' hands and because it survives well in the inanimate environment, cross-transmission in the complex ICU environment has become a substantial problem over the past decade. Patients in ICU are virtually an ideal substrate for VRE – often severely immunosuppressed – frequently encountering intercurrent infections, often requiring broad-spectrum antimicrobial therapy, and often hospitalized for extended periods of time.

In U.S. hospitals, and particularly in U.S. ICUs, the inanimate environment is likely a significant source of VRE transmission. Hayden and colleagues demonstrated that VRE was highly prevalent in the inanimate environment in their ICU and also subsequently demonstrated that reducing environmental contamination had a statistically significant effect on the spread of VRE in their ICU (60). As discussed elsewhere in this text, the increasing use of vancomycin (in great measure to treat infections resulting from the increasing prevalence of MRSA in U.S. healthcare institutions) has likely applied substantial antimicrobial pressure on enterococcal isolates from patients in U.S. ICUs, as well. To date, to my knowledge, no community reservoir for VRE has been identified in the US.

Some microorganisms produce glycopeptide compounds spontaneously and, of necessity, have resistance mechanisms "built in" to prevent auto-destruction. The possibility exists that the gene responsible for vancomycin resistance in enterococci may have initially come from one of these unusual microorganisms and then transmitted to the enterococcus, with subsequent selection of the resistant isolates resulting, at least in part, from the incredible pressure of antimicrobials administered to many chronically and critically ill patients in ICUs in the US (61).

Unlike the MRSA, the enterococcus is not a terribly aggressive pathogen. Nonetheless, owing to the dramatically immunosuppressed state of many twenty-first century critically ill patients, the frequency with which patients in ICU receive multiple courses of broad-spectrum antimicrobials, and the extent to which such patients are exposed to invasive techniques, these pathogens have become extremely common ICU pathogens, particularly in tertiary referral centers. By 1993, the prevalence of VRE had increased 20-fold in the ICUs of U.S. hospitals participating in the National Nosocomial Infections Study (NNIS) (62); however, a more recent publication suggests that the prevalence of VRE in NNIS ICUs had reached a plateau at approximately 28% (63).

Treatment of VRE infection remains difficult, although newer agents are becoming available. Agents currently marketed with efficacy against VRE include the streptogramins (e.g., synercid [quinupristin-dalfopristin]), oxazolidinone, linezolid, and the recently marketed glycylglycine agent, tigecycline. Whereas both synercid and linezolid have been shown to be relatively safe and effective, they are only bacteriostatic against enterococci (64), and VRE isolates resistant to each of these agents have been recovered. Whereas in vitro data evaluating tigecycline against VRE appear promising, clinical data have not yet been accumulated to demonstrate its clinical efficacy against VRE.

In terms of agents on the immediate horizon, daptomycin, a lipopeptide agent, has in vitro activity and is bactericidal against enterococci. To date, we have only limited clinical data about the efficacy of this agent in the treatment of serious VRE infections. Other agents in clinical trials include ramoplanin (a glycolipodepsipeptide), dalbavancin, and oritavancin (both glycopeptide antimicrobials) (65).

4.3 Resurgent C. difficile Enterocolitis

Antimicrobial-associated diarrhea is among the most frequent side effects resulting from antimicrobial therapy. C. difficile enterocolitis (initially described as "clindamycin-associated colitis") (66, 67) is an extremely common sequela of broad-spectrum antimicrobial therapy. Approximately 3% of healthy adults (68) and 14–40% of hospitalized patients are colonized with C. difficile (usually in the metabolically inactive spore form) (69–72). Historically, two toxins, A and B, are primarily involved in the pathogenesis of C. difficile-associated disease; however, recently a "binary toxin" has been recovered from approximately 6% of clinical isolates (73–80). The role of the "binary toxin" is uncertain, but in other Clostridial species, it is a significant virulence factor. In the past 3 years, we have observed a dramatic resurgence of C. difficile-associated disease, with both the rate of occurrence and the severity of the disease increasing in the United States (69, 73–81). In fact, data from the National Center for Health Statistics data suggest that the rate of C. difficile-associated infections in U.S. hospitals increased by 26% in 2001 (76). Further, the increase in disease that has been seen has been associated with a strain that has increased virulence as well as fluoroquinolone resistance. The increased virulence has included higher rates than anticipated of toxic megacolon, leukemoid reactions, severe hypoalbuminemia, colectomy, shock, and death (81). Several outbreaks of C. difficile-associated disease have occurred at large hospitals in the US and Canada over the past 6 years. Many, if not most, outbreaks of CDAD that have occurred were caused by a single strain that has been present in U.S. hospitals for more than 20 years. Curiously, until recently this strain has not been a cause of outbreaks. Although not a "new" strain, this organism may have gained a selective advantage due to the increasing use of fluoroquinolones (76). The strain also contains a mutated tcdC gene; this gene is thought to be responsible for "downregulation" of toxin production. Thus, the mutated gene may be less effective at downregulating toxin A and B production, resulting in increased levels of toxin production (76). Because of C. difficile's remarkable ability to persist in the environment, its resistance (at least in its spore form) to standard cleaning and disinfecting agents, and the substantial antimicrobial agent use among patients hospitalized in intensive care units, C. difficile has become one of the most challenging ICU pathogens to control.

4.4 Multiply Resistant A. baumannii

Another organism that has become a formidable problem for intensivists is the strictly aerobic, nonfermenting, Gram-negative coccobacillary rod known as A. baumannii. The organism we now know as A. baumannii has had a confusing taxonomic journey, having at one time or another in the not-so-distant past been classified in the following genera of microorganisms: Bacterium, Moraxella, Herellea, Mima, Achromobacter, and Alcaligenes (82). Some investigators even believed that these organisms were closely related to the Neisseriae. Differential biochemical and growth tests can now be used to identify 19 distinct species in the genus *Acinetobacter* and DNA hybridization studies suggest that there may be as many as 25. *A. baumannii*, perhaps the best known organism of this genus, has become a significant, emerging cause of healthcare-associated infections worldwide, and is a particular problem in both surgical and medical ICUs. *A. baumannii* has been estimated to be responsible for 2–10% of all Gram-negative infections in ICUs in both US and Europe (83). *A. baumannii* has been frequently and increasingly identified as a significant wound pathogen in U.S. troops returning from the Middle East with battlefield injuries (84). Significantly, *Acinetobacter* species are among the most commonly recovered Gram-negative rods from the hands of healthcare workers.

A. baumannii has the remarkable ability to develop durable antimicrobial resistance with alarming speed; resistance genes can be acquired from transposons, integrons, or plasmids carrying large clusters of resistance genes. Additionally, in several other respects *A. baumannii* is also a formidable pathogen. For example, atypical of most Gram-negative bacilli, *A. baumannii* is able to withstand long periods of desiccation and can therefore persist in the inanimate environment of the hospital ICU. In fact, *A. baumannii* has been found contaminating ventilators, mattresses, pillows, beds, gloves, pumps, and other electrical equipment in the ICU. For all of these reasons. *A. baumannii* is a particularly challenging ICU pathogen (8). The nosocomial reservoir for *A. baumannii* is unclear and may be quite diverse. Candidate reservoirs for this problematic pathogen include healthcare workers' hands and skin, hospital food, the inanimate hospital environment and hospital equipment, and even arthropods (85).

A. baumannii can be the responsible pathogen for several infectious syndromes in patients hospitalized in the ICU, including bacteremia, pneumonia (including ventilator-associated pneumonias), meningitis, urinary tract infection, as well as skin and soft-tissue infections (86). Data from participating hospitals in the NNIS suggest that the prevalence of *Acinetobacter* organisms among Gram-negative pathogens causing pneumonia in ICUs increased from 4.2% in 1986 to 7.0% in 2003 (87). Further, these same data document that resistance to the carbapenem antimicrobial, imipenem, among Acinetobacter isolates has increased from 0% to 42% in the same time period. Similarly, in the same time frame, resistance to ceftazidime has increased from 18% to 68% (87).

Because of the remarkable ability of these organisms to acquire multidrug resistance rapidly, the therapy of infections caused by *A. baumannii* is quite challenging. Colistin, an antimicrobial previously thought to be of historical interest only, has become one of the most commonly used agents for treatment of multiply resistant *A. baumannii* infection, though the frequent occurrence of nephrotoxicity with the use of this agent remains a major concern.

Tigecycline, the recently approved glycylglycine antimicrobial, has some activity against *A. baumannii*, though some carbapenem-resistant isolates may not be susceptible. Therapy must be individualized and must be guided by the antimicrobial susceptibility and the patient's clinical progress.

5 Measures to Prevent and Control Infection in the ICU

5.1 General Infection Control Measures

Several agencies and organizations have issued guidelines for controlling the spread of resistant pathogens in the healthcare setting (88, 89). Some of these guidelines are general in nature, whereas others address specific pathogens. The Society for Healthcare Epidemiology of America (SHEA) has issued guidelines that focus on the prevention of transmission of MRSA and VRE (88). Guidelines published by the Hospital Infection Control Practices Advisory Committee (HICPAC) from the Centers for Disease Control and Prevention (CDC) address preventing the spread of both Gram-positive (i.e., MRSA and VRE) as well as multiply resistant Gram-negative organisms (89). Recommendations for infection control interventions from these and other organizations will likely prove to be worthwhile in limiting the transmission of these and other resistant organisms in the healthcare setting. Principles designed to control the nosocomial spread of pathogens are described in detail in Chapter 93; however, some of these principles deserve special emphasis for addressing these important issues in the ICU. Among the infection control principles that have special relevance to the ICU setting are the following: (1) implementation of administrative controls; (2) ensuring antimicrobial stewardship in the ICU; and (3) use of special infection control interventions (e.g., cohorting, special microbial surveillance programs, decontamination strategies, molecular typing of organisms, etc.)

With respect to administrative controls, among the most important is the establishment of, and ensuring, strong administrative support for the creation of clear policies and procedures, grounded in science, that definitively delineate organizational expectations for techniques to be followed routinely in the management of specific infection syndromes. Several studies have argued that administrative engagement and support are critical to controlling the spread of resistant pathogens in the ICU (90–92). Several infection control interventions require substantial administrative investments, among them: (1) using technology (e.g., information systems) to provide important "real-time" data (e.g., alerts, warnings, feedback about adherence data, etc.) to healthcare providers at the point of care; (2) ensuring the provision of appropriate hospital infrastructure and supplies e.g., appropriate quantities of alcohol-based hand hygiene products, installation of dispensers throughout the ICU, ensuring appropriate numbers and placement of hand-washing sinks in the ICU, as well as appropriate placement of hand-washing sinks and alcohol-containing hand rub dispensers in the facility; (3) ensuring appropriate education and ongoing training of ICU staff; (4) providing appropriate staff and staffing levels to meet intensive care needs (93, 94); (5) ensuring the development and implementation of appropriate policies and procedures relating to infection control in the ICU (e.g., the appropriate use of masks, gowns, and gloves, and the appropriate use of contact isolation precautions for multiply resistant pathogens) and then also providing oversight to ensure adherence to these institutional infection control policies, procedures, and practices (see Tables 1 and 2) (89).

A second infection prevention principle that is worthy of emphasis for the ICU setting is antimicrobial stewardship. The potential for antimicrobial misuse and abuse is greater in the ICU than perhaps any other locus in the healthcare institution. Although rarely implemented as a single strategic intervention, several studies have demonstrated at least a temporal association between antimicrobial restriction and control of resistance (95–98). More recently, the resurgence of *C. difficile*-associated disease described above has been associated with increased fluoroquinolone use (74–77, 81, 87), and, at least in some settings, restriction of fluoroquinolone use has helped to limit the outbreak. Although a comprehensive discussion of antimicrobial stewardship is beyond the scope of this chapter, interventions to try to improve antimicrobial stewardship have used several different approaches. Fishman has categorized several types of interventions including education, formulary restriction, prior approval systems, streamlining empiric regimens, regimen cycling or rotation, the use of computer-assisted programs to provide relevant point of use information to the provider, and comprehensive programs that combine some or all of these strategies (discussed in detail in Ref. 99).

Education is a major aspect of the underpinning of any antibiotic stewardship program and includes both formal as well as personalized instruction. As noted above, formulary restriction can be effective and can allow consideration of costs, benefits, and untoward effect of candidate agents. The institution's formulary should be tailored to address current institutional endemic pathogens and current susceptibility patterns, and should be flexible enough to encompass new agents, as appropriate. So-called, "prior approval programs" (e.g., antibiotic order forms, required infectious diseases service consultation, automatic stop orders, and direct interactions with prescribers) can be effective (100), but are often viewed as intrusive by the medical staff. Prior approval programs also can improve clinical outcomes and reduce costs (99, 101). According to Fishman, streamlining is a strategy

that is infrequently used but could be beneficial in reducing the use of broad-spectrum antimicrobials as well as decreasing emergence of resistance. The broad-spectrum coverage that is provided by empiric therapy can and should be narrowed when a pathogen is identified. Although appealing intellectually, antibiotic cycling or antibiotic rotation (102–107) (reviewed in more detail in (99)) has, at least in my own view, yet to be definitively demonstrated to help reduce resistance. One review of this practice concluded that available evidence is as yet inadequate to recommend cycling as an important component of a stewardship program (107). Finally, computer decision support can provide the intensivist with the information she/he needs at the point of care (99). These programs have been used to address a number of prescribing issues. Several novel programs have been developed, and this field is growing rapidly.

A third infection control strategy or intervention that is worthy of additional discussion is the use of surveillance cultures for resistant pathogens. Whereas the SHEA guideline for managing MRSA and VRE has advocated for the broad-scale use of surveillance cultures (88), the recently issued HICPAC guideline stops short of such a recommendation (89). In fact, the importance and efficacy of using active microbiologic surveillance as an intervention to minimize transmission of resistant pathogens remains controversial. Whereas the strategy is intuitively appealing and has been shown to be effective in some models (108), as well as in some clinical venues (including ICU settings) (109), widespread use of this strategy is both costly and labor intensive. By screening all patients and identifying those colonized or infected with resistant pathogens, the intensivist can manage the affected patients aggressively with isolation precautions. A major problem with many of the studies that have used active surveillance cultures is that the strategy is not studied as an independent intervention. Almost all the published studies purporting to show a benefit of prospective surveillance cultures have implemented this strategy as one of several interventions in an outbreak setting. In all these studies, one cannot determine which, if any, of the interventions produced the benefit. The lack of well-controlled studies on the issue of active microbiologic surveillance has been the source of ongoing criticism of this intervention. In one cleverly designed study, investigators assessed the effect of daily microbiological surveillance cultures for *S. aureus* (including MRSA), but did not report either negative or positive culture results to the ICU staff (110). Nor did the investigators place patients identified as colonized with Staphylococci on isolation precautions. Nonetheless, these investigators demonstrated the absence of cross-transmission among patients in their ICU, despite the continual introduction of these pathogens during the study period. Interestingly, since the staff was not aware of the culture results, the results of the culture could have absolutely no impact on the lack of

Table 1 HICPAC Tier 1. General recommendations for routine prevention and control of multidrug-resistant organisms (MRDOs) in healthcare settings – reprinted from (89)

Administrative measures/ adherence monitoring	MDRO education	Judicious antimicrobial use	Surveillance	Infection control precautions to prevent transmission	Environmental measures	Decolonization
Make MDRO prevention/ control an organizational priority. Provide administrative support and both fiscal and human resources to prevent and control MDRO transmission. (IB)	Provide education and training on risks and prevention of MDRO transmission during orientation and periodic educational updates for HCP; include information on organizational experience with MDROs and prevention strategies. (IB)	In hospitals and LTCFs, ensure that a multi-disciplinary process is in place to review local susceptibility patterns (antibiograms), and antimicrobial agents included in the formulary, to foster appropriate antimicrobial use. (IB)	Use standardized laboratory methods and follow published guidelines for determining antimicrobial susceptibilities of targeted and emerging MDROs	Follow standard precautions in all healthcare settings. (IB)	Follow recommended cleaning, disinfection and sterilization guidelines for maintaining patient care areas and equipment	Not recommended routinely
Identify experts who can provide consultation and expertise for analyzing epidemiologic data, recognizing MDRO problems, or devising effective control strategies, as needed. (II)		Implement systems (e.g., CPOE, susceptibility report comment, pharmacy or unit director notification) to prompt clinicians to use the appropriate agent and regimen for the given clinical situation. (IB)	Establish systems to ensure that clinical micro labs (in-house and outsourced) promptly notify infection control or a medical director/designee when a novel resistance pattern for that facility is detected. (IB)	Use of Contact Precautions (CP): In acute care settings: Implement CP for all patients known to be colonized/infected with target MDROs. (IB)	Dedicate non-critical medical items to use on individual patients known to be infected or colonized with an MDRO.	
Implement systems to communicate information about reportable MDROs to administrative personnel and state/ local health departments. (II)		Provide clinicians with antimicrobial susceptibility reports and analysis of current trends, updated at least annually, to guide antimicrobial prescribing practices. (IB)	In hospitals and LTCFs: Develop and implement laboratory protocols for storing isolates of selected MDROs for molecular typing when needed to confirm transmission or delineate epidemiology of MDRO in facility. (IB)	In LTCFs: Consider the individual patient's clinical situation and facility resources in deciding whether to implement CP (II)	Prioritize room cleaning of patients on Contact Precautions. Focus on cleaning and disinfecting frequently touched surfaces (e.g., bed rails, bedside commodes, bathroom fixtures in patient room, doorknobs) and equipment in immediate vicinity of patient.	
Implement a multi-disciplinary process to monitor and improve HCP adherence to recommended practices for Standard and Contact Precautions. (IB)		In settings with limited electronic communication system infrastructures to implement physician prompts, etc., at a minimum implement a process to review antibiotic use. Prepare and distribute reports to providers. (II)	Establish laboratory-based systems to detect and communicate evidence of MDROs in clinical isolates (IB)	In ambulatory and home care settings, follow Standard Precautions (II)		

(continued)

Table 1 (continued)

Administrative measures/adherence monitoring	MDRO education	Judicious antimicrobial use	Surveillance	Infection control precautions to prevent transmission	Environmental measures	Decolonization
Implement systems to designate patients known to be colonized or infected with a targeted MDRO and to notify receiving healthcare facilities or personnel prior to transfer of such patients within or between facilities. (*IB*)			Prepare facility-specific antimicrobial susceptibility reports as recommended by CLSI; monitor reports for evidence of changing resistance that may indicate emergence or transmission of MDROs. (*IA/IC*)	In *hemodialysis units*: Follow dialysis-specific guidelines. (*IC*)		
Support participation in local, regional and/or national coalitions to combat emerging or growing MDRO problems. (*IB*)			Develop and monitor special-care unit-specific antimicrobial susceptibility reports (e.g., ventilator-dependent units, ICUs, oncology units). (*IB*)	No recommendation can be made regarding when to discontinue CP. (*Unresolved issue*)		
Provide updated feedback at least annually to healthcare providers and administrators on facility and patient-care unit MDRO infections. Include information on changes in prevalence and incidence, problem assessment and performance improvement plans. (*IB*)			Monitor trends in incidence of target MDROs in the facility over time to determine if MDRO rates are decreasing or if additional interventions are needed. (*IA*)	Masks are not recommended for routine use to prevent transmission of MDROs from patients to HCWs. Use masks according to Standard Precautions when performing splash-generating procedures, caring for patients with open tracheostomies with potential for projectile secretions, and when there is evidence for transmission from heavily colonized sources (e.g., burn wounds).		

Patient placement in hospitals and LTCFs:

When single-patient rooms are available, assign priority for these rooms to patients with known or suspected MDRO colonization or infection. Give highest priority to those patients who have conditions that may facilitate transmission, e.g., uncontained secretions or excretions. When single-patient rooms are not available, cohort patients with the same MDRO in the same room or patient-care area. (IB)

When cohorting patients with the same MDRO is not possible, place MDRO patients in rooms with patients who are at low risk for acquisition of MDROs and associated adverse outcomes from infection and are likely to have short lengths of stay. (II)

LTCF long-term care facilities, HCP healthcare professional, CPOE computerized practitioner order entry, HCW healthcare worker

Table 2 HICPAC Tier 2. Recommendations for Intensified MDRO control efforts – reprinted from (89)

Administrative measures/ adherence monitoring	MDRO education	Judicious antimicrobial use	Surveillance	Infection control precautions to prevent transmission	Environmental measures	Decolonization
Obtain expert consultation from persons with experience in infection control and the epidemiology of MDROS, either in-house or through outside consultation, for assessment of the local MDRO problem and guidance in the design, implementation and evaluation of appropriate control measures. (IB)	Intensify the frequency of educational programs for healthcare personnel, especially for those who work in areas where MDRO rates are not decreasing. Provide individual or unit-specific feedback when available. (IB)	Review the role of antimicrobial use in perpetuating the MDRO problem targeted for intensified intervention. Control and improve antimicrobial use as indicated. Antimicrobial agents that may be targeted include vancomycin, third-[d] generation cephalosporins, anti-anaerobic agents for VRE; third-generation cephalosporins for ESBLs; and quinolones and carbapenems. (IB)	Calculate and analyze incidence rates of target MDROs (single isolates/patient; location-, service-specific). (IB)	Use of contact precautions:	Implement patient-dedicated use of non-critical equipment. (IB)	Consult with experts on a case-by-case basis regarding the appropriate use of decolonization therapy for patients or staff during limited period of time as a component of an intensified MRSA control program. (II)
Provide necessary leadership, funding and day-to-day oversight to implement interventions selected. (IB)			Increase frequency of compiling, monitoring antimicrobial susceptibility summary reports. (II)	Implement Contact Precautions (CP) routinely for all patients colonized or infected with a target MDRO. (IA)	Intensify and reinforce training of environmental staff who work in areas targeted for intensified MDRO control. Some facilities may choose to assign dedicated staff to targeted patient care areas to enhance consistency of proper environmental cleaning and disinfection services. (IB)	When decolonization for MRSA is used, perform susceptibility testing for the decolonizing agent against the target organism or the MDRO strain epidemiologically implicated in transmission. Monitor susceptibility to detect emergence of resistance to the decolonizing agent. Consult with microbiologists for appropriate testing for mupirocin resistance, since standards have not been established.
Evaluate healthcare system factors for role in creating or perpetuating MDRO transmission, including staffing levels, education and training, availability of consumable and durable resources;			Implement laboratory protocols for storing isolates of selected MDROs for molecular typing; perform typing if needed. (IB)	Don gowns and gloves *before or upon entry* to the patient's room or cubicle. (IB)	Monitor cleaning performance to ensure consistent cleaning and disinfection of surfaces in close proximity to the patient and those	Do not use topical mupirocin routinely for MRSA decolonization of patients as a component of MRSA control programs in any healthcare setting. (IB)

communication processes, and adherence to infection control measures. (IB)

Update healthcare providers and administrators on the progress and effectiveness of the intensified interventions. (IB)

In LTCFs, modify CP to allow MDRO-colonized/infected patients whose site of colonization or infection can be appropriately contained and who can observe good hand hygiene practices to enter common areas and participate in group activities.

Develop and implement protocols to obtain active surveillance cultures from patients in populations at risk. (iB) (See recommendations for appropriate body sites and culturing methods.)

Conduct culture surveys to assess efficacy of intensified MDRO control interventions.

Conduct serial (e.g., weekly) unit-specific point prevalence surveys of the target MDRO to determine if transmission has decreased or ceased (IB)

Repeat point-prevalence culture surveys at routine intervals and at time of patient discharge or transfer until transmission has ceased. (IB)

likely to be touched by the patient and HCWs (e.g., bed rails, carts, bedside commodes, doorknobs, faucet handles) (IB).

Obtain environmental cultures (e.g., surfaces, shared equipment) only when epidemiologically implicated in transmission. (IB)

Vacate units for environmental assessment and intensive cleaning when previous efforts to control environmental transmission have failed. (II)

No recommendation is made for universal use of gloves and/or gowns. (Unresolved issue)

Implement policies for patient admission and placement as needed to prevent transmission of the problem MDRO. (IB)

Limit decolonization to HCP found to be colonized with MRSA who have been epidemiologically implicated in ongoing transmission of MRSA to patients. (IB)

No recommendation can be made for decolonization of patients who carry VRE or MDR-GNB.

(continued)

Table 2 (continued)

Administrative measures/adherence monitoring	MDRO education	Judicious antimicrobial use	Surveillance	Infection control precautions to prevent transmission	Environmental measures	Decolonization
			If indicated by assessment of the MDRO problem, collect cultures to assess the colonization status of roommates and other patients with substantial exposure to patients with known MDRO infection or colonization. *(IB)*	When single-patient rooms are available, assign priority for these rooms to patients with known or suspected MDRO colonization or infection. Give highest priority to those patients who have conditions that may facilitate transmission, e.g., uncontained secretions or excretions. When single-patient rooms are not available, cohort patients with the same MDRO in the same room or patient-care area. *(IB)*		
			Obtain cultures from HCP for target MDROs when there is epidemiologic evidence implicating the staff member as a source of ongoing transmission. *(IB)*	When cohorting patients with the same MDRO is not possible, place MDRO patients in rooms with patients who are at low risk for acquisition of MDROs and associated adverse outcomes from infection and are likely to have short lengths of stay. *(II)*		

Stop new admissions to the unit or facility if transmission continues despite the implementation of the intensified control measures. *(IB)*

Institute one or more of the interventions described below when 1) incidence or prevalence of MDROs are not decreasing despite the use of routine control measures; or 2) the *first* case or outbreak of an epidemiologically important MDRO (e.g., VRE, MRSA, VISA, VRSA, MDR-GNB) is identified within a healthcare facility or unit *(IB)* Continue to monitor the incidence of target MDRO infection and colonization; if rates do not decrease, implement additional interventions as needed to reduce MDRO transmission.

The CDC/HICPAC system for categorizing recommendations is as follows:

Category IA – Strongly recommended for implementation and strongly supported by well-designed experimental, clinical, or epidemiologic studies.

Category IB – Strongly recommended for implementation and supported by some experimental, clinical, or epidemiologic studies and a strong theoretical rationale.

Category IC – Required for implementation, as mandated by federal and/or state regulation or standard.

Category II – Suggested for implementation and supported by suggestive clinical or epidemiologic studies or a theoretical rationale.

No recommendation – Unresolved issue. Practices for which insufficient evidence or no consensus regarding efficacy exists.

transmission. The authors concluded that "reporting culture results and isolating colonized patients, as suggested by some guidelines, would have falsely suggested the success of such infection-control policies" (110).

The recently published HICPAC guideline advocates a sensible "two-tiered" approach to the management of resistant pathogens (89). The essence of each of these "tiers" is summarized in Tables 1 and 2, which are reprinted from these guidelines (89). The guideline suggests that the control of resistant pathogens is a dynamic process that requires a systematic approach tailored to the problem and the unique healthcare setting. In instances in which the practitioner is faced with the emergence of a resistant pathogen problem that cannot be controlled with standard or traditional infection control measures, additional control measures should be selected from a second set of interventions which include interventions from the following categories: administrative measures/adherence monitoring, staff education, antimicrobial stewardship, surveillance, infection control precautions, environmental measures, and decolonization (89). Decisions to increase control activities should be based on individual circumstance (89).

5.2 Syndrome-Specific Infection Control Measures

Whereas the principles outlined above relate to general infection control practices and procedures that have specific relevance to the ICU setting, specific interventions have also been developed to address the three major nosocomial infection syndromes frequently encountered in the ICU (discussed above).

5.2.1 Preventing Device-Associated Bacteremia in the ICU

Several strategies have been specifically directed at limiting the access of organisms to the intravascular device at the catheter insertion site. The use of sterile technique during insertion, attention to the detail of sterile technique when entering or manipulating the system, and rigorous attention to details of appropriate hand hygiene, all contribute to reductions in device-associated bacteremia rates in the ICU. Other techniques that have been shown repeatedly to be effective in reducing device-associated bacteremia rates include the use of maximal sterile barrier precautions during the process of catheter insertion, the use of cutaneous antisepsis with chlorhexidine, optimal insertion site selection (e.g., insertion in the subclavian vein is superior to the internal jugular or femoral veins), and frequent review of the need for

having the line in place, with prompt removal when it is no longer essential. The Institute for Healthcare Improvement advocated bundling these strategies as an approach to preventing device-associated infection in their "100,000 lives" campaign (111). Sites implementing this type of evidence-based approach experienced substantial success in reducing rates of device-associated bacteremia (111–115). Other techniques that have been suggested as effective in some, but not all, studies include the application of antiseptic ointment or cream at the insertion site, the use of special dressing materials (e.g., semipermeable membrane dressings, colloid dressing), and impregnating an implantable catheter's cuff with an antiseptic material.

Still further strategies have been suggested to reduce risk for infection at the catheter hub or junction, including the emphasis on hand hygiene; the development of protocols to ensure standard procedures for device management; emphasis on strict adherence to disinfection and system entry protocols for needleless systems; limiting system entry to instances that are essential to patient care; and the development of novel devices/approaches such as a hub that includes a connecting chamber filled with iodinated alcohol, a hub that is surrounded by povidone–iodine saturated sponge, the development of needleless connecting systems that have been designed to reduce infection risks, and the use of so-called "antibiotic locks" as a strategy for managing contaminated/infected devices.

Over the past several years, several ICUs have experienced increased device-associated infection rates that have been ascribed to the use of needleless intravenous device connectors. These devices were designed with two primary goals in mind – healthcare worker safety and device patency; infection control was not a primary consideration in the development of these devices. The first sets of these devices to be introduced were those with a split septum access port. One early study found that use of a needleless device was associated with increased risk for central catheter bacteremia (with a remarkable relative risk of 14.9), and also found that luminal fluid from device caps was significantly more likely to be culture-positive than fluid from protected needle devices (116). In a second paper, a retrospective cohort study of home infusion patients, Kellerman and colleagues observed increases in device-associated bacteremia rates of 80% after introducing a needleless system (117). In a subsequent study, higher device-associated infection rates were again associated with the use of a needleless system (118). In this latter study, an important finding was that nurses working with these catheters were unfamiliar with the system and their care and use practices often differed from manufacturer's recommendations (118). Needleless systems using mechanical valves were the next to be marketed. The rationale for the use of these devices was to decrease device occlusion (i.e., they have neutral pressure at disconnection). Newer devices have been designed to have positive displacement at disconnection, thereby reducing the need for flushing and fibrinolytics, the potential for device occlusion, the increased costs associated with catheter replacement, and, presumably, the costs associated with complications and their management. Even these newer devices have been associated with clusters of device-associated infection (119). These devices may contribute to the risk for device-associated infection in several ways. The clinician may not disinfect the device appropriately before use, the device may be difficult to disinfect effectively, or the clinician may not follow directions for use. These devices have several potential areas for contamination: the outside of the connector, the space around the mechanical device in the system, the "plunger" in the system (especially if it were to malfunction), and the opaque hub area. Although we have inadequate data to determine the factors contributing to the increased risks seen in these several studies, the primary issue is likely to be the inconsistent use of appropriate infection control procedures by ICU staff.

5.2.2 Preventing ICU-Associated Ventilator-Associated Pneumonia

Strategies have been developed to address the various pathogenetic mechanisms associated with risk for ventilator-associated pneumonia. To address the issues that relate to the rapid changes in hospitalized patients' microbial flora, some intensivists have emphasized the appropriate use of hand hygiene (and especially the continual use of alcohol-based hand hygiene products), the avoidance of the unnecessary use of antimicrobials, and the routine use of antimicrobial mouthwash (e.g., those containing chlorhexidine).

To address the risks associated with the endotracheal tube itself, noninvasive ventilation strategies have been developed, as well as approaches to decreasing the subglottic pooling of secretions. When possible, one should avoid nasotracheal or nasogastric intubation because of the risk for precipitating bacterial sinusitis that increases the risk for pneumonia. Staff should avoid unnecessary manipulation of ventilator circuitry/tubing, should assess the need for continued intubation at least daily, and should develop and adhere to weaning protocols. To address the issues relating to biofilm production, experimental endotracheal tubes coated with antiseptics/silver sulfadiazine and chlorhexidine in polyurethane or other materials are being evaluated. To minimize the risk for aspiration of gastric contents, the head of the patient's bed should be elevated to 45°. In addition, staff should judiciously use enteral nutrition and antimicrobials and should avoid procedures that are associated with gastric distention.

Other factors that are clearly associated with reduced risks for ventilator-associated pneumonia include maintenance of appropriate ICU staffing levels and administering stress bleeding prophylaxis only when truly indicated. Strategies that have been suggested to work in some, but not all, settings include lubrication of the endotracheal tube cuff, selective gastrointestinal (GI) decontamination with antimicrobials, and short courses of parenteral prophylactic antimicrobials in selected patients (i.e., those who will be intubated for short periods of time).

5.2.3 Preventing Infection in Immunocompromised Patients in the ICU

Preventing healthcare-associated infections among severely immunocompromised patients hospitalized in the ICU is a substantial challenge. For the myriad reasons outlined in the pathogenesis section above, preventing infections in this population is formidable. Basically, the intensivist and the ICU staff must pay attention to the details of all aspects of infection control, emphasizing hand hygiene, administrative controls, aggressive early diagnosis, appropriate empiric therapy, maintenance of a high index of suspicion for yeast and filamentous fungal infection, appropriate antibacterial and antifungal chemoprophylaxis, and maintenance of constant vigil for the development of infection caused by one or more of the aggressive resistant pathogens described above, keeping in mind that the source of these resistant pathogens may be the patient, a provider, or the healthcare environment. Such immunosuppressed patients are at substantially increased risk for many of the pathogens described above – MRSA, VRE, *Acinetobacter baumannii*, and other multidrug-resistant (MDR) organisms.

Other strategies that may be of use in preventing infections in immunocompromised patients in certain settings include the use of a totally protected environment and selective decontamination of oral and gastrointestinal flora (thereby protecting the patient's anaerobic flora).

In the final analysis, in the ICU, staff must maintain a constant vigil for resistant pathogens. Hand hygiene, using alcohol-based hand hygiene preparations, is of crucial importance in this setting. Use of these products was associated with a 41% decrease in healthcare-associated infections in one ICU (120). Other key issues for managing these patients include maintaining constant and consistent attention to every detail of infection control procedures and practices, decreasing devices and device days, as well as controlling and judiciously using antimicrobials.

References

1. Agvald-Ohman C, Lund B, Hjelmqvist H, Hedin G, Struwe J, Edlund C. ICU stay promotes enrichment and dissemination of multiresistant coagulase-negative staphylococcal strains. Scand J Infect Dis 2006;38(6–7):441–447

2. National Nosocomial Infections Surveillance (NNIS) System Report, data summary from January 1992 through June 2004, issued October 2004. Am J Infect Control 2004;32(8):470–485

3. Bonten MJ, Willems R, Weinstein RA. Vancomycin-resistant enterococci: why are they here, and where do they come from? Lancet Infect Dis 2001;1(5):314–325

4. Haddadin AS, Fappiano SA, Lipsett PA. Methicillin resistant Staphylococcus aureus (MRSA) in the intensive care unit. Postgrad Med J 2002;78(921):385–392

5. Chang S, Sievert DM, Hageman JC, et al. Infection with vancomycin-resistant Staphylococcus aureus containing the vanA resistance gene. N Engl J Med 2003;348(14):1342–1347

6. Tenover FC, Weigel LM, Appelbaum PC, et al. Vancomycin-resistant Staphylococcus aureus isolate from a patient in Pennsylvania. Antimicrob Agents Chemother 2004;48(1):275–280

7. Weigel LM, Clewell DB, Gill SR, et al. Genetic analysis of a high-level vancomycin-resistant isolate of Staphylococcus aureus. Science 2003;302(5650):1569–1571

8. Chastre J. Infections due to Acinetobacter baumannii in the ICU. Semin Respir Crit Care Med 2003;24(1):69–78

9. Bayram A, Balci I. Patterns of antimicrobial resistance in a surgical intensive care unit of a university hospital in Turkey. BMC Infect Dis 2006;6:155

10. Leroy O, d'Escrivan T, Devos P, Dubreuil L, Kipnis E, Georges H. Hospital-acquired pneumonia in critically ill patients: factors associated with episodes due to imipenem-resistant organisms. Infection 2005;33(3):129–135

11. Zarrilli R, Crispino M, Bagattini M, et al. Molecular epidemiology of sequential outbreaks of Acinetobacter baumannii in an intensive care unit shows the emergence of carbapenem resistance. J Clin Microbiol 2004;42(3):946–953

12. Jeena P, Thompson E, Nchabeleng M, Sturm A. Emergence of multi-drug-resistant Acinetobacter anitratus species in neonatal and paediatric intensive care units in a developing country: concern about antimicrobial policies. Ann Trop Paediatr 2001;21(3):245–251

13. Lepelletier D, Caroff N, Riochet D, et al. Role of hospital stay and antibiotic use on Pseudomonas aeruginosa gastrointestinal colonization in hospitalized patients. Eur J Clin Microbiol Infect Dis 2006;25(9):600–603

14. Brahmi N, Blel Y, Kouraichi N, et al. Impact of ceftazidime restriction on gram-negative bacterial resistance in an intensive care unit. J Infect Chemother 2006;12(4):190–194

15. Gould CV, Rothenberg R, Steinberg JP. Antibiotic resistance in long-term acute care hospitals: the perfect storm. Infect Control Hosp Epidemiol 2006;27(9):920–925

16. Ferrara AM. Potentially multidrug-resistant non-fermentative Gram-negative pathogens causing nosocomial pneumonia. Int J Antimicrob Agents 2006;27(3):183–195

17. Quinn JP. Pseudomonas aeruginosa infections in the intensive care unit. Semin Respir Crit Care Med 2003;24(1):61–68

18. Friedland I, Gallagher G, King T, Woods GL. Antimicrobial susceptibility patterns in Pseudomonas aeruginosa: data from a multicenter Intensive Care Unit Surveillance Study (ISS) in the United States. J Chemother 2004;16(5):437–441

19. Fridkin SK, Hill HA, Volkova NV, et al. Temporal changes in prevalence of antimicrobial resistance in 23 US hospitals. Emerg Infect Dis 2002;8(7):697–701

20. Nseir S, Di Pompeo C, Soubrier S, et al. First-generation fluoroquinolone use and subsequent emergence of multiple drug-resistant bacteria in the intensive care unit. Crit Care Med 2005;33(2):283–289

21. Henderson DK. Managing methicillin-resistant staphylococci: a paradigm for preventing nosocomial transmission of resistant organisms. Am J Med 2006;119(6 Suppl 1):S45–S52; discussion S62–S70

22. Williams RE. Healthy carriage of Staphylococcus aureus: its prevalence and importance. Bacteriol Rev 1963;27:56–71

23. Thompson RL, Cabezudo I, Wenzel RP. Epidemiology of nosocomial infections caused by methicillin-resistant Staphylococcus aureus. Ann Intern Med 1982;97(3):309–317

24. Foster TJ. The Staphylococcus aureus "superbug". J Clin Invest 2004;114(12):1693–1696

25. Sista RR, Oda G, Barr J. Methicillin-resistant Staphylococcus aureus infections in ICU patients. Anesthesiol Clin North America 2004;22(3):405–435, vi

26. Hidron AI, Kourbatova EV, Halvosa JS, et al. Risk factors for colonization with methicillin-resistant Staphylococcus aureus (MRSA) in patients admitted to an urban hospital: emergence of community-associated MRSA nasal carriage. Clin Infect Dis 2005;41(2):159–166

27. Troillet N, Carmeli Y, Samore MH, et al. Carriage of methicillin-resistant Staphylococcus aureus at hospital admission. Infect Control Hosp Epidemiol 1998;19(3):181–185

28. Cesur S, Cokca F. Nasal carriage of methicillin-resistant Staphylococcus aureus among hospital staff and outpatients. Infect Control Hosp Epidemiol 2004;25(2):169–171

29. Eveillard M, Martin Y, Hidri N, Boussougant Y, Joly-Guillou ML. Carriage of methicillin-resistant Staphylococcus aureus among hospital employees: prevalence, duration, and transmission to households. Infect Control Hosp Epidemiol 2004;25(2):114–120

30. Nulens E, Gould I, MacKenzie F, et al. Staphylococcus aureus carriage among participants at the 13th European Congress of Clinical Microbiology and Infectious Diseases. Eur J Clin Microbiol Infect Dis 2005;24(2):145–148

31. Devine J, Cooke RP, Wright EP. Is methicillin-resistant Staphylococcus aureus (MRSA) contamination of ward-based computer terminals a surrogate marker for nosocomial MRSA transmission and handwashing compliance? J Hosp Infect 2001;48(1):72–75

32. Oie S, Kamiya A. Survival of methicillin-resistant Staphylococcus aureus (MRSA) on naturally contaminated dry mops. J Hosp Infect 1996;34(2):145–149

33. Rutala WA, Katz EB, Sherertz RJ, Sarubbi FA, Jr. Environmental study of a methicillin-resistant Staphylococcus aureus epidemic in a burn unit. J Clin Microbiol 1983;18(3):683–688

34. Henderson DK, Baptiste R, Parrillo J, Gill VJ. Indolent epidemic of Pseudomonas cepacia bacteremia and pseudobacteremia in an intensive care unit traced to a contaminated blood gas analyzer. Am J Med 1988;84(1):75–81

35. Sitges-Serra A, Puig P, Jaurrieta E, et al. Hub colonization as the initial step in an outbreak of catheter-related sepsis due to coagulase negative staphylococci during parenteral nutrition. J Parenter Enteral Nutr 1984;8:668–672

36. Sitges-Serra A, Hernandez R, Maestro S, Pi-Suner T, Garces JM, Segura M. Prevention of catheter sepsis: the hub. Nutrition 1997;13(4 Suppl):30S–35S

37. Bauer TT, Torres A, Ferrer R, Heyer CM, Schultze-Werninghaus G, Rasche K. Biofilm formation in endotracheal tubes. Association between pneumonia and the persistence of pathogens. Monaldi Arch Chest Dis 2002;57(1):84–87

38. Adair CG, Gorman SP, Feron BM, et al. Implications of endotracheal tube biofilm for ventilator-associated pneumonia. Intensive Care Med 1999;25(10):1072–1076

39. Rumbak MJ. The pathogenesis of ventilator-associated pneumonia. Semin Respir Crit Care Med 2002;23(5):427–434

40. Safdar N, Crnich CJ, Maki DG. The pathogenesis of ventilator-associated pneumonia: its relevance to developing effective strategies for prevention. Respir Care 2005;50(6):725–739; discussion 39–41

41. Holzapfel L, Chevret S, Madinier G, et al. Influence of long-term oro- or nasotracheal intubation on nosocomial maxillary sinusitis and pneumonia: results of a prospective, randomized, clinical trial. Crit Care Med 1993;21(8):1132–1138

42. Ibanez J, Penafiel A, Raurich JM, Marse P, Jorda R, Mata F. Gastroesophageal reflux in intubated patients receiving enteral nutrition: effect of supine and semirecumbent positions. JPEN J Parenter Enteral Nutr 1992;16(5):419–422

43. Torres A, Serra-Batlles J, Ros E, et al. Pulmonary aspiration of gastric contents in patients receiving mechanical ventilation: the effect of body position. Ann Intern Med 1992;116(7):540–543

44. Spilker CA, Hinthorn DR, Pingleton SK. Intermittent enteral feeding in mechanically ventilated patients. The effect on gastric pH and gastric cultures. Chest 1996;110(1):243–248

45. Hofmeister CC, Stiff PJ. Mucosal protection by cytokines. Curr Hematol Rep 2005;4(6):446–453

46. Blot SI, Vandewoude KH, Hoste EA, Colardyn FA. Outcome and attributable mortality in critically ill patients with bacteremia involving methicillin-susceptible and methicillin-resistant Staphylococcus aureus. Arch Intern Med 2002;162(19):2229–2235

47. Cosgrove SE, Qi Y, Kaye KS, Harbarth S, Karchmer AW, Carmeli Y. The impact of methicillin resistance in Staphylococcus aureus bacteremia on patient outcomes: mortality, length of stay, and hospital charges. Infect Control Hosp Epidemiol 2005;26(2):166–174

48. Harbarth S, Rutschmann O, Sudre P, Pittet D. Impact of methicillin resistance on the outcome of patients with bacteremia caused by Staphylococcus aureus. Arch Intern Med 1998;158(2):182–189

49. Kaw R. Is MRSA more pathogenic in critically ill patients? Arch Intern Med 2003;163(6):739–740; author reply 740

50. Soriano A, Martinez JA, Mensa J, et al. Pathogenic significance of methicillin resistance for patients with Staphylococcus aureus bacteremia. Clin Infect Dis 2000;30(2):368–373

51. Yzerman EP, Boelens HA, Tjhie JH, Kluytmans JA, Mouton JW, Verbrugh HA. Delta APACHE II for predicting course and outcome of nosocomial Staphylococcus aureus bacteremia and its relation to host defense. J Infect Dis 1996;173(4):914–919

52. Saner FH, Heuer M, Rath PM, et al. Successful salvage therapy with tigecycline after linezolid failure in a liver transplant recipient with MRSA pneumonia. Liver Transpl 2006;12(11): 1689–1692

53. Silvia Munoz-Price L, Lolans K, Quinn JP. Four cases of invasive methicillin-resistant Staphylococcus aureus (MRSA) infections treated with tigecycline. Scand J Infect Dis 2006;38(11):1081–1084

54. Hiramatsu K, Hanaki H, Ino T, Yabuta K, Oguri T, Tenover FC. Methicillin-resistant Staphylococcus aureus clinical strain with reduced vancomycin susceptibility. J Antimicrob Chemother 1997; 40(1):135–136

55. Centers for Disease Control and Prevention. Staphylococcus aureus with reduced susceptibility to vancomycin – United States, 1997. MMWR Morb Mortal Wkly Rep 1997;46(33):765–766

56. Sieradzki K, Roberts RB, Haber SW, Tomasz A. The development of vancomycin resistance in a patient with methicillin-resistant Staphylococcus aureus infection. N Engl J Med 1999;340(7):517–523

57. Smith TL, Pearson ML, Wilcox KR, et al. Emergence of vancomycin resistance in Staphylococcus aureus. Glycopeptide-intermediate Staphylococcus aureus Working Group. N Engl J Med 1999;340(7):493–501

58. Noble WC, Virani Z, Cree RG. Co-transfer of vancomycin and other resistance genes from Enterococcus faecalis NCTC 12201 to Staphylococcus aureus. FEMS Microbiol Lett 1992;72(2):195–198

59. Centers for Disease Control and Prevention. Vancomycin-resistant Staphylococcus aureus – New York, 2004. MMWR Morb Mortal Wkly Rep 2004;53(15):322–323

60. Hayden MK, Bonten MJ, Blom DW, Lyle EA, van de Vijver DA, Weinstein RA. Reduction in acquisition of vancomycin-resistant enterococcus after enforcement of routine environmental cleaning measures. Clin Infect Dis 2006;42(11):1552–1560

61. Zirakzadeh A, Patel R. Vancomycin-resistant enterococci. colonization, infection, detection, and treatment. Mayo Clin Proc 2006;81(4):529–536

62. Centers for Disease Control and Prevention. Nosocomial enterococci resistant to vancomycin – United States, 1989–1993. MMWR Morb Mortal Wkly Rep 1993;42(30):597–599

63. Tenover FC, McDonald LC. Vancomycin-resistant staphylococci and enterococci: epidemiology and control. Curr Opin Infect Dis 2005;18(4):300–305

64. Torres-Viera C, Dembry LM. Approaches to vancomycin-resistant enterococci. Curr Opin Infect Dis 2004;17(6):541–547

65. Giamarellou H. Treatment options for multidrug-resistant bacteria. Expert Rev Anti Infect Ther 2006;4(4):601–618

66. Cohen LE, McNeill CJ, Wells RF. Clindamycin-associated colitis. JAMA 1973;223(12):1379–1380

67. Tedesco FJ, Stanley RJ, Alpers DH. Diagnostic features of clindamycin-associated pseudomembranous colitis. N Engl J Med 1974;290(15):841–843

68. Nakamura S, Mikawa M, Nakashio S, et al. Isolation of Clostridium difficile from the feces and the antibody in sera of young and elderly adults. Microbiol Immunol 1981;25(4):345–351

69. Marciniak C, Chen D, Stein AC, Semik PE. Prevalence of Clostridium difficile colonization at admission to rehabilitation. Arch Phys Med Rehabil 2006;87(8):1086–1090

70. Hota B. Contamination, disinfection, and cross-colonization: are hospital surfaces reservoirs for nosocomial infection? Clin Infect Dis 2004;39(8):1182–1189

71. Kyne L, Warny M, Qamar A, Kelly CP. Asymptomatic carriage of Clostridium difficile and serum levels of IgG antibody against toxin A. N Engl J Med 2000;342(6):390–397

72. Bartlett JG. Antibiotic-associated diarrhea. Clin Infect Dis 1992;15(4):573–581

73. Geric B, Carman RJ, Rupnik M, et al. Binary toxin-producing, large clostridial toxin-negative Clostridium difficile strains are enterotoxic but do not cause disease in hamsters. J Infect Dis 2006;193(8):1143–1150

74. Kazakova SV, Ware K, Baughman B, et al. A hospital outbreak of diarrhea due to an emerging epidemic strain of Clostridium difficile. Arch Intern Med 2006;166(22):2518–2524

75. Kuijper EJ, Coignard B, Tull P. Emergence of Clostridium difficile-associated disease in North America and Europe. Clin Microbiol Infect 2006;12 Suppl 6:2–18

76. McDonald LC, Killgore GE, Thompson A, et al. An epidemic, toxin gene-variant strain of Clostridium difficile. N Engl J Med 2005;353(23):2433–2441

77. Loo VG, Poirier L, Miller MA, et al. A predominantly clonal multi-institutional outbreak of Clostridium difficile-associated diarrhea with high morbidity and mortality. N Engl J Med 2005;353(23):2442–2449

78. Warny M, Pepin J, Fang A, et al. Toxin production by an emerging strain of Clostridium difficile associated with outbreaks of severe disease in North America and Europe. Lancet 2005;366(9491):1079–1084

79. Barbut F, Decre D, Lalande V, et al. Clinical features of Clostridium difficile-associated diarrhoea due to binary toxin (actin-specific ADP-ribosyltransferase)-producing strains. J Med Microbiol 2005;54(Pt 2):181–185

80. McEllistrem MC, Carman RJ, Gerding DN, Genheimer CW, Zheng L. A hospital outbreak of Clostridium difficile disease associated with isolates carrying binary toxin genes. Clin Infect Dis 2005;40(2):265–272

81. Bartlett JG. Narrative review: the new epidemic of Clostridium difficile-associated enteric disease. Ann Intern Med 2006;145(10):758–764

82. Hanlon GW. The emergence of multidrug resistant Acinetobacter species: a major concern in the hospital setting. Lett Appl Microbiol 2005;41(5):375–378

83. Richet H, Fournier PE. Nosocomial infections caused by *Acinetobacter baumannii*: a major threat worldwide. Infect Control Hosp Epidemiol 2006;27(7):645–646

84. *Acinetobacter baumannii* infections among patients at military medical facilities treating injured U.S. service members, 2002–2004. MMWR Morb Mortal Wkly Rep 2004;53(45): 1063–1066

85. La Scola B, Raoult D. *Acinetobacter baumannii* in human body louse. Emerg Infect Dis 2004;10(9):1671–1673

86. Jain R, Danziger LH. Multidrug-resistant Acinetobacter infections: an emerging challenge to clinicians. Ann Pharmacother 2004;38(9):1449–1459

87. McDonald LC. Trends in antimicrobial resistance in health care-associated pathogens and effect on treatment. Clin Infect Dis 2006;42 Suppl 2:S65–S71

88. Muto CA, Jernigan JA, Ostrowsky BE, et al. SHEA guideline for preventing nosocomial transmission of multidrug-resistant strains of *Staphylococcus aureus* and enterococcus. Infect Control Hosp Epidemiol 2003;24(5):362–386

89. Management of Multidrug-Resistant Organisms In Healthcare Settings, 2006. Centers for Disease Control and Prevention, 2006. (Accessed January 5, 2007, 2007, at http://www.cdc.gov/ncidod/dhqp/pdf/ar/mdroGuideline2006.pdf.)

90. Calfee DP, Farr BM. Infection control and cost control in the era of managed care. Infect Control Hosp Epidemiol 2002;23(7): 407–410

91. Haley RW, Cushion NB, Tenover FC, et al. Eradication of endemic methicillin-resistant *Staphylococcus aureus* infections from a neonatal intensive care unit. J Infect Dis 1995;171(3):614–624

92. Jochimsen EM, Fish L, Manning K, et al. Control of vancomycin-resistant enterococci at a community hospital: efficacy of patient and staff cohorting. Infect Control Hosp Epidemiol 1999;20(2):106–109

93. Grundmann H, Hori S, Winter B, Tami A, Austin DJ. Risk factors for the transmission of methicillin-resistant *Staphylococcus aureus* in an adult intensive care unit: fitting a model to the data. J Infect Dis 2002;185(4):481–488

94. Robert J, Fridkin SK, Blumberg HM, et al. The influence of the composition of the nursing staff on primary bloodstream infection rates in a surgical intensive care unit. Infect Control Hosp Epidemiol 2000;21(1):12–7

95. Marion ND, Rupp ME. Infection control issues of enteral feeding systems. Curr Opin Clin Nutr Metab Care 2000;3(5): 363–366

96. Rahal JJ, Urban C, Horn D, et al. Class restriction of cephalosporin use to control total cephalosporin resistance in nosocomial *Klebsiella*. JAMA 1998;280(14):1233–1237

97. Rahal JJ, Urban C, Segal-Maurer S. Nosocomial antibiotic resistance in multiple gram-negative species: experience at one hospital with squeezing the resistance balloon at multiple sites. Clin Infect Dis 2002;34(4):499–503

98. Rupp ME, Marion N, Fey PD, et al. Outbreak of vancomycin-resistant *Enterococcus faecium* in a neonatal intensive care unit. Infect Control Hosp Epidemiol 2001;22(5):301–303

99. Fishman N. Antimicrobial stewardship. Am J Med 2006;119 (6 Suppl 1):S53–S61; discussion S2–S70

100. John JF, Jr., Fishman NO. Programmatic role of the infectious diseases physician in controlling antimicrobial costs in the hospital. Clin Infect Dis 1997;24(3):471–485

101. Frank MO, Batteiger BE, Sorensen SJ, et al. Decrease in expenditures and selected nosocomial infections following implementation of an antimicrobial-prescribing improvement program. Clin Perform Qual Health Care 1997;5(4):180–188

102. Martinez JA, Nicolas JM, Marco F, et al. Comparison of antimicrobial cycling and mixing strategies in two medical intensive care units. Crit Care Med 2006;34(2):329–336

103. Raymond DP, Pelletier SJ, Sawyer RG. Antibiotic utilization strategies to limit antimicrobial resistance. Semin Respir Crit Care Med 2002;23(5):497–501

104. Warren DK, Hill HA, Merz LR, et al. Cycling empirical antimicrobial agents to prevent emergence of antimicrobial-resistant Gram-negative bacteria among intensive care unit patients. Crit Care Med 2004;32(12):2450–2456

105. Evans HL, Sawyer RG. Cycling chemotherapy: a promising approach to reducing the morbidity and mortality of nosocomial infections. Drugs Today (Barc) 2003;39(9):733–738

106. van Loon HJ, Vriens MR, Fluit AC, et al. Antibiotic rotation and development of gram-negative antibiotic resistance. Am J Respir Crit Care Med 2005;171(5):480–487

107. Brown EM, Nathwani D. Antibiotic cycling or rotation: a systematic review of the evidence of efficacy. J Antimicrob Chemother 2005;55(1):6–9

108. Bootsma MC, Diekmann O, Bonten MJ. Controlling methicillin-resistant *Staphylococcus aureus*: quantifying the effects of interventions and rapid diagnostic testing. Proc Natl Acad Sci U S A 2006;103(14):5620–5625

109. Shadel BN, Puzniak LA, Gillespie KN, Lawrence SJ, Kollef M, Mundy LM. Surveillance for vancomycin-resistant enterococci: type, rates, costs, and implications. Infect Control Hosp Epidemiol 2006;27(10):1068–1075

110. Nijssen S, Bonten MJ, Weinstein RA. Are active microbiological surveillance and subsequent isolation needed to prevent the spread of methicillin-resistant *Staphylococcus aureus*? Clin Infect Dis 2005;40(3):405–409

111. Jain M, Miller L, Belt D, King D, Berwick DM. Decline in ICU adverse events, nosocomial infections and cost through a quality improvement initiative focusing on teamwork and culture change. Qual Saf Health Care 2006;15(4):235–239

112. Warren DK, Yokoe DS, Climo MW, et al. Preventing catheter-associated bloodstream infections: a survey of policies for insertion and care of central venous catheters from hospitals in the prevention epicenter program. Infect Control Hosp Epidemiol 2006;27(1):8–13

113. Pronovost P, Needham D, Berenholtz S, et al. An intervention to decrease catheter-related bloodstream infections in the ICU. N Engl J Med 2006;355(26):2725–2732

114. Cosgrove SE. Evidence that prevention makes cents: Costs of catheter-associated bloodstream infections in the intensive care unit. Crit Care Med 2006;34(8):2243–2244

115. Warren DK, Cosgrove SE, Diekema DJ, et al. A multicenter intervention to prevent catheter-associated bloodstream infections. Infect Control Hosp Epidemiol 2006;27(7):662–669

116. Danzig LE, Short LJ, Collins K, et al. Bloodstream infections associated with a needleless intravenous infusion system in patients receiving home infusion therapy. JAMA 1995;273(23):1862–1864

117. Kellerman S, Shay DK, Howard J, et al. Bloodstream infections in home infusion patients: the influence of race and needleless intravascular access devices. J Pediatr 1996;129(5):711–717

118. Cookson ST, Ihrig M, O'Mara EM, et al. Increased bloodstream infection rates in surgical patients associated with variation from recommended use and care following implementation of a needleless device. Infect Control Hosp Epidemiol 1998;19(1): 23–27

119. Maragakis LL, Bradley KL, Song X, et al. Increased catheter-related bloodstream infection rates after the introduction of a new mechanical valve intravenous access port. Infect Control Hosp Epidemiol 2006;27(1):67–70

120. Rosenthal VD, Guzman S, Safdar N. Reduction in nosocomial infection with improved hand hygiene in intensive care units of a tertiary care hospital in Argentina. Am J Infect Control 2005;33(7):392–397

Chapter 90
Implications of Antibiotic Resistance in Potential Agents of Bioterrorism

Linda M. Weigel and Stephen A. Morse

1 Introduction

One of the latest challenges to global public health is the deliberate dissemination of a biological agent via a number of different routes, including air, water, food, and infected vectors, to affect the health of humans. U.S. Congress began to address this challenge by providing funding to the Centers for Disease Control and Prevention (CDC) to enhance the ability of the nation's epidemiology and laboratory systems to respond to the deliberate release of a biological agent (1). A Strategic National Stockpile (SNS, formerly called the National Pharmaceutical Stockpile) was also established to provide large quantities of essential medical materiel to states and communities during such an emergency. The SNS contains antibiotics as well as chemical antidotes, antitoxins, life-support medications, intravenous administration kits, airway maintenance supplies, and medical/surgical items (2). The broad-spectrum antibiotics in the SNS play an important role in providing postexposure prophylaxis and treatment for individuals exposed to or infected with a bacterial agent as a result of a deliberate release. The antibiotics in the SNS were selected, in part, for their effectiveness on the basis of the current data for antimicrobial susceptibility of each bacterial species. However, revelations during the last decade suggested that in the former Soviet Union, a priority of the offensive biological weapons program was the development of recombinant organisms that were resistant to common therapies (3–5). With the increased potential for deliberate dispersal of antimicrobial-resistant pathogens, determining the antimicrobial susceptibility of suspected agents of bioterrorism has become essential for selection and distribution of effective prophylactic or therapeutic treatments. The objective of this chapter is to examine issues concerning antimicrobial susceptibility testing and antimicrobial resistance in selected bacterial agents that have been identified for public health preparedness efforts.

1.1 Definitions

The use of biological agents is often characterized by the manner in which they are employed. For the purposes of this article, *biological warfare* has been defined as a specialized type of warfare conducted by a government against a target; *bioterrorism* has been defined as the threat or use of biological agents (or toxins) by individuals or groups motivated by political, religious, ecological, or other ideological objectives (6). Criminals may also be driven by psychological pathologies and may use biological agents. When criminals use biological agents for murder, extortion, or revenge it is called a *biocrime* (6). Terrorists are distinguished from criminals on the basis of motivation and objectives.

2 Threat Agents

Many biological agents can cause illness in humans, but not all are capable of affecting public health and medical infrastructures on a large scale (7). In order to bring focus to public health preparedness activities, the CDC convened a meeting of national experts to review the criteria for selecting bacterial, viral, and toxin agents that posed the greatest threat to civilians and to help develop a list of these agents for public health preparedness efforts. The considerations for inclusion on the "Critical Agents List" included the ability of the agent to be widely disseminated either by aerosol or by other means; the ability of the agent to be transmitted from person to person; the public's perception, correct or incorrect, associated with the intentional release of the agent; and special public health preparedness needs such as vaccines, therapeutics, enhanced surveillance, and

D.L. Mayers (ed.), *Antimicrobial Drug Resistance*,
DOI 10.1007/978-1-60327-595-8_90, © Humana Press, a part of Springer Science+Business Media, LLC 2009

L.M. Weigel (✉)
Antimicrobial Resistance Laboratory, Division of Healthcare Quality Promotion, Centers for Disease Control and Prevention, Atlanta, GA, USA
lweigel@cdc.gov

diagnostics (7). The Critical Agents List (1) includes viruses, toxins, and bacteria; however, because of its focus on antimicrobial resistance, this chapter will cover only the critical bacterial agents (Table 1). It is also important to recognize that no priority was assigned within the categories and that the list did not rank the probability of deliberate use of an agent.

As currently defined, Category A agents, which include some of the classic bacteria used for biological warfare, are high-priority organisms that are most likely to cause mass casualties if deliberately disseminated. Some of these bacteria have been responsible for epic plagues throughout human history (8, 9). Today, natural infections caused by the bacterial agents in Category A are uncommon in the United States. For example, prior to the bioterrorist attacks with letters carrying endospores of *Bacillus anthracis* in 2001, the last case of inhalational anthrax in the United States was in 1976 in a home craftsman from California, who died after being infected by endospores that were present on contaminated imported yarn containing goat hair (10). Thus, the rarity of these infections can present problems for bioterrorism preparedness owing, in part, to a lack of clinical awareness and expertise in laboratory diagnosis.

The bacterial agents in Category B also have some potential for large-scale dissemination, but generally cause less illness and fewer deaths than those in Category A. Some diseases caused by Category B agents are also exceedingly uncommon. For example, the first reported case of *Burkholderia mallei* infection (i.e., glanders) in the United States since 1949 occurred as the result of a laboratory exposure in a microbiologist with insulin-dependent diabetes (11). Despite the patient's history of working with *B. mallei*, both the clinical and laboratory diagnoses were delayed, highlighting the difficulties of identifying these rare infections. Many of the Category B agents have been weaponized in the past, or are being considered as weapons by some state-sponsored programs (3, 12). Some Category B agents could be used to contaminate food or water sources. In addition, many of these agents are relatively easy to obtain and therefore are more likely to be used in the setting of a biocrime or bioterrorism (13). Category C agents are emerging infectious diseases or agents with characteristics that could be exploited for deliberate dissemination. The only bacterial agent in Category C is multidrug-resistant *Mycobacterium tuberculosis*. This bacterial agent is not currently believed to present a high bioterrorism risk to public health. However, it could emerge as a future threat because it has characteristics, such as aerosol transmission and multidrug resistance, which could be exploited (14).

Table 1 Critical bacterial agents for public health preparedness[a]

Agent	Disease
Category A[b]	
Bacillus anthracis	Anthrax
Yersinia pestis	Plague
Francisella tularensis	Tularemia
Category B[c]	
Coxiella burnetii	Q fever
Brucella species	Brucellosis
Burkholderia mallei	Glanders
Burkholderia pseudomallei	Melioidosis
Subset of category B spread by food and water	
Salmonella spp.	Salmonellosis
Shigella dysenteriae	Bacillary dysentery
Escherichia coli O157:H7	Hemolytic uremic syndrome
Vibrio cholerae	Cholera
Category C[d]	
Multidrug-resistant *Mycobacterium tuberculosis*	Tuberculosis

[a]Modified from (1)
[b]Other Category A agents: Variola major, Filoviruses (e.g., Ebola and Marburg), Arenaviruses (e.g., Lassa and Junin), *Clostridium botulinum* neurotoxins
[c]Other Category B agents: Alphaviruses (e.g., Venezuelan, Eastern and Western encephalomyelitis viruses), Staphylococcal enterotoxin B, Ricin from *Ricinus communis*, *Clostridium perfringens* episilon toxin, *Cryptosporidium parvum*
[d]Other Category C agents: Yellow-fever virus, Tickborne encephalitis complex (flavi) viruses, Tickborne hemorrhagic fever viruses, Nipah and Hendra Complex viruses, Hantaviruses

3 Bioterrorism Preparedness and Response

3.1 Laboratory Response Network

Because there is only a small window of opportunity during which prophylaxis or other control measures can be implemented to reduce the morbidity and mortality associated with a bioterrorism event, the public health response must be rapid to be effective (15). The Laboratory Response Network (LRN) was created in order to facilitate the rapid identification of threat agents (16). The LRN was established in 1999 by the CDC, in concert with the Association of Public Health Laboratories (APHL) and with collaboration from the Federal Bureau of Investigation (FBI) and the United States Army Medical Research Institute of Infectious Diseases (USAMRIID) to address the extremely limited national infrastructure of diagnostic testing laboratories competent to deal with biological terrorism that existed at that time.

This national system is designed to link state and local public health laboratories with other advanced-capacity clinical, military, veterinary, agricultural, and water- and food-testing laboratories, including those at the federal level, building upon the existing interactions of nationwide public health laboratories and their complementary disease surveillance activities (17).

The LRN consists of laboratories that operate in either a sentinel or reference capacity, with the latter characterized by progressively stringent safety, containment, and technical proficiency capabilities (16). Sentinel laboratories are, for the most part, hospital and clinical laboratories because it is likely that in the aftermath of a covert bioterrorism attack, patients will seek care at widely dispersed hospitals, some of which would house such laboratories (17). Sentinel laboratories participate in the LRN by ruling out the presence of a crticial agent or referring suspected critical agents (Table 1) encountered in their routine work to a nearby LRN reference laboratory. Protocols and algorithms, which are available on the Internet (www.asm.org or www.bt.cdc.gov), have been developed to make this process as rapid as possible. Reference laboratories that perform confirmatory testing and characterization are primarily local and state public health laboratories, employing both biosafety level 2 (BSL-2) facilities where BSL-3 practices are observed (i.e., for culture and identification of *Mycobacterium tuberculosis*), public health laboratories with full BSL-3 facilities, and laboratories with the certified animal facilities that are necessary for performing the requisite mouse toxicity assay for the detection of botulinum toxin. The LRN reference laboratories use standard protocols and reagents for the identification, confirmation, and characterization of threat agents. Characterization of bacterial agents includes determining antimicrobial susceptibility and resistance. There are currently over 175 LRN reference laboratories in the United States, Canada, United Kingdom, and Australia.

There are two national LRN laboratories (CDC and USAMRIID) with BSL-4 facilities that are capable of handling extremely dangerous viral pathogens (e.g., Ebola, Variola major) for which other laboratories have insufficient safety facilities. These federal laboratories identify agents in specimens submitted by the reference laboratories, and can also identify recombinant (e.g., chimeras) or genetically engineered microorganisms that may not be recognizable by conventional isolation and identification methods.

3.2 Epidemiological Investigations

Bioterrorism events can be characterized by two types of scenarios: overt (announced) and covert (unannounced). The deliberate nature of an intentional release will often be obvious, as in the case of multiple mailed letters containing highly refined anthrax spores (18). The letter received and opened in a Senator's office in the Hart Senate Office Building is an example of an overt attack. The letter stated that the envelope contained anthrax spores and that the person opening the letter was going to die. First responders were called, the presence of spores of *Bacillus anthracis* was confirmed, and the exposed individuals were placed on antimicrobial prophylaxis consisting of ciprofloxacin or doxycycline (19, 20); no one in the Hart Senate Office Building developed anthrax. Some forms of bioterrorism may be more covert, such as the deliberate contamination of salad bars in the Dalles, Oregon, with *Salmonella typhimurium*, which sickened more than 751 persons (21).

The LRN has a dual function in that it has the ability to detect and respond not only to agents released intentionally but also to those that occur naturally, a capacity that warrants emphasis because it will generally not be known at the time of detection whether the outbreak is intentional or natural. A few examples involving the critical bacterial agents will suffice. In the first, the outbreak on Martha's Vineyard of primary pneumonic tularemia in 11 patients in the summer of 2000 may have indicated a deliberate aerosol release of *Francisella tularensis* type A. However, the epidemiologic investigation suggested that infection was associated with lawn mowing and brush cutting, activities that could aerosolize the organism from the environment (22). Second, the occurrence of plague in a couple visiting New York City in November 2002 was highly unusual and suggested the possibility of bioterrorism because these infections occurred outside the area where plague is endemic in the United States (23). On initial consultation with medical personnel, the couple reported that they had traveled from Santa Fe County, New Mexico, where routine surveillance conducted by the New Mexico Department of Health had identified *Yersinia pestis* in a dead wood rat and fleas collected several months earlier on their New Mexico property. One day after the patients were evaluated, the New Mexico Department of Health and CDC investigated the couple's New Mexico property and a nearby hiking trail where rodents and fleas were collected. The results of pulsed-field gel electrophoresis and multiple-locus variable-number tandem repeat assays (MLVA) on isolates from one of the patients and from seven flea pools suggested that the *Y. pestis* infection was most likely acquired on the couple's property. Third, the case of inhalation anthrax in a male drum maker who resided in New York City in February 2006 raised the specter of bioterrorism. However, the epidemiologic investigation determined that the source of exposure was spores on dried goat hides brought back from Côte d'Ivoire (24).

The epidemiological investigation may identify indicators, one or more of which were noted in the examples above, that raise the level of suspicion that an outbreak may have been caused intentionally (25). These epidemiologic clues include the following:

- A single case of disease caused by an uncommon agent (e.g., inhalation or cutaneous anthrax, glanders) without adequate epidemiologic explanation;
- The presence of an unusual, atypical, or antiquated strain of an agent or antibiotic resistance pattern;
- Higher morbidity and mortality in association with a common disease or syndrome, or failure of such patients to respond to usual therapy;
- Unusual disease presentation, such as inhalation anthrax or pneumonic plague;
- Disease with an unusual geographic or seasonal distribution (e.g., plague in a nonendemic area);
- An unexpected increase in the incidence of stable endemic disease, such as tularemia or plague;
- Atypical disease transmission through aerosols, food, or water, in a mode suggesting sabotage (i.e., no other possible explanation);
- Several unusual or unexplained diseases coexisting in the same patient without any other explanation;
- Unusual illness that affects a large, disparate population (e.g., respiratory disease in a large heterogeneous population may suggest exposure to an inhaled biologic agent);
- Illness that is unusual (or atypical) for a given population or age group (e.g., outbreak of measles-like rash in adults);
- Unusual pattern of death or illness among animals that is unexplained or attributed to an agent of bioterrorism that precedes or accompanies illness or death in humans;
- Unusual pattern of death or illness in humans that precedes or accompanies illness or death in animals, which may be unexplained or attributed to an agent of bioterrorism;
- Agents of an unusual illness isolated from temporally or spatially distinct sources that have a similar genotype;
- Simultaneous clusters of similar unusual illness in noncontiguous areas, domestic or foreign;
- Large numbers of unexplained diseases or deaths;
- Large numbers of ill individuals who seek treatment at about the same time (point source with compressed epidemic curve).

4 Critical Bacterial Agents

Vaccination has not been a major strategy in pre-event preparedness for the general population. Thus, it is imperative that the antimicrobial susceptibility patterns of suspected bacterial agents of bioterrorism be determined so that effective prophylactic or therapeutic treatment (Table 2) can be administered (26). However, all the bacterial agents in

Category A and many in Category B (Table 1) require BSL-3 containment and practices, which are usually not found in the sentinel and other clinical laboratories, but which are necessary for performing antimicrobial susceptibility studies. Many of these bacteria have intrinsic resistance to one or more antimicrobials. In addition, many of these bacterial agents can be genetically engineered by introduction of genes required for antimicrobial resistance (26) or selection of resistant mutants by in vitro passage on low levels of antimicrobial agents (27, 28). Thus, the antimicrobial susceptibility pattern of a microorganism encountered as a result of an intentional release is not necessarily predictable.

The deliberate introduction of antimicrobial resistance markers or selection of antimicrobial-resistant strains of critical bacterial agents is generally considered to be unethical. However, the introduction of antimicrobial resistance markers may be justifiable under certain circumstances (29). For example, DNA manipulation for genetic studies on virulence factors often requires the use of plasmids with antimicrobial resistance genes as markers for selection. In such cases, the antimicrobial resistance genes used should not confer resistance to antibiotics used for the treatment of infections caused by that organism (30). Nevertheless, laboratory mutants with resistance to antimicrobial agents used for treatment (e.g., ciprofloxacin) have been generated for studies on the molecular basis and for detection of fluoroquinolone resistance (27, 31, 32). Most laboratories use attenuated or avirulent strains for these purposes.

4.1 Detection of Resistance

Procedures for susceptibility testing may generate aerosols that pose a high risk of laboratory-acquired infections. Therefore, antimicrobial susceptibility testing of the critical bacterial agents should be performed only in designated LRN laboratories. Trained personnel, BSL-2 or BSL-3 laboratory facilities (depending on the organism), and personal protective equipment are required to work with these organisms. In addition to the hazards associated with the mechanics of performing susceptibility testing, BSL-3 working conditions contribute to difficulties in obtaining accurate and consistent results. Mohammed et al. (33) recognized this issue, commenting that visual evaluation of growth in broth microdilution assays or the ability to see single colonies or light films of growth on agar plates is complicated by the necessity of reading susceptibility results through the glass barrier of a biological safety cabinet. Visibility may be further compromised when laboratory personnel are using power-assisted respirators with face shields.

Susceptibility testing methods include disk diffusion, agar dilution, broth microdilution, and Etest. Many factors influence the test results. Among these are (1) inoculum density, which has been described as the single most important variable in susceptibility testing (34); (2) the pH, electrolyte concentration, and composition of the medium; (3) time and temperature of incubation; and (4) growth characteristics of the strain to be tested. This is because a typical susceptibility testing medium, such as Mueller-Hinton broth or agar, must be either enhanced with specific supplements (e.g., *Francisella*) or changed to a specific agar or broth medium (e.g., *Brucella*) to support growth of some critical bacterial agents. Not all procedures are appropriate for every species. For example, results of disk diffusion tests are not reliable for slow-growing organisms (34) such as *F. tularensis* and *Brucella* spp., and none of these in vitro culture methods supports the growth of *C. burnetii*.

The intrinsic resistance mechanisms in each species, the potential for additional naturally acquired resistance mechanisms among individual strains, and the possibility of engineered resistance are compelling reasons for susceptibility testing to guide therapy and prophylaxis in the event of a natural outbreak or intentional release of these organisms. Guidelines for broth dilution susceptibility testing of *B. anthracis*, *Brucella* spp., *B. mallei*, *B. pseudomallei*, *F. tularensis*, and *Y. pestis* are available in the Clinical and Laboratory Standards Institute (CLSI, formerly National Center for Clinical Laboratory Standards, NCCLS) document M100-S16. The guidelines provide testing conditions, quality control recommendations, and MIC (μg/mL) interpretations for susceptibility and resistance.

Interpretation of in vitro susceptibility data for facultative (e.g., *Brucella* spp. or *F. tularensis*) or obligate intracellular pathogens (e.g., *C. burnetii*) requires consideration of multiple factors that may affect the in vivo activity of the agent. These factors include the ability of the antimicrobial agent to enter an infected host phagocyte and the microenvironment within the eukaryotic intracellular space where the organism resides. The uptake and accumulation (pharmacokinetics) of the various classes of agents by phagocytes are dependent upon the chemical structure of the agent. The intracellular concentration of an antimicrobial agent is expressed as C_c/C_e, the ratio of the cellular (C_c) and extracellular (C_e) concentrations. Therefore, $C_c/C_e > 1$ indicates a higher concentration (accumulation) within the eukaryotic cells of the host. The slightly acidic cytosol prevents the intracellular accumulation of weakly acidic antimicrobial agents, such as β-lactams (35) and $C_c/C_e < 1$. However, even zwitterionic β-lactams (e.g., ampicillin) and many cephalosporins do not accumulate intracellularly, suggesting that additional factors are involved in the exclusion of β-lactams from intracellular cytosol and compartments (36). Macrolides, however, accumulate in many types of cells (37–41). This class of agents has a weakly basic character, which allows much higher concentrations to accumulate within the highly acidic (pH = 5)

phagolysosomes than in the cytosol (42, 43). Among the macrolides, C_c/C_e values at equilibrium range from 4 to 10 for erythromycin to 40–300 for azithromycin (36). Fluoroquinolones accumulate very quickly in cells (44–46), while aminoglycosides accumulate in the cell so slowly that early studies concluded that this class of antimicrobial agents did not enter eukaryotic cells (47). However, over a period of several days, aminoglycoside concentrations within macrophages have been shown to increase to 2–4 times the concentration outside the cell (48–50). There are limited data on the intracellular accumulation of tetracyclines (49, 51) or sulfonamides (52). It is important to note that the various methods used for determining the intracellular concentrations and, as a result, the C_c/C_e values may result in conflicting data between studies.

In addition to intracellular accumulation, the intracellular activity (pharmacodynamics) of an antimicrobial agent must be considered. Both the infecting microbe and the antimicrobial agent may exert unknown influences on the infected host cell (53). The pH within the cytosol or phagolysosome will affect the antimicrobial activity of some agents more than others. The general consensus is that fluoroquinolones, macrolides, and tetracyclines should have activity against intracellular bacteria and that β-lactams and aminoglycosides show little or no activity against intracellular bacteria. However, there are examples of β-lactam and aminoglycoside therapies that are known to be effective against intracellular infections. These include the use of β-lactams for the treatment of listeriosis and the use of aminoglycosides for the treatment of brucellosis, plague, tularemia, and tuberculosis (54–57).

4.1.1 Genomic Analysis for Determination of Possible Intrinsic Resistance

A number of genome sequences have been completed for the bacterial agents belonging to Category A and B and are publicly available (58). The annotated genomes can be searched for genes associated with resistance to antimicrobial agents (Table 3). The information that can be obtained in this manner is important but has limitations. Genome annotations are produced by computer algorithims to identify potential protein coding regions on the basis of the search of databases for sequence homology. Many of the genes thus identified have not been verified by laboratory methods. Also, in vitro susceptibility studies are necessary to ascertain whether potential resistance genes are expressed and functional. In addition, there may be considerable variability in the resistance genes among different strains, which is not reflected in the available genome sequence(s) of one or a few strains, and the available genome data may not reflect recent acquisition of antimicrobial resistance. Nevertheless, genomic data complements in vitro susceptibility data and may provide important information on mechanisms of resistance.

4.2 Bacillus anthracis

4.2.1 General Characteristics

B. anthracis, the etiologic agent of anthrax, is an aerobic, facultative anaerobic, spore-forming, nonmotile, nonhemolytic Gram-positive rod that grows rapidly (doubling time of 30 min) on most microbiologic media. The rod-shaped cells typically grow in long, bamboo-like chains that are characteristic of the organism. Optimal growth is achieved at 37°C, and growth does not occur at temperatures $\geq$ 43°C. B. anthracis cells are encapsulated in infected tissues and when grown with appropriate in vitro culture conditions.

Two plasmids, pXO1 and pXO2, are required for virulence. pXO1 encodes the genes required for production of lethal and edema toxins (59) and pXO2 encodes the genes for the antiphagocytic poly-D-glutamic acid capsule (60). Elevated temperature and CO_2 concentration are considered to be physiological signals for B. anthracis. Both toxin production and capsule formation are enhanced by growth in 5% CO_2 or in a medium supplemented with bicarbonate.

The CO_2/bicarbonate response is specific (not due to buffering capacity or decreased oxygen concentration) and results in a 20–25-fold increase in capsular gene transcription as well as a 5–8-fold increase in toxin production. Expression of toxin genes is further enhanced by growth of B. anthracis at 37°C.

B. anthracis is a pathogen of herbivores, and human infection is usually accidental, resulting from contact with contaminated meat or hides. In humans, the disease may present as cutaneous, inhalational, or gastrointestinal anthrax, based on the route of infection. Cutaneous anthrax occurs following introduction of spores through a wound in the skin. The lesion progresses from a papule to a characteristic eschar (a firm, dry, black lesion), which is accompanied by extensive edema. Antibiotics will not alter the progression of the lesion but will prevent systemic infection. Gastrointestinal anthrax may affect either the oropharynx area (resulting in sore throat, dysphagia, fever, and regional lymphadenopathy) or the intestines (characterized by nausea, vomiting, fever, and bloody diarrhea). In both cases, toxemia is rapidly followed by shock and death. The mortality rate of gastrointestinal anthrax is >50%, with death occurring 2–5 days after onset of symptoms. Inhalational anthrax is a rapidly fatal disease, with death occurring 2–7 days post exposure, depending on the number of organisms inhaled. Initial symptoms may be mild, but if left untreated a rapid succession of sudden shock, collapse, and death all occur within a matter of hours. At the time of death the blood may contain as many as 10^9 bacilli/mL in untreated patients (9).

4.2.2 Antimicrobial Susceptibility and Resistance

Intrinsic Resistance

The antimicrobials used for treatment of the various forms of anthrax and for post-exposure prophylaxis are listed in Table 2. Historically, penicillin has been the drug of choice for treatment of anthrax. Several susceptibility studies have been published (33, 62–65), most of which were conducted since the intentional release of B. anthracis in 2001 (Table 4). Comparison of the MICs determined by these studies has been difficult because there was no standardized testing method, nor were there any interpretive criteria available for B. anthracis. Most studies relied on breakpoints published for Staphylococcus aureus to interpret the data. Mohammed et al. (33) addressed this issue in a comparison of broth microdilution and Etest agar gradient diffusion methods and found that most of the results for the two methods were comparable, with the exception of penicillin. The Etest MIC result for a penicillin-resistant isolate of B. anthracis was consistently in the susceptible range, having 4–9 doubling dilutions difference when compared with the MIC from the broth microdilution method. The MIC results for other agents used for treatment or prophylaxis of anthrax, such as ciprofloxacin and doxycycline, indicate good in vitro activity against B. anthracis.

Although B. anthracis is generally susceptible to penicillin, penicillin-resistant strains as well as treatment failures with penicillin have been reported (66–68). Laboratory results with strains obtained from various sources estimate that the prevalence of naturally occurring penicillin-resistant B. anthracis ranges from 3 to 11.5% (64, 65). Two β-lactamase genes have been identified in the chromosome of B. anthracis, located approximately 900 kb apart (69). The bla1 gene, which encodes a group 2a penicillinase, is usually not expressed. The bla2 gene, which encodes a cephalosporinase similar to a group 3 Bacillus cereus metalloenzyme, is poorly expressed. The genes for both enzymes have been cloned and shown to confer resistance to β-lactams when expressed in E. coli (70). Further studies are required to fully explain the low levels of expression and activity found in most isolates of B. anthracis. In addition to the cephalosporinase, B. anthracis apparently has a high level of intrinsic resistance to both second- and third-generation cephalosporins, which is not associated with β-lactamase activity. Chen et al. (69) demonstrated that a laboratory-generated mutant of B. anthracis Sterne, lacking both bla1 and bla2, remained resistant to cefepime, ceftazidime, and cefpodoxime (MICs > 32, >128, >16 μg/mL, respectively). In vitro susceptibility results (Table 4) indicated that <10% of isolates tested were susceptible to cephalosporins (62).

B. anthracis is highly resistant to aztreonam (Table 4) and exhibits decreased susceptibility to macrolides such as erythromycin. Using susceptibility breakpoints for S. aureus,

Table 2 Antibiotics used in the treatment of infections caused by selected critical bacterial agents

Disease	Antibiotic	References
Anthrax	Ciprofloxacin[a]	(26, 27)
	Doxycycline[a]	
	Tetracycline[a]	
	Rifampin	
	Vancomycin	
	Penicillin[a]	
	Ampicillin	
	Chloramphenicol	
	Imipenem	
	Clindamycin	
	Clarithromycin	
	Amoxicillin	
	Meropenem	
	Levofloxacin	
	Penicillin G procaine	
Tularemia	Streptomycin[a]	(29)
	Gentamicin[a]	
	Doxycycline[a]	
	Tetracycline[a]	
	Chloramphenicol[a]	
	Ciprofloxacin[a]	
	Levofloxacin[a]	
Plague	Streptomycin[a]	(30)
	Gentamicin[a]	
	Doxycycline[a]	
	Tetracycline[a]	
	Ciprofloxacin[a]	
	Chloramphenicol[a]	
	Trimethoprim–sulfamethoxazole[a]	
Brucellosis	Doxycycline[a]	(31)
	Streptomycin[a]	
	Gentamicin	
	Rifampin	
	Trimethoprim–sulfamethoxazole[a]	
Glanders	Ceftazidime[a]	(32)
	Imipenem[a]	
	Doxycycline[a]	
	Tetracycline[a]	
Melioidosis	Ceftazidime[a]	(32, 33)
	Imipenem[a]	
	[a]Trimethoprim–sulfamethoxazole	
	Chloramphenicol	
	Doxycycline	
	Amoxacillin/clavulinic acid[a]	
Q Fever	Doxycycline	(34)
	Ciprofloxacin	
	Rifampin	
	Erythromycin	

[a]Interpretive guidelines for susceptibility or resistance available from CLSI (61)

Table 3 Antimicrobial resistance genes identified in the annotated genomes of category A and B bacterial agents[a]

Genome	Resistance genes
Bacillus anthracis[b]	Aminoglycosides
A0039	*aacC7*, aminoglycoside N-acetyltransferase
Ames	*str*, aminoglycoside 6-adenylyltransferase
Ames Ancestor	Aminoglycoside phosphotransferase
CNEVA 9066 (France)	β-Lactams
Kruger B	*bla1*, β-lactamase (penicillinase)
Sterne	*bla2*, β-lactamase (cephalosporinase)
Vollum	Metallo-β-lactamase family protein
Western N. America USA 6153	*mecR1*, methicillin resistance
	Chloramphenicol
	cat, chloramphenicol acetyltransferase
	bmr, chloramphenicol resistance protein
	Glycopeptides
	vanW, vancomycin B-type resistance protein
	vanZ, teicoplanin resistance
	Macrolides
	Macrolide 2-phosphotransferase
	Macrolide efflux protein
	Macrolide glycosyltransferase
	Tetracyclines
	tet(V), putative tetracycline efflux
	Others
	bacA-1, bacA-2, bacitracin resistance
	bmr1, bicyclomycin resistance
	fosB-1, fosmidomycin resistance
	vgaB, pristinamycin resistance
	emrA, multidrug resistance
	qac, quaternary ammonium compound resistance
	Multidrug resistance protein, Smr family
Brucella abortus 9–941	β-Lactams
	Putative β-lactamase
	Metallo-β-lactamase family proteins
	Macrolides
	Macrolide efflux protein
	Others
	fsr, fosmidomycin resistance
	qacH, quaternary ammonium compound resistance
Brucella melitensis Biovar Abortus	Aminoglycosides
	Aminoglycoside phosphotransferase
	β-Lactams
	β-Lactamase
	Metallo-β-lactamase family proteins
	Macrolides
	Macrolide efflux protein
	Tetracyclines
	tet(B), tetracycline efflux
	Others
	Multidrug resistance efflux protein
	norM, probable multidrug resistance
	Fosmidomycin resistance protein
	Florfenicol resistance protein
	Bleomycin resistance protein

(continued)

Table 3 (continued)

Genome	Resistance genes
	qacE, qacH, quaternary ammonium compound
	marC, multiple antibiotic resistance
	Bicyclomycin resistance
	fusB, fusC; fusaric acid resistance
Brucella melitensis 16M	Aminoglycoside
	Aminoglycoside phosphotransferase
	Chloramphenicol
	cat, chloramphenicol acetyltransferase
	Others
	emrB/qacA, macrolide efflux protein
	Florfenicol resistance
	fosB, fosfomycin resistance
	Multidrug resistance protein
	norM, putative multidrug resistance
Brucella suis 1330	Metallo-β-lactamase
	norM, putative multidrug resistance protein
	fsr, fosmidomycin resistance
	Fosfomycin resistance family protein
Burkholderia mallei ATCC 23344	Aminoglycosides
	aac(6´)-Iz, aminoglycoside 6-acetyltransferase
	β-lactams
	Metallo-β-lactamase
	penA (class A β-lactamase)
	Others
	Fosmidomycin resistance protein
	Fusaric acid resistance protein
	norM, putative multidrug resistance protein
Burkholderia pseudomallei 1710b	Aminoglycosides
	Aminoglycoside phosphotransferase
	β-Lactams
	β-Lactamase
	Metallo-β-lactamase
	oxa β-lactamase
	Macrolides
	macA, macB (macrolide-specific ABC-type efflux)
	Tetracyclines
	Tetracycline resistance protein, class A (efflux)
	Others
	Bleomycin resistance protein
	emrA, emrB; multidrug resistance
	Fsr, fosmidomycin resistance
	Fusaric acid resistance
	mdtA, mdtB, mdtC; multidrug resistance
	qacE, quaternary ammonium compound resistance
Burkholderia pseudomallei K96243	Aminoglycosides
	Aminoglycoside acetyltransferase
	β-Lactams
	β-Lactamase
	blaA (class A β-lactamase)
	oxa β-lactamase
	Metallo-β-lactamase
	Putative class B β-lactamase
	Tetracyclines
	Putative tetracycline efflux protein
	Others
	Bleomycin resistance protein
	emrB, multidrug resistance
	Fsr, fosmidomycin resistance

Genome	Resistance genes
	Fusaric acid resistance protein, putative
	mexB, putative multidrug resistance
	norM, multidrug resistance
	qacE, quaternary ammonium compound resistance
Francisella tularensis subsp. *tularensis* Schu 4	β-Lactams
	blaA (class A β-lactamase)
	β-Lactamase
	Metallo-β-lactamase (putative)
	Tetracyclines
	tet (multidrug transporter)
	Others
	Bcr/cflA, drug resistance transporter
	Fusaric acid resistance protein, putative
Coxiella burnetii RSA 493	Aminoglycosides
	aacA4, aminoglycoside 6-acetyltransferase
	β-Lactams
	β-Lactamase
	Metallo-β-lactamase family protein
	Others
	Multidrug resistance protein
Yersinia pestis CO92	β-Lactams
	ampG, ampE, ampD β-lactamase induction proteins
	Macrolides
	Macrolide efflux protein, putative
	Others
	bacA, bacitracin resistance, putative
	bicR/bicA, probable drug resistance translocator
	emrA, emrB, emrD-2; multidrug resistance
	marC, multidrug resistance
	qacE, quaternary ammonium compound resistance
	tcaB, multidrug resistance
	vceA/vceB, multidrug resistance
Yersinia pestis KIM	Others
	bacA, bacitracin resistance protein
	bcr, bicyclomycin resistance
	emrA, emrD-2, *emrE* multidrug resistance
	farB, drug resistance translocase
	Fosmidomycin resistance protein
Yersinia pestis Biovar Medievalis 91001	β-Lactams
	ampD1, ampE, ampG, ampG1 (β-lactamase induction proteins)
	β-Lactamase
	Metallo- β-lactamase family proteins
	Predicted Zn-dependent β-lactamase
	Others
	bcr, bicyclomycin resistance
	bssH bicyclomycin resistance (sulfonamide resistance)
	emrA/emrB, multidrug resistance
	Fusaric acid resistance
	marC2, multiple antibiotic resistance
	qacE, quaternary ammonium compound resistance
	ydeF, putative multidrug resistance

[a] J. Craig Venter Institute, www.jcvi.org/cmr; formerly TIGR–CMR, The Institute for Genomic Research–Comprehensive Microbial Resource at www.cmr.tigr.org

[b] Identified genes, gene copy numbers, and chromosomal locations vary among strains of *B. anthracis*

Table 4 Selected antimicrobial susceptibility studies by Etest, broth microdilution, and agar dilution for *Bacillus anthracis*

Antimicrobial agent	Doganay and Aydin (62)[a], agar dilution, n = 22		Mohammed et al. (33)[b], broth microdilution, n = 65		Coker et al. (63)[c], Etest, n = 25		Cavallo et al. (64)[d], agar dilution, n = 96		Turnbull et al. (65)[e], Etest, n = 76	
	MIC[f] range	% S-I-R[g]	MIC range	% S-I-R	MIC range	% S-I-R	MIC Range	% S-I-R	MIC range	% S-I-R
Amikacin	0.03 to 0.06	100-0-0					0.125 to 16	88.5-0-11.5		
Amoxicillin	0.015 to 003	ND								
Amox/clav	0.015 to 0.015	100-0-0							0.016 to 0.5	100-0-0
Azithromycin									1 to 12	26-64-10
Aztreonam	>128	0-0-100	4 to 32	22-78-0			1 to >128	0-0-100		
Cefaclor					0.125 to 0.75	100-0-0				
Cefotaxime	8 to 32	4.5-13.5-82							3 to >32	1-1-98
Cefoxitin							1 to 64	74-15.3-10.7		
Ceftazidime	128 to 256	4.5-0-95.5								
Ceftriaxone	16 to 32	9-50-41					4 to 64	0-100-0		
Cefuroxime	16 to 64	4.5-9-86.5			6 to 48	4-76-20				
Cephalexin					0.38 to 2	100-0-0				
Cephalothin							0.125 to 32	83.2-12.2-4.6		
Chloramphenicol	1 to 2	100-0-0	2 to 8	100-0-0			1 to 4	100-0-0		
Ciprofloxacin	0.03 to 0.06	100-0-0	0.03 to 0.12	100-0-0	0.032 to 0.38	100-0-0	0.03 to 0.5	100-0-0	0.032 to 0.094	100-0-0
Clindamycin	0.5 to 1	95.5-4.5-0	≤0.5 to 1	94-6-0			0.125 to 1	100-0-0		
Doxycycline					0.094 to 0.38	100-0-0	0.125 to 0.25	100-0-0		
Erythromycin			0.5 to 1	3-97-0			0.5 to 4	95.4-4.6-0	0.5 to 1	15-85-0
Gatifloxacin							0.125 to 0.125	100-0-0		
Gentamicin	0.03 to 0.25	100-0-0					0.125 to 0.5	100-0-0	0.064 to 0.5	100-0-0
Imipenem							0.125 to 2	0-0-100		
Levofloxacin							0.03 to 1	100-0-0		
Nalidixic acid							0.125 to 32	94.8-4.2-1		
Ofloxacin	0.03 to 0.06	100-0-0					0.06 to 2	99-1-0		
Penicillin			≤0.06 to 128	97-0-3	≤0.016 to 0.5	88-0-12	0.125 to 16	88.5-0-11.5	≤0.016 to >32	97-0-3
Pefloxacin	0.125 to 0.5	100-0-0					0.03 to 1	100-0-0		
Piperacillin							0.25 to 32	99-1-0		
Rifampin	1 to 4	ND	≤0.25 to 0.5	100-0-0			0.125 to 0.5	99-1-0		
Streptomycin							0.5 to 2	100-0-0		
Teicoplanin							0.125 to 0.5	100-0-0		
Tetracycline	0.25 to 1	100-0-0	0.03 to 0.06	100-0-0					0.016 to 0.094	100-0-0
Tobramycin	0.25 to 1	100-0-0			0.25 to 1.5	100-0-0				
Vancomycin	0.25 to 1	95.5-4.5-0	0.5 to 2	100-0-0			0.25 to 2	100-0-0	0.75 to 5	99-1-0

[a]Mueller–Hinton agar, 37°C/overnight (62); n number of strains
[b]Cation-adjusted Mueller–Hinton broth, 35°C/16–24h (33)
[c]Tryptic soy agar with 5% sheep blood, 37°C/overnight (63)
[d]Mueller–Hinton agar, 37°C/18h (64)
[e]Mueller–Hinton agar, 36°C/18–20h (65)
[f]MIC, minimal inhibitory concentration in μg/mL
[g]S- susceptible; I- intermediate; R- resistant: based on breakpoints for S. aureus (Interpretive criteria for ciprofloxacin, doxycycline, penicillin, and tetracycline available from CLSI for B. anthracis since 2003)

two studies (33, 65) found 97% and 85% of the isolates to be intermediate for erythromycin. A strain of *B. anthracis* from Korea was reported to possess the *ermJ* macrolide resistance determinant (71), which, if expressed, would confer resistance to macrolides, lincosamides, and streptogramin B. However, the MICs for these antimicrobial agents were not included in the report.

B. anthracis is naturally resistant to trimethoprim and sulfamethoxazole (72). The organism appears to be susceptible to rifampin in vitro; however, in an in vivo murine model, treatment with rifampin did not significantly increase the survival rate of infected mice (73). There have been no reports of naturally occurring *B. anthracis* with resistance to aminoglycosides, doxycycline, or fluoroquinolones. However, *B. anthracis* has been shown to acquire resistance determinants in its natural environment, the rhizosphere of grass plants (74); and coexisting soil-dwelling bacteria are known to harbor an extensive reservoir of resistance determinants (75). Thus, the potential for natural acquisition of additional antimicrobial resistance genes should not be overlooked.

The complete genome sequence has been determined for numerous strains of *B. anthracis* including strains A0039, Ames, Ames Ancestor, Sterne, Vollum, Western North America USA6153, CNEVA 9066 (France), and Kruger B http://cmr.jcvi.org/ (J. Craig Venter Institute, formerly The Institute for Genomic Research, TIGR). A search of the annotated sequences revealed numerous potential resistance genes in each strain (Table 3). In addition to the known β-lactamase genes, *bla1* and *bla2*, putative resistance determinants for aminoglycosides, chloramphenicol, macrolides, and a tetracycline were noted. As is the case with penicillin, the presence of a resistance determinant does not necessarily confer the resistance phenotype. For example, genes for chloramphenicol acetyltransferase (*cat*) and a chloramphenicol resistance protein (*bmr*) have been identified in the genomes of all the strains that have been sequenced (Table 3), yet results of in vitro susceptibility studies show that this organism remains susceptible to chloramphenicol (Table 4). The gene and/or the encoded protein may be incomplete or nonfunctional, or mutations in the regulatory elements controlling transcription or translation may prevent or limit expression.

Engineered Resistance

Resistance to several antimicrobial agents has been genetically introduced, or resistant mutants have been selected by in vitro passage. For example, fluoroquinolone-resistant mutants have been selected in vitro by serial passages on media with increasing concentrations of fluoroquinolones (27, 28, 31, 32, 76). Point mutations in the resistant organisms were found in the quinolone resistance-determining regions (QRDR) of *gyrA*,

parC, and *gyrB*. MICs were increased by 16- to 2,048-fold for ofloxacin, ciprofloxacin, levofloxacin, and moxifloxacin (77). In Gram-positive bacteria, such as *S. aureus* and *Streptococcus pneumoniae*, the preferred target for most fluoroquinolones is *parC* (78). However, first-step mutants of *B. anthracis* harbored point mutations in *gyrA* and second-step mutants acquired either a mutation in *parC* or an additional mutation in *gyrA*. The resulting amino acid substitutions within the QRDR were in the same position and with similar changes to those found in other Gram-positive bacteria. For GyrA, the most frequent change observed was Ser85-Leu and for ParC, Ser81-Phe (or Tyr). Amino acid changes detected at the Glu89 position of GyrA were highly variable (28, 32, 77).

Tetracycline resistance has been transferred to *B. anthracis* by the introduction of plasmids or transposons. Resistance to tetracycline, doxycycline, and minocycline was reported following introduction of pBC16, a plasmid that was originally obtained from *B. cereus* strain GP7 (79–81). Pomerantsev and Staritsyn (81) introduced a recombinant plasmid, pCET, which encodes the *tet*(L) gene, into the Russian anthrax vaccine strain STI-1. The *tet*(L) gene confers resistance to tetracycline but not to minocycline or glycylcyclines (82). Resistance to tetracyclines has also been transferred to *B. anthracis* following transposon mutagenesis using Tn*916* (83) and Tn*917* (84). Strains with point mutations resulting in streptomycin and rifampin resistance have been isolated following UV mutagenesis (84).

A multidrug-resistant strain of *B. anthracis* was engineered by Stepanov et al. (85) by the introduction of a plasmid, pTEC, into the Russian vaccine strain STI-1. The new strain, designated STI-AR, was resistant to penicillin, rifampin, tetracycline, chloramphenicol, macrolides, and lincosamides. Stable inheritance of the plasmid and resistance phenotype was confirmed for this strain.

Other resistance genes that have been transferred to *B. anthracis* include *ermC* on pE194, which encodes resistance to macrolides (81); *aad9* on a recombinant plasmid designated pDC, which encodes resistance to spectinomycin (87); and, chloramphenicol acetyltransferase (pC194/*cat*), which confers resistance to chloramphenicol (80).

4.3 *Yersinia pestis*

4.3.1 General Characteristics

Y. pestis, the etiologic agent of plague, is an aerobic, nonmotile, bipolar staining, Gram-negative coccobacillus, and is a member of the family Enterobacteriaceae. The organism grows relatively slowly, forming small colonies after 24–48 h. *Y. pestis* grows on most laboratory media (88) over a wide range of temperatures, with optimal growth at 28°C. To achieve the visible growth required for broth microdilution susceptibility testing, incubation for up to 48 h may be required.

Plague is a zoonotic disease. The classic model of the transmission *Y. pestis* from fleas to mammals was described by Bacot in 1915. In this model, the vector was the oriental rat flea (*Xenopsylla cheopis*). Ingestion of *Y. pestis* by the fleas during a blood meal from an infected animal results in infection of the flea. In *X. cheopis*, *Y. pestis* multiplies in the alimentary canal and eventually clumps of bacteria form, blocking attempts to feed by ingesting another blood meal. In this model, transmission results when the infected flea attempts to feed on another animal or human. Contaminated mouth parts or regurgitation of infected material results in infection of the new host. Twelve to sixteen days are required for the flea infection to progress to the point where the blockage results in an infectious vector, a time frame that is not consistent with the rapid spread of plague during epizootics or pandemics. Recent reports suggest that *Y. pestis* can be transmitted by unblocked fleas in other models. Eisen et al. (89) investigated the transmission of plague from *Oropsylla montana*, a flea that infests squirrels and is the primary vector of *Y. pestis* to humans in North America. These fleas rarely became blocked, were immediately infectious, and efficiently transmitted *Y. pestis* for 4 days following an infected blood meal. The dynamics of this flea model are consistent with the rapid rates of transmission necessary to support enzootic and epizootic spread of *Y. pestis*.

Animal reservoirs of *Y. pestis* include many rodents, especially rats, as well as squirrels, and prairie dogs. The most common type of human infection, bubonic plague, is characterized by bubos (acute lymphadenitis) that result from spread of the organism from the flea bite through the bloodstream to the lymph nodes where it grows in large numbers. However, human plague may also present as pneumonia or septicemia, or as meningitis (90).

In humans and animals *Y. pestis* is a facultative intracellular organism. While largely destroyed by polymorphonuclear (PMN) white blood cells, *Y. pestis* cells that are engulfed by monocytes will grow intracellularly and become resistant to phagocytosis by both types of phagocytes (55).

4.3.2 Antimicrobial Susceptibility and Resistance

Intrinsic Resistance

Mortality rates from plague are high in the absence of antimicrobial therapy. Fortunately, most isolates of *Y. pestis* are susceptible to antimicrobial agents that are active against Gram-negative bacteria. The antimicrobial agents used for the treatment of the various forms of *Y. pestis* infection are listed in Table 2. *Y. pestis* appears to be susceptible to β-lactams in vitro (Table 5), but penicillin and cephalosporins are considered to be ineffective for therapy (55). This difference may be due to the facultative intracellular nature of *Y. pestis* or to the expression of resistance genes (Table 3) in the human host. Streptomycin is the drug of choice for treatment of plague, but the availability of this agent is limited (95, 96). Gentamicin is an acceptable substitute (MIC_{90} = 0.5–1 µg/mL, Table 5). Both doxycycline and ciprofloxacin have been shown to be effective therapeutic agents.

In 1997 a multidrug-resistant strain of *Y. pestis* was isolated from a patient in Madagascar (97). This isolate was resistant to many of the drugs recommended for therapy and prophylaxis. The resistance phenotypes and associated genes included ampicillin, TEM-1 β-lactamase; chloramphenicol, *catI;* kanamycin, *aph(3′)-I;* streptomycin and spectinomycin, *aad(3″);* sulfonamides, *sulI;* tetracycline and minocycline, *tet*(D). A 150-kb broad-host-range conjugative plasmid, pIP1202, most likely originating from Enterobacteriaceae, was found to be responsible for the multidrug resistance. The plasmid was highly transferable in vitro, raising concerns that the incidence of multidrug-resistant *Y. pestis* may increase in future outbreaks of plague.

High-level resistance to streptomycin, an agent used for the treatment of plague in many countries outside the United States, has recently been reported for another clinical isolate of *Y. pestis* from Madagascar (98). The resistance determinant was encoded on a 40-kb conjugative plasmid, pIP1203, that transferred to other strains of *Y. pestis* at high frequencies. Molecular analysis identified the resistance genes as *aph(3″)-Ib* and *aph(6)-Id. Y. pestis* strains harboring the multidrug resistance plasmid pIP1202 and the streptomycin resistance plasmid pIP1203 were of different ribotypes. Furthermore, pIP1202 and pIP1203 belonged to different plasmid incompatibility groups. These results indicate that these two strains arose independently and that there are at least two different resistance plasmids present in strains of *Y. pestis* found in Madagascar.

Wong et al. (94) reported resistance to rifampin and imipenem in 20% of 92 *Y. pestis* isolates from diverse sources. However, all the strains were susceptible to antimicrobial agents recommended for treatment and prophylaxis. *Y. pestis* is usually highly susceptible to trimethoprim, although published reports from Russia indicate that resistance to trimethoprim is a natural marker for a variant of *Y. pestis* recovered from voles (99).

The DNA sequences of the complete genomes of numerous strains of *Y. pestis* have been determined. These include *Y. pestis* strains CO92, KIM, and biovar Medievalis 91001 http://cmr.jcvi.org/ (J. Craig Venter Institute, formerly The Institute for Genomic Research, TIGR). Putative resistance genes listed in the annotation of the genome sequence (Table 3) included β-lactamase genes, a macrolide-specific efflux system, and a sulfonamide resistance gene.

Table 5 Selected antimicrobial susceptibility studies for *Yersinia pestis*

Antimicrobial agent	Bonacorsi et al. (91)[a] Agar dilution n = 18		Smith et al. (92)[b] Agar dilution n = 78		Frean et al. (93)[c] Agar dilution n = 100		Wong et al. (94)[d] Etest n = 92		Frean et al. (95)[e] Agar dilution n = 28	
	MIC range[f]	MIC90	MIC range	MIC90	MIC range	MIC90	MIC range	MIC90	MIC range	MIC90
Amoxicillin	0.12 to 0.5	0.5			≤0.03 to 0.25	0.12				
Ampicillin			0.125 to 0.5	0.5			0.094 to 0.38	0.38		
Azithromycin			4 to 32	32						
Cefotaxime	≤0.03	0.03			≤0.03	≤0.03				
Cefixime							0.006 to 0.032	0.023		
Ceftazidime							0.016 to 0.19	0.125		
Ceftriaxone	≤0.03	0.03	0.008 to 0.031	0.031			0.006 to 0.032	0.023		
Chloramphenicol			0.5 to 4	4	0.06 to 2.0	1	0.25 to 4.0	2		
Ciprofloxacin	0.25 to 1	1	0.008 to 0.031	0.062					0.016 to 0.031	0.031
Clarithromycin									4 to 32	>32
Doxycycline			0.25 to 1	1	≤0.03 to 4.0	1	0.125 to 2.0	1.5	0.25 to 0.5	0.5
Erythromycin					≤0.03 to >16	16			16 to 32	32
Gentamicin	0.25 to 1	0.5	0.25 to 1	1			0.19 to 1.0	0.75		
Imipenem							0.094 to >32	>32		
Levofloxacin					≤0.03 to 0.06	≤0.03				
Ofloxacin	0.06 to 0.12	0.12	0.031 to 0.25	0.25	≤0.03 to 0.12	≤0.03				
Penicillin			0.25 to 2	2						
Rifampin			2 to 8	8	≤0.03 to 8.0	8	2 to 32	16		
Streptomycin	2 to 8	4	4 to 8	4	≤0.03 to 2.0	0.5	1.5 to 4	3		
Tetracycline			0.5 to 4	4	≤0.03 to 2.0	2				
TMP-SMX			0.5/2 to 1/32	1/16	≤0.03/0.59 to 0.06/1.18	0.06/1.18	0.012 to 0.047	0.032		

[a] Mueller–Hinton agar, 28°C/48 h (91)
[b] Mueller–Hinton agar (92)
[c] No information on agar or incubation (93)
[d] Mueller–Hinton agar with sheep blood, 35°C/overnight (94)
[e] 28°C/48 h (95)
[g] MIC minimal inhibitory concentration (μg/mL)
[h] TMP–SMX trimethoprim–sulfamethoxazole

Engineered Resistance

DNA manipulation for genetic studies of *Y. pestis* often requires the introduction of plasmids with antimicrobial resistance genes as markers for selection. Most laboratories use the KIM strain of *Y. pestis*, which is avirulent because of the loss of the Lcr (low-Ca^{2+} response) plasmid. Laboratory mutants of *Y. pestis* with resistance to ciprofloxacin have been generated for studies on the detection of fluoroquinolone resistance. Serial passage on media containing increasing concentrations of ciprofloxacin led to increases in the MIC of at least 40-fold among spontaneous mutants of *Y. pestis* KIM 5 (100). As with most Gram-negative species, the first-round mutations were localized to the gene for DNA gyrase A in which point mutations were detected in codons for two amino acids at positions Ser83-Ile (or -Arg), and Gly81 Asp (or -Cys). Only first-round mutants were selected in this study, so the importance of topoisomerase IV (*parC*) mutations, which are usually detected in second-round mutants of Gram-negative bacteria, is not known.

Russian scientists have purportedly developed antibiotic-resistant strains of *Y. pestis* as biological weapons (8). Ryzhoko et al. reported on the use of β-lactamase-producing strains containing plasmids RP-1 (TEM-2), R57b (OXA-3), and R40a (resistance to carbenicillin) (101). Further studies by this group employed the use of an avirulent strain, *Y. pestis* 363 Monr, with resistance to the aminoglycosides streptomycin, kanamycin, gentamicin, and amikacin (102). Mutant strains with resistance to rifampicin (strain Rifr) and nalidixic acid (strain Nair) also have been described. The Nair mutants were cross-resistant to the fluoroquinolones ciprofloxacin, ofloxacin, pefloxacin, and lomefloxacin (102, 103). A study reported in 2004 mentions the use of strains designated as *Y. pestis* EV Rifr R(SmTc) and *Y. pestis* 231 R(SmTc), both of which are apparently resistant to streptomycin and tetracyclines (104). Another report indicates that aminoglycoside (gentamicin–kanamycin) resistance genes were transferred to *Y. pestis* by transduction using a P1-type bacteriophage (105).

4.4 *Francisella Tularensis*

4.4.1 General Characteristics

Several biotypes or subspecies of *F. tularensis* have been described. *F. tularensis* subspecies *tularensis* (type A), *holarctica* (type B), *mediasiatica*, and *novicida* have been reported to be genetically homogeneous; however, these subspecies differ in both their virulence and their geographical distribution (106). For humans, the most virulent type is *F. tularensis* subsp. *tularensis*, the etiologic agent of tularemia. Culture of this microorganism in vitro presents a high risk of laboratory-acquired infection. The organism is a small, pleomorphic, aerobic, Gram-negative coccobacillus that stains poorly. Growth is very slow and requires an agar medium with numerous supplements including cysteine, cystine, and glucose. The optimal growth temperature is 37°C. Single colonies may require 2–3 days to appear, and therefore may be overgrown by other bacteria before detection.

F. tularensis is widely found in animal reservoirs. Tularemia, also known as rabbit fever or deerfly fever, results from transmission of *F. tularensis* to humans by biting arthropods, contact with infected animals, or exposure to contaminated aerosols, food, or water (107). The low infectious dose, which is estimated to be ten organisms by aerosol (108), and the potential for widespread dispersion make *F. tularensis* an agent of concern for bioterrorism.

4.4.2 Antimicrobial Susceptibility and Resistance

Intrinsic Resistance

The antimicrobial agents that are commonly used to treat the various forms of tularemia are listed in Table 2. Because *F. tularensis* is a facultative intracellular bacterium that resides and replicates inside host cells, usually macrophages, susceptibility data (Table 6) do not necessarily correlate with effective therapy. Antimicrobial agents that are bactericidal in vitro may be bacteriostatic in vivo. Relapse following antimicrobial therapy is not uncommon and may be attributable to the protective intracellular location of the microorganism.

F. tularensis is inherently resistant to most β-lactam antibiotics (including penicillin, cephalosporins, carbapenems) and to azithromycin (107, 111), and is usually resistant to vancomycin and sulfonamides (112) (Table 6). The use of cephalosporins, for which MIC data indicate excellent activity against *F. tularensis* in vitro, has resulted in treatment failures (113). The genomic sequence of *F. tularensis* subsp. *tularensis* Schu 4 and strains of *F. tularensis* subsp. novicida, *F. tularensis* subsp. holarctica, and *F. tularensis* subsp. mediasictica have been completed (www.ncbi.nlm.nih.gov). The annotation of open reading frames indicates the presence of genes that encode class A β-lactamase and metallo-β-lactamase enzymes (Table 3). Mutagenesis studies suggest that one of the *bla* genes (*blaA*) is either not expressed or has little activity; expression of the other *bla* gene (*blaB*) does not account for the full measure of resistance to β-lactams (114). Other factors such as cell membrane permeability or targets (penicillin-binding proteins) with low affinity for β-lactam antimicrobial agents may contribute to this resistance phenotype. A *tet* gene described as a multidrug transporter was also noted in the genome annotation.

Table 6 Selected antimicrobial susceptibility studies for *Francisella tularensis*

Antimicrobial agent	Johansson et al. (109)[a] Etest, n = 24		Ikaheimo et al. (110)[b] Etest, n = 38		Baker et al. (111)[c] Broth microdilution, n = 15	
	MIC range (4)	MIC$_{90}$	MIC range	MIC$_{90}$	MIC range	MIC$_{90}$
Ampicillin					>8	>8
Azithromycin	0.064 to 2	ND	>256	>256		
Aztreonam					4.0 to >32	>32
Cefotaxime					≤0.12 to 4.0	4
Cefoxitin					≤0.25 to 16	8
Cefpirome			>256	>256		
Ceftazidime			>256	>256	≤0.5 to 1.0	≤0.5
Ceftriaxone			>32	>32	0.5 to 16	8
Cephalothin					≤0.25 to 8.0	>8
Chloramphenicol	0.25 to 1	ND	0.125 to 0.5	0.38	≤0.25 to 4.0	1
Ciprofloxacin	0.016 to 0.064	ND	0.008 to 0.023	0.016		
Clindamycin					1.0 to >2.0	>2
Doxycycline	0.125 to 2	ND				
Erythromycin	0.125 to 2	ND			0.5 to 2.0	2
Gentamicin	0.032 to 0.25	ND	0.38 to 1.5	1	0.25 to 2.0	2
Imipenem			>32	>32		
Levofloxacin	0.016 to 0.064	ND	0.008 to 0.023	0.016		
Linezolid	1 to 16	ND				
Meropenem			>32	>32		
Methicillin					≤0.12 to >4	>4
Oxacillin					≤0.06 to >2	>2
Penicillin					4.0 to >8	>8
Piperacillin					≤0.5 to >64	>64
Piperacillin–tazobactam			>256	>256		
Rifampin	0.125 to 2	ND	0.094 to 0.38	0.25	≤0.03 to 1.0	1
Streptomycin	0.032 to 2	ND	0.25 to 4.0	4	≤0.5 to 4.0	4
Tetracycline			0.094 to 0.5	0.38	≤0.25 to 2.0	2
Tobramycin			0.5 to 2.0	1.5	≤0.12 to 4.0	2
Vancomycin					>16	>16

[a]The study included 20 human isolates and 4 animal isolates; 8 isolates of *F. tularensis tularensis*, each from a different state in the United States, and 16 isolates of *F. tularensis holarctica*; on Mueller-Hinton II agar supplemented with 1% isoVitaleX and on cysteine heart agar supplemented with 9% chocolatized sheep blood; 37°C/48 h/ambient air. MICs for subspecies *tularensis* and *holarctica* were similar for each agent tested (109)
[b]All isolates were identified as *F. tularensis*; cysteine heart agar supplemented with 2% hemoglobin; 35°C in 5% CO$_2$, overnight or for two nights (110)
[c]Strains were selected from the Centers for Disease Control collection; most isolates were from the southeastern and southwestern areas of the Untied States. Cation-adjusted Mueller–Hinton broth supplemented with 0.1% glucose, 2% IsoVitaleX; 35°C/5% CO$_2$ for 24 h (111)

Engineered Resistance

Numerous plasmid vectors have been developed for the study of *F. tularensis*. Many of these are derived from a cryptic plasmid, pFNL10, originally isolated from the *F. novicida*-like strain F6168. Recombination with pBR328 produced a derivative, pFNL100, that conferred resistance to ampicillin, tetracycline, and chloramphenicol and was stably inherited by *F. tularensis* (115). Additional constructs have produced stable plasmids with various combinations of the resistance genes. A hybrid plasmid, pSKEFT5, derived from pFNL10 and encoding the resistance gene for chloramphenicol was developed for mutagenesis of *F. tularensis*. Shuttle vectors have also been constructed for use in either *E. coli* or *F. tularensis*. These vectors confer resistance to either tetracycline and chloramphenicol (116) or to kanamycin and either tetracycline or ampicillin (117). pOM1, also derived from pFNL10, is a 4.4-kb plasmid that encodes *tet*(C) for tetracycline resistance (118).

In addition to plasmids, Lauriano et al. (119) described an allelic exchange method using linear polymerase chain reaction (PCR) products that include the *ermC* gene, which, after introduction and recombination, result in *F. tularensis* strains that are resistant to erythromycin.

4.5 Burkholderia pseudomallei

4.5.1 General Characteristics

B. pseudomallei is a small, motile, irregular staining, Gram-negative bacillus, and is also a facultative intracellular pathogen. *B. pseudomallei* grows well on simple media, including nutrient, blood, and MacConkey agars, but it does not grow on deoxycholate citrate or Salmonella–Shigella agars. After overnight incubation on nutrient agar at 37°C, the colonies are 1–2 mm in diameter. Culture and manipulation of *B. pseudomallei* present a risk to laboratory personnel; all procedures involving live cultures must be performed in a BSL-3 laboratory. A natural saprophyte, it is found in soil and water. Human infection, melioidosis, usually occurs by entry of the organism through skin abrasions, although aerosol inhalation or ingestion is also possible. The disease is endemic to Southeast Asia and Northern Australia. Melioidosis is difficult to treat, requiring prolonged courses of antimicrobial agents. The clinical response is slow, and relapse is common.

4.5.2 Antimicrobial Susceptibility and Resistance

Intrinsic Resistance

The therapeutic agents used to treat the various forms of melioidosis are listed in Table 2. *B. pseudomallei* is usually susceptible to carbapenems, β-lactam–β-lactamase inhibitor combinations, ceftazidime, sulfamethoxazole, and tetracyclines (Table 7) (123–127). *B. pseudomallei* is intrinsically resistant to many aminoglycosides, β-lactams, fluoroquinolones, and macrolides (120). A multidrug resistance efflux system, AmrAB-OprA, specific for aminoglycosides and macrolides, is encoded on the chromosome (120, 127). Genome sequence analysis of *B. pseudomallei* K96243 has revealed the presence of at least three β-lactamase genes, encoding class A, C, and D enzymes (Table 3). Chloramphenicol-resistant strains have been recognized since 1988 (124). In a study of 199 clinical isolates from Thailand, fewer than 20% of the strains were susceptible to trimethoprim–sulfamethoxazole and kanamycin (128). The emergence of resistance to doxycycline, ceftazidime, amoxicillin/clavulanic acid, and SMX/TMP has been documented during prolonged therapy (123).

The genome sequences of several *B. pseudomallei* strains including 170b and K96243 have been completed (http://cmr.jcvi.org/) ((J. Craig Venter Institute, formerly The Institute for Genomic Research, TIGR) www.tigr.org). In the annotation of genes, both strains have numerous gene sequences identified as β-lactamases, metallo-β-lactamase family proteins, macrolide efflux proteins, and a putative tetracycline efflux protein (Table 3). A gene identified as an aminoglycoside phosphotransferase was identified in strain 1710b, and an aminoglycoside acetyltransferase in strain K96243.

Engineered Resistance

Resistance to several antimicrobial agents has been engineered by Russian scientists by introduction of natural and recombinant plasmids (129). Abaev et al. (129) reported efficient and stable transfer of naturally occurring plasmids into *B. pseudomallei*: RSF1010 (streptomycin and sulfonamide resistance), pSa (*aacA4* – gentamicin and kanamycin resistance, *aad2* – streptomycin and spectinomycin resistance, *sul1* – sulfonamide resistance), RP4 (*aphA* – aminoglycoside resistance, *tetA* and *tetB* – tetracycline resistance), and R15 (resistant determinants not described). In the same study, derivatives of RSF1010 were not successfully maintained. Plasmid pOV13, containing the genes for streptomycin, kanamycin, and tetracycline resistance, was transferred into *Burkholderia* spp. by Zakharenko et al. (130).

4.6 Burkholderia mallei

4.6.1 General Characteristics

B. mallei, the etiologic agent of glanders, is a small, nonmotile, aerobic, Gram-negative bacillus. It grows less well than *B. pseudomallei* on nutrient agar, forming colonies 0.5–1 mm in diameter in 18 h at 37°C. In vitro growth of *B. mallei* presents a risk to laboratory personnel; all procedures involving live cultures must be performed in a BSL-3 laboratory. The organism is genetically very similar to *B. pseudomallei*, but it has evolved as an obligate parasite of equines. At one time glanders was widespread throughout the world, but the disease has been essentially eliminated from equine populations in the United States and Canada. Although glanders is now rarely seen in humans, the infection can be fatal and, like melioidosis, treatment is prolonged and clinical cures are difficult to achieve.

B. mallei was used as a biological weapon during the American Civil War, World War I, and World War II (131). Both *B. mallei* and *B. pseudomallei* have qualities that make them a concern for biological weapon use. These qualities include high infectivity, dissemination into the environment where they will survive for long periods, and have the capacity to cause severe disease and high mortality.

4.6.2 Antimicrobial Susceptibility and Resistance

Intrinsic Resistance

Very few studies of *B. mallei* antimicrobial susceptibility have been published, which probably reflects both the

Table 7 Selected antimicrobial susceptibility studies for *Burkholderia pseudomallei*

Antimicrobial agent	Yamamoto et al. (124)[a] Agar dilution n = 97		Smith et al. (169)[b] Agar dilution n = 100		Sookpranee et al. (128)[c] Agar dilution n = 199		Ashdown (126)[d] Broth microdilution n = 100	
	MIC range	MIC$_{90}$	MIC range	MIC$_{90}$	MIC range	MIC$_{90}$	MIC range	MIC$_{90}$
Ampicillin					0.25 to >512	32		
Amp/sul					0.25 to 128	8		
Amoxicillin							>64	>64
Amox/clav			0.5 to 8	4			2 to >64	4
Penicillin	0.39 to 3.13	1.56						
Pipercillin					0.25 to 16	2	1 to 4	2
Cefepime	3.13 to 50	12.5						
Cefotaxime	0.78 to 12.5	3.13					2 to 8	8
Ceftazidime	0.39 to 3.13	1.56	0.25 to 32	2	0.125 to 16	2	1 to 8	4
Ceftriaxone							2 to 8	8
Imipenem	0.2 to 1.56	0.78	0.12 to 1	0.5	0.06 to 4	0.5	0.25 to 2	1
Meropenem	0.39 to 3.13	0.78	0.25 to 1	1				
Aztreonam	6.25 to 50	25			8 to >256	32	2 to 16	8
Nalidixic acid	3.13 to >200	50						
Ofloxacin	0.78 to 12.5	6.25						
Ciprofloxacin	0.78 to 6.25	3.13			0.125 to 16	8	0.5 to 16	8
Tetracycline	0.78 to 12.5	12.5						
Minocycline	0.78 to 3.13	3.13						
Chloramphenicol	6.25 to >200	25						
Rifampin	3.13 to 25	25						
SXT	0.78 to 25	12.5						

[a]Human isolates: 27 from Ubon-Rajathanee, Thailand (1989); 70 from Nonthaburi, Thailand (1981–1989); Medium: Mueller–Hinton agar, incubated 37°C/20h, (124)
[b]Human isolates from Ubon Ratchatani, Thailand collected during 1991–1992 (169)
[c]Human isolates from Khon Kaen, Thailand; Mueller–Hinton agar (128)
[d]Human isolates from northern Australia, Mueller–Hinton broth (126)

scarcity of clinical isolates and the hazardous nature of this microorganism. The genome sequence of *B. mallei* ATCC 23344 has been completed (131) and genes associated with antimicrobial resistance have been identified. These include a Class A β-lactamase, *ampD*, multidrug efflux genes of the *emrB/qacA* and *bcr/cfiA* families, and an aminoglycoside resistance gene, *aac6´-Iz* (Table 3). The genomic data support the results of phenotypic studies, showing that *B. mallei* is intrinsically resistant to many antimicrobial agents including β-lactams, macrolides, and aminoglycosides (Table 8). Although most strains are highly resistant to ampicillin, the combination of ampicillin with a β-lactamase inhibitor such as clavulanic acid results in very low MICs in vitro. The percentage of gentamicin-resistant strains varies from 0 to 19% (122). Some antimicrobial agents that are active against *B. mallei* in vitro are clinically ineffective, most likely because of the intracellular location of the organism. Ceftazidime has been used successfully for treatment of glanders; however, a resistant isolate has been reported (132). *B. mallei* is usually susceptible to imipenim, doxycycline, and minocycline. Many strains are susceptible to erythromycin but resistant to clindamycin.

Engineered Resistance

Studies of the pathogenesis and genetics of *B. mallei* have often included the introduction of plasmids with antimicrobial resistance markers. These include resistance to gentamicin, kanamycin, streptomycin, tetracycline, chloramphenicol, trimethoprim, and bleomycin. The development of a multidrug-resistant strain by Russian scientists has been reported; however, the resistance genes that were introduced were not specified (3). Abaev et al. (129) described successful introduction of natural plasmids RSF1010, pSA, R15, and RP4 in *B. mallei* (as described above for *B. pseudomallei*). Unlike *B. pseudomallei*, several derivatives of these plasmids were stably maintained in *B. mallei*.

4.7 *Brucella* spp.

4.7.1 General Characteristics

Brucella spp., the etiologic agents of brucellosis, are small Gram-negative coccobacilli. These nonmotile, strictly aerobic organisms are facultative intracellular bacteria that grow

Table 8 Selected antimicrobial susceptibility studies for *Burkholderia mallei*

Antimicrobial agent	Thibault et al. (120)[a] Agar dilution n = 15		Heine et al. (121)[b] Broth microdilution		Etest n = 11		Kenny et al. (122)[c] Broth microdilution n = 17	
	MIC range[d]	MIC_{90}	MIC range	MIC_{90}	MIC range	MIC_{90}	MIC range	MIC_{90}
Amikacin	1 to 128	64	0.5 to 4	2	0.25 to 1	0.5		
Gentamicin	0.125 to 128	128	0.25 to 1	0.5	0.047 to 0.125	0.094	0.063 to 0.5	0.5
Streptomycin			2 to 8	4				
Tobramycin			0.25 to 16	0.5				
Clindamycin	>128	>128						
Azithromycin			0.25 to 1	1	0.094 to 0.75	0.5	0.25 to 16	4
Erythromycin	0.25 to 2	1						
Clarithromycin			4 to 16	4				
Ofloxacin	0.125 to 32	2	0.5 to 8	8	0.023 to 3	1	0.5 to 8	8
Ciprofloxacin	0.5 to 16	4	≤0.03 to 4	1	0.008 to 0.5	0.25	0.25 to 8	8
Levofloxacin	0.125 to 4	1						
Amoxicillin	16 to 128	64	>64	>64				
Amox/clav	0.125 to 8	4	1 to 4	4	0.125 to 0.5	0.25	1 to 8	8
Ampicillin			32 to 64	64	2 to 16	6	1 to >64	>64
Piperacillin	0.125 to 8	8	1 to 8	8	0.125 to 1	0.38	4 to 16	16
Imipenem	0.125 to 0.5	0.5	0.12 to 1	0.25	0.064 to 0.19	0.125	0.125 to 0.25	0.25
Ceftazidime	1 to 4	2	1 to 6	4	0.125 to 1	0.5	2 to 16	8
Cefotaxime	0.5 to 32	16	4 to 6	16				
Cefotetan			16 to >64	32	2 to 32	16		
Cefoxitin	4 to >128	>128						
Cefuroxime			32 to 64	64	1.5 to 16	6	8 to >64	>64
Cefazolin			32 to >64	>64				
Ceftriaxone			16 to 64	16	1 to 32	12		
Aztreonam	4 to 128	64	32 to >64	32	2 to 32	12		
Sulfamethoxazole			0.25 to >64	16			1 to >64	>64
Co-trimoxazole	1 to 4	4	0.25 to 64	32	0.003 to 0.25	0.125	0.063 to >64	>64
Trimethoprim			1 to 32	16			0.125 to 64	32
Doxycycline	0.125 to 0.5	0.25	≤0.5	0.12	≤0.016 to 0.094	0.032	0.125 to 4	2
Rifampin	0.25 to 16	4	2 to 16	8			1 to 16	16
Chloramphenicol	0.125 to 8	4	4 to 64	32	0.25 to 24	8	1 to 64	>64
Quinupristin–dalfopristin			1 to 32	32				

[a] Selected strains from China, Turkey, Hungary, Iran, and India collected over a period of 1920–1966 from man and animals; Mueller–Hinton agar, 37°C/48 h (120)

[b] Seven NCTC strains and four ATCC strains; broth microdilution in cation-adjusted Mueller–Hinton broth; 37°C/overnight; Etest on Mueller–Hinton agar incubated 37°C/18–24 h (121)

[c] Ten ATCC strains and seven strains from Central Veterinary Laboratories, Weybridge, UK. Broth microdilution in cation-adjusted Mueller–Hinton broth, 37°C/36 h (122)

[d] MIC, minimal inhibitory concentration in μg/mL

slowly and require complex media containing serum or blood. Many strains require CO_2 for growth. Currently, seven species are recognized on the basis of host preferences and pathogenicity: *B. melitensis* (goats, sheep), *B. abortus* (cattle), *B. suis* (swine), *B. canis* (dogs), *B. ovis* (sheep), *B. neotomae* (rodents), and *B. maris* (marine mammals). These bacteria are highly infectious and are distributed worldwide. Infection with *B. melitensis*, the most virulent species for humans, may be acquired by inhalation, consumption of contaminated food, or contact with infected animals. If acquired during pregnancy, the infection leads to early or mid-term abortion. Rare instances of person-to-person transmission have been recorded, either by sexual contact (133) or by transfer of tissue, including blood and bone marrow (134). Laboratory-acquired brucellosis with

B. melitensis, *B. abortus*, *B. suis*, and *B. canis* is a significant problem and results from accidental ingestion, inhalation, injection, and mucosal and skin contamination. Procedures involving *Brucella* cultures should be performed in a BSL-3 laboratory. Extended combination antimicrobial therapy is required, and relapse frequently occurs following treatment.

4.7.2 Antimicrobial Susceptibility and Resistance

Intrinsic Resistance

The antimicrobial agents used to treat brucellosis are listed in Table 2. The recommended regimens include combinations of doxycycline and an aminoglycoside such as streptomycin or gentamicin, or doxycycline and rifampin for 30–45 days. In vitro, *Brucellae* are usually susceptible to tetracyclines, aminoglycosides, fluoroquinolones, and rifampin (Table 9) (135–137). Erythromycin ($MIC_{90} > 8$) and vancomycin ($MIC_{90} > 16$) generally have poor activity (135, 138). As with other intracellular bacteria, the in vivo efficacy of antimicrobials may not correspond with in vitro test results. Additional factors include penetration and accumulation of the agent within the host cell and the effect of low pH in the phagolysosome where the organism resides. A multidrug efflux pump, NorMI, has been identified in *B. melitensis* ((139) and Table 3). The substrate profile for this type of pump includes fluoroquinolones (140). Although the clinical impact, if any, has yet to be established, efflux mechanisms may reduce susceptibility to an antimicrobial agent, allowing time for selection of mutations that increase the level of resistance. Genome sequences are available for several strains including *Brucella abortus* 9–941, *B. melitensis* 16M, *B. suis* 1330, and a strain identified as *B. melitensis* biovar Abortus (http://cmr.jcvi.org/) (J. Craig Venter Institute, formerly The Institute for Genomic Research, TIGR). Resistance genes have been identified in these genome annotations (Table 3). The putative resistance genes differed among the species. Several efflux systems were detected in *B. melitensis*, but none in *B. suis*. Macrolide and tetracycline resistance genes were also noted in the *B. melitensis* genome, but not *B. suis*. However, the *B. suis* sequence included β-lactamase genes and a chloramphenicol resistance determinant not found in the *B. melitensis* genome.

Engineered Resistance

Russian reports document the introduction of antimicrobial resistance genes in *Brucella*. The plasmid pOV13, which confers resistance to streptomycin, tetracycline, and kanamycin, was described as being stably inherited by *Brucella*, as well as *Pseudomonas* spp. (i.e., *Burkholderia*) (130). *B. abortus* strain 19-BA was mutated to rifampicin resistance and then transformed with the plasmid pOV1. The resulting strain was resistant to rifampicin, tetracycline, doxycycline, ampicillin, and streptomycin (141).

4.8 Coxiella burnetii

4.8.1 General Characteristics

C. burnetii, the etiologic agent of Q fever (named for query fever, a fever of unknown origin), is a small, Gram-variable coccobacillus from the family Rickettsiaceae. This organism is an obligate intracellular parasite that grows only in cytoplasmic vacuoles of animal cells, primarily macrophages. *C. burnetii* can be grown in tissue cultures but not on laboratory media. The most rapid cell culture method, the shell vial technique, takes 7–10 days (142). Small colony variants (SCVs) of *C. burnetii*, which resemble chlamydial elementary bodies, are common and apparently represent a stage of the developmental cycle (143). SCVs are highly resistant to heat, drying, and chemicals such as 10% bleach, 5% Lysol,

Table 9 Selected antimicrobial susceptibility studies for *Brucella melitensis*

Antimicrobial agent	Baykam et al. (170)[a] Etest n = 37		Akova et al. (171)[b] Broth microdilution n = 43		Trujillano-Martín et al. (172)[c] Agar dilution n = 160	
	MIC range[d]	MIC_{90}	MIC range	MIC_{90}	MIC range	MIC_{90}
Co-trimoxazole	0.047 to 3.0	1.5				
Ceftriaxone	0.125 to 1	0.5				
Doxycycline	0.016 to 0.094	0.064	≤0.125 to 8	≤0.125	0.12 to 0.25	0.25
Rifampin	0.19 to 1.5	1.0	1 to 32	2	0.5 to 1	1
Erythromycin			0.5 to 256	128		
Azithromycin			≤0.126 to 4	1		
Streptomycin			0.25 to 8	2	4 to 16	8
Ciprofloxacin	0.064 to 0.50	0.19	≤0.125 to 8	2	0.25 to 1	1
Ofloxacin			≤0.125 to 4	1	1 to 2	2

[a]Human blood isolates collected between 2000 and 2003, Ankara, Turkey. Medium: Mueller–Hinton agar supplemented with 5% sheep blood; incubated 35°C/48 h (170)
[b]Human isolates from blood or bone marrow, collected between 1991 and 1994, Ankara, Turkey. Medium: Mueller–Hinton broth supplemented with 1% PoliVitex, adjusted to pH 7.0, incubated 35°C/48 h (171)
[c]Human blood isolates collected during 1997, Salamanca, Spain. Medium: Mueller–Hinton agar supplemented with 1% hemoglobin and 1% PoliVitex (172)
[d]MIC, minimal inhibitory concentration in µg/mL

and 5% formalin (144). SCVs have been shown to survive pasteurization and can survive for months in milk or dried feces. *C. burnetii* cells, including SCVs, are highly infectious as an aerosol. Natural infections are usually transmitted by ticks, mites, and body lice. The infectious dose for humans is about ten organisms (145). Q fever may present either as an acute infection, usually febrile pneumonia or hepatitis, or as a persistent, chronic disease that often includes endocarditis. The environmental stability of the organism and the low infectious dose are the reasons for this agent to be considered as a potential bioweapon (146, 147).

4.8.2 Antimicrobial Susceptibilities and Resistance

Methodology

Historically, susceptibility studies of *C. burnetii* were performed with infected embryonated eggs or with cell cultures (148, 149). The organism replicates to high numbers, but the doubling time is estimated to be 12–20 h (150). These culture methods are labor and time intensive and are not easily adaptable for multiple antimicrobial agents. Two alternative methods are now in use. The shell vial assay (151) is a modified cell culture technique that facilitates testing of multiple antibiotics. The second method, quantitative real-time PCR, detects the number of copies of a *C. burnetii*-specific gene in the culture to estimate the growth (152, 153). Both of these methods require 6–7 days of bacterial growth in cell cultures.

The centrifugation–shell vial technique employs a shell vial (manufactured by Sterilin, Felthan, England) containing human embryonic lung (HEL) fibroblast cell monolayer. The inoculum of *C. burnetii* is added and subjected to low-speed centrifugation (700 g) to bring the bacteria in contact with the HEL monolayer. After 6 days of growth to allow 30–50% of the cells to become infected, the cell culture medium is replaced with a medium containing a specific concentration of an antimicrobial agent. The medium/antimicrobial solution is replaced daily during 6 days of incubation at 37°C in 5% CO_2. Cell numbers are determined by indirect immunofluorescence using anti-*C. burnetii* rabbit serum and fluorescently labeled goat-anti-rabbit antibodies. The number of *C. burnetii* cells in the test are compared with positive and negative controls (HEL cell cultures with and without *C. burnetii* infection, respectively) to determine whether the strain is susceptible (absence of infected cells), intermediate, (fewer than 10% cells infected), or resistant (normal growth in presence of antibiotic).

Brennan and Samuel (152) reported on the determination of antimicrobial susceptibility of *C. burnetii* by real-time PCR. In this method, the antimicrobial dose response curve is based on the number of copies of the *com1* gene from *C. burnetii* as determined semiquantitatively by real-time PCR. A similar method was used by Boulos et al. (153) using the gene for superoxide dismutase (*sod*). Both studies used murine macrophage cell lines that were infected with *C. burnetii*. A standard curve of the number of gene copies was established by real-time PCR for *C. burnetii*-infected cells grown without antibiotics. The effect of antimicrobials on the growth of *C. burnetii* was determined by the difference in the number of gene copies in the presence of the antibiotic when compared with the growth curve of the control culture.

Intrinsic Resistance

Doxycycline is the treatment of choice for the acute form of Q fever, although fluoroquinolones appear to be useful as an alternative (154). Treatment of persistent infections is problematic and requires extended therapy, and relapse may occur after antimicrobial agents are withdrawn. Combination therapy consisting of doxycycline with either ofloxacin or rifampin for a period of 3 years has been recommended as treatment. The use of hydroxychloroquine, an alkalinizing compound of the phagolysosome vacuole, has also been recommended to achieve bactericidal activity (155, 156). Results from representative susceptibility studies using the methods described above are shown in Table 10.

The genome sequence of *C. burnetii* (Nine Mile phase I, RSA 493 strain) has been completed (159). Gene sequences for putative β-lactamase and metallo-β-lactamase family proteins have been identified in the annotated genome (Table 3). Both genes are located on the chromosome. There is also an aminoglycoside acetyltransferase identified as *aacA4*. Different strains of *C. burnetii* are genetically heterogeneous with variations in both chromosomal and plasmid DNA. There is usually a single plasmid in *C. burnetii*. However, among strains there are considerable differences in the size (34 to >50 kb) and the gene arrangement of the plasmid. There are reports of significant differences in the susceptibility profiles of distinct isolates (157, 160) and also in isolates from acute vs. chronic disease (161). These data suggest that susceptibility testing of *C. burnetii* isolates may be beneficial to selection of appropriate antimicrobial therapy.

Engineered Resistance

Although the requirement for growth in tissue cultures and the slow generation time have limited genetic studies of *C. burnetii*, fluoroquinolone-resistant mutants have been selected in vitro. Two reports indicate that MICs of 8–16 µg/mL of ciprofloxacin (162) and 32–64 µg/mL pefloxacin (163) were attained by in vitro selection. Tetracycline-resistant strains have also been developed in laboratory studies (164).

Table 10 Selected antimicrobial susceptibility studies of *C. burnetii*

Antimicrobial agent	Raoult et al. (157) S, I, -R n = 13, shell-vial assay[a]	Boulos et al. (153) range of MICs in µg/mL, n = 2		Gikas et al. (158) 1998, range of MICs in µg/mL, n = 8, shell vial assay[c]
		Real-time PCR	IFA[b]	
Amikacin	R (13)			
Amoxicillin	R (13)			
Ciprofloxacin	S (5); I (8)	2 to 4[c]	4 to 8	4 to 8
Clarithromycin				2 to 4
Chloramphenicol	S (10); I (3)			
Co-trimoxazole	S (13)	8 to 16	8	
Doxycycline	S (13)	2 to 4	1 to 2	1 to 2
Erythromycin	I (7); R (6)	2 to 4	4 to 8	
Gentamicin		>10	>10	
Ofloxacin	S (12); I (1)	2	1 to 2	1 to 2
Rifampin	S (13)	4	2	
Tetracycline	S (13)			

[a]S, susceptible (no growth); I, intermediate (reduced growth); R, resistant (normal growth)
[b]IFA, immunofluorescence antibody assay
[c]Range of MICs in µg/mL

5 Conclusions and Future Considerations

Antimicrobial resistance remains an important factor to be considered in efforts to prepare and respond to the intentional release of an infectious agent. While the antimicrobial susceptibility of the bacterial agent is a concern for infections resulting from either a naturally occurring outbreak or bioterrorism, there is a growing concern that genetic engineering could be used to make a normally susceptible microorganism resistant to one or more of the antimicrobial agents commonly used for therapy. Conventional antimicrobial susceptibility testing requires time to isolate a pure culture of the organism and 1–3 days (depending on the organism) for growth in susceptibility tests. Rapid detection of potential resistance is essential for effective therapeutic and prophylactic treatment. To address this concern, molecular assays involving standard and real-time PCR are being developed, which will detect the presence of resistance determinants in 2–4 h (165, 166). Mutations associated with fluoroquinolone resistance can also be detected by rapid DNA sequence analysis or hydridization assays such as microarrays. Because the resistance determinant may be unknown or not previously found in a particular organism, oligonucleotide microarrays are being developed that can identify all known resistance determinants (167, 168). As new technologies become available, the rapid tests may become widely used. The availability of annotated genomes has provided information on resistance genes that are present in the sequenced strains. However, conventional susceptibility testing will remain necessary to determine the clinical significance of these resistance genes and to detect new mechanisms of resistance as they emerge and spread through microbial populations.

References

1. Khan AS, Morse S, Lillibridge S. Public-health preparedness for biological terrorism in the USA. Lancet 2000;356(9236):1179–1182
2. Strikas RA, Sinclair MF, Morse SA. Centers for Disease Control and Prevention's bioterrorism preparedness program. In: Pilch RF, Zilinskas RA, eds. Encyclopedia of Bioterrorism Defense. Hoboken, NJ: Wiley-Liss; 2005
3. Alibek K, Handleman S. Biohazard. New York: Random House; 1999
4. Lindler LE, Choffnes E, Korch GW. Definition and overview of emerging threats. In: Lindler LE, Lebeda FJ, Korch GW, eds. Biological Weapons Defense: Infectious Diseases and Counterbioterrorism. Totowa, NJ: Humana; 2005
5. Ainscough M. Next generation bioweapons: Genetic engineering and biowarfare. In: Davis J, Schneider B, eds. The Gathering Biological Warfare Storm, 2nd edn. Maxwell Air Force Base, AL: USAF Counterproliferation Center; 2002:253–288
6. Carus WS. Bioterrorism and Biocrimes: The Illicit Use of Biological Agents Since 1900. Amsterdam: Fredonia books; 2002
7. Rotz LD, Khan AS, Lillibridge SR, Ostroff SM, Hughes JM. Public health assessment of potential biological terrorism agents. Emerg Infect Dis 2002;8(2):225–230
8. Orent W. Plague: The Mysterious Past and Terrifying Future of the World's Most Dangerous Disease. New York: Free Press; 2004
9. Turnbull PCB. Anthrax history, disease, and ecology. In: Koehler TM, ed. Anthrax, Current Topics in Microbiology and Immunology. Berlin: Springer-Verlag; 2002
10. Suffin SC, Carnes WH, Kaufmann AF. Inhalation anthrax in a home craftsman. Hum Pathol 1978;9(5):594–597
11. Srinivasan A, Kraus CN, DeShazer D, et al. Glanders in a military research microbiologist. N Engl J Med 2001;345(4):256–258
12. Miller J, Engelberg S, Broad W. Germs: Biological Weapons and America's Secret War. New York: Simon & Schuster; 2001
13. Kolavic SA, Kimura A, Simons SL, Slutsker L, Barth S, Haley CE. An outbreak of *Shigella dysenteriae* type 2 among laboratory workers due to intentional food contamination. JAMA 1997;278(5):396–398
14. Moran GJ. Threats in bioterrorism. II: CDC category B and C agents. Emerg Med Clin North Am 2002;20(2):311–330

15. Kaufman AF, Meltzer MI, Schmid GP. The economic impact of a bioterrorist attack: are prevention and postattack intervention programs justifiable. Emerg Infect Dis 1997;3:83–94

16. Morse S, Kellogg RB, Perry S, et al. Detecting biothreat agents: the Laboratory Response Network. ASM News 2003;69:433–437

17. Gilchrist MJR. A national laboratory network for bioterrorism: Evolution from a prototype network of laboratories performing routine surveillance. Mil Med 2000;165(Suppl 2):28–31

18. Jernigan JA, Stephens DS, Ashford DA, et al. Bioterrorism-related inhalational anthrax: the first 10 cases reported in the United States. Emerg Infect Dis 2001;7(6):933–944

19. Hsu VP, Lukacs SL, Handzel T, et al. Opening a Bacillus anthracis-containing envelope, Capitol Hill, Washington, D.C.: the public health response. Emerg Infect Dis 2002;8(10):1039–1043

20. Shepard CW, Soriano-Gabarro M, Zell ER, et al. Antimicrobial postexposure prophylaxis for anthrax: adverse events and adherence. Emerg Infect Dis 2002;8(10):1124–1132

21. Torok TJ, Tauxe RV, Wise RP, et al. A large community outbreak of salmonellosis caused by intentional contamination of restaurant salad bars. JAMA 1997;278(5):389–395

22. Feldman KA, Enscore RE, Lathrop SL, et al. An outbreak of primary pneumonic tularemia on Martha's Vineyard. N Engl J Med 2001;345(22):1601–1606

23. Imported plague – New York City, 2002. MMWR Morbid Mortal Wkly Rep 2003;52:725–728

24. Inhalation anthrax associated with dried animal hides: Pennsylvania and New York City, 2006. MMWR Morb Mortal Wkly Rep 2006;55:280–282

25. Treadwell TA, Koo D, Kuker K, Khan AS. Epidemiologic clues to bioterrorism. Public Health Rep 2003;118(2):92–98

26. Tenover FC. Antimicrobial susceptibility testing of bacterial agents of bioterrorism: strategies and considerations. In: White DG, Alekshun MN, McDermott PF, eds. Frontiers in Antimicrobial Resistance: A Tribute to Stuart B. Levy. Washington, DC: ASM Press; 2005

27. Athamna A, Athamna M, Abu-Rashed N, Medlej B, Bast DJ, Rubinstein E. Selection of Bacillus anthracis isolates resistant to antibiotics. J Antimicrob Chemother 2004;54(2):424–428

28. Price LB, Vogler A, Pearson T, Busch JD, Schupp JM, Keim P. In vitro selection and characterization of Bacillus anthracis mutants with high-level resistance to ciprofloxacin. Antimicrob Agents Chemother 2003;47(7):2362–2365

29. Biotechnology Research in an Age of Terrorism. Washington, DC: The National Academies Press; 2004

30. Agerso Y, Jensen LB, Givskov M, Roberts MC. The identification of a tetracycline resistance gene tet(M), on a Tn916-like transposon, in the Bacillus cereus group. FEMS Microbiol Lett 2002;214(2):251–256

31. Brook I, Elliott TB, Pryor HI, II, et al. In vitro resistance of Bacillus anthracis Sterne to doxycycline, macrolides and quinolones. Int J Antimicrob Agents 2001;18(6):559–562

32. Grohs P, Podglajen I, Gutmann L. Activities of different fluoroquinolones against Bacillus anthracis mutants selected in vitro and harboring topoisomerase mutations. Antimicrob Agents Chemother 2004;48(8):3024–3027

33. Mohammed MJ, Marston CK, Popovic T, Weyant RS, Tenover FC. Antimicrobial susceptibility testing of Bacillus anthracis: comparison of results obtained by using the National Committee for Clinical Laboratory Standards broth microdilution reference and Etest agar gradient diffusion methods. J Clin Microbiol 2002;40(6):1902–1907

34. Acar JF, Goldstein FW. Disk susceptibility test. In: Lorian V, ed. Antibiotics in Laboratory Medicine, 4th ed. Baltimore, MD: Williams & Wilkins; 1996:1–51

35. Wilkinson GR. Pharmacokinetics: the dynamics of drugs absorption, distribution and elimination. In: Hardman JG, Limbird LL, eds. The Pharmacological Basis of Therapeutics. New York: McGraw Hill Medical Publishing Division; 2001:3–30

36. Carryn S, Chanteux H, Seral C, Mingeot Leclercq MP, Van Bambeke F, Tulkens PM. Intracellular pharmacodynamics of antibiotics. Infect Dis Clin North Am 2003;17(3):615–634

37. Mandell GL, Coleman E. Uptake, transport, and delivery of antimicrobial agents by human polymorphonuclear neutrophils. Antimicrob Agents Chemother 2001;45(6):1794–1798

38. Martin JR, Johnson P, Miller MF. Uptake, accumulation, and egress of erythromycin by tissue culture cells of human origin. Antimicrob Agents Chemother 1985;27(3):314–319

39. Miller MF, Martin JR, Johnson P, Ulrich JT, Rdzok EJ, Billing P. Erythromycin uptake and accumulation by human polymorphonuclear leukocytes and efficacy of erythromycin in killing ingested Legionella pneumophila. J Infect Dis 1984;149(5):714–718

40. Tyteca D, Van Der Smissen P, Van Bambeke F, et al. Azithromycin, a lysosomotropic antibiotic, impairs fluid-phase pinocytosis in cultured fibroblasts. Eur J Cell Biol 2001;80(7):466–478

41. Anderson R, Van Rensburg CE, Joone G, Lukey PT. An in-vitro comparison of the intraphagocytic bioactivity of erythromycin and roxithromycin. J Antimicrob Chemother 1987;20 Suppl B:57–68

42. Ohkuma S, Poole B. Fluorescence probe measurement of the intralysosomal pH in living cells and the perturbation of pH by various agents. Proc Natl Acad Sci U S A 1978;75(7):3327–3331

43. de Duve C, de Barsy T, Poole B, Trouet A, Tulkens P, Van Hoof F. Commentary. Lysosomotropic agents. Biochem Pharmacol 1974;23(18):2495–2531

44. Easmon CS, Crane JP. Uptake of ciprofloxacin by macrophages. J Clin Pathol 1985;38(4):442–444

45. Carlier MB, Scorneaux B, Zenebergh A, Desnottes JF, Tulkens PM. Cellular uptake, localization and activity of fluoroquinolones in uninfected and infected macrophages. J Antimicrob Chemother 1990;26 Suppl B:27–39

46. Garcia I, Pascual A, Ballesta S, Perea EJ. Uptake and intracellular activity of ofloxacin isomers in human phagocytic and non-phagocytic cells. Int J Antimicrob Agents 2000;15(3):201–205

47. Bonventre PF, Hayes R, Imhoff J. Autoradiographic evidence for the impermeability of mouse peritoneal macrophages to tritiated streptomycin. J Bacteriol 1967;93(1):445–450

48. Van der Auwera P, Matsumoto T, Husson M. Intraphagocytic penetration of antibiotics. J Antimicrob Chemother 1988;22(2):185–192

49. Hand WL, King-Thompson NL, Steinberg TH. Interactions of antibiotics and phagocytes. J Antimicrob Chemother 1983;12 Suppl C:1–11

50. Maurin M, Raoult D. Use of aminoglycosides in treatment of infections due to intracellular bacteria. Antimicrob Agents Chemother 2001;45(11):2977–2986

51. Najar I, Oberti J, Teyssier J, Caravano R. Kinetics of the uptake of rifampicin and tetracycline into mouse macrophages. In vitro study of the early stages. Pathol Biol (Paris) 1984;32(2):85–89

52. Berneis K, Boguth W. Distribution of sulfonamides and sulfonamide potentiators between red blood cells, proteins and aqueous phases of the blood of different species. Chemotherapy 1976;22(6):390–409

53. Pallister CJ, Lewis RJ. Effects of antimicrobial drugs on human neutrophil–microbe interactions. Br J Biomed Sci 2000;57(1):19–27

54. Solera J, Martinez-Alfaro E, Espinosa A. Recognition and optimum treatment of brucellosis. Drugs 1997;53(2):245–256

55. Perry RD, Fetherston JD. Yersinia pestis – etiologic agent of plague. Clin Microbiol Rev 1997;10(1):35–66

56. Enderlin G, Morales L, Jacobs RF, Cross JT. Streptomycin and alternative agents for the treatment of tularemia: review of the literature. Clin Infect Dis 1994;19(1):42–47

57. Meyers BR. Tuberculous meningitis. Med Clin North Am 1982;66(3):755–762

58. Morse SA, Budowle B. Microbial forensics: application to bioterrorism preparedness and response. Infect Dis Clin North Am 2006;20(2):455–73, xi

59. Mikesell P, Ivins BE, Ristroph JD, Dreier TM. Evidence for plasmid-mediated toxin production in *Bacillus anthracis*. Infect Immun 1983;39(1):371–376

60. Green BD, Battisti L, Koehler TM, Thorne CB, Ivins BE. Demonstration of a capsule plasmid in *Bacillus anthracis*. Infect Immun 1985;49(2):291–297

61. CLSI. Performance Standards for Antimicrobial Susceptibility Testing; Sixteenth Informational Supplement. Wayne, PA: Clinical and Laboratory Standards Institute; 2006

62. Doganay M, Aydin N. Antimicrobial susceptibility of *Bacillus anthracis*. Scand J Infect Dis 1991;23(3):333–335

63. Coker PR, Smith KL, Hugh-Jones ME. Antimicrobial susceptibilities of diverse *Bacillus anthracis* isolates. Antimicrob Agents Chemother 2002;46(12):3843–3845

64. Cavallo JD, Ramisse F, Girardet M, Vaissaire J, Mock M, Hernandez E. Antibiotic susceptibilities of 96 isolates of *Bacillus anthracis* isolated in France between 1994 and 2000. Antimicrob Agents Chemother 2002;46(7):2307–2309

65. Turnbull PC, Sirianni NM, LeBron CI, et al. MICs of selected antibiotics for *Bacillus anthracis, Bacillus cereus, Bacillus thuringiensis,* and *Bacillus mycoides* from a range of clinical and environmental sources as determined by the Etest. J Clin Microbiol 2004;42(8):3626–3634

66. Bradaric N, Punda-Polic V. Cutaneous anthrax due to penicillin-resistant *Bacillus anthracis* transmitted by an insect bite. Lancet 1992;340(8814):306–307

67. Lalitha MK, Thomas MK. Penicillin resistance in *Bacillus anthracis*. Lancet 1997;349(9064):1522

68. McSwiggan DA, Hussain KK, Taylor IO. A fatal case of cutaneous anthrax. J Hyg (Lond) 1974;73(1):151–156

69. Chen Y, Tenover FC, Koehler TM. Beta-lactamase gene expression in a penicillin-resistant *Bacillus anthracis* strain. Antimicrob Agents Chemother 2004;48(12):4873–4877

70. Materon IC, Queenan AM, Koehler TM, Bush K, Palzkill T. Biochemical characterization of beta-lactamases Bla1 and Bla2 from *Bacillus anthracis*. Antimicrob Agents Chemother 2003;47(6):2040–2042

71. Kim HS, Choi EC, Kim BK. A macrolide-lincosamide-streptogramin B resistance determinant from *Bacillus anthracis* 590: cloning and expression of *ermJ*. J Gen Microbiol 1993;139(3):601–607

72. Barrow EW, Bourne PC, Barrow WW. Functional cloning of *Bacillus anthracis* dihydrofolate reductase and confirmation of natural resistance to trimethoprim. Antimicrob Agents Chemother 2004;48(12):4643–4649

73. Navashin SM, Fomina IP, Buravtseva NP, Nikitin AV, Ivanitskaya LP. Combined action of rifampicin and peptidoglycan in experimental anthracic infection [Abstract 115]. In: 18th International Congress on Chemotherapy. Stockholm: American Society of Microbiology Press; 1993

74. Saile E, Koehler TM. *Bacillus anthracis* multiplication, persistence, and genetic exchange in the rhizosphere of grass plants. Appl Environ Microbiol 2006;72(5):3168–3174

75. D'Costa VM, McGrann KM, Hughes DW, Wright GD. Sampling the antibiotic resistome. Science 2006;311(5759):374–377

76. Choe CH, Bouhaouala SS, Brook I, Elliot TB, Knudson GB. In vitro development of resistance to ofloxacin and doxycycline in *Bacillus anthracis* Sterne. Antimicrob Agents Chemother 2000;44(6):1766

77. Bast DJ, Athamna A, Duncan CL, et al. Type II topoisomerase mutations in *Bacillus anthracis* associated with high-level fluoroquinolone resistance. J Antimicrob Chemother 2004;54(1):90–94

78. Hooper DC. Mechanisms of Quinolone Resistance. In: Hooper DC, Rubinstein E, eds. Quinolone Antimicrobial Agents, 3rd ed. Washington, DC: ASM Press; 2003:41–67

79. Pomerantsev AP, Shishkova NA, Marinin LI. [Comparison of therapeutic effects of antibiotics of the tetracycline group in the treatment of anthrax caused by a strain inheriting *tet*-gene of plasmid pBC16]. Antibiot Khimioter 1992;37(4):31–34

80. Ruhfel RE, Robillard NJ, Thorne CB. Interspecies transduction of plasmids among *Bacillus anthracis, B. cereus,* and *B. thuringiensis*. J Bacteriol 1984;157(3):708–711

81. Pomerantsev AP, Staritsyn NA. [Behavior of heterologous recombinant plasmid pCET in cells of *Bacillus anthracis*]. Genetika 1996;32(4):500–509

82. Testa RT, Petersen PJ, Jacobus NV, Sum PE, Lee VJ, Tally FP. In vitro and in vivo antibacterial activities of the glycylcyclines, a new class of semisynthetic tetracyclines. Antimicrob Agents Chemother 1993;37(11):2270–2277

83. Ivins BE, Welkos SL, Knudson GB, Leblanc DJ. Transposon Tn*916* mutagenesis in *Bacillus anthracis*. Infect Immun 1988;56(1):176–181

84. Koehler TM. *Bacillus anthracis* genetics and virulence gene regulation. In: Koehler TM, ed. Anthrax. Berlin: Springer; 2002:144–161

85. Stepanov AV, Marinin LI, Pomerantsev AP, Staritsin NA. Development of novel vaccines against anthrax in man. J Biotechnol 1996;44(1–3):155–160

86. Pomerantsev AP, Sukovatova LV, Marinin LI. [Characterization of a Rif-R population of *Bacillus anthracis*]. Antibiot Khimioter 1993;38(8–9):34–38

87. Pomerantsev AP, Sitaraman R, Galloway CR, Kivovich V, Leppla SH. Genome engineering in *Bacillus anthracis* using Cre recombinase. Infect Immun 2006;74(1):682–693

88. Gutman LT. *Yersinia*. In: Joklik WK, Willett HP, Amos DB, Wilfert CM, eds. Zinsser Microbiology, 19th ed. Norwalk, CN: Appleton & Lange; 1988:493–501

89. Eisen RJ, Bearden SW, Wilder AP, Montenieri JA, Gage KL. Early-phase transmission of *Yersinia pestis* by unblocked fleas as a mechanism explaining rapidly spreading plague epizootics. Proc Natl Acad Sci USA 2006;103(42):15380–15385

90. Butler T. *Yersinia* infections: centennial of the discovery of the plague bacillus. Clin Infect Dis 1994;19(4):655–661

91. Bonacorsi SP, Scavizzi MR, Guiyoule A, Amouroux JH, Carniel E. Assessment of a fluoroquinolone, three beta-lactams, two aminoglycosides, and a cycline in treatment of murine *Yersinia pestis* infection. Antimicrob Agents Chemother 1994;38(3):481–486

92. Smith MD, Vinh DX, Nguyen TT, Wain J, Thung D, White NJ. In vitro antimicrobial susceptibilities of strains of *Yersinia pestis*. Antimicrob Agents Chemother 1995;39(9):2153–2154

93. Frean JA, Arntzen L, Capper T, Bryskier A, Klugman KP. In vitro activities of 14 antibiotics against 100 human isolates of *Yersinia pestis* from a southern African plague focus. Antimicrob Agents Chemother 1996;40(11):2646–2647

94. Wong JD, Barash JR, Sandfort RF, Janda JM. Susceptibilities of *Yersinia pestis* strains to 12 antimicrobial agents. Antimicrob Agents Chemother 2000;44(7):1995–1996

95. Frean J, Klugman KP, Arntzen L, Bukofzer S. Susceptibility of *Yersinia pestis* to novel and conventional antimicrobial agents. J Antimicrob Chemother 2003;52(2):294–296

96. Boulanger LL, Ettestad P, Fogarty JD, Dennis DT, Romig D, Mertz G. Gentamicin and tetracyclines for the treatment of human plague: review of 75 cases in New Mexico, 1985–1999. Clin Infect Dis 2004;38:663–669

97. Galimand M, Guiyoule A, Gerbaud G, et al. Multidrug resistance in *Yersinia pestis* mediated by a transferable plasmid. N Engl J Med 1997;337(10):677–680

98. Guiyoule A, Gerbaud G, Buchrieser C, et al. Transferable plasmid-mediated resistance to streptomycin in a clinical isolate of *Yersinia pestis*. Emerg Infect Dis 2001;7(1):43–48

99. Kravchenko AN, Mishan'kin BN, Ryzhkov V, et al. [Trimethoprim resistance – a differential trait of strains of *Yersinia pestis* from a variety of voles]. Mikrobiol Zh 1990;52(4):84–88

100. Lindler LE, Fan W, Jahan N. Detection of ciprofloxacin-resistant *Yersinia pestis* by fluorogenic PCR using the LightCycler. J Clin Microbiol 2001;39(10):3649–3655

101. Ryzhko IV, Samokhodkina ED, Tsuraeva RI, Shcherbaniuk AI, Pasiukov VV. [Experimental evaluation of prospects for the use of beta-lactams in plague infection caused by pathogens with plasmid resistance to penicillins]. Antibiot Khimioter 1998;43(11):11–15

102. Ryzhko IV, Shcherbaniuk AI, Skalyga E, Tsuraeva RI, Moldavan IA. [Formation of virulent antigen-modified mutants (Fra-, Fra-Tox-) of plague bacteria resistant to rifampicin and quinolones]. Antibiot Khimioter 2003;48(4):19–23

103. Ryzhko IV, Shcherbaniuk AI, Samokhodkina ED, et al. [Virulence of rifampicin and quinolone resistant mutants of strains of plague microbe with Fra+ and Fra- phenotypes]. Antibiot Khimioter 1994;39(4):32–36

104. Ryzhko IV, Tsuraeva RI, Moldavan IA, Shcherbaniuk AI. [Efficacy of plague prophylaxis with streptomycin, tetracycline, and rifampicin in simultaneous immunization of white mice by resistant EV NRIEG strain] Antibiot Khimioter 2004;49(1):17–21

105. Grebtsova NN, Lebedeva SA, Cherniavskaia AS. [Mutagenic effect during transduction of (Gm-Km)R markers of the R323 plasmid in *Yersinia pestis*]. Mol Gen Mikrobiol Virusol 1985(3):22–27

106. Thomas R, Johansson A, Neeson B, et al. Discrimination of human pathogenic subspecies of *Francisella tularensis* by using restriction fragment length polymorphism. J Clin Microbiol 2003;41(1):50–57

107. Ellis J, Oyston PC, Green M, Titball RW. Tularemia. Clin Microbiol Rev 2002;15(4):631–646

108. McCrumb FR. Aerosol Infection of Man with *Pasteurella tularensis*. Bacteriol Rev 1961;25(3):262–267

109. Johansson A, Urich SK, Chu MC, Sjostedt A, Tarnvik A. In vitro susceptibility to quinolones of *Francisella tularensis* subspecies *tularensis*. Scand J Infect Dis 2002;34(5):327–330

110. Ikaheimo I, Syrjala H, Karhukorpi J, Schildt R, Koskela M. In vitro antibiotic susceptibility of *Francisella tularensis* isolated from humans and animals. J Antimicrob Chemother 2000;46(2):287–290

111. Baker CN, Hollis DG, Thornsberry C. Antimicrobial susceptibility testing of *Francisella tularensis* with a modified Mueller-Hinton broth. J Clin Microbiol 1985;22(2):212–215

112. Vasi'lev NT, Oborin VA, Vasi'lev PG, Glushkova OV, Kravets ID, Levchuk BA. [Sensitivity spectrum of *Francisella tularensis* to antibiotics and synthetic antibacterial drugs]. Antibiot Khimioter 1989;34(9):662–665

113. Cross JT, Jacobs RF. Tularemia: treatment failures with outpatient use of ceftriaxone. Clin Infect Dis 1993;17(6):976–980

114. LoVullo ED, Sherrill LA, Perez LL, Reader MD, Pavelka M, S., Jr. Genetic analysis of beta-lactam antibiotic resistance in *Francisella tularensis*. In: Tularemia Workshop: University of Rochester Medical Center; 2005

115. Pavlov VM, Mokrievich AN, Volkovoy K. Cryptic plasmid pFNL10 from *Francisella novicida*-like F6168: the base of plasmid vectors for *Francisella tularensis*. FEMS Immunol Med Microbiol 1996;13(3):253–256

116. Norqvist A, Kuoppa K, Sandstrom G. Construction of a shuttle vector for use in *Francisella tularensis*. FEMS Immunol Med Microbiol 1996;13(3):257–260

117. Maier TM, Havig A, Casey M, Nano FE, Frank DW, Zahrt TC. Construction and characterization of a highly efficient *Francisella* shuttle plasmid. Appl Environ Microbiol 2004;70(12):7511–7519

118. Pomerantsev AP, Obuchi M, Ohara Y. Nucleotide sequence, structural organization, and functional characterization of the small recombinant plasmid pOM1 that is specific for *Francisella tularensis*. Plasmid 2001;46(2):86–94

119. Lauriano CM, Barker JR, Nano FE, Arulanandam BP, Klose KE. Allelic exchange in *Francisella tularensis* using PCR products. FEMS Microbiol Lett 2003;229(2):195–202

120. Thibault FM, Hernandez E, Vidal DR, Girardet M, Cavallo JD. Antibiotic susceptibility of 65 isolates of *Burkholderia pseudomallei* and *Burkholderia mallei* to 35 antimicrobial agents. J Antimicrob Chemother 2004;54(6):1134–1138

121. Heine HS, England MJ, Waag DM, Byrne WR. In vitro antibiotic susceptibilities of *Burkholderia mallei* (causative agent of glanders) determined by broth microdilution and E-test. Antimicrob Agents Chemother 2001;45(7):2119–2121

122. Kenny DJ, Russell P, Rogers D, Eley SM, Titball RW. In vitro susceptibilities of *Burkholderia mallei* in comparison to those of other pathogenic *Burkholderia* spp. Antimicrob Agents Chemother 1999;43(11):2773–2775

123. Jenney AW, Lum G, Fisher DA, Currie BJ. Antibiotic susceptibility of *Burkholderia pseudomallei* from tropical northern Australia and implications for therapy of melioidosis. Int J Antimicrob Agents 2001;17(2):109–113

124. Yamamoto T, Naigowit P, Dejsirilert S, et al. In vitro susceptibilities of *Pseudomonas pseudomallei* to 27 antimicrobial agents. Antimicrob Agents Chemother 1990;34(10):2027–2029

125. Smith MD, Wuthiekanun V, Walsh AL, White NJ. Susceptibility of *Pseudomonas pseudomallei* to some newer beta-lactam antibiotics and antibiotic combinations using time-kill studies. J Antimicrob Chemother 1994;33(1):145–149

126. Ashdown LR. In vitro activities of the newer beta lactam and quinolone antimicrobial agents against *Pseudomonas pseudomallei*. Antimicrob Agents Chemother 1988;32(9):1435–1436

127. Moore RA, DeShazer D, Reckseidler S, Weissman A, Woods DE. Efflux-mediated aminoglycoside and macrolide resistance in *Burkholderia pseudomallei*. Antimicrob Agents Chemother 1999;43(3):465–470

128. Sookpranee T, Sookpranee M, Mellencamp MA, Preheim LC. *Pseudomonas pseudomallei*, a common pathogen in Thailand that is resistant to the bactericidal effects of many antibiotics. Antimicrob Agents Chemother 1991;35(3):484–489

129. Abaev IV, Astashkin EI, Pachkunov DM, Stagis NI, Shitov VT, Svetoch EA. [*Pseudomonas mallei* and *Pseudomonas pseudomallei*: introduction and maintenance of natural and recombinant plasmid replicons]. Mol Gen Mikrobiol Virusol 1995(1):28–36

130. Zakharenko VI, Gorelov VN, Seliutina DF, Kulakov Iu K, Nenashev AV, Skavronskaia AG. [Functional properties of the pOV13 plasmid as a vector for DNA cloning in a broad spectrum of gram negative bacteria]. Mol Gen Mikrobiol Virusol 1990(1):22–26

131. Nierman WC, DeShazer D, Kim HS, et al. Structural flexibility in the *Burkholderia mallei* genome. Proc Natl Acad Sci U S A 2004;101(39):14246–14251

132. Dance DA, Wuthiekanun V, Chaowagul W, Suputtamongkol Y, White NJ. Development of resistance to ceftazidime and co-amoxiclav in *Pseudomonas pseudomallei*. J Antimicrob Chemother 1991;28(2):321–324

133. Mantur BG, Mangalgi SS, Mulimani M. *Brucella melitensis*-a sexually transmissible agent? Lancet 1996;347(9017):1763

134. Naparstek E, Block CS, Slavin S. Transmission of brucellosis by bone marrow transplantation. Lancet 1982;1(8271):574–575

135. Mortensen JE, Moore DG, Clarridge JE, Young EJ. Antimicrobial susceptibility of clinical isolates of *Brucella*. Diagn Microbiol Infect Dis 1986;5(2):163–169

136. Bosch J, Linares J, Lopez de Goicoechea MJ, Ariza J, Cisnal MC, Martin R. In-vitro activity of ciprofloxacin, ceftriaxone and five other antimicrobial agents against 95 strains of *Brucella melitensis*. J Antimicrob Chemother 1986;17(4):459–461

137. Trujillano-Martin I, Garcia-Sanchez E, Martinez IM, Fresnadillo MJ, Garcia-Sanchez JE, Garcia-Rodriguez JA. In vitro activities of six new fluoroquinolones against *Brucella melitensis*. Antimicrob Agents Chemother 1999;43(1):194–195

138. Mateu-de-Antonio EM, Martin M. In vitro efficacy of several antimicrobial combinations against *Brucella canis* and *Brucella melitensis* strains isolated from dogs. Vet Microbiol 1995;45(1):1–10

139. Braibant M, Guilloteau L, Zygmunt MS. Functional characterization of *Brucella melitensis* NorMI, an efflux pump belonging to the multidrug and toxic compound extrusion family. Antimicrob Agents Chemother 2002;46(9):3050–3053

140. Piddock LJ. Clinically relevant chromosomally encoded multidrug resistance efflux pumps in bacteria. Clin Microbiol Rev 2006;19(2):382–402

141. Gorelov VN, Gubina EA, Grekova NA, Skavronskaia AG. [The possibility of creating a vaccinal strain of *Brucella abortus* 19-BA with multiple antibiotic resistance]. Zh Mikrobiol Epidemiol Immunobiol 1991(9):2–4

142. Raoult D, Levy PY, Harle JR, et al. Chronic Q fever: diagnosis and follow-up. Ann N Y Acad Sci 1990;590:51–60

143. Samuel JE. Developmental cycle of *Coxiella burnetii*. In: Brun YV, Shimkets LJ, eds. Procaryotic Development. Washington, D.C.: ASM Press; 2000:427–440

144. Scott GH, Williams JC. Susceptibility of *Coxiella burnetii* to chemical disinfectants. Ann N Y Acad Sci 1990;590:291–296

145. Waag DM, Thompson HA. Pathogenesis and Immunity of *Coxiella Burnetii*. In: Lindler L, Lebeda FJ, Korch GW, eds. Biological Weapons Defense: Infectious Diseases and Counterbioterrorism. Totowa, NJ: Humana Press; 2005:185–207

146. Christopher GW, Cieslak TJ, Pavlin JA, Eitzen EM, Jr. Biological warfare. A historical perspective. JAMA 1997;278(5):412–417

147. Greenfield RA, Drevets DA, Machado LJ, Voskuhl GW, Cornea P, Bronze MS. Bacterial pathogens as biological weapons and agents of bioterrorism. Am J Med Sci 2002;323(6):299–315

148. Jackson ER. Comparative efficacy of several antibiotics on experimental rickettsial infections in embryonnated eggs. Antibiot Chemother 1951;1:231–235

149. Yeaman MR, Mitscher LA, Baca OG. In vitro susceptibility of *Coxiella burnetii* to antibiotics, including several quinolones. Antimicrob Agents Chemother 1987;31(7):1079–1084

150. Zamboni DS, Mortara RA, Freymuller E, Rabinovitch M. Mouse resident peritoneal macrophages partially control in vitro infection with *Coxiella burnetii* phase II. Microbes Infect 2002;4(6):591–598

151. Raoult D, Torres H, Drancourt M. Shell-vial assay: evaluation of a new technique for determining antibiotic susceptibility, tested in 13 isolates of *Coxiella burnetii*. Antimicrob Agents Chemother 1991;35(10):2070–2077

152. Brennan RE, Samuel JE. Evaluation of *Coxiella burnetii* antibiotic susceptibilities by real-time PCR assay. J Clin Microbiol 2003;41(5):1869–1874

153. Boulos A, Rolain JM, Maurin M, Raoult D. Measurement of the antibiotic susceptibility of *Coxiella burnetii* using real time PCR. Int J Antimicrob Agents 2004;23(2):169–174

154. Rolain JM, Maurin M, Raoult D. Bacteriostatic and bactericidal activities of moxifloxacin against *Coxiella burnetii*. Antimicrob Agents Chemother 2001;45(1):301–302

155. Raoult D, Houpikian P, Tissot Dupont H, Riss JM, Arditi-Djiane J, Brouqui P. Treatment of Q fever endocarditis: comparison of 2 regimens containing doxycycline and ofloxacin or hydroxychloroquine. Arch Intern Med 1999;159(2):167–173

156. Maurin M, Benoliel AM, Bongrand P, Raoult D. Phagolysosomal alkalinization and the bactericidal effect of antibiotics: the *Coxiella burnetii* paradigm. J Infect Dis 1992;166(5):1097–1102

157. Raoult D, Bres P, Drancourt M, Vestris G. In vitro susceptibilities of *Coxiella burnetii*, *Rickettsia rickettsii*, and *Rickettsia conorii* to the fluoroquinolone sparfloxacin. Antimicrob Agents Chemother 1991;35(1):88–91

158. Gikas A, Spyridaki I, Psaroulaki A, Kofterithis D, Tselentis Y. In vitro susceptibility of *Coxiella burnetii* to trovafloxacin in comparison with susceptibilities to pefloxacin, ciprofloxacin, ofloxacin, doxycycline, and clarithromycin. Antimicrob Agents Chemother 1998;42(10):2747–2748

159. Seshadri R, Paulsen IT, Eisen JA, et al. Complete genome sequence of the Q-fever pathogen *Coxiella burnetii*. Proc Natl Acad Sci U S A 2003;100(9):5455–5460

160. Yeaman MR, Baca OG. Mechanisms that may account for differential antibiotic susceptibilities among *Coxiella burnetii* isolates. Antimicrob Agents Chemother 1991;35(5):948–954

161. Yeaman MR, Roman MJ, Baca OG. Antibiotic susceptibilities of two *Coxiella burnetii* isolates implicated in distinct clinical syndromes. Antimicrob Agents Chemother 1989;33(7):1052–1057

162. Musso D, Drancourt M, Osscini S, Raoult D. Sequence of quinolone resistance-determining region of *gyrA* gene for clinical isolates and for an in vitro-selected quinolone-resistant strain of *Coxiella burnetii*. Antimicrob Agents Chemother 1996;40(4):870–873

163. Spyridaki I, Psaroulaki A, Aransay A, Scoulica E, Tselentis Y. Diagnosis of quinolone-resistant *Coxiella burnetii* strains by PCR-RFLP. J Clin Lab Anal 2000;14(2):59–63

164. Brezina R, Schramek S, Kazar J. Selection of chlortetracycline-resistant strain of *Coxiella burnetii*. Acta Virol 1975;19(6):496

165. Espy MJ, Uhl JR, Sloan LM, et al. Real-time PCR in clinical microbiology: applications for routine laboratory testing. Clin Microbiol Rev 2006;19(1):165–256

166. Ng LK, Martin I, Alfa M, Mulvey M. Multiplex PCR for the detection of tetracycline resistant genes. Mol Cell Probes 2001;15(4):209–215

167. Ivnitski D, O'Neil DJ, Gattuso A, Schlicht R, Calidonna M, Fisher R. Nucleic acid approaches for detection and identification of biological warfare and infectious disease agents. Biotechniques 2003;35(4):862–869

168. Burton JE, Oshota OJ, North E, et al. Development of a multi-pathogen oligonucleotide microarray for detection of *Bacillus anthracis*. Mol Cell Probes 2005;19(5):349–357

169. Smith MD, Wuthiekanun V, Walsh AL, White NJ. In-vitro activity of carbapenem antibiotics against beta-lactam susceptible and resistant strains of *Burkholderia pseudomallei*. J Antimicrob Chemother 1996;37(3):611–615

170. Baykam N, Esener H, Ergonul O, Eren S, Celikbas AK, Dokuzoguz B. In vitro antimicrobial susceptibility of *Brucella* species. Int J Antimicrob Agents 2004;23(4):405–407

171. Akova M, Gur D, Livermore DM, Kocagoz T, Akalin HE. In vitro activities of antibiotics alone and in combination against *Brucella melitensis* at neutral and acidic pHs. Antimicrob Agents Chemother 1999;43(5):1298–1300

172. Trujillano-Martin I, Garcia-Sanchez E, Fresnadillo MJ, Garcia-Sanchez JE, Garcia-Rodriguez JA, Montes Martinez I. In vitro activities of five new antimicrobial agents against *Brucella melitensis*. Int J Antimicrob Agents 1999;12(2):185–186

Chapter 91
Internet Resources on Antimicrobial Resistance

Matthew E. Falagas and Efthymia A. Karveli

1 Significance of Internet Resources on Antimicrobial Resistance

We recently put together a list of a number of World Wide Web (WWW) addresses of sites or pages of major international networks that present data regarding resistance to commonly used antimicrobial therapeutic agents. The relevant article was published and is an open access educational resource available at: http://www.journals.uchicago.edu/CID/journal/issues/v43n5/40114/40114.html(1). This chapter is mainly based on the published article (1); however, here we supplemented our compilation of the relevant WWW resources with a collection of internet links of representative major national networks/organizations including data on antimicrobial resistance.

Our lists of WWW resources of data from surveillance studies on antimicrobial resistance may be useful to practitioners, especially infectious disease specialists, as well as to scientists with a research interest in the field of antimicrobial resistance. Such educational and informative WWW resources are potentially helpful because of the growing problem of antimicrobial resistance that has become a significant public health concern worldwide (2). This refers practically to all types of pathogens, including viruses, bacteria, mycobacteria, fungi, and parasites. Previous studies have shown the impact of antimicrobial resistance on various outcomes including mortality, morbidity, and cost and length of hospitalization (3–5).

The Infectious Diseases Society of America (IDSA) and the European Society of Clinical Microbiology and Infectious Diseases (ESCMID) have recently published their concerns regarding the considerable proportion of clinical isolates that are resistant to most antimicrobial agents (6, 7). Among the various clinically important bacteria, *Staphylococcus aureus*, *Streptococcus pneumoniae*, *Enterococcus* spp., *Acinetobacter* spp., *Pseudomonas* spp., and *Klebsiella* spp. represent major pathogens that cause high incidence of infections and are resistant to treatment with antibiotics of many antimicrobial classes (8–12). Of particular concern recently is the increasing incidence of community-acquired methicillin resistant *Staphylococcus aureus* (MRSA) in most countries (13) as well as the epidemic of multidrug-resistant (MDR) *Acinetobacter baumannii* infections in several countries, especially in patients in the intensive care unit (ICU) setting (14).

When practicing medicine during this era of easy international travel, and because transfer of patients between hospitals in different countries is not rare, the clinician and, especially, the infectious disease specialist should have easily available epidemiological data regarding antimicrobial resistance. In addition, investigators studying various aspects of the problem of antimicrobial resistance also benefit enormously from the availability of such data. Thus, both clinicians and investigators benefit by knowing the proportion of clinical isolates that are resistant to various antimicrobial agents in their community, hospital, area, country, continent, as well as around the globe, because the cross-continental travel of both humans and goods causes the spread of antibiotic-resistant bacteria from one country to another.

Advances of modern technology, including the development of the Internet and the WWW, have given the opportunity to clinicians and researchers to have immediate access to continuously updated information in various scientific fields. Thus, the collection and update of ongoing surveillance antimicrobial resistance data from various sources has been made possible (15). As a useful guidance tool to practitioners and researchers, we sought to compile a list of major networks' Web pages/sites that provide valuable WWW links that offer additional information relevant to the problem of antimicrobial resistance.

M.E. Falagas (✉)
Alfa Institute of Biomedical Sciences (AIBS), Marousi, Greece
m.falagas@aibs.gr

D.L. Mayers (ed.), *Antimicrobial Drug Resistance*,
DOI 10.1007/978-1-60327-595-8_91, © Humana Press, a part of Springer Science+Business Media, LLC 2009

2 Methodology of WWW Resource Selection

We gathered information regarding the relevant WWW resources by making use of internet search engines (Google, AltaVista, and Yahoo). We used as key words the abbreviated names of major antimicrobial surveillance systems/projects that were known to us (i.e., MYSTIC, GSMART, SENTRY, PROTEKT, NNIS, VICNISS, INSPEAR, ANSORM, STRAMA, DANMAP, etc.). Also, we performed searches of the PubMed database, *Current Contents*, and the WWW for information regarding additional relevant sources by using the following key words: resistance, antimicrobial resistance, surveillance, network, program, and project. In addition, we reviewed the information provided in the initially identified sources to find additional WWW links that contained data relevant to antimicrobial resistance.

We chose to include in our lists dependable English-language Web pages, which we categorized into three groups: those that presented antimicrobial resistance data from major international networks; those that presented antimicrobial resistance data from major national networks; and those that provided links to other international surveillance organizations/associations that study antimicrobial resistance. Regarding the first group of Web pages, those that were finally presented in our assessment were selected from a very extensive catalog, by the criterion of providing international surveillance data (more than two countries involved). In the second group we included representative major national network Web sites. For both groups, strong selection criteria were comprehensive and evidence-based information, as well as ease of access to that information. In the third group we included link-providing Web pages from the most commonly visited Web sites by infection experts.

Although we managed, through our gathering strategy, to review most of the major international and national networks' Web sites/pages, it is inevitable that some were overlooked, while for some others we decided that they did not fulfill the criteria to be enlisted.

3 Internet Resources on Antimicrobial Resistance from Major International Networks

In Table 1, we list 24 Web pages/sites of 19 major international networks that present data of antimicrobial resistance, either as interactive database or as reports of international antimicrobial resistance surveillance systems. We accessed each of the Web addresses and verified that they contain data from surveillance studies on antimicrobial resistance.

4 Internet Resources on Antimicrobial Resistance from Major National Networks

In Table 2, a catalog of 11 representative major national network Web pages, which present data of drug-resistant microorganisms either in the form of interactive databases or as annual surveillance reports, is shown. We could verify that the Web addresses presented in the table are easily accessible and contain comprehensive and valuable antimicrobial resistance information.

5 Internet Links on Antimicrobial Resistance from Major Networks

In Table 3, we present 11 major networks' Web pages/sites providing numerous of valuable Web links to international organisms/associations that conduct research on antimicrobial resistance and/or suggest guidelines for infection control as well as for prudent use of antibiotics. We accessed each of the links included in this table and verified that they contain information relevant to the field of antimicrobial resistance.

6 Limitations in the Selection of Relevant Internet Resources

The goal of our effort was to provide to clinicians and investigators immediate access to a collection of WWW resources that include updated information regarding the antimicrobial resistance patterns of clinical isolates from patients of various parts of the world. We acknowledge that the lists we present are far from exhaustive. Rather, they should be regarded as a subset of relevant WWW resources that include readily available information on antimicrobial resistance.

We need to highlight the significance of the numerous national antimicrobial resistance surveillance projects that are monitoring the resistance pattern of clinical isolates from patients, within the borders of each country. The investigators related to some of these projects report their national-level data in scientific publications. In addition, a small amount of data related to these efforts is included in regional Web sites. Although the presentation of each and every one of the various Web sites of the national antimicrobial surveillance networks of each country would be valuable, it was considered beyond the scope of this chapter.

We believe that efforts for the continuous update of information of databases reporting the findings of surveillance

Table 1 Summary of major international networks' Web pages/sites presenting data of antimicrobial resistance

Title/subject	Web address	Contents/objective	Source
Antimicrobial resistance information bank (AR info-bank)	http://rhone.b3e.jussieu.fr/arinfobank/	Central page of "Antimicrobial resistance information bank" Web site	WHO (World Health Organization)
Antimicrobial resistance data	http://rhone.b3e.jussieu.fr/arinfobank/ResistanceDataSearch.php	Resistance data from published documents only included. Focused on a limited number of bacterial species and antimicrobial agents	WHO
Drug resistance	http://www.who.int/drugresistance/en/	Information on malaria, tuberculosis, HIV/AIDS	WHO
The European Antimicrobial Resistance Surveillance System	http://www.rivm.nl/earss/	E. coli; E. faecalis, E. faecium, K. pneumoniae, P. aeruginosa, S. aureus, S. pneumoniae	EARSS (European Antimicrobial Resistance Surveillance System)
MYSTIC (Meropenem Yearly Susceptibility Test Information Collection – 100 centres worldwide) database	http://www.mystic-data.org/	Interactive database; provides resistance data and statistics on several bacteria regarding several antimicrobial agents, since 1997	AIM (Academy for Infection Management)
Infectious disease surveillance Surveillance resources links	http://www.cdc.gov/ncidod/osr/site/surv_resources/data_reports.htm	Available infectious disease surveillance data and reports (by name of surveillance system, by common disease name, by disease topic)	CDC (Centers for Disease Control and prevention)
Infectious disease surveillance Emerging infections programs in the USA	http://www.cdc.gov/ncidod/osr/site/eip/sites.htm	Emerging infections programs in the USA	CDC
Antimicrobial resistance in the healthcare setting	http://www.cdc.gov/ncidod/dhqp/ar.html	Drug-resistant organisms, prevention and control, campaigns, lab practices	CDC
NARMS (National Antimicrobial Resistance Monitoring System for enteric bacteria)	http://www.cdc.gov/narms/	NARMS highlights and annual reports	CDC for NARMS
NARMS	http://www.fda.gov/cvm/narms_pg.html	NARMS data, presentations, publications	FDA (Food and Drug Administration) for NARMS
Project ICARE (Intensive Care Antimicrobial Resistance Epidemiology) publications	http://www.sph.emory.edu/ICARE/publications.php	Published data on antimicrobial resistance in the healthcare system generated from Project ICARE	Rollins School of Public Health of Emory university (RSPH)
ENARE (European Network for Antimicrobial Resistance and Epidemiology)	http://www.enare.org/publications.html	Peer-reviewed publications about resistance by ENARE members since 2003	Eijkman-Winkler Institute for Medical Microbiology, University Hospital Utrecht
The "Alexander network" Web site	http://www.alexandernetwork.com/DesktopDefault.aspx	Local and regional data from surveillance studies conducted on over 150 different pathogens in 54 countries	The Alexander Network
NARSA (Network on Antibiotic Resistance in S. aureus)	http://www.narsa.net/content/default.jsp	Web site on S. aureus	U.S. National Institute of Health; U.S. National Institute of Allergy and Infectious Diseases
ROAR (Reservoirs Of Antibiotic Resistance network)	http://www.roarproject.org/	Registration required for database access. ROAR publications available	APUA (Alliance for the Prudent use of Antibiotics)
ARMed (Antimicrobial Resistance surveillance and control in the Mediterranean region)	http://www.slh.gov.mt/armed/default1.asp	E. coli, E. faecalis E. faecium, K. pneumoniae, P. aeruginosa, S. aureus, S. pneumoniae	ARMed Project/St. Luke's Hospital, Malta

(continued)

Table 1 (continued)

Title/subject	Web address	Contents/objective	Source
ESAC (European Surveillance of Antibiotic Consumption)	http://www.esac.ua.ac.be/main.aspx?c = *ESAC2 &n = 21600	Among others, interesting interactive database on antibiotic consumption in the European countries	DG/SANCO (Directorate-General, Health and consumer protection, European commission)
ESAR (European Surveillance of Antimicrobial Resistance)	http://www.esbic.de/esbic/ind_esar.htm	The Web site provides results of overall resistance. (Has not been informed since 1999)	ESCMID (European society of clinical microbiology and infectious diseases)
PNC Euro (Pneumococcal disease in Europe)	http://www.ktl.fi/pnceuro/	Study on *Streptococcus pneumoniae* (Pnc) in four European countries	The Finnish National Public Health Institute
HELICS (Hospital in Europe, Link for Infection Control through Surveillance)	http://helics.univ-lyon1.fr/helicshome.htm	Available online final reports on resistance (a) in intensive care unit settings and (b) in surgical site infections	IPSE (Improving Patient Safety in Europe – Supported by the European Union DG/Sanco)
Annual report of the monitoring/surveillance network for resistance to antibiotics 2003	http://www.paho.org/english/ad/dpc/cd/amr-lima-2004.htm	Annual report 2003. Also, links to communicable diseases prevention and control	PAHO (Pan American Health Association) WHO
ANSORP (Asian Network for the Surveillance Of Resistant Pathogens)	http://www.ansorp.org/	Publications provided online	ARFID (Asian-Pacific Research Foundation of Infectious Diseases)
Resistance surveillance Web site	http://www.bsacsurv.org/	Data on antimicrobial resistance for respiratory tract infections as well as bacteremias	BSAC (British Society for Antimicrobial Chemotherapy – Data from UK and Ireland)
ProMED-mail	http://www.promedmail.org/pls/promed/f?p = 2400:1000	The global electronic reporting system for outbreaks of emerging infectious diseases and toxins, open to all sources	ISID (International Society for Infectious Diseases)

Table 2 Summary of representative major national networks' Web pages/sites presenting data of antimicrobial resistance

Country	Title/subject	Web page address	Source of information	Contents
Australia	Communicable disease surveillance systems annual reports	http://www.health.gov.au/internet/wcms/publishing.nsf/Content/annual+reports-2	Australian Government. Department of health and Ageing	Provides the annual reports of the Australian surveillance systems
Canada	Canadian Integrated Program for Antimicrobial Resistance Surveillance (CIPARS)	http://www.phac-aspc.gc.ca/cipars-picra/index.html	Government of Canada. Public health agency of Canada	Provides CIPARS annual reports
Denmark	DANMAP: the Danish Integrated Antimicrobial Resistance Monitoring and Research Program	http://www.danmap.org/	Statens Serum Institute	DANMAP annual reports
France	RES-ONERBA: Results and Networks	http://www.onerba.org/rubrique.php3?id_rubrique = 17	ONERBA: (Observatoire National de l' Epidemiologie de la Resistance aux Antibiotics.) French National Observatory for Epidemiology of Bacterial Resistance to Antimicrobials	Interactive Database and Library of publications
Germany	German Network for Antimicrobial Resistance Surveillance	http://www.genars.de/	German association of Hygiene and Microbiology, German Association of Chemotherapy, German Association of Infection	(The site's English version is under construction)
Great Britain	Resistance – Surveillance Web site	http://www.bsacsurv.org/	BSAC: British society for Antimicrobial Chemotherapy	Focuses on respiratory infections and bacteremia
Greece	WHONET Greece: The Greek system for surveillance of antimicrobial resistance	http://www.mednet.gr/whonet/	Department of Hygiene & Epidemiology, Department of Microbiology Medical School, Athens University	Interactive database
Japan	Infectious diseases surveillance center (IDSC)	http://idsc.nih.go.jp/index.html	Japanese National Institute of Infectious Diseases (NIID)	Infectious agents surveillance monthly reports
Russia	Antimicrobial resistance map of Russia	http://www.antibiotic.ru/map/eng/	The Institute of Antimicrobial Chemotherapy, the Department of Clinical Pharmacology of the Smolensk State Medical Academy and All-Russia Drug Information Network Centers	Interactive database
Sweden	STRAMA: Swedish Strategic Program for the Rational use of Antimicrobial Agents and Surveillance of Resistance	http://en.strama.se/dyn//,92,4.html	The Swedish Reference Group for Antibiotics (SRGA), the Medical Products Agency, the National Board of Health and Welfare, the Swedish Institute for Infectious Disease Control (SMI) and others	Provides surveillance data as well as link to interactive database
USA	CDC surveillance systems and published data	http://www.cdc.gov/drugresistance/surveillance.htm	CDC: centers for disease control and prevention/ Department of health and human services	Links and publications of U.S. National Surveillance Systems

Countries are presented in alphabetical order

Table 3 Summary of major networks' Web pages/sites providing valuable Web links on antimicrobial resistance

Title/subject	Web address	Contents/objective	Source
Antibiotic/antimicrobial resistance related links	http://www.cdc.gov/drugresistance/links.htm	Extensive list of links to U.S. national and also international on antimicrobial resistance	CDC (centers for disease control and prevention)
Infectious disease surveillance. Surveillance resources quick links	http://www.cdc.gov/ncidod/osr/site/surv_resources/quick-links.htm	Links to available published data on surveillance/resistance in alphabetical order	CDC
Antimicrobial resistance information bank. Links	http://rhone.b3e.jussieu.fr/arinfobank/links.php	Web links to international surveillance associations	WHO (World Health Organisation)
National/international networks on antimicrobial resistance	http://www.rivm.nl/earss/links/	Provides links to national and international networks' Web pages on antibiotic resistance	The Dutch institute for public health and the environment (RIVM)
Antibiotic resistance archives	http://www.antibioresistance.be/Links.html	Provides links to Web pages on antibiotic resistance. (At the time of our search some were inaccessible)	Belgian Service of Biosafety and Biotechnology
Antimicrobial resistance	http://www.hpa.org.uk/infections/topics_az/antimicrobial_resistance/menu.htm	Related topics and links	HPA (Health Protection Agency, UK)
SSAC (Scandinavian Society for Antimicrobial Chemotherapy). Links	http://www.srga.org/SSAC/links/links.html	Links to Scandinavian and other international organizations that study antimicrobial resistance	SSAC
Related communicable diseases surveillance links	http://www.health.gov.au/internet/wcms/publishing.nsf/Content/cda-cdilinks.htm-copy2	Links to Australian and to international Web sites of organisms and associations studying antimicrobial resistance	Australian government, department of health and ageing
Antibiotic resistance resources	http://www.antibiotic.ru/en/ar/links.shtml	Provides links to Web pages on antibiotic resistance (at the time of our search some were inaccessible)	Institute of antimicrobial chemotherapy and department of clinical pharmacology, Smolensk state medical academy, Russia
Antimicrobial resistance	http://www.idlinks.com/antimicrobial_resistance.htm	Provides links to Web pages on antibiotic resistance. (At the time of our search some were inaccessible)	IDLINKS (Infectious Diseases Links) The communication center for infectious diseases
Antimicrobial resistance	http://www.geis.fhp.osd.mil/GEIS/SurveillanceActivities/AntimicrobialResistance/antimicrobialRes.asp	Mostly provides links on published documents on antimicrobial resistance	DoD–GEIS (US Department of Defence–Global Emerging Infections System)

studies of antimicrobial resistance should be encouraged and supported financially. The toll of infections due to MDR pathogens is too high to ignore the significance of various types of studies on antimicrobial resistance.

as well as to scientists with a research interest in the field of antimicrobial resistance.

Acknowledgment This chapter is based on an article of ours published in *Clinical Infectious Diseases* (1).

7 Conclusion

Advances of modern technology, including the development of the Internet and the WWW, have given the opportunity to clinicians and researchers to have immediate access to continuously updated information in various scientific fields. We tried to compile a list of WWW resources of data from surveillance studies on antimicrobial resistance that may be useful to practitioners, especially infectious disease specialists,

References

1. Falagas ME, Karveli EA. World Wide Web resources on antimicrobial resistance. Clin Infect Dis 2006; 43(5):630–633
2. Zhang R, Eggleston K, Rotimi V, et al. Antibiotic resistance as a global threat: evidence from China, Kuwait and the United States. Global Health 2006; 2:6
3. Falagas ME, Bliziotis IA, Siempos II. Attributable mortality of *Acinetobacter baumannii* infections in critically ill patients: a systematic review of matched cohort and case-control studies. Crit Care 2006; 10(2):R48

4. Ang JY, Ezike E, Asmar BI. Antibacterial resistance. Indian J Pediatr 2004; 71:229–239

5. Myrianthefs PM, Kalafati M, Samara I, et al. Nosocomial pneumonia. Crit Care Nurs Q 2004; 27:241–257

6. Struelens MJ, Van Eldere J. Conclusion: ESCMID declaration on meeting the challenges in clinical microbiology and infectious diseases. Clin Microbiol Infect 2005; 11 Suppl 1:50–51

7. Talbot GH, Bradley J, Edwards JE, et al. Bad bugs need drugs: an update on the development pipeline from the antimicrobial availability task force of the infectious diseases society of America. CID 2006; 42:657–668

8. Styers D, Sheehan DJ, Hogan P, et al. Laboratory-based surveillance of current antimicrobial resistance patterns and trends among *Staphylococcus aureus*: 2005 status in the United States. Ann Clin Microbiol Antimicrob 2006; 5:2

9. Johnson DM, Stilwell MG, Fritsche TR, et al. Emergence of multidrug-resistant *Streptococcus pneumoniae*: report from the SENTRY Antimicrobial Surveillance Program (1999–2003). Diagn Microbiol Infect Dis 2006; 56:69–74

10. Hoffman-Roberts HL, C Babcock E, Mitropoulos IF. Investigational new drugs for the treatment of resistant pneumococcal infections. Expert Opin Investig Drugs 2005; 14:973–995

11. Thomson JM, Bonomo RA. The threat of antibiotic resistance in Gram-negative pathogenic bacteria: beta-lactams in peril! Curr Opin Microbiol 2005; 8:518–524

12. Peterson LR. Squeezing the antibiotic balloon: the impact of antimicrobial classes on emerging resistance. Clin Microbiol Infect 2005; 11 Suppl 5:4–16

13. Moran GJ, Krishnadasan A, Gorwitz RJ, Fosheim GE, McDougal LK, Carey RB, Talan DA; EMERGEncy ID Net Study Group. Methicillin-resistant *S. aureus* infections among patients in the emergency department. N Engl J Med 2006;355(7):666–674

14. Falagas ME, Karveli EA. The changing global epidemiology of *Acinetobacter baumannii* infections: a development with major public health implications. Clin Microbiol Infect 2007; 13(2):117–119

15. Woodall JP. Global surveillance of emerging diseases: the ProMED-mail perspective. Cad Saude Publica 2001; 17 Suppl: 147–154

Index

Printed in the United States of America